8th Edition

DARBY'S
COMPREHENSIVE REVIEW OF
Dental Hygiene

Christine M. Blue, DHSc, MS, BSDH

Associate Professor and Director
Division of Dental Hygiene, School of Dentistry
University of Minnesota
Minneapolis, Minnesota

ELSEVIER

ELSEVIER

3251 Riverport Lane
St. Louis, Missouri 63043

DARBY'S COMPREHENSIVE REVIEW OF DENTAL HYGIENE   978-0-323-31671-2

Library of Congress Cataloging-in-Publication Data

Mosby's comprehensive review of dental hygiene.
   Darby's comprehensive review of dental hygiene/[edited by] Christine M. Blue. – Eighth edition.
     p. ; cm.
   Comprehensive review of dental hygiene
   Preceded by Mosby's comprehensive review of dental hygiene/[edited by] Michele Leonardi Darby.
7th ed. c2012.
   Includes bibliographical references and index.
   ISBN 978-0-323-31671-2 (hardcover : alk. paper)
   I. Blue, Christine M., editor. II. Title. III. Title: Comprehensive review of dental hygiene.
   [DNLM: 1. Dental Prophylaxis–Examination Questions.   2. Dental Prophylaxis–Outlines. WU 18.2]
   RK60.7
   617.6'01–dc23
                              2015037283

Content Strategist: Kristin Wilhelm
Content Development Manager: Billie Sharp
Associate Content Development Specialist: Samantha Dalton
Publishing Services Manager: Patricia Tannian
Senior Project Manager: Cindy Thoms
Design Direction: Ashley Miner

Printed in China
Last digit is the print number: 9   8   7   6   5   4   3   2   1

Jeanne M. Anderson, BSDH, MPA
Adjunct Professor
Division of Dental Hygiene
University of Minnesota
Minneapolis, Minnesota

Brenda Armstrong, BSDH, MDH
Assistant Professor
Dental Hygiene Department
Dixie State University
St. George, Utah

Stephen C. Bayne, MS, PhD
Professor and Chair
Cariology, Restorative Sciences, and
    Endodontics
School of Dentistry
University of Michigan
Ann Arbor, Michigan

**Christine French Beatty, RDH, BS,
    MS, PhD**
Professor Emeritus
Dental Hygiene
Texas Woman's University
Denton, Texas

Connie E. Beatty, RDH, MS
Assistant Professor
Division of Dental Hygiene
Department of Dental Medicine
University of New Mexico
Albuquerque, New Mexico

Denise M. Bowen, RDH, MS
Professor Emeritus
Department of Dental Hygiene
Idaho State University
Pocatello, Idaho

**Charlene B. Dickinson, RDH,
    BSDH, MS**
Assistant Clinical Professor
Dental Hygiene
Texas Woman's University
Denton, Texas

**Barbara Leatherman Dixon, RDH,
    BS, MEd**
Assistant Professor
University of Utah School of Dentistry
Salt Lake City, Utah
Dental Hygiene Board Examiner
WREB, CDCA

Jill S. Gehrig, RDH, MA
Dean Emeritus
Division of Allied Health and Public Service
    Education
Asheville-Buncombe Technical Community
    College
Asheville, North Carolina

JoAnn R. Gurenlian, RDH, MS, PhD
Professor and Graduate Program Director
Dental Hygiene
Idaho State University
Pocatello, Idaho

**Elena Bablenis Haveles, BS Pharmacy,
    PharmD, RPh**
Adjunct Associate Professor of
    Pharmacology
School of Dental Hygiene
Old Dominion University
Norfolk, Virginia

Gwen L. Hlava, RDH, MS
Professor and Chairman
Dental Hygiene
University of Nebraska Medical Center
College of Dentistry
Lincoln, Nebraska

Laura Jansen Howerton, RDH, MS
Instructor
Dental Hygiene
Wake Technical Community College
Acquisition Technologist
Carolina OMF Imaging
Raleigh, North Carolina

Olga A.C. Ibsen, RDH, AAS, BS, MS
Adjunct Professor
Department of Oral and Maxillofacial
    Pathology, Radiology, and Medicine
New York University College of Dentistry
New York, New York
Adjunct Professor
Fones School of Dental Hygiene
University of Bridgeport
Bridgeport, Connecticut

Kim T. Isringhausen, BSDH, MPH
Associate Professor, Chair
Oral Health Promotion and Community
    Outreach
Virginia Commonwealth University
School of Dentistry
Richmond, Virginia

Todd N. Junge, RDH, BS
Assistant Professor
Dental Hygiene
University of Nebraska Medical Center
Lincoln, Nebraska

**Leslie Koberna, RDH, BSDH, MPH/
    HSA, PhD**
Associate Clinical Professor
Dental Hygiene Program
Texas Woman's University
Denton, Texas

**Lisa F. Harper Mallonee, BSDH, MPH,
    RD, LD**
Associate Professor
Dental Hygiene
Baylor College of Dentistry
Texas A&M University
Dallas, Texas

Laura Mueller-Joseph, EdD, RDH
Associate Provost
Professor Dental Hygiene
Farmingdale State College of New York
Farmingdale, New York

Darnyl M. Palmer, RDH, MS
Clinical Instructor
Department of Dental Hygiene
Georgia State University
Dunwoody, Georgia

John M. Powers, PhD
Clinical Professor of Oral Biomaterials
Restorative Dentistry and Prosthodontics
University of Texas School of Dentistry
    at Houston
Houston, Texas
Senior Vice President and Senior Editor
The Dental Advisor
Dental Consultants, Inc.
Ann Arbor, Michigan

Maureen Dotzel Savner, MS, RDH
Professor of Dental Hygiene
Dental Health Department
Luzerne County Community College
Mountain Top, Pennsylvania

Jessica Peek Scott, RDH, DHSc
Department Chair of Allied Health
    Sciences
Allied Health
Central Carolina Community College
Sanford, North Carolina

M. Anjum Shah, BSDH, MS
Assistant Professor and Chair of Dental
   Hygiene Program Admissions
Oral Health Promotion and
   Community Outreach
Dental Hygiene Program
Virginia Commonwealth University
Richmond, Virginia

Rebecca A. Sroda, MS
Dean
Health Sciences
South Florida State College
Avon Park, Florida

Susan Lynn Tolle, BSDH, MS
Professor, University Professor
School of Dental Hygiene
Old Dominion University
Norfolk, Virginia

Pamela Zarkowski, JD, MPH, BSDH
Provost and Vice President for Academic
   Affairs
Professor in the Department of Patient
   Management
School of Dentistry
University of Detroit Mercy
Detroit, Michigan

SUBJECT MATTER CONSULTANTS (CHAPTER 18)

Margaret J. Fehrenbach, RDH, MS
Oral Biologist and Dental Hygienist
Adjunct Instructor
Bachelor of Applied Science Degree
Dental Hygiene Program
Seattle Central College
Educational Consultant and Dental
   Science Writer
Seattle, Washington

Demetra Daskalos Logothetis, RDH, MS
Professor Emeritus and
Professor and Graduate Program Director
Department of Dental Medicine
School of Medicine
University of New Mexico
Albuquerque, New Mexico

The transforming health care environment, new knowledge gained through research, and the need for evidence-based education and practice serve as the prime forces guiding the development of the eighth edition of *Darby's Comprehensive Review of Dental Hygiene*. Publishing a book that comprehensively reviews the foundation for dental hygiene competencies is a challenge. Demographic, societal, and educational trends, issues surrounding access to care for all citizens, and new health care delivery and finance systems require successful dental hygienists to possess competence in the biological, social, behavioral, and dental hygiene sciences and in general education. The book and the accompanying Evolve website offer a complete learning package to:

- assist individuals in reviewing the theory, skills, and judgments required on national, regional, and state dental hygiene board examinations;
- prepare dental hygienists for reentry into professional dental hygiene roles—clinician, educator, advocate, researcher, and administrator/manager;
- provide educators with salient information used for course and curriculum development and outcomes assessment.

"CLIENT" VS. "PATIENT"

Throughout the book, "client" (instead of "patient") is used predominantly because the term is congruent with the profession's disease prevention, health promotion, and wellness focus. Most important, the term "client" conveys dental hygiene's partnership with consumers and communities inclusive of individuals, families, and target groups who are fast becoming the focus of community-based dental hygiene practice. Both the American Dental Hygienists' Association and the Canadian Dental Hygienists' Association have embraced the term "client" in their policies and actions. When the client is debilitated by disease or disability, the term "patient" is used.

A special effort was made to design testlets for the community oral health content and case-based questions that include client health; dental, pharmacologic, and cultural history; and dental charts, radiographs, and photographs. Other multiple-choice test items mimic the various types used on the actual National Board Dental Hygiene Examination.

ORGANIZATION

The eighth edition of *Darby's Comprehensive Review of Dental Hygiene* is divided into 22 independent, interrelated chapters. Chapter 1 provides guidance and confidence-boosting recommendations for anyone preparing for a board examination. Emphasis is on understanding board examinations, test-taking strategies, and trends in standardized board examinations. Chapters 2 to 22 cover subject areas found on the National Board Dental Hygiene Examination and contain theoretical and applied information in an outline format. End-of-chapter review questions, with rationales on Evolve, explain why the correct answer is appropriate and why each incorrect choice is wrong. The rationales for the correct and incorrect answers provide an additional strategy for efficient board preparation. This information enables the reviewer to assess both decision making and judgment in integrating professional knowledge, and facilitates mastery of each chapter's content, further increasing the likelihood of success on examination day.

Internet links and a comprehensive index that enables users to locate information quickly and easily are included. Illustrations and the appendices minimize the need to search alternative sources; however, reference lists and website resources are provided for those who desire more in-depth study or enrichment.

SIMULATED NATIONAL BOARD DENTAL HYGIENE EXAMINATIONS/ELECTRONIC RESOURCES

Resources for Students and Faculty

Providing four simulated National Board Dental Hygiene Examination—style exams gives you and your students the practice opportunities needed to ensure test-taking confidence and exam-day success. The examinations are located on the Evolve companion site (see inside front cover for access information), and students have the ability to take each exam in practice and study modes. Practice mode displays the answer and rationale after the student answers each question, whereas exam mode mimics a realistic testing experience with timer functionality and end-of-exam results and feedback. Questions are scrambled each time, and students can take them as many times as they want. In addition, faculty members who have adopted this text can enroll students into their class to monitor progress, publish class syllabi and lecture notes, and enable communication with and among students.

ACKNOWLEDGMENTS

Almost everyone can recall a special individual - a tough but caring coach, a friend who went beyond the call of duty - someone who left an imprint on us for the rest of our lives. For me, that individual is Michele Darby. So first, I want to pay tribute to her, the creator of this work. I would not have had the wonderful career in dental hygiene education if it were not for Michele. As her graduate student, she taught me how to be a teacher, a writer, and a researcher. She inspired me with her vision of what the dental hygiene profession could become and we know now her vision was way ahead of its time. Throughout my professional career, Michele continued to be a wonderful mentor to me, always taking the time to listen and help whenever I needed it. She so often encouraged me to lead change, to take on challenges. And, when she could hear my reluctance, she calmly said, "You can do it" and "make it better." Michele taught me to strive for excellence in all I do. I am both honored and humbled to carry on as editor of this book for Michele.

I would like to express my sincere appreciation to those who helped make this edition of *Darby's Comprehensive Review of Dental Hygiene* a reality. Detailed outlines, board questions, answers, and rationales were developed by renowned experts identified in the table of contents. Comments and suggestions from students, faculty, and returning dental hygienists who have used the book are embodied in this edition. The exemplary work of these contributors has made *Darby's Comprehensive Review of Dental Hygiene* a board-preparation experience that is second to none.

My special thanks go to Kristin Wilhelm, Content Strategist; Billie Sharp, Content Development Manager; Samantha Dalton, Associate Content Development Specialist; and Cindy Thoms, Senior Project Manager, who facilitated the many steps of the publication process at Elsevier. Also acknowledged are the authors, corporations, and publishers who granted permission to use quotes, concepts, photographs, figures, and tables. Since the work of those who contributed to the earlier editions remains central to this revision, I want to gratefully acknowledge their efforts, particularly the work of Dr. Eleanor Bushee and Linda E. DeVore, whose competence and good humor as oral health professionals, teachers, administrators, colleagues, and friends will forever be missed, and Marilyn Beck, Dr. Marcia Brand, Kristin Calley, Patricia Regener Campbell, Karen Caspers, Marie A. Collins, Patricia Damon-Johnson, Judith A. Davidson, Dr. Catherine C. Davis, Mary-Catherine Dean, Susann Duncan, Diane M. Frazier, Jacquelyn L. Fried, Barbara Heckman, Jan Shaner Greenlee, Charlotte Hangorsky, Kara Hansen, Beverly Entwistle Isman, Dr. Donald E. Isselhard, Sandra Kramer, Mary M. Lee, Shirley Kuhn, Kathy Macciocca, Sally Mauriello, Susan Schwartz Miller, Cara Miyasaki, Dr. Marlene Moss-Klyvert, Lynn Ray, Dr. Peggy Reep, Dr. Lindsay Rettie, Danielle Leigh Ryan, Michelle Sensat, Dr. Lynn Utecht, Venkat Varkala, Nancy Webb, K. Cy Whaley, and Susan Zimmer. Without the earlier contributions of these talented people, the current edition of *Darby's Comprehensive Review of Dental Hygiene* would not be possible.

The eighth edition appropriately has a new title, that being *Darby's Comprehensive Review of Dental Hygiene*, and I dedicate this edition to Michele—a person who made a lasting imprint on my life.

Christine Blue

CONTENTS

1 Preparing for National, Regional, and State Dental Hygiene Board Examinations, 1
Barbara Leatherman Dixon

2 Histology and Embryology, 16
Maureen Dotzel Savner

3 Anatomy and Physiology, 53
Brenda Armstrong

4 Head and Neck Anatomy and Physiology, 107
Kim T. Isringhausen

5 Clinical Oral Structures, Dental Anatomy, and Root Morphology, 129
Jeanne M. Anderson

6 Oral and Maxillofacial Radiology, 152
Laura Jansen Howerton

7 General Pathology, 177
JoAnn R. Gurenlian

8 Oral Pathology, 193
Olga A.C. Ibsen

9 Microbiology and Immunology, 256
Jessica Peek Scott

10 Infection Control and Prevention of Disease Transmission in Oral Health Care, 300
Darnyl M. Palmer

11 Pharmacology, 325
Elena Bablenis Haveles

12 Biochemistry, Nutrition, and Nutritional Counseling, 360
Lisa F. Harper Mallonee

13 Biomaterials, 394
Stephen C. Bayne, John M. Powers

14 Periodontics, 427
Denise M. Bowen

15 Dental Hygiene Process of Care, 458
Laura Mueller-Joseph

16 Strategies for Oral Health Promotion and Disease Prevention and Control, 490
M. Anjum Shah

17 Periodontal Instrumentation for Assessment and Care, 518
Jill S. Gehrig, Rebecca A. Sroda

18 Management of Pain and Anxiety, 547
Gwen L. Hlava, Todd N. Junge

19 Dental Hygiene Care for Clients with Special Care Needs, 567
Susan Lynn Tolle

20 Community Oral Health Planning and Practice, 619
Christine French Beatty, Connie E. Beatty, and Charlene B. Dickinson

21 Medical Emergencies, 688
Leslie Koberna

22 Ethical and Legal Issues, 707
Pamela Zarkowski

Appendix A: Medical Terminology, 743
Appendix B: Professional Organizations of Interest to Dental Hygienists, 746
Appendix C: American Dental Hygienists Association and Canadian Dental Hygienists Association codes of Ethics, 748

Preparing for National, Regional, and State Dental Hygiene Board Examinations

Barbara Leatherman Dixon

Preparing for board examinations requires deliberate planning, study and review, time management, organization of information and schedules, and a positive "can-do" attitude. Conscientious dental hygienists will organize a plan for success well in advance and will be prepared to satisfy board requirements with confidence in their professional knowledge and skills. This book is a guide through the evidence-based knowledge on which dental hygiene practice is based. Systematic use of this book enables one to reinforce professional education, integrate concepts and ideas from many dental hygiene educators, and identify subject areas in which additional study is warranted.

The introductory chapter is a primer in navigating the licensure system—whether a new graduate, a practicing dental hygienist who is moving to another licensing jurisdiction, or a dental hygienist returning to practice after a lapse of activity—to prepare for both didactic and clinical board examinations. A dental hygienist must master all subject matter and skills necessary for practice; therefore, each subsequent chapter focuses on different aspects of such knowledge and skills. Success on board examinations also relies on being psychologically, emotionally, and physically prepared to demonstrate competence. It is essential to become thoroughly familiar with the format, logistics, and requirements of any preparatory examination for licensure.

This chapter discusses the multi-faceted licensure structure and explains the roles and interactions of the numerous organizations within the system. Information on both the National Board Dental Hygiene Examination (NBDHE) and clinical board examinations is provided. The chapter concludes with an overview of this review book, including its purpose and organization, as well as instructions on how to use the text effectively.

DENTAL HYGIENE LICENSURE

In the United States, licensure falls under the authority of an individual state or jurisdiction. Licensure of dental hygienists is a means of regulation to protect the public from unsafe practice of the profession and unqualified individuals. Each state has a *state practice act* that defines the practice of dental hygiene, establishes educational and testing requirements for licensure, sets parameters for enforcement of the law within that jurisdiction, and creates a state board of dentistry or dental hygiene to serve in accordance with the statute. A certificate for successful completion of an examination is *not* authorization to practice. Beginning practice without a license is illegal. Dental hygiene licensure requirements vary from state to state, but almost every state has the following three requirements:

- Graduation from a dental hygiene program accredited by the Commission on Dental Accreditation (CODA) or, based on reciprocity, by the Commission on Dental Accreditation of Canada (CDAC)
- Successful completion of the NBDHE
- Successful completion of a regional or state clinical board examination

Recognition of an accrediting agency is a governmental function. In health care fields with a domain of specialized education, accreditation is conducted by a dedicated agency within the profession. In dentistry, the U.S. Department of Education (USDE) has recognized the CODA of the American Dental Association (ADA) as the official accrediting body for schools of dentistry, dental hygiene, dental assisting, and dental laboratory technology. The CODA is also listed in the publications of accreditation agencies by the Council for Higher Education Accreditation (CHEA). A diploma, certificate, associate's degree, or baccalaureate degree in dental hygiene indicating graduation from an accredited program is an essential component for licensure that is based on the accreditation system carried out under the auspices of the CODA. States that provide for licensure of a dental hygienist from a non-accredited school generally require evidence of an educational program approved by the state board. The NBDHE is developed and administered by the Joint Commission on National Dental Examinations (JCNDE). Client-based clinical examinations are conducted by five regional testing agencies (Boxes 1-1 and 1-2). Currently three regional testing agencies (CITA, NERB, and SRTA) administer the American Board of Dental Examiners (ADEX) dental hygiene licensure examination. ADEX is strictly a *test development* corporation; it does not administer any examinations. The licensure boards of California, Delaware, and the Virgin Islands of the United States administer independent examinations. Clinical examinations accepted for initial dental hygiene licensure are shown in Figure 1-1.

A license is applicable only within the geographic boundaries of the issuing state. However, most states have provisions for granting dental hygiene licensure by credentials or endorsement. Requirements generally include an active license in good

---

BOX 1-1 Membership in the Five Regional Testing Agencies in the United States*

CITA
Alabama
Kentucky
Louisiana
North Carolina
West Virginia
Puerto Rico

CRDTS
Alabama
Colorado
Georgia
Hawaii (dental hygiene only)
Illinois
Iowa
Kansas
Minnesota
Missouri
Nebraska
New Mexico
North Dakota
South Carolina
South Dakota
Washington
West Virginia
Wisconsin
Wyoming

NERB
Connecticut
District of Columbia
Florida
Hawaii
Illinois
Indiana
Kentucky
Maine
Maryland
Massachusetts
Michigan
Mississippi
Missouri
Nevada

New Hampshire
New Jersey
New Mexico
New York
Ohio
Oregon
Pennsylvania
Rhode Island
Vermont
West Virginia
Wisconsin

SRTA
Arkansas
Kentucky
Mississippi
South Carolina
Tennessee
Virginia
West Virginia

WREB
Alaska
Arizona
California (dental only)
Hawaii (dental hygiene only)
Idaho
Illinois
Kansas
Kentucky
Missouri
Montana
Nevada
New Mexico
North Dakota
Oklahoma
Oregon
Texas
Utah
Washington
West Virginia
Wyoming

*CITA, Council of Interstate Testing Agencies; *CRDTS*, Central Regional Dental Testing Service, Inc.; *NERB*, Northeast Regional Board of Dental Examiners, Inc.; *SRTA*, Southern Regional Testing Agency, Inc.; *WREB*, WREB: A National Dental and Dental Hygiene Testing Agency.

BOX 1-2 Regional Testing Agencies and Contact Information*

Central Regional Dental Testing Service, Inc. (CRDTS)
Central Regional Dental Testing Service, Inc.
1725 Gage Boulevard
Topeka, KS 66604-3333
Phone: 785-273-0380
Fax: 785-273-5015
www.crdts.org

Council of Interstate Testing Agencies (CITA)
1003 High House Road, Suite 101
Cary, NC 27513
Phone: 919-460-7750
Fax: 919-460-7715
www.citaexam.com

Northeast Regional Board of Dental Examiners, Inc. (NERB)
Northeast Regional Board of Dental Examiners, Inc.
8484 Georgia Avenue, Suite 900
Silver Spring, MD 20910
Phone: 301-563-3300
Fax: 301-563-3307
www.nerb.org

Southern Regional Testing Agency, Inc. (SRTA)
Southern Regional Testing Agency, Inc.
4698 Honeygrove Road, Suite 2
Virginia Beach, VA 23455
Phone: 757-318-9082
Fax: 757-318-9085
www.srta.org

WREB: A National Dental and Dental Hygiene Testing Agency
23460 North 19th Avenue, Suite 210
Phoenix, AZ 85027
Phone: 602-944-3315
Fax: 602-371-8131
www.wreb.org

*Current information about examination policies, procedures, criteria, locations, dates, registration, and frequently asked questions can be accessed at the respective agency's website.

---

standing, recent practice experience, graduation from an accredited program, successful completion of the NBDHE, and successful completion of a clinical examination. Specifics differ from state to state and are subject to change. For example, some states only accept NBDHE results within the last 5 years, or limit recognition of clinical board examination scores to those from particular testing agencies.

Applicants for dental hygiene licensure must contact the individual state licensing board for current requirements and information. The American Association of Dental Boards (AADB)

website (http://www.dentalboards.org/states/index.htm) features a map of the United States with direct links to state board offices. State board websites are also readily accessible through an online search listing the state and "dental/dental hygiene board."

STATE BOARDS OF DENTISTRY OR DENTAL HYGIENE AND PROFESSIONAL ASSOCIATIONS

State boards of dentistry or dental hygiene are governmental agencies that control and manage dental hygiene licensure in accordance with laws adopted by the legislature of the states. Boards have the power or influence to grant, deny, and revoke licenses. Board members are charged with the following duties:
- Enforcing the state practice act and its rules and regulations
- Conducting or recognizing examinations for competence

Clinical Examinations Accepted for Initial Dental Hygiene Licensure*

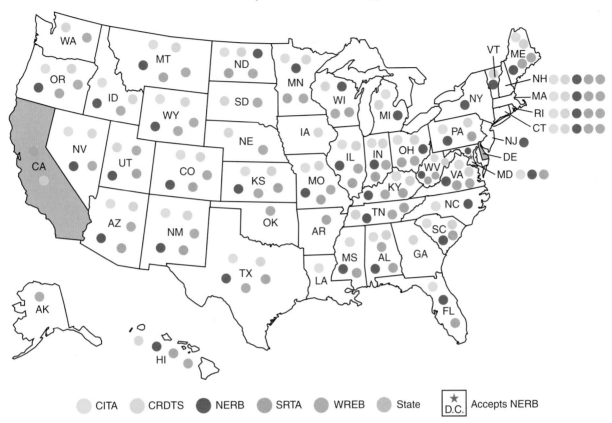

| CITA | CRDTS | NERB | SRTA | WREB | State | ★ D.C. | Accepts NERB |

Please note that this information does not include examinations accepted within a restricted span of years or with passing scores other than those set by the testing agency. Recognizing jurisdictions and licensing requirements are subject to change. Examinees are encouraged to contact the State Board where they seek licensure to confirm information.

*Initial Licensure is defined as the state licensure sought immediately following graduation from an accredited dental hygiene program.

FIG 1-1 Clinical examinations accepted for initial dental hygiene licensure.

- Reviewing and investigating complaints concerning unlawful or unprofessional conduct by licensees

Significant variations exist from jurisdiction to jurisdiction in regulatory board organizational structure, in scope of power and authority, and even in title. For the purpose of clarity in this text, the term *state board* or *state board of dentistry* is used to refer to the *regulatory body* in a respective legal jurisdiction that is empowered to determine prerequisites for licensure and issue licenses to practice dental hygiene.

Frequently, licensure candidates and even licensed practitioners confuse the state board with the state professional association. Although strong ties may exist between a state board and the state professional association, distinct legal differences exist between these two bodies. The state board of dentistry is a *governmental agency,* established by law, which functions as an arm of the state legislature to regulate the practice of dentistry and/or dental hygiene. Its sole purpose is to protect the public from incompetent or unethical practitioners. In contrast, a state dental hygiene or dental association is a *voluntary organization* of practitioners, who join together to advance the profession and promote the oral health of the public.

Practitioners need to understand both this distinction and the interaction between state boards and professional associations. Professional associations *do not* determine requirements for licensure or regulate practice; this is founded by law and implemented through state boards. Professional associations do, however, initiate programs and research projects, and propose legislative changes that may ultimately be incorporated into the legal requirements for practice. In most states, state board members are appointed by the governor. Alabama, Nebraska, North Carolina, Oklahoma, and the District of Columbia are the exceptions, with designation through election by members of the profession or through appointment by another governmental body. Typically, professional associations nominate and influence these appointments.

All states have some form of dental hygiene representation on the board. Recent years have seen a trend toward self-regulation, with the establishment of separate dental hygiene state boards and advisory committees. Currently, 18 states have varying degrees of self-regulation for dental hygienists (Arizona, California, Connecticut, Delaware, Florida, Iowa, Maine, Maryland, Michigan, Missouri, Montana, Nevada, New Hampshire, New Mexico, Oklahoma, Oregon, Texas, and Washington). In Canada, over 99% of dental hygienists are self-regulated (in all provinces except Prince Edward Island and the three territories).

The legislative and political arenas in dentistry are constantly changing, as are technologic advancements in health. As a result, revision to state practice acts—including the definitions of *dental hygiene* and the scope of practice—is ongoing. Likewise, as the standards of competence in dental hygiene are redefined in terms of requisite professional skills and knowledge, examinations undergo continual updating. Although this places demands on the individual practitioner, the educational system, and the agencies responsible for evaluating competence, it is the pathway for the advancement of professional standards, increasing access to care and improving the oral health status of populations. State practice acts charge the state board with conducting or sanctioning both didactic and clinical examinations to determine competence for entry into the profession. Some state laws even define the examination content and specify a passing score. The majority of practice acts authorize the state board to recognize multiple examinations (see Figure 1-1). Although other agencies are part of the licensure process, the fundamental authorization to recognize qualifications for licensure lies with the individual state regulatory board.

JOINT COMMISSION ON NATIONAL DENTAL EXAMINATIONS

The JCNDE is the agency responsible for the development and administration of the NBDHE. It includes a 15-member panel of representatives, as follows:
* American Dental Association, ADA (3)
* American Dental Education Association, ADEA (3)
* American Association of Dental Boards, AADB (6)
* American Dental Hygienists Association, ADHA (1)
* Public Member (1)
* American Student Dental Association, ASDA (1)

A standing committee of the JCNDE, the Committee on Dental Hygiene (CDH), consists of five dental hygienists (including the ADHA Commissioner)—two educators and two practitioners and a dental hygiene student representative appointed by the ADHA—plus one Commissioner from the ADA, the ADEA, and the AADB. The CDH's responsibilities relate primarily to the NBDHE and include the following:
* Examination content and specifications
* Test construction procedures, including nomination of test constructors
* Information to publicize or explain the testing program
* Examination regulations that affect dental hygiene examinees
* Matters pertaining to finances, the ADA and the Joint Commission Bylaws, and the Joint Commission Standing Rules that affect the NBDHE

The Commission has final authority to act on committee recommendations, but historically, the CDH has been the guiding force of the dental hygiene examination program.

NATIONAL BOARD DENTAL HYGIENE EXAMINATION

Examination Format

The NBDHE is designed to "assess the ability of an examinee to understand important information from biomedical, dental, and dental hygiene sciences, and to apply such information in a problem-solving context."[1] The examination is computer based and includes approximately 350 multiple-choice items in independent, case-based, and testlet formats. The NBDHE is a comprehensive examination with two components. Component A presents 200 discipline-based items in three major areas, as follows:
* Scientific basis for dental hygiene practice
* Provision of clinical dental hygiene services
* Community health/research principles

Component B presents 150 case-based items, which relate to 12 to 15 dental hygiene patient cases. Case material includes dental and health histories, dental charting, radiographs, and clinical photographs. Every examination includes one or more of the following patient types: geriatric, adult–periodontitis, pediatric, special needs, and medically compromised. The case-based items address knowledge, skills, and judgments necessary for the following:
* Assessing client characteristics
* Obtaining and interpreting radiographs
* Planning and managing dental hygiene care
* Performing periodontal procedures
* Using preventive agents
* Providing supportive treatment services
* Professional responsibility

The NBDHE tests the examinee's ability to apply the essential knowledge and skills as a beginning safe practitioner to solve oral health care problems and answer questions related to dental hygiene care. The examination is based on practice competencies underlying entry-level dental hygiene practice as defined by the ADEA, the ADHA, the *Accreditation Standards* published by the CODA, and other communities of interest. As part of its validity analyses to verify that the examination content supports these competencies, the JCNDE conducts a nationwide practice survey every 5 years. For more information, read the *NBDHE Technical Report* available on the ADA's website, http://www.ada.org/~/media/JCNDE/pdfs/nbdhe_technical_report.ashx. The *NBDHE Test Specifications* document, accessible in the *National Board Dental Hygiene Examination Guide,* is the blueprint for test development. The outline lists the specific categories of subject matter included in the examination, with an itemization of the number of items devoted to each area. It should be referenced as a guide for study and review.

Examination items are written and selected by test construction committees in accordance with the NBDHE Dental Hygiene Test Specifications. The test construction committees are composed of individuals who represent locations across the country and are selected on the basis of their expertise in six areas: (1) basic sciences, (2) radiology, (3) periodontics,

(4) dental hygiene curriculum, (5) clinical dental hygiene, and (6) community dental health. Test construction committees author new examination items and develop new cases, revise and clone test items, create multiple versions of the examination, and review examination drafts before publishing. Committees strive toward higher cognitive levels—understanding, application, and reasoning—in test development.

Item Format

The multiple-choice items on the NBDHE consist of a stem, which poses a problem, and a list of three to five possible responses. The stem is usually either a question or an incomplete statement. Key words in the stem such as *best, most, first, not, except,* or *least* are usually highlighted or italicized. Only one response is correct or clearly the best choice by universally accepted standards of care.

A variety of item formats are used in the NBDHE. Descriptions of formats as well as sample items from the *National Board Dental Hygiene Examination Guide* are provided next.

Completion

As indicated by the name, *completion* items necessitate the correct completion of a theory or idea. For example:

The sensation of touch, pain, pressure, or temperature is determined by the:
a. Specific nerve fiber stimulated
b. Method of stimulation of a nerve fiber
c. Degree of myelinization of a nerve fiber
d. Strength of the stimulation to a nerve fiber
e. Frequency of the stimulation to a nerve fiber

Question

A *question* item poses a problem or set of circumstances. Response choices include only one best answer. For example:

Which of the following is innervated by the phrenic nerve?
a. Diaphragm
b. Abdominal muscles
c. Sternocleidomastoid muscle
d. Internal intercostal muscles
e. External intercostal muscles

Negative

A *negative* item is characterized with words such as *except, least,* or *not* in the stem. These key words are emphasized by capitalization, italics, or both. For example:

Each of the following is affected by saliva EXCEPT one. Which one is the *exception*?
a. Swallowing
b. Dental caries
c. Oral microflora
d. Protein digestion
e. Carbohydrate breakdown

Paired True-False

In a *paired–true–false* item, the stem consists of two sentences on the same topic. The examinee is asked to determine whether the statements are true or false. For example:

Protection from excessive exposure to radiation is aided by use of aluminum filters and a lead diaphragm. The filters reduce the amount of soft radiation reaching the patient's face, and the diaphragm controls the area exposed.
a. Both statements are TRUE.
b. Both statements are FALSE.
c. The first statement is TRUE, the second is FALSE.
d. The first statement is FALSE, the second is TRUE.

Cause and Effect

In *cause-and-effect* items, the stem includes a statement and a reason joined by the word "because." This item requires judgment of both the accuracy and the relationship between the two statements. First, the examinee should determine whether each statement is correct or incorrect and then how the statements are related. For example:

A traumatic injury can cause the pulp space to calcify because the accident can trigger odontoclasts into accelerated activity.
a. Both the statement and the reason are correct and related.
b. Both the statement and the reason are correct but NOT related.
c. The statement is correct, but the reason is NOT.
d. The statement is NOT correct, but the reason is correct.
e. NEITHER the statement NOR the reason is correct.

Testlet

Testlet items are used for testing knowledge and application of community health and research principles; they are also used in the case-based section of the examination. A short scenario describing a situation, event, or problem is followed by a set of associated multiple-choice items. For example:

A dental hygienist employed at a public health clinic in a rural county of the United States is assigned the project of developing a preventive dental health program for a subgroup of the population.

Community Profile
The primary employers in this county have been coal-mining companies. The unemployment rate in the county has increased by 32% since the closing of the coal mines.

The median age of the population is 46 years. In the county, there are five general dentists, three dental hygienists, and one public health–centered dental clinic. The clinic employs a full-time dentist and dental hygienist. The public health clinic sees low-income children and senior citizens on a sliding-fee schedule.

The dental hygienist employed by the public health clinic conducts dental screenings for the kindergarten (K) students each year. The mean deft (decayed, extracted, filled teeth) scores for the K students for the last 3 years are $d = 1.02$, $e = 0.87$, and $f = 4.22$.

The community does not have water fluoridation because of multiple water sources. The state funds a 0.2% sodium fluoride rinse program in grades K through 5. The state mandates that a dentist or a dental hygienist perform

Continued

deft/dmft (decayed, missing, filled teeth)/DMFT and Gingival Index (GI) scoring on all students in grades 1, 2, 3, 5, 7, and 10. On a yearly basis, all pathology is brought to the parent's attention and referred to a dental professional.

1. Which population group is dentally underserved in this community?
   a. Adult age
   b. Geriatric age
   c. Adolescent age
   d. Early-childhood age
   e. Elementary school age

2. What would be the next step for the dental hygienist to take in program planning after selecting the target population?
   a. Appraise the program.
   b. Define goals for the program.
   c. Compile data on the target group population.
   d. Develop educational components.
   e. Identify manpower resources in the community.

3. Each of the following is perceived as a barrier to dental care for this community EXCEPT one. Which one is the *exception*?
   a. Geographic isolation
   b. Lack of water fluoridation
   c. Maldistribution of providers
   d. Lack of affordable services
   e. Loss of income and insurance

4. What can be stated about the deft scores of the kindergarten students?
   a. Early exfoliation
   b. High decay rate
   c. Increased referrals
   d. Late eruption pattern
   e. Treatment needs are being met.

5. How often should the fluoride rinse for grades K through 5 be performed?
   a. Daily
   b. Weekly
   c. Monthly
   d. Three times a week
   e. Based on the caries rate of the child

Case Based

The *case-based* portion of the examination presents 12 to 15 dental hygiene patient cases, including social, medical, and dental histories; a chief complaint; dental and periodontal charting; radiographs; and clinical photographs. Items based on observations and judgments about the client's clinical conditions and needs follow. These items may be presented in any of the test formats previously described.

Examples of cases and other items are provided in the NBDHE samples at the end of this book and on the Evolve website. Sample Examination Items can also be accessed from the ADA/JCNDE website.

National Board Dental Hygiene Examination Eligibility and Application

Eligibility for the NBDHE requires qualification through one of the following stipulations:

- A student in an accredited dental hygiene program is eligible when certified by the program director to be prepared for the examination.
- A graduate of an accredited dental hygiene program is eligible following the JCNDE's receipt of evidence of graduation.

- A graduate of a non-accredited program is eligible only if the program is deemed equivalent to an accredited program by an independent auditing agency (e.g., length of study, curriculum content, hours of clinical instruction).
- A dental student from an accredited dental school is eligible if the dean of that school certifies that the student has completed the equivalent of a dental hygiene program.
- A dentist is eligible if the National Board Dental Examination (NBDE) eligibility requirements have been met.

Applications must be submitted electronically to the Joint Commission. The steps involved in the application process include the following:

- Read the *NBDHE Guide* before applying
- Obtain a Dental Personal Identifier Number (DENTPIN) from the ADA. The DENTPIN is a unique number to identify students and examinees for secure reporting, transmission of test scores, and tracking of academic data in the educational system of the United States.
- Apply for the examination. Confirm and agree to the rules and regulations. Include requests for score reporting to state boards where seeking licensure. If applicable, submit appropriate documentation of a disability to support an appeal for testing accommodation. Also, indicate whether the NBDHE was previously taken.
- After processing the application, the Joint Commission will send notification of eligibility.
- Schedule an appointment to take the examination at a Pearson VUE Testing Center. The computer-delivered NBDHE is scheduled and administered on an individual basis year-round.

Examination Day

Candidates for the NBDHE must present two original, current forms of identification (ID) to the testing center, as follows.

- One government-issued ID with a photograph and signature
- One secondary ID with a signature

No personal items (e.g., cell phones, study materials, backpacks or purses, watches, "good luck charms," food or water bottles) are allowed in the secure testing area. The testing schedule begins with an optional 15-minute tutorial. Three and a half hours are allowed for the first session, Component A (200 discipline-based items), and 4 hours are allowed for the second session, Component B (150 client case-based items). An optional 1-hour break is scheduled between the sessions. Examinees may provide feedback in a 15-minute post-examination survey on completion of the examination and will receive a *Notice of Completion* before leaving the testing center.

Examination Results

The examinee's total score is calculated by the number of correct answers selected. On the NBDHE, there is no penalty for selecting an incorrect response. The total score is converted to a scale score, ranging from 49 to 99, which adjusts for any minor differences in difficulty across NBDHE forms. A score of 75 represents the minimum passing score. The NBDHE is "criterion referenced," that is, the minimum passing score is determined by experts through standard setting activities to ensure that scores accurately and fairly reflect the entry-level practitioner's ability to solve oral health care problems and to answer items relating to dental hygiene practice on the examination. Detailed specifics on the scoring system are outlined in the Technical Report on the Joint Commission's website. All examination results are audited for decision accuracy of the pass/fail point before being reported.

Results on the NBDHE are reported as pass/fail only. The status of "pass" is reported if a standard score of 75 or higher is achieved. The status of "fail" is reported if a standard score below 75 is achieved. For remediation purposes, examinees who fail receive numerical scores for each of the major subject areas covered on the test. Official results are available approximately 3 weeks after the examination. The examinee receives an individual score report, and by virtue of signing the NBDHE application, express permission is granted to give the dental hygiene program director a score report as well. Reports are sent directly to state licensing boards specified on the examinee's application.

Examinees who have passed the NBDHE may not retake the examination unless required by a state board or regulatory jurisdiction. An unsuccessful examinee may reapply after 90 days from the date of the previous examination attempt. After three failures, the examinee must wait 12 months before reapplying. Examination attempts on or after January 1, 2012, are restricted by the JCNDE's 5 Years/5 Attempts Eligibility Rule, which mandates examinees must pass the examination within 5 years of their first attempt or five examination attempts, whichever comes first.

Ethical and Legal Issues

The Joint Commission maintains a program to identify any irregularities or cheating on the examination. As professionals, applicants for the NBDHE are obliged to uphold ethical standards of behavior. All examinees are expected to pass the examination on individual merit, without assistance or prior knowledge of examination items. The National Board's *Rules of Conduct* are regulations that prohibit retaining or sharing test items so that no examinee has an unfair advantage. Maintaining the confidentiality of the examination protects the integrity of the examination process and ensures valid outcomes in determining satisfactory achievement to practice safely and responsibly. Violating the Confidentiality Agreement by distributing or seeking unreleased examination items is a legal infraction with stiff penalties, including voiding of examination results and civil liability or criminal penalties or both. In some cases, misconduct is reported to school or licensing authorities. Unethical conduct carries the risk of delay, denial, or loss of licensure. When the Joint Commission discovers, or is informed, that a breach of examination regulations has occurred, the examinee's results are withheld or invalidated. In some cases, the examinee must wait up to 2 years to be considered eligible for retesting.

In addition to unauthorized access, or the written or oral distribution of confidential exam content, other irregularities include the following:
- Falsifying information on the application
- Attempting to take the examination for someone else
- Bringing prohibited items (e.g., pens, cell phones, candy/gum, medicines, religious items) to the test center or the testing area
- Creating a disturbance of any kind
- Taking unscheduled breaks during the examination

Study the rules of conduct in the *NBDHE Guide,* and follow all regulations.

The JCNDE's systematic security control procedures to identify and investigate irregularities preserve the examination's legitimacy.

Preparing for the National Board Dental Hygiene Examination

Studying for a comprehensive, high-stakes licensure examination is intensive and unique from studying for other tests. The following are suggested steps in preparing for the NBDHE:

1. Organize a study plan 4 to 6 months in advance to allow an orderly, progressive review without undue pressure.
2. Obtain the NBDHE Guide and application materials provided by the JCNDE. Study the information thoroughly to gain a clear understanding of the examination's format, design, and administration. View the online tutorial for the NBDHE at http://www.pearsonvue.com/nbdhe/.
3. Obtain a copy of the most recently released NBDHE items from the Joint Commission. Released examinations, protected by copyright and available for a fee, are valuable as examples. However, retired examinations may contain out-of-date subject material and should not be relied on as the sole study activity. Simulated board examinations, such as the ones in this text and on the Evolve website, may also prove beneficial during review.
4. Outline areas of weakness. Be guided by school experience, as indicated by grades or difficulty in certain subjects and by the items from the released or simulated examinations missed or marked as questionable. Dental hygienists who have been out of school or practice for some period should focus on basic science material and any developments in dental technology or procedures that have expanded or changed evidence-based practice since graduation.
5. Gather a personal resource library for reference throughout the review process. Properly used, this book should be the mainstay study guide; directions for its use are included at the end of this chapter. This book is designed to direct a comprehensive review of dental hygiene, provide questions to assess mastery of the subject material, and offer documentation for correct and incorrect responses. This review book may be supplemented with textbooks, class notes, pertinent journal articles, and websites for further study in focused areas. Ensure all textbooks and reference materials are current resources. The JCNDE does not approve or recommend any particular texts or review courses. Programs or conferences that profess to be "National Board Review Courses" are not affiliated in any way with the JCNDE.
6. If considering a study club, recruit three to five colleagues whose study habits, personal style, and self-discipline complement group efforts for collaboration. Otherwise, study alone.

BOX 1-3   Tips for Managing Examination Anxiety

- Be well prepared. Nothing boosts confidence like good advance preparation.
- Study over several weeks. Do not rely on last-minute cramming.
- Maintain a positive attitude when preparing for the examination.
- Get physical exercise prior to the test day—it will help reduce stress.
- Eat nutritious foods, and get plenty of rest in the days leading up to the examination.
- Avoid negative thoughts and messages. Anxiety is contagious.
- Plan a relaxing activity the evening before the examination.
  On the day of the examination:
- Allow plenty of time for traffic, parking challenges, and bad weather.
- Dress comfortably, and layer clothing in case the room temperature is too hot or too cold.
- Bring the admission card and proper identification to the examination site.
- Leave study materials and cell phones at home or outside the examination center.
- Stay relaxed. If nervous, take a few deep breaths, and keep focused.
- Read the directions slowly and carefully. Follow all instructions.

---

7. If a study group is formed, do not rely exclusively on someone else for your preparation for the examination. Organize a schedule and procedures for operation. Content areas can be assigned to individuals for specific study and research, and then members of the group can pool information and notes. Discussion of items or content areas can contribute to the review process.

8. Create an orderly system to guide the review, and establish target dates to complete each area. Set deadlines for the review of each chapter in this book. Alternatively, organize review around the NBDHE test specifications. Another option is to assess and prioritize perceived needs. The point is to plan a system of review with goals and deadlines to monitor progress.

9. Launch, and then stay with the plan. If progress slows, assess the obstacles and make modifications to continue comprehensive review. Aim to complete study at least 3 to 5 days before the examination date.

10. Take positive steps to manage examination anxiety (Box 1-3).

Fundamental Guidelines for Taking Multiple-Choice Tests

A system for reading and responding to test items facilitates performance. Some general strategies for dealing with multiple-choice examination items follow:

A. Read the stem of the item carefully and completely before looking at the responses.
   1. Determine what the item is asking; identify key words; and try to formulate the answer before looking at the responses.
   2. Consider each response carefully, and determine whether the response is appropriate and complete.
   3. Immediately eliminate responses that are obviously incorrect; attempt to narrow the choices to no more than two.
   4. For combination items, consider only those choices confidently known to be correct.
   5. When the choices have been narrowed as much as possible and the correct answer is still not clear, make an educated guess.

B. Exercise caution in selecting any response that contains words such as *always, never, none, all,* or *every.* Unconditional responses are frequently incorrect.

C. Look for the answer that *best* applies to the conditions presented in the item.
   1. Avoid selecting responses based on isolated rules, are applicable only to certain locales or regions, or refer to procedures and techniques not universally accepted.
   2. If the item asks for an immediate action, such as the *first* thing one would do, all the options may be correct. The *best* answer would be based on identified priorities and conditions stipulated in the item.

D. The approach to case-based items encompasses a slightly different strategy.
   1. Case-based items require time to read and assimilate pertinent information; good time management is of critical importance. Before beginning a case-based section, estimate a reasonable amount of time that can be dedicated to each case and still complete the entire examination (divide the total time allowed by the number of cases in the section). If a case requires extra time, confidently answer as many items as possible, then flag remaining items and return to them when the other cases have been finished.
   2. When beginning a case, review *all* of the case material—client history; health, dental, and pharmacologic histories; chief complaint; clinical charts; radiographs; and photographs. Make a mental note of significant findings, and begin formulating a concept of specific problems or concerns about the case before attempting to answer the test items. Answering items *before* reviewing all the case material will result in overlooking important aspects of the case and subsequent incorrect responses.
   3. A well-constructed case *requires* referencing the case material to make clinical decisions and respond to the items. Before marking a response, consider what information is essential to answer an item correctly and where that information is documented in the case. For example, an item on an artifact in a radiograph may require looking only at a specific radiograph to determine the nature of the artifact. In contrast, an item on clinical attachment loss may necessitate review of periodontal probing depths, radiographs, and perhaps clinical photographs or client history. Items asking for disease classification or appropriate care plans are more likely to require consideration of *all* available information before responding.

E. Watch for grammatical clues. A well-edited item will offer responses that are grammatically consistent with the stem. If the item indicates a plural response, all the options should be in plural form. Any response that is incompatible with the flow of the question may be an indication of an incorrect response.

F. Take heed of the words *not, least,* and *except* in the item's stem. Read the stem carefully.

G. Carefully review questions that include "all of the above" or "none of the above." These responses impose broadly inclusive and exclusive conditions.

H. Avoid becoming upset over challenging items. Negativity and obsessing over a past difficult item affect the ability to concentrate on the current item. Also, remember, on any given test, up to 10% of the items are "seeded" or pretest items that will not count toward the final score.

Future Trends in the National Board Testing Program

In its mission to develop and conduct reliable, state-of-the-art examinations that assist regulatory boards in making valid decisions regarding licensure of dental hygienists and dentists, the JCNDE periodically incorporates modifications to its policies for the fair and secure administration of its examinations. Website and software updates enable the electronic release of secured score reports to examinees, dental hygiene schools, and state boards. In addition to an expanded and more robust item bank, as well as ongoing forensic analyses to audit quality control and monitor trends in examinee performance, actions to enhance examination security and reduce stress on the item pool are continually under investigation.

CLINICAL TESTING

The emphasis of the examinations conducted by regional and state boards is on evaluating entry-level clinical competence. The methodology for assessing clinical ability involves hands-on clinical treatment of clients. In addition, some testing agencies include a computer-delivered clinical simulation component. Testing agencies are obliged to adhere to published psychometric guidelines such as those from the AADB, the American Psychological Association (APA), the National Council on Measurement in Education (NCME), the American Educational Research Association (AERA), and others in the development and administration of their examinations. Committees of examiners and educators collaborate to determine the appropriate criteria, standards, and technical aspects of clinical testing. Examination content and format are similar among regional and state board examinations. An examinee's performance on the examination is reported to any of the regulatory state boards accepting that particular examination (see Figure 1-1 and Box 1-1.) Every state has a practice act, which delineates all provisions for licensure, including the authority for approval of performance on an examination as meeting its requirements for licensure to practice. A license *must* be obtained before beginning practice.

Regional examining boards are corporate agencies composed of individual dental and dental hygiene state boards. Regional agencies have no authority over state boards and cannot implement policy that supersedes the statutory powers of its member state boards. The state board makes the determination to accept the results of the regional board as satisfaction of its requirements for licensure. A regional agency consists of states that have opted to standardize clinical testing requirements and pool resources to develop and administer reliable clinical examinations. Regional examinations are developed with the consensus of the member states (see Boxes 1-1 and 1-2).

The membership of regional testing agencies fluctuates as states join or withdraw. Many states belong to more than one regional board, whereas other states belong to a single regional board but accept the examination results of one or more of the others (see Box 1-1 and Figure 1-1). The five existing regional testing agencies are similar in their organization and structure. Each maintains an office and employs staff separate from any of its member state board headquarters (see Box 1-2). A board of directors, steering committee, or general membership is responsible for determining agency policies and managing finances. A second key organizational element is an examination review committee or panel. Each member of a state board is represented in this group, which may include a dental hygiene program director or faculty member representing the region's educational institutions. The examination review committee oversees analysis, development, and administration. At present, two regional testing agencies, NERB and SRTA, administer the ADEX dental hygiene examination; CITA administers the ADEX dental examination only. As an organization whose exclusive purpose is *examination development,* ADEX formulates examination content, scoring, and criteria for the testing agencies that elect to administer it. Member state boards participate in ADEX examination development and approval. A list of member state boards, information on governance, and an overview of the dental and dental hygiene examinations are available on the ADEX website, www.adex.org. However, specific inquiries about the ADEX examination are directed to the administering testing agencies.

For jurisdictions conducting an independent examination, the state board is the testing agency.

EXAMINER SELECTION AND TRAINING

Typically, state board member dental hygienists and dentists serve as examiners. The pool of examiners for regional testing agencies comes primarily from its member state boards. Most state boards also have the authority to designate additional examiners; these appointed examiners are licensed practitioners who meet the testing agency's defined requirements. The number of examiners assigned to an examination is based on the examination agency's administrative protocols. Testing dates and sites are scheduled in advance by the examining agency. Training programs for examiners vary but typically emphasize standardization and grading exercises to calibrate examiners in the evaluation of examination criteria. Examiners do not use their personal criteria to assess examinee performance. Most testing agencies have some type of *examiner performance review system* to monitor scoring and ensure compliance with the agency's standards. The objective is to achieve an accurate and uniform assessment of clinical competence.

EXAMINATION ADMINISTRATION

Most clinical board examinations are administered anonymously or in a double-blind manner. Examinees are identified only by a number and are kept segregated from examiners.

Clients are brought to the examiners' clinics; examinees are not present when the examiners conduct their evaluations. The purpose of this practice is to eliminate any potential for examiner bias based on an examinee's personality, race, gender, religion, or personal background. Evaluations are focused solely on clinical performance. Curious examinees might be tempted to seek information from their clients for perceived outcomes about the grading assessments. Examiners typically are prohibited from sharing any information on scoring, so making assumptions based on the reports of clients, who generally understand little about the examination process, will only lead to misinformation and erroneous conclusions.

CLINICAL FACILITIES

Testing agencies use school clinical facilities to administer board examinations. Schools release their facilities for the days of the examination. Accommodating examination requirements entails scheduling adjustments, loss of clinic income, and increased demands on faculty and staff. Most schools charge a "school use fee" for services and supplies. This cost is added to the examination fee.

If testing will take place in an unfamiliar facility, visit the site before the testing date, if possible. Most testing agencies schedule an orientation session and clinic tour before the day of examination. The clinical facility is *not* under the management and control of the board examiners, and the school may have its own institutional requirements, or record keeping, for which the examinee is responsible. After an examination application has been processed, most testing agencies will mail examination-related documents as well as an information package from the school that includes a description of the clinic facilities, a list of provided supplies, emergency and infection control protocols, compatibility of handpieces, instrument rental policies, and so on. Equipment rental is handled through the testing site. Many schools have maintenance personnel on call during the examination to handle school equipment breakdown.

Concerns must be directed to the appropriate source. The testing site, or school, deals with questions about the facilities; the testing agency addresses questions about the examination itself; and the state board attends to jurisprudence and licensure applications.

EXAMINATION INSTRUMENTS

Because examiners are calibrated with select instruments, testing agencies are likely to require specific instruments for the examination. Although such requirements may present some inconvenience, they are vital to help ensure standardization in the examination process. Typically, instrument requirements pertain only to the examining instruments (e.g., mirror, explorer, periodontal probe). Handpiece and instrument selection for performing treatment are left to the examinee's discretion. Most clinical examinations allow the use of power scaling devices.

If the required instruments are unfamiliar, obtain them and practice with them in advance. Reference the instrument's task analysis, seek guidance in correct adaptation and usage, or do both.

Instruments should be in excellent condition and *sharp*. Examiners may request replacements if instruments are incorrect or defective. Have extra sets of sterile instruments in case a client is not accepted or an instrument is dropped.

EXAMINATION FORMS

Forms are an important consideration in charting, record keeping, and documentation required for the examination. Numerous systems for charting and for taking client histories exist. Obtain examination forms (or facsimiles) in advance, and study them carefully. Practice using them. If forms are not available prior to the examination, take the time to read and review them at the examination site to understand how to use the forms *before* beginning any charting procedures. When charting procedures are part of the examination, their function is to measure an examinee's ability to recognize and record oral conditions; copying from previous notes is considered an exam violation and may be grounds for dismissal. Familiarity with examination forms will help avoid confusion and facilitate recording of data on clinical judgments in the appropriate places. Follow exactly instructions on *how* and *when* to complete the forms.

EXAMINER SELECTION AND TRAINING

Classification of Oral Conditions of Clients

The selection of a board client is the single most important factor in preparing for and successfully completing a clinical examination. Testing agencies detail specific oral conditions as criteria for client acceptability, including the number of teeth and surfaces that must have subgingival calculus, and acceptable ranges of sulcular probing depths. Most examinations require a client with "moderate" to "heavy" subgingival calculus deposits. Clients exhibiting only plaque biofilm or supragingival deposits are probably inadequate to present a valid test of the examinee's skills. A client with grossly heavy calculus or severe periodontal disease is likely too difficult for the purposes of a clinical examination.

Testing agencies develop and maintain highly defined and precise criteria in an effort to equalize difficulty in the examination.

CLIENT RECRUITMENT

Testing agencies do not provide clients. This responsibility belongs to the examinee. Some schools assist their students in client recruitment and may allow examinees who are not students to screen clients before a board examination. Ultimately, however, *it is the responsibility of the examinee to present an appropriate client*. Examiners make the final decision regarding acceptability. Dental hygiene educators and other licensed practitioners are not calibrated to testing agency standards. Client selection is integral to the examination; it is part of the test. Success or failure on the examination often hinges on submitting a client who meets the criteria—this crucial decision must not be delegated to an instructor or other licensed dental professionals. It is risky to present a marginally qualifying client or to *design* the treatment selection by prescaling in hopes of an "easier" examination. Having a client rejected results in enormous stress on the examinee, grading penalties or failure of the examination, the loss of treatment time, or all these consequences.

Historically, examinees have exhibited incredible resourcefulness in recruiting clients. Family and friends are primary sources. The college campus or one's personal dentist or dental hygienist also serves as a potential client source. Students and staff at hospitals are frequently recruited. Many examinees have contacted local police and fire stations. Sometimes, graduating classes organize a collective effort to recruit clients, as well as backup clients, for the entire class. Examinees have been known to advertise online or in local newspapers to obtain clients. Some examinees have resorted to literally "beating the streets." Stories of bizarre and unprofessional methods of client recruitment are directly proportional to the examinees' desperation. Stress can be avoided by beginning a search for clients well in advance of the examination. Maintain professionalism in all contacts with potential clients. The pressures of a high-stakes board examination do not supersede ethical considerations. A client's personal, oral, and systemic health needs extend beyond the day of the examination and therefore must be given due consideration. Most testing agencies require some type of "continuing care" form to advise the client of additional treatment that may be necessary but not provided during the examination.

Client selection is dictated by the testing agency's defined criteria. Criteria may stipulate requirements for age; systemic health status; minimum number of teeth; combination of molars, premolars, and incisors; calculus deposits; periodontal conditions; radiographs; and more. The requirements also include informed consent from the client for treatment, confidentiality, and adherence to universal precautions for infection control. Carefully review *all* prerequisites before recruiting clients.

In addition to published criteria, take into consideration the attitude and cooperativeness of the client. Ascertain the client's pain threshold and tolerance to treatment procedures. Advise the client of the time commitment. Clinical examinations usually require long treatment sessions, waiting periods, and evaluation and instrumentation by multiple examiners. If clients are not adequately prepared for the demands of the examination, difficult situations can develop. Refusing to cooperate, threatening to leave, and actually leaving the examination are potential scenarios that must be circumvented. Advise the client of the purposes of the examination, its importance to your future career, the treatment that will be provided, the examiners' role, the examination schedule, and delays that may arise. When clients understand the purpose and format of the board examination, most are supportive of the profession's efforts to ensure the competence of practitioners and are appreciative of the dental hygiene care to be received.

Finding the "perfect" client who satisfies all criteria is challenging. It is prudent to recruit more than one client for backup purposes. Inform these clients that they may not be needed for the examination, but if willing, they may be able to sit for

another examinee. Stay in contact with any clients who have been recruited. Confirm the time and date, transportation or parking arrangements, and exact meeting locations.

CLINICAL EXAMINATION FORMATS

Clinical examinations provide a reliable third-party assessment of examinees' client-focused skills and judgments. Each testing program has distinct examination protocols, procedures, requirements, and forms. Examinees preparing to take a clinical examination *must contact the testing agency responsible for administering the examination* to obtain its test specifications (see Box 1-2). This chapter provides only a general overview.

Four basic categories of clinical competencies are typically included in regional and state clinical examinations: (1) appropriate client and treatment selection, (2) calculus detection and removal, (3) oral and head and neck assessment, and (4) tissue management. Components within these areas may include dental and periodontal charting, extraoral and intraoral examination, charting the location of subgingival deposits, and removal of extrinsic stain, plaque, and supragingival calculus. Root debridement and removal of subgingival calculus are universal requirements. As previously noted, specific requirements for case difficulty vary among examinations. All regional examinations mandate a treatment submission of a minimum of six teeth; some require the teeth to be in one quadrant but allow for a limited number of additional teeth. Client acceptability criteria also include a specific number of "qualifying" subgingival deposits. Typically, the number of anterior teeth that may be included in the treatment submission is limited, and a certain number of posterior teeth in proximal contact must be included. Examiners evaluate the treatment selection. If the client does not meet the criteria, at a minimum, points are deducted; at a maximum, client rejection results in failure of the examination.

Some examination requirements, although potentially affecting the examination outcome, are not actually scored. Acceptable client age and health criteria are prime examples of "nongraded" requirements. Acceptable probing depths are another such requirement. Diagnostic-quality radiographs must be submitted with the client, although the radiographs may not be a graded feature. Some agencies require a full-mouth series or panograph x-ray film (exposed within 3 years), and bitewing radiographs (exposed within 1 year). Others require only periapicals and bitewings (within 1 year) of the teeth in the treatment submission. Radiographs of "nondiagnostic quality" will result in point deductions, negative impact on client acceptance and the ability to continue the examination, or both.

Allotted clinic time is another variable factor. Most board examinations place specific time limits for the completion of assignments. If an examinee has one or more treatment selections rejected, it is likely that a point deduction, loss of treatment time, failure of the examination, or all these consequences will be incurred.

Pain management for the client is addressed by various means. Most testing agencies permit administration of local anesthetic agents by the examinee in compliance with the host school's state practice act. Testing agency protocols range from confirmation of formal education in administration of local anesthesia to successful completion of an examination on local anesthesia delivery. Some agencies also have provisions for "qualified" licensed practitioners to administer the local anesthesia. Generally, clients must be accepted for treatment prior to administering anesthetics. Verify the authorization for the delivery of local anesthetics with the testing agency and the regulatory board *before* the examination.

In addition to client-based testing in the clinic, some regional testing agencies utilize assessment on simulated patient cases at computer testing centers or at school testing sites. The knowledge, skills, and judgments necessary to provide competent entry-level dental hygiene care are evaluated in a standardized examination. Both the physical client-based section and the simulation section must be passed for successful completion of the examination.

EXAMINATION RESULTS

No uniform scoring system for regional or state board clinical examinations exists. Scoring is linked to the content and design of each examination. In general, clinical board examinations use a system of "weighting" to emphasize the importance or recognize the complexity of certain skills sets and treatment procedures. For example, dental hygiene practice surveys show that competency in scaling and root planing is more critical than competency in stain removal. Consequently, in examination development, when both components are measured, scaling and root planing are weighted with more point value than is stain removal. An examinee should strive to demonstrate competence in all skills that are evaluated in an examination but may choose to concentrate time and effort on each area in proportion to the weighted significance built into the examination.

The testing agency must be contacted for all performance criteria and the defined cutoff point separating acceptable performance from unacceptable performance (see Box 1-2).

ETHICAL AND LEGAL ISSUES

Because professional conduct and ethical behavior are central to the practice of dental hygiene, all testing agencies have stipulations for penalties, such as point deduction or immediate failure of the examination for infractions. Examples of improper and/or unethical conduct include, but are not limited to, the following:

- Violating standards as defined in the *Examination Guide*
- Evidence of dishonesty or misrepresentation during the application or course of the examination
- Misappropriation or damage of equipment during the examination
- Treatment of teeth other than those approved or assigned by examiners
- Receiving assistance from another practitioner or using unauthorized aids
- Altering examination records or radiographs
- Improper record keeping or failure to properly document anesthetic use

- Breach of infection control standards
- Causing excessive tissue trauma
- Rude or abusive behavior
- Continuing to work after the established cutoff time
- Disregard for client welfare or comfort
- Use of cell phones, cameras, or electronic devices

Examinees found to have engaged in improper or unethical conduct may be denied reexamination for 1 full year. Testing agencies reserve the right to take other reasonable actions as deemed appropriate. Infractions are reportable to all state licensing jurisdictions, the examinee's school, other testing agencies, and professional organizations. Examinees failed for dishonesty may be permanently ineligible for licensure.

Preparing for Regional or State Clinical Board Examinations

Contact the state board office to obtain a licensure application. Note all requirements, including which board examinations are accepted and any related conditions or restrictions. Consult the current state dental practice act as well as the rules and regulations for this information. Some jurisdictions require successful completion of local anesthesia, nitrous oxide, and restorative examinations in addition to the dental hygiene examination. Prepare a scheduled timeline for satisfying all licensure requirements. List pertinent examination dates, as well as the testing agency's published time frame for releasing examination results.

1. Obtain the testing agency's examination schedule, application forms, *Examination* Guide, and any official information pertaining to the examination. Most testing agencies have this information available online. Read the information carefully at least twice. Do this several months before the examination.

2. Review all the application material, and flag the desired examination's application deadline. Note examination requirements, including eligibility and documentation that must be provided, client requirements, instruments, and supplies.

3. Assemble the credentials necessary to sit for the examination. These credentials may include school transcripts, the NBDHE score, a copy of the diploma, current cardiopulmonary resuscitation (CPR) certification, evidence of malpractice or liability insurance, and a passport-quality photograph. Retain copies of everything.

4. Check the testing agency's website for *Frequently Asked Questions*. This section can provide insights and coping strategies to enhance confident preparation.

5. Begin searching for eligible clients. Present prospective clients with a clear and professional explanation of the client's role as well as your own in the examination.

6. For examinees still in school, many dental hygiene programs conduct "mock boards" as a trial practice run. Additional clinical experience with clients whose difficulty level is commensurate with board requirements is likely to be helpful as well.

7. Practicing dental hygienists can set up clinical simulations of board requirements using the examination's specified

oral conditions and time constraints to evaluate clinical skills through critical self-assessment.

8. For dental hygienists who have been out of practice, most dental and dental hygiene schools offer continuing education programs. Review courses need to be investigated and pursued well before the examination date.

9. Obtain the required examination instruments, and practice using them.

10. Obtain examination forms before the test, and become familiar with them. If unavailable, study the Forms section of the *Examination Guide.*

11. Be observant of the tooth-numbering system used in the examination—it must be applied accurately. Noncompliance can result in charting errors or incorrectly identifying which teeth are assigned by examiners.

12. A few days before the examination, prepare your clinic attire, and organize instruments and supplies. Confirm arrangements with the client(s) regarding time, date, location, and relevant directions. Check in with the client again the night before the examination.

13. If taking the examination at an unfamiliar testing site, tour the clinical facilities before the examination.

14. Plan to arrive at the testing site on time, taking into consideration traffic and parking difficulties as well as the time required for locating the operatory, setting up, and orienting to the clinic. Avoid starting the day feeling rushed and distracted.

15. At the examination, listen closely to instructions, and read thoroughly all materials provided. Failure to read and follow instructions is a common denominator in problems experienced by examinees.

16. *Relax,* and concentrate on the high-quality dental hygiene care that you are able to provide because of your professional education and experience. Test-coping mechanisms are provided in Box 1-3 and on the websites presented in the Website Information and Resources table at the end of this chapter.

Future Trends in Clinical Examinations and Licensure

In response to a growing demand for greater portability of credentials in dental hygiene and dentistry, most states long ago implemented licensure by credentials for active practitioners. Increasingly, many states now not only accept results of multiple clinical examinations for initial licensure (see Figure 1-1), but also are members of multiple testing agencies (see Box 1-1). An outcome of this overlap is increased competition for the market share among the testing agencies. In states where more than one examination is accepted for initial licensure, schools have a choice of which examination to host. Regional agencies have amped up public relations efforts and communications with state boards, educators, and students, touting candidate-friendly measures, sensitivity to escalating examination fees, and modifications to exam content and scoring, to gain a strategic advantage. This competition may result in enhancements to the examination process and, with the cross-pollination of examiners, who examine for multiple agencies, could result in an exchange of best practices and more standardized exam procedures.

Debate continues on the appropriateness of the use of humans in clinical examinations. As the National Council on Radiation Protection and Measurement (NCRP) Report #145 states, "Administrative use of radiation to provide information not related to the health of the patient shall not be permitted." A cohort of educators, students, and some state boards advocate discontinuation of the use of humans, citing both ethical and practical reasons. Some examination agencies have incorporated computer-delivered "simulation exercises," in addition to client-based testing, for the evaluation of clinical skills. It is generally agreed that a dental hygiene examination constructed, directed, and administered by dental hygienists, based on current and relevant scientific evidence, both benefits the dental hygiene community and provides protection of the public.

Most testing agencies utilize electronic scoring systems to augment efficiency in compiling and releasing examination scores, thus facilitating obtaining licensure in a timely manner. Software tracking of statistical data on examiner scoring and validation can be used to improve examiner training. Some testing agencies are reluctant to publish information on examiner calibration and therefore guard this information.

International Requirements

In our global culture, interest in working outside the United States is increasingly appealing. International licensure requirements vary significantly. A dental hygienist contemplating employment in another country should contact the ADHA, the ADA, and the International Federation of Dental Hygienists (IFDH) for pertinent information and potential connections. The IFDH has compiled a database with detailed requirements for working as a dental hygienist in the following 28 countries:

- Australia
- Austria
- Canada
- Czech Republic
- Denmark
- Fiji
- Finland
- Germany
- Ireland
- Israel
- Italy
- Japan
- Korea
- Latvia
- Malta
- Nepal
- Netherlands
- New Zealand
- Norway
- Portugal
- Russia
- Slovakia
- South Africa
- Spain
- Sweden
- Switzerland
- United Kingdom
- United States

The information is available by clicking the "Working Abroad" tab and then the county of choice on the IFDH website (http://www.ifdh.org/work_abroad.html). In addition to these countries, other nations known to have formal dental hygiene education programs and dental hygiene practice include the following:

- Bahrain
- Hong Kong
- Jamaica
- Jordan

- Kuwait
- Lithuania
- New South Wales
- Nicaragua
- Nigeria
- Puerto Rico
- Queensland
- Saudi Arabia

Individual resources or personal contacts within the country of destination should also be pursued.

As a starting point, collect documentation of all credentials, including passports or visas, school transcripts, diplomas, licenses, board examination scores, and employment history. Some countries require language proficiency before certification is granted; others require an employment contract *before* issuing a work permit. Most countries require proof of graduation from an accredited school and successful completion of cognitive and clinical or case-based board examinations; other counties request merely "reporting to employer."[2]

Special citation is warranted of the National Dental Hygiene Certification Board of Canada (NDHCB), which was established in 1994 in response to a priority concern of Canadian dental hygienists for portability of licensure. The NDHCB examination consists of 200 multiple-choice items designed to assess the requisite knowledge and skills for entry into practice. It is accepted for licensure by all provinces, except Quebec. Clinical practice evaluations are conducted by Canadian dental hygiene regulatory authorities only for graduates of nonaccredited dental hygiene programs.

The NDHCB delivers its examinations in both English and French, three times annually (January, May, and September) at computerized writing centers in numerous cities throughout Canada. Examination information can be obtained directly from the NDHCB using the following contact information:

National Dental Hygiene Certification Board
1929 Russell Road, Suite 322
Ottawa, Ontario K1G 4G3
Canada
Phone: 613-260-8156
Fax: 613-260-8511
General inquiries: exam@ndhcb.ca; http://www.ndhcb.ca/en/about.php

The rigors of a country's requirements appear to be strongly correlated with the number of dental hygienists in the country, how long dental hygiene has been established, and the size and strength of its educational system.

CONTENT AND ORGANIZATION OF THIS REVIEW BOOK

This book presents a review, in outline form, of basic, dental, dental hygiene, and clinical sciences. Each review outline is followed by related questions that test the reader's knowledge of concepts, principles, and theories underlying the practice of dental hygiene.

Each chapter contains a section on Evolve entitled "Answers and Rationales," which provides justification for the correct answer and every response in the review questions covering the subject matter. The rationale supporting the correct answer and explanations for incorrect responses are specified. By reviewing these rationales, the reader will be able to confirm facts and reinforce knowledge. An example is provided below.

REFERENCES

1. American Dental Association: *National board dental hygiene examination guide,* Chicago, 2014, American Dental Association, Commission on National Board Dental Examinations.
2. Johnson PM: International profiles of dental hygiene 2007: a 21-nation comparison, *Int Dent J* 59(2):63–77, 2009.

Website Information and Resources

Source	Website Address	Description
State University of New York at Buffalo	http://ub-counseling.buffalo.edu/stresstestanxiety.shtml	Causes of examination anxiety; physical signs and effects of examination anxiety; how to reduce examination anxiety; an anxiety checklist and goal-setting strategies
University of Illinois at Chicago, Academic Center for Excellence	http://www.uic.edu/depts/ace/strategies.shtml	"College Study Strategies & Study Tips" section; extensive information on time management, studying, lectures and reading, taking examinations, and controlling stress
Dartmouth	http://www.dartmouth.edu/~acskills/success/stress.html	Advice on coping with examination anxiety and stress; comprehensive recommendations for examination preparation and test taking
Massachusetts Institute of Technology	http://web.mit.edu/uaap/learning/test/anxiety.html	Detailed sections on time management, tooling and studying, and mastering tests
University of Michigan	http://www.lsa.umich.edu/advising/academicsupport/strategiesforsuccess/preppingfortests/overcomingtestanxiety	Tips on time management and test preparation; strategies for staying motivated; detailed section on "Collaborating with Peers," including guidelines for leading a study group

CHAPTER 1 REVIEW QUESTION

Answers and Rationales to Chapter Review Questions are available on this text's accompanying Evolve site. See inside front cover for details.

evolve

1. **An isolated radiopaque area in the periodontal ligament space is observed on a client's radiographs. This radiopaque structure is most likely a/an:**
   a. Denticle
   b. Cementicle
   c. Epithelial rest
   d. Cementum spur
   e. Exostosis of alveolar bone

How to Use This Book in Studying

A. Review one section of the content at a time. Study the material outlined in the section. Refer to other textbooks, websites, and references to research additional details if any area is unclear.

B. After reviewing the content, answer the review questions that immediately follow. As each question is answered, write a few words about why that response is correct; justify the response selected. If your response is a guess, make a special mark to identify it as such. This will enable ready identification of areas that need further review and clarification. Remember to analyze a question, narrow the choices, and select the correct or best answer.

C. Score yourself using the answers provided on the Evolve website. If the item was answered correctly, compare the reason noted for selecting that answer with the listed rationales.

For each item answered incorrectly, review the correct answer and its rationale. Go back to the chapter pertaining to that subject, and research information in your reference material. Carefully review all the questions and rationales for the items identified as guesses to ensure mastery of the material.

D. After an interval of several days or weeks, review the chapters and answer the questions again. If the same items are missed, further study of that content material is necessary.

Completion of the Review Process

Board examinations can be attempted with confidence and success after completing the comprehensive review presented in this book; assessing areas of strength and weaknesses with the aid of the chapter review questions; reinforcing concentrated study of particular material pinpointed by the review; becoming familiar with the board examination process, protocol, and purpose; and following instructions for preparation. Preparation for board examinations actually begins with the accredited dental hygiene program's first class and continues throughout the educational process. This book is designed to present a cohesive, comprehensive review of that professional educational base, to reinforce existing knowledge, and to provide guidance for areas requiring more concentrated study.

2 | CHAPTER

Histology and Embryology

Maureen Dotzel Savner

During the process of care, a dental hygienist must distinguish normal structures, variants of normal structures, and developmental abnormalities from pathology. A clear sense of developmental processes and tissue histology provides the background for competent assessment and evaluation.

Knowledge of tissue components and embryologic tissue origin supports an understanding of the physiologic changes that take place during the course of disease progression. This knowledge also provides insight into how tissue is capable of responding to a pathologic condition. This chapter contains basic general histologic information, with a focus on oral tissue components and oral and facial development. A clinician uses this knowledge to formulate a dental hygiene care plan, evaluate the outcomes of treatment, and make appropriate referrals to dentists and physicians when necessary.

GENERAL HISTOLOGY

Cells

A. Smallest structures and functionally self-contained units in the body; they vary in size, shape, and surface, depending on functional specialization (Figure 2-1)
B. Cells possess similar common physiologic properties that permit:
   1. Excitability
      a. Change in the environment stimulates the cell to bring about a response to adapt to a change
      b. Example—nerve cells conduct impulses
   2. Synthesis
      a. Cells must have the ability to form substances that produce products to aid in the body's function
      b. Example—glands synthesize and secrete products to aid bodily functions
   3. Membrane transport
      a. Fluids, chemical elements, and compounds must have the ability to move both in and out of cells
      b. Example—nutrients are transported across the epithelial lining of the gastrointestinal tract
   4. Reproduction
      a. Cells must have the ability to preserve the species by giving rise to offspring
      b. Example—union of a sperm and ovum can lead to the formation of an offspring

C. The building blocks of tissues in the body are attached to each other and to noncellular surfaces by cell junctions; the structures of various types of cell junctions depend on location and function; the types of junctions are:
   1. Desmosomes—cell-to-cell attachments; this type of attachment is found between ameloblasts (enamel-forming cells) and cells of the stratified squamous epithelium that lines the oral cavity
   2. Tight junctions—cells attach to each other by fusion of their cell membranes; adjacent odontoblasts (dentin-forming cells) form tight junctions that prevent substances in the pulp from passing into the dentin
   3. Gap junctions—contain a channel that runs between cells for communication of cell electrical impulses and passage of molecules; this type of junction is present among some odontoblasts, allowing them to coordinate their activity
   4. Hemidesmosome—the attachment of a cell to a noncellular surface; the basal layer cells of stratified squamous epithelium attach to the basement membrane by hemidesmosomes; this attachment mechanism is present in the epithelial attachment to the tooth; the epithelial attachment refers to the basal lamina and hemidesmosomes that connect the junctional epithelium of the soft tissue to the tooth surface
D. Cells are surrounded by a cell membrane that separates them from the extracellular environment; cell membrane encloses all components of the cell:
   1. Cytoplasm
   2. Organelles
   3. Inclusions
   4. Nucleus

Specialization

A. Differentiation
   1. Cells that recognize one another will group together
   2. Cancer cells do not recognize each other
B. Organization of chemicals
   1. Chemicals appear early in the development of the embryo
   2. Endocrine substances are produced by one type of cell and can affect other types of cells
C. Cells → tissues → organs → organ systems

Dermis   Basal   Superficial
              cells   cells

FIG 2-1 Typical cell. (From Chiego DJ: *Essentials of oral histology and embryology: a clinical approach,* ed 4, St Louis, 2013, Mosby.)

Cell Membrane

A. Referred to as plasma membrane or plasmalemma; usually too thin to be seen with a light microscope; average width is approximately 7 nanometers (nm); considered selectively permeable because it controls passage of materials into and out of the cell

1. It surrounds the cell and is semi-permeable, allowing some substances to pass through it and others to be excluded
2. Its permeability may vary selectively by porous openings
3. Selective permeability characteristics
   a. Protecting cell from external environment
   b. Permitting entrance and exit of selected substrates
   c. Using active transport, passive transport, or facilitated diffusion
4. Its composition is a 3:2 ratio of proteins to lipids; lipids and proteins are the major components
5. Its structure is trilaminar, with a bipolar membrane and a central core of lipids between two layers of protein
6. The 0.8-nm pores in the surface allow diffusion of small, lipid-insoluble substances

B. Trilaminar structure composed of two facing layers of lipid molecules, into which large globular proteins are inserted (Figure 2-2)

Cytoplasm

A. Translucent, aqueous, homogeneous gel enclosed in the cell by the cell membrane; organelles and inclusions are suspended in the cytoplasmic gel
B. All metabolic activities of the cell occur in the cytoplasm, including:
1. Assimilation (digestion)
2. Synthesis of substances such as proteins, proteoglycans, and glycoproteins
3. A transport medium in which all nutrients and metabolites are carried from one organelle to another
4. Presence of enzymes and electrolytes, in which specific metabolic reactions take place (e.g., glycolysis)

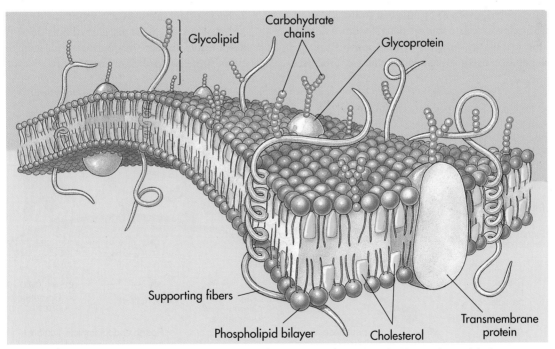

FIG 2-2 Fluid mosaic model. Schematic, three-dimensional view of the fluid mosaic model of membrane structure. The lipid bilayer provides the basic structure and serves as a relatively impermeable barrier to most water-soluble molecules. (Modified from Patton KT, Thibodeau GA: *Structure and function of the human body,* ed 15, St Louis, 2016, Elsevier.)

Nucleus

A. Controls the two major functions of the cell
   1. Chemical reactions—synthesizing activities; determines nutrient needs
   2. Stores genetic information of the cell
B. Genetic information stored in chromosomes for cell duplication; chromosomal deoxyribonucleic acid (DNA); the human nucleus contains 46 chromosomes
C. Chromosomes are visible only during cell division, when they become long, coiled strands; at other times, chromosomal material is dispersed in granular clumps of material called *chromatin*
D. Each nucleus contains one or more round, dense structures referred to as the *nucleolus* (plural, *nucleoli*); these produce ribosomal ribonucleic acid (RNA)—protein plus RNA; the nucleus also is surrounded by a nuclear membrane and contains nuclear matrix with chromosomes

Synthesis Activities

A. Three types of RNA are necessary for protein synthesis:
   1. Messenger RNA (mRNA)—copies of short segments of DNA, the genetic code
      a. mRNA can be compared with a tape that contains all the genetic information of proteins, but it must pass through the ribosomes attached to the endoplasmic reticulum (ER)
      b. As the tape passes through the ribosomes, transfer RNA (tRNA) adds the exact amino acid to the newly forming proteins (Figure 2-3)
   2. tRNA—carrier of specific amino acids (building blocks of proteins)
   3. Ribosomal RNA (rRNA)—found floating freely in the cytoplasm (polyribosomes) or attached to the ER
B. Protein synthesis also can occur on polyribosomes floating freely in the cytoplasm; proteins synthesized on the free polyribosomes are used in cellular metabolic processes; proteins synthesized on the ribosomes attached to the ER are transported out of the cell

Inclusions

A. Transitory, nonliving metabolic byproducts found in the cytoplasm of the cell
B. May appear as lipid droplets, carbohydrate accumulations (e.g., mucopolysaccharides), or engulfed foreign substances

Lysosomes

A. Membrane-bound organelles responsible for the breakdown of foreign substances that are engulfed by the cell by the process of phagocytosis or pinocytosis
B. Produced by a budding process from the Golgi complex, lysosomes form spherical vesicles containing powerful degradative or hydrolytic enzymes; enzymes are first produced by the ER and then transported to the Golgi complex
C. During phagocytosis, lysosomes fuse with engulfed substances to form a secondary vesicle; the vesicle with digestive materials may remain in the cell as a residual body or may be discharged outside of the cell
D. Vitamins A and E and zinc are important stabilizers for the lysosome's membrane

Golgi Complex

A. The structure consists of stacks of closely spaced membranous sacs, in which newly formed proteins are concentrated and prepared for export out of the cell (Figure 2-4)
   1. Small membrane-bound vesicles pinch off from the Golgi complex and form secretory granules (newly formed proteins)
   2. Secretory granules attach to the inside of the cell membrane and are then discharged outside of the cell
B. Responsible for secreting to the external environment a variety of proteins synthesized on the ER

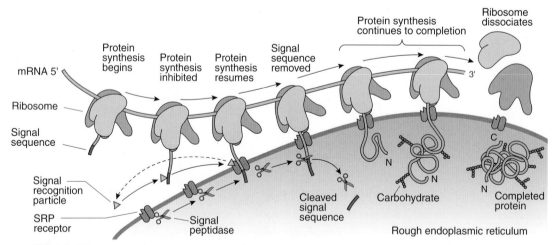

FIG 2-3 Ribosomes showing protein synthesis on rough endoplasmic reticulum. Messenger RNA is being passed through ribosomes on endoplasmic reticulum, where transfer RNA becomes incorporated in protein (being formed) that is assembled in the ribosome. (From Gartner LP, Hiatt JL: *Color textbook of histology*, ed 3, St. Louis, 2007, Saunders.)

FIG 2-4 Golgi complex. **A,** Schematic representation of the Golgi complex showing a stack of flattened sacs, or cisternae, and numerous small membranous bubbles, or secretory vesicles. **B,** Transmission electron micrograph showing the Golgi complex highlighted with color. (From Patton KT: *Anatomy and physiology,* ed 9, St Louis, 2016, Elsevier.)

C. Major site of membrane formation and recycling
D. Storage site for newly synthesized proteins
E. Site for packaging and transporting many cell products (e.g., polysaccharides, proteins, lipids)
F. Synthesis site for lysosomes
G. Also involved in the production of large carbohydrate molecules and lysosomes

Mitochondria

A. Membranous structure bounded by inner and outer cell membranes; the membranes contain enzyme complexes in a particular array (e.g., tricarboxylic acid cycle enzymes)
   1. The inner part is formed into folds (cristae) that extend, like shelves, inside the mitochondria to provide an additional work surface area for the organelle
   2. More than one mitochondrion is usually present in a cell; the number depends on the amount of energy required by the cell
B. This structure provides the chief source of energy for the cell ("powerhouse of the cell" by oxidation of nutrients) through enzymatic breakdown of fats, amino acids, and carbohydrates; transforms the chemical energy bond of nutrients into the high-energy phosphate bonds of adenosine triphosphate (ATP)
C. A single cell may contain 50 to 2500 mitochondria, depending on the cell's energy needs (Figure 2-5)

Endoplasmic Reticulum

A. Extensive membranous system found throughout the cytoplasm of the cell; composed of lipoprotein membranes existing in the form of connecting tubules and broad,

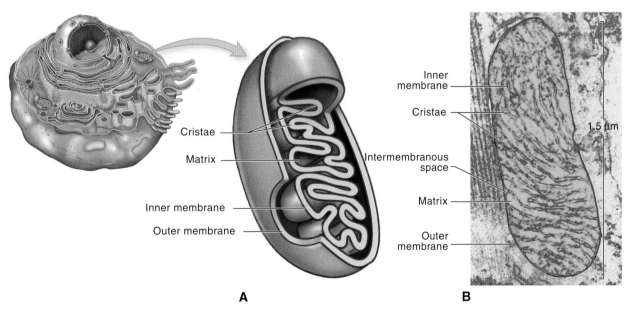

FIG 2-5 Mitochondrion. **A,** Cutaway sketch showing outer and inner membranes. Note the many folds (cristae) of the inner membrane. **B,** Transmission electron micrograph of a mitochondrion. Although some mitochondria have the capsule shape shown here, many are round or oval. (From Patton KT: *Anatomy and physiology,* ed 9, St Louis, 2016, Elsevier.)

flattened sacs (cisternae); the outer membrane may or may not be covered with ribosomes; the two types are:

1. Granular or rough-surfaced endoplasmic reticulum (RER)
   a. Contains ribosomes that are attached to the cytoplasmic side of the membrane
   b. Site of protein synthesis
2. Agranular or smooth-surfaced endoplasmic reticulum (SER)
   a. No ribosomes are present
   b. Site of steroid synthesis

B. The membrane system functions to synthesize, circulate, and package intracellular and extracellular materials
C. Proteins are synthesized on ribosomes attached to the ER and are transported to the Golgi complex for packaging
D. The system contains enzymes involved in a variety of metabolic activities (e.g., lipogenesis, glycogenesis)
E. SER has a number of diverse roles and is found in a variety of cell types

Filaments and Tubules

A. Thread-like structures approximately 7 to 10 nm thick; thicker filaments are the same as those seen in muscle (protein myosin strands) and have been associated with contractility in cells
B. Microfilaments act as a support system for the cell cytoskeleton
C. Bundles of microfilaments form tonofibrils and become part of the attachment apparatus (desmosomes) between cells

Microtubules

A. Delicate tubes, 20 to 27 nm wide, found in cells that are undergoing mitosis and alterations in cell shape (cell morphology)
B. Microtubules have an internal support function, particularly in long cellular processes such as neurites or odontoblastic processes
C. Microtubules have the capacity to direct intracellular transport through the cytoplasm

Centrioles

A. Cylindrical structures composed of microtubule-like components
B. Centrioles function in cell replication and the formation of cellular extensions

Internal Environment and Homeostasis

A. Extracellular fluid
   1. Fluid mass that circulates outside and between cells
   2. Extracellular fluid composition must be regulated exactly:

$$[Na^+] = 142\,mEq/L$$
$$[K^+] = 5\,mEq/L$$
$$[Cl^-] = 103\,mEq/L$$
$$[Ca^{+2}] = 5\,mEq/L$$
$$pH = 7.4$$

B. Intracellular fluid
   1. Fluid located inside the cells of the body
   2. Intracellular fluid composition must be regulated exactly:

$$[Na^+] = 10\,mEq/L$$
$$[K^+] = 141\,mEq/L$$
$$[Cl^-] = 4\,mEq/L$$
$$[Ca^{+2}] = <1\,mEq/L$$
$$pH = 7.0$$

C. Homeostasis—the delicate balance maintained between the two fluid compositions

Transport through the Cell Membrane

A. Diffusion
   1. Definition—continuous movement of molecules among one another in liquids or gases
   2. Molecules may move across a membrane
   3. Direction of diffusion of a substance is from a region of high concentration to a region of low concentration, which is the *diffusion gradient*
   4. If equal amounts of a substance are placed at either end of a chamber such as a cell, they diffuse toward each other, and the net rate of diffusion equals zero
B. Osmosis
   1. Definition—process of net diffusion of water through a semi-permeable membrane caused by a concentration difference
   2. Osmotic pressure—pressure that develops in a solution as a result of the net osmosis into that solution; pressure is affected by the number of dissolved particles per unit volume of fluid
   3. Isotonic solution—when placed on the outside of a cell, will not cause osmosis (e.g., 0.9% sodium chloride)
   4. Hypertonic solution—when placed on the outside of a cell, will cause osmosis out of the cell (e.g., greater than 0.9% sodium chloride) and lead to crenation (shrinking) of the cell
   5. Hypotonic solution—when placed on the outside of a cell, will cause osmosis into the cell (e.g., less than 0.9% sodium chloride) and lead to cell lysis
C. Active transport
   1. Process used by a cell when large quantities of a substance are needed inside the cell and only a small amount of the substance is present in the extracellular fluid
   2. Involves pumping the substance against its concentration gradient
   3. Uses a carrier system and energy (ATP)
   4. Keeps sodium extra-cellularly (sodium pump) and potassium intra-cellularly; important for the transmission of nerve impulses
   5. Almost all monosaccharides are actively transported into the body
D. Phagocytosis—movement of a solid particle into the cell
   1. Cell wall invaginates around the particle
   2. Pinches off from the rest of the membrane and floats inward
E. Pinocytosis—movement of fluid into a cell; similar to phagocytosis, except that the cell invaginates around fluid

CELL REPLICATION

A. Mitosis—process of cell replication (Figure 2-6)
   1. Interphase
      a. The genetic material of each chromosome replicates
      b. Chromosomes are dispersed as chromatin material in the nucleus
   2. Prophase
      a. Chromosomes coil and contract; each chromosome consists of a pair of strands called *chromatids*, which are held together by a centromere
      b. The nuclear envelope disappears
      c. The centriole divides, and the two centrioles move to opposite poles of the cell
      d. Spindle fibers develop
   3. Metaphase
      a. Chromatids line up at the center
      b. Spindle fibers attach at the centromere
      c. The centromere replicates, allowing the separation of chromatids
   4. Anaphase
      a. Spindle fibers pull the new chromosomes to opposite poles of the cell
   5. Telophase
      a. A nuclear membrane forms around each set of chromosomes
      b. Centrioles replicate in each cell

Concepts Relating to Dental Tissues

A. All calcified dental tissues are produced by secretory cells that require a great amount of energy in producing their organic matrices, which become calcified; organelles such as mitochondria play an important role in providing energy
B. Mitochondria have been associated with the calcification (mineralization) process that occurs in dental tissues
C. Cell organelles help maintain tissues after the initial formation by the cell; fibroblasts (i.e., connective tissue cells that are present in all tooth tissues except enamel) contain increased numbers of cell organelles; these additional organelles aid fibroblasts in their synthesizing and secretory functions

Basic Tissues

A. At the beginning of human development, individual cells multiply and differentiate to perform specialized functions; groups of cells with similar morphologic characteristics and functions come together and form tissues
B. Tissue components
   1. Cells
   2. Intercellular substance—a product of living cells; a medium for the passage of nutrients and waste within the tissue; the amount of substance varies with different tissues
   3. Tissue fluid—blood plasma that diffuses through capillary walls; the fluid carries nutrients to the intercellular substance and waste materials to capillaries

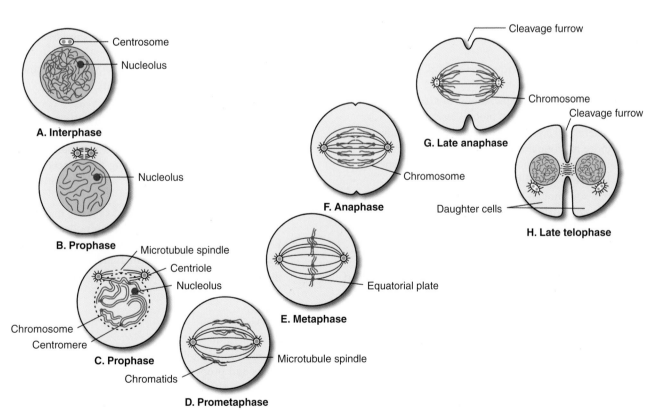

FIG 2-6 Phases of mitosis. (From Chiego DJ: *Essentials of oral histology and embryology: a clinical approach,* ed 4, St Louis, 2013, Mosby.)

C. Tissues in the human body can be classified into four types:
1. Epithelial tissue
2. Connective tissue
3. Nerve tissue
4. Muscle tissue
D. Each of the four basic tissues may be further subdivided into several variations

Epithelial Tissue

A. Main categories
1. Surface epithelia
2. Glandular tissue
B. The epithelium consists exclusively of cells held together by specialized cell junctions (minimal intercellular material is present between cells); cells rest on an underlying connective tissue, the *basement membrane*
C. Epithelial cells (keratinocytes) form continuous sheets (tissues) and perform the following functions:
1. Protection—covering all outer surfaces of the body (e.g., skin)
2. Absorption—forming the lining of all inner surfaces of the body (e.g., digestive tract)
3. Secretion—forming glands (glandular tissue)
D. Epithelial tissue varies, depending on function—it may have surface specializations on its free surfaces
1. Microvilli—for absorption
2. Cilia—for surface transportation
E. Replicates through mitosis
Surface Epithelia
A. The epithelium is classified according to:
1. The shape of the most superficial cells
   a. Squamous (flat)
   b. Cuboidal (cubical)
   c. Columnar (tall, narrow—cylindrical or prismatic)
2. Number of cell layers present
   a. One cell layer—simple; found in areas of little or no friction (e.g., lining of blood vessels)
   b. Several cell layers—stratified; capable of withstanding more functional use (e.g., mucous membranes)
B. Combined characteristics allow for six different types of epithelia (Figure 2-7) and locations:
1. Simple squamous—found in the walls of vessels
2. Simple cuboidal—lines the ovaries
3. Simple columnar—lines the intestines and the cervix of the uterus
4. Stratified squamous—lines the oral cavity
5. Stratified cuboidal and
6. Stratified columnar—line the large ducts of the major salivary glands
C. Other, intermediate forms of epithelium
1. Pseudo-stratified columnar (e.g., trachea)—appears stratified but is, in fact, only one layer
2. Transitional (e.g., urinary tract)—resembles both stratified squamous and stratified cuboidal epithelia
D. Other cell types found in the epithelium
1. Melanocytes—produce melanin (pigmentation); intensity of brown skin color is not caused by the difference

in the number of melanocytes present but by the difference in the rate of melanin production, the size of pigment granules, and the length of time of their preservation
2. Inflammatory cells—transient cells usually associated with inflammation
3. Langerhans cells—antigen-presenting cells
4. Merkel cells—mechano-receptors
E. The epithelium lining the oral cavity (oral mucosa) and the skin (dermis) is an example of stratified squamous epithelium
Glandular Tissue
A. Most glands develop from the epithelium; the epithelial basal cell grows downward into the underlying connective tissue
B. Types
1. Exocrine
   a. Serous; mucous or seromucous secretions
   b. Ducts carry secretions
      (1) Simple—nonbranching duct
      (2) Compound—branching duct
2. Endocrine
   a. Hormone secretions directly into the bloodstream
   b. The bloodstream carries secretions; no ducts

Connective Tissue
Connective Tissue Proper
A. All connective tissue proper develops from the embryonic mesenchyme; contains large amounts and various types of intercellular material and few cells; highly vascular; has two main functions:
1. Provides mechanical and biologic support (supports organs and other structures)
2. Provides pathways for metabolic substances and thus aids in the distribution of nutrients
B. Types of connective tissue
1. Bone—hard and calcified; serves supportive and protective functions
2. Cartilage—firm but flexible; serves a supportive function
3. Reticular—network of branching fibers; acts as a filter; loose and elastic; provides a connection between structures
4. Bone marrow—site where blood cells are manufactured
5. Lymphoid tissue (tonsils and lymph nodes)
6. Fat or adipose (special type of connective tissue composed of fat cells)—located under the skin; provides insulation
7. Dental tissues
   a. Pulp
   b. Dentin
   c. Cementum
C. Types of connective tissues—differ in composition of cell products and proportions of products present
1. Dense connective tissue—consists predominantly of heavy, tightly packed collagen fibers; main function is to resist tension; this dense collagenous connective tissue is present in the gingiva

CELL SHAPES   SIMPLE   STRATIFIED

FIG 2-7 Classification of epithelia according to morphologic shape and number of cell layers. (From Patton KT: *Anatomy and physiology*, ed 9, St Louis, 2016, Elsevier.)

2. Loose connective tissue—collagen and reticulin fibers extending in all directions; the main function is to provide biologic support and fill the spaces between organs and tissues

Connective Tissue Components

A. Cells
   1. Types of cells normally present
      a. Fibroblasts—produce the fibrous matrix and ground substance of connective tissue
      b. Macrophages—capable of digestive activity
      c. Mast cells—contain vesicles filled with heparin and histamine
      d. Mesenchymal cells—primitive cells with the capability of differentiating into various connective tissue cells; they play a key role in the replacement of connective tissue lost as a result of injury or disease
   2. Cells that are normally in the bloodstream but move in and out of the blood vessels into surrounding connective tissue when needed (wandering cells)
      a. Monocytes
      b. Polymorphonuclear leukocytes
      c. Lymphocytes
      d. Plasma cells

B. Fibrous matrix
   1. Matrix of connective tissue composed of some or all of the following fibers:
      a. Collagen fibers—consist of three long polypeptide chains coiled in a left-handed helix to form a tropocollagen unit, which is assembled in a "quarter-stagger" model outside of the cell; fibers are highly resistant to tension and are part of the anchoring mechanism by which the connective tissue attaches the basement membrane (see Figure 2-20, *B*); the most abundant fibers found in connective tissue
      b. Reticulin fibers—comparable with collagen fibers in their protein composition; usually found in the border areas between connective tissue and other tissues
      c. Elastic fibers—consist of long fibrous proteins that differ in composition from collagen; are the branching fibers responsible for recoiling tissues when they are stretched
      d. Oxytalan fibers—resemble elastic fibers in morphology and chemical composition; are believed to be immature elastic fibers

C. Ground substance
   1. Amorphous substance that consists of many large, highly organized carbohydrate chains attached to long protein cores (e.g., proteoglycans)
   2. Molecular structure and composition are responsible for the ground substance's resistance to compression, or compressive loading, from any direction

Types (Cartilage and Bone)
Cartilage
A. Cartilage and bone are sister tissues, both highly specialized forms of connective tissue, whose intercellular substances have assumed particular properties that allow them to perform support functions
   1. Very "bouncy," resilient tissue that is specialized to resist compression; has a gel-like matrix in which the ground substance predominates over the intercellular matrix
   2. Relatively avascular tissue
   3. In humans, most of the embryonic skeleton is preformed as hyaline cartilage that is eventually replaced by bone (during endochondral ossification); depending on the location and loading pattern imposed on the cartilage, it may specialize to form fibrous or elastic cartilage
   4. All mature cartilage is surrounded by the perichondrium, a fibrous connective tissue, which serves a biomechanical function; it acts as an attachment site for muscles and tendons
B. Cartilage, as with all types of connective tissue, has three components:
   1. Cells—chondroblasts and chondrocytes
   2. Fibrous matrix—type II collagen fibers and, in some cases, elastic fibers
   3. Ground substance—proteoglycans, which have a protein core with side chains of chondroitin sulfate and keratan sulfate (glycosaminoglycans); because of the chemical nature and organization of proteoglycans, the ground substance can readily bind and hold water, which allows the tissue to assume a gelatinous nature that can resist compression and also permit some degree of diffusion through the matrix
C. Types
   1. Hyaline cartilage
      a. Found in the adult human
         (1) Covering articular surfaces of movable long bones
         (2) Forms the skeletal support parts of:
            (a) Trachea
            (b) Larynx
            (c) External ear
            (d) Nasal septum
            (e) Ends of ribs
      b. Most abundant type of cartilage; forms the embryonic skeleton in humans; is best suited to resist compression; appears as a homogeneous, translucent tissue because its intercellular matrix dominates its collagenous fibers; the major type of fiber in collagen

2. Fibrous cartilage (fibrocartilage)
   a. Has a very sparse amount of intercellular substance dominated by collagen fibers, which are in such proportion that they are visible through a light microscope and are seen running between the chondrocytic cells in the cartilage
   b. Resembles tendons except for the presence of the chondrocytes enclosed in lacunae
   c. Usually found in areas that are subjected to both compression and tension, as in:
      (1) Intervertebral disc
      (2) Temporomandibular joint of older adults
      (3) Pubic symphysis
3. Elastic cartilage
   a. In areas that are in need of elastic recoil, hyaline cartilage becomes highly specialized, and elastic fibers are added to its intercellular matrix, as in:
      (1) External ear
      (2) Epiglottis
   b. Elastic fibers are highly branched and form a delicate fibrous matrix, often obscuring the intercellular substance; fibers can be seen only through a light microscope when stained with a specific elastic stain

Bone
A. A specialized vascular connective tissue composed of a mineralized organic matrix; the inorganic component of bone is hydroxyapatite:

$$Ca_{10}(PO_4)_6(OH)_2$$

B. Two main functions:
   1. Provides skeletal support and protection of soft tissues
   2. Acts as a reservoir for calcium and phosphorus ions; when these two ions drop below a critical level in the blood (100 mg of calcium per 100 mL of blood, and 600 mg of phosphorus per/100 mL of blood), they can be withdrawn from the bone
C. Characteristic of all bones
   1. Compact bone—dense bone that appears as a continuous solid mass
   2. Trabecular (cancellous or spongy) bone—composed of a central medullary cavity filled with either red or yellow marrow and with intervening spicules of bone (trabeculae); these trabeculae act to reinforce bone by increasing in number with increased function
D. Bone morphology
   1. Bone-forming cells (osteoblasts) are produced from undifferentiated mesenchymal cells of the periosteum, the endosteum, and the periodontal ligament
      a. The periosteum is the connective tissue that covers the outer aspects of bone
      b. The endosteum is a more delicate connective tissue lining the inner aspects of bone, the trabeculae, and Volkmann's canals (canals of the bone containing blood vessels)
      c. The periodontal ligament is specialized periosteum because it covers the outer aspects of the alveolar bone;

it is also capable of forming bone and of forming cells that produce cementum (cementoblasts)

2. Osteoblasts become incorporated into bone during their formation; they occupy a space called a *lacuna* (plural, *lacunae*)

3. Lacunae are connected to each other by means of a system of canals named *canaliculi*; these canals house the cytoplasmic extension of the osteocytes and provide a means for the transport of vascular components

4. Both compact and trabecular mature bones are formed in layers, or *lamellae*. Lamellae are found in three distinct types of arrangements present in all mature human bones (Figure 2-8):

   a. Concentric, or haversian system, bone makes up the bulk of compact bone; it consists of lamellae arranged in concentric circles around a blood vessel (haversian canal) to form an osteon. An osteon, which consists of this concentrically arranged bone and haversian canal, is the basic metabolic unit of bone

   b. Interstitial lamellae fill the space between the concentric circles of the haversian system bone

   c. Lamellar bone is not arranged in concentric circles and is found on the surfaces of most bones. This bone is further defined by its location. When found on the outer aspects or the circumference of the bone underneath the periosteum, it is referred to as *circumferential*, or *(sub)periosteal, bone*; when found on the surfaces of trabeculae or the inner aspect of compact bone, it is referred to as *(sub)endosteal bone*

E. Bone tissue

1. Bone, as with all connective tissues, has three main components:

   a. Cells
      (1) Osteoblasts—bone-forming cells
      (2) Osteoclasts—bone-resorbing cells
      (3) Osteocytes—osteoblasts that are embedded in the lacunae of bone matrix and that maintain bone tissue

   b. Fibrous matrix—collagen fibers (type I), which are the dominant component of bone matrix

   c. Ground substance—proteoglycans containing chondroitin sulfates and seeded with the mineral salt hydroxyapatite

2. Bone is formed by osteoblasts developed in one of two ways:

   a. Intramembranous ossification—mesenchymal cells move closer together (condensation), differentiate into osteoblasts, and begin to deposit bone matrix; this is how the maxilla and the mandible are formed

   b. Endochondral ossification—future bone is preformed in a cartilage model that is eventually resorbed and replaced by new bone formed by osteoblasts (Figure 2-9)
      (1) Cartilage must undergo two important changes before being resorbed and replaced by new bone:
         (a) Chondrocytic hypertrophy
         (b) Calcification of the cartilage model
      (2) Endochondral ossification is the process by which all long bones in the human body are formed
         (a) Bone growth in length—occurs in the cartilaginous epiphyseal growth plate
         (b) Bone growth in diameter—occurs in the cellular layer of the fibrous covering of connective tissue periosteum, which produces a periosteal bone collar on the outer bone surface

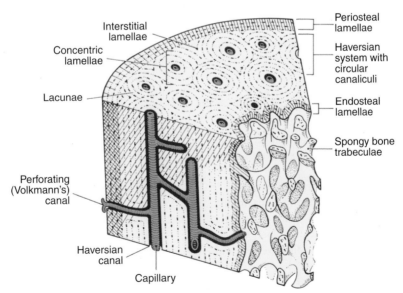

FIG 2-8 Microscopic morphology of bone tissue. Haversian system bone is composed of lamellae arranged in concentric circles around a canal. Interstitial bone fills the space between the concentric circles. Circumferential lamellar bone is found on the outer aspects of compact bone; endosteal lamellar bone covers the inner aspect of compact bone. Spongy bone is composed of trabeculae and marrow cavity. (From Avery JK, Chiego DJ: *Essentials of oral histology and embryology: a clinical approach*, ed 3, St Louis, 2006, Mosby.)

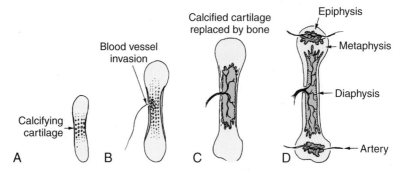

FIG 2-9 Stages of endochondral bone formation in long-bone growth. **A,** Original hyaline cartilage is calcified in the center of the diaphysis. **B,** Blood vessel invades the center of the shaft. **C,** The marrow space appears in the center of the shaft, and bone forms around the diaphysis. **D,** Bone formation continues in the shaft, and secondary ossification sites appear in the heads (epiphyses) of the bones. A disc of cartilage remains between bone forming in the head and the shaft (epiphyseal line). (From Chiego DJ: *Essentials of oral histology and embryology: a clinical approach,* ed 4, St Louis, 2013, Mosby.)

F. Structure of long bones (macroscopic)
  1. The typical long bone is composed of:
    a. Diaphysis (shaft)—thick compact bone forming a hollow cylinder with a central marrow cavity; this is the primary center of ossification in a long bone
    b. Epiphyses (ends)—spongy bone covered by a thin layer of compact bone; these are the secondary growth centers
    c. Metaphysis—transitional region between the epiphyses and the diaphysis, where the cartilage growth plate is located
    d. All articular surfaces of long bones are covered by articular cartilage
  2. While active, the epiphyseal growth plate usually has four zones, proceeding from first to last:
    a. Primary spongiosa with resorption
    b. Hypertrophy and provisional calcification
    c. Proliferation
    d. Resting zone (see Figure 2-9)

Blood and Lymph

A. Vascular system
  1. Develops embryonically from mesenchymal cells that come together and form delicate tubular structures composed of endothelial cells
  2. Consists of the heart, blood vessels, and lymphatics
    a. Is a closed system that runs from the heart to the organs of the body and back to the heart
    b. Between the heart and the organs, the blood vessels branch progressively into finer and finer vessels and finally enter the organs
      (1) Here a delicate network of capillaries forms, called the *capillary bed*—the most essential part of the vascular system
      (2) Exchanges of gases and substances occur in this capillary bed
    c. Blood is then carried back to the heart via larger vessels, the veins

  3. Functions
    a. Carries nutrients, oxygen, and hormones to all parts of the body
    b. Carries metabolic waste products to the kidneys
    c. Transports inflammatory cells and antibodies
    d. Maintains a constant body temperature
B. Lymph vessels empty into filtering organs (nodes) and generally flow toward larger lymph vessels, the thoracic duct, and the right lymphatic duct; lymph enters the venous branches of the circulatory system

Blood Vessels

A. Arteries—the largest of the blood vessels; walls are composed of:
  1. A thick layer of smooth muscle cells
  2. Elastic tissue—the largest amount is found in the large arteries close to the heart
B. Veins—usually accompany arteries but carry blood in the opposite direction
  1. Walls are composed of:
    a. A layer of endothelial cells
    b. A connective tissue layer
    c. Occasionally a few smooth muscle cells
  2. Veins contain about 70% of total blood volume of the body at any given time
C. Capillaries—the simplest of the blood vessels in the structure
  1. Walls consist of a simple layer of endothelial cells and a basal lamina
  2. Usually, the diameter of a capillary lumen is so small that only one blood cell at a time can pass through it
  3. Capillaries form a barrier between blood and tissues
  4. Transport of substances occurs at the capillary level through:
    a. Pores in the endothelial wall of the capillary
    b. Openings between adjacent endothelial cells
    c. Pinocytotic vesicles formed by the wall of the capillary

Microvasculature

A. Composed of the smallest arteries and veins located in the capillary bed

1. At the end of the arterioles is a preferential channel that has several side branches entering the capillary bed
2. Blood passes through the capillary bed from the arterial side to the venous side

B. Selective openings and closings of the capillary bed occur in the microvasculature to ensure regulation of the amount of blood throughout the body at any given time

Blood Components

A. Cells
   1. Red blood cells—erythrocytes; most numerous
   2. White blood cells—leukocytes (granular and nongranular)
   3. Platelets—cell fragments of a specific cell type found in red bone marrow; have no nuclei
B. Plasma—liquid portion of blood

Functions of Blood Cells

A. Red blood cells (erythrocytes) contain hemoglobin, which carries oxygen from lungs to tissues
B. White blood cells (leukocytes) function chiefly to fight infection, to scavenge foreign invaders, and to repair injured tissue
   1. Granular leukocytes
      a. Polymorphonuclear neutrophils (PMNs)—first line of defense against bacterial invasion
      b. Eosinophils—involvement in allergic reactions
      c. Basophils—antigen involvement
   2. Nongranular leukocytes
      a. Monocytes—can become macrophages in connective tissue
      b. Lymphocytes—produce antibodies
C. Platelets—promote blood clotting

Lymphatic System

A. Made up of a series of vessels that carry excess tissue fluid from the capillaries to filtering organs such as lymph nodes on the return to the bloodstream
B. Lymph nodes are found along the lymphatic pathway
   1. Consist of masses of lymph tissue that serve as a filtering system for the body
   2. The tonsils and the spleen are both filtering organs for the body
   3. Swollen and palpable lymph nodes may indicate that an infection is present somewhere in the body
C. The function of lymph is to protect and maintain the internal fluid environment of the body

Nerve Tissue

A. Main functions of the nervous system
   1. Directs and maintains the complex internal environment of the body
   2. Integrates and interprets incoming stimuli and directs appropriate responses at a conscious or unconscious level
B. The nervous system can be classified as follows:
   1. Central nervous system (CNS)
   2. Peripheral nervous system (PNS)
   3. Autonomic nervous system (ANS)
C. Afferent nerves transmit impulses (sensations) from the periphery to the CNS (sensory input); efferent nerves

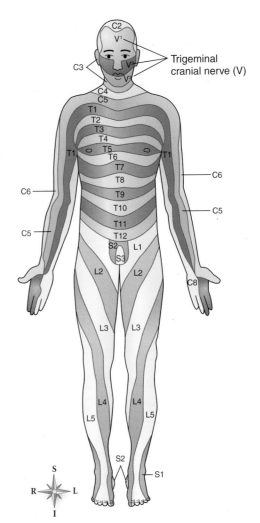

FIG 2-10 Cross section of a spinal cord showing pathways used to transmit nerve impulses from the periphery to the central nervous system. (From Patton KT: *Anatomy and physiology*, ed 9, St Louis, 2016, Elsevier.)

transmit impulses (commands) from the CNS to muscles and other organs (motor output) (Figure 2-10)

D. Divisions of the nervous system
   1. Central nervous system
      a. Includes the brain and the spinal cord
      b. Main functions:
         (1) Receives incoming information at a conscious or unconscious level (sensory)
         (2) Integrates outgoing responses (motor) that are transmitted to various parts of the brain and the spinal cord
   2. Peripheral nervous system
      a. Composed of 31 pairs of spinal nerves and 12 pairs of cranial nerves
      b. All nerves transmit information to and from the CNS
      c. Contains both sensory and motor nerves (neurons)
   3. Autonomic nervous system (Figure 2-11)
      a. Controls, regulates, and coordinates visceral activities (digestion, body temperature, blood pressure, and glandular secretions) at an unconscious level

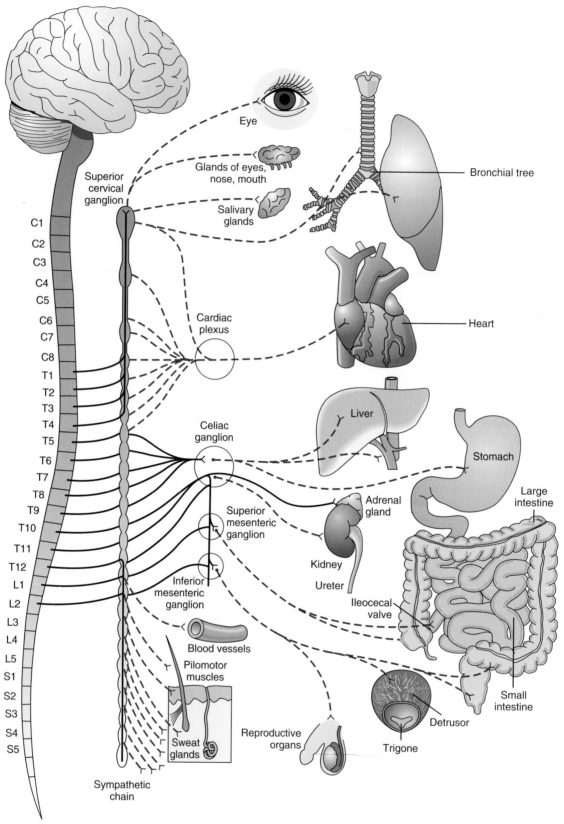

FIG 2-11 Distribution of sympathetic nerves. (From Copstead LC, Banasik JL: *Pathophysiology,* ed 5, St Louis, 2014, Elsevier.)

b. Is further subdivided into:
    (1) Sympathetic division—acts to regulate and mobilize activities during emergency or stress (flight activities); activities that require high outputs of energy produce an accelerated heart rate and increase in blood pressure
    (2) Parasympathetic division—works in the opposite manner of the sympathetic division; stimulates activities that restore or conserve energy (e.g., decreased heart rate, constricted pupils, contraction of ciliary muscle)
    (3) These two divisions are seen as acting reciprocally rather than antagonistically

Structural Components

A. Neurons (Figure 2-12)
  1. Structural components of nerve tissue
  2. Receive and transmit information
  3. Highly specialized cells consisting of:
    a. Cell body—contains the nucleus and organelles; located in the ganglia in the CNS and the PNS
    b. One or more cytoplasmic extensions
      (1) Dendrites—conduct impulses toward the cell body
      (2) Axons—conduct impulses away from the cell body
  4. Classified according to the number of cell processes (Figure 2-13):
    a. Multi-polar neurons—located in the CNS and autonomic ganglia; usually, one process is the axon and the other processes are the dendrites

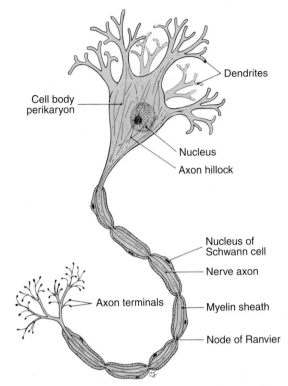

FIG 2-12 Neuron with its cell body, axon, dendrites, and synaptic relationships with the muscle tissue and another neuron. (From Avery JK, Chiego DJ: *Essentials of oral histology and embryology: a clinical approach*, ed 3, St Louis, 2006, Mosby.)

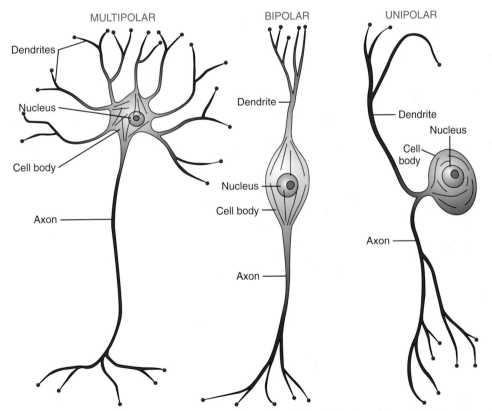

FIG 2-13 Classification of neurons based on the location of the cell body and the relative length and number of dendrites and axons. (From Copstead LC, Banasik JL: *Pathophysiology*, ed 5, St Louis, 2014, Elsevier.)

b. Unipolar neurons—have a short cell process that leaves the cell body and divides into two long branches; one branch goes to the CNS, and the other goes to the PNS (sensory neurons)

5. Interneurons—lie within the CNS; receive and link sensory and motor impulses to bring about appropriate responses in the body

B. Glial cells—provide structural support and nourishment for the neurons; Schwann cells in the PNS and satellite cells in the ganglia

Definitions

A. *Synapse*—an area that occurs between two neurons or between a neuron and its effector (muscle or gland); found between the cell surfaces are:
   1. Synaptic cleft—intercellular space separating a presynaptic and postsynaptic membrane
   2. Presynaptic membrane—situated before the synapse
   3. Postsynaptic membrane—situated after the synapse

B. *Neurotransmitters*—chemicals released from the neuron as electrical impulses travel along the axon and reach the terminal end
   1. Neurotransmitters increase the permeability of the cell membranes; impulses are relayed to the effector; impulses can be excitatory or inhibitory
   2. Two-membrane junctions
   3. Types of neurotransmitters
      a. Acetylcholine—secreted by cholinergic fibers
      b. Norepinephrine—secreted by adrenergic fibers

C. *Myelin sheath*—fatty layer surrounding the axon of the nerve
   1. Myelinated—contains a fatty sheath
   2. Unmyelinated—contains no fatty sheath

D. *Neurilemma*—continuous sheath that encloses the segmented myelin sheath of some nerves

E. *Neuroglia*—extremely soft tissue that supports the nervous tissue of the brain and the spinal cord

F. *Free nerve endings*—end portions of afferent (sensory) axons no longer covered by a supportive Schwann cell; found in:
   1. Dental pulp
   2. Oral epithelium

G. *Encapsulated nerve endings*—composed of several portions of afferent axons surrounded by a capsule of several Schwann cells without a myelin sheath and some connective tissue; they are associated with:
   1. Touch perception (Meissner's corpuscles) found in the lamina propria of the oral mucosa
   2. Periodontal ligament

Cranial Nerves

See the section titled "The Nervous System" in Chapters 3 and 4.

A. Twelve pairs of cranial nerves originate from the brain
   1. Cranial nerves transmit information to the brain from the special sensory receptors and regulate the functions of:
      a. Smell
      b. Sight
      c. Hearing
      d. Taste
   2. Cranial nerves bring impulses from the CNS to the voluntary muscles of:
      a. Eyes
      b. Mouth (masticatory muscles)
      c. Face (facial expression)
      d. Tongue (swallowing and speech)
      e. Larynx

B. In oral health care, a local anesthetic agent is injected into a sensory peripheral nerve; it diffuses through the nerve fibers and blocks the transmission of impulses to the brain in an area of several teeth or in a localized area of soft tissue (see the section "Characteristics and Physiology of Pain" in Chapter 18).

Muscle Tissue

A. Composed mainly of cells called *muscle fibers,* which have differentiated from the embryonic mesenchyme and have become highly specialized in contracting (shortening)

B. Contracting ability of muscle fibers is a result of large amounts of actin and myosin, which are intracellular, contractile protein filaments

C. The three muscle tissue types are:
   1. Skeletal (striated) muscle
      a. Under conscious control; referred to as *voluntary muscle*
      b. Has rapid, short, strong contractions; requires a great deal of energy
      c. Innervated by motor nerves
      d. Skeletal muscles of the head region:
         (1) Muscles of mastication
         (2) Muscles of facial expression
      e. Muscle attachments are possible because of the connective tissues surrounding the muscle, bone, or cartilage; connecting tissues of the muscle run directly into the periosteum, cover the bone or perichondrium, cover the cartilage or perimysium, or cover the muscle. The exact nature of the attachment depends on the site and function of the muscle. The intermediate structures may be:
         (1) Tendons
         (2) Ligaments
         (3) Aponeuroses
      f. Muscles that change the shape of the tongue by their contractions are attached on both sides to the lamina propria of the oral mucosa of the tongue
   2. Smooth muscle
      a. Under the control of the ANS and not under conscious control
      b. Contractions are slow and can be maintained over a long period without the use of much energy
   3. Cardiac muscle
      a. Has some of both skeletal (striated) and smooth muscle characteristics
      b. Is involuntary; has fast, powerful contractions
      c. Purkinje fibers—specialized cells present in heart muscle that act like nerves to conduct messages through the heart
      d. Bundle of His—a band of specialized cardiac muscle fibers

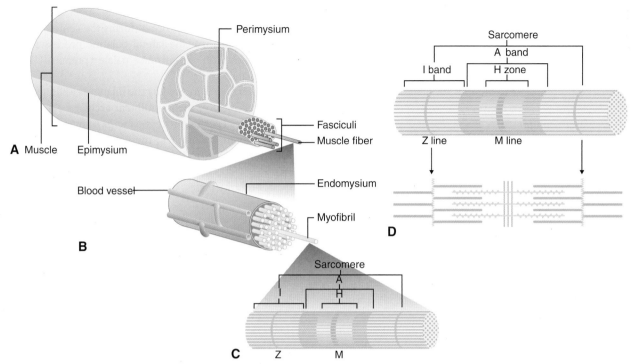

FIG 2-14 Muscle fiber. **A,** The epimysium runs continuously with the endomysium and the perimysium. **B,** The arrangement of fasciculi varies among muscles. **C,** The banding pattern apparent on microscopic inspection of a muscle cell results from the organized structure of the proteins (myofibrils) of the contractile apparatus. **D,** Thick and thin filaments are organized into contractile units called sarcomeres. (From Copstead LC, Banasik JL: *Pathophysiology*, ed 5, St Louis, 2014, Elsevier.)

Muscle Contraction

A. Muscle can be stimulated to contract by one nerve or by many nerves
B. Each striated muscle contains bundles of highly organized contractile proteins called *myofibrils*; each myofibril consists of regularly arranged protein filaments: actin and myosin (Figure 2-14)
C. Protein filaments are attached to a Z band; the section of a myofibril between two Z bands is called a *sarcomere,* which is the contractile unit
D. As a muscle unit contracts, actin and myosin filaments slide past each other, shorten the length of the individual sarcomere (sliding mechanism), and cause total shortening of the muscle fiber

GENERAL EMBRYOLOGY

A. All human development begins by fertilization, the union of a female germ cell (ovum) and a male germ cell (sperm)
B. Each germ cell contains 23 chromosomes (haploid number); during the process of fertilization, the number of chromosomes is restored to 46 (diploid number)
C. The developing organism, called the zygote, goes through a series of mitotic divisions
  1. Morula—16 to 32 cells, appearance resembles that of a mulberry
  2. Blastocele—a central cavity with an embryonic pole
  3. Blastocyst—thin-walled hollow ball of cells that attaches to and embeds in the uterine wall
    a. Two distinct layers become visible:
      (1) Epiblast (ectoderm) layer
      (2) Hypoblast (endoderm) layer
    b. These two layers constitute the embryonic disc, which will give rise to the future embryo
D. Three distinct periods in human development:
  1. Period of the ovum (first week)—fertilized ovum develops an embryonic disc
  2. Embryonic period (second week to eighth week)—most of the organs and organ systems develop
    a. A period of differentiation
    b. At the end of this period, a recognizable individual has developed
    c. Most congenital malformations occur during this time
  3. Fetal period (third month to ninth month)—growth of existing structures takes place
E. Development of some facial and oral structures is dependent on a group of cells (neural crest cells) derived from the ectoderm as the neural tube is forming; these cells migrate cephalad and interact with the cephalic ectoderm and mesoderm to result in the development of:
  1. Facial skeleton—Meckel's cartilage
  2. Neck skeleton—hyoid bone
  3. Connective tissue components
  4. Tooth development

F. Neural crest cells migrate into each of the branchial arches and surround the existing mesoderm; in each arch, the following components develop:
   1. Cartilage rod (skeleton of each arch)—first branchial arch, Meckel's cartilage
   2. Muscular component—second branchial arch, facial musculature
   3. Vasculature component
   4. Nerve component—first branchial arch, trigeminal nerve
G. On the internal aspect of the branchial arches are corresponding pharyngeal pouches that give rise to:
   1. External auditory meatus
   2. Pharyngotympanic tube
   3. Palatine tonsils
   4. Parathyroid glands

Facial Development

A. Initiation of the development of the oral cavity occurs in the third prenatal week (embryonic period) and is complete in the twelfth week
B. The future facial region is located among the bulging forebrain, the frontal nasal process, and the developing heart
C. At the beginning of the fourth week, five facial swellings, called branchial arches, appear on the embryo
   1. Located between the first branchial arch and the frontal process (forebrain) is the oral stomodeum (primitive oral cavity) (Figure 2-15); the stomodeum is the first sign of facial development
   2. The stomodeal ectoderm invaginates until it comes in contact with the primitive foregut; the stomodeum and the foregut are initially separated by the buccopharyngeal membrane, which is composed of the ectoderm and the endoderm. It is located in the region that will eventually house the palatine tonsils
   3. Rathke's pouch—a small invagination in the roof of the stomodeum; deepens into the brain and forms the anterior lobe of the pituitary gland
   4. The maxilla and the mandible develop from the first branchial arch
   5. The second to fifth branchial arches are involved in development of the neck
D. On the lower aspect of the frontal process, nasal pits (nostrils) arise from nasal placodes (see Figure 2-15, B) and separate the lower frontal process into:
   1. Medial nasal process (area between the nasal pits); this gives rise to:
      a. The center of the nose and the nasal septum
      b. The globular process that develops into:
         (1) The center of the upper lip (philtrum)
         (2) The primary palate (premaxilla)—the anterior portion of the palate
   2. Lateral nasal processes (area to the right and left of the nasal pits) that form the sides of the nose
E. Maxillary processes arise from the superolateral border of the first branchial arch; they grow:
   1. Downward to merge with the mandibular processes and form the closure at the corner of the mouth
   2. Medially to form the sides of the upper lip, which unite with the globular process (forms the center of the lip)
   3. Inward to form the lateral palatine processes that fuse together with the primary palate (premaxilla) to form the palate
F. The lower face is formed by the bilateral swellings (mandibular processes) of the mandibular arch
G. Several facial or oral processes merge or fuse together during development; incomplete merging or fusing can result in cleft formation—cleft lip or cleft palate
   1. A cleft lip occurs more often on the left side, more frequently in males, and at the end of the second month in utero
   2. A cleft palate occurs more often in females
   3. Cleft lips and cleft palates can occur as isolated defects, meaning a cleft lip can occur without a cleft palate; most cleft palates occur in combination with a cleft lip

Palatal Development

A. The globular process develops as medial nasal processes grow downward and gives rise to:
   1. The philtrum of the upper lip
   2. The primary palate (premaxillary process), which carries the incisor tooth buds
B. During the sixth week of embryonic life, two lateral palatine processes (palatal "shelves") develop from each side of the maxilla and lie vertically on each side of the tongue (these palatal shelves form the secondary palate)
C. During the seventh week of embryonic life, the developing tongue drops down, and the vertical lateral palatine processes flip up, assume a horizontal position, and fuse with the primary palate
D. Where the two palatal processes (shelves) fuse in the midline, trapped epithelium between the two processes may result in epithelial remnants, which may produce cysts
E. The right and left lateral palatine processes (palatal shelves) fuse with each other at the midline; anteriorly, they fuse with the primary palate in an area between the right and left laterals and the right and left canines
   1. A cleft palate occurs at the end of the third month in utero
   2. Failure of fusion can occur at any of these lines of fusion
   3. A cleft in the alveolar ridge could occur unilaterally (on one side) or bilaterally (on both sides); this cleft occurs between the lateral and the canine, so the lateral incisor is the tooth most often missing or malformed
   4. The right and left lateral palatal processes can fail to fuse with each other at the midline, and the oral cavity would be open to the nasal cavity

Tongue Development

During the fourth week of embryonic life, the tongue develops from several swellings arising on the internal aspect of branchial arches 1 to 4 (pouches); these swellings eventually merge and form the body and root of the tongue.
A. Branchial arch 1—two lateral swellings and one medial swelling (tuberculum impar) merge to form the body of the tongue

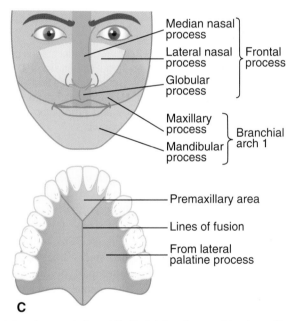

FIG 2-15 Facial development. **A** and **B,** Facial development begins with the outgrowth of branchial arches. Note the relationship of the oral stomodeum to the heart and the developing face. Nasal pits develop from the frontal nasal process and grow to become nostrils. The nasal pits separate the frontal nasal process into the medial nasal process and the right and left lateral nasal processes. **C,** Note the developmental processes and the lines of fusion on the adult face illustration. (**B** from Chiego DJ: *Essentials of oral histology and embryology: a clinical approach,* ed 4, St Louis, 2013, Mosby.)

B. Branchial arches 2, 3, and part of 4—copula merge to form the base of the tongue
C. Branchial arch 4—site where the epiglottis is formed
D. Thyroid gland—develops from an invagination of ectoderm in the area of the foramen cecum of the tongue; the thyroid gland eventually migrates down to its position in the neck; thyroid tissue that remains entrapped in the tissue of the tongue may result in a developmental abnormality known as *lingual thyroid nodule*

ORAL HISTOLOGY

Tooth Development

A. Begins in the seventh week of embryonic life with the 20 primary teeth; continues until the late teens with sequential exfoliation of the primary dentition and development and eruption of the secondary dentition—the 32 permanent teeth
B. Tissues of the tooth

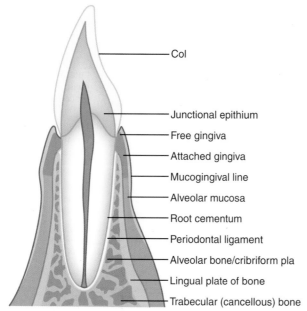

FIG 2-16 Four tissues of the tooth: enamel, cementum, dentin, and pulp. The periodontal ligament and alveolar bone are supporting tissues; junctional epithelium is the area where the enamel or cementum of the tooth and the epithelium of the gingival tissue form an attachment.

1. Each tooth consists of four tissues (Figure 2-16):
   a. Enamel—calcified
   b. Cementum—calcified
   c. Dentin—calcified
   d. Pulp—uncalcified
2. All tissues of the tooth are specialized forms of connective tissue, except enamel
3. Each tooth is the product of two tissues that interact during tooth development:
   a. Mesenchyme (ectomesenchyme)—derived from neural crest cells
   b. Epithelium—oral epithelium derived from the ectoderm
C. Involves two major events:
   1. Morphodifferentiation—shaping of the tooth
   2. Cytodifferentiation—cells differentiating into specific tissue-forming cells:
      a. Ameloblasts—enamel-forming cells
      b. Cementoblasts—cementum-forming cells
      c. Odontoblasts—dentin-forming cells
      d. Fibroblasts—pulp-forming cells (also capable of differentiating into a chondroblast, collagenoblast, or osteoblast)

Morphodifferentiation

A. Oral epithelium and underlying ectomesenchyme are responsible for shaping the tooth
   1. Both primary and permanent tooth germs go through the same stages of development
   2. The oral epithelium grows down into the underlying ectomesenchyme; small areas of condensed mesenchyme form future tooth germs

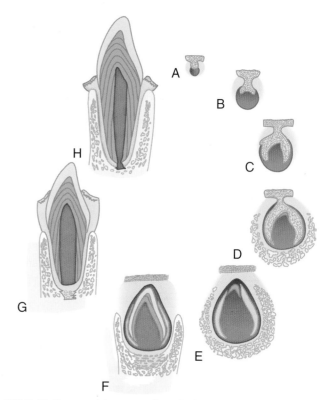

FIG 2-17 Sequential stages of tooth development. **A,** Bud stage. **B,** Cap stage. **C,** Bell stage. **D,** Dentinogenesis. **E,** Amelogenesis. **F,** Appositional dentin and enamel. **G,** Eruption and root development. **H,** Functional stage. (From Chiego DJ: *Essentials of oral histology and embryology: a clinical approach,* ed 4, St Louis, 2013, Mosby.)

B. Stages (Figure 2-17)
   1. Bud stage—condensed areas of ectomesenchymal cells that are continuous with the oral epithelium; connection between the two is referred to as the *dental lamina*
   2. Cap stage—future shape of the tooth becomes evident; cells specialize to form the enamel organ
   3. Bell stage—final stage of morphodifferentiation; in the latter part of this stage, cytodifferentiation begins in the enamel organ
   4. Dentinogenesis—origin or initial stages of dentin formation
   5. Amelogenesis—differentiated cells begin initial enamel formation
   6. Apposition stage—formation of dental tissue matrix; this matrix will then undergo maturation or calcification
   7. Eruption and root development
   8. Functional stage—the tooth is fully erupted in the mouth

Cytodifferentiation

A. Stages of cytodifferentiation and morphodifferentiation overlap; both epithelial and mesenchymal components of the tooth germ become organized
   1. Epithelial components become the enamel organ, which is organized into four distinct cell layers (Figure 2-18):
      a. Outer enamel epithelium (OEE)—outlines the shape of the future developing enamel organ on the

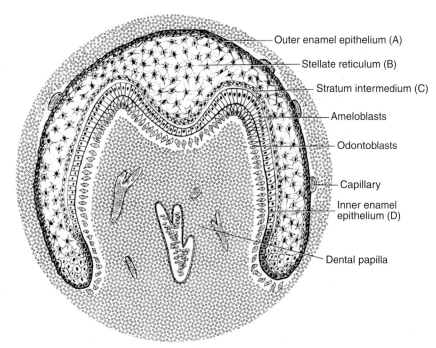

FIG 2-18 The four distinct layers of the enamel organ. **A,** Outer enamel epithelium. **B,** Stellate reticulum. **C,** Stratum intermedium. **D,** Inner enamel epithelium. (Modified from Avery JK, Chiego DJ: *Essentials of oral histology and embryology: a clinical approach,* ed 3, St Louis, 2006, Mosby.)

outer surface; composed of small cuboidal cells, one cell layer thick

b. Inner enamel epithelium (IEE)—innermost layer of the enamel organ on the concave side of the developing tooth germ; this will become the future enamel-producing cells, the ameloblasts; composed of cuboidal-type cells, one cell layer thick

c. Stratum intermedium (STI)—flat, supporting, squamous-type cells, two to three cell layers thick, lying on top of the inner enamel epithelial cells

d. Stellate reticulum (STR)—mechanically and nutritionally supporting cells that fill the bulk of the developing enamel organ; are star shaped with large amounts of intercellular space between them

2. Mesenchymal components become subdivided into:

a. Dental sac (follicle)—surrounds the developing tooth germ and provides cells that will form the periodontal ligament, which in turn will produce the cementum and the alveolar bone proper

b. Dental papilla—condensed ectomesenchyme located on the concave side of the enamel organ; peripheral cells facing the IEE will differentiate into odontoblasts (dentin-forming cells)

c. The center of the dental papilla will become the dental pulp

B. Tooth development depends on a series of sequential cellular interactions between the epithelial and mesenchymal components of the tooth germ

1. First interaction—between the oral epithelium and the mesenchyme; the ectomesenchyme instructs the epithelium to grow down into the ectomesenchyme and shape the tooth

2. Second interaction—signal given by cells of the inner enamel epithelium (preameloblasts) to the mesenchymal cells on the periphery of the dental papilla to differentiate into odontoblasts and begin the deposition of dentin

3. Third interaction—as soon as odontoblasts begin to deposit dentin, preameloblasts become true secreting ameloblasts and begin the deposition of enamel

4. Fourth interaction—occurs with the development of root dentin and cementum

Dentin and Enamel Formation

A. Both enamel-forming and dentin-forming cells are polarized, tall, columnar, secreting cells; just before ameloblasts and odontoblasts begin to deposit enamel and dentin, organelles, especially the mitochondria, increase in number; organelles move to the basal nonsecretory end of the cell; both cells require tremendous amounts of energy for the production of their calcified tissues

B. All dentin and enamel formation begins at the dento-enamel junction (DEJ) of the cup or the incisal edge of the tooth and continues in an apical direction

C. The permanent tooth germ grows off the primary (deciduous) tooth germ by an epithelial attachment similar to dental lamina, called *successional lamina*; this applies to all the developing permanent teeth except the first, second, and third molars; these develop from the dental lamina, which continues to grow back in oral arches

D. Dentin formation

1. Odontoblasts produce collagen fibers that unravel to produce a fibrous connective tissue matrix (fibrillar matrix) of predominantly collagen fibers with a rich proteoglycan ground substance; dentinal tissue is calcified by the

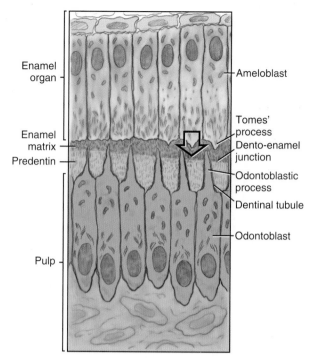

FIG 2-19 Odontoblasts and ameloblasts with their cell extensions. Tall, secretory odontoblast with its cell extension (odontoblastic extension). Tall, secretory ameloblast with its cell extension (Tomes' process). (From Fehrenbach MJ, Popowics T: *Illustrated dental embryology, histology, and anatomy*, ed 4, St Louis, 2016, Elsevier.)

deposition of the crystals of the calcium salt hydroxyapatite into the matrix

2. Each odontoblast has a long cell extension, the odontoblastic process, left behind in the calcified dentin and enclosed in a dentinal tubule (Figure 2-19)
3. Dentin remains a vital tissue throughout the life of the tooth; in a vital tooth, cells continue to produce dentin when needed

E. Enamel formation
1. Ameloblasts produce an enamel matrix with protein components called *amelogenins* and *enamelins*; the matrix is calcified immediately by the deposition of the crystals of the calcium salt hydroxyapatite
2. Ameloblasts deposit enamel; each ameloblast has a secretory process called *Tomes' process*; Tomes' process has a six-sided pyramidal shape and is responsible for prism-shaped microscopic patterns of enamel rods; unlike the odontoblastic process, Tomes' process is not left behind embedded in the calcified tissue (see Figure 2-19)
3. When the tooth emerges into the oral cavity, the enamel has no vital cells associated with the tissue; enamel is not a true tissue like other dental tissues and is incapable of tissue growth or repair; once formed, the mineral substance cannot be physiologically withdrawn from the tooth
4. A final product of the ameloblasts is the primary enamel cuticle, a calcified coating on the enamel surface
5. Secondary cuticle—a noncalcified coating; a product of the reduced enamel organ

6. Nasmyth's membrane consists of the primary enamel cuticle and the secondary enamel cuticle; this membrane on the newly erupted tooth can easily pick up extrinsic stain

F. Dento-gingival junction formation
1. After the enamel formation is complete, remains of the enamel organ (OEE, IEE, STI, and STR) come together to form the reduced enamel epithelium
2. Reduced enamel epithelium—plays an important role in the formation of the dento-gingival junction as the tooth emerges into the oral cavity

G. Cementum formation
1. Formation of root dentin and cementum follows after the formation of the crown of the tooth is complete
2. *Hertwig's root sheath* is formed by the joining of the outer enamel epithelium and the inner enamel epithelium; the sheath continues to grow down, shapes the root of the tooth and the formation of root dentin, and is followed by differentiation of cells from the dental sac; these cells produce:
   a. Cementum
   b. Periodontal ligament
   c. Alveolar bone proper

Soft Tissue of the Oral Cavity
Oral Mucosa
A. Oral epithelium (Figure 2-20)
1. Covered by a layer of the stratified squamous epithelium that:
   a. Acts as a mechanical barrier
   b. Protects the underlying tissues
2. Three types of stratified squamous epithelia are found in the oral cavity:
   a. Orthokeratinized
      (1) Effective as a mechanical protector and barrier against fluids
      (2) Least common of the three types
      (3) Layers
         (a) Basal cell layer—deepest layer
         (b) Prickle cell layer (stratum spinosium)
         (c) Granular layer—contains the keratohyaline granules, the precursor to keratin
         (d) Keratinized layer (stratum corneum)—contains degenerative cells with no nuclei or organelles; cells are filled with keratin, become hard (cornified), and are eventually lost from the surface epithelium
   b. Nonkeratinized
      (1) Functions as a selective barrier; acts as a cushion and as protection against mechanical stress and wear
      (2) Layers
         (a) Basal cell layer
         (b) Prickle cell layer
         (c) Outer surface of nonkeratinized cells (squamae); no distinctly recognizable layer above the prickle cell layer; superficial cells in the outermost layer undergo a gradual increase in size; look empty but are filled with fluid

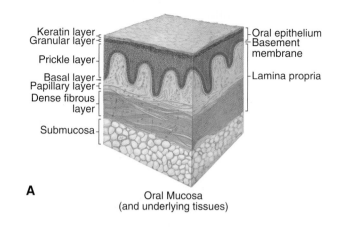

A

Oral Mucosa
(and underlying tissues)

B

FIG 2-20 Basic structure of the oral epithelium. **A,** Two basic tissues comprise the oral mucosa: the oral epithelium and connective tissue. Connective tissue is composed of a papillary layer and a reticular layer. A submucosal layer may or may not be present, depending on the location of the oral mucosa. Note the arrangement of rete ridges (or pegs) and connective tissue papillae. **B,** Basal lamina interface between oral epithelium and connective tissue. Note the hemidesmosomes with attachment plaque between epithelial cells and the basal lamina. (From Fehrenbach MJ, Popowics T: *Illustrated dental embryology, histology, and anatomy,* ed 4, St Louis, 2016, Elsevier.)

sacs; cells act as a cushion and are firmly attached to each other
c. Parakeratinized
(1) Intermediate form of the epithelium located between the orthokeratinized and nonkeratinized oral mucosa
(2) Layers
(a) Basal cell layer
(b) Prickle cell layer
(c) Keratinized layer—no distinct granular layer present; gradually becomes filled with keratin; nuclei and other cell organelles remain until the cell becomes cornified, and then they are eventually lost
3. The stratified squamous epithelium is constantly renewed by mitosis at the basal cell layer; turnover time ranges from 5 to 16 days
B. Connective tissue—referred to as *lamina propria*
1. Subdivided into two layers:
a. Papillary layer—directly under the epithelial layer; tattoo dye is injected into this portion of tissue
b. Reticular layer—dense fibrous layer located under the papillary layer; wrinkles in the skin occur because of degradation of the reticular layer

2. Forms a mechanical support system and carries
a. Blood vessels
b. Nerves
C. Submucosa
1. Layer of loosely organized connective tissue
2. Present only in areas that require a high degree of compressibility and flexibility (e.g., cheeks, soft palate)
3. When present, submucosa is located between the lamina propria and areas of muscle tissue
D. Interface
1. Area of interdigitation between the oral epithelium and connective tissue
2. Epithelial extensions into connective tissue (lamina propria) are called *ridges* or *rete pegs* (see Figure 2-20, *A*)
3. Connective tissue extensions into overlying epithelium are called *connective tissue papillae*
4. Corrugated arrangement
a. Increases the surface area between the two tissues
b. Increases the strength of the junction between the two tissues
c. Decreases the distance between the blood supply and the epithelium, which does not have its own blood supply; blood vessels are carried to the epithelium in connective tissue through connective tissue papillae
d. This rete peg arrangement is found in healthy attached gingiva, the stippling of which is caused by this arrangement; healthy sulcular epithelium does not have rete pegs
E. Basement membrane (see Figure 2-20, *B*)
1. Located between oral epithelium and connective tissue
2. Noncellular
3. Produced partly by epithelial cells and connective tissue cells
4. Composed of two layers:
a. The basal lamina is primarily the product of epithelial cells and can be further divided into two layers:
(1) The clear layer adjacent to the epithelium is the lamina lucida
(2) The denser layer closer to the connective tissue is the lamina densa and is about 20 to 70 nm thick; it contains some type IV collagen fibers that are produced by the connective tissue
b. Reticular lamina is found below the basal lamina and is much thicker than the basal layer; it contains collagen fiber produced by connective tissue cells and plays a role in anchoring the basal lamina to the underlying connective tissue
5. Epithelial cells form hemidesmosome attachments to the basal lamina (see Figure 2-20)
F. Clinical changes in the oral mucosa
1. Inflammation, friction, heat, and chronic irritation produce changes in the degree of keratinization
a. Inflammation causes a reduction in keratinization
b. Friction, heat, and chronic irritation cause an increase in keratinization
c. Increased keratinization causes tissue appearance to be lighter or whitish; in areas of the mouth that have

minor salivary glands, such as the soft palate, increased keratin may obstruct the gland openings, producing the appearance of red dots on hyperkeratinized tissue (nicotine stomatitis)

2. The appearance of the oral mucosa changes in response to pathologic, dermatologic, systemic, allergic, and localized factors

Classifications of Mucosa

A. Masticatory—gingiva, hard palate (orthokeratinized epithelial covering)
1. Histologic structure
   a. Keratinized stratified squamous epithelium; rete pegs—projections into the underlying connective tissue
   b. No submucosa; no salivary glands
   c. Fibrous connective tissue; gingival fibers
2. Clinical appearance
   a. Coral pink; influenced by vascularity, the thickness and degree of keratinization of the epithelium, and the presence of pigment cells
   b. Texture—stippled, the result of the rete peg arrangement
   c. Consistency—firm, caused by the fibrous content (mostly collagen) of the underlying connective tissue
B. Lining—lips, cheeks, floor of mouth, ventral surface (underside) of tongue, soft palate, alveolar mucosa (nonkeratinized epithelial covering)
1. The floor of the mouth is the thinnest part of the nonkeratinized squamous epithelial lining mucosa (100 μm)
2. Connective tissue of the lining mucosa has more elastic fiber than that of the masticatory mucosa; fluid disperses readily in this area, making it an ideal site for local anesthetic injections

Specialized Mucosa of the Tongue

A. Specialized covering found only on the top of the tongue; covered with lingual papillae
B. Epithelial layer—stratified squamous epithelium that varies in thickness and degree of keratinization
C. Taste buds are epithelial organs of special sense (taste); most taste buds are found on lingual papillae; isolated buds may be found on the soft palate and on the walls of the pharynx
D. Connective tissue papillae form specialized lingual papillae
1. Fungiform papillae—located on the dorsal aspect of the tongue; mushroom shaped; a single taste bud may be present on the top surface
2. Filiform papillae—most abundant of papillae; found covering the entire top surface of the tongue; have no taste buds; elongated in cases of "hairy" tongue
3. Circumvallate papillae—large papillae located in a V-shaped groove at the base of the tongue; encircled by a deep groove; mushroom shaped; taste buds are located on their sides; small salivary glands (Ebner's glands) empty into surrounding grooves of taste buds
4. Foliate papillae—located along the sides of the tongue, near the base; taste buds may be located on only one of the sides
E. No submucosa is present

Tissues of the Tooth
Dentin

A. Mature dentin composition
1. Chemical composition
   a. Organic matter, 18%
   b. Inorganic matter, 70%
   c. Water, 12%
2. Tissue composition
   a. Cells—odontoblasts
   b. Fibrous material—collagen fibers (type I)
   c. Ground substance—proteoglycans and glycoproteins
3. Calcification—deposition of crystals of the calcium salt hydroxyapatite in the dentin, fibrous matrix, and ground substance
B. Process of dentogenesis
1. Dentin begins to form in the late bell stage of the developing tooth germ (see Figure 2-17)
2. Newly differentiated odontoblasts deposit the dentin matrix; odontoblastic processes become surrounded by predentin (a newly deposited, uncalcified dentin matrix); predentin becomes calcified as cells deposit more dentin; predentin is adjacent to the pulp in young teeth
3. Each cell process in mature calcified dentin is enclosed in a dentinal tubule (Figure 2-21)
   a. Dentinal tubules can run from the DEJ to the periphery of the dental pulp, where cell bodies of odontoblasts are located

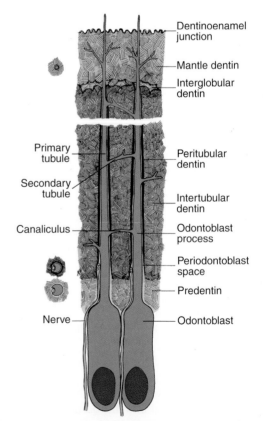

FIG 2-21 Odontoblastic process with its cell process enclosed in dentinal tubule. (From Chiego DJ: *Essentials of oral histology and embryology: a clinical approach*, ed 4, St Louis, 2014, Elsevier.)

b. Tubules follow a primary S-shaped curve (pathway) and secondary S-shaped curves along the length of the tubules
  (1) Primary S-shaped curves are caused by the movement of odontoblasts from a wider area to a narrower area, which produces crowding of the odontoblasts; because of the S-shaped–curved movement, odontoblasts adjust to the new crowding while moving back toward the dental pulp
  (2) Secondary S-shaped curves are seen along the length of the dentinal tubule as small waves in the tubules, about 4 μm apart; may possibly be reflecting changes in the movement of the odontoblasts during night and day
c. Tubules tend to have more branching at their terminal ends in the crown of the tooth than in root dentin; root dentin has more lateral branching, with fewer primary S-shaped curves
d. Higher tubular density in peripheral dentin makes teeth particularly sensitive when exposed, almost as sensitive as the dentin near the pulp
e. The diameter of tubules changes during the process of dentin formation; the widest dentinal tubules are found in children and are about 4 μm wide
4. The first layer of dentin immediately adjacent to the DEJ is called *mantle dentin*; the remainder of the deposited dentin is called *circumpulpal dentin* (around the pulp)
  a. Mantle dentin
    (1) The layer of dentin that is about 10 to 30 μm thick
    (2) Differs from circumpulpal dentin because in addition to collagen fibers normally found in dentin, it contains a second group of thicker and heavier collagen fibers
      (a) These fibers are deposited perpendicular to the DEJ
      (b) These heavier collagen fibers are referred to as *Korff's fibers*
    (3) Mantle dentin is less calcified than is circumpulpal dentin
  b. Circumpulpal dentin
    (1) Contains finer collagen fibers than does mantle dentin
    (2) Fibers are deposited parallel to the DEJ
5. Dentin that forms immediately around the odontoblastic process is called *peritubular dentin*
  a. Forms a sheath around each odontoblastic process about 1 μm thick
  b. Consists of a matrix of delicate collagen fibers
  c. Is highly calcified
  d. Is the first dentin to be decalcified by bacterial enzymes when exposed to caries
6. The remainder of dentin is called *intertubular dentin*
  a. Consists of large, coarse collagen fibers
  b. The matrix is less calcified than that of peritubular dentin
  c. Produced first by the odontoblast; then the odontoblast produces its peritubular dentin

7. Once dentin is deposited, it does not undergo any remodeling
C. Types
  1. Primary dentin—refers to dentin deposited before completion of the apical foramen
  2. Secondary dentin—refers to dentin formed after completion of the apical foramen; tends to be more calcified than primary dentin; forms at a slower rate
  3. Reactive (reparative) dentin—forms rapidly in localized areas where dental tubules have been exposed to external traumas such as:
    a. Dental caries
    b. Attrition or bruxism (enamel has been mechanically worn away)
    c. Thermal extremes
  4. Sclerotic dentin—forms when the dentinal fibers have degenerated and the tubules become filled with calcium salts
  5. Dead tracts—dentinal tubules that remain unfilled after dentinal fiber degeneration
  6. Interglobular dentin—small areas of unmineralized dentin near the DEJ
  7. Tomes' granular layer—small unmineralized areas of dentin beneath the cementum (may play a role in root sensitivity)
D. Sensory conduction
  1. Nerves associated with dentin are located in the dental pulp, but it is believed that they monitor the changes in the environment of odontoblasts, which allows for the perception of pain
  2. When dentinal tubules become exposed to the outside environment, a direct contact is made with the dental pulp; fluid in open, exposed tubules begins to evaporate, and the movement of fluid caused by evaporation may stimulate the nerves closest to odontoblasts to produce pain (dentinal hypersensitivity) (see the section "Control of Dentinal Hypersensitivity" in Chapter 16)

Pulp Tissue
A. Structure
  1. Most centrally located tissue in the tooth
  2. Loose connective tissue
  3. Cells
    a. Fibroblasts—undifferentiated mesenchymal cells
    b. Histiocytes—found along blood vessels; sometimes referred to as *macrophages* when filled with ingested materials
    c. Lymphocytes—when present, tend to be near the odontoblastic layer
    d. Cells present in diseased pulp include monocytes, polymorphonuclear leukocytes, eosinophils, and plasma cells
    e. No fat cells are present
  4. Structural arrangement
    a. The outer periphery of the pulp gives rise to the odontoblastic cell layer

    b. The layer subjacent to the odontoblastic layer is called the *cell-free zone,* or the *zone of Weil*

    c. Next to the cell-free zone is a relatively cell-rich zone

    d. The core of the pulp is centrally located

B. Functions

  1. Nutritive functions—very rich blood supply that forms a capillary plexus surrounding odontoblasts

  2. Formative function—peripheral layer of pulp cells gives rise to odontoblasts

  3. Sensory function—naked nerve fibers travel as free nerve endings and make contact with odontoblasts

  4. Protective function—the pulp can respond to stimuli that occur outside the tooth; response may trigger the formation of reactive dentin

C. Blood supply and nerves

  1. Blood vessels enter the pulp through the apical foramen; one or more small arterioles form a rich capillary plexus under the odontoblastic layer; exchange of nutrients occurs across the capillary wall

  2. Two types of nerve fibers enter the pulp:

    a. Autonomic nerve fibers—only the sympathetic autonomic nerve fibers are present; they regulate blood flow in the vessels

    b. Afferent nerve fibers—come from the second and third branches of the trigeminal nerve; they lose their myelin sheath and terminate as free nerve endings in close association with odontoblasts; it is thought that the presence of free nerve endings is responsible for the perception of pain by the dental pulp

D. Pulp changes

  1. Changes resulting from aging

    a. As the tooth ages, the amount of collagen fibers increases and the number of reticulin fibers decreases; in addition, the ground substance loses considerable water

    b. The pulp becomes less cellular and more fibrous

    c. The size of the pulp decreases because of the continued deposition of dentin

  2. Small calcified bodies, called *denticles,* may be present

    a. The three types of denticles are:

      (1) True denticles—form during tooth development in the root; have dentinal tubules in their structure; odontoblasts are present on the periphery

      (2) False denticles—form when the components of the pulp start to degenerate; calcify and grow into irregular calcified bodies; dentinal tubules are not usually present

      (3) Diffuse calcifications—occur in diseased pulp in many locations; are likely to grow and cause problems

    b. Both true and false denticles may be loose in the dental pulp, attached to the dentin wall, or embedded in the dentin tissue

    c. Calcified structures in the pulp appear radiopaque on radiographs

Comparison of Pulp and Dentin

A. Dentin and the dental pulp are closely related functionally and developmentally; both are products of the dental papilla (derived from neural crest cells)

B. Two major differences exist between these tissues:

  1. The pulp is a loose, noncalcified connective tissue; dentin is a highly specialized, calcified connective tissue

  2. The pulp is a very vascular tissue; dentin is avascular

C. Dentin and the pulp form the bulk of the fully developed tooth

D. During tooth development, the peripheral cells of the dental papilla differentiate into odontoblasts and form dentin, while the core of the dental papilla becomes the pulp

Enamel

A. Composition

  1. Most highly calcified of all the dental tissues

  2. Composed mainly of inorganic calcium salt and hydroxyapatite, with a small amount of protein material and water in the matrix

    a. Inorganic component, 95%

    b. Organic component, 1%

    c. Water, 4%

B. Process of amelogenesis

  1. Enamel formation, as with dentin formation, begins in the late bell stage of tooth development

  2. Shortly after the deposition of dentin, the inner enamel epithelial cells of the enamel organ become secretory ameloblasts

    a. Ameloblasts begin to deposit the enamel matrix, which is mineralized almost immediately

    b. Ameloblasts have tall columnar cell bodies that appear hexagonal in cross section

    c. The secretory process of the ameloblast is the shovel-shaped Tomes' process discussed earlier; the shape of the process is closely related to the form of the structural units that make up the fully developed enamel tissue

  3. Ameloblasts pass through two main stages while depositing enamel:

    a. Secretory stage—ameloblasts deposit the enamel matrix, which contains both organic and inorganic components

    b. Resorbing stage—ameloblasts remove most of the water and organic components from the matrix

  4. Enamel maturation begins before the completion of enamel formation

    a. First, very thin and needle-like hydroxyapatite crystals are deposited in the matrix

    b. During the process of enamel maturation, the crystals increase in all dimensions, which is made possible by the continual removal of water and organic components from the matrix

    c. The hydroxyapatite crystals in enamel are four times larger than those in bone, dentin, and cementum

FIG 2-22 Enamel rod, the basic unit of enamel. **A,** Relationship of the rod to enamel. **B,** Scanning electron micrograph of enamel showing head *(H)* and tail *(T)*. (**B** from Fehrenbach MJ, Popowics T: *Illustrated dental embryology, histology, and anatomy*, ed 4, St Louis, 2016, Elsevier.)

C. Enamel rods—structural units of enamel
   1. Enamel is composed of tightly packed masses of hydroxyapatite crystals called *enamel rods,* or *prisms*
   2. Rod formation is related to the shape of the Tomes' process and the orientation of crystals as they are deposited by ameloblasts
   3. The prisms are rod-shaped structures that run from the DEJ to the outer edge of the enamel surface
   4. They are stacked in interlocking rows, one on top of the other; the stacking arrangement causes the rods to appear as keyhole-shaped prisms when viewed in cross section, with the top of the keyhole facing the occlusal or incisal edge of the tooth and the tail facing the cervical portion; four ameloblasts contribute to form one keyhole (Figure 2-22)
   5. The average width of an enamel rod is approximately 4 μm; the rods are narrower near the DEJ and wider near the outer surface of the enamel
   6. The crystals in the head region of the rod are oriented with their long axis parallel to the long axis of the rod; in the tail region, crystals are perpendicular to the long axis of the rod
   7. Adjacent rods are separated from each other by rod sheaths approximately 0.1 to 2.0 μm wide; they can be

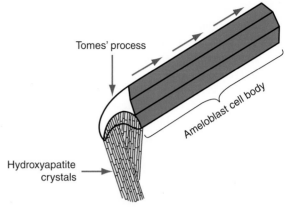

FIG 2-23 Ameloblast depositing hydroxyapatite crystals from the Tomes' process. Note the angular change in the orientation of crystals being deposited, which accounts for the rod sheath around the head of the rod. (Modified from Dr. Marlene Klyvert, Columbia University, School of Dental and Oral Surgery, New York.)

observed in the head region of the rods but are not as clearly defined in the tail region; and they are produced by an abrupt change in the angulation (orientation) of the crystals as they are deposited by the moving ameloblast (Figure 2-23)
   8. Rodless enamel may be found near the DEJ and the outer surface of the enamel
   9. The rods are perpendicular to the outer surface of the enamel; near the cervix of the tooth, they tend to be oriented apically; toward the inner third of the enamel, groups of rods curve but then straighten out to form right angles with the enamel surface
D. Microscopic structures
   1. Bands of Hunter-Schreger—alternating light and dark bands; perpendicular to the DEJ; manifest as a result of enamel rod curvature
   2. Stripes of Retzius—narrow brown lines that extend diagonally from enamel rods; on the tooth surface, they end in shallow furrows known as *perikymata*
   3. Enamel lamellae—cracks that occur during enamel crystallization
   4. Enamel tufts—hypomineralized inner ends of some enamel rods; located in the DEJ area
   5. Enamel spindles—terminal portions of dentinal fibers that extend across the DEJ into the enamel
E. Clinical importance
   1. Dental procedures performed on enamel
      a. Application of fluoride—because enamel is semipermeable, fluoride ions are attracted to the hydroxyapatite crystals; fluoride also changes hydroxyapatite into fluorapatite; the tooth becomes more resistant to acids produced by bacteria
      b. Acid etching of enamel—the structure of enamel (rods and rod sheaths) allows acid to penetrate it for a limited distance (30 μm), and the acid attacks the mineral at the periphery of the sheaths; the acid thus creates a rough enamel surface, which helps bonding materials

adhere more readily; the acid may attack the rod core and produce the same effect

   c. Cavity preparations—all rods are supported by dentin; margins will fail if enamel is left unsupported

  2. Tetracycline stains

   a. Appear clinically as dark bands through enamel, especially near the cervix of the tooth where enamel is thin

   b. Caused by the administration of tetracycline (antibiotic) during the formation of teeth

   c. Tetracycline binds chemically to organic and inorganic components of bone and dentin

   d. The resulting darkened area shows through enamel, making the fully developed tooth appear unattractive

   e. Stains are difficult to bleach out; affected teeth may need crowns or veneers, but only for aesthetic purposes

  3. Pits and fissures in enamel

   a. Are often present in less calcified areas

   b. Form where ameloblasts become crowded between adjacent areas (cusps), resulting in incomplete maturation of enamel

   c. Place teeth at increased risk for dental caries

   d. Require the application of dental sealants to prevent caries and arrest incipient caries

Cementum

A. General properties and functions

  1. Calcified connective tissue that covers the roots of teeth; in conjunction with the alveolar bone proper and the periodontal ligament, forms the attachment apparatus of the teeth, allowing the teeth to become suspended in the jaw

  2. Derived from the dental sac (dental follicle)

  3. Resembles bone in structure and composition; major differences are:

   a. Bone is a vascularized tissue

   b. Cementum is avascular

  4. Least mineralized of the calcified tissues of the tooth

B. Mature cementum composition

  1. Chemical composition

   a. Organic components, 23%

   b. Inorganic components, 65%

   c. Water, 12%

  2. Tissue composition

   a. Cells—cementoblasts, cementocytes

   b. Fibrous matrix—collagen fibers (type I); dominant component of the tissue, 90%

   c. Ground substance—proteoglycans

C. Process of cementogenesis (Figure 2-24)

  1. After crown formation is complete, the epithelial root sheath (Hertwig's root sheath) begins to grow down

   a. Shapes the root of the tooth

   b. Induces the formation of root dentin

  2. After the first root dentin is deposited, the root sheath breaks down; cells from the dental sac migrate onto the newly deposited dentin and differentiate into cementoblasts

D. Mature cementum (fibrous matrix)

  1. Very little cementum is deposited on the developing root until the tooth reaches functional occlusion (only

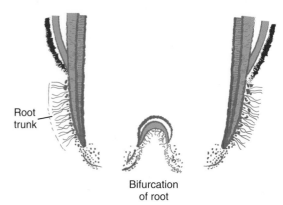

FIG 2-24 Relationship of the epithelial root sheath to the forming root and the formation of cementum.

approximately two thirds of the root has been formed when the tooth erupts)

  2. Cores of fibers remain uncalcified in the calcified cementum; referred to as *Sharpey's fibers*

E. Cellular and acellular cementum (Figure 2-25)

  1. Acellular cementum (primary cementum)

   a. Cervical half of the tooth is covered with a thin layer of cementum, approximately 10 μm thick

   b. Does not contain any embedded cementocytes (cementoblasts) in lacunae

   c. Forms at a slower rate than does cellular cementum

   d. Does not increase during the life of the tooth

   e. Appears to be involved more in maintenance than in the production of the tissue

   f. Contains less inorganic matrix than does cellular cementum

   g. Better calcified than cellular cementum

  2. Cellular cementum (secondary cementum)

   a. Apical portion of the tooth is covered with cellular cementum, reaching a thickness of 100 to 150 μm

   b. Contains cementocytes trapped in the lacunae of the tissue

   c. Deposited throughout the life of the tooth

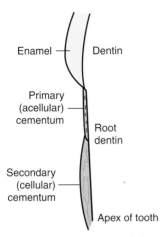

FIG 2-25 Relationship of the primary acellular cementum to the secondary (cellular) cementum, or root of tooth. Note the thickness of the cellular cementum near the tooth apex.

    d. Deposited at intervals (pauses), producing arrest lines—highly calcified lines similar to those seen in bone tissue

F. Abnormalities
  1. Reversal lines
    a. May be present in cementum as in bone tissue
    b. Reflect resorption of tissue (remodeling)
    c. Resorption of cementum does not occur as frequently as in bone tissue; when it does occur, it is usually associated with:
      (1) Extreme orthodontic movement of the teeth
      (2) Trauma to teeth
  2. Cementicles
    a. Small, abnormal calcified bodies occasionally found in the periodontal ligament
    b. Result of cellular debris (i.e., degenerating remnants of the epithelial root sheath)
    c. May be found:
      (1) Attached to the cementum surface
      (2) Free in the periodontal ligament
      (3) Embedded in the cementum of the root
  3. Hypercementosis
    a. Local abnormal thickening of parts of the cementum
    b. Usually found in the apical region, occurring on one or all of the teeth
    c. May be seen in cases of:
      (1) Chronic inflammation of the tooth
      (2) Loss of an antagonist tooth (no opposing tooth in the jaw)
      (3) Additional eruption; compensatory cementosis takes place
      (4) Tooth becoming fused with the surrounding alveolar bone proper

Cemento-Enamel Junction

A. Three types of cemento-enamel relationships can occur during the development of the tooth:
  1. Cementum meets enamel edge to edge—occurs in approximately 76% of all teeth

  2. Cementum overlaps a small part of enamel—occurs in approximately 14% of all teeth
  3. Cementum is ditched with no exposed dentin—occurs in approximately 10% of all teeth

B. Cemento-enamel relationships occur when root-cementum development begins; this is related to the timing of the disruption (breakdown) of the epithelial root sheath and allows the cells from the dental sac to differentiate and begin depositing cementum

C. Differentiation of root dental papillae into odontoblasts is mediated by a cell-to-matrix type of inductive interaction (between the basal lamina of Hertwig's root sheath and the undifferentiated root dental papilla)

D. Differentiation of dental sac cells into cementoblasts is mediated by a cell-substrate type of inductive interaction between sac cells and newly deposited dentin

E. Practicing dental hygienists should use caution during instrumentation in areas where cementum is thin or absent; conservation of tooth structure is recommended

F. Recession of gingiva and loss of clinical attachment may also leave exposed cementum or dentin, creating root sensitivity and increased risk of root caries

Supporting Tissues
Alveolar Bone

A. The part of the bony maxilla and mandible, the alveolar process, in which teeth are suspended in alveoli (bony sockets)

B. Existence or presence of alveolar bone is totally dependent on the presence of dental roots; when teeth do not develop and erupt, alveolar bone does not develop; when teeth are extracted, alveolar bone is resorbed

C. Formed during the development and eruption of teeth; developing teeth, primary or permanent, are located in bony crypts in the bone of the maxilla or of the mandible

D. Has the same biophysical and chemical properties as other bone tissue in the body; has the same basic components as other connective tissue
  1. Cells—osteoblasts, osteocytes, osteoclasts
  2. Fibrous matrix—collagen fibers are the dominant component; calcified by deposition of the calcium salt hydroxyapatite into the matrix
  3. Ground substance—proteoglycans

E. Gross anatomy of a mature bone socket (Figure 2-26)
  1. Each tooth is suspended in its own alveolus (socket), with each alveolus having the same structure and anatomy
    a. Outer cortical (compact lamellar) plate of bone—faces the cheek and lips (buccal)
    b. Inner cortical (compact lamellar) plate of bone—faces the tongue and palate (lingual)
    c. Spongiosa—cancellous bone sandwiched between the cortical plates of bone
  2. Alveolar bone proper—the part of the alveolus directly facing the root of the tooth; follows the general outline of the root; sometimes referred to as the *cribriform plate*, or lamina dura
    a. Cribriform plate

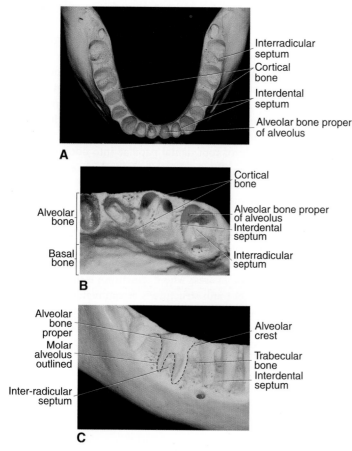

A

B

C

FIG 2-26 Components of alveolar bone. **A,** Mandibular arch of the skull with teeth removed. **B,** Portion of the maxilla of a skull with teeth removed. **C,** Cross section of mandible with teeth removed. (From Fehrenbach MJ, Popowics T: *Illustrated dental embryology, histology, and anatomy,* ed 4, St Louis, 2016, Elsevier.)

(1) Contains numerous small openings; allows blood vessels and nerves in the periodontal ligament and bone to communicate
(2) Consists of two layers of bone:
   (a) Compact lamellar bone
   (b) Layer of bundle bone into which the periodontal fibers insert themselves; the cores of the fibers remain uncalcified in the calcified tissues of bone or cementum, called Sharpey's fibers
b. *Lamina dura* is purely a radiographic term based on this area appearing more radiopaque on radiographs; it is not more calcified than the rest of the bone socket; rather, the opacity is caused by the two-dimensional view of the compact bone in the area
c. Alveolar bone proper that forms sockets around multiple-rooted teeth consists of the cribriform plates of both the roots and some spongy bone, called *inter-radicular alveolar bone*
d. The alveolar bone proper between teeth consists of the cribriform plates of both the teeth and some spongy bone, called *interdental alveolar bone*

e. Spongiosa is composed of small trabeculae of bone with large, narrow spaces between the trabeculae
3. The alveolar bone proper (cribriform plate) is the only essential part of the bone socket; spongiosa and outer and inner cortical plates of bone are not always present; spongiosa may be absent, and outer and inner cortical plates may be fused together
4. Trabeculae of the spongiosa reflect functional forces or loading patterns imposed on teeth; the pattern changes when the forces are altered; two principal directions of the trabeculae are parallel and perpendicular to the direction of the imposed forces; trabecular bone orientation can be observed on radiographs; the number of trabeculae increases with increased function
5. Orthodontic movement of teeth always causes remodeling of the alveolar bone proper to accommodate movement of teeth; it affects the insertion of periodontal ligament fibers in the bundle bone but is a localized type of resorption; when the bundle bone is redeposited, fibers become firmly attached again; with pressure, bone is resorbed; when tension is applied, bone formation occurs
6. Radiographs of teeth may be used to show the height or slope (or both) of the interdental bone septum, which may reflect periodontal disease or other disease; the crest of the alveolar bone is usually between 0.75 and 1.49 mm from the cemento-enamel junction
7. The periosteum is a dense connective tissue layer on the outer portion of bone and is active in bone formation
8. The endosteum lines the inner aspects (medullary cavity) of bone
F. Alveolar bone is constantly remodeled by means of resorption and formation; this makes it the least stable of periodontal tissues
1. Alveolar bone is affected by function, age-related and disease-related changes, hormones, and other systemic and host factors
2. Remodeling affects the height, contour, and density of alveolar bone

Periodontal Ligament

A. A specialized form of connective tissue derived from the dental sac that contributes to the attachment of teeth
B. Consists of groups of fiber bundles called *gingival fibers* and principal fiber bundles; areas of loose connective tissue, blood vessels, and nerves are present between principal fiber bundles; areas of loose connective tissue are called *interstitial spaces*
C. Tissue components
1. Fibroblasts of the periodontal ligament (PDL) are responsible for the production of the fibrous matrix and the ground substance; they are continually engaged in synthetic activities, rebuilding and producing new fibers to be incorporated into existing fibers, which are constantly being remodeled; PDL has a very fast turnover rate

2. Ground substance—proteoglycans
3. The fibrous matrix is the dominant component of the PDL
   a. The fibers are collagen and oxytalan, with a few elastic fibers associated with blood vessels
   b. The fibers are arranged in dense bundles inserted into the alveolar bone proper and cementum
   c. The fibers are arranged into two groups:
      (1) Gingival fiber groups (Figure 2-27, *B*)
         (a) Dento-gingival fibers—extend from the cervical cementum to the free gingiva and from the cervical cementum to the lamina propria of the gingiva, over the alveolar crest
         (b) Dento-periosteal fibers—extend from cervical cementum over the alveolar crest to the periosteum of the cortical plates of bone
         (c) Trans-septal fibers—extend from the cementum of the tooth to the adjacent tooth, over the alveolar crest
         (d) Circular fibers—extend horizontally around the most cervical part of the root and insert into the cementum and lamina propria of the gingiva and the alveolar crest
      (2) Principal fiber groups (see Figure 2-27, *A*)

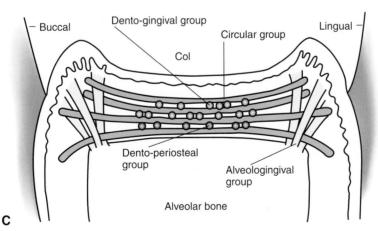

FIG 2-27 Connective tissue fibers. **A,** Principal fiber groups of the periodontal ligament. **B,** Gingival fiber groups. **C,** Gingival ligament fibers in the col area. (Modified from Nanci A: *Ten Cate's oral histology: development, structure, and function,* ed 8, St Louis, 2013, Elsevier.)

(a) Alveolar crest fibers—extend from cervical cementum and insert themselves into the alveolar crest

(b) Horizontal fibers—extend at right angles to the long axis of the root of the tooth in a horizontal plane from alveolar bone to cementum; found in the cervical third of the root

(c) Oblique fibers—slant occlusally from cementum to alveolar bone; most abundant of the fiber bundles; start at the apical two thirds of the root

(d) Apical fibers—radiate from apical cementum into alveolar bone

(e) Inter-radicular fibers (seen only in multiple-rooted teeth)—extend from the cementum in the furcation area of the tooth to the inter-radicular alveolar bone

    d. Sharpey's fibers—the terminal portion of a PDL fiber that is embedded in bone and cementum

    e. Fiber groups are oriented to give the tooth optimal resistance to all types of functional loading patterns

(1) Circular fibers resist rotational movements of the tooth (see Figure 2-27, C)

(2) Alveolar crest and apical fibers resist pull of the tooth from its socket

(3) Trans-septal fibers connect all teeth and maintain the integrity of the dental arches

    f. Elastic fibers in the PDL do not contribute to the support of the tooth; the role of the oxytalan fibers is not clear

D. Blood vessels

  1. The blood supply of the PDL is very rich and highly developed, more than in any other connective tissue; blood vessels are found in the interstitial spaces of the ligament

  2. Each tooth, with its PDL and alveolar bone, has a common blood supply; a small artery branches off the main artery that supplies the jaw and enters the following:

    a. Apical foramen of the tooth, which supplies the pulp of the tooth

    b. Periodontal ligament, which supplies the areas all around the tooth

    c. Alveolar bone of the tooth

  3. Once blood vessels enter the pulp chambers, they are isolated from surrounding tissues, but vessels supplying the PDL and alveolar bone are richly interconnected through openings in the cribriform plate

E. Nerves

  1. The PDL contains two types of nerves:

    a. Autonomic—sympathetic fibers that travel with blood vessels; these regulate blood flow to the tissues

    b. Afferent sensory fibers—mostly myelinated nerves from the branches of the second and third divisions of the trigeminal nerve (fifth cranial nerve)

  2. Two types of nerve endings are found in the PDL:

    a. Free, unmyelinated nerve endings—responsible for pain sensation

    b. Encapsulated nerve endings—responsible for registering pressure changes

F. The width of the PDL varies with the functional forces placed on the tooth and at different levels of the root (apex and cervix)

  1. The width is greater in young adults (0.21 mm) than in older adults (0.15 mm)

  2. The width is greater near the cervical and apical areas than in the middle of the root

  3. Minimal movement (rotations) of any tooth occurs around the axis in the middle of the root; greatest movement occurs near the apex and the cervix, accounting for the difference in the width of the PDL along the root

  4. The width is related to the amount of function and cellularity; an actively functioning tooth has a slightly wider PDL and more cellularity than does a nonfunctioning tooth

G. Abnormalities

  1. Cementicles

  2. Epithelial rests (cell rests of Malassez)

    a. Remnants of the epithelium from the root sheath that did not disintegrate; formed from a cluster of epithelial cells surrounded by a basement membrane

    b. In most cases, these rests are harmless, but they have the potential to become cystic

  3. Untreated periodontal disease can result in damage to the supporting apparatus of the tooth and eventual loss of the tooth

Dento-Gingival Junction

A. The area on the tooth where enamel and the epithelium form a junction; with aging, the junction is displaced more apically between cementum and the epithelium

B. First established as the tooth emerges into the oral cavity (Figure 2-28)

  1. Developing tooth is covered with reduced enamel epithelium (REE), consisting of:

    a. A layer of outer enamel epithelial cells

    b. Remnants of the stratum intermedium cell layers

    c. Stellate reticulum

    d. Postsecretory ameloblasts

  2. Basal cells of oral epithelium covering the emerging tooth and outer layer of cells of the REE begin to proliferate and soon grow together to form one continuous unit; as the tooth emerges through the combined epithelia, it forms the initial dento-gingival junction on the enamel of the tooth

C. Dento-junctional epithelium

  1. Gingival epithelium that faces the tooth

  2. Composed of nonkeratinized stratified squamous epithelium without rete pegs and divided into:

    a. Sulcular epithelium

(1) Found occlusally at the same height as the free gingiva

(2) The sulcus forms a shallow pocket around the tooth, about 0.5 mm deep

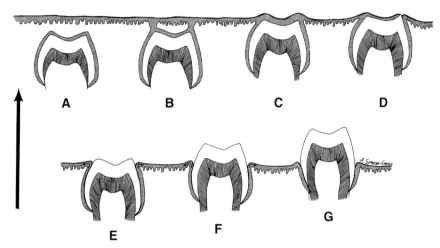

FIG 2-28 Tooth emerging into the oral cavity. Note that the reduced enamel epithelium covering the tooth joins the oral epithelium. The reduced enamel epithelium will form the initial junctional epithelium. **A,** Crown penetrating bone and connective tissue. **B,** Contact of crown with oral epithelium. **C,** Fusion of epithelia. **D,** Thinning of the epithelium. **E,** Rupture of the epithelium. **F,** Crown emergence. **G,** Occlusal contact. (From Avery JK, Chiego DJ: *Essentials of oral histology and embryology: a clinical approach,* ed 3, St Louis, 2006, Mosby.)

(3) In the disease state, the sulcus deepens and exhibits rete pegs and ulcerations

b. Junctional epithelium (see Figures 2-28 and 2-29)

(1) Begins at the base of the sulcus

(2) Firmly attached to the tooth, enamel, cementum, or all by hemidesmosomes

(3) Located between two basal laminae

(a) One basal lamina faces the enamel surface

(b) The second basal lamina faces the connective tissue of the gingiva

(c) Basal laminae are continuous at the base of the junctional epithelium (Figure 2-29)

3. A membrane called the *primary cuticle* intervenes between the basal lamina of the junctional epithelium and the tooth surface

a. The primary cuticle is formed during the late stages of eruption of the tooth

b. The composition of the cuticle is not known, but the cuticle thickens with aging

4. The newly erupted tooth is covered with a thin, delicate membrane (Nasmyth's membrane)

a. Will float off the tooth surface if placed in a 10% solution of hydrochloric acid

b. Contains some cells of the REE and the dental cuticle

FIG 2-29 The epithelial attachment is the part of the junctional epithelium that attaches the junctional epithelium to the tooth surface. Note that the outer external basal lamina is continuous with the inner basal lamina, and between them are the cells of the junctional epithelium. (From Fehrenbach MJ, Popowics T: *Illustrated dental embryology, histology, and anatomy,* ed 4, St Louis, 2016, Elsevier.)

5. In the area of the dento-gingival junction, the junctional epithelium has the capacity to repair itself

6. The site of the dento-gingival junction is easily invaded by microorganisms and is the area where periodontal disease often begins

For a review of the histology, see the listings in the Website Information and Resources table.

Website Information and Resources

Source	Website Address	Description
University of Pennsylvania and Temple University, 1999	http://www.dental.pitt.edu/informatics/periohistology/en/guin01m.htm	Histology slides of periodontal tissues and quiz questions
	http://www.youtube.com/watch?v=zLiV-b1jS28	A video describing tooth development
University of North Carolina at Chapel Hill	http://www.med.unc.edu/embryo_images/	Images and text on normal and abnormal human embryology

SUGGESTED READINGS

Bath-Balogh M, Fehrenbach MJ: *Dental embryology, histology and anatomy,* ed 3, St Louis, 2011, Saunders.

Chiego D: *Essentials of oral histology and embryology, a clinical approach,* ed 4, St Louis, 2014, Elsevier.

Finkelstein M: *Oral histology image index,* The University of Iowa, http://www.healthcare.uiowa.edu/anatomy/dental/oralhist/OHMAC/index.html. Accessed October 8, 2014.

Galil, KA: *Anatomy and histology quizzes,* University of Western Ontario Department of Anatomy and Cell Biology: http://www.drgalil.ca. Accessed October 8, 2014.

Ibsen OAC, Phelan JA: *Oral pathology for the dental hygienist,* ed 6, St Louis, 2014, Saunders.

CHAPTER 2 REVIEW QUESTIONS

Answers and rationales to chapter review questions are available on this text's accompanying Evolve site. See inside front cover for details.

evolve

Use Case A to answer questions 1 to 16.

Use Case B to answer questions 17 to 31.

CASE A

Synopsis of Patient History
Age: 22
Sex: F
Height: 5′7″
Weight: 148 lbs

Vital Signs
Blood pressure: 110/55
Pulse rate: 68
Respiration: 14

1. Under the care of a physician: ____YES x NO
2. Has or had the following conditions:
   Rheumatic fever or rheumatic heart disease ____YES x NO
   Congenital heart disease or heart murmur ____YES x NO
   Heart attack ____YES x NO
   Angina pectoris ____YES x NO
   Hypertension ____YES x NO
   Diabetes mellitus ____YES x NO
   Hepatitis ____YES x NO
   Bleeding disorder ____YES x NO
   Fainting spells, seizures, or epilepsy ____YES x NO
   Asthma ____YES x NO
3. Allergies (medication, food) x YES ____NO
   Allergic to: Penicillin
   Other:

Current Medications
Anticoagulants ____YES x NO
Insulin ____YES x NO
Antibiotics ____YES x NO
Aspirin ____YES x NO
Nitroglycerin ____YES x NO
High blood pressure ____YES x NO
Corticosteroids ____YES x NO
Oral contraceptives x YES ____NO
Other: NA
Smoke or use tobacco products ____YES x NO

Medical History
Patient is a healthy 22-year-old girl with a history of a penicillin allergy.

Dental History
Patient reports for most recall appointments. She uses fluoride toothpaste and a soft toothbrush. She flosses sporadically. Her chief complaint is halitosis.

Social History
Patient lives with mother and younger brother.

She is a college student.

Chief Complaint
Gums bleed when she brushes. It also hurts to brush at times.

Supplemental Oral Examination Findings
Extraoral and Intraoral Findings
The extraoral and intraoral exam reveals a tattoo on her neck and labial mucosa and a white-coated tongue.

Gingival Examination
The gingiva is erythematous with localized areas appearing bright red. The margins are rolled and in some areas irregular. The papillary shape is bulbous. The texture is smooth and the consistency spongy.

Dentition
It is noted that she has pitting on all central incisors. Proximal caries are recorded on the maxillary molars.

Radiographic Findings
There is no bone loss. There is an interproximal area of decay on the mesial tooth #3 and the distal of #14.

Deposits
There is generalized heavy marginal and interproximal plaque. There is generalized extrinsic yellow stain but no calculus.

Peridontal Charting
There is generalized bleeding on probing. The probing depths are within normal limits, with the exception of 4-mm probing depths on the mesial of teeth #4 and #13. There is no attachment loss.

Use Case A to answer questions 1 to 16, as needed.

1. **What type of epithelial tissue is found in the area of the labial mucosa?**
   a. Simple squamous epithelium
   b. Simple cuboidal epithelium
   c. Stratified squamous epithelium
   d. Stratified cuboidal epithelium
   e. Stratified columnar epithelium

2. **The tissue of the labial mucosa is considered what type of mucosa?**
   a. Masticatory
   b. Lining
   c. Specialized

3. **What type of epithelium is found on the neck?**
   a. Nonkeratinized stratified columnar
   b. Nonkeratinized stratified squamous
   c. Keratinized stratified columnar
   d. Keratinized stratified squamous
   e. Nonkeratinized simple squamous

4. **Epithelial tissues are characterized by:**
   a. Much intercellular substance and few cells
   b. No intercellular substance
   c. Little intercellular substance and many cells
   d. Intercellular substance in surface layer only

5. **The last visible layer is nonkeratinized stratified epithelium is:**
   a. Basal cell layer
   b. Prickle cell layer
   c. Granular layer
   d. Corneum layer

6. **The cells of the outer layer of keratinized stratified squamous epithelium:**
   a. Undergo constant mitosis
   b. Contain large amounts of melanin
   c. Are shaped like stars
   d. Contain large amounts of keratin
   e. Have several nuclei

7. **Continuous replacement of cells is characteristic of which type of epithelium?**
   a. Simple squamous
   b. Stratified squamous
   c. Pseudo-stratified columnar
   d. Stratified transitional
   e. Simple cuboidal

8. **If the epithelium undergoes continuous cellular replacement, why does the client's tattoo remain?**
   a. The tattoo ink keeps the surface cells from sloughing
   b. The ink is placed in the spinosium layer
   c. The ink is placed in the basal layer
   d. The ink is placed in the papillary layer of the connective tissue
   e. The ink is placed in the reticular layer of connective tissue

9. **The client has a white coating on her tongue. The papillae that are coated are:**
   a. Filiform
   b. Fungiform
   c. Foliate
   d. Circumvallate

10. **The tissue of the tongue labial mucosa is considered what type of mucosa?**
    a. Masticatory
    b. Lining
    c. Specialized

11. **In the oral cavity, one way in which lining mucosa differs from masticatory mucosa is that:**
    a. Lining mucosa contains more muscle fibers
    b. Masticatory mucosa contains glands
    c. Lining mucosa has no submucosa
    d. Lining mucosa is not keratinized

12. **The anterior portion, or body, of the tongue develops from the:**
    a. Second branchial arch
    b. Maxillary process
    c. Mandibular process
    d. Globular process
    e. Rathke's pouch

13. **The client claims the pitting on all her central incisors has always been present. She is told it is a condition called "enamel hypoplasia," a disturbance during the formation of enamel. It can occur as a result of:**
    a. Poor odontoblastic activity during matrix formation
    b. Childhood diseases during the calcification stage
    c. Too much fluoride during the calcification stage
    d. Poor deposition of the enamel matrix and not its actual calcification

14. **Enamel is derived from the:**
    a. Outer enamel epithelium
    b. Inner enamel epithelium
    c. Stellate reticulum
    d. Stratum intermedium
    e. Reduced enamel epithelium

15. **The client is told the caries on her maxillary molars has progressed into the dentin. Caries in the dentin of the tooth progresses through the:**
    a. Interglobular dentin
    b. Dentinal tubule
    c. Secondary dentin
    d. Predentin
    e. Sclerotic dentin

16. **Dentin is a product of the:**
    a. Dental lamina
    b. Dental papilla
    c. Dental organ
    d. Dental cuticle
    e. Dental sac

CASE B

Synopsis of Patient History
Age: 55
Sex: F
Height: 5'3"
Weight: 160 lbs

Vital Signs
Blood pressure: 140/85
Pulse rate: 68
Respiration: 15

1. Under the care of a physician: x   YES   ___NO
   Condition: High blood pressure
2. Has or had the following conditions:
   History of infective endocarditis   x   YES   ___NO
   Congenital heart disease or heart murmur   ___YES   x   NO
   Heart attack   ___YES   x   NO
   Angina pectoris   ___YES   x   NO
   Hypertension   ___YES   x   NO
   Diabetes mellitus   ___YES   x   NO
   Hepatitis   ___YES   x   NO
   Bleeding disorder   ___YES   x   NO
   Fainting spells, seizures, or epilepsy   ___YES   x   NO
   Asthma   ___YES   x   NO
3. Allergies (medication, food)   x   YES   ___NO
   Allergic to: Penicillin, epinephrine
   Other: _____

Current Medications
Anticoagulants   ___YES   x   NO
Insulin   ___YES   x   NO
Antibiotics   ___YES   x   NO
Aspirin   ___YES   x   NO
Nitroglycerin   ___YES   x   NO
High blood pressure   x   YES   ___NO
Procardia
Corticosteroids   ___YES   x   NO
Oral contraceptives   ___YES   x   NO
Other: NA
Smoke or use tobacco products: x   YES   ___NO
Cigarettes (two packs per day)

Medical History
Patient is a 55-year-old woman with a history of infective endocarditis. She needs to be premedicated for dental treatment. She is currently controlling her high blood pressure with Procardia. She has a history of a cleft of the alveolar process and a cleft lip.

Dental History
Patient smokes two packs of cigarettes per day. She has tried to quit twice. She complains of bleeding gums. Her chief complaint is sensitivity in the area of her maxillary right premolars. She is a mouth breather. She brushes twice a day and uses mouth rinse. She uses mints at work for her breath.

Social History
Patient lives with husband and dog. She works as a bartender.

Chief Complaint
Appearance of teeth and gums

Supplemental Oral Examination Findings
Extraoral and Intraoral Findings
There is slightly visible scarring in the area of the lip repair and nicotine stomatitis.

Dentition
It is noted that she has some missing maxillary teeth.
Pit and fissure caries on teeth #31 and #18.

Radiographic Findings
There is mild to moderate bone loss in the mandibular incisor area and around all posterior teeth.

Deposits
Moderate generalized tobacco stain.
Generalized moderate supragingival and subgingival calculus and plaque.

Periodontal Findings
Recession around the maxillary right premolars, but the gingiva in this area is firm and stippled. She has a small zone of attached gingival tissue in this area. All other areas reveal papillary and marginal inflammation.

Use Case B to answer questions 17 to 31, as needed.

17. **When a cleft of the alveolar process is present, it occurs between the:**
    a. First and second premolars
    b. Central incisors
    c. Lateral incisor and canine
    d. Canine and first premolar
    e. Central and lateral incisor

18. **Which statement is correct?**
    a. Cleft lip occurs more frequently on the left
    b. Cleft lip and palate always occur together
    c. Cleft palate is more common in boys
    d. Cleft lip and palate are hereditary
    e. Cleft lip occurs equally in boys and girls

19. **In the development of the oral cavity, the fusion of the embryonic processes that form the palate is usually completed by the:**
    a. End of the fifth month in utero
    b. End of the fifth week in utero
    c. End of the second month in utero
    d. End of the third month in utero

20. **Which of the following structures does NOT fuse with the rest during palate formation?**
    a. Nasal septum
    b. Lateral nasal process
    c. Right palatine process
    d. Premaxillary process
    e. Left palatine process

21. During palatal fusion, epithelial cells may become entrapped in the line of fusion. These cells may later contribute to the formation of:
    a. Teeth
    b. A cleft palate
    c. Cleft lips
    d. Cysts

22. A cleft lip occurs when the maxillary process fails to fuse with the:
    a. Palatine process
    b. Lateral nasal process
    c. Globular process
    d. Mandibular process
    e. Opposing maxillary process

23. With a cleft palate, the tooth that is most often missing or malformed is the:
    a. Central incisor
    b. Lateral incisor
    c. Canine
    d. First premolar
    e. Second premolar

24. The client has root sensitivity in the area of the maxillary right premolars, where there is gingival recession. The client's sensitivity in this area is most likely related to:
    a. Fluid entering the sulcular epithelium
    b. Fluid entering the rodless enamel
    c. Fluid entering the dentinal tubules
    d. Fluid entering the lacuna of the cementum

25. The tooth sensitivity around the premolars is attributed to the nerve sensation of the:
    a. Cementum
    b. Dentin
    c. Pulp
    d. Gingiva

26. The stippled texture of the gingiva may be attributed to:
    a. Keratinization
    b. Connective tissue projections
    c. Presence of submucosa
    d. Optimal blood supply
    e. Pigmentation

27. The firm consistency of the gingiva is a result of the:
    a. Collagenous nature of the lamina propria
    b. Rete peg arrangement
    c. Keratinization
    d. Vascularity
    e. Pigmentation

28. The color of the gingiva is affected by all the following EXCEPT:
    a. Vascularity
    b. Rete peg arrangement
    c. Keratinization
    d. Thickness
    e. Pigmentation

29. Attached gingiva extends from the mucogingival junction to the:
    a. Free gingival margin.
    b. Bottom of the pocket.

c. Cemento-enamel junction.
    d. None of the above

30. Healthy attached gingiva contains:
    a. Circular fibers
    b. Rete pegs
    c. Connective tissue papilla
    d. Fibroblasts
    e. All the above

31. Attached gingiva is composed of:
    a. Keratinized stratified squamous epithelium
    b. Nonkeratinized stratified squamous epithelium
    c. Keratinized simple squamous epithelium
    d. Pseudo-stratified columnar epithelium
    e. Nonkeratinized simple squamous epithelium

32. The embryonic origin of all connective tissue is:
    a. Mesenchyme
    b. Fascia
    c. Endoderm
    d. Ectoderm
    e. Epithelium

33. The site of muscle contraction is called the:
    a. Sarcomere
    b. I band
    c. H zone
    d. A band
    e. Z line

34. The three types of muscle tissue are:
    a. Skeletal, smooth, and striated voluntary
    b. Cardiac, striated involuntary, and smooth
    c. Nonstriated involuntary, cardiac, and skeletal
    d. Striated involuntary, smooth, and cardiac

35. Bone formation that follows a cartilage pattern is called:
    a. Endochondral
    b. Intramembranous
    c. Mesenchymal
    d. Intercellular
    e. Osteoblastic

36. The part of the neuron that conducts impulses toward the cell body is called the:
    a. Dendrite
    b. Neurilemma
    c. Axon
    d. Myelin sheath
    e. Neuroglia

37. An attachment plaque between a cell and a noncellular surface is called a:
    a. Desmosome
    b. Tight junction
    c. Hemidesmosome
    d. Gap junction

38. The buccopharyngeal membrane is composed of:
    a. Mesoderm and endoderm
    b. Ectoderm and mesoderm
    c. Ectoderm, mesoderm, and endoderm
    d. Ectoderm and endoderm

39. Rathke's pouch is the embryonic origin of the:
    a. Thyroid gland
    b. Palate

    c. Globular process

    d. Pituitary gland

    e. Nasal septum

40. **In the area of the foramen cecum, epithelium invaginates deep into the tissues and will eventually become the:**
    a. Pituitary gland
    b. Lingual salivary gland
    c. Submandibular salivary gland
    d. Trachea
    e. Thyroid gland

41. **What separates the root and body of the tongue?**
    a. Lingual frenum
    b. Median groove
    c. Fungiform papillae
    d. Third branchial arch
    e. Circumvallate papillae

42. **Tooth crown development begins during the:**
    a. Preeruptive stage
    b. Eruptive stage
    c. Prefunctional eruptive stage
    d. Posteruptive stage

43. **The cementum is derived from the:**
    a. Reduced enamel epithelium
    b. Dental papilla
    c. Outer enamel epithelium
    d. Dental sac
    e. Alveolar bone

44. **Hertwig's epithelial root sheath is derived from the:**
    a. Inner enamel epithelium
    b. Reduced enamel epithelium
    c. Primary enamel cuticle
    d. Rests of Malassez
    e. Periodontal ligament

45. **The basement membrane of the developing tooth will become the:**
    a. Cemento-enamel junction
    b. Primary enamel cuticle
    c. Dentino-cemental junction
    d. Secondary enamel cuticle
    e. Dentino-enamel junction

46. **Which relationship between cementum and enamel at the CEJ *cannot* occur?**
    a. Enamel overlaps cementum
    b. Enamel and cementum just meet
    c. Enamel and cementum do not meet
    d. Cementum overlaps enamel

47. **Remnants of Hertwig's epithelial root sheath found in the periodontal ligament of a functioning tooth are called:**
    a. Enamel pearls
    b. Rests of Malassez
    c. Denticles
    d. Cementicles
    e. Intermediate plexuses

48. **The mandible and maxilla are formed through what type of bone formation?**
    a. Endochondral
    b. Intramembranous
    c. Circumferential
    d. Lamellar

49. **During cellular mitosis, what is the phase during which the chromatids are held together by a centromere and the nuclear membrane disappears?**
    a. Interphase
    b. Prophase
    c. Telophase
    d. Metaphase
    e. Anaphase

50. **A decrease in the width of the periodontal ligament is most likely caused by:**
    a. Hyperfunction
    b. Hypofunction
    c. Occlusal trauma
    d. Inflammation

Anatomy and Physiology

Brenda Armstrong

Anatomy and physiology are subjects that focus on the structure, organization, and function of the human body. Dental hygienists use knowledge of anatomy and physiology most often during client assessment, treatment, and evaluation; during oral radiographic and pathologic examinations; and for the administration of local anesthetic agents. This knowledge also allows a dental hygienist to determine whether clients are functioning within normal limits, deviating from the normal, or presenting with structures that are ectopic. Moreover, this knowledge enables dental hygienists to link systemic and oral disease. This chapter covers basic concepts: definitions of terms, cell structure and function, and body systems, including the skeletal, muscular, nervous, circulatory, lymphatic, digestive, endocrine, urinary, and reproductive systems.

BASIC CONCEPTS

Anatomy

A. Study of the structure of an organism and the relationships of its parts; derived from the Greek word meaning "the act of cutting up"
B. Dissection is the principal technique used to isolate and study the structural components of the body
C. Branches of anatomy
   1. Gross anatomy—study of structures that can be identified with the naked eye (see Chapter 4)
   2. Microscopic anatomy—study of cells (cytology) and tissues (histology) (see Chapter 2)
   3. Developmental anatomy (embryology)—study of human growth and development (see Chapter 2)

Physiology

Study of body functions—how the body parts work

Levels of Organization

See Figure 3-1.
   The intricate human body is organized in a hierarchical order from simple to complex. The levels of organization discussed below culminate in the total organism, the human body.
A. Chemical level—organization of chemical structure separates living and nonliving material; atoms, molecules, and macromolecules result in living matter

B. Organelle level—organelles are structures made of molecules and organized to perform specific functions; allow the cell to perform vital functions; types include:
   1. Endoplasmic reticulum
   2. Golgi apparatus
   3. Mitochondria
   4. Peroxisomes
   5. Proteasomes
C. Cellular level—cells comprise the basic structural and functional units of an organism; the smallest living units in the human body
   1. Nucleus surrounded by cytoplasm within a limiting membrane
   2. Differentiate to perform unique functions
D. Tissue level—groups of cells and materials surrounding them that work together to perform a particular function
   1. Four major tissue types:
      a. Epithelial tissue
      b. Connective tissue
      c. Muscle tissue
      d. Nervous tissue
E. Organ level—different types of tissues joined together to form body structures
   1. Each organ has a unique size, shape, appearance, and placement in the body (e.g., stomach, heart, liver, lungs, brain)
F. System level—related organs that have a common function (e.g., digestive system breaks down and absorbs molecules in food; organs include the mouth, salivary glands, pharynx, esophagus, stomach, liver, gallbladder, pancreas, small intestine, and large intestine)
G. Organism level—all the systems of the body combine to make up an organism

Anatomic Nomenclature

Basic terms are needed to communicate regions and directions of the body. The anatomic position provides a reference point for all other terms (see the section on "Anatomic Nomenclature" in Chapter 4).
A. Anatomic position—erect body position with arms at the sides and palms upward
B. Plane or section—imaginary flat surfaces that pass through the body (Figure 3-2)

FIG 3-1 Levels of organization. (From Patton KT, Thibodeau GA, Douglas MM: *Essentials of anatomy and physiology,* St Louis, 2012, Mosby)

FIG 3-2 Directions and planes of the body. (Patton KT, Thibodeau GA, Douglas MM: *Essentials of anatomy and physiology,* St Louis, 2012, Mosby.)

1. Sagittal plane—vertical plane dividing the body into right and left sides; midsagittal plane bisects the body at the exact midline
2. Frontal plane—divides the body or organ into anterior and posterior portions (may also be called the *coronal plane*)
3. Transverse plane—divides the body or organ into superior and inferior portions (may also be called *cross-sectional,* or *horizontal, plane*)

Body Cavities

The human body contains two major cavities, the dorsal cavity and the ventral cavity. These two cavities are then sectioned into smaller cavities that contain internal organs. The dorsal body cavities are in the back part of the body. The ventral body cavities are on the front side of the trunk (Figure 3-3 and Table 3-1).

A. Dorsal cavity
  1. Cranial cavity—formed by the cranial bones of the skull; contains the brain
  2. Vertebral cavity—formed by the vertebrae; contains the spinal cord
B. Ventral cavity
  1. Thoracic (chest) cavity comprises the upper portion
    a. Pericardial cavity—contains the heart
    b. Pleural cavities—contain the lungs

    c. Mediastinum—mass of tissue between pleural cavities; contains all thoracic viscera except the lungs; includes the heart, esophagus, trachea, and several large blood vessels
  2. Abdominopelvic cavity
    a. Upper (abdominal) cavity contains the stomach, spleen, liver, gallbladder, small intestine, and most of the large intestine
    b. Lower (pelvic) cavity contains the bladder, rectum, sigmoid, and reproductive organs

CELLS

All living creatures or organisms are made up of one or more cells. Cells in a multi-cellular organism have the ability to regenerate to sustain life. As structural and functional units of the body, cells develop characteristics and functionality, resulting in a large variety of cells in the body (see the section on "General Histology" in Chapter 2).

Cellular Structure

See Figure 3-4.
A. Plasma or cell membrane
  1. Surrounds and contains the cytoplasm of a cell; composed of proteins and lipids

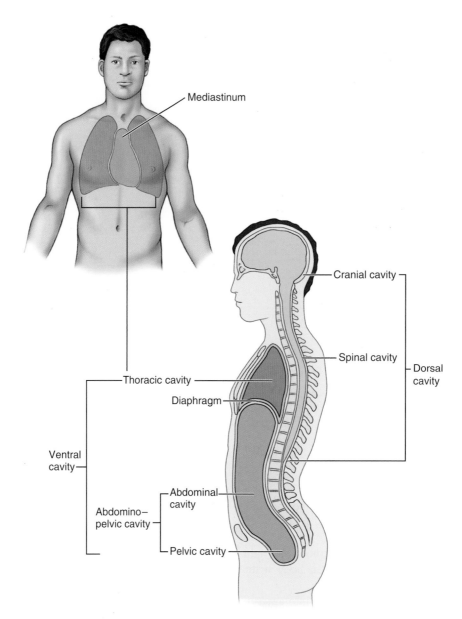

FIG 3-3 Major body cavities. (Patton KT, Thibodeau GA: *Mosby's handbook of anatomy and physiology,* ed 2, St Louis, 2014, Mosby.)

2. Selective permeability characteristics
   a. Protects cell from external environment
   b. Permits the entrance and exit of selected substrates
   c. Membrane proteins have several functions—channels and transporters are integral proteins that help specific solutes across the membrane; receptors serve as cellular recognition sites; some membrane proteins are enzymes
3. Basic framework—lipid bilayer; two layers of phospholipids, cholesterol, and glycolipids
B. Cytoplasm—all cellular contents between the plasma membrane and the nucleus; includes:
   1. Cytosol—fluid portion of cytoplasm; site of many chemical reactions for the cell's existence
   2. Cytoskeleton—network of several kinds of protein filaments that extend throughout the cytoplasm; structural framework for the cell; generates movement

3. Organelles—specialized cellular structures with characteristic shapes and specific functions
C. Ribosomes
   1. Free ribosomes—not attached to other organelles; synthesize proteins used inside the cell
   2. Bound ribosomes—attached to the endoplasmic reticulum (ER); form rough ER; synthesize proteins destined for use in the plasma membrane or for export from cell
D. Endoplasmic reticulum—network of membranes that form flattened sacs called *cisterns*; arranged in parallel rows within the cytoplasm of a cell; contains enzymes involved in a variety of metabolic activities
   1. Rough ER (granular)
      a. Contains ribosomes
      b. Site of protein synthesis
   2. Smooth ER (agranular)
      a. No ribosomes present

TABLE 3-1	Organs in the Ventral Body Cavities
Areas	**Organ**
Thoracic	
Right pleural cavity	Right lung
Mediastinum	Heart
	Trachea
	Right and left bronchi
	Esophagus
	Thymus gland
	Aortic arch and thoracic aorta
	Venae cavae
	Various lymph nodes and nerves
	Thoracic duct
Left pleural cavity	Left lung
Abdominopelvic Cavity	
Abdominal cavity	Liver
	Gallbladder
	Stomach
	Pancreas
	Intestines
	Spleen
	Kidneys
	Ureters
Pelvic cavity	Urinary bladder
	Female reproductive organs
	Uterus
	Uterine tubes
	Ovaries
	Male reproductive organs
	Prostate gland
	Seminal vesicles
	Part of vas deferens
	Part of large intestine (sigmoid colon and rectum)

    b. Synthesizes certain lipids and carbohydrates

    c. Contains enzymes that release glucose into the bloodstream and inactivate or detoxify a variety of drugs and potentially harmful substances, including alcohol, pesticides, and carcinogens

E. Golgi complex

    1. Stack of 3 to 20 flattened membranous sacs (cisterns)

    2. Within the cisterns, proteins are modified, sorted, and packaged into vesicles for transport to different destinations

F. Lysosomes

    1. Membrane-enclosed vesicles that form in the Golgi complex

    2. Contain digestive enzymes

    3. Function is the digestion of worn-out organelles (autophagy) and self (autolysis)

G. Mitochondria

    1. Ellipsoid bodies that consist of two membranes containing enzyme complexes in a particular array (e.g., tricarboxylic acid cycle enzymes)

    2. Function as the "powerhouse of the cell" by transforming the chemical energy bond of nutrients into the high-energy phosphate bonds of adenosine triphosphate

    3. A single cell may contain 50 to 2500 of these organelles, depending on the cell's energy needs

H. Nucleus

    1. Consists of a double nuclear membrane, nuclear pores (control the movement of substances into and out of nucleus), nucleoli (produce ribosomes), and deoxyribonucleic acid (DNA)

I. Peroxisomes

    1. Function to eliminate toxic substances from intercellular fluid

A

B

FIG 3-4 Typical, or composite, cell. **A,** Artist's interpretation of cell structure. **B,** Color-enhanced electron micrograph of a cell. Both show the many mitochondria, known as the "power plants of the cell." Note also the innumerable dots bordering the endoplasmic reticulum. These are ribosomes, the cell's "protein factories." (From Patton KT, Thibodeau GA: *Anthony's textbook of anatomy and physiology,* ed 20, St Louis, 2013, Elsevier.)

J. Proteasomes
1. Remove abnormal and misfolded proteins
2. Destroy specific normal proteins that are no longer needed

Movement of Substances through Cell Membranes

See Tables 3-2 and 3-3.

A. Passive transport processes—do not require energy expenditure of the cell membrane
1. Diffusion—a passive process
   a. Molecules spread through the membranes
   b. Molecules move from an area of high concentration to an area of low concentration (down a concentration gradient)
   c. Eventually a state of equilibrium is reached
   d. Membrane channels—pores in cell membranes through which specific ions or small water-soluble molecules can pass
2. Simple diffusion—substances diffuse across a membrane in one of two ways: lipid-soluble substances diffuse through the lipid bilayer, ions diffuse through pores
3. Osmosis
   a. Diffusion of water through a selectively permeable membrane (limits diffusion of at least some solute particles); results in gain of volume on one side of the membrane and loss of volume on the other side of the membrane

b. A solution containing solute particles that cannot pass through a membrane exerts osmotic pressure on the membrane
c. Potential osmotic pressure—maximum pressure that could develop in a solution when it is separated from pure water by a selectively permeable membrane; knowledge of potential osmotic pressure allows the prediction of the direction of osmosis and resulting change of pressure
   (1) Isotonic—when two fluids have the same potential osmotic pressure
   (2) Hypertonic (higher pressure)—cells placed in solutions that are hypertonic to intracellular fluid shrivel as water flows out of cells by osmosis faster than it enters
   (3) Hypotonic (lower pressure)—a solution that has a lower concentration of solutes than the cytosol inside the cell; water molecules enter the cells by osmosis faster than they leave
4. Facilitated diffusion (carrier-mediated passive transport)
   a. Movement of molecules made more efficient by the action of specific transport mechanisms in the plasma membrane; facilitated by channel proteins or carrier proteins
   b. Transports substances down a concentration gradient
   c. Substances moved by facilitated diffusion include glucose, fructose, galactose, urea, and some vitamins

TABLE 3-2 Passive Transport Processes

Process		Description	Examples
Simple diffusion		Movement of particles through the phospholipid bilayer or through channels from an area of high concentration to an area of low concentration—that is, down the concentration gradient	Movement of carbon dioxide out of all cells; movement of sodium ions into nerve cells as they conduct an impulse
Channel-mediated passive transport (facilitated diffusion)		Diffusion of particles through a membrane by means of channel structures in the membrane (particles move down their concentration gradient)	Diffusion of sodium ions into nerve cells during a nerve impulse
Osmosis		Diffusion of water through a selectively permeable membrane in the presence of at least one impermanent solute	Diffusion of water molecules into and out of cells to correct imbalances in water concentration
Carrier-mediated passive transport (facilitated diffusion)		Diffusion of particles through a membrane by means of carrier structures in the membrane (particles move down their concentration gradient)	Movement of glucose molecules into most cells

Art from Patton KT, Thibodeau GA, Douglas MM: *Essentials of anatomy and physiology,* St Louis, 2012, Mosby.

TABLE 3-3   Active Transport Processes

Pumping	Movement of solute particles from an area of low concentration to an area of high concentration (up the concentration gradient) by means of an energy-consuming pump structure in the membrane	In muscle cells, pumping of nearly all calcium ions to special compartments—or out of a cell
Phagocytosis	Movement of cells or other large particles into a cell by trapping it in a section of plasma membrane that pinches off to form an intracellular vesicle; type of endocytosis	Trapping of bacterial cells by phagocytic white blood cells
Pinocytosis	Movement of fluid and dissolved molecules into a cell by trapping them in a section of plasma membrane that pinches off to form an intracellular vesicle; type of endocytosis	Trapping of large protein molecules by some body cells
Exocytosis	Movement of proteins or other cell products out of a cell by fusing a secretory vesicle with a plasma membrane	Secretion of the hormone prolactin by pituitary cells

Art from Patton KT, Thibodeau GA, Douglas MM: *Essentials of anatomy and physiology,* St Louis, 2012, Mosby.

5. Filtration
   a. Passage of water and permeable solutes through a membrane by the force of hydrostatic pressure; occurs most often in capillaries
   b. Small molecules travel down a hydrostatic pressure gradient and through a sheet of cells; results in the separation of large and small particles
B. Active transport processes—require the expenditure of metabolic energy by the cell
   1. Active transport
      a. Process that moves substances against a concentration gradient (from an area of low concentration to an area of high concentration)
      b. Opposite of diffusion
      c. Substances moved by "pumps," for example, calcium pumps and sodium-potassium pumps
   2. Endocytosis and exocytosis—allow substances to enter or leave the interior of a cell without actually moving through its plasma membrane
      a. Endocytosis—process by which the plasma membrane "traps" some extracellular material and brings it into the cell in a vesicle; the two basic types are:
         (1) Phagocytosis (cell eating)—large particles are engulfed by the plasma membrane and enter the cell in vesicles; vesicles fuse with lysosomes, where particles are digested
         (2) Pinocytosis (cell drinking)—the plasma membrane folds inward, forming a pinocytic vesicle containing a droplet of extracellular fluid; the vesicle detaches from the plasma membrane and enters the cytosol
      b. Exocytosis—process by which large molecules, notably proteins, can leave the cell, even though they are too large to move through the plasma membrane; large molecules are enclosed in membranous vesicles and then pulled to the plasma membrane by the cytoskeleton, where the contents are released
         (1) Provides a way for new material to be added to the plasma membrane

Cell Metabolism

A. Metabolism—chemical reactions in a cell
   1. Catabolism—breaking of large molecules into smaller ones; usually releases energy
   2. Anabolism—building of large molecules from smaller ones; usually consumes energy
B. Role of enzymes
   1. Enzymes—chemical catalysts, reducing activation energy needed for a reaction
   2. Regulate cell metabolism
   3. Chemical structure of enzymes
      a. Proteins of a complex shape

b. Active site—where the enzyme molecule fits the substrate molecule; lock-and-key model

4. Enzyme nomenclature
    a. Enzymes usually have an "-ase" suffix; the first part of the word often signifies the substrate or the type of reaction catalyzed
    b. Oxidation-reduction enzymes—known as *oxidases, hydrogenases,* and *dehydrogenases*; energy release depends on these enzymes
    c. Hydrolyzing enzymes—hydrolases, for example, digestive enzymes
    d. Phosphorylating enzymes—phosphorylases or phosphatases; add or remove phosphate groups
    e. Carboxylases and decarboxylases—add or remove carbon dioxide
    f. Mutases or isomerases—rearrange atoms within a molecule
    g. Hydrases—add water to a molecule without splitting it

5. Functions of enzymes
    a. Regulate cell functions by regulating metabolic pathways; specific in their actions
    b. Chemical and physical agents called *allosteric effectors* alter enzyme action by changing the shape of the enzyme molecule, for example:
        (1) Temperature
        (2) Hydrogen ion (H^+) concentration (pH)
        (3) Ionizing radiation
        (4) Cofactors
        (5) End products of certain metabolic pathways
    c. Most catalyze chemical reactions in both directions
    d. Continually being destroyed and replaced
    e. Many are first synthesized as inactive proenzymes

C. Catabolism—breakdown of larger molecules to smaller molecules.
    1. Energy is needed to function and is obtained from the foods we eat; the most efficient way for cells to harvest energy stored in food is through *cellular respiration,* a catabolic pathway for the production of adenosine triphosphate (ATP), a high-energy molecule expended by working cells
    2. Cellular respiration is what cells do to break up sugars into a form that the cell can use as energy
    3. There are three main stages of cellular respiration: glycolysis, the citric acid cycle, and electron transport
        a. Glycolysis
            (1) The cellular degradation of the simple sugar glucose to yield pyruvic acid, with ATP as an energy source
            (2) Pathway in which glucose is broken apart into two pyruvic acid molecules to yield a small amount of energy (which is transferred to ATP and nicotinamide adenine dinucleotide [NADH])
            (3) Includes many chemical steps (reactions that follow one another), each regulated by specific enzymes
            (4) Can occur aerobically or anaerobically, depending on whether oxygen is available
            (5) Occurs within the cytosol (outside the mitochondria)
        b. Citric acid cycle (Krebs cycle)
            (1) Pyruvic acid (from glycolysis) is converted into acetyl coenzyme A (CoA) and enters the citric acid cycle after losing carbon dioxide (CO_2) and transferring some energy to NADH
            (2) A cyclic sequence of reactions that occurs inside the inner chamber of a mitochondrion; the acetyl splits from the CoA and is broken down, yielding CO_2 and energy (in the form of energized electrons), which is transferred to ATP, NADH, and flavin adenine dinucleotide (FADH2)
        c. The electron transport system (ETS)
            (1) Energized electrons are carried by NADH and FADH2 from glycolysis and the citric acid cycle to electron acceptors embedded in the cristae of the mitochondrion
            (2) As electrons are shuttled along a chain of electron-accepting molecules in the cristae, their energy is used to pump accompanying protons (H^+) into the space between mitochondrial membranes
            (3) Protons flow back into the inner chamber through carrier molecules in the cristae; their energy of movement is transferred to ATP
            (4) Low-energy electrons coming off the ETS bind to oxygen and rejoin their protons, forming water (H_2O)

D. Anabolism—the opposite of catabolism; involves making larger molecules out of smaller molecules
    1. Anabolism allows the body to grow new cells and maintain all the tissues
    2. Protein synthesis is an example of a central anabolic pathway as biologic cells generate new proteins (protein synthesis pathway is outlined below)
    3. DNA (see the section on "Genetics" in Chapter 7)
        a. A double-helix polymer (composed of nucleotides); functions to transfer the information encoded in genes, which directs protein synthesis
        b. Gene—a segment of a DNA molecule that consists of approximately 1000 pairs of nucleotides; contains the code for synthesizing one polypeptide
    4. Transcription
        a. Messenger ribonucleic acid (mRNA) forms along a segment of one strand of DNA
        b. Noncoding introns are removed, and the remaining exons are spliced together to form the final edited version of the mRNA copy of the DNA segment
    5. Translation
        a. After leaving the nucleus and being processed, mRNA associates with a ribosome in the cytoplasm
        b. Transfer ribonucleic acid (tRNA) molecules bring specific amino acids to the mRNA at the ribosome; the type of amino acid is determined by the fit of a specific tRNA's anticodon with an mRNA's codon
        c. As amino acids are brought into place, peptide bonds join them, eventually producing an entire polypeptide chain

6. Processing—enzymes in the ER and Golgi apparatus link polypeptides into whole protein molecules or process them in other ways

Cell Growth and Reproduction

A. Cell growth and reproduction of cells are the most fundamental of all functions in a living being; together they constitute the life cycle of the cell
  1. Cell growth—depends on the use of the genetic information in DNA to make structural and functional proteins for cell survival
  2. Cell reproduction—ensures that genetic information is passed from one generation to the next
B. Cell growth
  1. Production of cytoplasm—more cell material is made, including growth and replication of organelles and plasma membrane; a largely anabolic process
  2. DNA replication
     a. Replication of the genome prepares the cell for reproduction; mechanics similar to RNA synthesis
     b. DNA replication
        (1) DNA strand uncoils, and strands come apart
        (2) Along each separate strand, a complementary strand forms
        (3) The two new strands are called *chromatids* (attached pairs); their point of attachment is called a *centromere*
  3. Growth phase of the cell's life cycle—subdivided into the first phase (G1), the DNA synthesis phase (S), and the second growth phase (G2)
C. Cell reproduction
  1. Mitosis—process of organizing and distributing nuclear DNA during cell division; cells reproduce by splitting themselves into two smaller daughter cells (see the section on "Cell Replication" and Figure 2-6 in Chapter 2)
  2. Meiosis—germ cell division; produces gametes (sperm and oocytes), the cells needed to form the next generation of sexually reproducing organisms
D. Regulating the cell's life cycle
  1. Cyclin-dependent kinases (CDKs)—activating enzymes that drive the cell through the phases of its life cycle
  2. Cyclins—regulatory proteins that control the CDKs and "shift" them to start the next phase; important in cancer pathways

TISSUES

Cells that have a similar structure and function make up a tissue. Tissues working together configure, connect, and hold together organs. The study of tissues is referred to as histology (see the sections on "Concepts Relating to Dental Tissues," "Basic Tissues," "Epithelial Tissue," "Connective Tissue," "Blood and Lymph," "Nerve Tissue," and "Muscle Tissue" in Chapter 2).

Body Membranes
A. Thin tissue layers that cover surfaces, line cavities, and divide spaces or organs

B. Epithelial membranes are the most common
  1. Cutaneous membranes (skin)
     a. Primary organ of the integumentary system
     b. One of the most important organs
     c. Comprises approximately 16% of body weight
  2. Serous membranes
     a. Parietal membranes—line closed body cavities
     b. Visceral membranes—cover visceral organs
     c. Pleura—surround the lung and line the thoracic cavity
     d. Peritoneum—covers the abdominal viscera and lines the abdominal cavity
  3. Mucous membranes (see the section on "Soft Tissue of the Oral Cavity" and Figure 2-21 in Chapter 2)
     a. Line and protect orifices that open to the exterior of the body, for example, anus, vagina, and oral cavity
     b. Line ducts and passageways of respiratory and digestive tracts
C. Connective tissue membranes
  1. Have smooth and slick synovial membranes to reduce friction between opposing surfaces in a movable joint; contain no epithelial components
  2. Synovial membranes—line bursae and the spaces between the bones in joints; secrete synovial fluid

SYSTEMS OF THE BODY AND THEIR COMPONENTS

The Integumentary System
The integumentary system is made up the skin, hair, nails, and glands that provide a protective barrier for the internal environment of the body from the external physical and biologic world.
A. Functions—regulation of body temperature, protection, sensation, excretion, immunity, synthesis of vitamin D
B. Parts
  1. Epidermis—thin outer portion composed of keratinized stratified squamous epithelium
     a. Components include keratin, melanin, Langerhans cells, Merkel cells
     b. Four layers:
        (1) Stratum basale
        (2) Stratum spinosum
        (3) Stratum lucidum
        (4) Stratum corneum
  2. Dermis—deeper, thicker, connective tissue
     a. Components include collagen and elastic fibers that give skin its extensivity and elasticity; dermal papillae that produce fingerprints and facilitate gripping objects; corpuscles of touch (Meissner's corpuscles); and nerve endings that are sensitive to touch
     b. One layer
C. Skin color—from melanin, carotene, and hemoglobin pigments
D. Accessory structures—hair, skin glands, and nails
  1. Hair—threads of fused, dead keratinized cells that have a protective function
     a. Consist of a shaft above the surface, a root that penetrates the dermis and subcutaneous layer, and a hair follicle

2. Sebaceous glands—usually connected to hair follicles; absent in palms and soles of feet; produce sebum, which moistens hair and waterproofs skin
3. Sudoriferous glands—produce perspiration; carry waste to the skin's surface; assist in maintaining body temperature
4. Nails—hard keratinized epidermal cells covering terminal portions of fingers and toes; the principal parts are body, free edge, root, lunula, cuticle, and matrix

Tissues and Membranes of the Body

A. Epithelial tissues
   1. Form membranes that contain and protect the internal fluid environment
   2. Absorb nutrients
   3. Secrete products that regulate functions involved in homeostasis
B. Connective tissues
   1. Hold organs and systems together

2. Form structures that support the body and permit movement
C. Muscle tissues—work with connective tissues to permit movement
D. Nervous tissues—work with glandular epithelial tissue to regulate body function

The Skeletal System

The skeletal system contributes about 20% of body weight. It comprises the bones and cartilages, ligaments, and tendons related to the bones. Bones are rigid living organisms that furnish the framework of the body while protecting soft body parts. In addition to providing sites for muscle attachment, the skeletal system enables bones and muscle to work together for movement. It also contributes to blood cell formation and storage of inorganic ions (calcium salts, sodium, magnesium, potassium, and carbonate) (Figure 3-5; see the section on "Connective Tissue" in Chapter 2.)

FIG 3-5 Skeleton. **A,** Anterior view. **B,** Posterior view. (From Solomon EP: *Introduction to human anatomy and physiology,* ed 2, St Louis, 2008, Saunders.)

A. Functions of the skeletal system
   1. Provides rigid support system
   2. Provides protection; for example, cranial bones protect the brain
   3. Serves as a source and a sink for calcium; involved in the formation of blood cells (hemopoiesis)
   4. Basis of attachment of muscles; allows movement
B. Types of bones
   1. Classified by shape
      a. Long bones
      b. Short bones
      c. Flat bones
      d. Irregular bones
   2. Sutural bones—found between the sutures of certain cranial bones
C. Parts of a long bone
   1. Diaphysis—shaft
   2. Epiphyses—ends
   3. Articular cartilage—layer of hyaline cartilage that covers the articular surfaces of epiphyses; cushions jolts and blows to bone
   4. Periosteum—white fibrous membrane that covers bone; contains cells that form and destroy bone, blood vessels; point of attachment for ligaments and tendons
   5. Medullary (marrow) cavity
      a. Tube-like hollow space in the diaphysis
      b. Filled with narrow marrow in adult
   6. Endosteum—epithelial membrane that lines the medullary cavity
D. Bone tissue
   1. Most distinctive form of connective tissue
   2. Extracellular components are hard and calcified
   3. Rigidity allows its supportive and protective functions
   4. Tensile strength nearly equal to cast iron at less than one-third the weight
   5. Bone matrix composition
      a. Inorganic salts
         (1) Hydroxyapatite—highly specialized chemical crystals of calcium and phosphate contribute to the hardness of bone
         (2) Slender needle-like crystals oriented to resist stress and mechanical deformation
         (3) Magnesium and sodium are also present
      b. Organic matrix
         (1) Ground substance—composite of collagenous fibers and an amorphous mixture of protein and polysaccharides; secreted by connective tissue cells
         (2) Adds to the overall strength and resilience of bone

Microscopic Structure of Bone

See the section on "Bone" and Figure 2-9 in Chapter 2.
A. Compact bones' microstructures
   1. Osteons, or haversian systems—cylinder-shaped structural units (living bone cells are located in these units); constitute the structural framework of compact bone; surround canals that run lengthwise through bone and are connected by transverse Volkmann's canals; permit the delivery of nutrients and removal of waste products
   2. Four types of structures make up each osteon:
      a. Lamellae—concentric, cylinder-shaped layers of calcified matrix
      b. Lacunae—small spaces containing tissue fluid; bone cells are located between the hard layers of the lamellae
      c. Canaliculi—ultra-small canals radiating in all directions from the lacunae and connecting them to each other and to the haversian canal
      d. Haversian canal—extends lengthwise through the center of each osteon; contains blood vessels and lymphatic vessels
B. Cancellous (spongy) bone
   1. No osteons in cancellous bone; instead, it has trabeculae
   2. Nutrients are delivered and waste products removed by diffusion through tiny canaliculi
   3. Bony spicules are arranged along the lines of stress, enhancing the bone's strength
C. Blood supply
   1. Bone cells are metabolically active and need a blood supply, which comes from the bone marrow in the internal medullary cavity of cancellous bone
   2. Blood vessels, lymphatic vessels, and nerves from the periosteum penetrate bone by way of Volkmann's canals; connect with vessels in the haversian canals
D. Types of bone cells
   1. Osteoblasts—bone-forming cells found in all bone surfaces; synthesize and secrete osteoid, an important component of ground substance; collagen fibrils line up in the osteoid and serve as a framework for the deposition of calcium and phosphate
   2. Osteoclasts—giant multi-nucleate cells that contain powerful lysosomal enzymes that destroy bone matrix (resorption); contain large numbers of mitochondria and lysosomes
   3. Osteocytes—mature bone cells; maintain metabolism such as exchange of nutrients and wastes with the blood

Bone Marrow

A. Myeloid tissue—specialized type of soft, diffuse connective tissue found in the medullary cavities of long bones and in the spaces of spongy bone; site for the production of blood cells
B. Two types of marrow occur during a person's lifetime:
   1. Red marrow
      a. Found in virtually all bones in an infant or child's body; in an adult, red marrow found in ribs, bodies of the vertebrae, humerus, pelvis, and femur
      b. Produces red blood cells
   2. Yellow marrow
      a. As an individual ages, red marrow is replaced by yellow marrow
      b. Marrow cells become saturated with fat and are no longer active in blood cell production

c. Yellow marrow can revert to red marrow during times of decreased blood supply, for example, anemia, exposure to radiation, and certain diseases

Regulation of Blood Calcium Levels

A. The skeletal system serves as a reservoir for approximately 98% of body calcium reserves
1. Helps maintain the constancy of blood calcium
    a. Calcium is mobilized in and out of blood during bone remodeling
    b. During bone formation, osteoblasts remove calcium from blood and lower circulating levels
    c. During breakdown of bone, osteoclasts release calcium into blood and increase circulating levels
2. Homeostasis of calcium ion concentration essential for:
    a. Bone formation, remodeling, and repair
    b. Blood clotting
    c. Transmission of nerve impulses
    e. Maintenance of skeletal and cardiac muscle contraction

Divisions of the Skeleton

A. Axial skeleton—made up of 80 bones of the head, neck, and torso
B. Appendicular skeleton—made up of 126 bones that form the appendages to the axial skeleton; the upper and lower extremities

Axial Skeleton

A. Skull (see Chapter 4)
B. Vertebral column (Figure 3-6)
1. Consists of 24 vertebrae plus the sacrum and the coccyx
2. Segments of the vertebral column
    a. Cervical vertebrae (7)
    b. Thoracic vertebrae (12), T1 to T12 are stronger than cervical vertebrae; have facets for articulating with the ribs
    c. Lumbar vertebrae (5), L1 to L5 are the largest and strongest vertebrae; well adapted for the attachment of large back muscles
    d. Sacrum (5 fused vertebrae)—provides strong foundation for pelvic girdle
    e. Coccyx (4 or 5 fused vertebrae)—articulates with the sacrum
3. Characteristics of vertebrae
    a. All vertebrae, except the first, have a flat, rounded body anteriorly and centrally, a spinous process posteriorly, and two transverse processes laterally
    b. All vertebrae except the sacrum and the coccyx have a vertebral foramen
    c. The first cervical vertebra, the atlas, supports the head
    d. The second cervical vertebra, the axis, has an upward projection (dens) to allow the rotation of the head
4. The vertebral column as a whole articulates with the head, ribs, and iliac bones
5. Individual vertebrae articulate with each other in joints between their bodies and between their articular processes

FIG 3-6 The vertebral column. (From Patton KT, Thibodeau GA: *Anthony's textbook of anatomy and physiology,* ed 20, St Louis, 2013, Elsevier.)

C. Sternum
   1. Dagger-shaped bone in the middle of the anterior chest wall made up of three parts:
      a. Manubrium—upper handle part
      b. Body—middle blade part
      c. Xiphoid process—blunt cartilaginous lower tip; ossifies during adult life
   2. The manubrium articulates with the clavicle and the first and second ribs
   3. Ribs join the body of the sternum, either directly or indirectly, by means of costal cartilages
D. Ribs
   1. Twelve pairs of ribs form the sides of the thoracic cavity
   2. Each rib articulates with the body and the transverse process of its corresponding thoracic vertebra
   3. From its vertebral attachment, each rib curves outward and then forward and downward
   4. Rib attachment to the sternum:
      a. Ribs 1 to 8 join a costal cartilage that attaches it to the sternum
      b. The costal cartilage of ribs 8 to 10 indirectly joins the cartilage of the rib above to the sternum (false ribs)
      c. Ribs 11 and 12 are floating ribs, because they are not attached to the sternum

Appendicular Skeleton

A. Upper extremity (Figure 3-7)
   1. Consists of the bones of the shoulder girdle, upper arm, lower arm, wrist, and hand
   2. Shoulder girdle
      a. Made up of the scapula and the clavicle
      b. The clavicle forms the only bony joint with the trunk (sternoclavicular joint)
      c. At its distal end, the clavicle articulates with the acromion process of the scapula
   3. Humerus (Figure 3-8)
      a. Longest bone of the upper arm
      b. Articulates proximally with the glenoid fossa of the scapula and distally with the radius and the ulna
   4. Ulna (Figure 3-9)
      a. Long bone found on the little finger side of the forearm
      b. Articulates proximally with the humerus and the radius and distally with the fibrocartilaginous disc
   5. Radius (Figure 3-9)
      a. Long bone found on the thumb side of the forearm
      b. Articulates proximally with the capitulum of the humerus and the radial notch of the ulna; articulates distally with the scaphoid and lunate carpals of the wrist
   6. Carpal bones (Figure 3-10)
      a. Eight small bones that form the wrist; bound closely and firmly by ligaments; arranged in two transverse rows:
         (1) Top row made up of the pisiform, the triquetrum, the lunate, and the scaphoid
         (2) Bottom row made up of the hamate, the capitate, the trapezoid, and the trapezium
      b. Joints between the radius and carpals allow wrist and hand movements

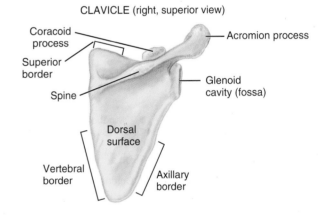

FIG 3-7 Right scapula and clavicle. (From Applegate E: *The anatomy and physiology learning system,* ed 2, St Louis, 2011, Saunders.)

      c. Carpal tunnel—concavity formed by the pisiform and the hamate (on the ulnar side) and the scaphoid and the trapezium (on the radial side), through which the median nerve passes; narrowing of the carpal tunnel gives rise to carpal tunnel syndrome
   7. Metacarpal bones
      a. Form the framework of the hand
      b. The thumb metacarpal forms the most freely movable joint with the carpals
      c. The heads of the metacarpals (knuckles) articulate with the phalanges
   8. Phalanges—bones of the fingers
B. Lower extremity
   1. Consists of the bones of the hip, thigh, lower leg, ankle, and foot

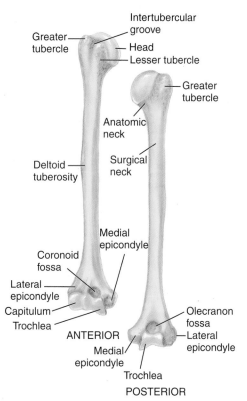

FIG 3-8 Humerus (upper arm). (Modified from Applegate E: *The anatomy and physiology learning system,* ed 4, St Louis, 2011, Saunders.)

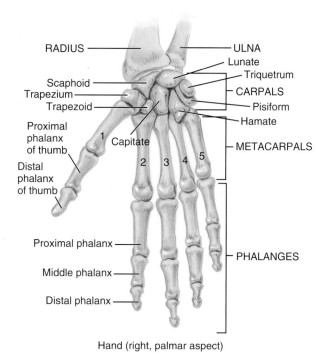

Hand (right, palmar aspect)

FIG 3-10 Bones of the hand and wrist. (From Patton KT, Thibodeau GA, Douglas MM: *Essentials of anatomy and physiology,* St Louis, 2012, Mosby.)

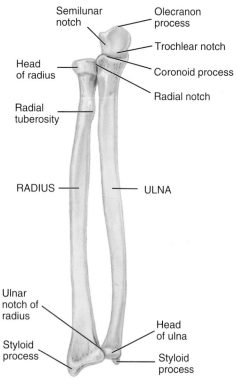

FIG 3-9 Radius and ulna (lower arm). (Modified from Applegate E: *The anatomy and physiology learning system,* ed 4, St Louis, 2011, Saunders.)

2. The pelvic girdle is made up of the sacrum and the two coxal (hip) bones bound tightly by strong ligaments
   a. A stable circular base that supports the trunk and attaches the lower extremities to the axial skeleton
   b. Each coxal bone is made up of three fused bones:
      (1) Ilium—largest and uppermost part
      (2) Ischium—strongest and lowermost part
      (3) Pubis—anterior and inferior part
3. Femur—longest and heaviest bone in the body (Figure 3-11)
4. Patella—kneecap; small triangular bone in front of the joint between the femur and the tibia
5. Tibia
   a. Larger bone of the leg; bears the weight of the body
   b. Articulates proximally with the femur to form the knee joint
   c. Articulates distally with the fibula and the talus of the ankle
6. Fibula
   a. Smaller, more laterally and deeply placed of the two shin bones
   b. Articulates with the tibia
7. Foot (Figures 3-12 and 3-13)
   a. The structure is similar to that of the hand, with adaptations for supporting weight
   b. Foot bones are held together to form spring arches
      (1) Tarsus (ankle)—contains seven bones: calcaneus (heel bone), talus (ankle bone), cuneiforms, cuboid, and navicular

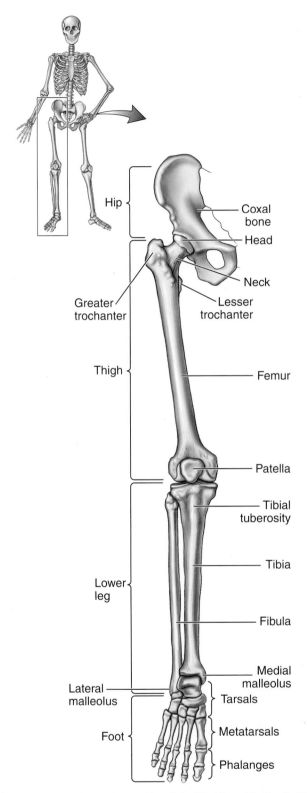

FIG 3-11 Bones of the thigh and leg. (Modified from Herlihy B: *The human body in health and illness,* ed 5, St Louis, 2015, Elsevier.)

Labels in figure:
Hip
Coxal bone
Head
Neck
Greater trochanter
Lesser trochanter
Thigh
Femur
Patella
Tibial tuberosity
Tibia
Lower leg
Fibula
Medial malleolus
Lateral malleolus
Tarsals
Foot
Metatarsals
Phalanges

Joints

A. Classification of joints
    1. Structural—based on the presence or absence of synovial cavity and type of connecting tissue; classified as fibrous, cartilaginous, or synovial

    2. Functional—based on the degree of movement permitted; joints may be synarthroses (immovable), amphiarthroses (slightly movable), or diarthroses (freely movable)

B. Fibrous joints (Figure 3-14)
    1. Bones held together closely by fibrous connective tissue
        a. Syndesmoses—joints in which ligaments connect two bones
        b. Sutures—found only in the skull; tooth-like projections from adjacent bones interlock with each other
        c. Gomphoses—found between the root of the tooth and the alveolar process of the mandible or the maxilla

C. Cartilaginous joints (Figure 3-15)
    1. Bones held together by hyaline cartilage or fibrocartilage; allow little motion
        a. Synchondroses—hyaline cartilage present between articulating bones
        b. Symphysis—joints in which a pad or disc of fibrocartilage connects two bones

D. Synovial joints
    1. Structures of synovial joints (Figure 3-16)
        a. Joint capsule—sleeve-like casing around the ends of bones, which binds them together
        b. Synovial membrane—membrane lining the joint capsule; secretes synovial fluid
        c. Articular cartilage—hyaline cartilage covering the articular surfaces of the joint cavity
        d. Menisci (articular discs)—pads of fibrocartilage located between articulating bones
        e. Bursae—sac-like body cavities; reduce friction in joints
        f. Ligaments—strong cords of dense white fibrous tissue; hold the bones of a synovial joint more firmly together (temporomandibular joint [TMJ] has three ligaments)

    2. Types of synovial joints
        a. Uniaxial joints—permit movement around only one axis and in only one plane
            (1) Hinge joints—the articulating ends of bones form a hinge-shaped unity that allows only flexion and extension
            (2) Pivot joints—a projection of one bone articulates with a ring or notch of another bone
        b. Biaxial joints—permit movements around two perpendicular axes in two perpendicular planes
        c. Saddle joints—the articulating ends of bones that resemble reciprocally shaped miniature saddles, for example, thumbs
        d. Condyloid (ellipsoidal) joints—a bony projection that fits into an elliptical socket
        e. Multi-axial joints—permit movements around three or more axes in three or more planes
            (1) Ball-and-socket (spheroid) joints—most movable joints; the ball-shaped head of one bone fits into a concave depression, for example, shoulder
            (2) Gliding joints—relatively flat articulating surfaces that allow limited gliding movements along various axes, for example, neck

FIG 3-12 The foot. **A,** Bones on the right foot viewed from above. Tarsal bones consist of cunei-forms, navicular, talus, cuboid, and calcaneus. **B,** Posterior aspect of the right ankle skeleton and inferior aspect of the right foot skeleton. **C,** X-ray film of the left foot showing prominent sesamoid bones near the distal end (head) of the first metatarsal bone of the great toe. (From Patton KT, Thi-bodeau GA: *Anthony's textbook of anatomy and physiology*, ed 20, St Louis, 2013, Elsevier.)

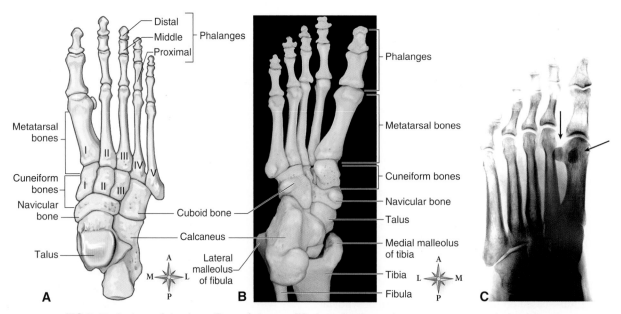

FIG 3-13 Arches of the foot. (From Solomon EP: *Introduction to human anatomy and physiology*, ed 2, St Louis, 2008, Saunders.)

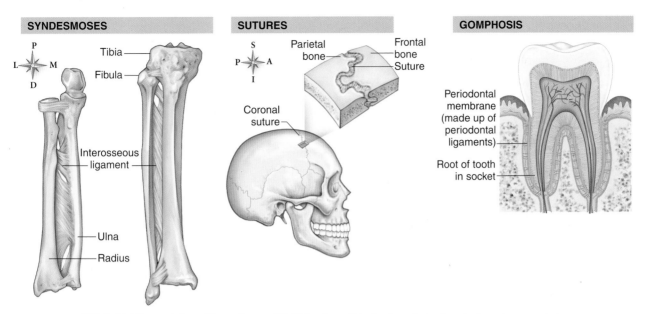

FIG 3-14 Fibrous joints. (From Patton KT, Thibodeau GA: *Anthony's textbook of anatomy and physiology*, ed 20, St Louis, 2013, Elsevier.)

Muscular System

The muscular system makes up about 40% of body weight and comprises more than 600 muscles. The muscular system acts together with the skeletal system to provide form, contours, and movement. The three types of muscle are cardiac, smooth, and skeletal.

Anatomy of the Muscular System

See Figure 3-17.
A. Muscle tissue has five key functions:
  1. Producing body movements
  2. Stabilizing body positions
  3. Regulating organ volume
  4. Moving substances within the body
  5. Producing heat
B. Characteristics
  1. Excitability—ability of muscle fibers (and neurons) to respond to a stimulus and convert it into an action potential
  2. Contractibility—ability to contract (shorten and thicken)
  3. Extensibility—ability to be stretched
  4. Elasticity—ability to return to original shape after contraction or extension
C. Types
  1. Skeletal muscle—mostly attached to bones; striated and voluntary
  2. Cardiac muscle—forms most of the walls of the heart; striated and involuntary
  3. Smooth muscle—located in viscera; participates in internal processes

Skeletal Muscle Structure

See Figure 3-18.
A. Connective tissue components (may become a tendon or an aponeurosis)

  1. Endomysium—delicate connective tissue membrane that covers specialized skeletal muscle fibers
  2. Perimysium—tough connective tissue binding fascicles together
  3. Epimysium—coarse sheath covering the muscle as a whole
B. Size, shape, and fiber arrangement
  1. Size—ranging from extremely small to large masses
  2. Shape—variety of shapes, such as broad, narrow, long, tapering, short, blunt, triangular, quadrilateral, or irregular, and as flat sheets or bulky masses
  3. Arrangement—variety of arrangements; the direction of fibers is significant because of its relationship to function
C. Attachment of muscle
  1. Origin—point of attachment that does not move when the muscle contracts
  2. Insertion—point of attachment that moves when the muscle contracts
D. Muscle actions
  1. Most movements produced by the coordinated actions of several muscles; some muscles in the group contract while others relax
    a. Prime mover (agonist)—muscles that directly perform a specific movement
    b. Antagonist—when contracting, directly oppose prime movers; relax while the agonist is contracting to produce movement; provide precision and control during contraction of prime movers
    c. Synergists—contract at the same time as prime movers do; facilitate prime mover actions to produce a more efficient movement
    d. Fixator muscles—stabilize joints
E. Lever systems—bones serve as levers, and joints serve as fulcrums; the muscle applies a pulling force on a bone lever at the point of the muscle's attachment to the bone, causing the insertion bone to move about its joint fulcrum

SYNCHONDROSES

Ribs

Sternum

Costosternal synchondrosis

Costal cartilage

Epiphyseal plate (hyaline cartilage)

Long bone

SYMPHYSES

Pubic symphysis

Vertebral disk

FIG 3-15 Cartilaginous joints. (From Patton KT and Thibodeau GA: *Anthony's textbook of anatomy and physiology,* ed 20, St Louis, 2013, Elsevier.)

Femur

Patella

Joint cavity (filled with synovial fluid)

Synovial membrane

Lateral meniscus

Tibia

Articular cartilage

Capsule

FIG 3-16 Structure of synovial joints. (From Herlihy B: *The human body in health and illness,* ed 5, St Louis, 2015, Elsevier.)

C. Muscles of the pelvic floor—support structures in the pelvic cavity

Upper Limb Muscles

A. Muscles acting on the shoulder girdle—muscles that attach the upper extremity to the torso; located anteriorly (chest) or posteriorly (back and neck); allow extensive movement

B. Muscles that move the upper arm—the shoulder is a synovial joint allowing extensive movement in every plane of motion

C. Muscles that move the forearm—found proximal to the elbow and attached to the ulna and radius

D. Muscles that move the wrist, hand, and fingers—located on the anterior or posterior surfaces of the forearm

Lower Limb Muscles

A. The pelvic girdle and the lower extremity function in locomotion and maintenance of stability

B. Muscles that move the thigh and the lower leg

C. Muscles that move the ankle and the foot

1. Extrinsic foot muscles—located in the leg; exert their actions by pulling on tendons that insert on bones in the ankle and foot; responsible for dorsiflexion, plantar flexion, inversion, and eversion

2. Intrinsic foot muscles—located within the foot; responsible for flexion, extension, abduction, and adduction of the toes

Posture

A. Maintaining body posture is an important function of muscles

B. Good posture—body alignment that favors function and requires the least muscular work to maintain, keeping the body's center of gravity over its base

Head and Neck Muscles See the section on "The Muscular System" and Figure 4-4 in Chapter 4.

A. Muscles of facial expression—unique in that at least one point of attachment is to the deep layers of the skin over the face or neck

B. Muscles of mastication—responsible for chewing movements

C. Muscles that move the head—paired muscles on either side of the neck that are responsible for head movements

Trunk Muscles

A. Muscles of the thorax—critical in respiration

B. Muscles of the abdominal wall—arranged in three layers, with fibers in each layer running in different directions to increase strength

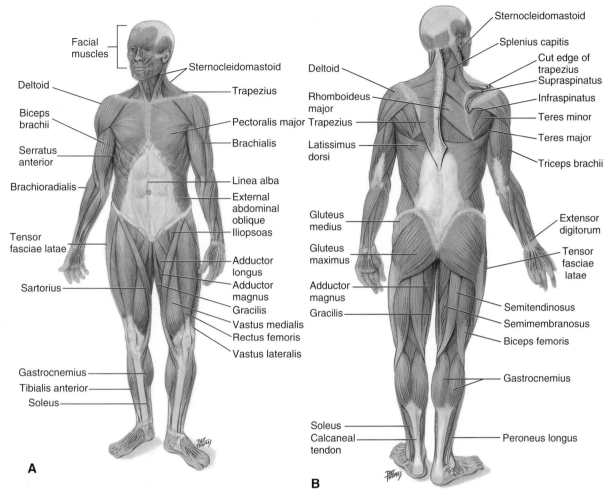

FIG 3-17 General overview of the body musculature. **A,** Anterior view. **B,** Posterior view. (Modified from Applegate E: *The anatomy and physiology learning system,* ed 4, St Louis, 2011, Saunders.)

C. How posture is maintained:
   1. Muscles exert a continual pull on bones in the opposite direction from gravity
   2. Structures other than muscle and bone have a role in maintaining posture
      a. The nervous system—responsible for the existence of muscle tone and for the regulation and coordination of the amount of pull exerted by individual muscles
      b. Respiratory, digestive, excretory, and endocrine systems all contribute to maintain posture

Function of Skeletal Muscle

A. Overview of muscle cells
   1. Muscle cells are called *fibers* because of their thread-like shape
   2. Sarcolemma—plasma membrane of muscle fibers
   3. Sarcoplasmic reticulum
      a. A network of tubules and sacs found within muscle fibers
      b. The membrane of the sarcoplasmic reticulum continually pumps calcium ions from the sarcoplasm and stores the ions within sacs
   4. Muscle fibers contain many mitochondria and several nuclei
   5. Myofibrils—numerous fine fibers packed close together in the sarcoplasm
   6. Sarcomere
      a. The segment of myofibril between two successive Z lines
      b. Each myofibril consists of many sarcomeres
      c. The contractile unit of muscle fibers
   7. Striated muscle
      a. Dark stripes are called *A bands*; the light H zone runs across the midsection of each dark A band
      b. Light stripes are called *I bands*; the dark Z line extends across the center of each light I band
   8. T tubules
      a. Transverse tubules that extend across the sarcoplasm at right angles to the long axis of the muscle fiber
      b. Formed by the inward extension of the sarcolemma
      c. The membrane has ion pumps that continually transport calcium ions inward from the sarcoplasm
      d. Allow electrical impulses traveling along the sarcolemma to move deeper into the cell

A

B

FIG 3-18 Structure of a muscle organ. (From Patton KT, Thibodeau GA: *Anthony's textbook of anatomy and physiology*, ed 20, St Louis, 2013, Elsevier.)

9. Triad
   a. Triplet of tubules; a T tubule is sandwiched between two sacs of the sarcoplasmic reticulum; allows an electrical impulse traveling along a T tubule to stimulate the membranes of adjacent sacs of the sarcoplasmic reticulum
B. Myofilaments
   1. Each myofibril contains thousands of thick and thin myofilaments
   2. Four different types of protein molecules make up myofilaments:
      a. Myosin
         (1) Makes up almost all the thick filament

(2) Myosin "heads" are chemically attracted to actin molecules; known as *cross-bridges* when attached to actin
      b. Actin—globular protein that forms two fibrous strands twisted around each other to form the bulk of the thin filament
      c. Tropomyosin—protein that blocks the active sites on actin molecules
      d. Troponin—protein that holds tropomyosin molecules in place
   3. Thin filaments attached to both Z lines of a sarcomere and extend partway toward the center
   4. Thick myosin filaments are not attached to Z lines
C. Mechanism of contraction
   1. Excitation and contraction
      a. A skeletal muscle fiber remains at rest until stimulated by a motor neuron
      b. Neuromuscular junction—motor neurons connect to the sarcolemma at the motor endplate
      c. Neuromuscular junction—synapse where neurotransmitter molecules transmit signals
      d. Acetylcholine—neurotransmitter released into the synaptic cleft, which diffuses across the gap, stimulates receptors, and initiates an impulse in the sarcolemma
      e. A nerve impulse travels over the sarcolemma and inward along T tubules to trigger the release of calcium ions
      f. Calcium binds to troponin, causing the tropomyosin to shift and expose the active sites on actin
      g. Sliding filament theory
         (1) When active sites on actin are exposed, myosin heads bind to them
         (2) Myosin heads bend, pulling the thin filaments past them
         (3) Each head releases itself, binds to the next active site, and pulls again
         (4) The entire myofibril becomes shortened
   2. Relaxation
      a. Immediately after calcium ions are released, the sarcoplasmic reticulum begins actively pumping them back into sacs
      b. Calcium ions are removed from troponin molecules, ending the contraction
   3. Energy sources for muscle contraction
      a. Hydrolysis of ATP yields the energy required for muscular contraction
      b. ATP binds to the myosin head to perform the work of pulling the thin filament during contraction
      c. Muscle fibers continually synthesize ATP from the breakdown of creatine phosphate
      d. Catabolism by muscle fibers requires glucose and oxygen
      e. At rest, excess oxygen (O_2) in the sarcoplasm is stored by myoglobin
         (1) Red fibers—muscle fibers with high levels of myoglobin

(2) White fibers—muscle fibers with minimal myoglobin

f. Aerobic respiration occurs when adequate O_2 is available

g. Anaerobic respiration occurs when low levels of O_2 are available and results in the formation of lactic acid

h. Skeletal muscle contraction produces excess heat that can be used to maintain body temperature

Function of Skeletal Muscle Organs

A. Motor unit

1. Motor unit—comprises the motor neuron and the muscle fibers to which it is attached

2. Some motor units can consist of only a few or numerous muscle fibers

3. Generally, with a smaller number of fibers in a motor unit, more precise movements are possible; the larger the number of fibers in a motor unit, the more powerful is the contraction

B. Twitch contraction

1. A quick jerk of a muscle that is produced as a result of a single, brief threshold stimulus (generally occurs only in experimental situations)

2. Three phases:

a. Latent phase—the nerve impulse travels to the sarcoplasmic reticulum to trigger the release of calcium

b. Contraction phase—calcium binds to troponin, and the sliding of filaments occurs

c. Relaxation phase—the sliding of filaments ceases

C. Treppe—the "staircase phenomenon"

1. Gradual, step-like increase in the strength of a contraction; observed in a series of twitch contractions that occur 1 second apart

2. Eventually, the muscle responds with less forceful contractions, and the relaxation phase becomes shorter

3. If the relaxation phase disappears completely, a contracture (abnormal shortening of muscle tissue that can cause disability) occurs

D. Tetanus—smooth, sustained contractions

1. Multiple-wave summation—multiple twitch waves are added together to sustain muscle tension for a longer time

2. Incomplete tetanus—very short periods of relaxation occur between peaks of tension

3. Complete tetanus—twitch waves fuse into a single, sustained peak

E. Muscle tone

1. Tonic contraction—continual, partial contraction of a muscle

2. At any one time, a small number of muscle fibers within a muscle contract, producing tightness of muscle tone

3. Muscles with less tone than normal are *flaccid*

4. Muscles with more tone than normal are *spastic*

5. Muscle tone is maintained by negative feedback mechanisms

F. Principle of graded strength

1. Skeletal muscles contract with varying degrees of strength at different times

2. Factors that contribute to the phenomenon of graded strength:

a. Metabolic condition of individual fibers

b. Number of muscle fibers contracting simultaneously; the greater the number of fibers contracting, the stronger the contraction

c. Number of motor units recruited

d. Intensity and frequency of stimulation

3. Length-tension relationship

a. The maximal strength that a muscle can develop bears a direct relationship to the initial length of its fibers

b. A shortened muscle's sarcomeres are compressed; therefore the muscle cannot develop much tension

c. An overstretched muscle cannot develop much tension because the thick myofilaments are too far from the thin myofilaments

d. The strongest maximal contraction is possible only when the skeletal muscle has been stretched to its optimal length

4. Stretch reflex

a. The load imposed on a muscle influences the strength of a skeletal contraction

b. The body tries to maintain a consistency of muscle length in response to increased load

c. Maintains a relatively constant length as the load is increased up to a maximum sustainable level

G. Isotonic and isometric contractions

1. Isotonic contraction

a. Contraction in which the tone or tension within a muscle remains the same as the length of the muscle changes

(1) Concentric—the muscle shortens as it contracts

(2) Eccentric—the muscle lengthens as it contracts

b. *Isotonic* means "same tension"

c. All the energy of contraction is used to pull on the thin myofilaments and thereby change the length of a fiber's sarcomeres

2. Isometric contraction

a. Contraction in which muscle length remains the same while muscle tension increases

b. *Isometric* means "same length"

3. Body movements occur as a result of both types of contractions

Function of Cardiac and Smooth Muscle Tissue

A. Cardiac muscle (also known as *striated involuntary muscle*)

1. Found only in the heart; forms bulk of the walls of each chamber

2. Contracts rhythmically and continuously to maintain a constant blood flow

3. Resembles skeletal muscle but has specialized features related to its role in continuous pumping of blood

a. Each cardiac muscle contains parallel myofibrils

b. Cardiac muscle fibers form strong, electrically coupled junctions (intercalated discs) with other fibers; individual cells also exhibit branching

c. Syncytium—continuous, electrically coupled mass; important for coordinating muscle contractions

d. Cardiac muscle fibers form a continuous, contractile band around the heart chambers and conduct a single impulse across a virtually continuous sarcolemma

e. T tubules are larger and form dyads with a rather sparse sarcoplasmic reticulum

f. Cardiac muscle sustains each impulse longer than does skeletal muscle; therefore, impulses cannot come rapidly enough to produce tetanus

g. Cardiac muscle does not run low on ATP and does not experience fatigue

h. Cardiac muscle is self-stimulating

B. Smooth muscle
1. Smooth muscle is composed of small, tapered cells with single nuclei
2. T tubules are absent; only a loosely organized sarcoplasmic reticulum is present
3. Calcium comes from outside the cell and binds to calmodulin instead of troponin to trigger a contraction
4. No striations are present because both the thick and the thin myofilaments have an arrangement different from that in skeletal or cardiac muscle fibers; myofilaments are not organized into sarcomeres
5. Two types of smooth muscle tissue:
   a. Visceral muscle (single unit)
      (1) Gap junctions join smooth muscle fibers into large, continuous sheets
      (2) Most common type; forms a muscular layer in the walls of hollow structures such as the digestive, urinary, and reproductive tracts
      (3) Exhibits autorhythmicity, which produces peristalsis
   b. Multi-unit
      (1) Does not act as a single unit; is composed of many independent cell units
      (2) Each fiber responds only to input from nerves

The Nervous System

The nervous system is primarily composed of the brain, the spinal cord, nerves, and ganglia. Along with the endocrine system, the nervous system regulates and maintains homeostasis. It allows the human body to communicate, integrate, and regulate body functions vital for living. Subdivisions of the nervous system aid in the understanding of structure, direction of information flow, and motor output or motor function (see the section on "Nerve Tissue" in Chapter 2).

A. Two main subsystems (Figure 3-19):
1. The central nervous system (CNS)—consists of the brain and the spinal cord
2. The peripheral nervous system (PNS)—includes all nervous tissue outside the CNS; contains the nerves to and from the body wall

B. Other divisions of the nervous system
1. Direction of information flow
2. *Afferent* consists of incoming sensory pathways
3. *Efferent* consists of outgoing motor pathways
4. Control of effectors
5. The somatic nervous system (SNS) carries information to the somatic effectors (skeletal muscle)

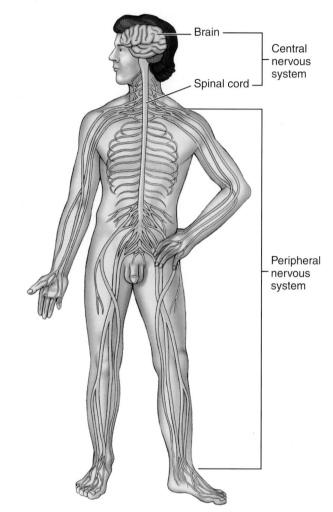

FIG 3-19 The nervous system. (From Herlihy B: *The human body in health and illness,* ed 5, St Louis, 2015, Elsevier.)

6. The autonomic nervous system (ANS) carries information to the autonomic effectors (e.g., cardiac and smooth muscle, glands, adipose tissue)

C. Functions
1. Sensory—detection of different types of stimuli both inside and outside the body
   a. Afferent or sensory neurons—carry information from the PNS to the CNS
2. Integrative—processing of sensory information by analyzing and storing some of it and by making decisions regarding appropriate responses; interneurons carry out this function
3. Motor—responses to integrative decisions
   a. Efferent or motor neurons carry information from the CNS to the PNS

D. The central nervous system
1. Brain—housed within the skull; contains about 100 billion neurons
2. Spinal cord—contains about 100 million neurons; is connected directly to the brain and is protected by the vertebral column

3. Source of thoughts, emotions, memories; source of most nerve impulses that stimulate muscles to contract and glands to secrete

4. Communication to and from CNS accomplished by:
   a. Cranial nerves
   b. Spinal nerves
   c. Ganglia—small clusters of neuronal cell bodies that relay signals traveling along cranial and spinal nerves
   d. Enteric plexuses—in the walls of the organs of the gastrointestinal (GI) tract; help regulate the digestive system

E. The peripheral nervous system
   1. Subdivisions
      a. The somatic nervous system
         (1) Sensory neurons—convey information to the CNS from the somatic receptors in the head, body wall, and limbs and also from the receptors for the special senses of vision, hearing, taste, and smell
         (2) Motor neurons—conduct impulses from the CNS to skeletal muscles only; motor responses are voluntary
      b. The autonomic nervous system (ANS)
         (1) Sympathetic division (thoracolumbar) involves motor (afferent) nerves from the ANS
         (2) Parasympathetic division (craniosacral)
      c. The enteric nervous system
         (1) "Brain of the GI system"
         (2) Enteric motor neurons govern the contraction of GI tract smooth muscle, secretions of the GI tract organs (e.g., acid secretions by stomach), and activity of GI tract endocrine cells

Cellular Organization

Nervous System Structure See Figure 3-20 and the section on "Nerve Tissue" and Figures 2-13 and 2-14 in Chapter 2.

A. Each neuron (nerve cell) consists of a cell body containing a nucleus

B. Dendrite—sends impulses toward the cell body or to a muscle or gland

C. Axon—conducts nerve impulses away from the cell body

D. Neuroglia—specialized tissue cells that support neurons, attach neurons to blood vessels, produce the myelin sheath around the axons of the CNS, carry out phagocytosis, and retain the ability to undergo mitosis

E. Myelin—fatty substance around axons; provides insulation and increases the speed of nerve conduction; deposited by Schwann cells in layers in the PNS
   1. Neurilemma—outermost layer of the Schwann cell
   2. Nodes of Ranvier—located between myelin segments; unmyelinated
   3. Oligodendrocytes myelinate CNS axons

F. White matter consists of aggregations of myelinated processes from many neurons

G. Gray matter contains the neurons, dendrites, and axon terminals of unmyelinated axons and neuroglia; forms an H-shaped inner core in the spinal cord that is surrounded by white matter; a superficial shell of gray matter covers the cerebrum and the cerebellum

H. The nervous system exhibits plasticity—the capability to change on the basis of experiences; limited ability to regenerate

I. Axons and dendrites that are associated with a neurilemma in the PNS may undergo repair if the cell body is intact, Schwann cells are functional, and scar tissue does not form too rapidly

Action Potentials See the section on "Characteristics and Physiology of Pain" in Chapter 18.

A. Neurons communicate by means of nerve action potentials (impulses)

B. Generation of action is dependent on:
   1. The presence of special types of ion channels and the existence of a resting membrane potential
   2. Membrane potential—a difference in electrical charge across the plasma membrane; a cell that has a membrane potential is said to be *polarized*
   3. A nerve impulse results from the concentration of two ions on the inside and outside of the nerve

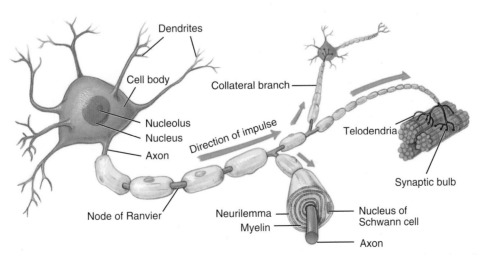

FIG 3-20 Structure of a typical neuron. (From Applegate E: *The anatomy and physiology learning system*, ed 4, St Louis, 2011, Saunders.)

4. Resting membrane potential—the outside surface of plasma membrane has a positive charge; the inside surface has a negative charge; the resting membrane in neurons is ≈ 70 millivolts (mV)

5. During an action potential, voltage-gated sodium (Na^+) and potassium (K^+) channels open in sequence; opening of voltage-gated Na^+ channels results in depolarization, followed by the loss and reversal of membrane polarization (from -70 mV to $+30$ mV); then, the opening of voltage-gated K^+ channels allows repolarization, the recovery of the resting membrane potential

6. According to the "all-or-none" principle, if a stimulus is strong enough to generate an action potential, the impulse generated is of a constant size; a stronger stimulus does not generate a larger impulse

7. During the absolute refractory period, another impulse cannot be generated; during the relative refractory period, an impulse can be triggered only by a supra-threshold stimulus

8. Nerve impulse conduction that occurs as a step-by-step process along an unmyelinated axon is called *continuous conduction*; in *salutatory conduction,* a nerve impulse "leaps" from one node of Ranvier to the next along a myelinated axon

9. Axons with larger diameters conduct impulses faster than those with smaller diameters; myelinated axons conduct impulses faster than unmyelinated axons

Synaptic Transmission

A. Neurons communicate with each other and with effectors at synapses in a series of events known as *synaptic transmission*

B. Two types of synapses:
   1. Electrical synapses—gap junctions allow ions to flow from one cell to another
   2. Chemical synapses—neurotransmitter is released from a presynaptic neuron into the synaptic cleft and then binds to receptors on the postsynaptic plasma membrane

C. Types of neurotransmitters
   1. Excitatory neurotransmitter—depolarizes the membrane of the postsynaptic neuron to bring the membrane potential closer to threshold
   2. Inhibitory neurotransmitter—hyperpolarizes the membrane of the postsynaptic neuron

D. The postsynaptic neuron integrates excitatory and inhibitory signals in a process called *summation* and then responds accordingly

E. The neurotransmitter is removed from the synaptic cleft in three ways: diffusion, enzymatic degradation, and reuptake by neurons or neuroglial cells

F. Important neurotransmitters include acetylcholine, gamma-aminobutyric acid (GABA), glycine, norepinephrine, epinephrine, dopamine, serotonin, neuropeptides, and nitric oxide

Spinal Cord

See Figure 3-21; see also Figure 2-11 in Chapter 2.

A. Location—in the vertebral canal; extends from the foramen magnum of the occipital bone of the skull to the superior border of the second lumbar vertebrae in the vertebral column; approximately 40 to 45 cm (16 to 18 inches)

B. Meninges—three layers of connective tissue coverings that extend around the spinal cord and the brain
   1. Dura mater—outermost of three layers
   2. Arachnoid—middle layer composed of collagen and elastic fibers
   3. Pia mater—inner layer composed of collagen and elastic fibers that adhere to the surface of the spinal cord and brain; contains numerous blood vessels

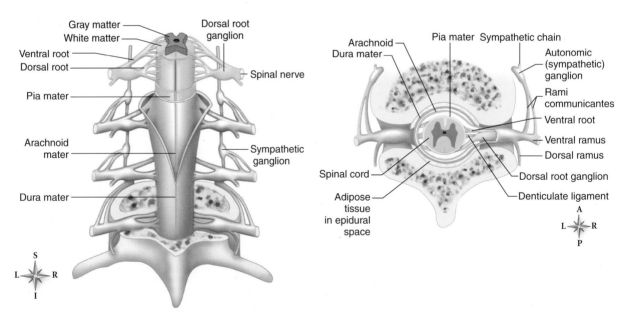

FIG 3-21 Coverings of the spinal cord. (From Patton KT, Thibodeau GA: *Anthony's textbook of anatomy and physiology,* ed 20, St Louis, 2013, Elsevier.)

C. Spinal cord does not run the entire length of the vertebral column; nerves called *cauda equina* arise from the lowest portion of a cord and angle down the vertebral canal

D. Functions

1. White matter tracts in the spinal cord are pathways for nerve impulse conduction; sensory impulses flow from the periphery to the brain, and motor impulses flow from the brain to the periphery

2. Gray matter receives and integrates incoming and outgoing information

3. Spinal reflexes—fast automatic responses to sensory impulses that enter the spinal cord via spinal nerves

4. Reflex arc—pathway followed by nerve impulses that produce a reflex

   a. Somatic reflex—reflex involving involuntary contraction of skeletal muscles (e.g., knee-jerk reflex)

   b. Withdrawal reflex—causes immediate withdrawal of a limb from a source of injury before awareness of pain

   c. Autonomic reflex—reflexes involving smooth muscle, cardiac muscle, and glands (e.g., swallowing, urinating)

E. Spinal nerves

1. Thirty-one pairs of spinal nerves; each has a dorsal (afferent) root and a ventral (efferent) root

2. Named and numbered according to the region and level of the vertebral column from which they emerge

3. Emerge from the spinal cord to form plexuses along the cord, except in the thoracic region

   a. The cervical plexus (C1 to C4) innervates muscles, skin, posterior head, neck, upper shoulders, and diaphragm

   b. Brachial plexus (C5 to T1) nerves supply upper limbs, neck, and muscles

      (1) Radial—lateral side of the arm

      (2) Medial—middle portion of the arm

      (3) Ulnar—medial side of the arm

   c. T2 to T12 comprise the intercostal nerves; do not form a plexus

   d. Lumbosacral plexus—includes L1 to S4

      (1) Lumbar portion—first four lumbar nerves contribute to the femoral nerve; supplies abdominal wall, external genitals, and part of lower limbs

      (2) Sacral portion—sacral nerves, the last lumbar nerve, and the coccygeal nerve supply the pelvis and legs; contribute to the sciatic nerve (longest nerve in the body)

Brain

See Figure 3-22.

A. Principal parts—brain stem (consists of the medulla oblongata, pons, and midbrain), diencephalon (consists of the thalamus and hypothalamus), cerebrum, and cerebellum

B. Supplied with oxygen and nutrients by the cerebral arterial circle, or circle of Willis

1. Any interruption of the oxygen supply may permanently damage or kill brain cells

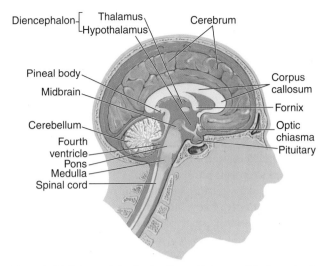

FIG 3-22 Divisions of the brain. (From Solomon EP: *Introduction to human anatomy and physiology,* ed 2, St Louis, 2008, Saunders.)

2. Glucose deficiency may produce dizziness, convulsions, and unconsciousness

C. The blood-brain barrier (BBB) limits the passage of certain materials from the blood into the brain

D. The brain is protected by cranial bones, meninges, and the cerebrospinal fluid

1. Cranial meninges are continuous with the spinal meninges (dura mater, arachnoid, and pia mater)

2. Cerebrospinal fluid (CSF)—formed in the choroid plexuses; circulates continually through the subarachnoid space, ventricles, and central canal; protects the brain and spinal cord by serving as a shock absorber; delivers nutritive substances from the blood and removes wastes

E. Medulla oblongata (also called *medulla*)—is continuous with the upper part of the spinal cord

1. Contains regions for regulating heart rate, diameter of blood vessels, respiratory rate, swallowing, coughing, vomiting, sneezing, and hiccupping

2. The vestibulocochlear, accessory, vagus, and hypoglossal nerves originate at the medulla

F. Pons—connects the spinal cord to the brain; links parts of the brain to one another; relays impulses related to voluntary skeletal movements from the cerebral cortex to the cerebellum

1. Contains two regions that control respiration

2. The trigeminal, abducens, facial, and vestibular branches of the vestibulocochlear nerves originate at the pons

G. Midbrain—conveys motor impulses from the cerebrum to the cerebellum and the spinal cord, and transmits sensory impulses from the spinal cord to the thalamus

H. Reticular formation—net-like arrangement of gray and white matter extending throughout the brain stem; alerts the cerebral cortex to incoming sensory signals; helps regulate muscle tone

I. Diencephalon—consists of the thalamus and the hypothalamus
   1. Thalamus—contains nuclei that serve as relay stations for sensory impulses to the cerebral cortex; provides crude recognition of pain, temperature, touch, pressure, and vibration
   2. Hypothalamus—located below the thalamus; controls and integrates the ANS and pituitary gland; functions in rage and aggression; controls body temperature; regulates food and fluid intake; maintains consciousness and sleep patterns
J. The reticular activating system—functions in arousal (awakening from deep sleep) and consciousness (wakefulness)
K. Cerebrum—largest part of the brain; the cortex contains convolutions, fissures, and sulci
   1. Cerebral lobes—frontal, parietal, temporal, and occipital
   2. White matter under the cerebral cortex consists of myelinated axons extending in three principal directions
   3. Sensory areas receive and interpret sensory impulses; motor areas govern muscular movement
   4. Contains tissues associated with emotional and intellectual processes
   5. Generates brain waves measurable by electroencephalogram (EEG), which may be used to diagnose epilepsy, infections, and tumors
L. Basal ganglia—paired masses of gray matter in the cerebral hemispheres that control muscle movements
M. The limbic system—found in cerebral hemispheres and the diencephalon; functions in the emotional aspects of behavior and memory
N. Hemispheres of the brain
   1. Left hemisphere—receives sensory signals from and controls the right side of the body; more important for language, numerical and scientific skills, and reasoning
   2. Right hemisphere—receives sensory signals from and controls the left side of the body; more important for musical and other artistic awareness, spatial and pattern perception, recognition of faces, emotional content of language, and generating mental images of sight, sound, touch, taste, and smell
O. Cerebellum—occupies the inferior and posterior aspects of the cranial cavity; consists of two hemispheres with a cerebellar cortex of gray matter and an interior of white matter tracts; attaches to the brain stem by three pairs of cerebellar peduncles; coordinates skeletal muscles and maintains normal muscle tone and body equilibrium

Cranial Nerves

See the section on "The Nervous System" in Chapter 4.
A. Twelve pairs of cranial nerves originate from the brain
B. As with spinal nerves, cranial nerves are part of the PNS

The Autonomic Nervous System

A. Regulates smooth muscle, cardiac muscle, and certain glands; usually operates without conscious control by the centers in the brain, in particular by the hypothalamus

B. Two principal divisions—sympathetic and parasympathetic; most organs have dual innervation; in general, nerve impulses from one division stimulate excitation, and impulses from the other division cause inhibition
   1. Sympathetic (thoracolumbar division)—sympathetic ganglia are classified as sympathetic trunk ganglia (lateral to the vertebral column) and prevertebral ganglia (anterior to the vertebral column)
   2. Parasympathetic—parasympathetic ganglia are called *terminal ganglia*; located near or within visceral effectors
   3. Neurons of preganglionic autonomic neurons are myelinated; those of postganglionic autonomic neurons are unmyelinated
C. Functions
   1. Cholinergic neurons release acetylcholine (ACh); adrenergic neurons release norepinephrine (NE)
   2. Activation of the sympathetic division causes widespread responses; the "fight-or-flight" response
   3. Activation of the parasympathetic division produces more restricted responses that typically are concerned with "rest-and-digest" activities

Special Senses

A. Sensation—conscious or subconscious awareness of external and internal conditions of the body; for a sensation to occur, three conditions must be satisfied:
   1. A stimulus, or change in environment, capable of activating certain sensory neurons must occur
   2. A sensory receptor must convert the stimulus to nerve impulses
   3. The nerve impulses must be conducted along a neural pathway from the sensory receptor to the brain
B. Components of the eye (Figure 3-23)
   1. Conjunctiva—thin mucous membrane that covers the front of the eye and lines the eyelid
   2. Lacrimal glands—located bilaterally on the outer borders of the orbital cavity; secrete about 1 milliliter (mL) of fluid per day; contain lysozyme to destroy bacteria
   3. Nasolacrimal duct—carries fluid away from the gland
   4. Iris—the colored part of the eye that is a circular diaphragm; regulates the amount of light that enters the eye
   5. Pupil—where light enters the eye; black in color
   6. Lens—biconvex disc without blood
   7. Sclera—white covering on the anterior aspect of the eye
   8. Vitreous body—colloid inside of the eyeball; maintains the shape
   9. Optic disc—located on the posterior surface of the eyeball; contains no rods or cones, only optic nerves
   10. Retina—contains cones in its center (fovea) and rods on the outer periphery; process of forming an image on the retina is similar to a camera producing a picture:
       a. Light rays are bent as they enter the eye
       b. The lens adjusts to the amount of light
       c. Light rays are converged on the fovea
       d. Rays cause changes in the chemistry of rods and cones
       e. Optic nerve sends impulses to the occipital lobes of the brain

FIG 3-23 Horizontal cross section of the eye. (From Patton KT, Thibodeau GA, Douglas MM: *Essentials of anatomy and physiology*, St Louis, 2012, Mosby.)

FIG 3-24 The ear. (From Patton KT, Thibodeau GA, Douglas MM: *Essentials of anatomy and physiology*, St Louis, 2012, Mosby.)

C. Hearing and equilibrium (Figure 3-24)
   1. The external ear consists of an ear flap
   2. The middle ear is separated by the tympanic membrane (eardrum); contains the ossicles (malleus, incus, and stapes) and the eustachian tube (to equalize pressure)
   3. The inner ear contains the vestibule, the cochlea, and semicircular canals
      a. Cranial nerve VIII innervates this structure
      b. Small hairs detect various frequencies and pitches; impulses are sent to the temporal lobes of the brain
      c. Semi-circular canals maintain equilibrium

D. Tongue
   1. Cranial nerve VII provides sensory fibers to the anterior two thirds of the tongue, including fungiform and foliate papillae; sensations of sweet, sour, and salty tastes are detected
   2. Cranial nerve IX provides sensations of taste to the posterior one third of the tongue's circumvallate papillae; the bitter taste is detected there
   3. Food must be in solution in the mouth before taste buds can transfer the information to the brain
   4. Most taste sensations are made up of various combinations of the four basic tastes
E. Olfactory sense
   1. Stimulates hairs (cilia) that are sensitive to slight odors
   2. On each side of the nose, bundles of slender, unmyelinated axons of olfactory receptors extend through holes in the cribriform plate of the ethmoid bone
   3. These bundles of axons form cranial nerve I, the olfactory nerve; they terminate in the brain in olfactory bulbs, which are located inferior to the frontal lobes of the cerebrum
   4. Within the olfactory bulbs, the axon terminals of olfactory receptors synapse with the dendrites and cell bodies of the next neurons in the olfactory pathway
   5. The axons of the neurons extending from the olfactory bulb form the olfactory tract
   6. The olfactory tract projects into the primary olfactory area in the temporal lobe, where the conscious awareness of smell begins
F. Tactile sensation (Table 3-4)
   1. Meissner's corpuscles—receptors that control the sensation of touch
   2. Pacinian corpuscles—receptors that control the sensation of pressure
   3. Ruffini's corpuscles—receptors that control the sensation of heat
   4. Krause's end bulbs—receptors that control the sensation of cold
   5. Nociceptors—sensory receptors for pain; during tissue irritation or injury, release of chemicals such as prostaglandins stimulates nociceptors
G. Proprioceptive sensations—inform consciously and subconsciously; sense the degree of muscle contraction, amount of tension present in tendons, position of joints, and orientation of head and equilibrium

The Endocrine System

A. The endocrine system is a collection of glands, each of which secretes different types of hormones that regulate metabolism, growth and development, tissue function, sexual function, reproduction, sleep, mood, and other processes
B. Communication, integration, and control of body processes is accomplished by secreting cells that send hormone molecules through the blood to specific target cells contained in target tissues or target organs
   1. Works in conjunction with the nervous system to achieve and maintain homeostasis
   2. The neuroendocrine system—interaction of the endocrine and nervous systems to perform similar functions
C. Endocrine glands—"ductless glands"; many are made of glandular epithelium whose cells manufacture and secrete hormones; a few endocrine glands are made of neurosecretory tissue; widely scattered throughout the body

Hormones

A. Function of hormones—regulate most cells to stimulate a physiologic activity; work more slowly and last longer than neurotransmitters; carried to almost every point in the body
B. Classification of hormones
   1. Classification by general function
      a. Tropic hormones—target other endocrine glands and stimulate their growth and secretion
      b. Sex hormones—target reproductive tissues
      c. Anabolic hormones—stimulate anabolism in target cells
   2. Classification by chemical structure
      a. Steroid hormones
         (1) Synthesized from cholesterol
         (2) Lipid soluble; can easily pass through plasma membrane of target cells
         (3) Examples include cortisol, aldosterone, estrogen, progesterone, and testosterone
      b. Nonsteroid hormones—synthesized primarily from amino acids
      c. Protein hormones—long, folded chains of amino acids (e.g., insulin, parathyroid hormone)
      d. Glycoprotein hormones—protein hormones with carbohydrate groups attached to the amino acid chain
      e. Peptide hormones—smaller than protein hormones; short chain of amino acids (e.g., oxytocin, antidiuretic hormone)
      f. Amino acid derivative hormones—each is derived from a single amino acid molecule
         (1) Amine hormones—synthesized by modifying a single molecule of tyrosine; produced by neurosecretory cells and by neurons (e.g., epinephrine, norepinephrine)
         (2) Amino acid derivatives produced by the thyroid gland; synthesized by adding iodine to tyrosine
C. Mechanism of action
   1. General principles
      a. Hormones signal a cell by binding to the specific receptors of a target cell in a "lock-and-key" arrangement
      b. Different hormone-receptor interactions produce different regulatory changes within the target cell through chemical reactions
      c. Combined hormone actions
         (1) Synergism—combinations of hormones acting together have a greater effect on a target cell than the sum of the effects that each would have if acting alone

TABLE 3-4 Classification of Somatic Sensory Receptors

By Structure	By Location and Type	By Activation Stimulus	By Sensation or Function
Free Nerve Endings			
Nociceptors	Both exteroceptors and visceroceptors—most body tissues	Almost any noxious stimulus; temperature change; mechanical	Pain; temperature; itch; tickle; stretching
Merkel discs	Exteroceptors	Light pressure; mechanical	Discriminative touch
Root hair plexuses	Exteroceptors	Hair movement; mechanical	Sense of "deflection" hair movement

Nociceptors

Merkel discs

Root hair plexuses

Encapsulated Nerve Endings			
Touch and Pressure Receptors			
Meissner's corpuscle	Exteroceptors; epidermis, hairless skin	Light pressure, mechanical	Discriminative touch; low-frequency vibration
Krause's corpuscle	Mucous membranes	Mechanical; thermal	Touch; low-frequency vibration
Ruffini's corpuscle	Dermis of skin, exteroceptors	Mechanical; thermal	Crude and persistent touch
Pacinian corpuscle	Dermis of skin, joint capsules	Deep pressure, mechanical	Deep pressure; high-frequency vibration; stretch
Stretch Receptors			
Muscle spindles	Skeletal muscle	Stretch, mechanical	Sense of muscle length
Golgi tendon receptors	Musculotendinous junction	Force of contraction and tendon stretch, mechanical	Sense of muscle tension

Meissner's corpuscle

Krause's end bulb

Ruffini's corpuscle

Pacinian corpuscle

Intrafusal fibers

Muscle spindles

Golgi tendon receptors

Modified from Patton KT, Thibodeau GA: *Anthony's textbook of anatomy and physiology,* ed 20, St Louis, 2013, Elsevier.

(2) Permissiveness—when a small amount of one hormone allows a second one to have its full effects on a target cell

(3) Antagonism—one hormone produces the opposite effects of another hormone; used to fine-tune the activity of target cells with great accuracy

d. Endocrine glands produce more hormone molecules than needed; unused hormones are quickly excreted by the kidneys or broken down by metabolic processes

2. Mechanism of steroid hormone action

a. Steroid hormones are lipid soluble, and their receptors are normally found within the target cell

b. After a steroid hormone molecule has diffused into the target cell, it binds to a receptor molecule to form a hormone-receptor complex

c. Mobile receptor hypothesis—the hormone passes into the nucleus, where it binds to a mobile receptor and activates a certain gene sequence to begin transcription of mRNA; newly formed mRNA molecules move into the cytosol, associate with ribosomes, and begin synthesizing protein molecules that produce the effects of the hormone

d. The amount of steroid hormone present determines the magnitude of the target cell's response

e. Because transcription and protein synthesis take time, responses to steroid hormones are often slow

3. Mechanisms of nonsteroid hormone action

a. Second messenger mechanism—also known as the *fixed-membrane-receptor hypothesis*

(1) A nonsteroid hormone molecule acts as a "first messenger" and delivers its chemical message to receptors that are fixed in the plasma membrane of the target cell

(2) The message is then passed by way of a G-protein into the cell where a "second messenger" triggers the appropriate cellular response

(3) The second messenger mechanism produces target cell effects that differ from steroid hormone effects in several important ways:

(a) The effects of the hormone are amplified by a cascade of reactions

(b) The second messenger mechanisms include inositol trisphosphate (IP_3), guanosine monophosphate (GMP), and calcium calmodulin

(c) The second messenger mechanism operates much more quickly than the steroid mechanism

b. Nuclear receptor mechanism—small iodinated amino acids (T_4 and T_3) enter the target cell and bind to receptors associated with a DNA molecule in the nucleus; this binding triggers transcription of mRNA and synthesis of new enzymes

D. Regulation of hormone secretion

1. Usually part of a negative feedback loop called an *endocrine reflex*; the simplest regulatory mechanism is when an endocrine gland is sensitive to the physiologic changes produced by its target cells

2. Regulated by a hormone produced by another gland

3. May be influenced by the input of the nervous system; this fact emphasizes the close functional relationship between the two systems

Prostaglandins

A. Function of prostaglandins

1. Unique group of lipid molecules (20-carbon fatty acid with 5-carbon ring); serve important, widespread integrative functions, but do not meet the usual definition of a hormone; tend to integrate activities of neighboring cells

2. Called *tissue hormones* because the secretion is produced in a tissue and diffuses only a short distance to other cells within the same tissue

B. Structural classes of prostaglandins

1. Prostaglandin A (PGA)—intra-arterial infusion resulting in an immediate drop in blood pressure accompanied by an increase in regional blood flow to several areas

2. Prostaglandin E (PGE)—regulation of red blood cell deformability and platelet aggregation; regulation of hydrochloric acid secretion in the GI tract

3. Prostaglandin F (PGF)—causes uterine contractions; affects intestinal motility; required for normal peristalsis

Pituitary Gland

A. The function of pituitary gland is divided by two separate glands:

1. The anterior pituitary gland: secretory cells produce growth hormone, prolactin, and a number of tropic hormones

2. The posterior pituitary gland: serves as a storage site for antidiuretic hormone and oxytocin

B. Structure of the pituitary gland

1. Also known as *hypophysis,* the "master gland"

2. Size: 1.2 to 1.5 cm

3. Located on the ventral surface of the brain within the skull

4. Infundibulum—stem-like stalk that connects the pituitary to the hypothalamus

5. Composed of two separate glands, the adenohypophysis (anterior pituitary gland) and the neurohypophysis (posterior pituitary gland)

C. Adenohypophysis (anterior pituitary)

1. Divided into two parts:

a. Pars anterior—forms the major portion of the adenohypophysis

b. Pars intermedia

2. Tissue is composed of irregular clumps of secretory cells supported by fine connective tissue fibers and surrounded by a rich vascular network

3. Three types of cells can be identified by their stain affinity:

a. Chromophobes—do not stain

b. Acidophils—stain with acidic stains

c. Basophils—stain with basic stains

4. Five functional types of secretory cells:

a. Somatotrophs—secrete GH

b. Corticotrophs—secrete ACTH

c. Thyrotrophs—secrete TSH

d. Lactotrophs—secrete prolactin

e. Gonadotrophs—secrete LH and FSH

D. Hormones secreted by the adenohypophysis

1. Growth hormone (GH); also known as *somatotropin* (STH)

   a. Promotes growth of bone, muscle, and other tissues by accelerating amino acid transport into the cells

   b. Stimulates fat metabolism by mobilizing lipids from storage in adipose cells and speeding up the catabolism of lipids after they have entered another cell

   c. Shifts cell chemistry away from glucose catabolism and toward lipid catabolism as an energy source; this leads to increased blood glucose levels

   d. Functions as an insulin antagonist; vital to maintaining the homeostasis of blood glucose levels

2. Prolactin (PRL); also known as *lactogenic hormone*

   a. Produced by acidophils in the pars anterior

   b. Promotes breast development during pregnancy in anticipation of milk secretion; stimulates lactation after delivery

3. Tropic hormones—have a stimulating effect on other endocrine glands; four principal tropic hormones are produced and secreted by the basophils of the pars anterior:

   a. Thyroid-stimulating hormone (TSH), or thyrotropin—promotes and maintains the growth and development of the thyroid; causes the thyroid to secrete its hormones

   b. Adrenocorticotropic hormone (ACTH), or adrenocorticotropin—promotes and maintains normal growth and development of the cortex of the adrenal gland; stimulates the adrenal cortex to secrete some of its hormones

   c. Follicle-stimulating hormone (FSH)—stimulates primary graafian follicles to grow toward maturity in females; also stimulates follicle cells to secrete estrogens; in males, stimulates the development of the seminiferous tubules of the testes and maintains spermatogenesis

   d. Luteinizing hormone (LH)—stimulates the formation and activity of the corpus luteum of the ovary in females; the corpus luteum secretes progesterone and estrogens when stimulated by LH; LH also supports FSH in stimulating the maturation of follicles; in males, LH stimulates the interstitial cells in the testes to develop and secrete testosterone

   e. FSH and LH are called *gonadotropins* because they stimulate the growth and maintenance of the gonads

4. Control of secretion in the adenohypophysis

   a. The hypothalamus secretes releasing hormones into the blood, which are then carried to the hypophyseal portal system; through negative feedback, the hypothalamus adjusts the secretions of the adenohypophysis, which then adjusts the secretions of the target glands, which in turn adjust the activity of their target tissues

   b. The hypophyseal portal system carries blood from the hypothalamus directly to the adenohypophysis, where the target cells of the releasing hormones are located;

releasing hormones influence the secretion of hormones by acidophils and basophils

c. Under stress, hypothalamus translates nerve impulses into hormone secretions by endocrine glands, creating a neuroendocrine link

E. Neurohypophysis (posterior pituitary)

1. Serves as storage and release site for antidiuretic hormone (ADH, vasopressin) and oxytocin (OT), which are synthesized in the hypothalamus

2. ADH and OT are released into blood; controlled by nervous stimulation

3. Antidiuretic hormone

   a. Prevents the formation of a large volume of urine, thereby helping the body conserve water

   b. Causes the tubules in the kidney to resorb water from urine

   c. Dehydration triggers the release of ADH

4. Oxytocin—has two actions:

   a. Causes the release of milk from the lactating breast; regulated by the positive feedback mechanism; PRL cooperates with OT

   b. Stimulates the contractions of uterine muscles during childbirth; regulated by positive feedback mechanism

Pineal Gland

A. Function of pineal glands

1. A member of the nervous system because it receives visual stimuli; also a member of the endocrine system because it secretes hormones

2. Supports the body's biologic clock

   a. Principal pineal secretion is melatonin

B. Structure of pineal glands

1. Tiny, pinecone-shaped structure located on the dorsal aspect of the brain's diencephalon

Thyroid Gland

See the section on "Glands of the Head and Neck Region" and Figure 4-8 in Chapter 4.

A. Function of the thyroid gland

1. Increases metabolic rate and essential for growth and development; crucial for brain development in children

2. Influences body temperature

B. Structure of the thyroid gland

1. Two large lateral lobes and a narrow connecting isthmus; located in the neck, on the anterior and lateral surfaces of the trachea, just below the larynx

2. A thin, worm-like projection of thyroid tissue, often extends upward from the isthmus

3. The weight of the thyroid in an adult is approximately 30 grams (g)

4. Composed of follicles

   a. Small hollow spheres

   b. Filled with thyroid colloid that contains thyroglobulins

C. Thyroid hormone

1. Two different hormones:

   a. Triiodothyronine (T_3)—contains three iodine atoms; considered to be the principal thyroid hormone; T_3 binds efficiently to the nuclear receptors in target cells

b. Tetraiodothyronine (T_4), or thyroxine—contains four iodine atoms; approximately 20 times more abundant than T_3; its major importance is its role as a precursor to T_3

2. The thyroid gland stores considerable amounts of a preliminary form of its hormones before secreting them

3. Before being stored in the colloid of follicles, T_3 and T_4 are attached to globulin molecules to form thyroglobin complexes

4. On release, T_3 and T_4 detach from globulin and enter the bloodstream

5. Once in the blood, T_3 and T_4 attach to plasma globulins and travel as a hormone-globulin complex

6. T_3 detaches from plasma globulin as it nears the target cells; T_4 also detaches, but to a lesser extent

7. Thyroid hormone—helps regulate the metabolic rate of all cells, cell growth, and tissue differentiation; it is said to have a "general" target

D. Calcitonin

1. Produced by the thyroid gland in the parafollicular cells

2. Influences the processing of calcium by bone cells by decreasing blood calcium levels and promoting the conservation of the hard bone matrix

3. Parathyroid hormone acts as antagonist to calcitonin to maintain calcium homeostasis

Parathyroid Glands

A. Function of the parathyroid glands

1. Control calcium in the blood by stimulating bone breakdown, increasing calcium absorption in the digestive tract, and decreasing loss of calcium in the urine

B. Structure of the parathyroid glands

1. Four or five parathyroid glands are embedded in the posterior surface of the thyroid's lateral lobes

2. Tiny, rounded bodies within thyroid tissue formed by compact, irregular rows of cells

C. Parathyroid hormone (PTH, parathormone)

1. An antagonist to calcitonin; acts to maintain calcium homeostasis

2. Acts on bone and the kidneys

a. Causes more bone to be dissolved, yielding calcium and phosphate, which enter the bloodstream

b. Causes phosphate to be secreted by the kidney cells into urine to be excreted

c. Increases the intestinal absorption of calcium by stimulating the kidney to produce active vitamin D

Adrenal Glands

A. Function of the adrenal glands

1. Work with the hypothalamus and pituitary gland to stimulate and produce hormones that influence metabolism, body characteristics, ability to cope with physical and emotional stress, and aids in the regulation of sodium and potassium levels

B. Structure of the adrenal glands

1. Located on top of the kidneys like caps

2. Made up of two portions:

a. Adrenal cortex—the outer part of the gland; produces hormones that are vital to life, such as cortisol, which regulates metabolism and the body's response to stress, and aldosterone, which helps regulate blood pressure

b. Adrenal medulla—produces nonessential hormones, such as adrenaline, which helps the body react to stress

C. Adrenal cortex

1. All cortical hormones are steroids; known as *corticosteroids*

2. Composed of three distinct layers of secreting cells:

a. Zona glomerulosa—outermost layer, directly under the outer connective tissue capsule of the adrenal gland; secretes mineralocorticoids

b. Zona fasciculata—middle layer; secretes glucocorticoids

c. Zona reticularis—inner layer; secretes small amounts of glucocorticoids and gonadocorticoids

3. Mineralocorticoids—important role in regulating sodium levels

a. Aldosterone

(1) The only physiologically important mineralocorticoid; its primary function is to maintain sodium homeostasis in blood by increasing sodium resorption in the kidneys

(2) Increases water retention; promotes the loss of potassium and hydrogen ions

(3) Secretion is controlled by the renin-angiotensin mechanism and by blood potassium concentration

b. Glucocorticoids

(1) Secreted by the zona fasciculata

(2) Examples include cortisol, cortisone, and corticosterone

(3) Affect every body cell

(4) Are protein mobilizing, gluconeogenic, and hyperglycemia inducing

(5) Tend to cause a shift from carbohydrate catabolism to lipid catabolism

(6) Essential for maintaining normal blood pressure by helping norepinephrine and epinephrine to have their full effect; cause vasoconstriction

(7) High blood concentration causes eosinopenia and marked atrophy of lymphatic tissues

(8) Act with epinephrine to bring about normal recovery from injury produced by inflammatory agents

(9) Secretion increases in response to stress

(10) Except during stress response, secretion is mainly controlled by a negative feedback mechanism involving ACTH from the adenohypophysis

4. Gonadocorticoids—sex hormones (androgens) released from the adrenal cortex

D. Adrenal medulla

1. Neurosecretory tissue—composed of neurons specialized to secrete their products into blood

2. Secretes epinephrine and norepinephrine, part of the class of nonsteroid hormones called *catecholamines*; both hormones bind to the receptors of sympathetic effectors to prolong and enhance the effects of sympathetic stimulation by the ANS

Pancreatic Islets

A. Function of pancreatic islets
1. From the liver, increases breakdown of glycogen to increase blood glucose levels
2. Decreases blood glucose by influencing uptake and use of the body's cells
B. Structure of the pancreatic islets
1. Elongated gland; its head lies in the duodenum; extends horizontally behind the stomach and touches the spleen
2. Composed of endocrine and exocrine tissues
   a. Islets of Langerhans—endocrine portion; each islet contains four primary types of endocrine glands joined by gap junctions:
      (1) Alpha cells (α-cells)—secrete glucagon
      (2) Beta cells (β-cells)—secrete insulin; account for up to 75% of all pancreatic islet cells
      (3) Delta cells (δ-cells)—secrete somatostatin
      (4) Pancreatic polypeptide cells (F- or PP-cells)—secrete pancreatic polypeptides
   b. Acini—exocrine portion; secretes a serous fluid containing digestive enzymes into the ducts draining into the small intestine
C. Pancreatic hormones—work as a team to maintain the homeostasis of food molecules
1. Glucagon—produced by α-cells; tends to increase blood glucose levels; stimulates gluconeogenesis in liver cells
2. Insulin—produced by β-cells; lowers the blood concentration of glucose and fatty acids; promotes their metabolism by tissue cells
3. Somatostatin—produced by δ-cells; primary role is regulating the other endocrine cells of pancreatic islets
4. Pancreatic polypeptide—produced by F-cells (PP-cells); influences the digestion and distribution of food molecules to some degree

Gonads

A. Testes
1. Paired organs within the scrotum in a male
2. Composed of seminiferous tubules and a scattering of interstitial cells
3. Testosterone—produced by interstitial cells; responsible for the growth and maintenance of male sexual characteristics; secretion is mainly regulated by gonadotropin levels in blood
B. Ovaries
1. Primary sex organs in a female
2. Set of paired glands in the pelvis that produce several types of sex hormones
   a. Estrogens—steroid hormones secreted by ovarian follicles; promote development and maintenance of female sexual characteristics
   b. Progesterone—secreted by the corpus luteum; maintains the lining of the uterus necessary for successful pregnancy
   c. Ovarian hormone secretion depends on the changing levels of FSH and LH from the adenohypophysis

Placenta

A. Tissues that form on the lining of the uterus as a connection between the circulatory systems of the mother and the developing fetus
B. Serves as a temporary endocrine gland; produces human chorionic gonadotropin, estrogens, and progesterone

Thymus Gland

A. Function of thymus gland
1. Important for immune system development and function
B. Structure of thymus gland
1. Located in the mediastinum just beneath the sternum
2. Large in children, begins to atrophy at puberty, and is a vestige of fat and fibrous tissue by old age
3. Considered to be primarily a lymphatic organ
4. Thymosin—isolated from thymus tissue; stimulates development of T cells

Gastric and Intestinal Mucosa

A. The mucous lining of the GI tract contains cells that produce both endocrine and exocrine secretions
B. GI hormones such as gastrin, secretin, and cholecystokinin-pancreozymin (CCK) play regulatory roles in coordinating the secretory and motor activities involved in the digestive process
C. Ghrelin—a hormone secreted by endocrine cells in the gastric mucosa; stimulates the hypothalamus to boost appetite; slows metabolism and fat burning; may be a contributor to obesity

Heart

A. Has a secondary endocrine role; hormone-producing cells produce the hormone atrial natriuretic peptide (ANP)
B. ANP opposes increases in blood volume or blood pressure; also an antagonist to ADH and aldosterone

The Cardiovascular System

The purpose of the cardiovascular system is to transport oxygen to all the tissues in the body and remove, from these same tissues, metabolic waste products. The cardiovascular system consists of three interrelated components: blood, the heart, and blood vessels.

A. Blood—a vital liquid that has three general functions:
1. Transportation—transports oxygen from the lungs to the cells throughout the body and carbon dioxide from the cells to the lungs; carries nutrients from the GI tract to body cells, heat and waste products away from cells, and hormones from endocrine glands to other body cells
2. Regulation—helps regulate the pH of body fluids; helps adjust body temperature; blood osmotic pressure also influences the water content of cells
3. Protection—blood clots in response to injury to protect against excessive blood loss; white blood cells protect against disease through phagocytosis and by producing antibodies; blood contains interferons, which also help protect against disease

FIG 3-25 Composition of whole blood. (From Patton KT, Thibodeau GA: *Anthony's textbook of anatomy and physiology*, ed 20, St Louis, 2013, Elsevier.)

B. Characteristics of blood
 1. Viscosity greater than that of water; temperature of 38°C (100.4°F); pH ranges between 7.35 and 7.45
 2. Blood constitutes about 8% of body weight in an adult
C. Components of blood (Figure 3-25)
 1. Consists of 55% plasma; 45% formed elements that include red blood cells (RBCs, erythrocytes), white blood cells (WBCs, leukocytes), and platelets
 2. Hematocrit—the percentage of RBCs in whole blood
 3. Plasma contains 91% water, 7% proteins, and 2% solutes
 4. Principal solutes include proteins (albumins, globulins, fibrinogen), nutrients, hormones, respiratory gases, electrolytes, and waste products
 5. Hemopoiesis—the formation of blood cells from pluripotent stem cells; occurs in red bone marrow
 6. Red blood cells—biconcave discs without a nucleus that contain hemoglobin
  a. Hemoglobin transports oxygen
  b. RBCs live for about 120 days; in terms of a normal blood count, a healthy male has about 4.7 to 6.1 million/mm³ RBCs; a healthy female has about 4.2 to 5.4 million/mm³ RBCs
  c. After phagocytosis of aged RBCs by macrophages, hemoglobin is recycled
  d. Erythropoiesis—RBC formation occurring in adult red bone marrow; stimulated by hypoxia, which stimulates the release of erythropoietin by the kidneys
 7. White blood cells—nucleated cells with two principal groups:
  a. Granular leukocytes (neutrophils, eosinophils, basophils)

  b. Agranular leukocytes (lymphocytes and monocytes)
  c. Function—to combat inflammation and infection; neutrophils and monocytes do so by phagocytosis
  d. Eosinophils combat the effects of histamine in allergic reactions and increase with allergies and parasites
  e. Basophils develop into mast cells that liberate heparin, histamine, and serotonin in allergic reactions that intensify the inflammatory response
  f. B cells (lymphocytes)—effective against bacteria and other toxins
  g. T cells (lymphocytes)—effective against viruses, fungi, and cancer cells
  h. WBCs usually live for only a few hours or a few days
  i. Normal blood contains 5000 to 10,000 WBCs/mm³
 8. Platelets—disc-shaped cell fragments without nuclei
  a. Formed from megakaryocytes; take part in hemostasis by forming a platelet plug
  b. Normal blood contains 150,000 to 450,000 platelets/mm³
D. Hemostasis—stoppage of bleeding
 1. Three mechanisms:
  a. Vascular spasm—when a blood vessel is damaged, the smooth muscle in its walls contracts immediately
  b. Platelet plug—when platelets come into contact with parts of a damaged blood vessel, their characteristics change drastically, and they come together to form a plug that helps fill the gap in the injured vessel
  c. Blood clotting—a series of reactions
   (1) Prothrombinase is formed
   (2) Conversion of prothrombin into thrombin

(3) Conversion of soluble fibrinogen into insoluble fibrin

2. Clot—a network of insoluble protein fibers (fibrin), in which formed elements of blood are trapped

3. Normal coagulation requires vitamin K and also involves clot retraction and fibrinolysis

4. Anticoagulants prevent clotting

5. Thrombosis—clotting in an unbroken blood vessel; a thrombus that moves from its site of origin is called an *embolus*

E. Blood groups

1. Surfaces of RBCs contain a genetically determined assortment of glycolipids and glycoproteins called *isoantigens*
   a. Based on the presence or absence of various isoantigens, blood is categorized into different blood groups
   b. Within a blood group, two or more different blood types may be present

2. ABO blood group system—based on isoantigens A and B
   a. Type A—red cells display only antigen A
   b. Type B—red cells display only antigen B
   c. Type AB—red cells display both antigens A and B
   d. Type O—red cells display neither antigen A nor B

F. Heart

1. Located in the space between the lungs, behind the sternum, in the thoracic cavity known as the *mediastinum*; size of a human fist; apex of the heart points down and to the left

2. Consists of four chambers: two atria and two ventricles (Figure 3-26)
   a. Blood from superior and inferior venae cavae fills the right atrium and passes into the right ventricle through the tricuspid valve (three flaps)
   b. From the right ventricle, the unoxygenated blood is sent to the lungs by passing through the semi-lunar valve and the pulmonary artery
   c. Oxygenated blood is sent from the lungs to the left atrium through the pulmonary veins; the left semi-lunar valve separates the left atrium from the pulmonary veins
   d. From the left atrium, blood flows through the mitral valve (two flaps) into the left ventricle
   e. Blood enters the circulation by passing through the left semi-lunar valve into the aorta

3. The heart walls consist of three layers:
   a. Visceral pericardium or epicardium
   b. Myocardium—heaviest covering
   c. Endocardium—smooth continuous covering
   d. All valves and chambers are lined by the endothelium

4. The valves of the heart are unique
   a. Atrioventricular (AV) valves—tough, fibrous tissue; open except when ventricles contract; hang into the ventricle like a leaf; held in place by chordae tendineae at the edge of the valves
      (1) Tricuspid AV valve—formed by three flaps

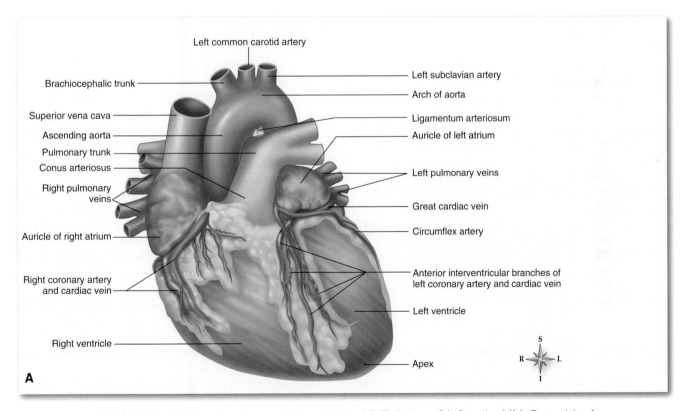

FIG 3-26 The heart and great vessels. (From Patton KT, Thibodeau GA, Douglas MM: *Essentials of anatomy and physiology*, St Louis, 2012, Mosby.)

(Continued)

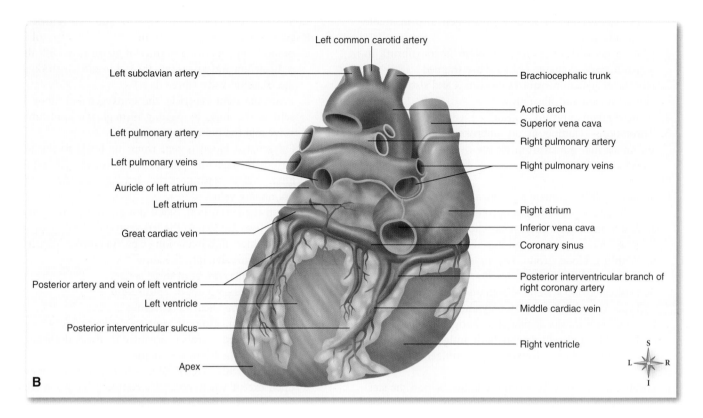

Left common carotid artery

Left subclavian artery

Left pulmonary artery

Left pulmonary veins

Auricle of left atrium

Left atrium

Great cardiac vein

Posterior artery and vein of left ventricle

Left ventricle

Posterior interventricular sulcus

Apex

Brachiocephalic trunk

Aortic arch

Superior vena cava

Right pulmonary artery

Right pulmonary veins

Right atrium

Inferior vena cava

Coronary sinus

Posterior interventricular branch of right coronary artery

Middle cardiac vein

Right ventricle

B

FIG 3-26, CONT'D

(2) Bicuspid AV valve (mitral valve)—formed by two parts
b. Semi-lunar (SL) valves—pressure opens them, and reverse pressure closes them; remain closed until ventricles contract
(1) Pulmonary SL valve—located at the right
(2) Aortic SL valve—located at the left
5. Heart rate averages 70 to 72 beats per minute; the heart cannot contract without nerve impulses; nerves regulate heart rate
a. Sinoatrial (SA) node—located in the walls of the right atrium near the superior vena cava; the heart beat begins there
(1) From there, the action current spreads out and passes down to the fibrous layer and stops
(2) The current goes through the AV node at the upper end of the interventricular septum
(3) Modified cardiac muscle divides into right and left branches
(4) Along the AV bundle, fibers pass out into the cardiac muscle (Purkinje fibers)
b. The action current consists of an impulse starting at the SA node, spreads to the atria, passes to the AV node, is picked up and sent down through all the cardiac fibers from Purkinje fibers, and ends by spreading over the ventricles; muscle contracts after the impulse spreads over the heart
(1) Purkinje fibers provide for uniform contraction

(2) If the AV node is blocked, ventricles will set up their own rhythm
6. Cardiac cycle—includes all the events associated with one heartbeat (Figure 3-27)
a. In a normal cardiac cycle, the two atria contract while the two ventricles relax; then, while the two ventricles contract, the two atria relax
(1) Systole—phase of contraction
(2) Diastole—phase of relaxation
b. Three phases of cardiac cycle (each cycle lasts about 0.8 second):
(1) Relaxation period—begins at the end of a cardiac cycle; ventricles start to relax, and all four chambers are in diastole; repolarization of ventricular muscle fibers initiates relaxation; as ventricles relax, pressure within them drops; when ventricular pressure drops below atrial pressure, AV valves open, and ventricular filling begins
(2) Contraction (atrial systole)—an action potential from the SA node causes atrial depolarization; atria contract and force the last 25% of blood into ventricles; AV valves are still open, and SL valves are closed
(3) Contraction (ventricular systole)—ventricular contraction pushes blood against AV valves, forcing them to shut; pressure inside chambers rises when left ventricular pressure surpasses aortic pressure; right ventricular pressure rises above

1 Atrial systole

2 Isovolumetric ventricular contraction

5 Passive ventricular filling

Cardiac cycle

3 Ejection

4 Isovolumetric ventricular relaxation

S
R   L
I

FIG 3-27 The cardiac cycle. (From Patton KT, Thibodeau GA: *Anthony's textbook of anatomy and physiology,* ed 20, St Louis, 2013, Elsevier.)

the pressure in the pulmonary trunk; both SL valves open, and ejection of blood from the heart begins; ejection continues until ventricles start to relax; ventricular pressure drops, SL valves close, and another relaxation period begins

   c. Heart sounds

     (1) First sound—AV valves close

     (2) Second sound—SL valves close

   d. Cardiac output—volume of blood ejected per minute from the left ventricle into the aorta; determined by:

     (1) Stroke volume (SV)—amount of blood ejected by the left ventricle during each contraction or beat; in a resting adult, stroke volume averages 70 mL, and heart rate is about 75 beats/min

     (2) Number of heartbeats per minute

     (3) Regulation of stroke volume depends on three factors:

       (a) Starling's law—the more the heart is stretched as it fills during diastole, the greater the force of contraction during systole

       (b) The forcefulness of the contraction of individual ventricular muscle fibers

       (c) The pressure required to eject blood from the ventricles

     (4) Regulation of heart rate—adjustments of heart rate are important in the short-term control of cardiac output and blood pressure; for example, during exercise, cardiac output rises to supply working tissues with increased amounts of oxygen and nutrients

       (a) The most important factors are the autonomic nervous system and the hormones epinephrine and norepinephrine released by adrenal glands

       (b) The regulation of the nervous system originates in the cardiovascular center in the medulla oblongata

       (c) Sympathetic impulses increase heart rate and force of contraction; parasympathetic impulses decrease heart rate

       (d) Sensory receptors help adjust heart rate; for example, baroreceptors (neurons sensitive to blood pressure) are strategically located in the arch of the aorta and carotid arteries; if an increase in blood pressure occurs, baroreceptors send nerve impulses along the sensory neurons that are part of the glossopharyngeal and vagus nerves (X) to the cardiovascular center; the center responds, and the result is a decrease in heart rate that lowers cardiac output, thus lowering blood pressure

     (5) Chemical regulation of heart rate

       (a) Epinephrine and norepinephrine enhance the heart's pumping effectiveness by increasing both heart rate and contraction force

       (b) Thyroid hormones also increase heart rate; a sign of hyperthyroidism is tachycardia

       (c) Ions—elevated blood levels of K^+ or Na^+ decrease heart rate and contraction force

The Circulatory System

The circulatory system contributes to the homeostasis of other body systems by transporting and distributing blood throughout the body to deliver oxygen, nutrients, and hormones and to carry away wastes.

A. Types of blood vessels

   1. Arteries—carry blood away from the heart to body tissues; walls have three layers of tissue surrounding a hollow space called the *lumen*

     a. Inner layer composed of endothelium

     b. Middle layer composed of smooth muscle and elastic tissue

     c. Outer layer composed mainly of elastic and collagen fibers

     d. Vasoconstriction—increase in sympathetic stimulation stimulates smooth muscle to contract, squeezing the vessel wall and narrowing the lumen

     e. Vasodilation—sympathetic stimulation decreases; smooth muscle fibers relax

   2. Arteriole—very small artery that delivers blood to capillaries

3. Capillaries—microscopic vessels that connect arterioles to venules; present near almost every body cell; permit the exchange of nutrients and wastes between the body's cells and blood; the number of capillaries varies with the metabolic activity they serve
    a. Because capillaries are so numerous, blood flows more slowly through them than through larger blood vessels
    b. Slow flow aids the prime mission of the entire cardiovascular system—to keep blood flowing through capillaries so that capillary exchange (movement of substances into and out of capillaries) can occur
    c. Methods of capillary exchange
        (1) Diffusion
        (2) Bulk flow (filtration and resorption)—capillary blood pressure "pushes" fluid out of capillaries into interstitial fluid (filtration); blood colloid osmotic pressure "pulls" fluid into capillaries from interstitial fluid (resorption)
4. Venules—small vessels that emerge from capillaries and merge to form veins; they receive blood from capillaries and empty blood into veins, which return blood to the heart
5. Venous return—volume of blood flowing back to the heart occurs because of the pumping action of the heart, aided by skeletal muscle contractions (skeletal muscle pump) and breathing (respiratory pump).
6. Hormonal regulation of blood pressure—several hormones regulate blood pressure and blood flow by altering cardiac output, changing vascular resistance, or adjusting the total blood volume
    a. Renin-angiotensin-aldosterone (RAA) system—when blood volume or blood flow to the kidneys decreases, certain cells in the kidneys secrete renin into the bloodstream
        (1) Renin and angiotensin together produce the hormone angiotensin II, which raises blood pressure by causing vasoconstriction
        (2) Angiotensin II also stimulates the secretion of aldosterone, which increases resorption of sodium ions (Na^+) and water by the kidneys; water resorption increases the total blood volume, which in turn increases blood pressure
    b. Epinephrine and norepinephrine—in response to sympathetic stimulation, the adrenal medulla releases these hormones, which in turn increase cardiac output by increasing the rate and force of heart contractions; also cause vasoconstriction of arterioles
B. Blood pressure—pressure exerted by blood on the walls of a blood vessel; generated by the contraction of ventricles (see the sections on "Health History Evaluation" in Chapter 15 and "Vital Signs" in Chapter 21)
    1. Blood pressure is highest in the aorta and in the large systemic arteries; it drops progressively as distance from the left ventricle increases
    2. An increase in blood volume increases blood pressure; a decrease in blood volume decreases blood pressure

3. Vascular resistance—the opposition to blood flow because of friction between blood and the walls of blood vessels; depends on the size of the blood vessel lumen, blood viscosity, and total length of the blood vessel
4. Neural regulation—the nervous system regulates blood pressure through negative feedback loops that occur as two types of reflexes, baroreceptor and chemoreceptor
    a. Baroreceptors—neurons sensitive to pressure; send impulses to the cardiovascular center to regulate blood pressure
    b. Chemoreceptors—neurons sensitive to concentrations of O_2, CO_2, and hydrogen ions (H^+); chemoreceptors detect changes in the blood levels of O_2, CO_2, and H^+ and in the veins in skin and abdominal organs
    c. Antidiuretic hormone—produced by the hypothalamus and released from the pituitary gland in response to dehydration or decreased blood volume; also causes vasoconstriction
    d. Atrial natriuretic peptide—released by cells in the atria of the heart; lowers blood pressure by causing vasodilation and by promoting loss of salt and water in urine, which reduces blood volume
5. *Autoregulation* refers to local adjustments of blood flow in response to physical and chemical changes in a tissue
C. Assessing circulation through pulse and blood pressure (see the section on "Health History Evaluation" and Table 15-5 in Chapter 15, and "Pulse, Blood Pressure, and Shock" and Figures 21-1 and 21-2 in Chapter 21)
    1. Pulse—alternative expansion and elastic recoil of an artery with each heartbeat
    2. Blood pressure—pressure exerted by blood on the walls of an artery when the left ventricle undergoes systole and then diastole
    3. Shock—failure of the cardiovascular system to circulate blood adequately or to deliver adequate amounts of O_2 and nutrients to meet the metabolic needs of cells
D. Circulatory route
    1. Systemic circulation—takes oxygenated blood from the left ventricle through the aorta to all parts of the body and returns deoxygenated blood to the right atrium
        a. Parts of the aorta include the ascending aorta, the arch of the aorta, and the descending aorta; each part gives off arteries that branch to supply the whole body
        b. Blood leaving the aorta and traveling through systemic arteries has a bright-red color; as it moves through the capillaries, it loses some of its O_2 and takes on CO_2 so that the blood in systemic veins has a dark-red color
    2. Pulmonary circulation—takes deoxygenated blood from the right ventricle to the air sacs of the lungs and returns oxygenated blood from the air sacs to the left atrium; allows blood to be oxygenated for systemic circulation; deoxygenated blood is returned to the heart through systemic veins; all veins of systemic circulation flow into the superior vena cava, inferior vena cava, or coronary sinus, which empty into the right atrium

3. Hepatic portal circulation—collects deoxygenated blood from the veins of the GI tract and spleen and directs it into the hepatic portal vein of the liver; allows the liver to extract, modify, and detoxify harmful substances in blood; the liver also receives oxygenated blood from the hepatic artery

The Lymphatic and Immune System

The primary purpose of the lymphatic and immune system is to aid in the body's resistance against disease. Primary functions include aborption of fats from the digestive system, transportation of fats and surplus interstitial fluid, and a defense system against attacking microorganisms and disease.

A. Components (Figure 3-28)
   1. Lymph
   2. Lymphatic vessels
   3. Structures and organs that contain lymphatic tissue (specialized reticular tissue containing large numbers of lymphocytes)
   4. Red bone marrow
B. Function
   1. Drains tissue spaces of excess interstitial fluid
   2. Transports dietary lipids (triglycerides, cholesterol, and lipid-soluble vitamins A, D, E, K) from the GI tract to blood

3. With the help of macrophages, protects the body from foreign invasion by microbes and cancer cells
4. The major difference between the interstitial fluid and lymph is location; when fluid bathes tissue cells, it is called *interstitial fluid,* or *intercellular fluid*; when it flows through lymphatic vessels, it is called *lymph*

C. Lymphatic vessels and lymph circulation
   1. Lymphatic vessels—begin as lymphatic capillaries in tissue spaces between cells; have thinner walls and more valves than veins
   2. Lymphatic capillaries—merge to form larger vessels, called *lymphatic vessels,* which ultimately converge into the thoracic duct or the right lymphatic duct
   3. Lymph flows from the interstitial fluid, to lymphatic capillaries, to lymphatic vessels, to lymph trunks, to the thoracic duct or right lymphatic duct, and to the subclavian veins, as a result of skeletal muscle contractions, respiratory movements, and the valves in the lymphatic vessels
      a. The milking action of skeletal muscle contractions compresses lymphatic vessels and forces lymph toward subclavian veins (skeletal muscle pump)
      b. Lymphatic vessels contain valves that ensure the one-way movement of lymph; lymph flow is also

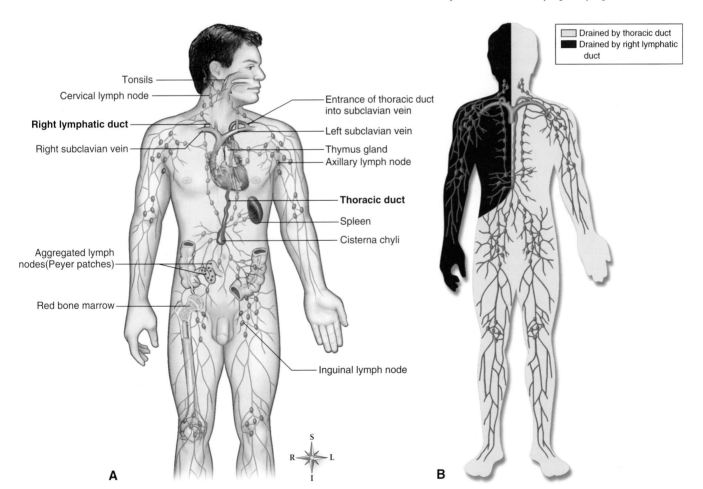

FIG 3-28 Components of the lymphatic system. (From Patton KT, Thibodeau GA, Douglas MM: *Essentials of anatomy and physiology,* St Louis, 2012, Mosby.)

maintained by pressure changes that occur during inhalation (respiratory pump); lymph flows from the abdominal region, where the pressure is higher, toward the thoracic region, where it is lower; when the pressures reverse during exhalation, valves prevent the backflow of lymph

   c. Edema—accumulation of the interstitial fluid in tissue spaces caused by an obstruction such as an infected lymph node, blockage of lymphatic vessels, injury, or inflammation (see the section on "Inflammation" in Chapter 7).

D. Lymphatic organs and tissues (see Table 9-9 and Figures 9-1 and 9-2 in Chapter 9)
  1. Primary lymphatic organs (red bone marrow)—sites where stem cells divide and mature into B cells and T cells
  2. Secondary lymphatic organs and tissues—lymph nodes, spleen, and lymphatic nodules; sites where most immune responses occur
  3. Thymus—a two-lobed organ located posterior to the sternum and medial to the lungs
    a. Site of T cell maturation
    b. Produces hormones
    c. Large in infants; after puberty, much of thymic tissue is replaced by fat and connective tissue; the gland continues to function throughout life
  4. Lymph nodes—approximately 600 bean-shaped organs located along lymphatic vessels; scattered throughout the body, both in superficial and deep locations; usually occur in groups (see the section on "Blood and Lymph" in Chapter 2; "The Lymphatic System" and Figure 4-7 in Chapter 4; and "Extraoral and Intraoral Assessment" and Figure 15-6 in Chapter 15)
    a. Contain B cells that develop into plasma cells, which secrete antibodies, T cells, and macrophages
    b. Function as filters of lymphatic fluid

The Immune System

The immune system comprises a wide variety of body reactions or responses to fight the invasion of pathogens. This is accomplished by detecting pathogens and differentiating them from the body's own healthy tissue. The defense mechanisms are categorized as either nonspecific or specific immunity, providing mechanical and chemical barriers, inflammatory responses, phagocytosis, antibodies, and many other means to protect the body (Figure 3-29; see the section on "Disease Barriers," Tables 9-8 and 9-9, and Figures 9-1 and 9-2 in Chapter 9).

A. Nonspecific (innate) immunity—mechanisms that provide general defense by acting against anything recognized as "not self" or foreign
B. Specific (adaptive) immunity—mechanisms that recognize specific threatening agents

Nonspecific Immunity

A. Species resistance—genetic characteristics of an organism or species that defend against pathogens
B. First line of defense—mechanical and chemical barriers, for example, skin, mucous membranes, sebum, mucus, enzymes, and hydrochloric acid in the stomach

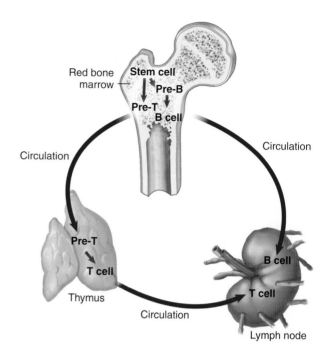

FIG 3-29 Lines of defense. (From Patton KT, Thibodeau GA: *Anthony's textbook of anatomy and physiology,* ed 20, St Louis, 2013, Elsevier.)

C. Second line of defense—inflammation (see Figure 3-29; see the sections on "Inflammation," "Acute Inflammation," and "Chronic Inflammation" in Chapter 7)
  1. Inflammatory response—tissue damage elicits responses to counteract injury and promote normalcy
  2. Phagocytosis—ingestion and destruction of microorganisms or other small particles by phagocytes, for example, neutrophils, macrophages, histiocytes in connective tissue, microglia in the nervous system, and Kupffer cells in the liver
D. Third line of defense—natural killer cells (lymphocytes that kill tumor cells and cells infected by viruses); method of killing cells: lysing cells by damaging plasma membranes
  1. Interferon—protein synthesized and released into the circulation by certain cells if invaded by viruses
  2. Complement—group of enzymes lyse cells when activated by either specific or nonspecific mechanisms

Specific Immunity

A. Specific immunity—part of the third line of defense consisting of lymphocytes; lymphocytes are densest where they develop in bone marrow, thymus gland, lymph nodes, and spleen; lymphocytes flow through the bloodstream, become distributed in tissues, and return to the bloodstream in a continuous recirculation; lymphocytes are named by the CD protein surface markers that the cells carry, for example, CD4 and CD cells (called the CD system)
B. Two classes of lymphocytes—B lymphocytes (B cells) and T lymphocytes (T cells)
  1. B cells—produce antibodies that attack pathogens (antibody-mediated immunity)

2. T cells—attack pathogens more directly (cell-mediated immunity)

B Cells and Antibody-Mediated Immunity See the section on "Disease Barriers" and Figure 9-1 in Chapter 9.

A. B cells develop in two stages:
   1. Pre-B cells develop by a few months of age
   2. The second stage occurs in lymph nodes and the spleen—activation of B cell when it binds to a specific antigen
   3. B cells serve as ancestors to antibody-secreting plasma cells
B. Antibodies—proteins (immunoglobulins) secreted by activated B cell; resist disease first by recognizing foreign abnormal substances
C. Antibody molecule—consists of two heavy and two light polypeptide chains; each molecule has two antigen-binding sites and two complement-binding sites; produces antibody-mediated immunity (humoral immunity) within plasma
D. Classes of immunoglobulin (Ig) (see Table 9-9 in Chapter 9)
   1. IgM—inactive B cells synthesize and insert themselves into their own plasma membranes; predominant class produced after initial contact with an antigen
   2. IgG—makes up 75% of antibodies in blood; predominant antibody of the secondary antibody response
   3. IgA—major class of antibody in external secretions of the mucous membranes, saliva, and tears
   4. IgE—role in immediate hypersensitivity reactions and parasitic infections
   5. IgD—small amount in blood; precise function unknown; thought to activate B cells
E. Complement—component of blood plasma consisting of several protein compounds; serves to kill foreign cells by cytolysis; causes vasodilation and enhances phagocytosis and other functions; complement protein 3 activated without antigen stimulation; produces full complement effect by binding to bacteria or viruses in presence of properdin
F. Clonal selection theory
   1. The human body contains many diverse clones of cells, each committed by its genes to synthesize a different antibody
   2. When an antigen enters the body, it selects the clone whose cells are synthesizing its antibody and stimulates them to proliferate and create more antibodies
   3. The clones selected by antigens consist of lymphocytes and are selected by the shape of antigen receptors on the lymphocyte's plasma membrane

T Cells and Cell-Mediated Immunity See the section on "Disease Barriers" and Figure 9-1 in Chapter 9.

A. T cells—lymphocytes that go through the thymus gland before migrating to the lymph nodes and spleen; function to produce cell-mediated immunity and regulate specific immunity in general
   1. Pre-T cells develop into thymocytes while in the thymus
   2. Thymocytes stream into blood and are carried to the T-dependent zones in the spleen and lymph nodes
B. T cells display antigen receptors on their surface membranes; the T cell is activated when an antigen (presented by a macrophage) binds to its receptors, causing it to divide repeatedly to form a clone of identical sensitized T cells
   1. Sensitized T cells go to the site where the antigen entered, bind to antigens, and release cytokines (lymphokines)
C. Killer T cells—release lymphotoxin to kill cells
D. Helper T cells—regulate the function of B cells
E. Suppressor T cells—suppress B cell differentiation into plasma cells

The Respiratory System

In order to maintain life, the body needs oxygen for metabolic processes. The respiratory system, working with the cardiovascular system, provides oxygen and removal of waste products. Air is filtered and warmed by the respiratory system while providing a mechanism for vocal communication. It aids in homeostasis of circulation, metabolism, electrolyte and water balance, and acidity of the blood.

A. The respiratory system functions as an air distributor and gas exchanger that supplies O_2 and removes CO_2 from cells, and warms, filters, and humidifies air (Figure 3-30)
   1. Alveoli serve as gas exchangers; all other parts of the respiratory system serve as air distributors
   2. Respiratory organs influence speech, homeostasis of body pH, and olfaction
B. Divided into two parts:

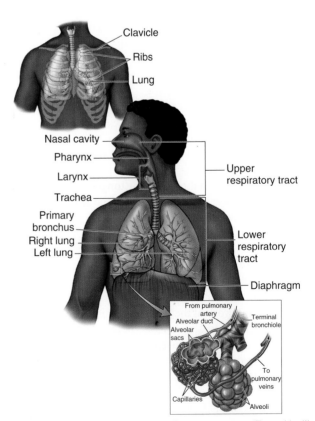

FIG 3-30 Structural plan of the respiratory system. (From Herlihy B: *The human body in health and illness,* ed 5, St Louis, 2015, Elsevier.)

1. Upper respiratory tract—organs located outside of the thorax and consist of the nose, nasopharynx, oropharynx, laryngopharynx, and larynx
2. Lower respiratory tract—organs located within the thorax and consist of the trachea, bronchial tree, and lungs
C. Accessory structures—oral cavity, rib cage, and diaphragm

Upper Respiratory Tract

See the section on "Osteology" in Chapter 4.
A. Nose—passageway for air traveling to and from the lungs; filters air, aids speech, and makes the sense of smell possible
   1. The external portion of the nose consists of a bony and cartilaginous frame covered by skin containing sebaceous glands; two nasal bones meet and are surrounded by frontal bone to form the roof; the floor of the nose is bound by the maxilla
   2. The internal nose (nasal cavity) lies over the roof of the mouth, separated by the palatine bones
      a. Cribriform plate—separates the roof of the nose from the cranial cavity
      b. Septum—separates the nasal cavity into right and left cavities; consists of four structures: the perpendicular plate of the ethmoid bone, the vomer bone, the vomeronasal cartilages, and the septal nasal cartilage
   3. Each nasal cavity is divided into three passageways: superior, middle, and inferior meatus
   4. Anterior nares—external openings to nasal cavities, open into the vestibule
   5. Nasal mucosa—a mucous membrane over which air passes; contains a rich blood supply
      a. Olfactory epithelium—specialized membrane containing many olfactory nerve cells and a rich lymphatic plexus
   6. Paranasal sinuses (see the section on "Paranasal Sinuses" in Chapter 4)
B. Pharynx (throat) (see the section on "Clinical Oral Structures" and Figures 5-1 and Table 5-1 in Chapter 5)
C. Larynx
   1. Located between the root of the tongue and the upper end of the trachea; functions as part of the airway to the lungs and produces the voice
   2. Consists of cartilages attached to each other by muscle; lined by a ciliated mucous membrane that forms two pairs of folds:
      a. Vestibular (false) vocal folds
      b. True vocal cords
   3. The framework of the larynx is formed by nine cartilages:
      a. Single laryngeal cartilages—the three largest cartilages: the thyroid cartilage, the epiglottis, and the cricoid cartilages
      b. Paired laryngeal cartilages—three pairs of smaller cartilages: the arytenoid, corniculate, and cuneiform cartilages
   4. Muscles of the larynx
      a. Intrinsic muscles both insert and originate within the larynx
      b. Extrinsic muscles insert in the larynx but originate on another structure

Lower Respiratory Tract

A. Trachea (windpipe)—extends from the larynx to the primary bronchi; furnishes part of the open airway to the lungs; obstruction causes death
B. Bronchi and alveoli
   1. The lower end of the trachea divides into two primary bronchi (one at the right and one at the left), which continue into each lung and then divide into secondary bronchi that branch into bronchioles, which then divide into alveolar ducts
   2. Alveoli—the primary gas exchange structures
      a. Respiratory membrane—the barrier between which gases are exchanged by alveolar air and blood; consists of the alveolar epithelium, the capillary endothelium, and their joined basement membranes
      b. Surfactant—a component of the fluid coating the respiratory membrane that reduces surface tension
   3. Bronchi and alveoli distribute air to the lung's interior
C. Lungs
   1. Cone-shaped organs extending from the diaphragm to above the clavicles; function in air distribution and gas exchange
      a. Hilum—slit on lung's medial surface, where primary bronchi and pulmonary blood vessels enter
      b. Base—the inferior surface of the lung; rests on the diaphragm
      c. Costal surface—lies against the ribs
      d. Left lung—divided into two lobes (superior and inferior)
      e. Right lung—divided into three lobes (superior, middle, and inferior)
      f. Lobes—further divided into functional units called *bronchopulmonary segments*
         (1) Ten segments in the right lung
         (2) Eight segments in the left lung
D. Thorax
   1. Part of the body between the neck and the abdomen; partially encased by the ribs and containing the heart and lungs
   2. Functions to bring about inspiration and expiration

Respiratory Physiology

The respiratory system includes pulmonary ventilation, gas exchange in the lungs and tissues, transport of gases by blood, and regulation of respiration.
A. Pulmonary ventilation (breathing)
   1. Mechanism
      a. Establishes two gas pressure gradients: in one gradient, the pressure within the alveoli of the lungs is lower than atmospheric pressure to produce inspiration; in the other, the pressure in the alveoli of the lungs is higher than atmospheric pressure to produce expiration
      b. Pressure gradients—established by changes in the size of the thoracic cavity through the contraction and relaxation of muscles
      c. Boyle's law—the volume of gas varies inversely with pressure at a constant temperature (expansion of the thorax results in decreased intrapleural pressure,

leading to a decreased alveolar pressure and causing air to move into the lungs)

2. Two components of respiration:
   a. Inspiration—contraction of the diaphragm produces inspiration; as the diaphragm contracts, the thoracic cavity enlarges; the ability of pulmonary tissues to stretch, which makes inspiration possible, is termed *compliance*
   b. Expiration—a passive process that begins when the inspiratory muscles are relaxed, decreasing the size of the thorax and increasing intrapleural pressure from about -6 mm Hg to a preinspiration level of -4 mm Hg
      (1) The pressure between the parietal and visceral pleurae is always less than atmospheric pressure
      (2) Elastic recoil—tendency of pulmonary tissues to return to a smaller size after having been stretched passively during expiration

3. Pulmonary volumes—amount of air moved in and out and air remaining; important for normal exchange of O_2 and CO_2 to take place
   a. Spirometer—instrument used to measure the volume of air
   b. Tidal volume (TV, V_T)—amount of air exhaled after normal inspiration
   c. Expiratory reserve volume (ERV)—largest volume of additional air that can be forcibly exhaled (normal ERV is 1.0 to 1.2 liters [L])
   d. Inspiratory reserve volume (IRV)—amount of air that can be forcibly inhaled after normal inspiration (normal IRV is 3.3 L)
   e. Residual volume—amount of air that cannot be forcibly exhaled (1.2 L)
   f. Pulmonary capacity—the sum of two or more pulmonary volumes
   g. Vital capacity—the sum of IRV + TV + ERV; depends on many factors, including the size of the thoracic cavity and posture
   h. Minimal volume—amount of air remaining after RV
   i. Functional residual capacity—amount of air at the end of a normal respiration
   j. Total lung capacity—sum of all four lung volumes; the total amount of air a lung can hold
   k. Anatomic dead space—air in passageways that does not participate in gas exchange
   l. Physiologic dead space—anatomic dead space plus the volume of any nonfunctioning alveoli (as in pulmonary disease)
   m. Alveolar ventilation—volume of inspired air that reaches the alveoli; alveoli must be properly ventilated for adequate gas exchange

B. Pulmonary gas exchange
   1. Once pulmonary ventilation (inhaled a breath of air) has occurred and the lungs are filled with air, the second stage of respiration takes place: pulmonary gas exchange occurs in the lungs between the alveoli and the blood; also referred to as "external respiration" because it involves the respiratory processes that have contact with the external environment

   2. Gas exchange in the lungs takes place between alveolar air and blood flowing through lung capillaries
      a. Four factors determine the amount of O_2 that diffuses into blood:
         (1) O_2 pressure gradient between alveolar air and blood
         (2) Total functional surface area of the respiratory membrane
         (3) Respiratory minute volume
         (4) Alveolar ventilation
      b. Structural facts that facilitate O_2 diffusion from alveolar air to blood
         (1) The walls of alveoli and capillaries form only a very thin barrier for gases to cross
         (2) Alveolar and capillary surfaces are large
         (3) Blood is distributed through capillaries in a thin layer so that each red blood cell comes close to alveolar air

C. How blood transports gases
   1. O_2 and CO_2 are transported as solutes and as parts of the molecules of certain chemical compounds
   2. Transport of O_2
      a. Hemoglobin—made up of four polypeptide chains (two α-chains, two β-chains), each with an iron-containing heme group; CO_2 can bind to amino acids in the chains, and O_2 can bind to iron in the heme groups
      b. Oxygenated blood contains about 0.3 mL of dissolved O_2 per 100 mL of blood
      c. Hemoglobin increases the O_2-carrying capacity of blood
      d. O_2 travels in two forms: as dissolved O_2 in plasma (PO_2) and associated with hemoglobin (oxyhemoglobin)
         (1) Increasing blood PO_2 accelerates the association of hemoglobin with O_2
         (2) Oxyhemoglobin carries the majority of the total O_2 transported by blood
   3. Transport of CO_2
      a. A small amount of CO_2 dissolves in plasma and is transported as a solute (10%)
      b. Less than one fourth of blood CO_2 combines with NH_2 (amine) groups of hemoglobin and other proteins to form carbaminohemoglobin (20%)
      c. The association of CO_2 with hemoglobin is accelerated by an increase in blood PO_2
      d. More than two thirds of the CO_2 in plasma is bicarbonate ions (HCO_3^-, 70%)

D. Systemic gas exchange
   1. Gas exchange in tissues takes place between arterial blood flowing through tissue capillaries and cells
      a. O_2 diffuses out of arterial blood because the O_2 pressure gradient favors its outward diffusion
      b. As dissolved O_2 diffuses out of arterial blood, blood PO_2 decreases, which accelerates oxyhemoglobin dissociation to release more O_2 to plasma for diffusion to cells
   2. CO_2 exchange between tissues and blood occurs in the opposite direction from O_2 exchange
      a. Bohr effect—increased PO_2 decreases the affinity between O_2 and hemoglobin
      b. Haldane effect—increased CO_2 loading is caused by a decrease in PO_2

E. Regulation of respiration
  1. Respiratory control centers—main integrators that are located in the brain stem and control the nerves that affect inspiratory and expiratory muscles
    a. Medullary rhythmicity center—generates the basic rhythm of the respiratory cycle
      (1) Consists of two interconnected control centers:
        (a) Inspiratory center, which stimulates inspiration
        (b) Expiratory center, which stimulates expiration
    b. The basic breathing rhythm can be altered by different inputs to the medullary rhythmicity center
      (1) Input from the apneustic center in the pons stimulates the inspiratory center to increase the length and depth of inspiration
      (2) Pneumotaxic center in the pons—inhibits the apneustic center and the inspiratory center to prevent overinflation of the lungs
  2. Factors that influence breathing—sensors from the nervous system provide feedback to the medullary rhythmicity center
    a. Changes in the partial pressure of oxygen (P_{O_2}) and carbon dioxide (P_{CO_2}) and the pH of arterial blood influence the medullary rhythmicity area
      (1) P_{CO_2} acts on the chemoreceptors in the medulla; an increase in P_{CO_2} results in faster breathing; a decrease results in slower breathing
      (2) A decrease in blood pH stimulates the chemoreceptors in the carotid and aortic bodies
      (3) Arterial blood P_{O_2} presumably has little influence if it stays above a certain level
    b. Arterial blood pressure controls breathing through the respiratory pressor reflex mechanism
    c. Hering-Breuer reflexes control respirations by regulating the depth of respirations and the volume of tidal air
    d. The cerebral cortex influences breathing by increasing or decreasing the rate and strength of respirations

The Digestive System

The digestive system is vital in preparing nutrients to be absorbed and utilized by body cells. The chemical and physical alteration of nutrients to aid in absorption is called *digestion*. The digestive system includes the digestive tract and other accessory organs (Figure 3-31).
A. System of organs that breaks down food into molecules small enough for cells to use; the two groups are:

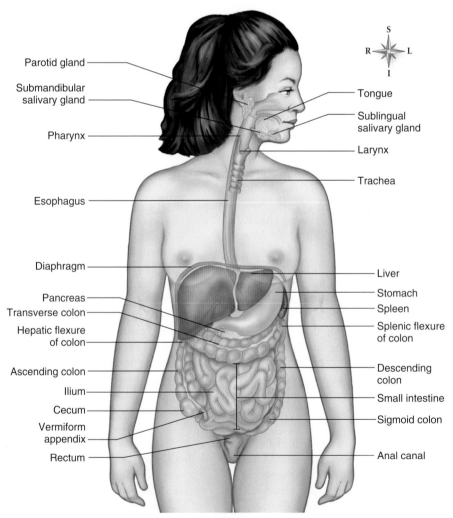

FIG 3-31 Location of digestive organs. (From Patton KT, Thibodeau GA, Douglas MM: *Essentials of anatomy and physiology,* St Louis, 2012, Mosby.)

1. Gastrointestinal tract—continuous tube that extends from the mouth to the anus; organs include the mouth, pharynx, esophagus, stomach, and small and large intestines
2. Accessory digestive organs—teeth, tongue, salivary glands, liver, gallbladder, and pancreas; teeth and tongue only accessory organs that come into direct contact with food

B. Functions
1. Ingestion—taking foods and liquids into mouth
2. Secretion—cells within the walls of the GI tract and accessory organs secrete a total of about 7 L of water, acid, buffers, and enzymes into the lumen of the tract
3. Mixing and propulsion—alternating contraction and relaxation of smooth muscle in the walls of the GI tract mix food and secretions and propel them toward the anus; motility is the ability of the GI tract to mix and move material along its length
4. Digestion—mechanical and chemical processes break down ingested food into small molecules
5. Absorption—entrance of ingested and secreted fluids, ions, and small molecules that are products of digestion into the epithelial cells lining the lumen of the GI tract; absorbed substances pass into blood or lymph and circulate to cells throughout the body
6. Defecation—wastes, indigestible substances, microorganisms, and digested materials that were not absorbed leave the body through the anus; the eliminated material is called feces

C. Organs
1. Mouth
   a. Formed by cheeks, palates, lips, and tongue, which aid mechanical digestion
   b. Fauces—opening from the mouth to the throat
   c. Tongue—composed of skeletal muscle covered with mucous membrane and forms the floor of the oral cavity; superior and lateral surfaces covered with papillae, some of which contain taste buds
   d. Salivary glands empty via ducts into the oral cavity; three pairs of parotid, submandibular, and sublingual glands; secrete saliva that lubricates food and starts the chemical digestion of carbohydrates (salivary amylase begins the digestion of starches in the mouth); salivation is entirely under the control of the nervous system
   e. Teeth—see the sections on "Dental Terminology" and "Dental Anatomy" in Chapter 5.
   f. Mastication—food is chewed, mixed with saliva, and shaped into a bolus
2. Pharynx
   a. Food that is swallowed passes from the mouth into the oropharynx
   b. From the oropharynx, food passes into the laryngopharynx
3. Esophagus
   a. Muscular tube that connects the pharynx to the stomach
   b. Swallowing—moves the bolus from the mouth to the esophagus, which passes the food bolus into the stomach by peristalsis; consists of a voluntary stage, a

pharyngeal stage (involuntary), and an esophageal stage (involuntary)
4. Stomach
   a. Is attached to the esophagus and ends at the pyloric sphincter
   b. Anatomic subdivisions: cardia, fundus, body, and pylorus
   c. Adaptations for digestion include rugae; glands that produce mucus, hydrochloric acid, a protein-digesting enzyme (pepsin), intrinsic factor, and gastrin; and a three-layered muscularis for efficient mechanical movement
   d. Mechanical digestion consists of mixing waves; chemical digestion consists of conversion of proteins into peptides by pepsin; mixing waves and gastric secretions reduce food to chyme
   e. Gastric secretion and motility are regulated by neural and hormonal mechanisms; parasympathetic impulses and gastrin cause the secretion of gastric juices; food in the small intestine, secretin, and cholecystokinin inhibit gastric secretion
   f. Gastric emptying
      (1) Stimulated in response to stretching; gastrin released in response to the presence of certain foods
      (2) Inhibited by reflex action and hormones (secretin and cholecystokinin)
   g. Impermeable to most substances; the stomach can absorb water, certain ions, drugs, and alcohol
5. Pancreas
   a. Connected to the duodenum by the pancreatic duct
   b. Pancreatic islets (islets of Langerhans)—secrete hormones; endocrine portion of the pancreas
   c. Acinar cells—secrete pancreatic juice; exocrine portion of the pancreas
   d. Pancreatic juice—contains enzymes that digest starch, glycogen, and dextrins (pancreatic amylase); proteins (trypsin, chymotrypsin, and carboxypeptidase); triglycerides (pancreatic lipase); and nucleic acids (nucleases)
6. Liver and gallbladder
   a. Liver—has left and right lobes; produces bile
   b. Gallbladder—a sac located in a depression under the liver; stores and concentrates bile

D. Layers of the GI tract
1. Basic arrangement from deep to superficial: mucosa, submucosa, muscularis, and serosa (visceral peritoneum)
2. The mucosa contains extensive patches of lymphatic tissue

The Urinary System

The function of the urinary system is not only to produce urine, but also to balance the composition of blood plasma. The primary organs of the urinary system are the kidneys, which control the homeostasis of water, electrolytes, and pH in body fluids. The accessory organs that aid in the excretion of waste are the ureters, urinary bladder, and urethra.

A. Kidneys—principal organs of the urinary system; accessory organs are ureters, urinary bladder, and urethra

B. Regulates content of blood plasma to maintain the "dynamic constancy," or homeostasis, of the internal fluid environment within normal limits

C. Anatomy of the urinary system—structure
   1. Kidneys (Figure 3-32)
      a. Shape, size, and location
         (1) Roughly oval, with a medial indentation; each kidney approximately $11 \times 7 \times 3$ cm

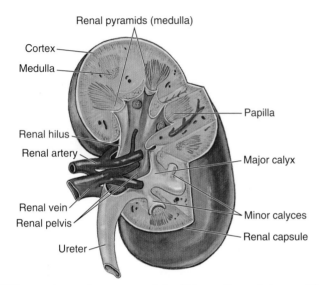

FIG 3-32 Internal structure of the kidney. (From Solomon EP: *Introduction to human anatomy and physiology*, ed 2, St Louis, 2008, Saunders.)

(2) The left kidney is often larger than the right; the right kidney is located slightly lower than the left
(3) The kidneys are located in the retroperitoneal position; lie on either side of the vertebral column between T12 and L3
(4) Superior poles of both kidneys extend above the level of the twelfth rib and the lower edge of the thoracic parietal pleura
(5) The renal fascia anchors the kidneys to surrounding structures; heavy cushion of fat surrounds each kidney
      b. Internal structures of the kidney
         (1) Cortex and medulla
         (2) Renal pyramids: constitute much of the medullary tissue
         (3) Renal columns: where cortical tissue dips into the medulla between the pyramids
         (4) Calyx: cup-like structure at each renal papilla that collects urine; the structures join together to form the renal pelvis
         (5) Renal pelvis: narrows as it exits the kidney to become the ureter
      c. Kidneys are highly vascular
   2. Renal artery: a large branch of the abdominal aorta; brings blood into each kidney (Figure 3-33)
   3. Interlobular arteries—the renal artery branches between the pyramids of the medulla; interlobular arteries extend toward the cortex, arch over the bases of the pyramids, and form arcuate arteries; from arcuate arteries, interlobular arteries penetrate the cortex

FIG 3-33 Circulation of blood through the kidney. (Modified from Applegate E: *The anatomy and physiology learning system*, ed 4, St Louis, 2011, Saunders.)

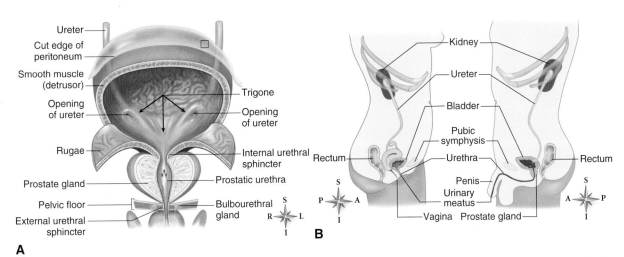

FIG 3-34 Structure and location of the urinary bladder. **A,** Frontal view of a dissected urinary bladder (male) in a fully distended position. **B,** Sagittal view of the female urinary system *(left)* and male urinary system *(right),* each showing a partially distended bladder. (From Patton KT, Thibodeau GA: *Anthony's textbook of anatomy and physiology,* ed 20, St Louis, 2013, Elsevier.)

4. Juxtaglomerular apparatus—located where the afferent arteriole brushes past the distal tubule; important for the maintenance of blood flow homeostasis by reflexively secreting renin when blood pressure in the afferent arteriole drops
5. Ureter—tube running from each kidney to the urinary bladder; composed of three layers: mucous lining, muscular middle layer, and fibrous outer layer
6. Urinary bladder (Figure 3-34)
   a. Collapsible, bag-like structure located behind the symphysis pubis; made mostly of smooth muscle tissue; lining forms rugae; can distend considerably
   b. Functions
      (1) Reservoir for urine before it is voided
      (2) Expels urine from the body with the aid of the urethra
   c. Mechanism for voiding
      (1) Voluntary relaxation of external sphincter muscle
      (2) Reflexive contraction of regions of the detrusor muscle
      (3) Urine forced out of bladder through the urethra
7. Urethra
   a. Small mucous membrane–lined tube; extends from the trigone to the exterior of the body
   b. In the female, lies posterior to the symphysis pubis and anterior to the vagina; approximately 3 cm long
   c. In the male, after leaving the bladder, passes through the prostate gland, where it is joined by two ejaculatory ducts; from the prostate, it extends to the base of the penis and then through the center of the penis and ends as the urinary meatus; approximately 20 cm long; the male urethra is part of the urinary system as well as the reproductive system
D. Microscopic structure of the nephron
   1. Nephrons—microscopic functional units; make up the bulk of the kidney; those located in the renal cortex are called *cortical nephrons*; those near the junction of the cortical and medullary layers are called *juxtamedullary nephrons*; each nephron is made up of various structures
      a. Renal corpuscle
      b. Bowman's capsule—cup-shaped mouth of the nephron
         (1) Formed by parietal and visceral walls, with a space between them
         (2) Pedicles in the visceral layer are packed closely together to form filtration slits; slit diaphragm prevents filtration slits from enlarging under pressure
         (3) Glomerulus—network of fine capillaries in Bowman's capsule; together called *renal corpuscle*; located in the cortex of the kidney
         (4) The basement membrane lies between the glomerulus and Bowman's capsule
         (5) Glomerular-capsular membrane—formed by the glomerular endothelium, the basement membrane, and the visceral layer of Bowman's capsule; function is filtration
      c. Proximal tubule—first part of the renal tubule nearest to Bowman's capsule; follows a winding, convoluted course; also known as *proximal convoluted tubule*
      d. Loop of Henle
         (1) Renal tubule segment just beyond proximal tubule
         (2) Consists of a thin descending limb, a sharp turn, and a thick ascending limb
         (3) Juxtamedullary nephron—a nephron with a loop of Henle that dips far into the medulla
         (4) Cortical nephron—a nephron with a loop of Henle that does not dip into the medulla but remains almost entirely within the cortex; constitutes about 85% of the total number of nephrons
      e. Distal tubule—convoluted tubule beyond the loop of Henle; also known as *distal convoluted tubule*
      f. Collecting duct
         (1) Straight tubule joined by the distal tubules of several nephrons

(2) Joins larger ducts; larger collecting ducts of one renal pyramid converge to form one tube that opens at a renal papilla into a calyx

E. Physiology of the urinary system—the kidneys are important organs with many functions in the body, including producing hormones, absorbing minerals, and filtering blood and producing urine

1. Functions of the kidneys

   a. Waste excretion—the kidneys filter out toxins, excess salts, and urea, a nitrogen-based waste created by cell metabolism

      (1) While filtering waste, kidneys measure out chemicals (e.g., sodium, phosphorus, potassium) and release these back to the blood to return to the body; in this way, kidneys regulate the body's level of these substances

      (2) Urea is synthesized in the liver and transported through the blood to the kidneys for removal

   b. Water level balance—kidneys are key in the production of urine

      (1) The kidneys react to changes in the body's water level throughout the day

      (2) As water intake decreases, the kidneys adjust accordingly and leave water in the body instead of helping to excrete it

   c. Blood pressure regulation—the kidneys need constant pressure to filter the blood

      (1) When it drops too low, the kidneys increase the blood pressure

      (2) One way is by producing a blood vessel–constricting protein (angiotensin) that also signals the body to retain sodium and water

      (3) Both constriction and retention help restore normal blood pressure

   d. Red blood cell regulation—when the kidneys do not receive enough oxygen, they send out a "distress call" in the form of *erythropoietin,* a hormone that stimulates the bone marrow to produce more oxygen-carrying RBCs

   e. Acid regulation—as cells metabolize, they produce acids

      (1) Foods eaten can either increase the acid in the body or neutralize it

      (2) To function properly, the body needs to keep a healthy balance of these chemicals, as is done by the kidneys

   f. Nephron—basic functional unit; forms urine through:

      (1) Filtration—movement of water and protein-free solutes from the plasma in the glomerulus into the capsular space of Bowman's capsule

      (2) Tubular resorption—movement of molecules out of the tubule and into peritubular blood

      (3) Tubular secretion—movement of molecules out of peritubular blood and into the tubule for excretion

2. Filtration—first step in blood processing that occurs in the renal corpuscles

   a. From the blood in glomerular capillaries, about 180 L of water and solutes filter into Bowman's capsule each day; takes place through the glomerular-capsular membrane

   b. Occurs because of the existence of a pressure gradient

   c. Occurs rapidly because of the increased number of fenestrations

   d. Glomerular hydrostatic pressure and filtration are related to systemic blood pressure

3. Tubular reabsorption—second step in urine formation; results from passive and active transport mechanisms from all parts of the renal tubules; major portion of resorption occurs in proximal tubules

   a. Tubular reabsorption in the proximal tubule—most water and solutes are recovered by blood, leaving only a small volume of tubule fluid to move on to the loop of Henle

      (1) Sodium—actively transported out of the tubule fluid and into blood

      (2) Glucose and amino acids—passively transported out of the tubule fluid by means of the sodium co-transport mechanism

      (3) Chloride, phosphate, and bicarbonate ions passively move into blood because of an imbalance of electrical charge

      (4) Water—movement of sodium and chloride into blood causes an osmotic imbalance, moving water passively into blood

      (5) Urea—approximately one half of urea passively moves out of the tubule; the remaining urea moves on to the loop of Henle

   b. Reabsorption in the loop of Henle

      (1) Water is reabsorbed from the tubule fluid, and urea is picked up from the interstitial fluid in the descending limb

      (2) Sodium and chloride are resorbed from the filtrate in the ascending limb, where the reabsorption of salt dilutes the tubule fluid and creates and maintains a high osmotic pressure of the medulla's interstitial fluid

4. Reabsorption in the distal tubules and collecting ducts

   a. The distal tubule resorbs sodium by active transport, but in smaller amounts than in the proximal tubule

   b. ADH—secreted by the posterior pituitary gland; targets the cells of distal tubules and collecting ducts to make them more permeable to water

   c. With the reabsorption of water in the collecting duct, urea concentration of the tubule fluid increases, causing urea to diffuse out of the collecting duct into the medullary interstitial fluid

   d. Urea participates in a countercurrent multiplier mechanism that, along with countercurrent mechanisms of the loop of Henle and the vasa recta, maintains the high osmotic pressure needed to form concentrated urine and avoid dehydration

5. Tubular secretion

   a. Tubular secretion—movement of substances out of blood and into the tubular fluid

   b. The descending limb of the loop of Henle secretes urea by diffusion

   c. Distal and collecting tubules secrete potassium, hydrogen, and ammonium ions

d. Aldosterone—hormone that targets the cells of distal and collecting tubules; causes increased activity of sodium-potassium pumps

e. Secretion of hydrogen ions increases with increased H^+ concentration in blood

6. Regulation of urine volume

a. ADH influences water reabsorption; as water is resorbed, the total volume of urine is reduced by the amount of water removed by the tubules; ADH reduces water loss

b. Aldosterone—secreted by the adrenal cortex; increases the absorption of sodium by the distal tubule, raising the sodium concentration of blood and thus promoting the reabsorption of water

c. Atrial natriuretic peptide—secreted by specialized atrial muscle fibers; promotes the loss of sodium through urine; opposes aldosterone, causing the kidneys to resorb less water and thereby produce more urine

d. Tubuloglomerular feedback mechanism—maintains constant glomerular filtration rate (GFR) by regulating resistance in afferent arterioles; protects kidney GFR function from rapid blood pressure variations; dependent on macula densa cells and the juxtaglomerular apparatus; may influence the renin-angiotensin mechanism

e. Myogenic mechanism—rapid and effective regulation of GFR through changes in the contraction and relaxation of afferent arteriole smooth muscle

f. Related to the total amount of solutes other than sodium excreted in urine; generally, the more solutes present, the higher the volume of urine

7. Urine composition—approximately 95% water with several substances dissolved in it, for example:

a. Nitrogenous wastes—result of protein metabolism; for example, urea, uric acid, ammonia, and creatinine

b. Electrolytes—mainly the ions sodium, potassium, ammonium, chloride, bicarbonate, phosphate, and sulfate; amounts and types of minerals vary with diet and other factors

c. Toxins—during disease, bacterial poisons leave the body in urine

d. Pigments—especially urochromes

e. Hormones—high hormone levels may spill into the filtrate

f. Abnormal constituents such as blood, glucose, albumin, casts, or calculi

The Reproductive System

The primary function of the reproductive system is to produce offspring. Other systems in the endocrine system function to maintain homeostasis, whereas the reproductive system is vital for survival of the species. The primary reproductive organs are the gonads (ovaries and testes), producing gametes (egg or sperm) and hormones. All other organs in the reproductive system are considered secondary and function to nurture and transport the gametes and developing offspring.

Male

A. Testes

1. Two ovoid bodies that lie in the scrotum and are suspended in the inguinal region by the spermatic cord

2. Sperm—formed and stored in the seminiferous tubules of the testes

3. Testosterone—produced in the testes

4. The epididymis is adjacent to the testes in the scrotum

a. Acts as a storage reservoir for sperm along with the seminiferous tubules

b. Sperm may live for as long as 1 month in both the epididymis and the seminiferous tubules

5. If the testes fail to descend during infancy, the condition is referred to as cryptorchidism

B. Vas deferens

1. Conducts sperm from the epididymis to the urethra

2. Acts as a storage site for sperm

C. Urethra

1. Passageway for semen from the vas deferens through the penis

2. Passage for urine from the bladder through the penis

3. Ends at the urinary meatus, which is the opening in the glans penis through which urine and semen are excreted

D. Seminal vesicles

1. Membranous pouches located posterior to the bladder

2. Produce a secretion that contains fructose, amino acids, and mucus

3. Secrete mucoid material into the upper end of the vas deferens

E. Prostate gland

1. Located inferior to the bladder

2. Secretes an alkaline fluid to activate sperm

3. Secretes its milky fluid into the vas deferens

F. Bulbourethral glands (Cowper's glands)

1. Located inferior to the prostate gland

2. Secrete a mucous secretion into the urethra before ejaculation to aid in lubrication

G. Penis

1. Organ of copulation; divided into the shaft and the glans penis

a. Glans penis—most sensitive portion of the penis

b. The foreskin covers the glans penis (removed by circumcision)

2. Erectile tissue (corpus cavernosum) surrounds the penile urethra; causes erection when engorged with blood

H. Sperm

1. Spermatozoa formed in the testes

2. Contains head, neck, body, and tail

a. The head contains the genetic material of the male

b. The tail provides motility through flagellar movement

c. Sperm move through the female genital tract to seek the ovum at a velocity of approximately 1 to 4 mm per minute

3. Spermatogenesis

a. After a spermatogonium has been divided by mitosis for the last time, it increases in size and forms a primary spermatocyte

b. The primary spermatocyte is divided by meiosis to form the secondary spermatocyte, with a haploid number of chromosomes

c. Division of the secondary spermatocytes results in the formation of spermatoids

d. Spermatoids are transformed into motile cells called *spermatozoa*

I. Physiology of ejaculation

1. Erection—stiffening of a flaccid penis
2. Rhythmic peristalsis in the genital ducts during orgasm causes semen to be propelled through the epididymis, vas deferens, seminal ducts, and urethra
3. Semen—a thick, whitish fluid of high viscosity
   a. Between 2.5 and 5 mL are secreted at ejaculation
   b. Each milliliter contains 10 million to 150 million sperm
   c. Sperm usually move at about 3 mm per minute

J. Hormonal influences

1. Hormones are essential to the mechanism of reproduction and to the development and maintenance of secondary sex characteristics
2. The anterior pituitary gland secretes FSH and LH, which cause the growth and function of testes at puberty
3. Secondary sex characteristics in the male (appear during adolescence)
   a. Deepening of voice; widening of the musculature of the chest and shoulders
   b. Growth of facial and body hair

Female

A. Pelvis

1. Wider and shallower than the male's pelvis
2. Shaped like a funnel with a wide mouth
3. Divided into true and false pelvis by the inlet, or brim; the sacral promontory and ileopectineal lines are dividing points between true and false pelvis
4. Forms part of the birth canal
5. The perineum, vagina, muscles, and ligaments form the soft structures of the pelvis
   a. Retain pelvic organs in place
   b. During labor, the direct presenting part of the infant is forward

B. Ovaries

1. Flat, oval-shaped bodies about 2.5 cm long
2. Supported in the pelvis by the broad ligament and suspensory ligament
3. Three types of follicles in the ovaries:
   a. Primordial follicles contain a primary oocyte
      (1) Present at birth
      (2) Follicles complete their first maturation under the influence of FSH
   b. Growing follicles—contain a mature ovum and spaces that contain fluid
   c. Mature follicles—bulge from the surface of the ovary

C. Fallopian tubes (oviducts)

1. Lie in the folds of the broad ligaments
2. Fimbriae (finger-like projections) located at the ovarian ends; the isthmus portion is connected to the uterus

3. Important events occurring in the fallopian tube are fertilization of the ovum by a spermatozoon, segmentation, and formation of the blastocyst

D. Uterus

1. Hollow, pear-shaped organ with thick muscular walls; located behind the bladder and in front of the rectum
2. Divided into three parts:
   a. Fundus—rounded upper part
   b. Body—narrows from the fundus
   c. Cervix—tapering projection
3. Muscular layers
   a. Endometrium—one layer of ciliated columnar cells except for the lower one third of the cervical canal where it changes to stratified squamous epithelium; contains glands and a good blood supply
   b. Myometrium—contains smooth muscle and large blood vessels
   c. Exometrium—contains the pelvic peritoneum
4. Serves as the womb for a developing fetus

E. External genitalia

1. Vagina—female organ of copulation
   a. Passageway for menstrual flow
   b. Connects the uterus to the external surface (vaginal orifice)
   c. Serves as the birth canal
2. Mons pubis—rounded eminence in front of the pubic symphysis
3. Labia majora—two longitudinal folds; protect the inner vulva
4. Labia minora—two smaller inner folds; protect the clitoris
5. Clitoris
   a. Homologue of the penis in the male
   b. Increases in size with sexual stimulation

F. The perineum contains the structures found between the pubic symphysis and the coccyx

G. Mammary glands

1. Composed of compound alveolar glands
2. Secrete milk to the nipples under the influence of lactogenic hormone from the pituitary gland
3. Pigmented circular region (areolae surround the nipple)
4. Active glandular growth occurs during pregnancy to prepare mammary glands to produce milk (lactation)

H. Hormonal cycle

1. Begins at puberty and ends at menopause
2. FSH—secreted by the anterior pituitary gland; activates the primary graafian follicle; maturing follicle produces estrogen; causes the endometrium to become engorged with blood and prepares it to receive the fertilized ovum
3. Both hormones (FSH and estrogen) allow the ovum to mature
4. The mature ovum is released into the fallopian tube by a ruptured graafian follicle; LH assists ovulation; the follicle forms the corpus luteum and secretes progesterone
5. Increased progestogen levels reduce FSH and increase LH; cause the corpus luteum to secrete progesterone
   a. Stimulate the uterus to store glycogen and increase the uterine blood supply

b. The corpus luteum begins to involute as a result of lowered FSH levels

6. Menstrual cycle lasts 21 to 35 days
   a. Menstruation begins if the ovum is not fertilized
   b. If fertilization occurs, the placenta will secrete chorionic gonadotropin to maintain the corpus luteum; estrogens and progesterone continue to be secreted to maintain the rich vascular supply in the endometrium for the developing embryo

SUGGESTED READINGS

Applegate EJ: *The anatomy and physiology learning system,* ed 4, St Louis, 2011, Saunders.

Herlihy B: *The human body in health and illness,* ed 5, St Louis, 2014, Saunders.

Patton KT, Thibodeau GA: *Mosby's handbook of anatomy and physiology,* ed 2, St Louis, 2014, Mosby.

Patton KT, Thibodeau GA, Douglas MM: *Essentials of anatomy and physiology,* St Louis, 2012, Mosby.

CHAPTER 3 REVIEW QUESTIONS

Answers and rationales to chapter review questions are available on this text's accompanying Evolve site. See inside front cover for details.

evolve

1. **Which passive transport process enables the transfer of molecules into cells by a carrier molecule?**
   a. Channel mediated
   b. Facilitated diffusion
   c. Osmosis
   d. Simple diffusion

2. **Which active transport process requires metabolic cell energy to move substances against a concentration gradient?**
   a. Active transport pump
   b. Endocytosis
   c. Exocytosis
   d. Phagocytosis

3. **The dental hygienist created a client treatment plan by dividing the oral cavity at the midsagittal plane, or two dentition quadrants per client appointment (UR, upper right; UL, upper left; LR, lower right; LL, lower left). Which quadrants will be treated at each scheduled appointment?**
   a. Appointment one: UR and LR; Appointment two: UL and LL
   b. Appointment one: LR and LL; Appointment two: UR and UL
   c. Appointment one: UR and LL; Appointment two: UL and LR
   d. Appointment one: all anterior teeth; Appointment two: all posterior teeth

4. **Which epithelial membrane covers body cavities that open to the exterior of the body and are adapted for absorption and secretion?**
   a. Cutaneous
   b. Mucous
   c. Periosteal
   d. Synovial

5. **Which of the following BEST describes the functions of the hypodermis, or subcutaneous layer of the skin?**
   a. Forms ridges that make up fingerprints and footprints
   b. Serves as an attachment for skeletal muscle fibers
   c. Serves as a protection against microorganisms and dehydration
   d. Forms as a connection between the skin and underlying structures

6. **Which one of the following statements is NOT true about cancellous bone?**
   a. Arranged in crisscrossing branches or plates called trabeculae
   b. Provides structure for blood production
   c. Makes up 80% of the body's bone mass
   d. Located in the ends of long bones

7. **Which statement describes the importance and function of osteoblasts?**
   a. Creates bone resorption, allowing the movement of calcium from bone to blood
   b. Widens the bone through internal "sculpting"
   c. Helps in the regulation of blood calcium by increasing calcium levels
   d. Located on the undersurface of periosteum, and deposits bone

8. **Suzy, an RDH, has not maintained good ergonomics during her 20-year professional career as a dental hygienist and is experiencing paresthesias in her right-hand phalanges. This is most likely caused by:**
   a. Constriction of nerves in the carpal tunnel
   b. Constriction of nerves at the acromion process
   c. Constriction of blood supply at the radial tuberosity
   d. Constriction of blood supply at the coronoid process of the ulna

9. **What do the ulna, radius, and humerus have in common?**
   a. Articulate at the glenoid cavity
   b. Are part of the appendicular skeleton
   c. Are bony impressions that form joints
   d. Are distal to the tarsals

10. **Which classification of joints is between the radius and carpal bones?**
    a. Cartilaginous
    b. Fibrous
    c. Syndesmoses
    d. Synovial

11. The muscle action group that serves to stabilize joints is referred to as:
    a. Agonist
    b. Antagonist
    c. Fixator
    d. Synergist
12. Which type of muscle contraction is an example of concentric (isotonic) contraction?
    a. Biceps curl
    b. Setting an object down
    c. Sitting in a chair
    d. Walking down the stairs
13. Which muscle is found in the respiratory tract?
    a. Striated and voluntary
    b. Smooth
    c. Skeletal
    d. Striated and involuntary
14. Which muscle has an origin on the cheek bone and inserts on the corner of the mouth?
    a. Buccinator
    b. Frontalis
    c. Orbicularis oris
    d. Zygomaticus
15. Which muscle group moves the phalanges for the dental hygienist?
    a. Adductor
    b. Flexor and extensor carpi
    c. Flexor and extensor digitorum
    d. Supinator
16. Which nervous system structure has the ability to undergo mitosis, thus making its cells also vulnerable to cancer?
    a. Axon
    b. Dendrite
    c. Neuroglia
    d. Neuron
17. Which of the following is a function of myelin?
    a. Increases the speed of nerve conduction
    b. Transmit impulses away from the spinal cord or brain
    c. Transmit impulses to the spinal cord or brain
    d. Provides impulses toward the cell body
18. The period of time that the neuron is "recovering" from depolarization is referred to as:
    a. Absolute refractory period
    b. Refractory period
    c. Reverse polarization
    d. Salutatory conduction
19. All the following are descriptive of neurotransmitters EXCEPT:
    a. Classified by their function or chemical structure
    b. Facilitate synaptic transmission across the synaptic cleft
    c. Are inactivated by enzymes to prevent prolonged reactions
    d. Allow ions to flow from one cell to another as they are joined together

20. Spinal meningitis is an infection or inflammation of the connective tissue covering that includes all the following layers EXCEPT:
    a. Arachnoid
    b. Cauda equina
    c. Dura mater
    d. Pia mater
21. The area of the cerebrum most responsible for personality and emotional expression is the:
    a. Frontal lobe
    b. Occipital lobe
    c. Parietal lobe
    d. Temporal lobe
22. Which of the following would NOT be a response by the sympathetic nervous system?
    a. Constrict blood vessels
    b. Constrict iris of eye
    c. Dilate bronchial tubes
    d. Increase heart rate
23. The auditory area that extends from the middle ear down to the nasopharynx is called the:
    a. Auricle
    b. Basilar membrane
    c. Eustachian tube
    d. Tympanic membrane
24. All the following describe a steroid hormone EXCEPT:
    a. A mobile receptor in nucleus
    b. Chemical structure is made up of lipids
    c. Response time is 1 hour to several days
    d. Stored in secretory vesicles before release
25. Which *one* of the following is a function of the anterior pituitary gland?
    a. Produces growth hormone
    b. Secretes melatonin
    c. Stores and releases antidiuretic hormone
    d. Stores and releases oxytocin

CASE A

A 32-year-old woman has been diagnosed with hyperthyroidism. Her symptoms include nervousness, weakness, and heart palpitations whenever she tries to exert herself. Recently, she noticed that she even sweats at night.

Use Case A to answer questions 26 to 29.
26. Which of the following is one of the main actions of the thyroid gland?
    a. Increases breakdown of glycogen
    b. Increases heart rate and blood pressure
    c. Increases metabolic rate
    d. Increases sodium resorption and potassium secretion
27. Which of the following is a symptom manifested from high levels of thyroid hormone?
    a. Dry skin
    b. Increased heart rate
    c. Fatigue
    d. Unexplained weight gain

28. Which trophic hormone does the anterior pituitary gland secrete that is essential for the thyroid gland to secrete its hormones?
    a. ACTH
    b. FSH
    c. LH
    d. TSH

29. Which is the function of parathyroid hormone?
    a. Important for the promotion of breast development
    b. Increase the release of calcium into the blood by influencing bone and kidneys
    c. Inhibits the production of large amounts of urine
    d. Stimulates contraction of uterine muscles during labor

30. A dental hygiene client states on his medical history that he is experiencing polyuria and polydipsia. Which of the following hormones could be at decreased levels for this client?
    a. ADH
    b. Gonadotropin
    c. Prolactin
    d. TSH

31. Which blood protein account for 38% of plasma, functioning to transport lipids and antibodies for immunity?
    a. Albumin
    b. Fibrinogen
    c. Globulin
    d. Prothrombin

32. Which chamber of the heart pumps oxygen depleted blood into the lungs?
    a. Left atrium
    b. Left ventricle
    c. Right atrium
    d. Right ventricle

33. Which is the innermost layer of the heart and also lines the valves?
    a. Endocardium
    b. Epicardium
    c. Myocardium
    d. Pericardium

34. During a health history review, the client tells the RDH that she has stenosis of the aortic valve. This means that:
    a. Deoxygenated blood is not reaching the lungs
    b. The left ventricle could have hypertrophy
    c. The client has a diagnosis of mitral valve prolapse
    d. The right atrium is not working effectively

35. The four major factors that affect blood pressure include all the following EXCEPT:
    a. Blood volume
    b. Cardiac output
    c. Peripheral resistance
    d. Pulse points
    e. Viscosity

36. The acquired immunity response that results from a person contracting a disease and then recovering is called:
    a. Active artificial immunity
    b. Active natural immunity

    c. Passive artificial immunity
    d. Passive natural immunity

CASE B

A 23-year-old patient presents for an initial exam and prophylaxis. Her medical history is negative, but during the review, you learn that she is extremely nervous at dental visits and has avoided preventive care since she lived at home as a teenager. She appears anxious, and her vitals are slightly elevated from previous appointments (pulse 90; respiration 20; blood pressure 130/85). Following the assessment, a care plan is discussed, and you begin treatment for moderate gingivitis. During treatment, the patient then complains of not being able to "catch my breath." You recognize that this might be hyperventilation and a potential emergency.

Use Case B to answer questions 37 to 39.

37. During hyperventilation, a patient is breathing faster and deeper, eliminating more carbon dioxide than is produced. This results in respiratory alkalosis, or a decrease in the pH of the circulating blood.
    a. Both statements are TRUE.
    b. Both statements are FALSE.
    c. The first statement is TRUE; the second statement is FALSE.
    d. The first statement is FALSE; the second statement is TRUE.

38. What other physiologic effect(s) can result from the decrease of carbon dioxide?
    a. Reduction of calcium levels in the bloodstream
    b. Vasoconstriction of blood vessels and veins
    c. Reduced cardiac output and coronary blood flow
    d. All the above

39. What is the effect of the diaphragm relaxing during the breathing cycle?
    a. Air is let out of the lungs.
    b. The diaphragm contracts and drops.
    c. The volume of the thoracic cavity increases.
    d. Surfactants cause the alveoli to collapse.

40. A client presents for a dental hygiene appointment. On review of the medical history, the client reports that he frequently experiences dyspnea. This means that he is experiencing:
    a. Frequent urination
    b. Muscle fatigue
    c. Peripheral edema
    d. Shortness of breath

41. What is the function of the blood cell called a basophil?
    a. Phagocytosis
    b. Secretes antibodies
    c. Secretes heparin
    d. Transportation of respiratory gases

42. Which of the following is one of the openings found in the pharynx?
    a. Epiglottis
    b. Eustachian tube
    c. Glottis
    d. Paranasal sinus

43. **Aldosterone is a mineralocorticoid that functions to:**
    a. Support sodium homeostasis of the blood
    b. Break down proteins into amino acids
    c. Give male characteristics
    d. Increase the release of calcium in the blood

44. **Which portion of the small intestine makes up the uppermost division?**
    a. Ascending colon
    b. Duodenum
    c. Fundus
    d. Ileum

45. **Which of the following is NOT a function of the liver?**
    a. Detoxify substances
    b. Secrete bile
    c. Secrete insulin
    d. Store iron

46. **Which organ(s) of the digestive system include the mechanical process of deglutition?**
    a. Colon
    b. Pharynx
    c. Rectum
    d. Small intestine

47. **The structures of a kidney nephron include the following:**
    a. Bowman's capsule, loop of Henle, renal corpuscle
    b. Cortex, medulla, calyx
    c. Juxtaglomerular apparatus, renal artery, urinary bladder
    d. Urethra, Ureter, Interlobular arteries

48. **The three main functions of the kidneys include all the following EXCEPT:**
    a. Digestion
    b. Filtration
    c. Tubular reabsorption
    d. Tubular secretion

49. **Which hormone is secreted by the anterior pituitary gland and influences both male and female reproductive systems?**
    a. Adrenocorticotropin
    b. Follicle-stimulating hormone
    c. Prolactin
    d. Thyroid-stimulating hormone

CASE C

A 62-year-old man presents at an end-of-day appointment for an initial dental exam and prophylaxis. On review of his health history, you learn he is hypertensive with type 2 diabetes. In addition, he suffers from clinical depression. You record his vitals as blood pressure 150/95; pulse 72 beats per minute; and respiration 16 breaths per minute. Further questioning reveals that the patient did not eat lunch today and that he frequently experiences xerostomia.

Use Case C to answer questions 50 to 55.

50. **Which of the following medications taken by the client controls his hypertension?**
    a. Glipizide
    b. Hydrochlorothiazide
    c. Metformin
    d. Sertraline (Zoloft)

51. **Which of the following BEST describes this client's blood pressure?**
    a. Blood pressure rate is considered prehypertensive, and he should be encouraged to see a physician.
    b. Blood pressure rate is considered high, and he should be encouraged to see a physician.
    c. Blood pressure rate is considered too high, and he should not receive dental treatment until seen by a physician.
    d. Blood pressure is within normal limits.

52. **Which statement is TRUE regarding insulin secretion by pancreatic islets?**
    a. If blood glucose level is low, there is a decrease of glucagon secreted.
    b. If blood glucose level is low, there is an increase of insulin secreted.
    c. If blood glucose level is high, there is a decrease of insulin secreted.
    d. If blood glucose level is high, there is a decrease of glucagon secreted.

53. **During the initial exam, the client begins to exhibit unusual nervousness, complaining of blurry vision and a headache. On taking his vitals, you note that his heart rate has increased to 100 beats per minute. You use the glucometer, and his blood glucose is 68 mg/dL. Which statement BEST describes the situation?**
    a. The client's blood glucose is too high; defer elective treatment and refer to physician.
    b. The client's blood glucose is within normal limits; proceed with treatment plan.
    c. The client's blood glucose is too low; defer treatment and give carbohydrates.
    d. The client's blood glucose is within normal limits, but his heart rate needs to be addressed.

54. **Which statement BEST describes oral manifestations of xerostomia?**
    a. An operculum on tooth #17
    b. Raised lesion with a rough surface
    c. The floor of the mouth does not have a "pool" of saliva
    d. White, soft, elevated plaque on the mucosa that can be wiped away

55. **Rapid changes in chair position for this client should be avoided because:**
    a. Antihypertensive medications can produce orthostatic hypotension
    b. It might be disruptive to the patient, causing low blood sugar reactions
    c. The client's blood pressure could be elevated
    d. It may cause the patient to experience hypothyroid conditions

Head and Neck Anatomy and Physiology

Kim T. Isringhausen

For the dental hygienist, knowledge of the skeletal, muscular, circulatory, endocrine, and nervous systems within the head and neck is essential for client assessment and evaluation; radiologic examination and interpretation; identification of sources of infection and pathways of spread; and client referral for abnormal findings. An understanding of the nervous system will facilitate treatment planning and safe and effective delivery of local anesthesia by the dental hygienist.

ANATOMIC NOMENCLATURE

A. All references to body structures are made assuming the body is in anatomic position; *anatomic position* is the erect position of the body, arms at the sides, with head, eyes, and palms facing forward (Figure 4-1)
B. Planes—sections of the body divided by imaginary lines; the body may be sectioned in one of three planes:
   1. Sagittal plane—a vertical plane that passes through the body from front to back; divides the body into right and left regions
      a. Midsagittal or median plane—a sagittal plane passing through the midline of the body from front to back; divides the body into equal right and left sides
   2. Coronal or frontal plane—a vertical plane passing through the body from side to side; divides the body into front (anterior) and back (posterior)
   3. Transverse or horizontal plane—a horizontal plane dividing the body into upper (superior) and lower (inferior) parts
C. Directional terms—used to describe the location of one body structure in relation to another
   1. Anterior or ventral—structures toward or at the front of the body; in front
   2. Posterior or dorsal—structures toward or at the back of the body; behind
   3. Tongue surfaces—the ventral surface of the tongue is the bottom surface, toward the belly; and the dorsal surface of the tongue is the top surface, toward the back when the tongue is upright in the mouth with the tip of the tongue touching the palate
   4. Medial—structures toward or at midline of the body; inner side (e.g., eyes)
   5. Lateral—structures away from the midline of the body; outer side (e.g., ears)
   6. Contralateral—structures on opposite sides of the body
   7. Superficial—structures located toward the body surface
   8. Deep—structures located away from the body surface
   9. Proximal—closer to the point of attachment of a limb to the body trunk; closer to the shoulder or hip (e.g., the elbow is proximal to the wrist)
   10. Distal—farther from the point of attachment of a limb to the body trunk; farther from the shoulder or hip (e.g., the ankle is distal to the knee)
   11. Superior or cranial—structures toward the head; upper
   12. Inferior or caudal—structures away from the head; lower
   13. Apex—the narrow end or tip of a conical structure

OSTEOLOGY

A. Definition—the study of bones
B. Classification—bones are classified on the basis of shape (each shape has a distinct function), pattern of development (membranous, cartilaginous, or mixed), region (axial or appendicular), and structure (arrangement of material, compact or spongy)
C. Function—bone supports organs and structures; protects the soft tissues and organs of the body; enables movement by providing attachments for muscles and ligaments; and is involved in mineral storage and blood cell formation
D. Histology of bone (see the section on "Connective Tissue" in Chapter 2)
   1. Intramembranous ossification—one of two processes resulting in bone formation, no cartilage is present; begins as a fibrous membrane of collagen and blood vessels; osteoblasts form a sponge-like network of bony processes; (e.g., flat bones of the skull)
      a. Osteoblasts—bone-forming cells, form bone tissue; model bone
      b. Osteoclasts—bone-destroying cells, break down bone tissue; resorb bone
      c. Osteocytes—mature bone cell embedded in bone matrix; maintain bone; most abundant cells
   2. Endochondral ossification— one of two processes resulting in bone formation; cartilage is present as a precursor; cartilage is gradually replaced by bone produced by osteoblasts; (e.g., long bones)

FIG 4-1 Anatomic directions and planes of section. **A,** Sagittal. **B,** Frontal. **C,** Transverse. (From Herlihy B: *The human body in health and illness,* ed 5, St Louis, 2015, Elsevier.)

3. Cartilage—noncalcified, avascular, pliable connective tissue; three types of cartilage:
   a. Hyaline cartilage—most abundant, precursor to bone, facilitates smooth movement at joints
   b. Fibrocartilage—strongest, contains collagen fibers in its matrix, provides rigidity (e.g., intervertebral discs)
   c. Elastic cartilage—contains elastic fibers in its matrix; provides support and defines shape (e.g., external ear)
E. Descriptive terminology
   1. Bony prominences—an area where bone is immediately below the skin surface; usually landmarks for the attachment of muscles, ligaments, and tendons; *process* is a general term used to describe any prominence on the bony surface
      a. Condyle—a rounded articular process; forms joints
      b. Tuberosity—a large, rough, rounded process on the surface of bone for the attachment of connective tissue
      c. Tubercle or eminence—a small, rough, rounded process on the surface of bone for the attachment of connective tissue
      d. Arch—a bridge-like bony structure
      e. Cornu (plural, cornua)—a horn-like prominence
      f. Crest—a raised, prominent border or ridge; attachment for connective tissue, usually muscle
      g. Spine—a sharp, slender projection; higher than a crest; often a site for muscle attachment

   2. Bony depressions—on the surface of bones; provide for the passage of blood vessels and other soft tissue
      a. Notch—an indentation at the edge of the bone; an articulatory surface
      b. Sulcus (plural, sulci)—a channel-like, shallow depression or groove that usually accommodates a blood vessel, nerve, or tendon (plural, sulci)
      c. Fossa (plural, fossae)—a deeper depression on a bone surface, basin-like; can be an area for muscle attachment or articulating bone
      d. Sinus—a cavity within a bone
   3. Bony openings—occur primarily where blood vessels and nerves pass into or through the bone
      a. Foramen (plural, foramina)—a short, window-like opening in a bone; round hole (e.g., incisive foramen)
      b. Canal—a longer, tube-like opening in a bone (e.g., mandibular canal)
      c. Meatus—a type of canal or channel within the bone (e.g., internal acoustic meatus)
      d. Fissure—a narrow, slit-like opening between adjacent parts of bones forming a passageway for blood vessels and nerves (e.g., superior orbital fissure)
   4. Skeletal articulations—connections between bones that be movable or immovable
      a. Joints—articulation classified by the amount of movement allowed (e.g., immovable, slightly movable, free);

the temporomandibular joint (TMJ) is the only movable joint in the skull

b. Sutures—fibrous joints found on the skull where bones are held together, immovable

Axial Skeleton: Skull

Bones of the head are grouped into two categories—cranial bones and facial bones.

A. Cranial bones, or neurocranium (eight bones)—bones that surround the brain; four singular bones, two paired bones

1. Frontal bone (single bone) (Figure 4-2)
   a. Forms the forehead and the top portion of the orbits
   b. Contains the frontal sinuses
   c. Supraorbital ridges form the roof of the orbits
   d. Articulates with many of the cranial and facial bones; articulation with the parietal bones forms the coronal suture
   e. Landmarks include the supraorbital notch, the zygomatic process of the frontal bone, and the lacrimal fossa, which contains the tear-producing lacrimal gland

2. Parietal bones (paired bones) (see Figure 4-2)
   a. Constitute a large part of the vault and sides of the cranium

   b. Articulate with each other at the sagittal suture and with various bones to form the coronal, lambdoidal, and squamosal sutures of the skull

3. Temporal bones (paired bones)
   a. Form the lateral walls of the skull
   b. Articulate on each side of the skull with the zygomatic and parietal bones, the sphenoid and occipital bones, and the mandible
   c. Divided into three portions:
      (1) Squamous portion—largest portion; forms the zygomatic process of the temporal bone, which is a portion of the zygomatic arch; the zygomatic process contains the articular (mandibular) fossa and articular eminence, which articulate with the mandible; this area also forms the cranial portion of the TMJ
      (2) Tympanic portion—forms most of the external acoustic meatus; it is separated from the petrous portion by the petrotympanic fissure, through which the chorda tympani nerve emerges
      (3) Petrous portion—located inferiorly; contains the mastoid process that serves as an attachment for the sternocleidomastoid muscle; other landmarks

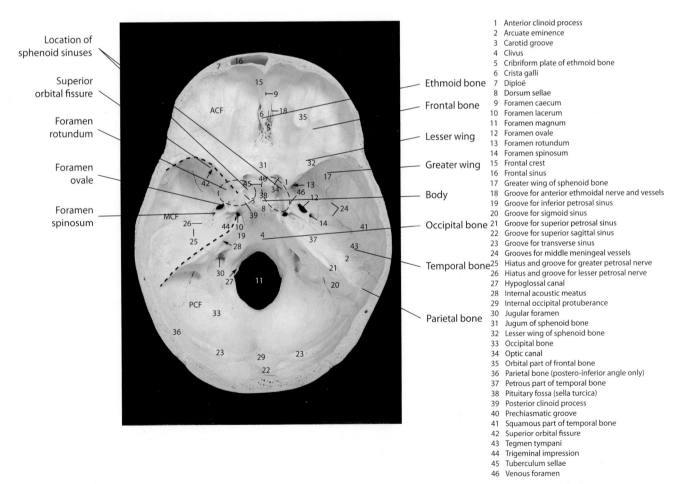

1 Anterior clinoid process
2 Arcuate eminence
3 Carotid groove
4 Clivus
5 Cribriform plate of ethmoid bone
6 Crista galli
7 Diploë
8 Dorsum sellae
9 Foramen caecum
10 Foramen lacerum
11 Foramen magnum
12 Foramen ovale
13 Foramen rotundum
14 Foramen spinosum
15 Frontal crest
16 Frontal sinus
17 Greater wing of sphenoid bone
18 Groove for anterior ethmoidal nerve and vessels
19 Groove for inferior petrosal sinus
20 Groove for sigmoid sinus
21 Groove for superior petrosal sinus
22 Groove for superior sagittal sinus
23 Groove for transverse sinus
24 Grooves for middle meningeal vessels
25 Hiatus and groove for greater petrosal nerve
26 Hiatus and groove for lesser petrosal nerve
27 Hypoglossal canal
28 Internal acoustic meatus
29 Internal occipital protuberance
30 Jugular foramen
31 Jugum of sphenoid bone
32 Lesser wing of sphenoid bone
33 Occipital bone
34 Optic canal
35 Orbital part of frontal bone
36 Parietal bone (postero-inferior angle only)
37 Petrous part of temporal bone
38 Pituitary fossa (sella turcica)
39 Posterior clinoid process
40 Prechiasmatic groove
41 Squamous part of temporal bone
42 Superior orbital fissure
43 Tegmen tympani
44 Trigeminal impression
45 Tuberculum sellae
46 Venous foramen

FIG 4-2 Superior view of the internal surface of the skull. (From Abrahams PH, Marks SC Jr, Hutchings RT: *McMinn's color atlas of human anatomy*, ed 6, St Louis, 2008, Mosby.)

include the styloid process, stylomastoid foramen, jugular notch, and internal acoustic meatus

4. Occipital bone (single bone) (see Figure 4-2)
   a. Forms the posterior portion of the skull
   b. Articulates with the parietal bones to form the lamb-doidal suture and temporal and sphenoid bones
   c. Foramen magnum is formed completely by occipital bone
   d. Jugular notches on both the occipital and the temporal bones form the jugular foramen
   e. Occipital condyles on each side form a movable articulation with the first cervical vertebrae (atlas)
   f. Occipital bone has paired hypoglossal canals that are openings for cranial nerve (CN) XII
5. Sphenoid bone (single bone)
   a. Articulates with the frontal, patietal, ethmoid, temporal, zygomatic, maxillary, palatine, vomer, and occipital bones
   b. Body of the sphenoid bone contains the sphenoid sinuses and the sella turcica, the seat of the pituitary gland, which supplies numerous hormones to the body
   c. Three paired processes: lesser wing of the sphenoid bone, greater wing of the sphenoid bone, and the pterygoid processes
   d. Lesser sphenoid wings—anterior process
      (1) Forms the top of the superior orbital fissure
      (2) Optic foramen—entrance point of CN II
   e. Greater sphenoid wings—lateral projections in the temporal area
      (1) Forms the inferior border of the superior orbital fissure
      (2) Infratemporal crest—union of the temporal and infratemporal surfaces
      (3) Foramen rotundum—maxillary division of CN V
      (4) Foramen ovale—mandibular division of CN V
      (5) Foramen spinosum—opening that gives passage to the middle meningeal artery
      (6) Superior orbital fissure—a cleft between the lesser and greater wings; transmits cranial nerves III, IV, and VI and the ophthalmic division of CN V
   f. Pterygoid process—long process projecting downward from the junction of the body and greater wing of the sphenoid bone; formed by two plates
      (1) Medial and lateral pterygoid plates—attachment points for pterygoid muscles
      (2) Pterygoid fossa—formed by divergence of the medial and lateral pterygoid plates
      (3) Hamulus—inferior termination of the medial pterygoid plate; also provides attachment for a tendon of the soft palate
6. Ethmoid bone (single bone) (see Figure 4-2)
   a. Single midline bone of the skull, anterior to the sphenoid
   b. Articulates with the sphenoid, frontal, lacrimal, and maxillary bones; joins the vomer inferoposteriorly
   c. Contains ethmoid sinuses
   d. Cribriform plate—horizontal plate with numerous openings for passage of olfactory nerves

   e. Crista galli—midline process of the ethmoid bone that serves as an attachment for the dura mater (meninges) of the brain
   f. Perpendicular plate—projects downward from the crista galli, assists in forming the nasal septum
   g. Superior and middle nasal conchae—located laterally in the nasal cavity; part of ethmoidal labyrinth; protect olfactory bulb and buffer sinuses

B. Facial bones, or viscerocranium (14 bones)— surround the face; two singular bones, six paired bones (Figure 4-3)
   1. Inferior nasal conchae (paired bones)
      a. Arise from the maxilla horizontally into the nasal cavity
      b. Responsible for airflow direction, humidification, and heating and filtering of inhaled air
   2. Nasal bones (paired bones) (see Figure 4-3)
      a. Form the bridge of the nose, articulating with each other
      b. Articulate with the maxillae, and the frontal and ethmoid bones
   3. Lacrimal bones (paired bones) (see Figure 4-3)
      a. Thin bones that form part of the medial wall of the orbit of the eye
      b. The nasolacrimal duct is located at the junction of the lacrimal and maxillary bones
      c. Fluid (tears) from the lacrimal gland is drained through this duct into the inferior nasal meatus
   4. Zygomatic bones (paired bones) (see Figure 4-3)
      a. Zygomatic arch (cheekbone)—composed of the temporal process of the zygomatic bone and the zygomatic process of the temporal bone
      b. Three processes are named for the bones with which the zygomatic bones articulate: frontal process, maxillary process, and temporal process
   5. Maxillae (paired bones)—fused; each has a body and four processes (see Figure 4-3)
      a. The body contains the maxillary sinus and forms the lower and medial rims of the orbits and the borders of the nasal cavity; other landmarks are:
         (1) Infraorbital foramen—originates as the inferior orbital fissure and becomes the infraorbital canal that carries the infraorbital nerve, the inferior ophthalmic vein, and the infraorbital artery; it is a landmark for the administration of local anesthesia (infraorbital nerve block) to achieve facial/pulpal anesthesia to the maxillary premolars, canines, and incisors
         (2) Canine fossa—inferior to the infraorbital foramen and distal to the roots of the maxillary canines
      b. The frontal process articulates with the frontal bone, forming the medial orbital rim with the lacrimal bone
      c. The alveolar process (see the section on "Supporting Tissues" in Chapter 2)
         (1) Less dense bone containing the roots of the maxillary teeth; thinner facially; less dense than mandibular alveolar process, making infiltration of local anesthesia more successful; may resorb completely in edentulous arch

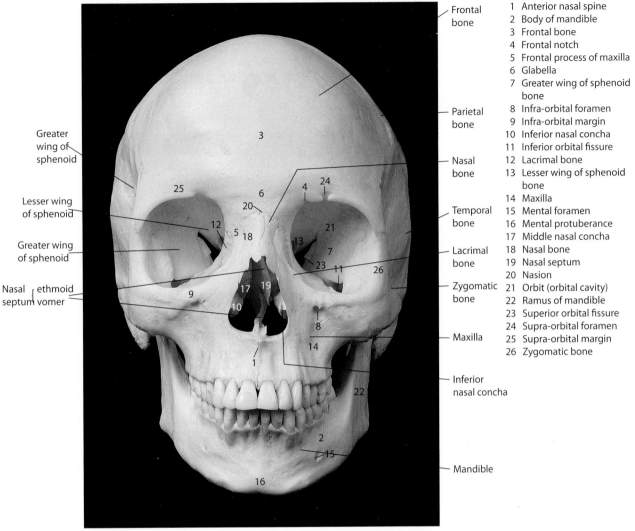

Frontal bone	1 Anterior nasal spine
	2 Body of mandible
	3 Frontal bone
	4 Frontal notch
	5 Frontal process of maxilla
	6 Glabella
	7 Greater wing of sphenoid bone
Parietal bone	8 Infra-orbital foramen
	9 Infra-orbital margin
	10 Inferior nasal concha
	11 Inferior orbital fissure
Nasal bone	12 Lacrimal bone
	13 Lesser wing of sphenoid bone
	14 Maxilla
Temporal bone	15 Mental foramen
	16 Mental protuberance
	17 Middle nasal concha
Lacrimal bone	18 Nasal bone
	19 Nasal septum
	20 Nasion
Zygomatic bone	21 Orbit (orbital cavity)
	22 Ramus of mandible
	23 Superior orbital fissure
	24 Supra-orbital foramen
Maxilla	25 Supra-orbital margin
	26 Zygomatic bone

Greater wing of sphenoid

Lesser wing of sphenoid

Greater wing of sphenoid

Nasal ethmoid septum vomer

Inferior nasal concha

Mandible

FIG 4-3 Anterior view of facial bones. (From Abrahams PH, Marks SC Jr, Hutchings RT: *McMinn's color atlas of human anatomy,* ed 6, St Louis, 2008, Mosby.)

(2) Sockets (alveoli) for maxillary teeth
(3) Canine eminence—a protuberance over the root of the maxillary canine
(4) Maxillary tuberosity— a soft tissue depression distal to the last maxillary molar; contains foramina for the passage of the posterior superior alveolar nerve; it is a landmark for the administration of local anesthesia (posterior superior alveolar nerve block) to achieve buccal/pulpal anesthesia for the maxillary molar teeth
d. Zygomatic process
(1) Articulates with the zygomatic bone
(2) Completes the infraorbital rim
e. Palatine processes
(1) Articulate with each other to form the anterior, major portion of the hard palate and the median palatine suture
(2) Contains the incisive foramen, a landmark for the administration of local anesthesia (nasopalatine nerve block) to the lingual of maxillary canines and incisors

6. Palatine bones (paired bones)
a. The horizontal plates of the palatine bones articulate with each other to form the posterior portion of the hard palate
b. Articulate with the maxillary and sphenoid bones
c. The vertical plates form part of the lateral walls of the nasal cavity and a small part of the orbital apex
d. Contain the greater palatine foramen, located at the apex of the maxillary second or third molar, a landmark for the administration of local anesthetic agent (greater palatine nerve block) to palatal soft tissues distal to the canine
7. Vomer (single bone)
a. Located in the midsagittal line; forms the posterior portion of the nasal septum
8. Mandible (single bone) (see Figure 4-3)
a. Largest, strongest, and only movable facial bone; articulates with the temporal bones on both sides
b. Body—curved, horizontal portion with two surfaces and two borders; landmarks include:
(1) Mental protuberance—the chin

(2) Symphysis—midline, faint ridge formed by fusion

(3) Alveolar process of the mandible—contains roots of mandibular teeth; less dense around mandibular incisors than posterior molars, allowing for improved infiltration of local anesthetic to anterior teeth; may resorb completely in edentulous arch

(4) Sockets (alveoli)—for mandibular teeth

(5) Mental foramen—located bilaterally on the external surface, below and between the first and second premolars; the landmark for the administration of local anesthesia (mental nerve block) to facial periodontium of mandibular premolars and incisors; also important landmark on radiographs, not to be confused with periapical or other lesions

(6) Genial tubercles—near the midline on the internal surface, provide points of muscle attachment

(7) Retromolar triangle—distal to the last mandibular molar

(8) Sublingual and submandibular fossae—shallow depressions on the internal surface, these fossae contain their corresponding salivary glands

c. Ramus—extends vertically and backward from the body of the mandible

(1) External oblique line—a crest on the external surface where the ramus joins the body of the mandible

(2) Mandibular foramen—located bilaterally on the internal surface; forms the opening of the mandibular canal and the exit for blood vessels and the inferior alveolar nerve; the landmark for the administration of local anesthesia (inferior alveolar nerve block) to the lingual periodontium and pulp of mandibular teeth, and the facial periodontium of mandibular anterior and premolar teeth

(3) Condyle—articulates with temporal bone, forming the movable part of the TMJ

(4) Lingula—a sharp bony spine overlapping the mandibular foramen, giving attachment to the sphenomandibular ligament

(5) Coronoid process—the superior margin, which forms the anterior border of the ramus and provides points of muscle attachment

(6) Coronoid notch—greatest concavity on the anterior border of the ramus; landmark for determining height of injection for the inferior alveolar nerve block

(7) Mandibular notch—concave area between the condyle and the coronoid process

C. Neck bones

1. Hyoid bone—U-shaped bone suspended in the neck; located superior and anterior to the thyroid cartilage; paired projections are the greater and lesser cornua for the attachment for many muscles and ligaments of the tongue and throat

2. Atlas—first cervical vertebra; its lateral masses articulate superiorly with the occipital condyles of the skull and inferiorly with the axis

3. Axis—second cervical vertebra; along with the atlas, the axis provides attachment points for many muscles responsible for the movement of the head

PARANASAL SINUSES

A. Air-filled, mucus-lined cavities in the bones of the skull that function to lighten the weight of the skull and act as sound resonators; the four paired sinuses are:

1. Frontal sinuses—frontal bone above the nasal cavity; drain into the middle nasal meatus

2. Sphenoid sinuses—body of sphenoid bone; drain into the superior nasal meatus

3. Ethmoid sinuses—small compartments in ethmoid bone: anterior and middle compartments drain into the middle meatus; posterior compartment drains into the superior meatus of the nasal cavity

4. Maxillary sinuses—largest, pyramid shaped, drain into the middle meatus; infection and diseases of these sinuses can cause complications of the maxillary posterior teeth

THE MUSCULAR SYSTEM

A. Descriptive terminology

1. Muscle tissue, one of the four classifications of body tissue, consists of specialized fibers for contraction; three types of muscle tissue are skeletal (voluntary), cardiac (involuntary), and smooth (involuntary); muscles in the head and neck region are skeletal muscles

2. Movement—muscles are under neural control to shorten or contract; contraction is the action of the muscle fibers

3. Origin—origin of a muscle is bone; less movable structure (e.g., sternocleidomastoid muscle originates on the clavicle and sternum)

4. Insertion—the structure muscle attaches to and tends to be moved by the contraction of the muscle (e.g., tendon); more movable structure; during muscle contraction the insertion moves toward the origin (e.g., sternocleidomastoid muscle inserts on the mastoid process of the temporal bone; when contracted, the head bends to the side)

B. Muscles of facial expression—most facial muscles are superficial, paired muscles originating in bone and inserting into skin; responsible for functions related to speech, emotional expression, and mastication; innervated by the seventh cranial, or facial, nerve; damage to this nerve results in facial paralysis

1. Epicranial muscle—scalp region; composed of two bellies, the frontal and occipital, which are connected by the epicranial aponeurosis; raise the eyebrows and scalp when a person shows surprise

2. Orbicularis oculi muscle—surrounds the eye; closes the eyelid

3. Corrugator supercilii muscle—superior to the orbicularis; wrinkles the forehead when a person frowns

4. Orbicularis oris muscle—encircles the mouth; closes lips

5. Buccinator muscle—anterior part of the cheek; functions to pull the mouth laterally, thereby shortening

the cheek, and as an aid in keeping food on the chewing surfaces of the teeth

6. Risorius muscle—mouth region; widens mouth when a person smiles broadly
7. Levator labii superioris muscle—upper lip; raises the upper lip
8. Levator labii superioris alaeque nasi muscle—upper lip; raises the upper lip and dilates the nose, as in sneering
9. Zygomaticus minor muscle—upper lip; raises the upper lip
10. Zygomaticus major muscle—angle of the upper lip; pulls the angle of the upper lip laterally, creating the appearance of a smile
11. Levator anguli oris muscle—angle of the mouth; elevates the angle of the mouth, as in smiling
12. Depressor anguli oris muscle—angle of the mouth; depresses the angle of the mouth, as when frowning
13. Depressor labii inferioris muscle—lower lip; lowers the lower lip to expose lower mandibular incisors
14. Mentalis muscle—chin area; raises the chin, narrows the vestibule near mandibular incisors
15. Platysma muscle—neck region; originates in the clavicle fascia and inserts in the region of the mandible and facial muscles of the mouth; pulls down the corners of the mouth, raises the skin of the neck

C. Muscles of mastication—four paired muscles, all inserting on the mandible; innervated by the mandibular division of the fifth cranial, or trigeminal, nerve; they are responsible for movement of the jaw: depression, elevation, protrusion, retraction, and lateral deviation
1. Masseter muscle—most superficial, largest, and strongest of the four muscles
    a. Originates on the zygomatic arch; originates from two heads, one superficial and one deep, and inserts on the lateral surface of the angle of the mandible
    b. Action—elevates the mandible, raising the lower jaw during closing
2. Temporalis muscle
    a. Originates from a fan-like attachment on the temporal fossa; inserts on the coronoid process of the mandible
    b. Action—when the entire muscle contracts, it elevates the mandible, raising the jaw; contraction of only the posterior portion causes retraction of the mandible
3. Medial (internal) pterygoid muscle (Figure 4-4)
    a. Originates from the pterygoid fossa; inserts on the medial surface of the angle of the mandible
    b. Action—elevates the mandible, raising the lower jaw
4. Lateral (external) pterygoid muscle; lies within the infratemporal fossa (see Figure 4-4)
    a. Originates from two heads: the superior head originates from the greater wing of the sphenoid bone; the inferior head originates from the lateral pterygoid plate of the sphenoid bone; both heads unite, passing posteriorly to insert on the anterior neck of the mandibular condyle at the pterygoid fovea
    b. Action—both heads working together protrude the mandible, which occurs during opening; when only

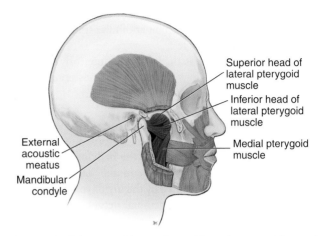

FIG 4-4 Medial pterygoid muscle and lateral pterygoid muscle with both heads of each muscle highlighted (inferior part of temporalis muscle, zygomatic arch, and most of the mandibular ramis have been removed). (From Fehrenbach MJ, Herring SW: *Illustrated anatomy of the head and neck*, ed 5, St Louis, 2017, Elsevier.)

one side is contracted, the jaw shifts to the opposite side, causing lateral deviation of the mandible; lateral pterygoid is the only muscle of mastication that depresses the mandible

D. Cervical muscles—superficial, paired, large, easily palpated muscles, both innervated by CN XI (accessory nerve)
1. Sternocleidomastoid muscle—large, well-defined muscle; important landmark for palpating lymph nodes
    a. Originates from the clavicle and sternum; inserts on the mastoid processes of the temporal bone
    b. Action—contraction of one side makes the head bend to the same side, turning the face to the opposite side; contraction of both muscles causes the head to flex forward
    c. Innervated by CN XI (accessory nerve)
2. Trapezius muscle—broad, superficial muscles covering lateral and posterior surfaces of the neck
    a. Originates from the occipital bone and the cervical and thoracic vertebrae; inserts on the clavicle and the scapula
    b. Action—lifts the clavicle and scapula, as when shrugging shoulders
    c. Innervated by CN XI (accessory nerve) and third and fourth cervical nerves

E. Hyoid muscles—all are attached to the hyoid bone; usually grouped as suprahyoid or infrahyoid muscles, depending on their relationship to the hyoid; aid in mastication and swallowing
1. Suprahyoid muscle group—located superior to the hyoid; act to raise the hyoid and the larynx during swallowing and depress the mandible during mastication
    a. Digastric muscle
        (1) Two separate bellies—anterior belly originates from the intermediate tendon on the hyoid bone and inserts near the symphysis of the mandible; posterior belly originates from the mastoid notch

and inserts on the intermediate tendon of the hyoid; form the submandibular triangles and submental triangle

    (2) Action—pulls the jaw back; anteriorly innervated by the mylohyoid nerve and posteriorly by the posterior digastric nerve

  b. Mylohyoid muscle

    (1) Originates from the inner surface of the mandible; unites with counterpart to form the floor of the mouth, and inserts on the body of the hyoid

    (2) Action—depresses mandible, helps elevate the tongue; innervated by the mylohyoid nerve, a division of CN V (trigeminal nerve)

  c. Stylohyoid muscle

    (1) Originates from the styloid process; inserts on the body of the hyoid; innervated by the stylohyoid branch of the seventh cranial, or facial, nerve

  d. Geniohyoid muscle

    (1) Originates from the genial tubercles on the mandible; inserts into the body of the hyoid

    (2) Innervated by CN XII (hypoglossal nerve)

2. Infrahyoid muscle group—act to depress the hyoid bone; all muscles in the group innervated by the second and third cervical nerves

  a. Sternothyroid muscle

    (1) Originates on the sternum; inserts on the thyroid cartilage

    (2) Depresses the thyroid cartilage and the larynx (but not the hyoid)

  b. Sternohyoid muscle

    (1) Originates on the sternum; inserts on the body of the hyoid

  c. Omohyoid muscle

    (1) Two separate bellies—inferior belly originates from the scapula and attaches to the tendon of the superior belly, which is the origin of the superior belly that inserts on the body of the hyoid

  d. Thyrohyoid muscle

    (1) Originates on the thyroid cartilage; inserts on the body and greater cornu of the hyoid

    (2) Raises the thyroid cartilage and larynx in addition to depressing the hyoid

F. Muscles of the tongue—all are innervated by CN XII (hypoglossal nerve); aid in speech, mastication, and swallowing; grouped into intrinsic and extrinsic muscles

1. Intrinsic tongue muscles

  a. Located entirely within the tongue; include the superior longitudinal, transverse, vertical, and inferior longitudinal muscles; considered by some to be one muscle; act together to change the shape of the tongue

2. Extrinsic tongue muscles

  a. All insert inside the tongue but originate elsewhere; their names indicate their origin; these muscles move the tongue

    (1) Genioglossus muscle—acts in the protrusion of the tongue, helps prevent airway obstruction; originates from the genial tubercles

    (2) Styloglossus muscle—acts in the retraction of the tongue; originates from the styloid process of the temporal bone

    (3) Hyoglossus muscle—depresses the tongue; originates on areas of the hyoid bone

TEMPOROMANDIBULAR JOINT

A. Description—a bilateral articulation between the articular fossa of the temporal bones (immovable) and condylar process of the mandible (movable); innervated by the mandibular division of the fifth cranial, or trigeminal, nerve; blood supply comes from the external carotid artery

B. Type of joint—a synovial joint by structure

C. Type of movement—gliding in the upper synovial cavities, rotating in the lower synovial cavities; the action allows for functions of speech and mastication

D. Structure of joint (Figure 4-5)

1. Articular (joint) capsule—completely surrounds the TMJ

2. Articular (joint) disc—a fibrous disc that divides the synovial cavity of the TMJ into superior and inferior synovial cavities; both cavities are filled with synovial fluid secreted by the articular capsule; perforation or displacement can cause TMJ problems

3. Temporomandibular joint ligament—located laterally on each joint, extending from the zygomatic arch to the posterior neck of the condyle; prevents posterior and inferior displacement of the mandible

4. Sphenomandibular ligament—located medially; extends from the spine of the sphenoid to the lingula of the mandible; the inferior alveolar nerve is located in the space between the mandibular ramus and the sphenomandibular ligament, making it an important landmark for the administration the inferior alveolar nerve block

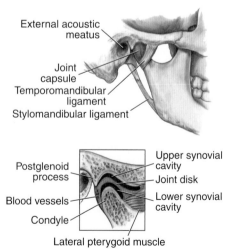

FIG 4-5 View of the temporomandibular joint depicting upper and lower synovial cavities and the joint disk. (From Avery JK, Chiego DJ: *Essentials of oral histology and embryology: a clinical approach*, ed 3, St Louis, 2006, Mosby.)

5. Stylomandibular ligament—located medially; runs from the styloid process of the temporal bone to the angle of the mandible; also assists in stabilizing the jaw; separates the submandibular salivary and parotid glands

THE CIRCULATORY SYSTEM

A. Classification and function
   1. Blood is classified as connective tissue and consists of two main components, plasma and formed elements (blood cells and platelets)
   2. Three main functions of blood:
      a. Transportation—transports gases (oxygen and carbon dioxide), nutrients, waste products of metabolism, hormones, and heat to the skin for maintenance of body temperature
      b. Regulation—sustains the pH of the body; maintains fluid balance
      c. Protection—defends the body against infections and blood loss
B. Four components of blood (see the section on "Blood and Lymph" in Chapter 2)
   1. Plasma—liquid portion of blood; consists of 90% water, the remaining mixture comprises proteins, glucose, hormones, and electrolytes; makes up more than half the total volume of blood
   2. Erythrocytes—red blood cells (RBCs) lack nuclei and have a biconcave shape; produce hemoglobin, which functions to transport oxygen (O_2) from the lungs to body tissues in exchange for carbon dioxide (CO_2); then delivered to the lungs
   3. Leukocytes—white blood cells (WBCs); much less numerous than RBCs; protect the body against infections
      a. Granulocytes—contain granules in their cytoplasm
         (1) Neutrophils are the first to respond to bacterial invasion; fight infection by the digesting bacteria (phagocytosis) and releasing enzymes that destroy bacteria; make up the majority of leukocytes
         (2) Eosinophils function in the destruction of allergens and release enzymes that destroy parasites
         (3) Basophils secrete histamine and heparin in allergic reactions, intensifying inflammatory reactions
      b. Agranulocytes—lack granules in their cytoplasm
         (1) Lymphocytes produce antibodies and provide immune response; second most abundant leukocyte
         (2) Monocytes reach sites of infection after neutrophils and can phagocytize more microbes than neutrophils; clean up cellular debris after an infection
   4. Platelets—thrombocytes; cell fragments that participate in blood clotting
C. Vascular system
   1. Arteries carry blood, typically oxygenated, away from the heart to arterioles and capillaries, which supply blood directly to the tissue
   2. Venules (smaller veins that drain capillaries) and veins carry blood, typically deoxygenated, to the heart

3. Arteries supply blood to all structures in their surrounding vicinity, and veins drain blood from all their regional structures
D. Descriptive terminology
   1. Anastomosis—connection between vessels by channels
   2. Arteriole—smaller artery that connects with a capillary
   3. Capillary—smaller blood vessel branching off an arteriole to supply blood directly to tissue
   4. Plexus—a congregation of multiple veins
   5. Venous sinus—blood-filled space between two layers of tissue
E. Arterial blood supply to the head and neck
   1. Common carotid and subclavian arteries supply the head and neck; pathways from the aorta to the head and neck differ on the right and left sides:
      a. Right side of the body—the right common carotid and right subclavian arteries arise from the brachiocephalic artery
      b. Left side of the body—the left common carotid and left subclavian arteries ascend directly from the aorta
      c. The subclavian artery terminates in the upper arm extremity
   2. Each common carotid artery ends by dividing into the internal carotid and external carotid arteries
      a. Internal carotid artery—enters the skull to the brain area
      b. External carotid artery—supplies the principal areas of the oral cavity and face
      c. Carotid sinus—just before the common carotid artery bifurcates; a swelling; most reliable arterial pulse in the body
   3. Anterior branches of the external carotid artery (Figure 4-6)
      a. Lingual artery—runs above the hyoid bone; supplies the floor of the mouth, the tongue, and the suprahyoid muscles; gives rise to the sublingual artery, which supplies the mylohyoid muscle, sublingual salivary gland, and mucous membranes of the floor of the mouth
      b. Facial artery—complicated path that runs over the submandibular gland, crossing the lower border of the mandible laterally, anterosuperioly near the angle of the mouth and alongside the nose terminating near the eye; supplies the muscles of the face in the oral, buccal, nasal, infraorbital, and orbital regions; branches from the facial artery are:
         (1) Ascending palatine artery—supplies the soft palate, palatine muscles, and palatine tonsils
         (2) Submental artery—supplies the submandibular lymph nodes, the submandibular salivary gland, and mylohyoid and digastric muscles
         (3) Inferior labial artery—supplies lower lip muscles of facial expression
         (4) Superior labial artery—supplies the upper lip tissues
   4. Medial branch of the external carotid artery
      a. Ascending pharyngeal artery—supplies the pharyngeal walls, where they form an anastomosis with the ascending palatine artery; supplies the soft palate and meninges of the brain

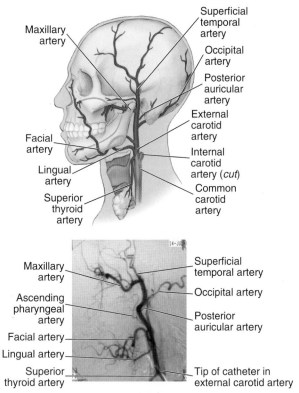

FIG 4-6 Carotid vasculature. Note the arteries branching from the external carotid artery. (From Reynolds PA, Abrahams PH: *McMinn's interactive clinical anatomy: head and neck,* ed 2, London, 2001, Mosby Ltd.)

5. Posterior branch of the external carotid artery
   a. Occipital artery—supplies the suprahyoid and sterno-cleidomastoid muscles as well as the scalp and meningeal tissue of this region
   b. Posterior auricular artery—supplies the inner ear and mastoid air cells
6. Terminal branches of the external carotid artery
   a. Superficial temporal artery—gives rise to smaller arteries supplying the temporalis muscle, the parotid salivary gland duct, and the scalp in the frontal and parietal regions
   b. Maxillary artery—three parts:
      (1) The first diverges from the external carotid artery near the neck of the condyle in the parotid gland; the second runs between the mandible and the sphenomandibular ligament anteriorly and through the infratemporal fossa superiorly; within the infratemporal fossa, this part of the maxillary artery gives off many branches:
         (a) Inferior alveolar artery—enters the mandibular canal by way of the mandibular foramen, along with the inferior alveolar nerve; supplies the mandibular teeth and the floor of the mouth and diverges into three branches
         (b) Mylohyoid artery—travels in mylohyoid groove; supplies the mylohyoid muscle and the floor of the mouth

(c) Mental artery—exits the mandibular canal by the mental foramen; supplies the chin region; forms an anastomosis with the inferior labial artery
(d) Incisive artery—remains in the mandibular canal, dividing into branches that supply the teeth, periodontium, and gingiva of the anterior mandibular region
(2) The second part of the maxillary artery also has muscle branches:
   (a) Deep temporal artery—supplies the temporalis muscle
   (b) Pterygoid artery—supplies the lateral and medial pterygoid muscles
   (c) Masseteric artery—supplies the masseter muscle
   (d) Buccal artery—supplies the buccinator muscle and buccal region
(3) After traversing the infratemporal fossa, the maxillary artery enters the pterygopalatine fossa as the third part:
   (a) Posterior superior alveolar artery—exits the infratemporal fossa and descends into the maxillary tuberosity; supplies the maxillary posterior teeth and periodontium and maxillary sinus
   (b) Infraorbital artery—branches off the maxillary artery in the pterygopalatine fossa; travels through the inferior orbital fissure, enters the infraorbital canal, giving off branches to the orbit, and then branches off as the anterior superior alveolar artery; it travels through the infraorbital foramen, exiting on the face
   (c) Anterior superior alveolar artery—travels down the maxillary sinus to supply the anterior maxillary teeth and the periodontium; forms an anastomosis with the posterior superior alveolar artery
   (d) Greater palatine and lesser palatine arteries—travel to the palate through the pterygopalatine canal and the greater and lesser foramina, supplying the hard and soft palates

F. Venous drainage of the head and neck
   1. Generalizations—the venous system originates as small venules, which become larger veins in the neck region that carry blood back to the heart; veins anastomose freely with one another; veins lack one-way valves, which would prevent backflow, they are easily involved in the spread of infections
   2. Internal and external jugular veins
      a. Internal jugular vein—drains the brain and most tissue of the head and neck
      b. External jugular vein—drains a small portion of extracranial tissue
   3. Facial vein—drains into the internal jugular vein
      a. Drains the veins from the tissues of the frontal region and orbit of the eye; communicates with the cavernous

venous sinus, which may become fatally infected through spread of dental infection

   b. Drains the veins of the lower lip, chin, and submandibular region

   c. Variations of the facial vein drain the tongue and floor of the mouth; sometimes drain indirectly into the facial vein or directly into the internal jugular vein

4. Retromandibular vein—formed by the superficial temporal and maxillary veins

   a. Posterior division—drains the temporal, maxillary, and posterior auricular areas and joins the external jugular vein

   b. Anterior division—joins the facial vein

5. Maxillary vein—originates in the infratemporal fossa; drains the pterygoid plexus, which drains the veins from the area served by the maxillary artery, such as the middle meninges, oral cavity, nose, and palate

6. Pterygoid plexus of veins—collection of vessels that form anastomoses with the facial and retromandibular veins located in the infratemporal fossa

   a. Drains portions of the face into the maxillary vein

   b. Drains the meninges of the brain

   c. Surrounds and protects the maxillary artery

   d. Can be pierced during the administration of a local anesthetic agent

   e. Can be involved in the spread of dental infections during improper administration of local anesthetic agent

7. External and internal jugular veins on both sides of the neck merge with the subclavian veins to form the brachiocephalic veins, which then drain into the superior vena cava, directly to the heart

THE LYMPHATIC SYSTEM

A. Function—part of the circulatory system; primary function is to help fight disease through ridding the body of toxins (Figure 4-7).

B. Descriptive terminology (see the section on "Blood and Lymph" in Chapter 2)

   1. Lymph—tissue fluid that drains into lymphatic vessels from surrounding regions

   2. Lymphatic vessels—a system of structures paralleling blood vessels that transport fluid (lymph) away from tissues; only carries fluid one direction, away

   3. Lymph nodes—oval shaped organs of lymphatic system clustered along connecting lymphatic vessels; contain lymphocytes that filter toxins from lymph; not visible or palpable during extraoral examination in a healthy patient

   4. Lymphadenopathy—an increase in size or consistency of lymphoid tissue; allows lymph node to be visualized and palpated; can indicate infection or disease

   5. Tonsils—masses of lymphoid tissue located in the oral cavity and pharynx, remove toxins

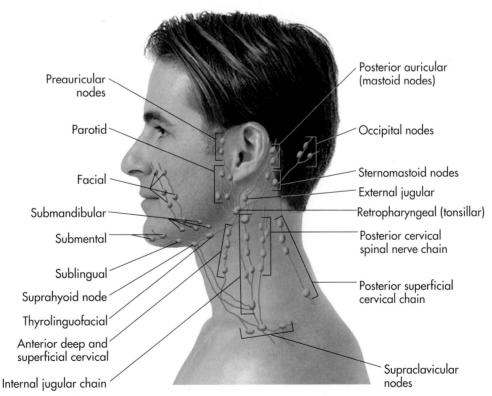

FIG 4-7 The lymphatic drainage system of the head and neck. If the group of nodes is often referred to by another name, the second name appears in parentheses. (From Ball JW, et al: *Seidel's guide to physical examination*, ed 8, St Louis, 2015, Elsevier.)

C. Superficial cervical lymph nodes
   1. Submental nodes
      a. Located beneath the chin near the midline
      b. Drain the chin, lower lip, floor of the mouth, mandibular incisors, and the apex of the tongue
      c. Empty into the submandibular nodes or superior deep cervical nodes
   2. Submandibular nodes
      a. Located along the inferior border of the mandible superficial to the submandibular gland
      b. Drain the cheek, upper, lip, anterior portion of the hard palate, the body of the tongue, and all teeth except maxillary third molars and mandibular incisors
      c. Empty into the superior deep cervical nodes
D. Deep cervical lymph nodes
   1. Superior deep cervical nodes
      a. Located deep beneath the sternocleidomastoid muscle, 2 inches (5 cm) below the ear
      b. Primary nodes for the drainage of the posterior nasal cavity, posterior hard palate, base of tongue, and maxillary third molars
      c. The jugulodigastric lymph node in this area is easily palpable in clients with tonsillar lymphadenopathy
      d. Empty into the inferior deep cervical nodes or directly into the jugular trunk
   2. Inferior deep cervical nodes
      a. Continuation of the superior deep cervical nodes, two inches above the clavicle
      b. Primary nodes for the drainage of the posterior part of the scalp and neck as well as part of the arm
      c. The inferior deep cervical node also communicate with the axillary lymph nodes, which can become involved in breast cancer
      d. Empty into the jugular trunk
E. Superficial lymph nodes of the head
   1. Occipital nodes
      a. Located in the occipital region on the posterior head; drain the occipital portion of the scalp
      b. Empty into the deep cervical nodes
   2. Three groups of nodes drain the external ear and lacrimal gland; all empty into the deep cervical nodes:
      a. Retroauricular nodes—located posterior to the ear; also drain adjacent region
      b. Anterior auricular nodes—located anterior to the ear; also drain adjacent region
      c. Superficial parotid nodes—located on the surface of the parotid gland; also drain adjacent region
   3. Facial nodes
      a. Located along the facial vein; subgroups include buccal and mandibular; all drain the skin where they are located
      b. Infections from teeth may cause lymphadenopathy, described as being "firm like a pea"
      c. Drain into submandibular nodes, which empty into deep cervical nodes
F. Deep lymph nodes of the head—all located too deep for palpation; include deep parotid and retropharyngeal nodes

G. Tonsils—not located along lymphatic vessels; drain into the superior deep cervical nodes
   1. Palatine tonsils—located between the anterior and posterior pillars, commonly referred to as "tonsils"
   2. Lingual tonsils—located on the dorsal surface of the base of the tongue
   3. Pharyngeal tonsils—located on the midline of the posterior wall of the nasopharynx, commonly referred to as "adenoids," enlarged in children
   4. Tubal tonsils—located in the nasopharynx, posterior to the openings of the auditory tube

GLANDS OF THE HEAD AND NECK REGION

A. General definition—a *gland* is an organ that secretes chemical substances for use in normal body functioning; two main types of glands:
   1. Exocrine glands—have ducts; empty directly to a body location where secretions will be used (e.g., salivary glands)
   2. Endocrine glands—have no ducts; empty directly into the circulatory system, which transports secretions to the region to be used (e.g., thyroid gland)
B. Exocrine glands of the head
   1. Major salivary glands—paired glands, have named ducts
      a. Parotid salivary gland—located on the surface of the masseter muscle behind the ramus of the mandible, anterior and inferior to the ear; has a superficial and deep lobe and is the largest salivary gland, but produces only 25% of the total salivary volume, mainly serous; the associated duct is the parotid, or Stensen duct; the duct pierces the buccinator muscle and opens opposite the second maxillary molar; the parotid papilla marks the opening of the duct
      b. Submandibular salivary gland—located medially underneath the angle of the mandible; the second largest salivary gland, providing 60% to 65% of the total salivary volume, mixed serous and mucous; the associated duct is the submandibular, or Wharton duct; the duct opens at the sublingual caruncle on the floor of the mouth; the submandibular gland is the most common salivary gland involved in salivary stone formation
      c. Sublingual salivary gland—located in the sublingual fossa, anterior to the submandibular gland; the smallest, most diffuse salivary gland, providing 10% of the total salivary volume, mixed serous and mucous; associated ducts are located along the sublingual fold, combine to form the sublingual or Bartholin duct
   2. Minor salivary glands—smaller and more numerous than major salivary glands
      a. Numerous small glands—located in oral cavity tissues such as the soft palate; buccal, labial, and lingual mucosa; and the floor of the mouth; most secrete mainly mucous fluid
      b. Von Ebner glands—located in the circumvallate lingual papillae of the dorsal surface of the tongue; only minor salivary gland that secretes serous fluid only

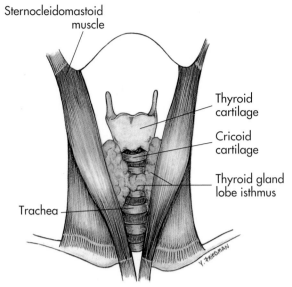

Sternocleidomastoid muscle

Thyroid cartilage

Cricoid cartilage

Thyroid gland lobe isthmus

Trachea

Y. FRIEDMAN

FIG 4-8 Anatomic position of the thyroid gland. (From Potter PA, et al: *Fundamentals of nursing,* ed 9, St Louis, 2017, Elsevier.)

3. Lacrimal glands—located in the lacrimal fossa of the frontal bone; secrete lacrimal fluid, or tears; the associated duct is the nasolacrimal duct, at the junction of the lacrimal and maxillary bones

C. Endocrine glands of the neck region
1. Thyroid gland—located below the hyoid bone; consists of two lobes connected by an isthmus; largest of the endocrine glands; secretes the hormone thyroxine, which regulates body metabolism; in a healthy patient, the thyroid gland moves with the thyroid cartilage when swallowing (Figure 4-8)
2. Parathyroid glands—located behind or within the thyroid gland; secrete parathyroid hormone, which regulates calcium metabolism and phosphorus uptake; not visible or palpable during examination
3. Thymus gland—located inferior to the thyroid in the upper part of the chest; secretes thymosin, which assists in the maturation of T cell lymphocytes, which play a role in the immune system of the body; shrinks after puberty

THE NERVOUS SYSTEM

A. Classification and function—a complex network of nerves and cells that coordinates voluntary and involuntary actions through transmission of information from one location to another; the nervous system controls all body functions essential to life
B. Descriptive terminology (see the section on "Nerve Tissue" in Chapter 2)
1. Neuron—a nerve cell that is the basic building block of the nervous system, specialized to transmit information; contains a nucleus, which holds genetic information; dendrites, which conduct impulses to the cell body; and axons, which conduct impulses away from the cell body
2. Nerve—a collection of neurons in the peripheral nervous system (PNS)
3. Synapse— connection that allows the transmission of nerve impulses between two neurons or between a neuron and an effector organ
4. Ganglion—a group of nerve cell bodies in the PNS
5. Afferent, or sensory, neurons carry nerve impulses toward the central nervous system (CNS) away from a body structure (e.g., information sent to the brain for analysis or action)
6. Efferent, or motor, neurons transmit carry nerve impulses away from the CNS toward a body structure (e.g., information sent to a muscle for activation)
C. The nervous system—two major divisions:
1. Central nervous system—comprises the brain and spinal cord
2. Peripheral nervous system—composed of nerves outside the CNS, such as sensory neurons carrying impulses to the CNS and motor neurons carrying messages from the CNS
   a. Autonomic nervous system (ANS)—responsible for control of body functions not consciously directed, such as respiratory rate, heart rate, and salivation; functions performed involuntarily and reflexively; two subdivisions of the ANS:
      (1) Sympathetic nervous system—prepares the body for stressful situations (e.g., increases heart rate, dilates airways); known as the "fight-or-flight" response; also slows body processes that are less important in emergencies, such as digestion (salivation) and urination
      (2) Parasympathetic nervous system—controls the body in ordinary situations (e.g., slows heart rate, decreases blood pressure); known as the "rest and digest" system; it generally conserves and restores body functions
D. Cranial nerves (12 pairs)—part of the PNS; designated with Roman numerals, for example, cranial nerves V, VI, and VII; provide afferent, efferent, or mixed impulses
1. Cranial nerve I (olfactory nerve)—afferent type; carries smell from the nasal mucosa to the brain; enters the skull through the cribriform plate of the ethmoid bone
2. Cranial nerve II (optic nerve)—afferent type; carries visual impulses from retina to the brain; enters the skull through the optic canal of the sphenoid bone
3. Cranial nerve III (oculomotor nerve)—efferent type; innervates muscles of the eye; exits the skull through the superior orbital fissure of the sphenoid bone
4. Cranial nerve IV (trochlear nerve)—efferent type; supplies one eye muscle; also exits the skull through the superior orbital fissure of the sphenoid bone
5. Cranial nerve V (trigeminal nerve)— largest cranial nerve, both efferent and afferent types; efferent component for the muscles of mastication and some cranial muscles; afferent component for the teeth, tongue, oral cavity, and most of the skin of the face and head; knowledge of CN V is critical for the successful administration of a local anesthetic agent (Tables 4-1 and 4-2; see Chapter 18, Management of Pain and Anxiety)

TABLE 4-1   Summary of Maxillary Injection Sites for Local Anesthetic Agent Administration

Landmark and Nerve	Injection	Teeth or Tissue Anesthetized
Maxillary tuberosity/ posterosuperior alveolar nerve of the maxillary branch of trigeminal nerve (second division, V_2)	Posterosuperior alveolar (PSA)	Maxillary first,* second, and third molars and related buccal tissues
Apex of second premolar/ middle superior alveolar nerve of V_2 (not present in all people)	Middle superior alveolar (MSA)	Maxillary first and second premolars; mesiobuccal root of maxillary first molar and buccal tissues
Apex of maxillary canine/ anterosuperior alveolar nerve of V_2	Anterosuperior alveolar (ASA)	Maxillary premolars, canines, and incisors and associated buccal tissues
Greater palatine foramen/ greater palatine nerve of V_2	Greater palatine (GP)	Palatal roots of maxillary molars and premolars and related lingual tissues
Incisive foramen/ nasopalatine nerve of V_2	Nasopalatine (NP)	Anterior portion of palate or lingual aspects of anterior maxillary teeth
Infraorbital foramen/ infraorbital nerve of V_2	Infraorbital (IO)	Facial aspects of anterior maxillary teeth and buccal aspects of the premolars

*In some cases, the mesiobuccal root is not innervated by the PSA nerve, but by the MSA nerve.

TABLE 4-2   Summary of Mandibular Injection Sites for Local Anesthetic Agent Administration

Landmark and nerve	Injection	Teeth or Tissue Anesthetized
Mandibular foramen/ inferior alveolar nerve of the mandibular branch of the trigeminal nerve (third division, V_3)	Inferior alveolar (IA)	Mandibular teeth to midline; buccal mucoperiosteum; mucous membrane anterior to mandibular fist molar; anterior two thirds of tongue and floor of oral cavity; lingual soft tissues
Mental foramen/inferior alveolar nerve; mental and incisive nerve branches of V_3	Mental block (MB) or incisive block (IB)	IB: mandibular premolars, canines, and incisors; lower lip and skin of chin; buccal mucous membrane anterior to the mental foramen MB: buccal mucous membranes anterior to mental foramen to midline; skin of lower lip and chin
Buccal tissue distal and buccal to the most distal molar/buccal nerve of V_3	Buccal block (LB)	Buccal periodontium and gingiva of mandibular molars

6. Three divisions or branches of the trigeminal nerve:
   a. Ophthalmic nerve, first division, or V_1—afferent nerve; carries information to the brain via the superior orbital fissure of the sphenoid bone for the conjunctiva, cornea, eyeball, orbit, forehead, and ethmoid and frontal sinuses; arises from three major nerves:
      (1) Frontal nerve—a merger of the supraorbital nerve (forehead and anterior scalp) and the supratrochlear nerve (bridge of the nose and medial part of the upper eyelid and forehead)
      (2) Lacrimal nerve—controls the upper eyelid, conjunctiva, and lacrimal gland; regulates the production of lacrimal fluid (tears)
      (3) Nasociliary nerve—several branches from the eyelids, sides of the nose, eyeball, nasal cavity, and paranasal sinuses
   b. Maxillary nerve, second division, or V_2—afferent nerves enter the skull through the foramen rotundum of the sphenoid bone to supply the maxillae and related skin, maxillary sinuses, nasal cavity, palate, and nasopharynx (Figure 4-9)
      (1) Zygomatic nerve—merger of two smaller nerves emerging from the lateral wall of the orbit that serve the skin of the cheek and the temple
      (2) Infraorbital (IO) nerve—formed from the merger of nerve branches from the upper lip, medial portion of the cheek, lower eyelid, and side of the nose; passes into the infraorbital foramen of the maxilla, which is the landmark for anesthetic injection of the infraorbital nerve block
      (3) Anterior superior alveolar (ASA) nerve—carries sensations from the dental branches in the pulp tissue of maxillary central incisors, lateral incisors, and canines and their associated tissues; forms a nerve network with interdental branches, which is the landmark for anesthetic injection of the anterior superior alveolar nerve block
      (4) Middle superior alveolar (MSA) nerve—carries sensations from the dental branches in the pulp tissue of the maxillary premolar teeth and mesial buccal root of the maxillary first molar, the

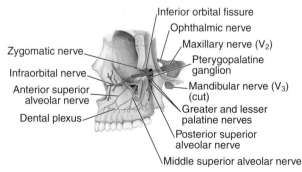

FIG 4-9 Lateral view of the skull (part of lateral wall of orbit has been removed) with branches of the maxillary nerve (V_2) highlighted. (From Fehrenbach MJ, Herring SW: *Illustrated anatomy of the head and neck*, ed 5, St Louis, 2017, Elsevier.)

associated periodontium, and buccal gingiva; forms a nerve network that is the landmark for anesthetic injection of the middle superior alveolar nerve block; the MSA is not present in all clients. In this case, the area is innervated by the ASA primarily and posterior superior alveolar nerves

(5) Posterior superior alveolar (PSA) nerve—carries sensations from the dental branches in the pulp tissue of the maxillary molars, periodontium, buccal gingiva, and the maxillary sinus; internal branches of the PSA nerve exit from several PSA foramina on the maxillary tuberosity, these foramina are landmarks for anesthetic injection of the posterior superior alveolar nerve block

(6) Greater palatine (GP) nerve, anterior nerve—carries sensations from the hard palate and posterior lingual gingiva; enters the greater palatine foramen near the maxillary second or third molar, which is the landmark for anesthetic injection of the greater palatine block

(7) Lesser palatine nerve, posterior nerve—carries sensations from the soft palate and palatine tonsil; enters the lesser palatine foramen where it joins the greater palatine nerve within the pterygopalatine canal

(8) Nasopalatine (NP) nerve—carries sensations from the anterior hard palate and lingual gingiva of maxillary anterior teeth; enters the incisive canal through the incisive foramen, which is the landmark for anesthetic injection of the nasopalatine block; the NP nerve travels along the nasal septum and communicates with the greater palatine nerve

c. Mandibular nerve, third division, or V_3—the only division containing both afferent and efferent types; largest of the trigeminal branches; enters the skull through the foramen ovale on the sphenoid bone (Figure 4-10)

(1) Buccal nerve, long buccal nerve—carries sensations from the cheek, buccal mucosa, and buccal gingiva of mandibular posterior teeth; the nerve crosses in front of the anterior border of the ramus between the two heads of the lateral pterygoid muscle, which is the landmark for anesthetic injection of the buccal nerve block

(2) Muscular branches—efferent (motor) nerves supplying the four muscles of mastication, deep temporal nerves, masseteric nerve, and lateral pterygoid nerve

(3) Auriculotemporal nerve—carries sensations from the ear and scalp; branches of this nerve innervate the parotid salivary gland through postganglionic parasympathetic fibers from the ninth cranial nerve (CN IX)

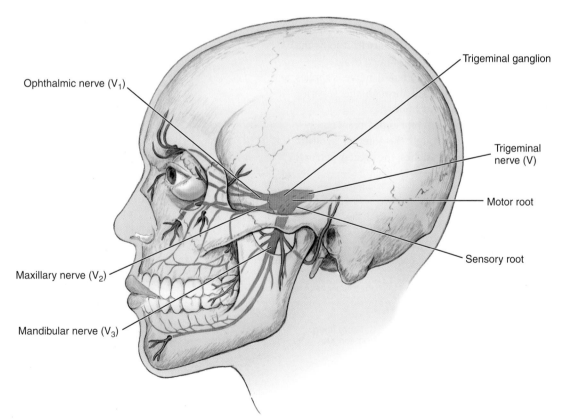

FIG 4-10 Pathway of the mandibular nerve (branch), or third division (V_3), of the trigeminal nerve is highlighted. *Inset* shows innervation coverage. (From Fehrenbach MJ, Herring SW: *Illustrated anatomy of the head and neck,* ed 5, St Louis, 2017, Elsevier.)

(4) Lingual nerve—carries sensations from the floor of the mouth, the lingual mandibular gingiva, and the body of the tongue; it communicates with CN VII (facial nerve) supplying parasympathetic fibers to the submandibular and sublingual salivary glands; because of its location in the floor of the mouth, it is often anesthetized when an inferior alveolar nerve block is administered

(5) Inferior alveolar (IA) nerve—carries sensations from mandibular teeth; it travels through the mandibular canal, along with the inferior alveolar artery and vein; exits the mandible through the mandibular foramen, which is the landmark for anesthetic injection of the inferior alveolar nerve block; it is a merger of the mental and incisive nerves

(a) Mental nerve—carries sensations from the chin, lower lip, and the labial mucosa of anterior teeth and premolars; enters the mental foramen between the premolars, which is the landmark for anesthetic injection of the mental nerve block

(b) Incisive nerve—carries sensations from the dental branches of the pulp tissue of the mandibular anterior teeth and premolars; merges with the mental nerve to form the inferior alveolar nerve and travels through the mandibular canal

(6) Mylohyoid nerve—a small efferent (motor) nerve branch that supplies the mylohyoid muscle and the anterior belly of the digastric muscle; it joins the inferior nerve entering the foramen ovale

7. Cranial nerve VI (abducens)—efferent nerve; supplies one eye muscle; exits the skull through the superior orbital fissure of the sphenoid bone

8. Cranial nerve VII (facial)—efferent and afferent components, leaves the brain through the internal acoustic meatus and gives off two branches, the greater petrosal and chorda typmpani (Figure 4-11)

a. Greater petrosal nerve—efferent nerve; fibers are carried through the pterygopalatine ganglion to the lacrimal gland, nasal cavity, and minor salivary glands of the hard and soft palate; the afferent nerve fibers also carry taste sensations from the palate

b. Chorda tympani nerve—parasympathetic efferent nerve supplying submandibular and sublingual salivary glands; has an afferent component carrying taste sensations for the body of the tongue

c. Facial nerve continues anteriorly, passing through the parotid gland, and separates into efferent branches supplying the muscles of facial expression in their respective areas; temporal, zygomatic, buccal, mandibular, and cervical branches (Figure 4-12)

d. Although the facial nerve passes into the parotid salivary gland, it does not innervate the gland; disease process in the parotid gland may be painful due to the proximity of the facial nerve

e. Knowledge of the facial nerve is important for avoidance of complications in the administration of local anesthesia

9. Cranial nerve VIII (vestibulocochlear nerve)—afferent nerve for hearing, supplied to the cochlea, and balance, supplied to the semicircular canals; enters the brain through the internal acoustic meatus of the temporal bone

10. Cranial nerve IX (glossopharyngeal nerve)—afferent and efferent nerve; carries sensory fibers from the back of the oropharynx, providing taste and sensation from

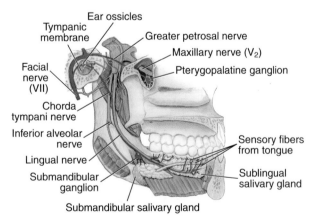

FIG 4-11 Pathway of the trunk of the facial nerve: greater petrosal nerve and chorda tympani nerve. Note relationship with the lingual nerve. (From Fehrenbach MJ, Herring SW: *Illustrated anatomy of the head and neck,* ed 5, St Louis, 2017, Elsevier.)

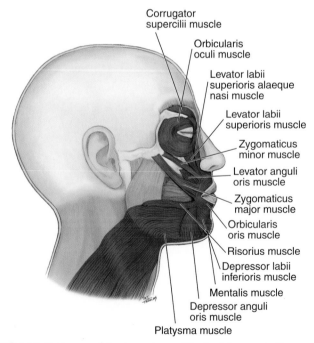

FIG 4-12 Pathway of the branches of the facial nerve to the muscles of facial expression. (Fehrenbach MJ, Herring SW: *Illustrated anatomy of the head and neck,* ed 5, St Louis, 2017, Elsevier.)

the base of the tongue; also controls gag reflex; the efferent innervation controls swallowing

11. Cranial nerve X (vagus nerve)—mixture of afferent and efferent nerves; the larger efferent component supplies the muscles of the soft palate, pharynx, larynx, and parasympathetic fibers to the organs in the thoracic and abdominal cavities; the smaller afferent component conveys to skin around the ear and taste sensation of the epiglottis

12. Cranial nerve XI (accessory nerve)—efferent nerve; impulses to the trapezius and sternocleidomastoid muscles, soft palate, and pharynx

13. Cranial nerve XII (hypoglossal nerve)—efferent nerve; innervates all muscles of the tongue; exits the skull through the hypoglossal canal of the occipital bone

Note: Cranial nerves IX, X, and XI are part of the pharyngeal plexus; all pass through the skull by way of the jugular foramen.

Website Information And Resources

Source	Web Address	Description
Laboratory Dissections of the Head and Neck/ Osteology of the Skull Laboratories	http://ect.downstate.edu/courseware/ haonline/labs/headneck.htm	Laboratory dissections of the head and neck, along with quiz questions
Digital library of anatomy information	http://www.anatomyatlases.org/ atlasofanatomy/index.shtml	Atlas of anatomy providing illustrations as representations of the human body, including bones, muscles, nerves, blood, and lymph vessels of the head and neck
Loyola University Medical Center, Chicago, Medical Education Network (images from the Visible Human Project)	http://www.meddean.luc.edu/lumen/ meded/grossanatomy/	Cross-sectional magnetic resonance imaging (MRI), computed tomography (CT), and cinematic images of human anatomy

■ CHAPTER 4 REVIEW QUESTIONS

Answers and rationales to chapter review questions are available on this text's accompanying Evolve site. See inside front cover for details.

evolve

1. **All references to body structures are made assuming the body is in anatomic position; *anatomic position* is the erect position of the body, arms at the sides, with head, eyes and palms facing forward.**
   a. Both statements are TRUE.
   b. Both statements are FALSE.
   c. The first statement is TRUE; the second statement is FALSE.
   d. The first statement is FALSE; the second statement is TRUE.

2. **The anatomic term that BEST describes the top surface of the tongue is:**
   a. Superior
   b. Inferior
   c. Ventral
   d. Dorsal

3. **Which of the following results in the formation of the flat bones of the skull?**
   a. Osteoclasts
   b. Osteocytes
   c. Intramembranous ossification
   d. Endochondral ossification

4. **Each of the following bones of the skull is considered a facial bone EXCEPT the:**
   a. Maxilla
   b. Occipital bone
   c. Zygomatic bone
   d. Lacrimal bone

5. **The articulation between the frontal bone and the parietal bone is the:**
   a. Coronal suture
   b. Sagittal suture
   c. Frontonasal suture
   d. Lambdoidal suture

6. **The petrous portion of the temporal bone contains the mastoid process. This process serves as an attachment for the trapezius muscle.**
   a. Both statements are TRUE.
   b. Both statements are FALSE.
   c. The first statement is TRUE; the second statement is FALSE.
   d. The first statement is FALSE; the second statement is TRUE.

7. **All three branches of which one of the following nerves passes through foramina on the sphenoid bone?**
   a. Facial nerve
   b. Glossopharyngeal nerve
   c. Hypoglossal nerve
   d. Trigeminal nerve

8. **Which of the following bones has paired canals that transmit cranial nerve XII, hypoglossal?**
   a. Sphenoid bone
   b. Occipital bone
   c. Maxilla
   d. Mandible

9. Which part of the temporal bone forms the cranial portion of the temporomandibular joint?
   a. Squamous part
   b. Tympanic part
   c. Zygomatic process
   d. Petrous part

10. In which of the following pairs is a movable articulation formed?
    a. Frontal bone with parietal bones
    b. Coronoid process with mandibular fossa
    c. Occipital condyles with first cervical vertebrae (atlas)
    d. Coronoid notch with mandibular fossa

11. Which of the following is a landmark on the sphenoid bone for the attachment of many of the muscles of mastication?
    a. Body of the sphenoid
    b. Lesser wing
    c. Greater wing
    d. Pterygoid process

12. Which of the following structures is perforated by foramina for the passage of olfactory nerves for the sense of smell?
    a. Sphenoid bone
    b. Maxillary tuberosity
    c. Cribriform plate
    d. Ethmoidal sinuses

13. All the following are paired facial bones EXCEPT the:
    a. Nasal bone
    b. Maxilla bone
    c. Zygomatic bone
    d. Vomer

14. An important landmark for local anesthesia lies posterior to the most distal maxillary molar. Identify the landmark and the nerve that passes through its foramina.
    a. Infraorbital foramen, infraorbital nerve
    b. Greater palatine foramen, greater palatine nerve
    c. Maxillary tuberosity, posterior superior alveolar nerve
    d. Incisive foramen, nasopalatine nerves

15. Infiltration of local anesthetic is more successful in mandibular anterior teeth than mandibular posterior teeth because:
    a. The alveolar process of the mandibular incisors is less dense
    b. The alveolar process of the mandibular incisors is denser
    c. The alveolar process of the mandibular incisors is absent
    d. The body of the mandible is less dense than the alveolar process

16. Which of the following landmarks on the ramus of the mandible serves as a landmark for determining the height of injection for the inferior alveolar nerve block?
    a. Coronoid process
    b. Mandibular notch
    c. Coronoid notch
    d. Lingula

17. Which of the following is an important landmark to note radiographically to avoid misinterpretation as an oral radiolucent lesion?
    a. Mental foramen
    b. Genial tubercles
    c. Mandibular foramen
    d. Mental protuberance

18. Infection of which of the following sinuses can cause discomfort and complications with the maxillary posterior teeth?
    a. Maxillary
    b. Ethmoid
    c. Sphenoid
    d. Frontal

19. When a skeletal muscle contracts to cause a given movement, the more movable end of attachment of the muscle is termed its:
    a. Origin
    b. Insertion
    c. Antagonist
    d. Synergist

20. All the following are muscles of facial expression EXCEPT the:
    a. Orbicularis oculi
    b. Buccinator
    c. Temporalis
    d. Mentalis

21. When contracted, which of the following muscles tightens and narrows the vestibule, making access to the facial aspect of the mandibular incisors difficult?
    a. Buccinator
    b. Mentalis
    c. Levator labii superioris
    d. Depressor labii inferioris

22. Which one of the following muscles of facial expression encircles the mouth and is responsible for closure of the lips?
    a. Orbicularis oris
    b. Buccinator
    c. Levator anguli oris
    d. Depressor anguli oris

23. The muscles of mastication consist of four paired muscles inserting on the mandible. The muscles of mastication are innervated by the mandibular division of cranial nerve V.
    a. Both statements are TRUE.
    b. Both statements are FALSE.
    c. The first statement is TRUE; the second statement is FALSE.
    d. The first statement is FALSE; the second statement is TRUE.

24. The muscle of facial expression that aids in mastication is the:
    a. Risorius
    b. Buccinator
    c. Mentalis
    d. Masseter

25. **Lateral deviation of the mandible occurs when:**
    a. The medial pterygoid muscle is contracted
    b. The digastric muscle is contracted
    c. One head of the lateral pterygoid muscle is contracted
    d. Both heads of the lateral pterygoid muscle are contracted

26. **Which of the following occurs when one side of the sternocleidomastoid muscle is contracted?**
    a. The head and neck bend to the same side.
    b. The head and neck bend to the opposite side.
    c. The head flexes and extends the neck.
    d. The head flexes and remains stable.

27. **Which of the following muscle groups elevate the hyoid bone?**
    a. Intrinsic tongue muscles
    b. Extrinsic tongue muscles
    c. Suprahyoid muscles
    d. Infrahyoid muscles

28. **All the following muscles of mastication elevate the mandible EXCEPT the:**
    a. Masseter
    b. Medial pterygoid
    c. Temporalis
    d. Lateral pterygoid

29. **During an oral examination, you ask the client to protrude the tongue. What muscle is necessary for this action?**
    a. Hypoglossus
    b. Genioglossus
    c. Palatoglossus
    d. Styloglossus

30. **Intrinsic tongue muscles are located entirely inside the tongue. These muscles act to change the shape of the tongue.**
    a. Both statements are TRUE.
    b. Both statements are FALSE.
    c. The first statement is TRUE; the second statement is FALSE.
    d. The first statement is FALSE; the second statement is TRUE.

31. **The muscle that unites with its counterpart to form the floor of the mouth is the:**
    a. Stylohyoid
    b. Digastric
    c. Mylohyoid
    d. Geniohyoid

32. **Taste sensations for the body of the tongue are provided by which of the following nerves?**
    a. Maxillary division of the trigeminal
    b. Mandibular division of the trigeminal
    c. Chorda tympani branch of the facial
    d. Greater petrosal branch of the facial

33. **Which of the following describes the type of movement achieved by the temporomandibular joint?**
    a. Gliding only
    b. Gliding and rotation
    c. Rotation only
    c. Gliding, rotation, and extension

34. **The articular fossa of the temporal bone articulates with the mandible at the temporomandibular joint at which landmark?**
    a. Articular eminence
    b. Articular fossa
    c. Zygomatic process of the temporal bone
    d. Condyle

35. **The temporomandibular joint is innervated by the:**
    a. Hypoglossal nerve
    b. Trigeminal nerve
    c. Facial nerve
    d. Accessory nerve

36. **All the following major salivary glands secrete mixed secretions EXCEPT the:**
    a. Parotid gland
    b. Submandibular salivary gland
    c. Sublingual salivary gland
    d. Von Ebner gland

37. **The parotid gland produces the least volume of saliva because it is the smallest salivary gland.**
    a. Both the statement and the reason are correct and related.
    b. Both the statement and the reason are correct but are NOT related.
    c. The statement is correct, but the reason is NOT correct.
    d. NEITHER the statement NOR the reason is correct.

38. **The sublingual caruncle:**
    a. Receives the parotid duct
    b. Receives the sublingual duct
    c. Receives the submandibular duct
    d. Receives the Bartholin duct

39. **A ligament associated with the temporomandibular joint is an important landmark for local anesthesia. Name the landmark and the nerve block.**
    a. Sphenomandibular ligament, inferior alveolar
    b. Sphenomandibular ligament, long buccal
    c. Stylomandibular ligament, long buccal
    d. Temporomandibular joint ligament, inferior alveolar

40. **Salivary glands in the soft palate (buccal, labial, and lingual mucosa) secrete mostly mucous fluid. Von Ebner glands located in the circumvallate lingual papillae secrete only serous fluid.**
    a. Both statements are TRUE.
    b. Both statements are FALSE.
    c. The first statement is TRUE; the second statement is FALSE.
    d. The first statement is FALSE; the second statement is TRUE.

41. **Which of the following glands secrete hormones to regulate calcium metabolism and phosphorus uptake?**
    a. Thymus
    b. Thyroid
    c. Parathyroid
    d. Adrenal

42. **Which of the following is NOT an exocrine gland of the head?**
    a. Parotid gland
    b. Lacrimal gland
    c. Von Ebner gland
    d. Thyroid gland

43. The thymus gland is an endocrine gland because it has an associated duct.
    a. Both the statement and the reason are correct and related.
    b. Both the statement and the reason are correct but are NOT related.
    c. The statement is correct, but the reason is NOT correct.
    d. NEITHER the statement NOR the reason is correct.

44. The salivary gland most often associated with salivary stone formation is the:
    a. Parotid
    b. Submandibular
    c. Sublingual
    d. Lacrimal

45. Which of the following glands is the *largest* salivary gland?
    a. Parotid
    b. Submandibular
    c. Sublingual
    d. Lacrimal

46. When examining a healthy client, this exocrine gland moves with its associated cartilage.
    a. Parotid gland
    b. Thymus gland
    c. Thyroid gland
    d. Parathyroid gland

47. The palatine tonsil is commonly enlarged in children. This tonsil is also referred to as the adenoids.
    a. Both statements are TRUE.
    b. Both statements are FALSE.
    c. The first statement is TRUE; the second statement is FALSE.
    d. The first statement is FALSE; the second statement is TRUE.

48. Which of the following lymph nodes is easily palpable in clients with tonsillar lymphadenopathy?
    a. Submental node
    b. Jugulodigastric node
    c. Jugulo-omohyoid node
    d. Accessory node

49. Pea-like firmness of the facial lymph nodes might indicate:
    a. Infection from adjacent teeth
    b. Infection from the upper lip
    c. Infection from tonsils
    d. Normal health

50. Which of the following lymph nodes drain the cheek, hard palate, tongue, and anterior nasal cavity?
    a. Submental nodes
    b. Submandibular nodes
    c. Facial nodes
    d. Occipital nodes

51. Which of the following lymph nodes empty into the jugular trunk?
    a. Deep cervical nodes
    b. Superficial nodes
    c. Submandibular nodes
    d. Facial nodes

52. Leukocytes are white blood cells that protect the body against infection. All the following are leukocytes EXCEPT:
    a. Neutrophils
    b. Eosinophils
    c. Basophils
    d. Erythrocytes

53. The most reliable arterial pulse in the body is located in the:
    a. Internal carotid artery
    b. External carotid artery
    c. Carotid sinus
    d. Lingual artery

54. Which of the following arteries supplies the muscles of mastication?
    a. Occipital artery
    b. Maxillary artery
    c. Facial artery
    d. Lingual artery

55. The facial vein communicates with the cavernous venous sinus; this sinus can become fatally infected through the spread of dental infection.
    a. Both statements are TRUE.
    b. Both statements are FALSE.
    c. The first statement is TRUE; the second statement is FALSE.
    d. The first statement is FALSE; the second statement is TRUE.

56. Which of the following facial arteries supplies the sub-mandibular salivary gland?
    a. Ascending palatine artery
    b. Submental artery
    c. Inferior labial artery
    d. Superior labial artery

57. Which one of the following statements is NOT true about the pterygoid plexus?
    a. Drains portions of the face into the maxillary vein
    b. Can be involved in the spread of dental infections by improper administration of local anesthesia
    c. Protects the maxillary artery
    d. Has valves that prevent backflow of blood

58. Dental infections can lead to serious complications, since veins in the head and neck generally lack valves that prevent the backflow of blood.
    a. Both the statement and the reason are correct and related.
    b. Both the statement and the reason are correct but are NOT related.
    c. The statement is correct, but the reason is NOT correct.
    d. NEITHER the statement NOR the reason is correct.

59. The central nervous system consists of the following:
    a. Sympathetic nervous system
    b. Parasympathetic nervous system
    c. Brain and spinal cord
    d. Nerves, receptors, muscles, and glands of the body

60. Nerves that carry impulses away from the brain or spinal cord to a body structure are known as:
    a. Synapse
    b. Ganglion
    c. Afferent
    d. Efferent

61. The sympathetic nervous system prepares the body for stressful situations, "fight or flight." Which of the following symptoms might a client with severe dental anxiety exhibit during the dental appointment?
    a. Decrease in blood pressure
    b. Increase in salivary flow
    c. Dental caries
    d. Increase in heart rate

62. Which of the following nerves is paired correctly with the tissue it innervates?
    a. Glossopharyngeal nerve, base of tongue
    b. Buccal nerve, buccinator muscle
    c. Hypoglossal nerve, extrinsic tongue muscles
    d. Facial nerve, parotid gland

63. All the following are branches of the maxillary division of the trigeminal nerve EXCEPT the:
    a. Infraorbital nerve
    b. Anterior superior alveolar nerve
    c. Auriculotemporal nerve
    d. Nasopalatine nerve

64. The only trigeminal nerve division carrying both afferent and efferent nerves is the:
    a. Ophthalmic
    b. Mandibular
    c. Maxillary
    d. Facial

65. Which of the following nerves is NOT always present in the oral cavity?
    a. Greater palatine
    b. Mental
    c. Middle superior alveolar
    d. Anterior superior alveolar

66. Damage to this nerve can result in facial paralysis or Bell palsy.
    a. Trigeminal
    b. Facial
    c. Buccal
    d. Hypoglossal

67. The facial nerve travels through the parotid gland; innervation of the parotid gland is provided by the facial nerve.
    a. Both statements are TRUE.
    b. Both statements are FALSE.
    c. The first statement is TRUE; the second statement is FALSE.
    d. The first statement is FALSE; the second statement is TRUE.

68. Which of the following nerves enters the skull through the foramen ovale?
    a. Ophthalmic
    b. Maxillary
    c. Mandibular
    d. Zygomatic

69. Knowledge of the trigeminal nerve is critical for the successful administration of a local anesthetic agent. Which of the following cranial nerves is the trigeminal nerve?
    a. I
    b. III
    c. IV
    d. V

70. Which of the following nerves is NOT part of the mandibular division of the trigeminal nerve?
    a. Buccal
    b. Mental
    c. Lacrimal
    d. Incisive

71. Which of the following nerves innervates the four muscles of mastication?
    a. Mandibular
    b. Maxillary
    c. Ophthalmic
    d. Trigeminal

72. Which of the following nerves is the largest of the trigeminal branches?
    a. Maxillary
    b. Facial
    c. Ophthalmic
    d. Mandibular

73. What is the purpose of synovial fluid in the synovial joint?
    a. Lubricates the joint
    b. Transports nutrients to the joint
    c. Prevents displacement of the joint
    d. Stabilizes the joint

74. The four muscles of mastication are the masseter, temporalis, medial pterygoid, and lateral pterygoid; these muscles of mastication are innervated by the cranial nerve VI.
    a. Both statements are TRUE.
    b. Both statements are FALSE.
    c. The first statement is TRUE; the second statement is FALSE.
    d. The first statement is FALSE; the second statement is TRUE.

75. All the following cranial nerves are part of the pharyngeal plexus and pass through the skull by way of the jugular foramen EXCEPT:
    a. Cranial nerve VI (abducens nerve)
    b. Cranial nerve IX (glossopharyngeal nerve)
    c. Cranial nerve X (vagus nerve)
    d. Cranial nerve XI (accessory nerve)

CASE A

Ms. Thomas, 49 years old, is a new patient at the dental office. Her health history and pharmacologic history reveal that she takes medications for hypertension and depression. She complains of thermal hypersensitivity on tooth #5. She reports brushing twice per day, using a soft toothbrush, and occasionally flossing. Ms. Thomas has a history of orthodontic appliances as a teenager. Her periodontal history reveals generalized severe chronic periodontitis with moderate subgingival calculus. She has generalized, moderate levels of plaque biofilm. The dental hygienist has planned for four quadrants of scaling and root planing and a reevaluation appointment 6 weeks after the initial treatment. She is missing teeth #1, #5, #12, #16, #17 #21, #28, and #32.

Use Case A to answer questions 76 to 82.

76. **Which of the following is mostly likely the swollen lymph node identified by the dental hygienist during an extraoral exam?**
    a. Occipital
    b. Posterior auricular
    c. Preauricular
    d. Submental

77. **Which of the following American Academy of Periodontology classifications would Ms. Thomas's periodontal condition be documented as?**
    a. AAP type I
    b. AAP type II
    c. AAP type III
    d. AAP type IV

78. **Which of the following premolars are often extracted before orthodontic treatment?**
    a. Teeth #1 and #16
    b. Teeth #5 and #12
    c. Teeth #6 and #11
    d. Teeth #20 and #29

79. **Which of the following local anesthetic agents would be a better choice for Ms. Thomas because of her hypertension?**

    a. Lidocaine hydrochloride with epinephrine
    b. Mepivacaine hydrochloride
    c. Benzocaine topical anesthetic
    d. Lidocaine without epinephrine

80. **To make sure that tooth #5 is anesthetized, which of the following nerves would be infiltrated during anesthesia?**
    a. Posterior superior alveolar
    b. Middle superior alveolar
    c. Anterior superior alveolar
    d. Nasopalatine

81. **Infiltration of all the following nerves would help anesthetize quadrant 1 EXCEPT the:**
    a. Greater palatine
    b. Mental
    c. Posterior superior alveolar
    d. Nasopalatine

82. **Which of the following would the dental hygienist NOT do during the reevaluation appointment?**
    a. Assess bleeding on probing
    b. Assess the gingival health
    c. Remove residual calculus
    d. Take four horizontal bitewings

Clinical Oral Structures, Dental Anatomy, and Root Morphology

Jeanne M. Anderson

The practice of dental hygiene is based on oral anatomy, a fundamental dental science. A thorough knowledge of oral anatomy provides the basis for assessing, diagnosing, planning, implementing, and evaluating clients during the dental hygiene process of care. Oral structures reflect oral and systemic health. Oral anatomy provides the basis for nonsurgical periodontal therapy, fluoride regimens, pit-and-fissure sealant placement, and patient education; all requiring imagery and tactile perception. The dental hygienist also uses oral anatomy to assess the relationship of teeth, both within and between the arches. These factors influence evidence-based decision making, care plans, professional recommendations, and referral to other health care practitioners.

CLINICAL ORAL STRUCTURES

Oral tissues are indicators of a client's oral and general health. Abnormal conditions can be recognized if the appearance of normal oral structures is known (Figures 5-1 to 5-8 and Table 5-1). Oral structures are identified according to their specific locations and functions. Generally, oral structures appear in shades of pink and may be pigmented in dark-complexioned individuals. In the oral cavity, the presence of melanin pigmentation is random, scattered, and unpredictable. Most importantly, the dental hygienist must be proficient in performing a clinical examination of the head and neck both extraorally and intraorally to detect variations of normal and abnormal conditions that may be indicators of overall health.

DENTAL TERMINOLOGY

A. Parts of a tooth (Figure 5-9; see the section on "Tissues of the Tooth" in Chapter 2)
  1. Crown
    a. Anatomic crown—part of the tooth covered by enamel
    b. Clinical crown—portion of the tooth that is unattached and visible in the oral cavity; determined by the location of the gingival margin
    c. Anatomic crown and clinical crown are the same when the marginal gingiva is at the junction of the cementum and enamel (CEJ)
  2. Root—part of the tooth covered by cementum; single root or multi-rooted

    a. Apex (plural, apices)—rounded end of the root
    b. Periapex (periapical)—area around the apex of a tooth
    c. Foramen (plural, foramina)—opening at the apex through which blood vessels and nerves enter
    d. Furcation—area of a two-rooted or three-rooted tooth where the root divides
      (1) Furcation entrance—area of opening into the furcation
      (2) Roof of the furcation—most coronal area of the furcation; the "ceiling" of a mandibular furcation; the base of a maxillary furcation
      (3) Interfurcal area/furcal area—area between the roots of a two-rooted or three-rooted tooth
    e. Root trunk—area from the cemento-enamel junction (CEJ) to the furcation
    f. Root concavity/depression—concave, vertical depression on the root; named by location: mesial, distal, and lingual; can be narrow or broad, shallow or deep; a concavity located within the furcation is called a *furcal concavity*
  3. Enamel—hardest calcified tissue covering the dentin in the crown of the tooth; 96% mineralized (inorganic); thinnest at the CEJ of permanent teeth
  4. Dentin—hard calcified tissue surrounding the pulp and underlying enamel and cementum; makes up the bulk of the tooth; 70% mineralized (inorganic)
  5. Cementum—bone-like calcified tissue covering the dentin in the root of the tooth; 50% mineralized (inorganic)
  6. Pulp—innermost, noncalcified tissue containing blood vessels, lymph, and nerves
    a. Pulp cavity—space containing the pulp; within the crown and root
    b. Pulp canal—portion of the pulp cavity in the root of the tooth
    c. Pulp chamber—portion of the pulp cavity in the crown of the tooth
    d. Pulp horns—pointed, crown-ward extensions of the pulp chamber tooth; generally, one horn per cusp on posterior teeth and one to three horns per cusp on anterior teeth
B. Junction of tooth tissues
  1. Cemento-enamel junction/cervical line—junction of cementum and enamel

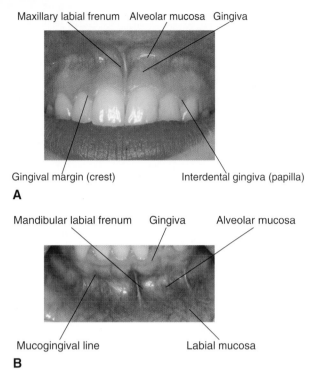

Maxillary labial frenum   Alveolar mucosa   Gingiva

Gingival margin (crest)   Interdental gingiva (papilla)

A

Mandibular labial frenum   Gingiva   Alveolar mucosa

Mucogingival line   Labial mucosa

B

FIG 5-1 Labial and oral mucosa. **A,** Maxillary. **B,** Mandibular.

Buccal mucosa   Parotid papilla   Mucobuccal fold   Buccal frenum

FIG 5-2 Buccal mucosa.

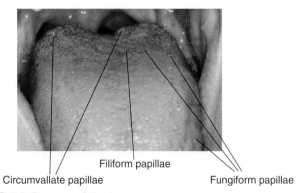

Circumvallate papillae   Filiform papillae   Fungiform papillae

FIG 5-3 Dorsum of the tongue.

Foliate papillae

Lingual tonsils

FIG 5-4 Lateral surface of the tongue.

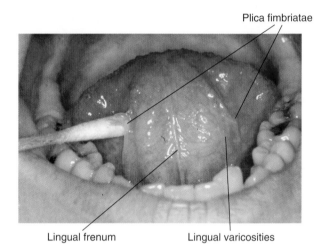

Plica fimbriatae

Lingual frenum   Lingual varicosities

FIG 5-5 Ventral surface of the tongue.

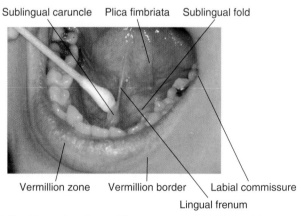

Sublingual caruncle   Plica fimbriata   Sublingual fold

Vermillion zone   Vermillion border   Labial commissure
                                        Lingual frenum

FIG 5-6 Ventral surface of the tongue and the floor of the mouth.

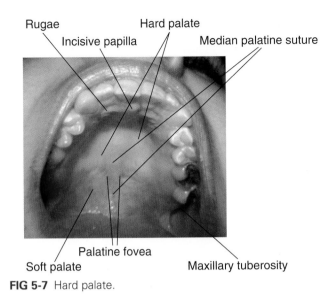

Rugae   Hard palate

Incisive papilla   Median palatine suture

Palatine fovea

Soft palate   Maxillary tuberosity

FIG 5-7 Hard palate.

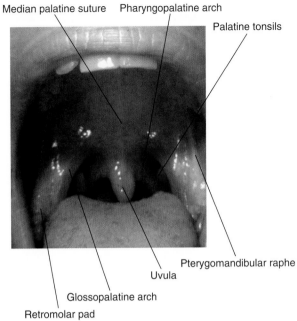

Median palatine suture   Pharyngopalatine arch

Palatine tonsils

Pterygomandibular raphe

Uvula

Glossopalatine arch

Retromolar pad

FIG 5-8 Soft palate and oropharynx.

TABLE 5-1	**Oral Structures**	
Structure	**Clinical Description**	**Clinical Consideration**
Lips, Cheeks, and Oral Mucosa (see Figures 5-1 and 5-2)		
Philtrum	Midline vertical depression of the skin between the nose and upper lip	Common location for cleft lip
Vermillion zone/border	Transitional area between the skin of the face and the oral mucosa of lips; medium pink in light-skinned individuals, and pigmented with melanin in dark-skinned individuals	Junction between vermillion zone and skin of face is a frequent site of herpetic lesions. The lower lip is a frequent site of oral cancer. Fordyce's granules or spots (small white spots of ectopic sebaceous material) may be present.
Labial commissure	Junction of upper and lower lips at the corner of the mouth	Frequent site of chafing, herpetic lesions, and cracking (angular cheilitis); avoid pulling with instrument handle.
Vestibule	Space between the teeth (alveolar processes) and the lips and cheeks	Frequent site of aphthous ulcers
Labial mucosa	Mucosal lining of the inner lip next to the anterior teeth; vascular; small elevations are external manifestation of numerous labial salivary glands	Frequent site of mucoceles, mucus-retention cysts, aphthous ulcers, and scars
Labial frenum (plural, frena) (maxillary and mandibular)	Fold of tissue at the midline (maxillary and mandibular) between the inner surface of the lip and the alveolar mucosa; attaches the lips to the mucosal tissue between central incisors.	Maxillary fold is sometimes overdeveloped, which results in a space between the central incisors, (diastema); frequently has an extra flap of tissue. If overextended onto the attached gingiva, mandibular fold may cause recession
Buccal mucosa	Mucous membrane lining of the inner cheek next to the posterior teeth	Frequent site of linea alba, cheek bites, and Fordyce's granules
Parotid papilla	Flap of tissue on the cheek opposite the maxillary first and second molars; contains the opening of Stensen duct, which carries saliva from the parotid gland	Large amounts of mainly serous saliva come from this duct; the opening can often be seen as a dark spot.
Buccal frena (muscle attachments)	Folds of epithelium between the cheek and attached gingivae (maxillary and mandibular) in the premolar area	Overextension may cause gingival recession. Movement of the frena aids in guiding food during mastication.
Mucobuccal fold	Fold between the alveolar and buccal or labial mucosa	The height of the mucobuccal fold is penetration site for injection techniques.
Alveolar mucosa	Thin movable mucosal lining covering alveolar bone; between the attached gingiva and the mucobuccal fold on the facial aspect of maxillary and mandibular arches and between the attached gingiva and the floor of the mouth on the lingual aspect of the mandibular arch	Very thin and fragile epithelium; frequent site of apthous ulcers

(Continued)

TABLE 5-1   Oral Structures—cont'd

Structure	Clinical Description	Clinical Consideration
Gingiva	Keratinized mucosa that surrounds teeth and alveolar bone. Attached gingiva: part attached to the alveolar bone Free gingiva: part that surrounds the necks of the teeth	Ideally, except for a narrow band around the necks of teeth, it is firmly attached to teeth and bone.
Mucogingival line or junction	A visible line where the pink, keratinized, attached gingiva meets the more vascular, nonkeratinized, looser alveolar mucosa	Found on maxillary facial and mandibular facial and lingual areas
Gingival margin or crest	The most coronal edge of keratinized gingiva	Can change positionally because of inflammation, recession, and attachment loss

Tongue (see Figures 5-3 to 5-6)

The tongue is a flat, muscular organ of speech, taste, mastication, and swallowing; the lateral border and undersurface are frequent sites of oral cancer; dorsum is the top surface covered by papillae (projections for taste); ventral is the underside of the tongue.

Median sulcus	Midline depression on the dorsum of the tongue	Presence and depth vary. Additional deep depressions are called *fissures* (a fissured tongue).
Fungiform papillae	Large, round, mushroom-shaped, red to dark-brown elevations scattered over the anterior third of the dorsum of the tongue (tip)	In dark-skinned individuals, these papillae may contain melanin pigmentation. Function in taste sensations of sweet, sour, and salty
Filiform papillae	Fringe-like, fine, keratinized projections concentrated in the middle third of the dorsum of the tongue	Readily collect plaque and stain Tongue with moving patches devoid of these papillae is called a *geographic tongue*.
Circumvallate papillae	From 8 to 12 large papillae arranged in an inverted V-shaped row posterior to filiform papillae	Function in the taste sensation of bitter Ducts of von Ebner salivary glands open around these papillae and secrete serous saliva.
Foliate papillae	Vertical ridges on the lateral borders of the tongue	Function in the taste sensation of sour May be a site of precancerous or cancerous findings (white or red areas, ulcers, masses, pigmentations)
Lingual tonsils	Mass of lymphoid tissue on the base of the tongue, posterior to circumvallate papillae	Difficult to observe; extend and move the tongue to the right and left to examine
Lingual frenum	Thin fold of epithelium attaching the undersurface of the tongue to the floor of the mouth	A short frenum limits movement (ankyloglossia, tongue-tied) and makes exposing radiographs and taking impressions difficult; if located too close to the mandibular central incisors, cause periodontal issues
Sublingual folds (plica sublingualis)	Two ridges of tissue on the floor of the mouth arranged in a V-shaped direction, from the lingual frenum to the base of the tongue	Contains Wharton duct from the submandibular (also called *submaxillary*) salivary gland, Bartholin duct, and the openings of the sublingual salivary glands Limited amounts of mixed saliva secreted there
Sublingual caruncle	Round elevation of the floor of the mouth on either side of the lingual frenum; contains the openings for both the submandibular and the sublingual salivary glands	Wharton duct carries large amounts of saliva from the submandibular salivary gland.
Lingual veins	Blue line on the undersurface of the tongue on either side of the lingual frenum	With age, these veins become more prominent in size and color; varicosities may be present.
Plica fimbriata	Delicate, fringe-like projections of the mucous membranes on the undersurface of the tongue, lateral to the lingual vein	May be dark colored, with more melanin pigmentation

Palate (see Figures 5-7 and 5-8)

Hard palate: the anterior two thirds of the roof of the mouth; soft palate: the posterior third of the roof of the mouth; a frequent site of oral cancer

Incisive papilla	Midline, elevated pad of tissue lingual to the maxillary central incisors	Often burned or traumatized when eating Protects the nasopalatine nerve, which enters through the underlying incisive foramen The palatal mucosa immediately lateral to the papilla is needle insertion site for nasopalatine nerve block anesthesia.
Rugae	Firm, irregular ridges of masticatory mucosa on anterior half of the hard palate branching off of the palatine raphe (see below)	If prominent, rugae may be burned or traumatized more easily. Functions include tactile sensation of food and aiding sounds in speech.
Palatine fovea		

TABLE 5-1	Oral Structures—cont'd	
Structure	**Clinical Description**	**Clinical Consideration**
	Small dimple on either side of the midline at the junction of the hard and soft palates	Touching area posterior to this may initiate the gag reflex. Site for the greater palatine nerve block
Palatal salivary duct openings	Small, dark spots scattered on the hard and soft palates	Represent the duct openings of minor palatal salivary glands
Palatine raphe	Hard, linear elevated ridge of tissue along the midline of the hard palate; external manifestation of the palatine suture, which joins the right and left maxillary and palatine bones	Excess bone (tori) or a deep depression may be present there. Site of hyperkeratinization or associated nicotine stomatitis
Maxillary tuberosity	Protuberance of alveolar bone distal to the last maxillary molar	Erupting third molar may be present there.
Tonsillar Region (see Figure 5-8)		
Retromolar area	Triangular area of bone and pad of movable tissue distal to the last mandibular molar	An erupting third molar may be present, and a flap of tissue (operculum) is often associated with infection in this area.
Pterygomandibular raphe	Fold of tissue from the retromolar area to an area near the maxillary tuberosity; separates the soft palate from the cheek; lies medial to the posterior border of the ramus of the mandible	Covers a ligament from the mandible to sphenoid bone Used as a guide for needle insertion for inferior alveolar nerve block
Anterior or glossopalatine arch	Thin fold of epithelium extending laterally and inferiorly from both sides (two pillars) of the soft palate to the base of the tongue	Marks the entry into the pharynx; the anterior boundary of the tonsillar recess
Posterior or pharyngopalatine arch	Thin fold of epithelium (two pillars) that is more posterior and narrower than the anterior arch	Marks the posterior boundary of the palatine tonsillar recess
Tonsillar recess	Recessed area between the anterior and posterior arches	May or may not contain palatine tonsils
Palatine tonsils	Globules of lymphoid tissue in the tonsillar recess	Vary greatly in size Not visible if removed or atrophied, or may be so large that the fauces is very narrow
Uvula	Fleshy tissue suspended from the midline of the posterior border of the soft palate	Closes the opening to the nasopharynx when swallowing Varies in size and shape
Pharyngeal tonsils	Globules of lymphoid tissue on the oropharyngeal wall	Nontechnical term is *adenoids*; appear as globules of reddish orange tissue. Mucosal secretions from the sinuses may be seen here.
Fauces or faucial isthmus	Isthmus (narrowing) of the space from the oral cavity into the pharynx; posterior border of the oral cavity	

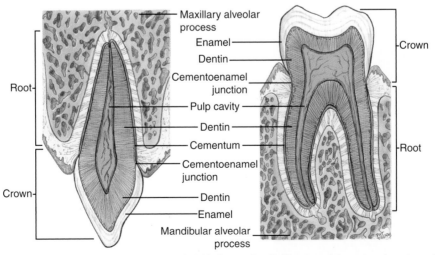

FIG 5-9 Parts of a molar. (From Fehrenbach MJ, Popowics T: *Illustrated dental embryology, histology, and anatomy,* ed 4, St Louis, 2016, Elsevier.)

2. Dento-enamel junction (DEJ)—junction of dentin and enamel
3. Cemento-dentin junction (CDJ)—junction of cementum and dentin

C. Tooth surfaces—axial surfaces are those parallel to the tooth long axis; facial, lingual, mesial, and distal
   1. Facial—surface toward the face
      a. Labial (toward the lips)—facial surfaces of anterior teeth
      b. Buccal (toward the cheeks)—facial surfaces of posterior teeth
   2. Lingual—surface toward the tongue; may also be called *palatal* for maxillary teeth
   3. Proximal—surface toward the adjacent tooth
      a. Mesial—proximal surface toward the midline
      b. Distal—proximal surface farthest from the midline
   4. Contact area—area that touches the adjacent tooth in the same arch; at the crest of curvature/height of contour in normal occlusion
   5. Incisal—surface of an incisor that is toward the opposite arch; the biting surface
   6. Occlusal—surface of a posterior tooth that is toward the opposite arch; the chewing surface; has elevations and depressions, complex anatomy of ridges, pits, and grooves (Figure 5-10)
   7. Features of biting or chewing surfaces
      a. Cusp—large, rounded, elevated area of enamel found on posterior teeth, usually named for its location
      b. Ridge—rounded, linear elevation of enamel
         (1). Marginal ridge—forms the mesial and distal borders of the lingual surface of anterior teeth and the occlusal proximal surfaces of posterior teeth (see Figure 5-10)
         (2) Triangular ridge—ridges on posterior teeth from the tip of the cusp to the central developmental groove; formed by the junction of two cuspal inclines

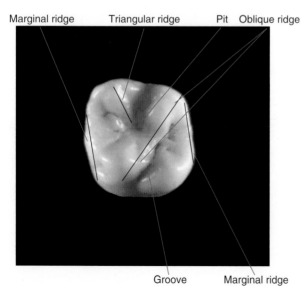

Marginal ridge   Triangular ridge   Pit   Oblique ridge

Groove   Marginal ridge

FIG 5-10 Occlusal anatomy.

         (3) Oblique ridge—two triangular ridges meeting in an oblique line; a characteristic of maxillary molars
         (4) Transverse ridge—two triangular ridges meeting in a faciolingual line (often on two-cusped premolars, molars) (see Figure 5-10)
         (5) Cingulum (plural, cingula)—large, rounded elevation of enamel on the linguocervical third of anterior teeth (the lingual developmental lobe) (Figure 5-11)
      c. Cuspal inclines—two surfaces of a cusp that slant or slope down and away from the crests of the triangular ridge toward developmental grooves
      d. Groove—narrow linear depression (see Figure 5-10)
         (1) Fissure—narrow crevice within a groove where fusion is incomplete; potential site for caries
         (2) Developmental groove/depression—groove or line that indicates the primary anatomic divisions (cusps, developmental lobes) of a crown
         (3) Supplemental groove—a less distinct groove that branches from a developmental groove
      e. Fossa (plural, fossae)—a depression on anterior teeth between marginal ridges on the lingual surfaces, and on occlusal surfaces of posterior teeth
      f. Pit—a sharp, pointed depression generally located at the junction of developmental grooves (fissures) or at their termination; narrow or wide; pits in primary teeth are not as deep as those in permanent teeth (see Figure 5-10)

D. Angles/junction of surfaces—a tooth has curved surfaces; therefore, no "corner" where one surface begins and another ends
   1. Line angle—the junction of two tooth surfaces; a transition area named for the surfaces that are involved (e.g., mesiobuccal, distolingual); each tooth has eight line angles
   2. Point angles—the junction of three tooth surfaces (e.g., mesiodisto-occlusal); each tooth has four point angles

E. Embrasure—the interproximal space between teeth that begins at the contact area and widens in facial, lingual, occlusal or incisal, and cervical/gingival directions; functions in deflecting food and reducing the forces placed on the periodontium during chewing; provides a self-cleaning area; the interproximal gingiva fills the cervical embrasure

DENTAL ANATOMY

A. Permanent dentition (Table 5-2)
   1. Humans are diphyodonts, with two sets of teeth in a lifetime—a primary dentition and a permanent dentition; span three dentition periods: primary, mixed/transitional, and permanent
   2. The permanent dentition consists of 32 teeth if all are present; arranged in four quadrants: maxillary right, maxillary left, mandibular left, and mandibular right (quadrants 1 to 4)
   3. Naming teeth—use this order: set, arch, side, type, class (e.g., permanent mandibular right second molar)

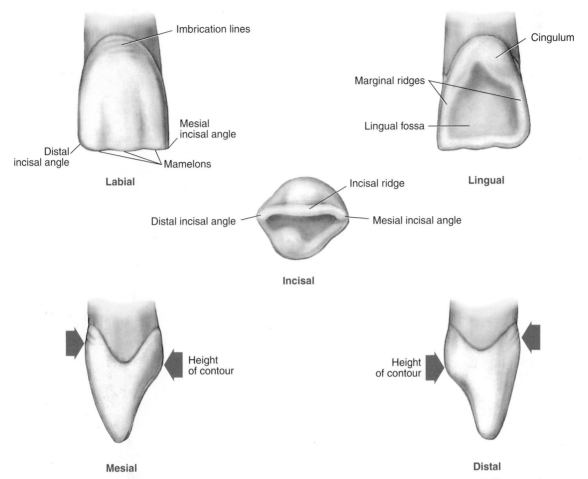

FIG 5-11 Lingual developmental lobe and cingulum. (From Fehrenbach MJ, Popowics T: *Illustrated dental embryology, histology, and anatomy*, ed 4, St Louis, 2016, Elsevier.)

B. Classes of teeth: incisors, canines, premolars, and molars; each quadrant (from the midline) has two incisors (central and lateral), one canine, two premolars (first and second), and three molars (first, second, and third); incisors and canines are anterior teeth; premolars and molars are posterior teeth
  1. Anatomic features of anterior teeth
    a. Incisors
      (1) Developmental lobes—developmental centers; anterior teeth are formed from four developmental lobes; posterior teeth have four or five lobes
      (2) Incisal ridge—found on incisors; function is cutting; newly erupted incisors have *mamelons*: three rounded elevations on the incisal ridge, delineating the three facial developmental lobes, which are usually worn away with normal function after eruption
      (3) Incisal angles—formed by the proximal surfaces and the incisal ridge; central incisor angles are sharper and more acute than lateral incisor angles, and mesioincisal angles are sharper than distoincisal angles
      (4) Maxillary lateral incisors vary the most in size and shape and may be congenitally missing or anomalous, as in the case of a peg lateral (smaller and more pointed)
    b. Canines—one in each quadrant; only teeth with one cusp; function in grasping and tearing
      (1) Considered the cornerstone of the dentition because of the long, large root, which is externally manifested by the canine eminence of maxillary alveolar bone
      (2) Have a prominent lingual ridge between two fossae; lingual anatomy is more prominent on maxillary canines
  2. Anatomic features of posterior teeth
    a. Premolars—two in each quadrant; first and second premolars; function in grinding
      (1) Generally have two cusps; the mandibular second premolar also typically has a three-cusped type
      (2) Have one root, except maxillary first premolars, which have two roots 60% of the time
      (3) Replace (succeed) primary molars when exfoliated
      (4) First premolars are frequently extracted for orthodontic reasons

TABLE 5-2   **Characteristics of the Crowns and Roots of Permanent Teeth**

Maxillary	Crown	Root(s)	Visual Characteristics
Central incisor	Largest of incisors The mesiodistal is greater than the faciolingual width. Distinct lingual anatomy; broad cingulum with tubercles The lingual surface (mesiodistal) is smaller than the facial surface because of proximal surface convergence.	One root, conical in shape Proximal root concavities uncommon Prominent incisal curvature of proximal cemento-enamel junctions Smallest root-crown ratio Cervical cross section is "rounded triangular" in shape with a flat mesial surface.	 Tooth #8
Lateral incisor	Similar to central but smaller, more slender; rounded incisal angles Cingulum is narrow, and a lingual pit is common.	One root, conical in shape The root is longer and more rounded than the central incisor. The root is 1⅓ times the length of the crown; may have a narrow lingual or palato-radicular groove extending from the crown to the root.	 Tooth #7
Canine	Single cusp formed by cusp ridges, facial and lingual ridges; one-third the length of the crown Lingual anatomy is distinct: large cingulum; lingual ridge between two lingual fossae; rarely has pits.	One long root, conical in shape Proximal root concavities; distal crown and root depression more significant Bulbous distal height of contour (HOC) may hinder access to the mesial surface of the first premolar. Cervical cross section is ovoid in shape. The root is 1½ times the length of the crown.	 Tooth #6
First premolar	Two cusps, facial longer and wider mesiodistally than the lingual; pentagonal shape from the occlusal with sharper angles on the facial cusp Occlusal: long central developmental groove; mesial and distal pits Mesial marginal ridge groove interrupts the mesial marginal ridge.	Two roots (40% have one root); one facial, one lingual Bifurcated in the apical to middle thirds; mesial and distal furcation entrances Prominent mesial concavity begins on the crown cervical to the mesial contact; extends apically to the furcation.	 Tooth #4
Second premolar	Two cusps of more equal length and width Occlusal outline is more rounded. Short central developmental groove; supplemental grooves No mesial crown concavity or groove	One root Proximal root concavities common; mesial root concavity not as pronounced as the first premolar Elliptical in cross section; broad proximally The root is 1¾ times the length of the crown.	 Tooth #5

TABLE 5-2   Characteristics of the Crowns and Roots of Permanent Teeth—cont'd

Maxillary	Crown	Root(s)	Visual Characteristics
First molar	Largest tooth faciolingually Rhomboidal occlusal view outline Oblique ridge from mesiolingual to distobuccal cusp Four cusps and one minor cusp on the mesiolingual cusp *(cusp of Carabelli)* An occlusal lingual groove ends with a pit on the lingual surface. Pits on occlusal, in mesial, central, and distal fossae. Lingual surface wider than facial surface due to large distolingual cusp (exception)	Three roots: mesiofacial, distofacial, and lingual; lingual root the longest Furcations on mesial, facial, and distal surfaces Root concavities: palatal surface of lingual root, mesial surface of mesiofacial root, and furcal surfaces (furcal concavities) Mesiofacial and distofacial root apices curve toward each other; resembles a pliers handle. Furcations begin gradually before the entrance, which is generally located near the junction of the cervical and middle third of the root; the mesial furcation is located more toward the lingual surface (mesiofacial root is broad in the faciolingual dimension). Root is 1¾ times the length of the crown.	Tooth #3
Second molar	Resembles the first molar, but is smaller; more rhomboidal from occlusal view Four cusps; distolingual cusp is smaller (lingual surface is narrower in the mesiodistal dimension) and sometimes absent. Pits in mesial, central, and distal fossae	Three roots: mesiofacial, distofacial, and lingual Roots are closer together; more distally oriented; less inter-radicular bone. Longer root trunk The root is 1¾ times the length of the crown.	Tooth #2
Third molar	Resembles the second molar, but varies frequently	May have three roots; varies frequently Roots frequently fused	

Mandibular	Crown	Root(s)	Visual Characteristics
Central and lateral incisors	Central incisor is the smallest tooth; symmetrical. Lateral incisor is slightly larger; asymmetrical. Sharp incisal angles Contact areas near the incisal ridge Lingual surface is concave, less distinct lingual anatomy. Lateral crown has a distal twist; incisal ridge is more lingually located on the distal, but cingulum is displaced toward the distal. More prominent distal concavity on lateral incisor	One root, wider faciolingually than mesiodistally Proximal root concavities are likely. Cervical cross section, elliptical in shape The root is 1½ times the length of the crown.	Tooth #25 Tooth #26

(Continued)

TABLE 5-2   Characteristics of the Crowns and Roots of Permanent Teeth—cont'd

Maxillary	Crown	Root(s)	Visual Characteristics
Canine	Cusp ridges and tip occupy ¼ to ⅕ of crown length. Lingual anatomy same as that of the maxillary canine, not as prominent Mesial surfaces of the crown and the root are in a straight line; mesial HOC more incisal than the maxillary canine.	One root, conical in shape Proximal root concavities are present. In cervical cross section, ovoid in shape, small lingual surface Occasionally is bifurcated into a facial and lingual root in apical third The root is 1½ times the length of the crown.	Tooth #27
First premolar	Two cusps: large facial with small, nonfunctional lingual Prominent transverse ridge, two pits, and a mesiolingual groove Crowns of all mandibular posterior teeth are inclined lingually.	One root, conical in shape In cervical cross section, may be ovoid or elliptical in shape May have a mesiolingual proximal root concavity The root is 1⅔ times the length of the crown.	Tooth #28
Second premolar	Bicuspidate (2) or tricuspidate (3) forms Two-cusped form: H-shaped or U-shaped groove pattern Three-cusped form: Y-shaped groove pattern with large facial cusp and smaller mesiolingual and distolingual cusps	One root, conical in shape In cervical cross section, may be ovoid or elliptical in shape The root is 1⅔ times the length of the crown. No significant root concavities	Tooth #29
First molar	Largest tooth mesiodistally Five cusps: mesiofacial, distofacial, distal, mesiolingual, and distolingual; Y-shaped occlusal groove pattern; extends onto facial surface and forms two facial grooves with a mesiofacial pit Occlusal pits in mesial, central, and distal fossae	Two roots, mesial is wider faciolingually and longer then the distal root. Furcations on facial and lingual surfaces; concavity before the furcation on facial surface begins just apical to cemento-enamel junction. Short root trunk; larger inter-radicular area Major proximal concavity and two root canals on the mesial root Cervical enamel projections may occur. The root is 1¾ times the length of the crown.	Tooth #30
Second molar	Similar to the first molar Four cusps: two facial and two lingual; "+"-shaped occlusal groove pattern; extends onto facial surface to form one groove and pit Occlusal pits in mesial, central, and distal fossae	Two roots, mesial and distal Roots are more likely to be closer together with a longer root trunk. Mesial root concavity is not as prominent. Roots are 1¾ times the length of the crown.	Tooth #31
Third molar	Similar to the second molar Varies greatly in form	Usually two roots Roots are short, frequently fused, and angled to the distal.	

b. Molars—three in each quadrant; named first, second, and third molars
   (1) Largest crown in the dentition both mesiodistally and faciolingually; shorter cervico-occlusally
   (2) Only teeth that do not replace primary teeth (non-succedaneous); erupt posterior to primary molars
   (3) The mandibular first molar is the first permanent tooth to erupt
   (4) Multi-cusped, with each having a distinct cusp-and-groove pattern
   (5) Maxillary molars have three roots; mandibular molars have two roots
   (6) The presence, size, and shape of third molars vary greatly, roots commonly fused

C. Tooth-numbering systems
   1. Universal Numbering System—Arabic numerals 1 to 32 to specify permanent teeth, beginning with the maxillary right third molar and ending with the mandibular right third molar.
   2. International Numbering System—a two-digit code: the first digit—1 to 4—designates the quadrant location; the second digit—1 to 8—designates the tooth, starting from the midline, from the central incisor to the third molar (e.g., 1-1 is the maxillary right central incisor)

D. General characteristics of tooth form
   1. Crest of curvature (crest of convexity) or height of contour (HOC)—the greatest curvature on each axial surface; four on each tooth
   2. All proximal surfaces narrow mesiodistally from the crest of curvature (HOC) to the CEJ (Figure 5-12)
   3. The proximal crest (HOC) convergence provides spacing for the interproximal gingiva and bone
   4. Contact area—ideally formed by the proximal HOC area, which functions to stabilize adjacent teeth and protect the interproximal gingiva
   5. Proximal crests (HOC) gradually move from the incisal third on incisors to the middle third on molars; as a general rule, the mesial crest is more incisal-occlusal than the distal crest
   6. Facial and lingual crests (HOC) are generally in the cervical third on anterior teeth, with the lingual HOC more in the middle third on premolars and molars; mandibular posteriors, especially molars, have their lingual HOC more toward the occlusal third
   7. Mesial cusp ridges are shorter than distal cusp ridges (except the maxillary first premolar); mesial outlines are straighter than distal outlines (Figure 5-13)

FIG 5-12 Apical convergence *(arrows)* of proximal surfaces.

FIG 5-13 Comparison of mesial *(M)* and distal *(D)* outlines.

FIG 5-14 Apical and incisal occlusal convergence *(arrows)* of facial and lingual surfaces.

FIG 5-15 Facial and lingual contours *(arrows)* and the proximal curvature of the cemento-enamel junctions. *L,* Lingual aspect.

   8. All facial and lingual surfaces converge toward the apex and toward the incisal-occlusal surface from the crests of curvature
      a. This convergence facilitates mastication (Figure 5-14)
      b. These contours deflect food away from the gingiva and facilitate the function of teeth (Figure 5-15)
   9. Cemento-enamel junctions
      a. The CEJ on the proximal surface curves toward the incisal-occlusal; more prominent on anterior teeth than on posterior teeth; curves more on the mesial surface than on the distal surface (see Figure 5-15)
      b. Maxillary CEJs curve more than mandibular
   10. Crown and root inclination—from a proximal view, the long axes of the crown and the root are in line, except for the mandibular posterior teeth crowns, which tilt lingually to the long axes of the root; this lingual inclination enables the intercuspal relationship of posterior teeth and the distribution of forces along their long axes (Figure 5-16)
   11. Proximal surfaces converge toward the lingual; this is most prominent on maxillary incisors and canines

FIG 5-16 Lingual inclination of mandibular posterior crowns.

    a. Lingual embrasures then are larger than facial embrasures

    b. The two exceptions are the mandibular second premolar, three-cusp type, and the maxillary first molar, because of its large distolingual cusp (Figure 5-17; see Table 5-2)

D. General characteristics of roots

  1. Root anatomy varies in size, shape, and number

  2. Teeth have one, two, or three roots; some roots may divide in the apical third

    a. One root—incisors, canines, maxillary second premolars, mandibular premolars

    b. Two roots—maxillary first premolars (buccal and lingual) and mandibular molars (mesial and distal)

    c. Three roots—maxillary molars (mesiobuccal, distobuccal, and lingual)

  3. Root trunk—area from the CEJ to the division of the roots

  4. Teeth with two or three roots have a root trunk with depressions that deepen until the trunk divides at the furcation

    a. Furcation—area where the root divides; complex anatomy within the furcation

    b. The more cervical the furcation, the more stable the tooth because of the divergence of roots with interradicular bone; first molars have the shortest root trunk

    c. Furcation involvement—loss of attachment of tissue and bone exists

    d. Furcations closer to the CEJ are more likely to become involved in periodontal disease, but are more accessible

    e. Individual roots are basically cone shaped, widest at the CEJ and converge (taper) to the apex; more root surface area is present in the cervical than apical third

    f. A cervical cross section of a tooth with one root shows three basic shapes (Figure 5-18; see Table 5-2), which may be slightly altered by the presence of root concavities

      (1) Triangular—maxillary incisors; have narrower mesiodistal dimension on the lingual surface

      (2) Ovoid (egg shaped)—canines and some mandibular premolars

      (3) Elliptical (oblong)—maxillary premolars, mandibular incisors, and some mandibular premolars

    g. A cervical cross section of molars follows the form of the crown, with depressions on most axial surfaces

    h. From a facial or lingual view, roots often have distal flexion; more reliably on posterior teeth

    i. Second-molar and third-molar roots are more likely to be closer together or fused, and distally inclined

    j. Variations in root form

      (1) Fused roots—no division or furcations

      (2) Supernumerary roots—extra roots

      (3) Dilaceration—unusual bending or root curvature

      (4) Hypercementosis—deposition of extra cementum

      (5) Enamel pearls—spherical enamel formed on cementum, usually near a furcation

      (6) Cervical enamel projections—CEJ curves more apically near a furcation

      (7) Bifurcational ridge—ridge of cementum between mesial and distal roots on mandibular molars

E. Clinical considerations of permanent tooth form—as a general rule, proximal surfaces of most teeth are more accessible from the lingual approach because of the convergence (tapering) of lingual teeth surfaces producing larger lingual embrasures

  1. Incisors

    a. Maxillary lingual anatomy is more prominent than mandibular lingual anatomy; however, plaque, calculus, and stain readily collect on mandibular lingual surfaces

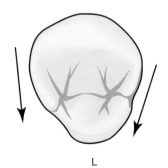

FIG 5-17 Lingual convergence *(arrows)* of proximal surfaces. *L,* Lingual aspect.

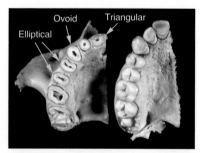

FIG 5-18 Root shapes as seen in cervical cross section: elliptical, ovoid, and triangular.

b. Repeated instrumentation on the narrow roots of mandibular incisors makes them subject to loss of structure, resulting in unsupported cervical enamel
c. Deep fossae and narrow dimensions of roots are difficult for instrumentation
d. Pits on maxillary lateral incisors more subject to caries

2. Canines
   a. Crown length, bulk, and long roots make these teeth very stable
   b. Prominent distal crown and root depression

3. Premolars
   a. Distinctive pit-and-groove patterns facilitate the identification of premolars
   b. Proximal root concavities, especially the mesial of the maxillary first premolar, make subgingival instrumentation difficult on the proximal surfaces
   c. Lingual inclination of mandibular premolar crowns makes instrumentation difficult
   d. Self-care more difficult with root depressions and lingual inclination

4. Molars
   a. Complex pit-and-groove patterns make molars susceptible to dental caries; sealants should be placed shortly after eruption
   b. Lingual inclination of mandibular molar crowns makes self-care and instrumentation difficult
   c. Maxillary molar furcations better accessed from the lingual approach because of locations
   d. Furcation involvement challenging for access; requires more time and possible surgical intervention

F. Primary/deciduous dentition
   1. The primary (deciduous) dentition consists of 20 teeth (5 per quadrant): 8 incisors, 4 canines, and 8 molars
   2. Numbering systems
      a. The Universal Numbering System uses capital letters (Figure 5-19): A through T for primary teeth, beginning with the maxillary right second primary molar and ending with the mandibular right second primary molar
      b. The International System uses a two-digit code: the first digit—5 to 8—designates the quadrant in the dentition, clockwise from the upper-right quadrant; the second digit—1 to 5—designates the tooth, from the central incisor to the second primary molar

   3. Set traits—the anatomy of primary teeth is similar to that of permanent teeth, except (Figure 5-20):
      a. Primary teeth are smaller in size than their permanent counterparts; primary molars are wider than the premolars *(leeway space)*
      b. Primary teeth are whiter than permanent teeth
      c. The crowns of primary teeth are shorter cervico-incisally/occlusally, with pronounced labial and lingual cervical ridges
      d. Occlusal tables of primary teeth narrower faciolingually (smaller intercuspal width), and the cuspal anatomy is not as pronounced as in permanent teeth (smaller intercuspal depth)
      e. Enamel thickness is more consistent and thinner: 0.5 to 1 mm thick, compared with that of permanent teeth, 2.5 mm
      f. Pulp chambers (relative to the size of the tooth) are larger, and pulp horns extend more occlusally than in permanent teeth; the amount of dentin is proportionately less

FIG 5-20 Comparison of dentitions. **A,** Comparison of primary and permanent anterior teeth. **B,** Comparison of primary second molars and permanent first molars.

FIG 5-19 Primary teeth, designated according to the Universal Numbering System; *F,* facial; *O,* occlusal.

g. Roots are slender and longer than in permanent teeth, approximately twice the length of the crown (larger root-crown ratio)
h. Molar root trunks are shorter (furcations closer to the CEJ); roots are more divergent to accommodate the developing premolar crown
i. Primary teeth have fewer anomalies and variations in tooth form
5. Class traits—anatomy of primary teeth (see Figure 5-19)
a. Incisors—resemble the outline of their permanent counterparts, except no mamelons on the incisal ridge and no pits on the lingual surface
b. Canines—resemble the outlines of their permanent counterparts; maxillary canine has a sharp cusp, wide and short; mesial cusp ridge is longer than the distal cusp ridge
c. Molars
(1) First primary molars—do not resemble any other teeth
(2) Have the same number and position of roots as that of permanent molars
(3) The CEJ on the mesial half of the buccal surface curves apically around a very prominent cervical ridge
(4) The maxillary first primary molar has an H-shaped groove pattern and usually has three to four cusps; somewhat resemble a maxillary premolar; the mesial cusps are the largest; a prominent cervical ridge is present
(5) The mandibular first primary molar has four cusps; the mesial cusps are larger, and the mesiolingual cusp is long, pointed, and angled toward the occlusal surface
(6) Second primary molars are larger than the first primary molars and resemble the form of the first permanent molar (isomorphic)

ERUPTION

A. General comments
1. *Eruption* frequently is defined as "the emergence of the tooth through the gingiva"
2. Also defined as the movements a tooth makes to attain and maintain a relationship with the teeth in the same and opposing arches; follows distinct stages:
a. Beginning of hard tissue formation
b. Enamel (crown) completion, after which actual tooth movement begins
c. Eruption; approximately 50% of the root is formed when eruption begins
d. Root completion
3. Ages at which eruption occurs are given in classic eruption tables
4. Sequential pattern (order) is more predictable than age of eruption
5. As a generalization, the mandibular tooth of a class (e.g., incisor, canine) emerges before the maxillary tooth of the same type, and the first before the second (e.g., the central incisor emerges before the lateral incisor)

B. Primary dentition development and eruption
1. A guide for the emergence of teeth into the oral cavity is provided in the following table:

	Mandibular	Maxillary
Central incisor	6 months	7½ months
Lateral incisor	7 months	9 months
Canine	16 months	18 months
First molar	12 months	14 months
Second molar	20 months	24 months

2. The order of eruption for primary tooth development is: central incisor, lateral incisor, first molar, canine, and second molar
3. Hard tissue formation begins in utero between 4 and 6 months
4. Crowns are completed between 1½ and 10 months of age
5. Roots are completed between 1½ and 3 years of age, 6 to 18 months after eruption
6. By 3 years of age, all primary teeth are erupted, and permanent teeth (except the third molars) are in some stage of development
7. Root resorption of a primary tooth is triggered by the pressure exerted by the developing permanent tooth; followed by primary tooth exfoliation in sequential patterns
C. Mixed/transitional dentition—period with both deciduous and permanent teeth present; begins with the eruption of the first permanent tooth (often the mandibular first molar) and ends with the exfoliation of the last primary tooth
1. Mixed/transitional dentition occurs between 6 and 12 years of age
2. Characteristics
a. Edentulous areas
b. Perception of disproportionately sized teeth
c. Varying clinical crown heights
d. Crowding
e. Enlarged and edematous gingiva
f. Enamel color variations between dentitions
D. Permanent dentition development and eruption
1. Succedaneous teeth replace primary teeth: incisors, canines, and premolars; nonsuccedaneous teeth are the permanent molars
2. Permanent tooth formation begins between birth and 3 years of age (except for the third molars)
3. The crowns of permanent teeth are completed between 4 and 8 years of age, at approximately one-half the age of eruption
4. The order of eruption in permanent tooth development follows:

Mandibular	Maxillary
First molar	First molar
Central incisor	Central incisor
Lateral incisor	Lateral incisor
Canine	First premolar
First premolar	Second premolar
Second premolar	Canine
Second molar	Second molar
Third molar	Third molar

5. A guide for the emergence of permanent teeth into the oral cavity follows:

	Mandibular	Maxillary
First molar*	6-7 years	6-7 years
Central incisor	6-7 years	7-8 years
Lateral incisor	7-8 years	8-9 years
Canine	9-10 years	11-12 years
First premolar	10-12 years	10-11 years
Second premolar	11-12 years	10-12 years
Second molar	11-13 years	12-13 years
Third molar	17-21 years	17-21 years

*First permanent tooth to erupt.

6. Roots of permanent teeth are completed between 10 and 16 years of age, 2 to 3 years after eruption

INTRA-ARCH AND INTERARCH RELATIONSHIPS

Each tooth has a relationship with adjacent teeth in the same and opposing arches. These relationships are influenced by size and shape of the maxilla, the mandible, the teeth themselves, spacing, and a variety of external factors, such as oral habits and dental disease.

A. Intra-arch relationship—the alignment of the teeth within an arch
   1. Position of teeth in the jaw
      a. Interproximal contacts—in an ideal alignment, teeth contact at their proximal crests of curvature (HOC); a continuous arch form is observed from an occlusal view
         (1) Anterior teeth contacts are in the middle of the faciolingual dimension
         (2) Posterior teeth contacts are facial of center in a faciolingual dimension
         (3) Some permanent dentitions have normal alignment with no contact
         (4) Primary dentitions often have developmental spacing in the anterior area; some have *primate spaces* between the primary maxillary lateral incisor and the canine and between the primary mandibular canine and the first molar (Figure 5-21)

FIG 5-21 Primary teeth showing primate spaces. **A,** Mandibular primate space between the canine and the first molar. **B,** Maxillary primate space between the lateral incisor and the canine. (Modified from Wilkins E: *Clinical practice of the dental hygienist,* ed 10, Philadelphia, 2008, Lippincott, Williams & Wilkins.)

b. Axial positioning—relationship of the long axis of individual teeth to an imaginary horizontal or median plane (mesiodistally and faciolingually); ideally, each tooth "sits" at an angle that best withstands the forces placed on it (Figure 5-22)
   (1) Most teeth are inclined facially, with the incisors having the greatest inclination
   (2) The mandibular posterior teeth tip lingually toward the median plane
c. Curves of the occlusal plane (a line connecting the cusp tips of canines, premolars, and molars)
   (1) Curve of Spee—from the buccal aspect in centric occlusion, the cusp tips of posterior teeth curve anteroposteriorly; for mandibular teeth, the curve is concave, and for maxillary teeth, it is convex (Figure 5-23, *A*)
   (2) Curve of Wilson—mediolateral curve connecting cusp tips of posterior mandibular teeth on opposite sides of the mouth (side to side); for mandibular teeth, the curve is concave because of their lingual tilt, and for maxillary molars, it is convex (Figure 5-23, *B*).
   (3) The matching curve is termed the *compensating curve*
2. Disturbances in intra-arch alignment
   a. Open contacts—sites where an interproximal space exists because proximal crests (HOC) do not meet; from developmental disturbances, missing teeth, oral habits, dental disease, or overdeveloped frena
   b. Positional variations, or versions—misplaced positioning of teeth from developmental disturbances, crowding, oral habits, dental caries, or periodontal disease; named for their positions: facioversion (facial of normal alignment), linguoversion, mesioversion, distoversion, supraversion (supraerupted), infraversion (undererupted), and torsiversion (rotated); interproximal contacts are often not normal

B. Interarch relationships—alignment between arches; can be viewed from a stationary (fixed) perspective and a dynamic (movable) perspective
   1. Stationary relationships
      a. Centric relationship—the most retruded position of the mandible, as in swallowing; muscles contract fully, not usually resulting in maximum tooth contact
      b. Centric occlusion—habitual occlusion where maximum tooth contact between arches (intercuspation) occurs (*note*: a normal physiologic rest position of the mandible during nonfunction)
         (1) Overjet (horizontal overlap)—the characteristic of maxillary teeth to overlap mandibular teeth in a horizontal direction; the maxillary arch is slightly larger; it functions to protect the narrow edge of incisors and to provide for an intercusping relationship of posterior teeth (Figure 5-24)
         (2) Overbite (vertical overlap)—the characteristic of the anterior maxillary teeth to overlap the anterior mandibular teeth in a vertical direction normally;

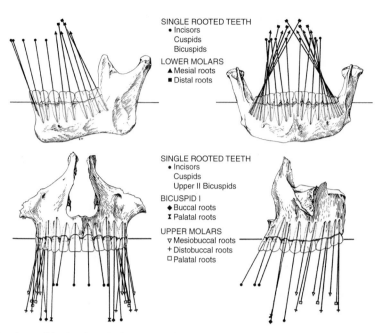

SINGLE ROOTED TEETH
• Incisors
  Cuspids
  Bicuspids
LOWER MOLARS
▲ Mesial roots
■ Distal roots

SINGLE ROOTED TEETH
• Incisors
  Cuspids
  Upper II Bicuspids
BICUSPID I
◆ Buccal roots
Ⅰ Palatal roots
UPPER MOLARS
▽ Mesiobuccal roots
+ Distobuccal roots
□ Palatal roots

FIG 5-22 Tooth positioning in relation to the horizontal plane. (From Dempster WT, Adams WJ, Duddles RA: Arrangement in the jaws of the roots of the teeth, *J Am Dent Assoc* 67:779, 1963.)

A

B

FIG 5-23 The curves of occlusion. **A,** Curve of Spee. **B,** Curve of Wilson. (From Berkovitz BKB, Holland GR, Moxham BJ: *Color atlas and textbook of oral anatomy, histology and embryology,* ed 2, London, 1992, Mosby–Year Book, Inc.)

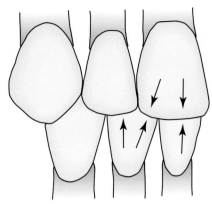

FIG 5-27 Interdigitation of teeth.

FIG 5-24 *Overjet,* the term used to describe the horizontal overlap of the anterior maxillary teeth on the anterior mandibular teeth.

facilitating the scissors-like cutting function of incisors (Figure 5-25)

(3) Intercuspation—the characteristic of posterior teeth to intermesh in a faciolingual direction; mandibular facial cusps and maxillary lingual cusps are centric cusps (supporting cusps) that contact interocclusally in the opposing arch (Figure 5-26)

    (a) Guiding cusps (maxillary facial and mandibular lingual) protect the teeth and tissues

(4) Interdigitation—the characteristic of each tooth to articulate with two opposing teeth (except for mandibular central incisors and maxillary last molars); a mandibular tooth occludes with its counterpart in the upper arch and the one mesial to it; a maxillary tooth occludes with its

FIG 5-25 *Overbite,* the term used to describe the vertical overlap of the anterior maxillary teeth on the anterior mandibular teeth.

FIG 5-26 Intercuspation of posterior teeth. Centric cusps have interocclusal contact with opposing teeth.

counterpart in the mandibular arch and the one distal to it (Figure 5-27)

c. Angle's classification of occlusion—using the first permanent molars, Edward H. Angle classified these relationships as follows (Figure 5-28):

    (1) Normal (ideal)—mesiobuccal groove of the mandibular first permanent molar aligns with the mesiobuccal cusp of the maxillary first permanent molar with no deviations in tooth positioning

    (2) Class I occlusion (orthognathic)—normal molar relationships with alterations in other characteristics of the occlusion, such as versions, crossbites, excessive overjets, or overbites

    (3) Class II malocclusion (retrognathic)—distal relationship of the mesiobuccal groove of the mandibular first permanent molar to the mesiobuccal cusp of the maxillary first permanent molar

        (a) Division 1—protruded anterior maxillary teeth

        (b) Division 2—one or more retruded anterior maxillary anterior teeth

    (4) Class III malocclusion (prognathic)—a mesial relationship of the mesiobuccal groove of the mandibular first permanent molar to the mesiobuccal cusp of the maxillary first permanent molar

d. Canines may also be used to classify occlusion when a molar is missing; class I canine relationship: cusp tip of the maxillary canine is facial to and between the mandibular canine and the first premolar

e. Occlusion in a primary dentition is assessed by the relationship of the distal terminus (surface) of second primary molars in centric occlusion; three relationships are possible: a flush terminal plane, a distal step, or a mesial step (Figure 5-29)

f. Mixed dentition represents a transitional stage of occlusal development; the initial contact of permanent first molars usually begins at age 7, and by 12 years of age, the final occlusion of the first molars is established

    (1) Distal-step primary dentitions always lead to a class II permanent molar occlusion

    (2) Exaggerated mesial-step primary dentitions lead to a class III permanent molar occlusion

FIG 5-28 Malocclusion classified using Angle's system. **A,** Angle's class I occlusion. **B,** Angle's class II malocclusion (division 1). **C,** Angle's class II malocclusion (division 2). **D,** Angle's class III malocclusion. (Modified from Berkovitz BKB: *Oral anatomy, histology and embryology,* ed 4, London, 2009, Elsevier Ltd.)

FIG 5-29 Terminus of second primary molars in centric occlusion. **A,** Flush terminal plane. **B,** Distal step. **C,** Mesial step.

(3) Development of occlusion from a flush terminus or a mild mesial-step primary dentition is variable but frequently leads to a class I first permanent molar relationship

2. Disturbances in interarch alignment
   a. Excessive overbite—the incisal edges of maxillary incisors extend to the cervical third of mandibular incisors
   b. Excessive overjet—horizontal overlap of maxillary teeth to mandibular teeth by more than 3 mm
   c. End-to-end relationships—edge-to-edge bite; anterior teeth meet at their incisal edges with no overjet or overbite; cusp-to-cusp bite in which posterior teeth meet cusp to cusp with no intercuspation
   d. Open bite—no incisal or occlusal contact between maxillary and mandibular teeth; teeth cannot be brought together, a space is created, may be caused by tongue thrust or thumb sucking
   e. Crossbites—altered normal faciolingual relationship between maxillary teeth and mandibular teeth; for anterior teeth, mandibular teeth are facial rather than lingual to maxillary teeth; for posterior teeth, normal intercuspation is not observed; numerous alterations are possible and result in maxillary or mandibular, buccal or lingual, or partial or total crossbites

3. Dynamic interarch relationships are a result of functional mandibular movements that start and end with centric occlusion during mastication
   a. Mandibular movements involve complex neuromuscular functions
      (1) Depression (opening)
      (2) Elevation (closing)
      (3) Protrusion (thrusting forward)
      (4) Retrusion (bringing back)
      (5) Lateral movements right and left; one side is always the working, or chewing, side; the opposite side is the nonworking, or balancing, side; ideally, these alternate during chewing
   b. Mandibular movements from centric occlusion are guided by maxillary teeth
      (1) Protrusion is guided by incisors; called *incisal guidance*
      (2) Lateral movements are guided by the canines on the working side in young, unworn dentitions (canine-protected occlusion); lateral movements may be guided by incisors and posterior teeth in worn dentitions
   c. As mandibular movements commence from a centric occlusion, posterior teeth should disengage in protrusion; on the balancing side, posterior teeth should disengage in lateral movement

d. If tooth contact occurs where teeth should be disengaged, occlusal interferences or premature contacts exist

SUMMARY OF TOOTH DIMENSIONS

A. Crowns
   1. From 7 to 11 mm cervico-incisally
   2. Anterior teeth are longer cervico-incisally (2 to 3 mm longer) than posterior teeth in both arches
   3. Smallest crown mesiodistally is the mandibular central incisor
   4. Maxillary first molar is the widest tooth faciolingually; mandibular first molar is the widest tooth mesiodistally
B. Roots
   1. From 12 to 17 mm in length
   2. Incisor roots are shortest
   3. Longest root is the maxillary canine
C. Ratio of root length to crown length is smaller in anterior teeth (root-to-crown ratio)
   1. Smallest ratio is the maxillary central incisor, where the root is only slightly longer
   2. Molars have a greater root-crown ratio because of short crowns cervico-occlusally
   3. Largest ratio is the mandibular first molar, where the root is 1.83 times longer

Website Information and Resources

Source	Website Address	Description
National Institute of Dental and Craniofacial Research	http://www.nidcr.nih.gov	Information and links related to awareness of craniofacial development and disorders; publications aimed at client/patient education are available.
Dental Hygiene Education Net	http://www.dhed.net/Site_Map.html	Links to both professional dental and dental hygiene organizations as well as numerous health care resource centers
		Dental anatomy information for professionals and clients/patients is available, as well as resources such as journals and research sites for and by dental hygienists.
Medscape from WebMD	http://emedicine.medscape.com	Numerous topics concerning oral health, including the oral examination, diseases of the oral cavity, and links to the Centers for Disease Control and Prevention (CDC) and other resources
Medline Plus	https://www.nlm.nih.gov/medlineplus/	Current health information, including a medical encyclopedia; a service of the U.S. National Library of Medicine and the National Institutes of Health

SUGGESTED READINGS

Bath-Balogh M, Fehrenbach MF: *Illustrated dental embryology, histology, and anatomy,* ed 4, St Louis, 2015, Saunders.

Beck M, Bryan L: Root morphology and instrumentation implications. In Darby ML, Walsh MM, editors: *Dental hygiene: theory and practice,* ed 3, Philadelphia, 2010, Saunders.

Nelson S: *Wheeler's dental anatomy, physiology, and occlusion,* ed 10, Philadelphia, 2014, Saunders.

Norton N: *Netter's head and neck anatomy for dentistry,* Philadelphia, 2012, Saunders.

Wilkins E: *Clinical practice of the dental hygienist,* ed 11, Philadelphia, 2012, Lippincott, Williams & Wilkins.

Woelfel JB, Scheid RC: *Dental anatomy: its relevance to dentistry,* ed 8, Baltimore, 2011, Lippincott, Williams & Wilkins.

Zwemer T, Thomas J, editors: *Mosby's dental dictionary,* ed 3, St Louis, 2014, Mosby.

CHAPTER 5 REVIEW QUESTIONS

Answers and rationales to review questions are available on this text's accompanying Evolve site. See inside front cover for details.

evolve

CASE A

Permanent Dentition

A 19-year-old woman presents for an initial dental hygiene appointment. Although she has had restorative procedures completed due to caries, she has not had prophylaxis for a few years. After a complete assessment, she is diagnosed with gingivitis and given oral self-care instructions. She has several questions about her bite and intraoral tissues, and she is concerned about her front teeth.

Use Case A and Figures 5-30 and 5-31 to answer questions 1 to 10.

1. **Several of this patient's maxillary anterior teeth show irregular incisal edges. What term is used to describe this wear?**
   a. Abfraction
   b. Abrasion
   c. Attrition
   d. Erosion
2. **From the lateral view of the maxillary left quadrant, there is a fracture of what feature of tooth #10?**
   a. Cervical area
   b. Mesioincisal angle
   c. Distoincisal angle
   d. Distal height of contour
3. **What term is used to describe the space between #10 and #11?**
   a. Diastema
   b. Leeway space
   c. Primate space
   d. Missing tooth
4. **Using the canine relationship, determine Angle's classification for this patient.**
   a. Class I occlusion
   b. Class II, division 1
   c. Class II, division 2
   d. Class III

5. **From the lateral view, which teeth do NOT have an ideal vertical overlap?**
   a. #4 and #5
   b. #11 and #12
   c. #13 and #14
   d. #21 and #22
6. **What term is used to describe this malocclusion?**
   a. Overjet
   b. Overbite
   c. End-to-end
   d. Crossbite
7. **During the clinical examination, you notice small round areas of pigmentation on the:**
   a. Commissure
   b. Vermillion zone
   c. Mucosal tissue
   d. Gingival margins
8. **From the occlusal view of the maxillary right quadrant (Figure 5-31), which tooth is malpositioned?**
   a. Canine
   b. First premolar
   c. Second premolar
   d. First molar

FIG 5-30 Lateral view, permanent dentition.

FIG 5-31 Occlusal view, permanent dentition.

9. The malpositioning of that tooth is called:
   a. Supraversion
   b. Torsiversion
   c. Infraversion
   d. Linguoversion

10. During the assessment, you note slight erythema at the anterior entrance to the tonsillar recess. Name this structure.
    a. Palatine raphe
    b. Fauces
    c. Pharyngopalatine arch
    d. Glossopalatine arch

CASE B

Mixed dentition

An 8½-year-old boy presents to your clinic for radiographs, examination, and prophylaxis. His mother is concerned about the appearance of his teeth and whether his permanent teeth are erupting on schedule.

Use Case B and Figure 5-32 to answer questions 11 to 17.

11. This patient's history of thumb sucking has caused malocclusion in the anterior of his mouth. This malocclusion is referred to as:
    a. Crossbite
    b. Open bite
    c. Overjet
    d. Edge-to-edge

12. Of the following, which of his permanent teeth are unerupted?
    a. #8, #9, and #10
    b. #23, #24, and #25
    c. #7, #10, and #26
    d. #23, #25, and #26

13. By what age would all permanent maxillary incisors normally be erupted?
    a. 4 to 5 years
    b. 5 to 6 years
    c. 6 to 7 years
    d. 8 years

14. Which tooth is malpositioned in linguoversion?
    a. #7
    b. #9
    c. #23
    d. #25

15. Which primary/deciduous mandibular incisor is still present?
    a. N
    b. O
    c. P
    d. Q

16. What explains the intraoral lesion present on the marginal gingiva of the maxillary arch?
    a. Apthous ulcer
    b. Abscess of the permanent tooth
    c. Eruption lesion
    d. Pericoronitis

17. Approximately how many millimeters of anterior overbite exist with this boy's occlusion?
    a. 0 mm
    b. 2 to 3 mm
    c. 4 to 5 mm
    d. More than 5 mm

18. Which of the following teeth would NOT be observed clinically in an 11-year-old child?
    a. Permanent lateral incisors
    b. Mandibular permanent canines
    c. Permanent central incisors
    d. Permanent second molars

FIG 5-32 Facial view, mixed dentition.

19. Which succedaneous teeth are usually present in a 7-year-old child?
    a. Mandibular first molars
    b. Mandibular central incisors
    c. Maxillary canines
    d. Mandibular canines

20. When comparing maxillary premolars, the maxillary first premolar has two cusps that are more equal in size than the second premolar, but the second premolar has a greater mesial depression on the crown and root.
    a. Both statements are TRUE.
    b. Both statements are FALSE.
    c. The first statement is TRUE; the second statement is FALSE.
    d. The first statement is FALSE; the second statement is TRUE.

21. Which of the following is TRUE of furcations on molars?
    a. A long root trunk places the furcation nearer to the cemento-enamel junction.
    b. Second molars have furcations more cervical than first molars.
    c. Third molars often have furcations in the cervical third of the root.
    d. Furcations increase the amount of attachment of bone and tissues.

22. When tooth J exfoliates, it will be replaced by:
    a. #5
    b. #12
    c. #13
    d. #21

23. Which of the following permanent teeth develops from five lobes?
    a. Maxillary premolar
    b. Mandibular canine
    c. Maxillary second molar
    d. Mandibular first molar

24. Performing root canal therapy would be most complex on this tooth because it usually has the most pulp canals.
    a. #12
    b. #14
    c. #20
    d. #28

25. In class I occlusion, normal wear can occur on all these structures EXCEPT:
    a. Incisal edges of mandibular incisors
    b. Mandibular canine cusp tips
    c. Maxillary lingual fossae
    d. Cervical areas

26. All the following are common sites for caries on a mandibular first molar EXCEPT:
    a. Occlusal pits and grooves
    b. Lingual developmental groove
    c. Interproximal contact areas
    d. Mesiofacial developmental groove

27. Radiographically, the density of this tooth tissue resembles that of caries.
    a. Pulp
    b. Dentin
    c. Cementum
    d. D. Enamel

28. For both arches, the *interproximal* heights of contour/crests of convexities follow this pattern.
    a. For incisors, heights of contour are in the middle third.
    b. For molars, heights of contour are in the occlusal third.
    c. The mesial height of contours are less incisal/occlusal than the distal height of contours.
    d. The mesial height of contours are more incisal/occlusal than the distal height of contours.

29. Which permanent tooth has the smallest root-to-crown ratio?
    a. Maxillary canine
    b. Mandibular first molar
    c. Maxillary central incisor
    d. Maxillary lateral incisor

30. What term is used to describe the extra spacing that exists to allow the permanent premolars adequate room to erupt?
    a. Primate spaces
    b. Leeway space
    c. Diastemas
    d. Interproximal space

31. Choose a trait that describes teeth in the maxillary arch.
    a. Fossae of incisors and canines have more distinct features.
    b. Crowns are wider mesiodistally than faciolingually.
    c. Premolars and molar crowns are inclined to the median.
    d. Interproximal curvatures of the CEJ are less than for mandibular teeth.

32. Comparing the maxillary canine with the mandibular canine, the maxillary canine has more prominent root depressions, whereas the mandibular canine has interproximal heights of contour more in the middle third of the cervico-incisal dimension.
    a. Both statements are TRUE.
    b. Both statements are FALSE.
    c. The first statement is TRUE, the second statement is FALSE.
    d. The first statement is FALSE, the second statement is TRUE.

33. Of the permanent teeth, which usually erupts out of sequence and may cause problems with spacing?
    a. Maxillary canine
    b. Mandibular canine
    c. Maxillary second premolar
    d. Mandibular second premolar

34. Of the following, during mastication of hard or hot food, all these structures of the palate may be injured EXCEPT:
    a. Rugae
    b. Median sulcus
    c. Alveolar process
    d. Incisive papilla

35. **When giving a supraperiosteal (infiltration) injection, into which area is the penetration site?**
    a. Pterygomandibular raphe
    b. Sublingual fold
    c. Mucobuccal fold
    d. Palatine fovea

36. **During a clinical examination, the patient presents with geographic tongue. This indicates the involvement of which papillae?**
    a. Fungiform
    b. Circumvallate
    c. Foliate
    d. Filiform

37. **Which of these structures provides openings into the mouth for two major salivary glands?**
    a. Parotid papilla
    b. Sublingual caruncle
    c. Palatal salivary duct
    d. Stensen duct

38. **Each cusp on a posterior tooth has one cusp ridge, but each posterior tooth has two marginal ridges.**
    a. Both statements are TRUE.
    b. Both statements are FALSE.
    c. The first statement is TRUE; the second statement is FALSE.
    d. The first statement is FALSE; the second statement is TRUE.

39. **For molars, which ridges extend from the cusp tip of each cusp to the grooves of the occlusal surface?**
    a. Triangular
    b. Marginal
    c. Facial
    d. Lingual

40. **For a buccal injection, choose the correct penetration site.**
    a. In the mucobuccal fold near the mental foramen
    b. Lateral to the retromolar pad near the most posterior molar
    c. In the mucobuccal fold posterior to the maxillary second molar
    d. Medial to the deep tendon of the temporalis muscle

41. **Which statement is TRUE of the mandibular first molar?**
    a. It usually has four cusps.
    b. It usually has two root canals.
    c. Its roots are close together.
    d. The mesial root is wider faciolingually than mesiodistally.

42. **Which of the following is NOT an anomaly of the maxillary incisors?**
    a. Peg lateral
    b. Shovel shape
    c. Supernumerary tooth
    d. Bifid/bifurcated root

43. **The curve of Spee is determined by the mediolateral curvature of the posterior occlusal surfaces, whereas the curve of Wilson is determined by the anteroposterior curvature of the occlusal surfaces.**
    a. BOTH statements are TRUE.
    b. BOTH statements are FALSE.
    c. The first statement is TRUE; the second statement is FALSE.
    d. The first statement is FALSE; the second statement is TRUE.

44. **Correct vertical overlap of teeth exists with which of the following relationships?**
    a. Mandibular anterior teeth overlap the maxillary anterior teeth facially.
    b. Mandibular lingual cusps fall within the occlusal table of maxillary teeth.
    c. Maxillary buccal cusps fall within the occlusal table of mandibular teeth.
    d. Maxillary buccal cusps overlap mandibular buccal cusps facially.

45. **Which of the following intraoral structures is NOT observed when lifting the tongue palatally?**
    a. Plica fimbriata
    b. Lingual frenum
    c. Philtrum
    d. Lingual veins

46. **Choose the CORRECT statement regarding axial positioning of teeth in the dental arches.**
    a. The mandibular posterior teeth crowns tip facially to the median plane.
    b. The incisors of both arches have the greatest inclination faciolingually.
    c. The premolars are at approximately 60 degrees to the horizontal plane.
    d. Maxillary teeth are more prone to axial deviation than mandibular teeth.

47. **What tooth surface is used to assess the occlusion in the primary occlusion?**
    a. Distal surface of the primary maxillary first molar
    b. Mesial surface of the primary maxillary first molar
    c. Distal surface of the primary mandibular second molar
    d. Mesial surface of the primary mandibular second molar

48. **All the following anatomic variations can occur within furcations and can complicate instrumentation EXCEPT:**
    a. Tubercles
    b. Cervical enamel projections
    c. Enamel pearls
    d. Bifurcational ridges

49. **Which permanent premolar can present with three different pit-and-groove patterns?**
    a. Maxillary first premolar
    b. Maxillary second premolar
    c. Mandibular first premolar
    d. Mandibular second premolar

50. **When comparing crown lengths to root lengths, the canines have the longest roots, whereas the third molars have the shortest crowns.**
    a. Both statements are TRUE.
    b. Both statements are FALSE.
    c. The first statement is TRUE; the second statement is FALSE.
    d. The first statement is FALSE; the second statement is TRUE.

6 | CHAPTER

Oral and Maxillofacial Radiology

Laura Jansen Howerton

Diagnostic dental radiographs are an important and necessary component of total patient care. Radiographic images enable the practitioner to see conditions that may otherwise go undetected. The goal of dental radiography is to obtain the highest-quality radiographic image while maintaining the lowest possible radiation exposure dose to the patient. The dental hygienist must be not only capable of producing diagnostic radiographs but also competent in interpretation skills.

Knowledge and skill in applying this information are critical for the safe use of ionizing radiation in the oral health care setting. This chapter emphasizes basic information on radiation, film processing, digital imaging, intraoral and extraoral techniques and errors, and radiographic interpretation.

GENERAL CONSIDERATIONS

Discovery of X-Radiation

A. Radiation—a form of energy carried through space in the form of waves or a stream of particles
B. Radiation characteristics
  1. Bundles of energy that have neither mass nor charge
  2. Travels at the speed of light (186,000 miles per second)
  3. Electromagnetic energies exist over a wide range of magnitudes, termed the *electromagnetic spectrum* (Figure 6-1)
  4. Interaction of radiation with biologic tissues causes change in the tissue due to ionization
  5. Electromagnetic spectrum is measured according to frequency, velocity, and wavelength
C. X-ray—a beam of energy that has the power to penetrate substances and record image shadows on receptors
D. Wilhelm Roentgen discovered the x-ray in 1895
  1. He was experimenting with vacuum tubes, photographic plates, and electrical currents
  2. Dr. Roentgen was awarded a Nobel Prize in physics

Radiation Physics

A. Ion—an atom that gains or loses an electron and becomes electronically unbalanced
B. Ionization— the process by which radiant energy removes an orbital electron from an atom to yield an ion pair
C. Ionizing radiation—radiation capable of producing ions; two types:
  1. Particulate radiation
    a. Tiny particles have both mass and energy, travel in straight lines at high speeds
    b. Examples: neutrons, protons, alpha and beta particles
  2. Electromagnetic radiation
    a. Electromagnetic radiation
    b. The propagation of wave-like energy without mass through space
    c. Arranged in an electromagnetic spectrum and measured according to frequency, velocity, and wavelength (see Figure 6-1)
      (1) Wavelength—distance from one crest of a wave to the next; the shorter the wavelength, the greater are the energy and penetrating ability of the radiation
      (2) Velocity—the speed of a wave
      (3) Frequency—number of wavelength crests passing a particular point per unit of time; the shorter the wavelength, the higher the frequency
      (4) Photon and quantum—a single unit or bundle of energy
      (5) Energy—ability to do work; electromagnetic radiation is measured in electron volts (eV)
D. X-ray machine
  1. Control panel—contains on/off switch exposure button and the controls to regulate the exposure factors (mA, kVp, time); modern x-ray machines may have preset exposure factors for various anatomic areas of the maxilla and mandible
  2. Extension arm—suspends the x-ray tubehead and houses electrical wires
  3. X-ray tubehead—lead-lined metal casing for the x-ray tube designed to prevent excessive radiation exposure and electrical shock
    a. Protects the x-ray tube
    b. Insulating oil surrounds x-ray tube and absorbs excess heat produced during x-ray production
    c. Transformers alter voltage of incoming electricity
    d. Aluminum discs filter the longer-wavelength x-rays
    e. Lead collimator restricts the size and shape of the x-ray beam
    f. Position-indicating device (PID) aims and shapes the x-ray beam; the longer PID produces an x-ray beam less divergent, decreases radiation exposure to client, and provides less image magnification

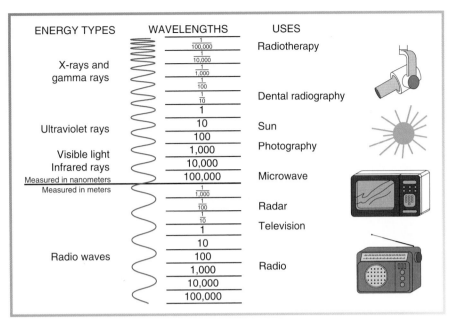

FIG 6-1 Electromagnetic energy spectrum. (From Iannucci JM, Howerton LJ: *Dental radiography: principles and techniques*, ed 4, St Louis, 2012, Elsevier Saunders.)

g. X-ray tube is the heart of the x-ray–generating system
  (1) Cathode
    (a) Negative electrode
    (b) Consists of a tungsten wire filament and molybdenum (focusing) cup
    (c) Supplies the electrons necessary to generate x-rays; milliamperage control (mA) regulates the step-down transformer, the quantity of x-rays produced, and heating of the filament
    (d) Because like charges repel, the electron beam is directed to a small area on the anode
  (2) Anode
    (a) Positive electrode
    (b) Consists of a tungsten plate fixed to a copper arm
    (c) The tungsten target serves as a focal spot and converts bombarding electrons into x-ray photons
    (d) Kilovoltage control (kVp) regulates the step-up transformer, voltage between cathode and anode, and speed of electrons
  (3) Aluminum filters are placed in the path of the x-ray beam to filter and selectively remove the low-energy, nonpenetrating x-rays from the beam
  (4) A lead collimator is positioned next to the aluminum filter to restrict the size and shape of the x-ray beam
E. Production of x-radiation (Figure 6-2)
  1. Control panel is activated by the on/off switch; appropriate mA, kVp, and time selections are chosen
    a. Milliamperage (mA)—allows for warming of the cathode filament and determines the number of electrons available for x-ray production; the higher the mA setting, the hotter the filament becomes, resulting in a greater number of available electrons
    b. Kilovoltage peak (kVp)—controls the current passing from cathode to anode; the higher the kVp setting, the greater the penetrating power and speed of acceleration of electrons from the cathode to the anode
    c. Exposure time establishes the time during which electrons are available for the bombardment of target material; the higher the time setting, the more electrons available for x-ray production
  2. Exposure button is pressed
    a. The heated filament provides electrons for x-ray production by *thermionic emission*, referred to as a "boiling off" of electrons; an electron cloud surrounding the filament is formed
    b. An electrical potential difference is created whereby electrons are attracted from the negative cathode to the positive anode
    c. The directional flow of electrons is influenced by the focusing cup of the cathode; electrons are repelled away from the negatively charged focusing cup; this mechanism controls the size and shape of the electron stream
    d. Less than 1% of the kinetic energy leaving the cathode is converted into x-ray energy; more than 99% of the energy leaving the cathode is converted into heat and absorbed by the insulating oil
F. Types of x-rays produced
  1. General (braking or "bremsstrahlung") radiation
    a. Produces 70% of x-ray photons by dental x-ray machines
    b. The accelerating electron passes near the nucleus of the target atom and is slowed down by the attraction of the nucleus

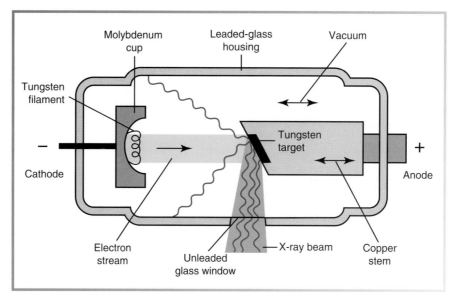

FIG 6-2 Diagram of x-ray tube. (From Iannucci JM, Howerton LJ: *Dental radiography: principles and techniques,* ed 5, St Louis, 2017, Elsevier.)

c. The slowing-down process results in the transference of the kinetic energy of the electron into x-ray energy

2. Characteristic radiation
   a. Can only occur at levels of 70 kVp or higher with a tungsten target; accounts for a small portion of x-rays produced by dental x-ray machines
   b. Occurs when an electron removes an orbital electron from the target atom
   c. During restabilization of the ionized atom, the movement of the outer-shell electron results in the transference of electron-binding energy into x-ray energy

G. Interactions of x-rays with matter
   1. Definitions
      a. Primary radiation—penetrating beam that is produced at the target anode; also termed *primary* or *useful beam*
      b. Secondary radiation—results from the interaction of primary radiation and matter
      c. Scatter radiation—one form of secondary radiation in which the direction of travel of the x-ray has been altered
   2. Interactions of x-ray photons and matter
      a. No interaction
         (1) The passing of x-ray photons through a material without any alteration of the photon or the material
         (2) Photons proceed to strike the image receptor
      b. Photoelectric effect
         (1) Results from an incident photon colliding with a tightly bound inner-shell electron
         (2) Incident photon ceases to exist; the electron is ejected as a recoil electron; ionization of the atom occurs
         (3) Accounts for approximately 30% of interactions

   c. Compton scatter
      (1) Results from an incident photon colliding with a loosely bound outer-shell electron
      (2) Incident photon gives up part of its energy in the ejection of the orbiting electron; ionization of the atom occurs
      (3) Accounts for approximately 62% of interactions
   d. Coherent scatter
      (1) The interaction of an incident photon passing near an outer-shell electron and being scattered without energy loss
      (2) Incident photon ceases to exist, and a new photon of identical energy is released from the electron; no ionization of the atom occurs
      (3) Accounts for approximately 8% of interactions

Characteristics of X-Radiation

A. Beam quality—the mean energy or penetrating ability of the x-ray beam
   1. Controlled by kVp; increasing the kVp will result in a higher-energy x-ray beam with increased penetrating ability
   2. Increasing the kVp will create a beam with shorter wavelength and higher frequency
   3. Density—the overall darkness of an image
      a. Increase kVp = increase density (darker)
      b. Decrease kVp = decrease density (lighter)
   4. Contrast—the differences between the dark and light areas on an image
      a. Increase kVp = low contrast (many shades of gray)
      b. Decrease kVp = high contrast (few shades of gray, mostly dark and light)

B. Beam quantity—the number of x-rays produced in the dental x-ray machine

1. Controlled by mA; determines the amount of electrons passing through the cathode filament
2. Increasing the mA will increase the number of x-rays produced and will also increase the temperature of the cathode filament
   a. Increase mA = increased density (darker)
   b. Decrease mA = decreased density (lighter)
   c. Milliamperage does not have an affect on image contrast
3. Exposure time also has an effect on the beam quantity; an increase in exposure time results in an increase in the number of x-rays produced
C. Beam intensity—the product of the quality and quantity of x-radiation; beam intensity is affected by kVp, mA, exposure time, and distance
   1. Increase kVp = increase beam intensity
   2. Increase mA = increase beam intensity
   3. Increase exposure time = increase beam intensity
   4. Increase distance = decrease beam intensity
      a. The distance between the source of radiation and the receptor has an influence on the intensity of the x-ray beam.
      b. The inverse square law is defined as "the intensity of radiation is inversely proportional to the square of the distance from the source of radiation"

$$\frac{Original\ intensity}{New\ intensity} = \frac{New\ distance^2}{Original\ distance^2}$$

      (1) As the distance between the source of radiation and an object increases, the intensity of the x-ray beam decreases
      (2) As the distance between the source of radiation and an object decreases, the intensity of the x-ray beam increases
      (3) For example, if the intensity of an x-ray beam is 400 mSv at 36 inches, at 72 inches the intensity is only one-fourth as great, or 100 mSv

RADIATION BIOLOGY AND PROTECTION

A. Radiation exposure
   1. Harmful to all living tissues; should be used cautiously
   2. Injury to cells, tissues, and organs occurs at the time of exposure but may take hours, days, or generations to manifest
   3. Two mechanisms of radiation injury are possible
      a. Radiation injury is caused by ionization
         (1) May cause a breakage in the molecule or a relocation of the atom in the molecule
         (2) Such changes may have a profound effect of structures of great importance, such as DNA
      b. Radiolysis of water
         (1) Yields free radicals that combine to form hydrogen peroxide (H_2O_2)
         (2) H_2O_2 is toxic to living tissues; its formation is an indirect, damaging effect of ionizing radiation
B. Characteristics of dose-response relationships
   1. Linear—the response is directly proportional to the dose
   2. Nonthreshold—any dose, regardless of its size, is expected to produce a response
   3. Threshold—from zero to a particular point, no response would be expected; above the threshold point, any dose will produce a response
C. Interactions of ionizing radiation with cells, tissues, and organs
   1. Stochastic effects—occur as a direct function of dose
   2. Nonstochastic effects—increase in severity with an increase in dose
   3. Genetic effects— not seen in the irradiated person but are passed to future generations
   4. Somatic effects—seen in the irradiated person but are not passed to future generations
   5. Short-term effects—associated with large amounts of radiation absorbed in a short time
   6. Long-term effects—associated with small amounts of radiation absorbed repeatedly over a long period of time
D. Sequence of radiation injury
   1. Latent period—the time between exposure to radiation and the appearance of the first observable clinical signs
   2. Period of injury—a variety of cellular injuries may occur
   3. Recovery period—not all cellular radiation injuries are permanent
   4. Cumulative effects—repeated radiation exposures can lead to problems with the health of the patient
E. Radiation effects on cells
   1. Not all cells respond to radiation in the same manner
   2. Several factors determine tissue sensitivity
      a. Mitotic activity—cells that divide frequently or undergo many divisions are more sensitive to radiation
      b. Cell differentiation—cells that are immature are more sensitive to radiation
      c. Cell metabolism—cells that have a higher metabolism are more sensitive to radiation
   3. Tissue and organ sensitivity
      a. Radiosensitive—a cell that is sensitive to radiation effects
         (1) Lymphatic (most sensitive)
         (2) Erythrocytes
         (3) Reproductive cells
      b. Radioresistant—a cell that is resistant to radiation effects
         (1) Nerve (most resistant)
         (2) Liver
         (3) Muscle
      c. Organ tissues considered critical for dental radiography are skin, thyroid gland, lens of the eyes, and bone marrow
      d. Continued low-dose exposure negatively affects the repair mechanism; overloading of the repair system by time or amount of exposure can result in somatic or genetic damage

Radiation Measurements and Sources

A. Two systems are used to define the radiation measurements: the older system, or traditional system (may be found in literature dated before 1985), and the newer or metric equivalent system known as International System of Units (SI)

B. The International Commission on Radiation Units and Measurements (ICRU) has established units for the measurement of radiation[1]

1. Radiation exposure—the measurement of ionization in air produced by x-rays
   a. Traditional unit of exposure is the roentgen (R)
   b. SI unit of exposure – defined as electrical charge per unit mass of air or coulomb per kilograms (C/kg)
   c. $1 \text{ R} = 2.58 \times 10^{-4}$ C/kg
      $1 \text{ C/kg} = 3.88 \times 10^3$ R
2. Radiation absorbed dose—the amount of radiation absorbed by a tissue
   a. Traditional unit is the radiation absorbed dose (rad)
   b. SI unit is the gray (Gy)
   c. 1 Gy = 100 rad
3. Dose equivalent—the measure of biologic effects produced by different types of radiation
   a. Traditional unit is the roentgen-equivalent man (rem)
   b. SI unit is the sievert (Sv)
   c. 1 Sv = 100 rem

C. Radiation risks and sources of radiation
1. Naturally occurring (or background) radiation constitutes 50% of the overall exposure to the United States population[2]
   a. Radon gas, the result of naturally occurring radionuclides found in soil (a *radionuclide* is an unstable atom that decays by emitting particles and energy from the nucleus to become electrically stable) accounts for 37% of the natural background radiation (Figure 6-3)
   b. Other terrestrial sources, cosmic radiation from outer space, and internal sources constitute another 13% of natural exposure
2. Medical applications account for 48% the overall exposure to the U.S. population[2]
   a. Computed tomography (CT) and nuclear medicine lead medical exposures by 24% and 12%, respectively
   b. Other conventional radiographs, including oral and maxillofacial radiography, constitute 5% of medical exposures
   c. Consumer products and industrial and occupational exposures account for the remaining 2% of total exposure to the U.S. population
3. *Exposure* is defined as the average annual effective dose equivalent of ionizing radiation
   a. Average annual effective dose equivalent of ionizing radiation to a member of the U.S. population is 6.2 millisieverts (mSv), up from 3.6 mSv in the early 1980s[2] (Figure 6-4)
   b. Significant increase largely arising from the increased use of large-dose medical imaging technologies

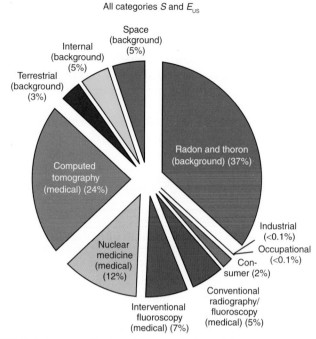

FIG 6-3 Annual effective dose equivalent of ionizing radiations. This chart illustrates the approximate percentage of exposure of the U.S. population to background and artificial radiations. (From www.NCRPonline.org.)

Radiation Protection

A. Before exposure
1. Proper prescribing of radiographs (Table 6-1)
   a. To limit the amount of radiation received by the patient, radiographs must be ordered on an individual basis, based on the patient need
   b. Evidence-based selection criteria is recommended[3]
2. Proper equipment must be used
   a. Filtration removes long-wavelength, less penetrating x-rays from the beam; dental x-ray machines operating at or below 70 kVp require 1.5-mm aluminum filtration; machines operating above 70 kVp require 2.5-mm aluminum filtration (Figure 6-5)
   b. Collimation restricts the size and shape of the x-ray beam; federal regulations require that the x-ray beam be collimated to a diameter of no more than 2.75 inches as it reaches the skin of the patient (Figure 6-6)
   c. The PID must be an open-ended, lead-lined cylinder; the longer the focal spot to object distance, the less divergent beam is created
B. During exposure
1. Use of the fastest image receptor
   a. Currently, "F" speed is the fastest speed intraoral film available
   b. Digital imaging further reduces patient exposure
2. Use of the lead apron and thyroid collar limits the amount of radiation received by the patient

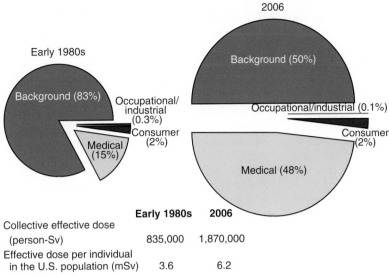

FIG 6-4 Comparison of effective dose equivalents. These charts illustrate the difference in approximate percentage of exposure of the U.S. population to background and artificial radiations in the early 1980s and 2006. (From www.NCRPonline.org.)

3. Beam alignment devices and proper technique also reduce the chances of retakes, thereby reducing unnecessary exposure to the patient

C. After exposure
   1. Correct film or sensor handling is necessary to produce diagnostic images
   2. Proper film processing and retrieval of digital images is necessary to produce diagnostic results

D. Operator protection
   1. The dental radiographer should remain behind a barrier during patient exposure
   2. If a structural wall or shield is not available, the radiographer should stand at least 6 feet away from the source of radiation and should be in a position at an angle of 90 to 135 degrees to the primary beam (Figure 6-7)

E. Maximum permissible dose (MPD)—defined by the National Council on Radiation Protection and Measurements (NCRP) as the maximum dose equivalent that a body is permitted to received within a specific period[2]
   1. The current MPD for occupationally exposed persons is 50 mSv/year
   2. The current MPD for nonoccupationally exposed persons is 5 mSv/year (one-tenth [1/10] the dose of the occupational radiation worker)

F. ALARA concept—individuals working with radiation should attempt to keep all radiation exposures "as low as reasonably achievable"

DENTAL X-RAY FILM

A. Film composition
   1. The base material (polyester) must possess the dimensional stability to withstand processing procedures and support the emulsion
   2. An adhesive is applied evenly to the base to provide for uniform attachment of emulsion to the base
   3. The emulsion consists of gelatin and silver halide crystals; gelatin suspends the silver halide crystals, which are sensitive to radiation and light
   4. A protective layer is applied to protect the emulsion from being scratched

B. Classifications of dental x-ray film
   1. *Intraoral* and *extraoral* film refer to the designated use of the film
      a. Intraoral film is placed inside the oral cavity (e.g., bitewing, periapical, or occlusal)
      b. Extraoral film is placed outside the mouth for exposure of larger areas of the head or skull (e.g., panoramic, cephalometric, skull)
   2. Film speed—the amount of radiation needed to produce an image with standard density
      a. Film speed is determined by the size of silver halide crystals in the emulsion, the thickness of the emulsion, and the presence of radiosensitive dyes
      b. Speed ranges used in dental radiography are designated from "D" (slowest) to "F" (fastest)
      c. E-speed intraoral film requires only 50% of the exposure of D-speed intraoral film; F-speed film requires only 77% of the exposure of E-speed film[4]
   3. Film size—various sizes are available for both intraoral and extraoral films
      a. Intraoral film
         (1) No. 0 size film—22 × 35 mm
         (2) No. 1 size film—24 × 40 mm
         (3) No. 2 size film—31 × 41 mm (standard film size)
         (4) No. 3 size film—27 × 54 mm
         (5) No. 4 size film—57 × 76 mm

TABLE 6-1   Guidelines for Prescribing Dental Radiographs

TYPE OF ENCOUNTER	CHILDREN		ADOLESCENT		ADULT
	Primary Dentition (before eruption of first permanent tooth)	Transitional Dentition (after eruption of first permanent tooth)	Permanent Dentition (before eruption of third molars)	Dentate or Partially Edentulous	Edentulous
New client* being evaluated for dental diseases and dental development	Individualized radiographic examination consisting of selected periapical views, occlusal views, or both; posterior bitewings if proximal surfaces cannot be visualized or probed Clients without evidence of disease and with open proximal contacts may not require a radiographic examination at this time.	Individualized radiographic examination consisting of posterior bitewings with panoramic examination or posterior bitewings and selected periapical images	Individualized radiographic examination consisting of posterior bitewings with panoramic examination or posterior bitewings and selected periapical images A full-mouth intraoral radiographic examination is preferred when the client has clinical evidence of generalized dental disease or a history of extensive dental treatment.		Individualized radiographic examination based on clinical signs and symptoms
Recare client* with clinical caries or at increased risk for caries[†]	Posterior bitewing examination at 6- to 12-month intervals if proximal surfaces cannot be examined visually or with a probe			Posterior bitewing examination at 6- to 18-month intervals	Not applicable
Recare client* with no clinical caries and not at risk for caries[†]	Posterior bitewing examination at 12- to 24-month intervals if proximal surfaces cannot be examined visually or with a probe		Posterior bitewing examination at 18- to 36-month intervals	Posterior bitewing exam at 24- to 36-month intervals	Not applicable
Recare client* with clinical periodontal disease	Clinical judgment as to the need for and type of radiographic images for the evaluation of periodontal disease. Imaging may consist of, but is not limited to, selected bitewing images, periapical images, or both, of areas where periodontal disease (other than nonspecific gingivitis) can be identified clinically.				Not applicable
Client for monitoring of growth and development	Clinical judgment as to the need for and type of radiographic images for evaluation, monitoring, or both, of dentofacial growth and development		Clinical judgment as to the need for and type of radiographic images for evaluation, monitoring, or both, of dentofacial growth and development Panoramic or periapical exam to assess developing third molars		Not usually indicated
Client with other circumstances, including, but not limited to, proposed or existing implants, pathology, needs, treated periodontal disease, and caries remineralization	Clinical judgment as to the need for and type of radiographic images for evaluation, monitoring, or both, in these circumstances				

*Clinical situations for which radiographs may be indicated include, but are not limited to the following. *Positive historical finding:* Previous periodontal or endodontic treatment, history of pain or trauma, familial history of dental anomalies, postoperative evaluation of healing, remineralization monitoring, presence of implants or evaluation for implant placement. *Positive clinical signs and symptoms:* Clinical evidence of periodontal disease; large or deep restorations; deep carious lesions; malposed or clinically impacted teeth; swelling; evidence of dental or facial trauma; mobility of teeth; fistula involving sinus tract; clinically suspected sinus pathology; growth abnormalities; oral involvement in known or suspected systemic disease; positive neurologic findings in the head and neck; evidence of foreign objects; pain, dysfunction, or both, of the temporomandibular joint; facial asymmetry; abutment teeth for fixed or removable partial prosthesis; unexplained bleeding; unexplained sensitivity of teeth; unusual eruption, spacing, or migration of teeth; unusual tooth morphology, calcification, or color; unexplained absence of teeth; clinical erosion.

[†]Factors increasing the risk for caries may include, but are not limited to the following: High level of caries experience or demineralization, history of recurrent caries, high titers of cariogenic bacteria, existing restoration(s) of poor quality, poor oral hygiene, inadequate fluoride exposure, prolonged nursing (bottle or breast), high-sucrose diet, poor familial oral health, developmental or acquired enamel defects, developmental or acquired disability, xerostomia, genetic abnormality of teeth, many multi-surface restorations, chemotherapy or radiation therapy, eating disorders, drug or alcohol abuse, irregular dental care.

FIG 6-5 Aluminum discs are placed in the path of the beam to filter out the low-energy, longer-wavelength x-rays that are harmful to the patient. (From Iannucci JM, Howerton LJ: *Dental radiography: principles and techniques*, ed 5, St Louis, 2017, Elsevier.)

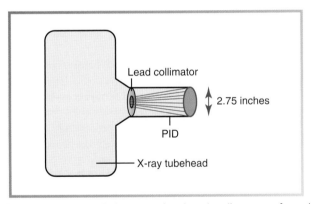

FIG 6-6 Federal regulations require that the diameter of a collimated x-ray beam be restricted to 2.75 inches at the patient's skin. (From Iannucci JM, Howerton LJ: *Dental radiography: principles and techniques*, ed 5, St Louis, 2017, Elsevier.)

C. Components of intraoral film packets
　1. Light-tight, leakproof wrapping protects film from light and moisture
　2. Black protective paper is used for additional protection of the film from light
　3. Lead foil is inserted between the black paper and the outer wrapping on the back side of the film packet; the purpose of the lead foil is to prevent backscattered radiation from fogging the film
　4. Single or double films are enclosed in the packet

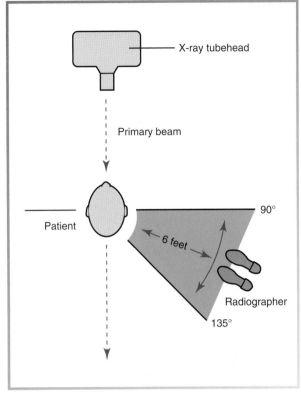

FIG 6-7 Operator protection guidelines suggest that the dental radiographer stand at an angle of 90 to 135 degrees to the primary beam. (From Iannucci JM, Howerton LJ: *Dental radiography: principles and techniques*, ed 5, St Louis, 2017, Elsevier.)

D. Intensifying screens used with extraoral film
　1. Housed inside a light-tight cassette
　2. Used as a component of the indirect imaging system to reduce client exposure to x-radiation for study of large anatomic areas
　3. Screen construction
　　a. Base material composed of polyester plastic
　　b. Reflective layer is coated onto the base material; redirects light toward the film to increase film efficiency
　　c. Phosphor layer composed of phosphorescent crystals; calcium tungstate emits blue light to expose the film; rare-earth crystals emit green light and respond more efficiently to reduce radiation exposure needed to produce the image
　　d. Protective coating is applied to phosphor layer
E. Film storage and protection
　1. Unexposed film must be stored away from heat, moisture, chemical vapors, and radiation; film should be stored in a cool, dry place
　2. Film has a limited shelf life and must be used before the expiration date

Dental X-Ray Image Characteristics

Table 6-2 summarizes the characteristics and respective influencing factors.

TABLE 6-2 Radiation Characteristics and Influencing Factors

Characteristics	Influencing Factors	Effect of Influencing Factors	Result
Sharpness	Focal spot size	Decrease focal spot size	Increase sharpness
	Film composition	Decrease crystal size	Increase sharpness
	Movement	Decrease movement	Increase sharpness
Magnification	Target-film distance	Increase target-film distance	Decrease magnification
	Object-film distance	Decrease object-film distance	Decrease magnification
Distortion	Object-film alignment	Object and film parallel	Decrease distortion
	X-ray beam alignment	Beam perpendicular to object and film	Decrease distortion

A. Radiolucent—refers to a portion of an image that is dark or black

B. Radiopaque—refers to a portion of an image that is light or white

C. Density—the overall darkness or blackness of an image
1. Increase kVp, increase density
2. Increase mA, increase density
3. Increase time, increase density

D. Contrast—the difference in the degrees of darkness between adjacent areas on an image
1. Increase kVp, low contrast (many shades of gray)
2. Decrease kVp, high contrast (many areas of black and white)

E. Sharpness—the capability of the image receptor to reproduce the distinct outlines of an object
1. The smaller the focal spot size, the sharper the image
2. The smaller the silver halide crystals in the film emulsion, the sharper the image
3. The less movement of the patient, tubehead, or film, the sharper the image

F. Magnification—a radiographic image that is larger than its actual size
1. The longer the target-to-receptor distance, the less image magnification produced
2. The shorter the tooth-to-receptor distance, the less image magnification produced

G. Distortion—a variation in the true size and shape of an object
1. Align the tooth and receptor parallel to each other to avoid distortion
2. Position the x-ray beam perpendicular to the tooth and receptor to avoid distortion

Dental X-Ray Film Processing

A. Manual film processing consists of five steps: development, rinse, fixation, rinse, and dry
1. Developer solution reduces the exposed silver halide crystals into black metallic silver and softens the emulsion
   a. Reducing agent (hydroquinone and elon) reduces the exposed silver halide crystals to black metallic silver
   b. Alkalizer (sodium carbonate) softens and swells the gelatin of the emulsion to allow the reducing agent to reach the silver halide crystals
   c. Preservative (sodium sulfite) slows the oxidation of the solution to prolong its life span
   d. Restrainer (potassium bromide) slows down the action of chemicals
2. A water bath is used to wash or rinse the film and stop the development process
3. Fixer solution removes the unexposed silver halide crystals from the emulsion and hardens the emulsion
   a. Clearing or fixing agent (sodium or ammonium thiosulfate) removes the unexposed or undeveloped crystals from the emulsion
   b. Acidifier (acetic acid) provides the required acidity so that the fixing solutions can work; stops the action of the developer
   c. Preservative (sodium sulfite) slows the solution's oxidation to prolong its life span
   d. Hardener (potassium aluminum) shrinks and hardens the emulsion
4. A water bath is used to wash the films and remove all chemicals
5. Films must be completely dried before handling for mounting or viewing
6. Total time involved for manual film processing: approximately 45 to 60 minutes

B. Equipment needed for manual film processing
1. Darkroom: to provide a completely darkened environment for film handling
2. Processing tanks: two insert tanks hold the developer and fixer solutions, while a master tank holds circulating water
3. A thermometer is needed to determine the temperature of the developer solution
   a. The optimum time/temperature for manual processing is 68°F (20°C) for 5 minutes
   b. Higher temperatures require shorter development time; cooler temperatures require longer development time
4. A timer, film hangers, and stirring paddles are also recommended for manual film processing

C. Automatic film processing consists of four steps: development, fixation, rinse, and dry
1. Films are carried from solutions to the dryer by a roller assembly
2. Processing solutions are highly concentrated to work quickly
3. Total time involved for automatic film processing: approximately 4 to 5 minutes

D. Equipment needed for automatic film processing
   1. Darkroom: to provide a completely darkened environment for film handling
      a. Some processors are equipped with daylight loaders
      b. Daylight loaders are light-shielded compartments that allow processing to be completed in a room with white light
   2. Automatic processor is built with a housing; film feed slot; roller film transporter; compartments for developer, fixer, and water; a drying chamber; and replenisher pumps
E. Darkroom design and requirements
   1. Light-tight room with a revolving light-sealed door, or door with an inside lock
   2. Safelight to allow sufficient illumination without exposing or damaging the film
      a. Low-wattage bulb of 7.5 or 15 watts
      b. Must be placed at least 4 feet from the work surface
      c. The GBX-2 filter is recommended because it is safe to use with both intraoral and extraoral films
   3. Overhead white light provides illumination for cleaning and stocking materials
   4. Adequate work space
F. Film duplication
   1. Copies of original radiographs may be needed for third-party payment, a change to another oral health care practitioner, referrals to specialists, or use in litigation
   2. The duplication of film requires the use of a film duplicator machine and specialized duplicating film

FILM-PROCESSING ERRORS

A. Fogged radiographs; appear gray and lack contrast (Figure 6-8)
   1. Improper safelighting in the darkroom
   2. Exposure to scatter radiation, heat, humidity, or chemical vapors
   3. Contaminated processing chemicals
   4. Old, expired, or damaged film

FIG 6-9 An overdeveloped film appears dark. (From Iannucci JM, Howerton LJ: *Dental radiography: principles and techniques,* ed 5, St Louis, 2017, Elsevier.)

B. Dark radiographs (Figure 6-9)
   1. Temperature of developer solution too high; developer solution too concentrated
   2. Excessive developing time used
   3. Inaccurate timer or thermometer
C. Light radiographs (Figure 6-10)
   1. Temperature of developer solution too cool; developer solution too weak
   2. Insufficient developing time
   3. Inaccurate timer or thermometer
D. Clear (blank) radiographs
   1. Film was not exposed to radiation; most common reason for a clear radiograph
   2. Film placed in fixer solution prior to developer solution
   3. Excessive washing, which causes the removal of film emulsion
E. Completely black radiographs are caused by the film being exposed to white light before processing

FIG 6-8 A fogged film appears gray and lacks detail and contrast. (From Iannucci JM, Howerton LJ: *Dental radiography: principles and techniques,* ed 5, St Louis, 2017, Elsevier.)

FIG 6-10 An underdeveloped film appears light. (From Iannucci JM, Howerton LJ: *Dental radiography: principles and techniques,* ed 5, St Louis, 2017, Elsevier.)

FIG 6-11 Fixer spots appear light or white. (From Iannucci JM, Howerton LJ: *Dental radiography: principles and techniques*, ed 5, St Louis, 2017, Elsevier.)

F. Radiographs with spots (Figure 6-11)
1. Developer splashing on film before processing causes dark or black spots
2. Fixer splashing on film before processing causes white or light spots
3. Water splashing on film before processing causes light spots
G. Yellow-brown stained radiographs
1. Insufficient fixing or washing times
2. Processing solutions are exhausted and must be replaced or replenished
H. Dark roller lines or marks
1. Dirty or contaminated processing chemicals cause dark lines to appear on automatically processed films
2. Dirty or contaminated automatic processor rollers may also cause roller marks
I. Static electricity artifacts (Figure 6-12)
1. Caused by the rapid removal of the film from the packet or the cassette when the humidity level is very low, such as during winter months
2. Yields black artifacts in tree-shaped streaks, smudges, or dots

FIG 6-12 Static electricity appears as black branching lines. (From Iannucci JM, Howerton LJ: *Dental radiography: principles and techniques*, ed 5, St Louis, 2017, Elsevier.)

QUALITY ASSURANCE

A. A quality control plan in dental radiography ensures the production of diagnostic-quality radiographs while minimizing radiation exposure through a plan of action; in addition, the means of testing and regulating x-ray equipment and procedures used to expose, process, and store radiographs are reviewed
B. Components of a quality control plan
1. Competence of radiographer
   a. Evaluation of radiographs for self-analysis of technique
   b. Peer review of radiographs for technique analysis
   c. Continuing education courses to maintain state-of-the-art practice
2. Equipment inspections by state and local radiation regulatory agencies
   a. Milliamperage, kilovoltage, timer accuracy
   b. Collimation and alignment of the x-ray beam
   c. Measures to avoid leakage radiation
   d. Mechanical support of the unit; may include tube drifting
   e. Penetrating quality of the beam tested by using the half-value layer (HVL); uses a material (usually aluminum) that reduces exposure by one-half when placed within path of radiation beam
3. Quality assurance procedures for film processing
   a. Periodic evaluation of the darkroom
      (1) Checks for light leaks
      (2) Coin test for safelight evaluation involves the placement of a coin on an unwrapped, unexposed film under a safelight for 2 to 3 minutes; if the outline of the coin is present on the processed film, corrective action is necessary
4. Creation of a reference or step-wedge radiograph to compare strengths of processing solutions; evaluates films for consistency in density and contrast
5. Periodic cleaning, maintenance, and daily monitoring of processing equipment
   a. Clean the automatic roller assembly and manual racks to prevent debris buildup and artifacts; schedule cleaning maintenance on the basis of usage
   b. Schedule preventive maintenance for optimal equipment operation
   c. Monitor solution temperatures daily
   d. Replenish solutions in accordance with the volume of films processed

DIGITAL IMAGING

A. Digital imaging is a filmless system in which a radiographic image is captured using a sensor, the image is broken down into electronic pieces and viewed and stored on a computer
1. Source of radiation—a conventional dental x-ray unit
2. Intraoral sensor—replaces the traditional dental x-ray film
3. Computer—converts the electronic signal received by the sensor; processes and stores the information

B. Methods of obtaining digital images
   1. Direct digital imaging
      a. Uses an x-ray machine, intraoral sensor, and computer
      b. The sensor contains a fiberoptic cable linked to the computer as it is placed into the mouth of the patient; the sensor is rigid, and patients may complain of the bulkiness
      c. Within seconds of exposure, the image appears on the computer monitor
   2. Indirect digital imaging
      a. Uses an x-ray machine, intraoral sensor, and computer
      b. The sensor is a reusable imaging plate coated with phosphors (often termed *PSP plate*); this sensor is thin and flexible, much like an intraoral film packet
      c. After exposure, the plate is scanned to convert the information into electronic files
      d. Because of the laser scanning step, this type of digital imaging is less rapid than direct digital imaging
C. Advantages of digital imaging[5]
   1. Superior resolution produces images with increased diagnostic capabilities
   2. Because of the sensitivity of the sensors, patients are exposed to less radiation than with traditional film
   3. Increased speed of image viewing leads to increased time efficiency in the dental office
   4. Because the image may be viewed on a computer monitor, patient education is enhanced
D. Disadvantages of digital imaging
   1. Initial expense of purchasing and setting up equipment may be costly
   2. Depending on the system used, sensor size and bulkiness may be an issue
   3. Infection control procedures may be difficult, especially with corded sensors
   4. Learning a new computer language may be problematic for the staff

RADIOLOGY TECHNIQUES: INTRAORAL AND EXTRAORAL

A. Adhering to shadow-casting principles produces diagnostic radiographic images
   1. Smallest focal spot possible
   2. Longest source-to-object distance possible (focal spot to tooth)
   3. Shortest object-to-receptor distance possible (tooth to receptor)
   4. Tooth and receptor should be in a parallel relationship
   5. X-ray beam should be perpendicular to the tooth and the image receptor
B. Angulation of the x-ray beam
   1. Vertical angulation refers to the position of the PID in the vertical plane
      a. Positive vertical angulation indicates the PID is pointing downward

      b. Negative vertical angulation indicates the PID is pointing upward
   2. Horizontal angulation refers to the position of the PID in the horizontal plane

Intraoral Radiographic Techniques
A. Paralleling
   1. Yields radiographs with a minimum of image distortion
   2. Minimizes the superimposition of adjacent oral structures
   3. Application of the paralleling technique
      a. The receptor is placed parallel to the long axis of the tooth
      b. The x-ray beam is directed perpendicular to the long axis of the tooth and the receptor
      c. The x-ray beam is directed perpendicular through interproximal spaces
      d. The x-ray beam is centered over the anatomic structures and the receptor
B. Bisecting the angle
   1. Applies the rule of isometry: the accurate length of the tooth is obtained if the x-ray beam is perpendicular to the imaginary bisector of the angle formed by the plane of the receptor and the long axis of the tooth (Figure 6-13)
   2. Allows for ease of receptor placement for certain patients with a small mouth, shallow palate, large tori, or gag reflex
   3. Application of the bisecting angle technique
      a. The receptor is placed against the teeth
      b. The x-ray beam is directed perpendicular to the imaginary bisector of the angle formed by the plane of the receptor and the long axis of the tooth
      c. The x-ray beam is directed perpendicular through interproximal spaces
      d. The x-ray beam is centered over the anatomic structures and the receptor

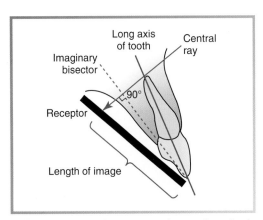

FIG 6-13 The image on the receptor is equal to the length of the tooth when the central ray is directed at 90 degrees to the imaginary bisector. A tooth and its image will be equal in length when two equal triangles are formed that share a common side (imaginary bisector). (From Iannucci JM, Howerton LJ: *Dental radiography: principles and techniques*, ed 5, St Louis, 2017, Elsevier.)

FIG 6-14 Periapical radiograph.

Types of Intraoral Radiographic Examinations

A. Periapical
1. Periapical examination demonstrates the entire tooth and surrounding bone (Figure 6-14)
2. Indications for periapical radiographs[3]
   a. Suspected periapical conditions
   b. Evidence of periodontal disease
   c. Injury or trauma to teeth
   d. Endodontic therapy
   e. Deep or large carious lesions
   f. Suspected impacted teeth
   g. Unusual eruption, malposition, or unexplained missing teeth
   h. Unexplained sensitivity or tooth mobility
   i. Unusual tooth morphology or color
   j. Dental implant evaluation

B. Bitewing
1. Bitewing radiographs demonstrate the anatomic crowns of maxillary and mandibular teeth as well as the height of alveolar bone (Figure 6-15)
2. Indications for bitewing radiographs[3]
   a. Suspected interproximal caries
   b. Defective restorations
   c. Early periodontal disease
3. Horizontal bitewing radiographs are considered the traditional placement; the long dimension of the receptor positioned horizontally
4. Bitewing radiographs may also be exposed by placing the receptor with the long dimension vertically; vertical bitewing radiographs are typically used with patients with periodontal disease because the vertical image increases the viewing area of alveolar bone

C. Occlusal
1. An occlusal radiograph demonstrates a large anatomic region or the entire arch; it is usually exposed in conjunction with other intraoral radiographs (Figure 6-16)
2. Indications for the exposure of occlusal radiographs[6]
   a. Image margins of large pathologic conditions
   b. Localization of objects (foreign or impactions)
   c. Injury or trauma to surrounding bone structure
   d. Suspected supernumerary teeth

FIG 6-16 Occlusal radiographs. **A,** Topographic maxillary occlusal radiograph. **B,** Topographic mandibular occlusal radiograph. **C,** Cross-sectional mandibular occlusal radiograph.

FIG 6-15 Bitewing radiographs. **A,** Long horizontal bitewing. **B,** Traditional horizontal bitewing. **C,** Vertical bitewing.

FIG 6-17 Full-mouth radiographic survey. (From Bird DL, Robinson DS: *Modern dental assisting,* ed 11, St Louis, 2015, Elsevier.)

e. Unexplained swelling or growth abnormality
f. Salivary stone detection
3. Occlusal radiographs may be prescribed for children, patients with limited jaw opening or those who cannot tolerate periapical receptor placement
D. Full-mouth survey (Figure 6-17)
1. A series of intraoral radiographs that reveal all the tooth-bearing areas of the maxilla and mandible
2. Usually a combination of periapical and bitewing radiographs
3. May include dentulous and edentulous areas

Types of Extraoral Radiographic Examinations

A. The panoramic radiograph is the most common extraoral exposure (Figure 6-18)
B. Provides an overall view of the maxilla, mandible, and surrounding structures; used to supplement intraoral images
C. Indications for the exposure of panoramic radiographs[6]

1. Impacted teeth
2. Eruption patterns; growth and development
3. Assessment of trauma
4. Examination of the extent of large lesions or pathologic conditions
D. Image production is created while the receptor and tubehead rotate around the patient
1. The image is produced through a process termed *tomography*
2. Tomography is a radiographic technique that permits visualization of structures in a chosen plane or layer while intentionally blurring the images above and below the selected plane
3. The zone in which structures are most clearly demonstrated is termed the *focal trough*
a. The size and shape of each focal trough varies, determined by the manufacturer of the panoramic machine
b. The focal trough is designed to accommodate the average-size maxilla and mandible

FIG 6-18 Panoramic radiograph.

E. Patient positioning is important in preparation of exposure of panoramic radiographs
   1. Follow the directions from the manufacturer for specific positioning guidelines for determining the location of the focal trough
   2. Insert the receptor into the cassette and panoramic unit
   3. Position the patient with the midsagittal plane perpendicular to the floor and the Frankfort plane parallel to the floor
   4. Instruct the patient to occlude on the bite stick or similar device and to hold still throughout the exposure
   5. Consult the manufacturer's instructions to select appropriate exposure settings
   6. Maintain pressure on the exposure button until the procedure is completed

RADIOGRAPHIC ERRORS: INTRAORAL AND EXTRAORAL

Intraoral Technique Errors[7]

A. Receptor placement
   1. Correct receptor placement is important for the production of diagnostic images
   2. Improper receptor placement includes not centering the receptor over the area of interest, inadequate coverage of the apical areas, and tipped occlusal/incisal edges (Figure 6-19)
B. Vertical angulation
   1. Too much or excessive vertical angulation causes foreshortened images (Figure 6-20)
   2. Too little or insufficient vertical angulation causes elongated images (Figure 6-21)
C. Horizontal angulation
   1. Correct horizontal angulation directs the central ray of the beam through the interproximal regions
   2. Incorrect horizontal angulation causes overlapping of the contact areas; the adjacent teeth appear overlapped onto each other (Figure 6-22)
D. Position-indicating device alignment problems
   1. If the PID is not aligned correctly and the x-ray beam is not centered over the receptor, a partial image is seen on the resultant image

FIG 6-19 Improper placement; no apices are seen on this periapical image. (From Iannucci JM, Howerton LJ: *Dental radiography: principles and techniques*, ed 5, St Louis, 2017, Elsevier.)

FIG 6-20 If the vertical angulation is too steep, the image of the tooth on the receptor is shorter than the actual tooth; the images are foreshortened. (From Iannucci JM, Howerton LJ: *Dental radiography: principles and techniques*, ed 5, St Louis, 2017, Elsevier.)

FIG 6-21 If the vertical angulation is too flat, the image of the tooth on the receptor is longer than the actual tooth; the images are elongated. (From Iannucci JM, Howerton LJ: *Dental radiography: principles and techniques*, ed 5, St Louis, 2017, Elsevier.)

   2. A clear, unexposed area is seen on the image known as a *cone-cut* (Figure 6-23)
E. Blurred images
   1. If the patient or tubehead is not still during exposure, blurred images will appear on the image (Figure 6-24)

FIG 6-22 Nondiagnostic bitewing image with overlapped interproximal contacts. (From Iannucci JM, Howerton LJ: *Dental radiography: principles and techniques*, ed 5, St Louis, 2017, Elsevier.)

FIG 6-23 A cone-cut is seen as a curved unexposed (clear) area on the radiograph. (From Iannucci JM, Howerton LJ: *Dental radiography: principles and techniques*, ed 5, St Louis, 2017, Elsevier.)

FIG 6-24 Movement results in a blurred image. (From Iannucci JM, Howerton LJ: *Dental radiography: principles and techniques*, ed 5, St Louis, 2017, Elsevier.)

2. Instruct patients to keep all movement to a minimum during x-ray exposure

F. Reversed film
   1. If the film is placed backward in the mouth and then exposed, a light image with a herringbone (or "tire track") pattern will appear (Figure 6-25)

FIG 6-25 A reversed film causes an image that appears light with a herringbone (or tire track) pattern. (From Iannucci JM, Howerton LJ: *Dental radiography: principles and techniques*, ed 5, St Louis, 2017, Elsevier.)

2. Since the primary beam penetrated the lead foil inside the packet before reaching the film, the image demonstrates a lighter appearance and the herringbone pattern

Extraoral Technique Errors[7]

A. Frankfort plane positioning errors
   1. If the chin is too low or tipped down, the mandibular incisor region will appear blurred, the condyles may not be visible, and an exaggerated smile line is seen on the image (Figure 6-26, *A*)
   2. If the chin is too high or tipped upward, the hard palate will be superimposed over the maxillary roots, the maxillary incisors will be blurred and magnified, and a reverse smile line is seen on the image (Figure 6-26, *B*)

B. Focal trough positioning errors
   1. Anterior teeth appear blurred and magnified in size if the dental arches are positioned too far back (posterior) in the focal trough (Figure 6-27, *A*)
   2. Anterior teeth will appear narrowed and diminished in size if the dental arches are positioned too far forward (anterior) in the focal trough (Figure 6-27, *B*)

C. Midsagittal plane errors
   1. If the head of the patient is not centered in the panoramic machine, the ramus and posterior teeth will be unequally magnified
   2. The side closest to the receptor will appear smaller, whereas the side farther away from the receptor will appear magnified

D. Cervical spine errors—if the patient is not standing or sitting up, the cervical spine will appear as a vertical radiopacity in the middle of the image

FIG 6-26 A, Chin positioned too far down; the Frankfort plane is angled downward. **B,** Chin positioned too far up; the Frankfort plane is angled upward.

FIG 6-27 A, Dental arches positioned too far posterior to the focal trough. **B,** Dental arches positioned too far anterior to the focal trough.

E. Lead apron errors—if the lead apron is placed too high on the neck of the patient, the apron will block the x-ray beam from reaching the receptor, and a radiopaque, cone-shaped artifact will obscure the mandible

F. Ghost images
  1. Any metallic object that remains in the head and neck region during panoramic radiography may cause a ghost image to appear
  2. Earrings, hearing aids, napkin chains, removable dental appliances, and hair clips are some examples of items that may cause a ghost image
  3. Ghost images are seen on the panoramic image on the opposite side of the original item, located higher than the original item, and indistinct or distorted

FILM MOUNTING

A. Purpose—film mounting provides a systematic approach for viewing and evaluating radiographs, with placement of radiographs in a holding device according to anatomic considerations
B. Mount construction—made of cardboard or plastic; available with windows for placement of radiographs in various number and size combinations
C. Mounting procedures
  1. Intraoral radiographs—labial mounting; recommended by the American Dental Association (ADA)
    a. Raised portion of the embossed dot is toward the radiographer
    b. The patient's left side is the radiographer's right side
    c. The orientation is that of the radiographer facing the patient
  2. Intraoral radiographs—lingual mounting
    a. Raised portion of the embossed dot is away from the radiographer
    b. The patient's left side is the radiographer's left side
    c. The orientation is that of the radiographer behind the patient
  3. Extraoral radiographs
    a. During exposure, side(s) under examination should be identified with a metal letter (R or L) placed on the cassette
    b. A commercial film identification imprinter can be used to label after exposure but before processing

RADIOGRAPHIC INTERPRETATION

A. Radiographic tooth anatomy (Figure 6-28)
  1. Enamel—outermost layer of the crown; radiopaque
  2. Dentin—found beneath the enamel and surrounds the pulp cavity; less radiopaque than enamel
  3. Pulp cavity—relatively radiolucent
  4. Alveolar bone—composed of cancellous and cortical bone; radiopaque
  5. Lamina dura—dense radiopaque line that surrounds the root of a tooth
  6. Periodontal ligament space—the space between the root of a tooth and the lamina dura; appears as a thin radiolucent line
B. Radiographic anatomic landmarks of the maxilla (Figure 6-29)

FIG 6-28 Tooth anatomy. *1,* Enamel. *2,* Dentin. *3,* Cementum. *4,* Pulp. *5,* Periodontal ligament space. *6,* Lamina dura. *7,* Alveolar crest. *8,* Trabeculae.

FIG 6-29 Radiographic anatomy of the maxillary arch. **A,** Maxillary anterior region. *1,* Incisive foramen. *2,* Median palatal suture. *3,* Nasal cavity (fossae). *4,* Nasal septum. *5,* Anterior nasal spine. *6,* Lateral (canine) fossa. *7,* Soft tissue outline of the nose (*dashed line*). *8,* Inferior nasal conchae. **B,** Maxillary posterior region. *9,* Maxillary sinus. *10,* Zygomatic process. *11,* Hanulus. *12,* Maxillary tuberosity. *13,* Floor of the maxillary sinus. *14,* Septa dividing the sinus. *15,* Coronoid process.

1. Incisive foramen—a hole in bone found at the midline of the anterior portion of the hard palate; oval radiolucency located between the maxillary central incisors
2. Lateral fossa (canine fossa) —diffuse radiolucency located between the maxillary lateral incisor and the canine
3. Median palatine suture—radiolucent line extending vertically between maxillary central incisors
4. Nasal fossae (nasal cavity)—two paired radiolucent compartments seen superior to the maxillary central incisors; outlined by the floor of the nasal cavity
5. Nasal septum—vertical bony radiopaque wall that divides the nasal cavity
6. Inferior nasal conchae—curved plates of bone that extend from the lateral walls of the nasal cavity; appear as a diffuse radiopacity within the nasal cavity
7. Anterior nasal spine—V-shaped radiopacity seen at the intersection of the floor of the nasal cavity and the nasal septum
8. Inverted Y—Y-shaped radiopacity seen at the intersection of the lateral wall of the nasal cavity and the anterior portion of the maxillary sinus
9. Maxillary sinus—paired cavities of bone seen as bilateral radiolucencies that originate at the maxillary canine region and extend posteriorly; outlined by a radiopaque wall or floor
10. Nutrient canals—tiny, tube-like passageways through bone that appear as thin radiolucent lines with radiopaque borders; may be seen within the maxillary sinus
11. Zygomatic process of the maxilla—J- or U-shaped radiopacity seen superior to the maxillary posterior teeth
12. Maxillary tuberosity—rounded prominence bone seen as a radiopaque bulge in the most posterior region of the maxilla
13. Hamulus—radiopaque spine located on the medial pterygoid plate seen posterior to the maxillary tuberosity
14. Lateral pterygoid plate—radiopaque extension of sphenoid bone; distinguished as separate from the maxillary tuberosity

C. Radiographic anatomic landmarks of the mandible (Figure 6-30)
1. Genial tubercles—circular radiopaque spines located inferior to mandibular central incisors
2. Lingual foramen—tiny opening in bone found on the internal surface of the mandible; small radiolucent dot seen in the center of the genial tubercles
3. Nutrient canals—tiny, tube-like passageways through bone that appear as thin radiolucent lines with

FIG 6-30 Radiographic anatomy of the mandibular arch. **A,** Mandibular anterior region. *1,* Genial tubercles. *2,* Lingual foramen. *3,* Mental ridge. *4,* Inferior border of the mandible. **B,** Mandibular posterior region. *5,* Mylohyoid ridge. *6,* External oblique ridge. *7,* Submandibular fossa. *8,* Mental foramen. *9,* Mandibular canal.

radiopaque borders; may be seen in the mandibular anterior region

4. Mental ridge—radiopaque ridge of bone that extends from the mandibular premolar region to the midline, extending upward
5. Mylohyoid ridge—radiopaque ridge of bone that extends downward and forward from the mandibular molar region; may be superimposed over the roots of the mandibular posterior teeth
6. Internal oblique ridge—radiopaque ridge of bone that extends downward and forward from the ramus; may continue as the mylohyoid ridge
7. External oblique ridge—radiopaque ridge of bone that ends at the anterior border of the ramus
8. Submandibular fossa—large radiolucent area in the posterior body of the mandible; represents the lingual depression corresponding to the location of the submandibular salivary gland
9. Mental foramen—a hole in bone found on the external surface of the mandible; seen as a round radiolucency in the area of the apical portion of the mandibular premolars
10. Mandibular canal—a tube-like passageway through bone; seen as a radiolucent horizontal canal with radiopaque borders that runs in the mandible below the apices of mandibular posterior teeth
11. Coronoid process of the mandible—a marked prominence of bone seen on the anterior portion of the mandible; this radiopacity is the only mandibular landmark to be viewed on maxillary posterior periapical images

D. Radiographic appearance of restorative materials (Figure 6-31)
1. Amalgam—completely radiopaque, irregular borders
2. Gold—completely radiopaque, smooth borders
3. Stainless steel crown (temporary crown)—slightly radiopaque with a "see-through" component
4. Porcelain crown—slightly radiopaque; thin radiopaque line represents cement

5. Porcelain-fused-to-metal crown—metal component is completely radiopaque; porcelain component is slightly radiopaque
6. Composite—radiolucent to radiopaque
7. Endodontic materials—guttapercha is slightly radiopaque; silver points are radiopaque
8. Orthodontic appliances—radiopaque bands, brackets, and wires representing the materials

E. Radiographic appearance of dental caries[7] (Figure 6-32)
1. Interproximal caries—seen as a radiolucent area at or just below the contact area
2. Occlusal caries—seen as a radiolucent area in the chewing surfaces of posterior teeth
3. Buccal or lingual caries—seen as a circular radiolucency in the buccal or lingual surface of a tooth
4. Root surface caries—seen as a radiolucent area that involves only the roots of teeth; usually preceded by bone loss or gingival recession
5. Recurrent caries—a radiolucent area seen below or adjacent to an existing restoration
6. Rampant caries—radiolucent areas seen in numerous teeth

FIG 6-32 Dental caries are evident on this bitewing image. (From Iannucci JM, Howerton LJ: *Dental radiography: principles and techniques*, ed 5, St Louis, 2017, Elsevier.)

FIG 6-31 Common restorative materials. *1,* Composite. *2,* Post-and-core restoration with a porcelain-fused-to-metal crown. *3,* Porcelain-fused-to-metal crown. *4,* Occlusal composite or temporary restoration. *5,* Amalgam. *6,* Porcelain-fused-to-metal crowns with endodontic material, silver points.

FIG 6-33 Dental caries and bone loss. *1,* Interproximal caries. *2,* Interproximal calculus deposits. *3,* Heavy calculus deposits. *4,* Severe bone loss.

F. Radiographic appearance of periodontal disease[7] (Figure 6-33)
   1. Bone loss
      a. Pattern—horizontal or vertical bone loss
      b. Distribution—localized or generalized bone loss

   c. Severity—slight, moderate, or severe bone loss
2. Classification of periodontal disease: ADA case types I, II, III, and IV

REFERENCES

1. International Commission on Radiation Units and Measurements, www.icru.org.
2. National Council on Radiation Protection and Measurements: *Ionizing radiation exposure of the population of the united states,* Report No 160, Bethesda, Md, 2009, NCRP.
3. American Dental Association, US Food and Drug Administration: *The selection of patients for dental radiographic examinations,* www.ada.org.
4. Radiation Safety in Dentistry, www.carestreamdental.com.
5. Van der Stelt PF: Better imaging: the advantages of digital radiography, *J Am Dent Assoc* 139:7S–13S, 2008.
6. Thomson EM, Johnson ON: *Essentials of dental radiography for dental assistants and hygienists,* ed 9, Upper Saddle River, NJ, 2012, Pearson Education, Prentice Hall.
7. Iannucci JM, Howerton LJ: *Dental radiography: principles and techniques,* ed 4, St Louis, 2012, Elsevier Saunders.

Website Information and Resources

Source	Website Address	Description
American Academy of Oral and Maxillofacial Radiology	http://www.aaomr.org	Promotes and advances the art and science of radiology in dentistry and provides a forum for communication among its members and to the health care community and the public
International Commission on Radiological Protection (ICRP)	http://www.icrp.org	Provides recommendations and guidance on all aspects of protection against ionizing radiation
National Council on Radiation Protection and Measurements (NCRP)	http://www.ncrponline.org	Dissemination of information and recommendations on protection against radiation
International Commission on Radiological Units and Measurements (ICRU)	http://www.icru.org	Develops and promulgates internationally accepted recommendations on radiation-related quantities and measurement procedures and references data for the safe and efficient application of ionizing radiation

CHAPTER 6 REVIEW QUESTIONS

Answers and rationales to review questions are available on this text's accompanying Evolve site. See inside front cover for details.

evolve

CASE A

An adult male patient presents to the dental office with a chief complaint of heat/cold sensitivity in his teeth, along with discontent of the appearance of the anterior crown. It has been 5 years since his last dental visit. Tooth #30 was recently avulsed due to advanced periodontal disease and trauma.

Use Case A and the panoramic radiograph in Figure 6-34 to answer questions 1 to 5.

1. **Which type of caries is visible on teeth #3 and #14?**
   a. Interproximal
   b. Occlusal
   c. Buccal/lingual
   d. Root

2. **Which type of caries is visible on tooth #29?**
   a. No caries are visible
   b. Interproximal

   c. Occlusal
   d. Root

3. **Which restorative material is seen on tooth #9?**
   a. Guttapercha and metal crown
   b. Silver points and all-porcelain crown
   c. Guttapercha and composite
   d. Post-and-core restoration

4. **The arrow is pointing to which radiopaque structure?**
   a. Internal oblique ridge
   b. Mandibular canal

FIG 6-34 Panoramic and occlusal view.

c. Condensing bone
d. Descending ramus

5. **In addition to the panoramic image, which intraoral radiographs would be most beneficial for the total care of this patient?**
   a. Maxillary and mandibular occlusal radiographs
   b. Four horizontal bitewing radiographs
   c. Four vertical bitewing radiographs
   d. A full-mouth series

Use Figure 6-35 to answer questions 6 and 7.

FIG 6-35

6. **All the anatomic landmarks may be viewed on this radiograph EXCEPT:**
   a. Incisive foramen
   b. Median palatal suture
   c. Maxillary torus
   d. Inferior nasal conchae

7. **The yellow arrow is pointing to a V-shaped radiopacity. What is this radiographic finding?**
   a. Anterior nasal spine
   b. Nasal septum

c. Nutrient canal
d. Root fracture

Use Figure 6-36 to answer questions 8 to 10.

FIG 6-36

8. **Which tooth has been extracted and is not visible on this periapical image?**
   a. #4
   b. #5
   c. #12
   d. #13

9. **Which tooth demonstrates interproximal caries?**
   a. Distal of maxillary premolar
   b. Mesial of maxillary first molar
   c. Distal of maxillary first molar
   d. Mesial of maxillary second molar

10. **Which restorative material is present on the maxillary first molar?**
    a. Amalgam
    b. Amalgam with base material
    c. Gold
    d. Composite

Use Figure 6-37 to answer questions 11 to 13.

FIG 6-37

11. Along with bone loss and calculus deposits, what other radiographic sign indicative of periodontal disease is present?
a. Furcation involvement
b. Cantilevered bridge
c. Root caries
d. Attachment loss

12. The cantilevered bridge is fabricated from what dental material?
a. Gold
b. Porcelain
c. Stainless steel
d. Porcelain-fused-to-metal

13. The arrow is pointing to which radiographic finding?
a. Zygomatic arch
b. Zygoma
c. Maxillary tuberosity
d. Scratched emulsion

Use Figure 6-38 to answer questions 14 and 15.

FIG 6-38

14. The overlapped contact area between teeth #18 and #19 was the result of:
a. Too much vertical angulation
b. Too little vertical angulation
c. Incorrect horizontal angulation
d. Improper receptor placement

15. The yellow arrow is pointing to which radiographic finding?
a. The identification dot
b. Submandibular fossa
c. Mental foramen
d. Periapical pathology

16. Which is an appropriate condition to expose a periapical radiograph?
a. Pulpitis
b. Slight bone loss
c. Amalgam overhang
d. Interproximal caries

17. Which would be an appropriate reason to expose an occlusal radiograph?
a. Mucocele
b. Salivary stones
c. Advanced bone loss
d. Temporomandibular joint (TMJ) disorder

18. Which is a suitable use of a panoramic radiograph?
a. Diagnosis of occlusal caries
b. Assessment of eruption patterns
c. Evaluation of periapical pathology
d. Measurement of periodontal bone loss

19. Which type of caries does NOT involve the enamel surface?
a. Root
b. Rampant
c. Recurrent
d. Interproximal

20. A male patient has been diagnosed with slight to moderate periodontitis. He declines the prescription of a full-mouth series due to concern with x-radiation. Which exposures would be appropriate to replace the intraoral periapical series?
a. Maxillary and mandibular occlusal radiographs
b. Panoramic
c. Four vertical bitewings
d. Four horizontal bitewings

21. Which exposure factor controls the penetrating power of the x-ray beam?
a. Time
b. Voltage
c. Milliamperage
d. Kilovoltage peak

22. Which speed of film is currently recommended by the American Dental Association (ADA) and the American Academy of Oral and Maxillofacial Radiology (AAOMR)?
a. C
b. D
c. E
d. F

23. Which error will produce a lighter radiographic image?
    a. Timer set too long
    b. Film exposed to light
    c. Fixer solution too weak
    d. Developer solution too warm
24. Your film exits the automatic processor completely clear. What is the most common reason for this appearance?
    a. Expired film
    b. Exposed to white light
    c. Not exposed to radiation
    d. Exposed backward in the mouth
25. The patient states that movement occurred during x-ray exposure. Which error will result on the image?
    a. Decreased distortion
    b. Increased sharpness
    c. Decreased sharpness
    d. Increased magnification
26. Where should the thermometer be kept for manual processing procedures?
    a. Water bath
    b. Fixer solution
    c. Developer solution
    d. Light-tight drawer inside the darkroom
27. Which agent is responsible for converting the exposed silver halide crystals to black metallic silver?
    a. Acetic acid
    b. Hydroquinone
    c. Sodium thiosulfate
    d. Ammonium thiosulfate
28. Which error produces a darker radiographic image?
    a. Fixer solution too cold
    b. Film left in the water rinse too long
    c. Film exposed backward in the mouth
    d. Film placed in fixer before developer solution
29. Which of the following is a quality control test used to monitor the strength of the developer solution?
    a. Coin test
    b. Light-leak check
    c. Step-wedge radiograph
    d. Half-value layer (HVL)
30. Which anatomic landmark will appear on an image of the mandibular anterior teeth?
    a. Mental ridge
    b. Mental foramen
    c. Mylohyoid ridge
    d. Mandibular canal
31. Which structure appears radiopaque on a dental radiograph?
    a. Dentin
    b. Air spaces
    c. Dental pulp
    d. Periodontal ligament space
32. Which periapical radiograph reveals the anatomic landmark referred to as the "inverted Y"?
    a. Maxillary canine
    b. Maxillary incisor
    c. Mandibular molar
    d. Mandibular incisor
33. Which cell is most sensitive to radiation exposure?
    a. Muscle
    b. Nerve
    c. Oral mucosa
    d. Bone marrow
34. A dental hygienist is working in a mobile dental unit and is asked to expose radiographs. No wall is present in the small x-ray room. What is the minimum distance in feet that the hygienist should stand from the source of x-radiation?
    a. 4
    b. 6
    c. 8
    d. 10
35. Which statement is correct for the production of the most diagnostic image?
    a. The receptor is placed as close as possible to the tooth.
    b. The shortest PID length is used.
    c. The receptor is placed as far away from the tooth as possible.
    d. The x-ray beam is positioned parallel to the long axis of the tooth.
36. Which of the following is MOST likely to cause a ghost image to appear on a panoramic radiograph?
    a. Cervical spine
    b. Hearing aid
    c. Dental implant
    d. Tongue
37. Which item remains stationary during panoramic exposure?
    a. Patient
    b. Film
    c. Tubehead
    d. Cassette
38. All the following landmarks may be viewed on a maxillary incisor periapical image EXCEPT:
    a. Nasal cavity
    b. Anterior nasal spine
    c. Inferior conchae
    d. Lingual foramen
39. What is the first stage of radiation injury?
    a. Period of injury
    b. Cumulative effects
    c. Latent period
    d. Period of recovery
40. Which restorative materials have the same radiographic appearance?
    a. Gold and amalgam
    b. Porcelain and stainless steel crown
    c. Guttapercha and silver points
    d. Composite and porcelain-fused-to-metal crown
41. Why is a filter placed inside the dental x-ray tubehead?
    a. To eliminate scatter radiation
    b. To reduce high-energy electrons
    c. To narrow the size and shape of the x-ray beam
    d. To remove long-wavelength photons

42. **All the following situations may cause film fogging EXCEPT:**
    a. Films stored for several years
    b. Films stored near a heat source
    c. Films left in an area exposed to x-radiation
    d. Films left in the fixing solution too long

43. **Which ingredient is the clearing agent found in the fixer solution?**
    a. Potassium alum
    b. Ammonium thiosulfate
    c. Acetic acid
    d. Hydroquinone

44. **In the bisecting-angle technique, the central ray of the x-ray beam is directed perpendicular to what plane?**
    a. Long axis of the tooth
    b. Long axis of the receptor
    c. Angle formed by the intersection of the long axis of the tooth and receptor
    d. Angle formed by the intersection of the occlusal plane and the tooth

45. **Which is the standard film size?**
    a. 0
    b. 1
    c. 2
    d. 4

46. **A person standing 2 feet from a source of radiation receives a dose of 2 rad. What would be the dose for a person standing 4 feet from the source of radiation?**
    a. 0.5 rad
    b. 1.0 rad
    c. 2.0 rad
    d. 4.0 rad

47. **What is the primary factor in the determination of the contrast of an image?**
    a. kVp
    b. Exposure time
    c. Source-to-receptor distance
    d. mA

48. **The size of the focal spot inside the x-ray tubehead determines which radiographic characteristic?**
    a. Sharpness
    b. Distortion
    c. Density
    d. Magnification

49. **In what part of the x-ray tube does thermionic emission occur?**
    a. Positive anode
    b. Positive cathode
    c. Negative anode
    d. Negative cathode

50. **X-rays belong to which category of radiation?**
    a. Particulate
    b. Alpha
    c. Beta
    d. Electromagnetic

General Pathology

JoAnn R. Gurenlian

Concepts of general pathology relate to multiple facets of dental hygiene care. Inflammatory diseases significantly affect the oral cavity, and research continues to focus on the linkages among inflammatory processes, systemic diseases, and oral diseases. Advances in genomics contribute to our understanding of the genetic basis of oral health conditions and their treatment. Individuals vary in their genetic makeup and thus their response to microbial challenges, injury, risk factors, and treatments. Dental hygienists use genomic information to assess clients for periodontal and other disease risks and will use genetics in planning effective care and evaluating therapeutic outcomes in the near future.

This chapter reviews major concepts related to inflammation, wound healing, and repair; genetics; and the differential diagnostic process that enables dental hygienists to integrate the biologic basis of health and disease into client care and acquire skills in diagnostic decision making.

INFLAMMATION[1-3]

A. A host response to cellular injury that consists of vascular responses, migration and activation of leukocytes, and systemic reactions
B. Cellular injury may occur because of trauma, genetic defects, physical and chemical agents, tissue necrosis, foreign bodies, immune reactions, and infections
C. A protective response designed to rid the body of the initial cause of cell injury and the consequences of that injury, paving the way for a return to normal structure and function
D. Inflammatory response consists of a vascular reaction and a cellular reaction
  1. Reactions are mediated by chemical factors derived from plasma proteins or cells
  2. Reactions are produced in response to or activated by the inflammatory stimulus
E. Cardinal signs of inflammation
  1. Rubor (redness)—caused by increased vascularity
  2. Tumor (swelling)—caused by exudation of fluid; synonymous with edema or increased fluid in the interstitial space
  3. Calor (heat)—caused by a combination of increased blood flow and the release of inflammatory mediators
  4. Dolor (pain)—caused by the stretching of pain receptors and nerves by inflammatory exudates and by the release of chemical mediators

  5. Functio laesa (loss of function)—caused by a combination of the previous signs
F. Types of inflammation
  1. Acute
    a. Characterized by rapid onset and short duration
    b. Manifests with exudation of fluid and plasma proteins and emigration of leukocytes, mainly neutrophils
  2. Chronic
    a. Sustained inflammatory reaction characterized by longer duration
    b. Histologic manifestation identified by the presence of lymphocytes and macrophages, blood vessels, fibrosis, and tissue necrosis
G. Cells involved in inflammation (Figure 7-1)
  1. Neutrophil or polymorphonuclear leukocyte (PMN)
    a. First cell to emigrate to the site of injury
    b. Primary cell involved in acute inflammation
    c. Capable of phagocytosis
  2. Monocyte or macrophage
    a. Second white blood cell (WBC) to emigrate to injured tissue, where it becomes a macrophage
    b. Capable of phagocytosis; helper during the immune response
    c. Produces potent vasoconstrictive mediators (prostaglandins, leukotrienes, platelet-activating factor, and inflammatory cytokines), which maintain chronic inflammation
  3. Lymphocytes and plasma cells—involved in both chronic inflammation and immune response
  4. Eosinophils—involved in immune reactions and parasitic infections
  5. Mast cells
    a. Involved in both acute and chronic inflammatory reactions (releasing chemical mediators) and in immune responses
    b. Important in regulating vascular permeability and bronchial smooth muscle tone, especially in allergic hypersensitivity reactions

Acute Inflammation

A. Vascular changes (Figure 7-2)
  1. Transient vasoconstriction of arterioles caused by neurogenic reflex lasting several seconds to minutes

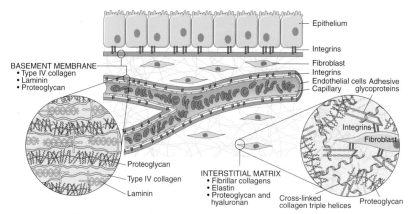

FIG 7-1 Components of acute and chronic inflammatory responses: circulating cells and proteins, cells of blood vessels, and cells and proteins of the extracellular matrix. (From Kumar V, Abbas AK, Fausto N, Aster JC: *Robbins and Cotran pathologic basis of disease*, ed 8, Philadelphia, 2010, Saunders.)

FIG 7-2 Major local manifestations of acute inflammation, compared with normal. *1*, Vascular dilation and increased blood flow (causing erythema and warmth). *2*, Extravasation and deposition of plasma fluid and proteins (edema). *3*, Leukocyte emigration and accumulation at the site of injury. (From Kumar V, Abbas AK, Fausto N, Aster JC: *Robbins and Cotran pathologic basis of disease*, ed 8, Philadelphia, 2010, Saunders.)

2. Vasodilation
   a. First involves arterioles, then results in the opening of new capillary beds
   b. Results in increased blood flow, which causes heat and redness, known as *hyperemia*
   c. Induced by chemical mediators such as histamine and nitric oxide on vascular smooth muscle
3. Increased permeability of microvasculature
   a. An exudate of protein-rich fluid escapes into extravascular tissue, resulting in edema
   b. Proposed mechanisms to explain the leakage of endothelium in inflammation to allow this response:
      (1) Formation of endothelial gaps in venules elicited by chemical mediators
         (a) Usually reversible
         (b) Lasts 15 to 30 minutes
      (2) Direct endothelial injury resulting in endothelial cell necrosis and detachment
         (a) Occurs in severe burns or lytic bacterial infections
         (b) Sustained for several hours
         (c) Venules, capillaries, and arterioles affected
      (3) Delayed prolonged leakage
         (a) Begins after a delay of 2 to 12 hours
         (b) Lasts for several hours or days
         (c) Involves venules and capillaries
         (d) Caused by thermal injury, radiation, and certain bacterial toxins
      (4) Leukocyte-mediated endothelial injury
      (5) Increased transcytosis across the endothelial cytoplasm
      (6) Leakage from new blood vessels until new endothelial cells mature and form intercellular junctions
4. Concentration of red blood cells (RBCs) in small vessels and increased viscosity of blood, known as *stasis*
5. Leukocytes, mainly neutrophils, accumulate along the vascular endothelium (margination); the endothelium

becomes lined by leukocytes ("pavementing"); leukocytes adhere to the endothelium and, soon after, migrate through the vascular wall into interstitial tissue (*diapedesis* or emigration)

    a. Neutrophils predominate in the inflammatory infiltrate during the first 6 to 24 hours

    b. Neutrophils are replaced by monocytes in 24 to 48 hours

B. Chemotaxis

  1. Chemical attraction of leukocytes to emigrate in tissues

  2. Exogenous agents are bacterial products

  3. Endogenous chemoattractants

    a. Components of the complement system, particularly C5a

    b. Products of the lipoxygenase pathway, such as leukotriene B_4 (LTB_4)

    c. Cytokines, such as interleukin-8 (IL-8)

C. Phagocytosis

  1. Recognition and attachment

    a. Mannose receptors and scavenger receptors bind and ingest microbes

    b. Phagocytosis is greatly enhanced by *opsonins*, specific proteins such as immunoglobulin G (IgG) antibodies, fragments of the complement protein C3, and plasma lectins, which are recognized by specific receptors on leukocytes

  2. Engulfment

    a. Extensions of the cytoplasm flow around the particle to be engulfed, resulting in the complete enclosure of the particle within a phagosome created by cell's plasma membrane

    b. Neutrophils and monocytes become degranulated during this process

  3. Killing and degradation

    a. Eliminate infectious agents and necrotic cells

    b. After the killing, acid hydrolases degrade the microbes within phagolysosomes

    c. pH drops to between 4 and 5

  4. Release of leukocyte products

    a. Include lysosomal enzymes, reactive oxygen intermediates, and products of arachidonic acids such as prostaglandins and leukotrienes

    b. These products may cause endothelial injury and tissue damage

    c. If unchecked, this leukocyte infiltrate becomes harmful and is associated with many chronic systemic diseases

    d. Also produce growth factors that aid in repair after tissue injury

  5. Apoptosis—defined as programmed cell death, used by the body to eliminate old cells

    a. After phagocytosis, neutrophils undergo apoptotic cell death and are then ingested by macrophages

D. Chemical mediators (Table 7-1)

  1. General principles

    a. Originate from plasma proteins or from cells

     (1) Plasma-derived mediators such as complement proteins and kinin are in precursor form and must be activated

     (2) Cell-derived mediators such as histamine, prostaglandins, and cytokines come from mast cells, platelets, neutrophils, and monocytes/macrophages

    b. Production of active mediators is triggered by microbial products or by host proteins

    c. Mediators perform their activities by binding to specific receptors on target cells, performing direct enzymatic activity, or mediating oxidative damage

    d. Once activated, most mediators are short-lived, but cause harmful effects

TABLE 7-1   Actions of the Principal Mediators of Inflammation

Mediator	Principal Sources	Actions
Cell Derived		
Histamines	Mast cells, basophils, platelets	Vasodilation, increased vascular permeability, endothelial activation
Serotonin	Platelets	Vasodilation, increased vascular permeability
Prostaglandins	Mast cells, leukocytes	Vasodilation, pain, fever
Leukotrienes	Mast cells, leukocytes	Increased vascular permeability, chemotaxis, leukocyte adhesion and activation
Platelet-activating factor	Leukocytes, mast cells	Vasodilation, increased vascular permeability, leukocyte adhesion, chemotaxis, degranulation, oxidative burst
Reactive oxygen species	Leukocytes	Killing of microbes, tissue damage
Nitric oxide	Endothelium, macrophages	Vascular smooth muscle relaxation, killing of microbes
Cytokines (tumor necrosis factor [TNF], interleukin 1 [IL-1])	Macrophages, endothelial cells, mast cells	Local endothelial activation (expression of adhesion molecules); fever, pain, anorexia, hypotension; decreased vascular resistance (shock)
Chemokines	Leukocytes, activated macrophages	Chemotaxis, leukocyte activation
Plasma Protein Derived		
Complement products (C5a, C3a, C4a)	Plasma (produced in liver)	Leukocyte chemotaxis and activation, vasodilation (mast cell stimulation)
Kinins	Plasma (produced in liver)	Increased vascular permeability, smooth muscle contraction, vasodilation, pain
Proteases activated during coagulation	Plasma (produced in liver)	Endothelial activation, leukocyte recruitment

From Kumar V, Abbas AK, Fausto N Aster JC: *Robbins and Cotran pathologic basis of disease*, ed 8, Philadelphia, 2010, Saunders.

2. Vasoactive amines
    a. Histamine
        (1) Found in mast cells, blood basophils, and platelets
        (2) Causes dilation of the arterioles and increases the permeability of venules; constricts large arteries
    b. Serotonin
        (1) Present in platelets and certain neuroendocrine cells
        (2) Causes increased permeability during immunologic reactions
3. Plasma proteins
    a. Complement system
        (1) Consists of 20 component proteins found in greatest concentration in plasma; primary function is defense against microbes
        (2) Causes increased vascular permeability, chemotaxis, and *opsonization* (the process by which certain cells are made more susceptible to phagocytosis)
        (3) C3 and C5 are the most important inflammatory mediators of the complement components
            (a) Vascular phenomenon created by C3a, C5a, and to a lesser extent, C4a; stimulate histamine release from mast cells; called *anaphylatoxins* because they have similar effects in the reaction of anaphylaxis
            (b) Leukocyte adhesion, chemotaxis, and activation occur through C5a as a chemotactic agent for neutrophils, monocytes, eosinophils, and basophils
            (c) Phagocytosis enhanced by C3b, which acts as opsonin to facilitate foreign bodies being more efficiently engulfed by phagocytosis
            (d) Acquired or congenital deficiencies of specific complement components or regulatory proteins result in increased susceptibility to infectious agents and a propensity for autoimmune diseases associated with circulating immune complexes (e.g., systemic lupus erythematosus, pyogenic infections, hereditary angioedema)
    b. Kinin system
        (1) Generates vasoactive peptides from plasma proteins called *kininogens* by the action of proteases known as *kallikreins*
        (2) Bradykinin increases vascular permeability; causes the contraction of smooth muscle, dilation of blood vessels, plasma extravasation, cell migration, inflammatory cell activation and inflammatory-mediated pain responses
        (3) Is triggered by the activation of Hageman factor (factor XII of the intrinsic clotting pathway)
        (4) Is short-lived; quickly inactivated by the enzyme kininase
    c. Clotting system
        (1) Induces the formation of thrombin, fibrinopeptides, and factor XII, which have inflammatory properties
        (2) Activated by substances released during tissue destruction, such as collagen, proteinases, kallikrein, and bacterial endotoxins
        (3) Prevents the spread of infection and inflammation; localizes microorganisms at the site of phagocytosis; helps clot formation to stop bleeding and for repair, chemotaxis of neutrophils, and increased permeability of vessels
4. Other mediators
    a. Arachidonic acid
        (1) A lipid mediator that is a short-range hormone; is formed rapidly and acts locally
        (2) Produces prostaglandins, leukotrienes, and lipoxins
            (a) Prostaglandins (e.g., PGE_2, PGD_2, PGF_{2a}, PGI_2) and thromboxane A_2 (TXA_2), are most important in inflammation, causing increased permeability, the chemotactic effects of other mediators, and vasodilation resulting in edema as well as pain and fever in inflammation
            (b) Pathway initiating these prostaglandins occurs by two different enzymes, COX-1 and COX-2
                [1] Cyclooxygenase-1 (COX-1) produces prostaglandins that are involved in inflammation and also maintains homeostasis, protecting the gastrointestinal mucosal lining, regulating water/electrolyte balance, stimulating platelet aggregation, and maintaining resistance to thrombosis on vascular endothelial cell surfaces
                [2] Cyclooxygenase-2 (COX-2) stimulates the production of prostaglandins involved in the inflammatory reactions previously noted and may play a role in normal homeostasis
            (c) Leukotrienes cause intense vasoconstriction, bronchospasm, and increased vascular permeability; important in the pathogenesis of bronchial asthma
            (d) Lipoxins are synthesized by platelets and neutrophils; inhibit leukocyte recruitment, neutrophil chemotaxis, and adhesion to the endothelium; may play a role in resolving inflammation
            (e) Resolvins inhibit leukocyte recruitment and activation by inhibiting the production of cytokines; aspirin may work by stimulating the production of resolvins
            (f) Platelet-activating factor (PAF) causes platelet stimulation, vasoconstriction, bronchoconstriction, vasodilation, and increased venular permeability; far more potent than histamine; increased leukocyte adhesion to endothelium; chemotaxis, degranulation, and oxidative burst; also boosts synthesis of other mediators, such as serotonin, causing changes in vascular permeability

(g) Tumor necrosis factor (TNF) and interleukin-1 (IL-1)

[1] Two major cytokines that mediate inflammation and are produced primarily by macrophages

[2] Responsible for endothelial activation, which induces the synthesis of endothelial adhesion molecules and chemical mediators, producing enzymes associated with matrix remodeling and increasing the surface thrombogenicity of endothelium

[3] Induces the systemic acute-phase responses of infection and injury, including fever, loss of appetite, release of neutrophils, corticotropin, and corticosteroids

[4] TNF—responsible for the hemodynamic effects of septic shock; regulates body mass and contributes to *cachexia* (wasting away), which is part of some infections and diseases

(h) Chemokines—small proteins that act as chemoattractants for leukocytes and control the normal migration of cells through various tissues

(i) Nitric oxide (NO)—released from endothelial cells; causes vasodilation by relaxing vascular smooth muscle; microbicidal; a mediator of host defense against infection

(j) Lysosomal components of leukocytes

[1] Neutrophils and monocytes, contain lysosomal granules; granules contain a variety of enzymes used for phagocytosis (e.g., lysozyme, collagenase, alkaline phosphatase, elastase)

[2] These enzymes are destructive and, if unchecked, can potentiate further inflammation and tissue damage

(k) Oxygen-derived free radicals may be released from leukocytes following a phagocytic event and are potent mediators

[1] Can be damaging to the host, causing endothelial cell damage and increased vascular permeability, inactivation of antiproteases, and injury to other cell types, such as parenchymal cells and RBCs

b. Neuropeptides

(1) Include substance P and neurokinin A

(2) Play a role in the initiation and propagation of inflammatory response

E. Outcomes of inflammation

1. Complete resolution
2. Healing by connective tissue replacement
3. Abscess
4. Lymphadenitis
5. Progression of tissue response to chronic inflammation

Chronic Inflammation

A. Causes

1. Persistent infections

2. Prolonged exposure to potentially toxic agents
3. Autoimmunity

B. Characteristics

1. Infiltration with macrophages, lymphocytes, and plasma cells
2. Tissue destruction, a hallmark of chronic inflammation
3. Attempts at healing by connective tissue replacement and fibrosis

C. Cells involved

1. Macrophages, lymphocytes, plasma cells, eosinophils, mast cells, and fibroblasts
2. Produce granulomatous inflammation, characterized by focal accumulation of activated macrophages that develops an epithelioid appearance, and fibrosis
3. Products of these cells eliminate injurious agents and help initiate repair, but are also responsible for much of the tissue injury in chronic inflammation

D. Role of lymphatics

1. Secondary line of defense that monitors the extravascular fluids
2. Help drain edema from the extravascular space

E. Systemic effects of inflammation—acute-phase response or the systemic inflammatory response syndrome (SIRS)

1. Fever—produced in response to pyrogens that act by stimulating prostaglandin synthesis
2. Acute-phase proteins, including C-reactive protein (CRP), fibrinogen, and serum amyloid A protein (SAA) increase during the inflammatory process

a. Bind to microbial cell walls; act as opsonin and fix complement

b. Prolonged activation causes secondary amyloidosis in chronic inflammation

c. Elevated CRP used as a marker for increased risk of myocardial infarction in persons with coronary artery disease

3. Leukocytosis

a. Common feature in bacterial infections resulting in elevated to extremely high levels of different types of leukocytes, depending on the type of infection

b. Normal count of WBCs is 4000 to 10,000/mm^3 in blood

c. In an inflammatory reaction, particularly with an infection, WBC count can increase to 15,000 or 20,000 and sometimes to extremely high levels exceeding 40,000/mm^3

4. Sepsis

a. In severe bacterial infections, large quantities of cytokines, particularly TNF and IL-1, cause thrombosis and coagulation

b. Eventually, hypoglycemia and cardiovascular failure occur, resulting in septic shock

c. Multiple organs can be affected by inflammation and intravascular thrombosis, resulting in organ failure

F. Systemic disease affected by chronic inflammation

1. Cardiovascular disease
2. Cancer
3. Diabetes mellitus

4. Asthma
5. Chronic obstructive pulmonary disease (COPD)
6. Alzheimer's disease
7. Periodontal diseases

REGENERATION AND WOUND HEALING[1-3]

A. Definitions
   1. Regeneration—growth of cells and tissues to replace lost structures; favored when the matrix composition and architecture are unaltered
   2. Healing—a tissue response to a wound, inflammatory process, or cell necrosis in organs that cannot regenerate; involves either regeneration or scar formation (Figure 7-3)
B. General concepts
   1. Involves a complex process that includes a number of steps
      a. A thrombus (clot) is formed at the site of injury; scab results from the drying of the exposed surfaces of the clot; forms a barrier to invading microorganisms.
      b. An inflammatory response caused by the initial injury
      c. Proliferation of parenchymal and connective tissue cells
      d. Formation of new blood vessels (angiogenesis) and granulation tissue (transient, specialized tissue of repair)
      e. Synthesis of extracellular matrix (ECM) proteins and collagen deposition
      f. Tissue remodeling
      g. Wound contraction
      h. Acquisition of wound strength
   2. Repair process—a combination of regeneration and scar formation influenced by local and systemic factors that may inhibit or prolong the wound-healing process

   a. Local factors
      (1) Size, location, and type of wound
      (2) Persistent infection
      (3) Early movement
      (4) Foreign material
      (5) Ionizing radiation
   b. Systemic factors
      (1) Blood supply
      (2) Metabolic factors (e.g., diabetes)
      (3) Corticosteroids
      (4) Cytotoxic drugs
      (5) Nutritional deficiencies
   3. Generally, repair begins early in inflammation—formation of granulation tissue, which is a hallmark of healing
      a. Pink, soft, granular appearance on the surface of wounds
      b. Formation of new small blood vessels and proliferation of fibroblasts
      c. New vessels tend to leak; edematous
      d. Amount of granulation tissue that forms depends on the size of the wound and the intensity of the inflammation
C. Angiogenesis (new blood vessels formed through preexisting vessels)
   1. Occurs from the branching and extension of adjacent blood vessels and the recruitment of endothelial progenitor cells (EPCs) from bone marrow
   2. Angiogenesis from adjacent blood vessels occurs through the vasodilation and increased permeability of existing vessels, degradation of ECM, migration of endothelial cells, maturation of endothelial cells and remodeling into capillary tubes, and recruitment of periendothelial cells to support endothelial tubes and to form the mature vessel

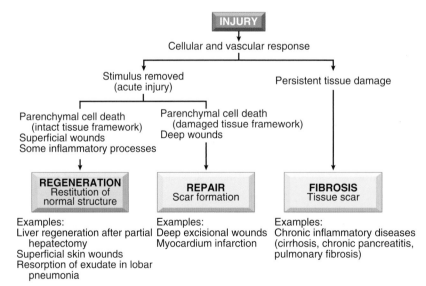

FIG 7-3 Repair responses after injury and inflammation. Repair after acute injury has several outcomes, including normal tissue restitution and healing with scar formation. Healing in chronic injury involves scar formation and fibrosis. (From Kumar V, Abbas AK, Fausto N, Aster JC: *Robbins and Cotran pathologic basis of disease*, ed 8, Philadelphia, 2010, Saunders.)

3. Growth factors such as vascular endothelial growth factor (VEGF) support adult tissues undergoing angiogenesis
4. Directed migration of endothelial cells—controlled by ECM proteins, including integrins, matricellular proteins, and proteinases

D. Scar formation—three processes occur: emigration and proliferation of fibroblasts in the site of injury, deposition of ECM, and tissue remodeling
   1. Fibroblast emigration and proliferation
      a. Migration of fibroblasts to the site of injury and their proliferation triggered by growth factors that come from platelets, inflammatory cells, and activated endothelium
   2. ECM deposition
      a. Fibroblasts deposit increased amounts of ECM
      b. Fibrillar collagens form a major portion of connective tissue in repair sites; help develop the strength of the healing wound
      c. Fibroblasts begin forming 3 to 5 days after injury and continue for several weeks
      d. Growth factors that stimulate fibroblasts also stimulate ECM synthesis
      e. Granulation tissue is converted into a scar composed of fibroblasts, dense collagen, fragments of elastic tissue, and other ECM components; richly vascularized granulation tissue transforms into a pale, avascular scar
   3. Tissue remodeling
      a. Degradation of ECM components causes tissue remodeling; achieved through matrix metalloproteinases (MMPs)
      b. MMPs are produced by fibroblasts, macrophages, neutrophils, synovial cells, and some epithelial cells
         (1) MMP secretion is induced by certain growth factors, physical stress, and phagocytosis; inhibited by steroids and other growth factors
         (2) MMPs degrade matrix proteins at the site of injury, allowing reorganization of the tissue capable of influencing cell growth and apoptosis

E. Cutaneous wound healing (Figure 7-4)
   1. Healing by primary intention—primary union (e.g., surgical incision and placement of sutures)
      a. Narrow incisional space fills with clotted blood, a clot forms, and a scab covers the surface of the wound; the clot stops the bleeding and acts as a scaffold for migrating cells
      b. Within 24 hours, neutrophils appear at the margins of the incision and move toward the clot
      c. In 24 to 48 hours, epithelial cells move from the wound edges and fuse in the midline beneath the scab to close the wound; a basement membrane is formed
      d. Within 3 days, neutrophils are replaced by macrophages, and granulation tissue forms
         (1) Collagen fibers begin to form in the margins of the incision
         (2) Epithelial cells proliferate and thicken the epidermal layer
      e. By day 5, the incisional space is filled with granulation tissue

      (1) Collagen fibers become more abundant and start to bridge the incision
      (2) A mature epidermal architecture with surface keratinization appears
      f. During week 2, proliferation of collagen and fibroblasts continues
         (1) The inflammatory process has largely dissipated
         (2) Blanching begins as the incisional scar forms
      g. By week 4, the scar is composed of connective tissue and an intact epidermis; the tensile strength of the wound increases
   2. Healing by secondary intention—secondary union (e.g., wounds with separated edges)
      a. Abundant granulation tissue grows in from the margin to complete the repair
      b. The inflammatory reaction is more intense because of the presence of a larger clot and more necrotic debris and exudates that must be removed from the defect
      c. Wound contraction occurs in larger surface wounds because of myofibroblasts that have the characteristics of smooth muscle cells
      d. Substantial scar formation and thinning of the epidermis occurs
   3. Healing by tertiary intention (delayed primary closure)
      a. Reserved for highly contaminated wounds
      b. Contaminated wound is initially treated with repeated debridement and either topical or systemic antibiotics to control infection
      c. Once wound is ready for closure, surgery is performed (suturing, skin graft replacement, flap)

F. Wound strength
   1. Tissues recover approximately 70% to 80% of tensile strength over a 3-month period compared with intact skin
   2. Recovery of wound strength comes from an excess of collagen synthesis over collagen degradation during the first 2 months of healing and from structural modifications of collagen fibers after collagen synthesis is complete

G. Complications of cutaneous wound healing
   1. Deficient scar formation leading to wound dehiscence or ulceration—often seen after abdominal surgery and in lower extremity wounds in patients with peripheral vascular disease, diabetes, or severe atherosclerosis
   2. Excessive scar formation
      a. Raised scar (hypertrophic scar, keloid)
      b. Scar grows beyond the boundaries of the original wound and does not regress (keloid)
   3. Contracture
      a. Exaggeration of the normal contraction process of wound healing, resulting in the deformity of the wound and surrounding tissues
      b. Common after serious burn injuries; can affect joint mobility

H. Fibrosis
   1. Processes that occur in cutaneous scar formation because of extensive deposition of collagen; similar to the fibrosis

HEALING BY PRIMARY INTENTION   HEALING BY SECONDARY INTENTION

24 hours

- Scab
- Neutrophils
- Clot

3 to 7 days

- Mitoses
- Granulation tissue
- Macrophage
- Fibroblast
- New capillary

Weeks

- Fibrous union

Wound contraction

FIG 7-4 Steps in wound healing by primary intention *(left)* and secondary intention *(right)*. Note large amounts of granulation tissue and wound contraction in healing by secondary intention. (From Kumar V, Abbas AK, Aster JC: *Robbins and Cotran pathologic basis of disease*, ed 9, Philadelphia, 2015, Elsevier.)

associated with chronic inflammatory diseases (e.g., rheumatoid arthritis, cirrhosis); a major component of diseases that involve ongoing injury

2. Characterized by the persistence of initial stimuli for fibrosis or the development of immune and autoimmune reactions that sustain the synthesis and secretion of growth factors and other biologically active molecules

3. May cause permanent dysfunction

REGENERATIVE MEDICINE[4]

A. Stem cells
  1. Characterized by self-renewal abilities and the capacity to generate differentiated cells; stem cells from bone marrow and basal layer of epidermis provide a renewal source of epidermal and dermal cells that can form new blood vessels and epithelium and regenerate skin structures
    a. Autogenous stem cells—derived from the individual being treated
    b. Allogenous stem cells—derived from other individuals
    c. May be totipotent, multipotent, or unipotent
    d. Process of differentiation is known as *plasticity* or *transdifferentiation*
  2. Types (Table 7-2)
    a. Embryonic stem cells
      (1) Pluripotent and can generate all tissue of the body
      (2) Isolated from inner cell mass of blastocytes

TABLE 7-2 Types of Stem Cells

Type of Stem Cell	May Differentiate to:
Embryonic	Any type of cell
Amniotic fluid derived	Cartilage cells
	Fat cells
	Bone cells
	Muscle cells
	Endothelial cells
	Neuron-like cells
	Liver cells
Umbilical cord	Liver cells
	Skeletal muscle cells
	Neural tissue
	Immune cells
Bone marrow–derived mesenchymal	Bone cells
	Cartilage cells
	Muscle cells
	Fat cells
	Neuron-like cells
	Pancreatic islet beta-cells
Tooth derived	Neural cell lineages
	Bone cells
	Cartilage cells
	Muscle cells
	Fat cells
	Pancreatic islet beta-cells
Adipose derived	Fat cells
	Cartilage cells
	Muscle cells
	Neuronal cells
	Bone cells
Induced pluripotent stem cells	Any type of cell, potentially

From Mao JJ: Stem cells and the future of dental care, *NY State Dent J* 74 (2):20-24, 2008.

(3) May be used in the future for the treatment of organs affected by diabetes, neurologic defects, myocardial infarction, and liver damage
b. Adult stem cells or somatic stem cells
(1) More restricted capacity to generate different cell types
(2) Potential for adult stem cells to be reprogrammed into pluripotent cells similar to embryonic stem cells
(3) Found in skin, lining of intestine, cornea, brain, and hematopoietic tissue (e.g., bone marrow, umbilical cord)
3. Types of adult stem cells
a. Induced pluripotent stem cells (iPs)—adult cells that behave similar to embryonic cells
b. Amniotic fluid–derived stem cells (AFSCs)
(1) Isolated from the aspirates of amniocentesis during genetic screening
(2) Capacity to differentiate into multiple lineages, such as chondrocytes, adipocytes, osteoblasts, myocytes, endothelial cells, neuron-like cells, and live cells

c. Umbilical cord blood stem cells (UCBSCs)
(1) Derived from the blood of the umbilical cord
(2) Differentiate into cells that resemble liver cells, skeletal muscle, neural tissue, pancreatic cells, immune cells, and mesenchymal stem cells
d. Bone marrow–derived stem cells (BMSCs)
(1) Consists of both hematopoietic stem cells and stromal cells (mesenchymal stem cells) that generate bone, cartilage, other connective tissues, and fat
(2) Most common commercially available stem cells
e. Adipose-derived stem cells (ASCs)
(1) Derived from lipectomy or liposuction aspirates
(2) Differentiate into adipocytes, chondrocytes, myocytes, and neuronal and osteoblastic lineages; may provide hematopoietic support
f. Dental stem cells
(1) Develop from material created during the development of the nervous system and can differentiate into neural cell lines
(2) Sources include primary teeth, permanent third molars, or extracted healthy permanent teeth and periodontal ligament
(3) Have been transdifferentiated in the laboratory to form bone, nervous tissue, and pancreatic islet beta-cells that produce insulin
(4) Current animal studies are exploring applications to regenerate bone, cartilage, skin, nerve and brain tissues, adipose, and heart and muscle tissues
(5) Dental application may include tooth, root, jaw, and salivary gland regeneration and cranial bone repair

GENETICS[2,5]

A. General concepts
1. Almost all health-related conditions (except trauma) have a genetic component; common diseases such as cardiovascular disease, dyslipidemia, diabetes, and cancer, as well as dental caries, periodontitis, oral cancer, cleft lip, and craniofacial abnormalities, are associated with genetic factors
2. Draft sequencing of the human genome has been completed; provides information about biologic inheritance and health consequences
3. Genome—all the deoxyribonucleic acid (DNA) of a given organism
4. Genomics—the study of all the genes in the genome, their extensive DNA sequences, and their interactions
5. Gene—a segment of DNA that contains instructions for making a specific protein or proteins required by the human body; found in succession along the length of chromosomes; humans have 20,000 to 25,000 genes
6. About 99.5% of DNA sequences are shared among humans; the diversity of humans is encoded in approximately 0.5% of human DNA; this 0.5% represents 15 million base pairs

7. Chromosomes—thread-like structures in the nucleus of a cell; made of DNA and structural proteins; human cells other than egg and sperm have 46 chromosomes (23 pairs); egg and sperm cells have 23 chromosomes
8. Molecular biology has resulted in the development of recombinant DNA technology that has allowed the isolation and characterization of genes through cloning, production of human biologically active agents, study of gene therapy, and development of molecular probes to aid in disease diagnosis

B. Mutations
  1. Mutations represent permanent changes in the DNA code; they can be beneficial, neutral, or harmful
    a. Four letters of the DNA code: A=adenine, T=thymine, C=cytosine, and G=guanine; one letter can be changed, deleted, or added; entire pieces of code can be spelled backward, cut and pasted, or cut short, which can change the form and function or the end protein product in the body
    b. The impact of a mutation depends on the environment in which it is expressed
    c. Classification of mutations
      (1) Genome mutations—involve the loss or gain of whole chromosomes, resulting in monosomy or trisomy
      (2) Chromosome mutations—rearrangement of genetic material that gives rise to structural changes in the chromosome; most are incompatible with survival
      (3) Submicroscopic gene mutations—represent the vast majority of mutations associated with hereditary diseases; may result in a partial or complete deletion of a gene or may affect a single base

C. Single-gene disorders
  1. Autosomal dominant inheritance
    a. An affected person usually has an affected parent
    b. An affected person has a 50% chance of passing the trait to an offspring
    c. Both genders are equally likely to be affected, and both can transmit the condition
    d. Dominant traits are usually seen in multiple, successive generations
  2. Additional characteristics of autosomal dominant disorders
    a. Some affected persons do not have affected parents; the disorder is caused by new mutations involving either the egg or the sperm and seems to occur in the germ cells of older fathers
    b. Some inherit the mutant gene but are phenotypically normal (called *reduced* or *incomplete penetrance*)
    c. If the trait is seen in all individuals but is expressed differently among them, the phenomenon is called *variable expressivity*; combinations of these traits can be less or more severe among individuals even within the same family
    d. In many conditions, onset is delayed, and symptoms do not appear until adulthood

    e. Biochemical mechanism is either loss-of-function mutations or gain-of-function mutations; the effects of these mutations depend on the nature of the enzyme protein affected
    f. Examples of autosomal dominant disorders
      (1) Huntington's disease
      (2) Neurofibromatosis
      (3) Polycystic kidney disease
      (4) Von Willebrand disease
      (5) Marfan syndrome
      (6) Ehlers-Danlos syndrome
      (7) Osteogenesis imperfecta
      (8) Familial hypercholesterolemia
  3. Autosomal recessive inheritance
    a. Both genders equally likely to be affected
    b. Disease often found in siblings; affected individuals often have unaffected parents
    c. Offspring of the affected person are carriers of the gene mutation
    d. If a child is born to two carrier parents and is not affected, a two-thirds chance of the child being a carrier is present
    e. Carriers are usually not clinically affected
    f. Two carrier parents have a 25% chance with each conception to have an affected child
    g. Onset is frequently early in life
    h. In many cases, enzyme proteins are affected by a loss of function
    i. Examples of autosomal recessive disorders
      (1) Cystic fibrosis
      (2) Phenylketonuria
      (3) Sickle cell anemia
      (4) Thalassemias
      (5) Congenital adrenal hyperplasia
      (6) Neurogenic muscular atrophies
      (7) Spinal muscular atrophy
  4. X-linked recessive inheritance
    a. Primarily affects males
    b. Sons of carrier females have a 50% chance of receiving the gene and expressing that trait or condition
    c. Carrier females may show no disease trait or mild symptoms only
    d. No male-to-male transmission
    e. Affected males transmit the genes to all daughters but not to their sons; all daughters are carriers
    f. Uncles and cousins may also be affected
    g. Examples of X-linked recessive disorders
      (1) Duchenne muscular dystrophy
      (2) Hemophilia A and B
      (3) Chronic granulomatous disease
      (4) Glucose-6-phosphate dehydrogenase (G6PD) deficiency
      (5) Agammaglobulinemia
      (6) Diabetes insipidus
      (7) Fragile X syndrome
  5. Biochemical and molecular basis of single-gene disorders

a. The genetic defect may lead to the formation of an abnormal protein as reduction in the output of gene product

b. The pattern of inheritance is related to the type of protein affected by the mutation

c. The mechanisms are classified into four categories:
   (1) Enzyme defects and their consequences
   (2) Defects in membrane receptors and transport systems
   (3) Alterations in structure, function, or quality of nonenzyme proteins
   (4) Mutations resulting in unusual reactions to drugs—pharmacogenetics

6. Disorders with multifactorial inheritance
   a. Result from the combined actions of environmental influences and two or more mutant genes having additive effects
   b. The greater the number of inherited deleterious genes, the more severe the expression of the disease
   c. Risk is greater in siblings of persons having severe expressions of the disorder
   d. Frequency of concordance for identical twins is 20% to 40%
   e. Examples of disorders with multifactorial inheritance
      (1) Cleft lip, cleft palate, or both
      (2) Congenital heart disease
      (3) Coronary heart disease
      (4) Hypertension
      (5) Gout
      (6) Diabetes mellitus
      (7) Pyloric stenosis

7. Diagnosis of genetic diseases—requires examination of genetic material through cytogenetic analysis or molecular analysis
   a. Cytogenetic analysis involves *karyotyping*, an organized graphic representation of the chromosomes in a single cell
      (1) Normal human karyotypes show 23 pairs of chromosomes, numbered from larger to smaller
      (2) The twenty-third pair comprises the sex chromosomes (XX = female, XY = male)
      (3) Karyotypes are described using a shorthand notation, with the total number of chromosomes listed first, followed by the sex chromosome complement, and then a description of the abnormalities in ascending numerical order
   b. Prenatal chromosome analysis should be offered to individuals at risk; can be performed on cells obtained by amniocentesis, on chorionic villus biopsy, or on umbilical cord blood
   c. Postnatal chromosome analysis can be performed on peripheral blood lymphocytes in cases of multiple congenital anomalies, unexplained mental retardation or developmental delay, suspected genetic disorders such as Turner syndrome or fragile X syndrome, infertility, or multiple spontaneous abortions

d. Recombinant DNA technology is also used for the diagnosis of inherited diseases because it is highly sensitive; tests are not dependent on a gene product produced only in certain specialized cells
   (1) Testing performed through either direct gene diagnosis using polymerase chain reaction (PCR) analysis or indirect DNA diagnosis through linkage analysis, which involves studying several relevant family members
   (2) 0.1 μL of blood or cells scraped from the buccal mucosa is sufficient for PCR analysis
   (3) Salivary DNA-PCR used to evaluate periodontal status
      (a) MyPerioPathSM identifies the type and quantity of 13 periodontopathic bacteria
      (b) MyPerioIDSM PST determines if the patient is genetically predisposed to periodontal disease by evaluating IL-1 polymorphism
      (c) Perio Predict Genetic Risk Test identifies genetic predisposition to periodontal disease (www.PerioPredict.com)

e. Identifying molecular genetic signatures for acquired diseases
   (1) Diagnosis and management of cancer
      (a) Detection of tumor-specific acquired mutations and cytogenic alterations that are hallmarks of specific tumors
      (b) Determination of clonality as an indicator of neoplastic condition
      (c) Identification of specific gene alterations that can direct therapeutic choices
      (d) Determination of treatment efficacy
      (e) Determination of Gleeve-resistant forms of chronic myeloid leukemia or gastrointestinal stromal tumors
   (2) Diagnosis and management of infectious diseases
      (a) Detection of microorganisms and specific genetic material for definitive diagnosis (i.e., human immunodeficiency virus [HIV], human papillomavirus [HPV], herpes simplex virus [HSV])
      (b) Identification of specific genetic alterations in the genomes of microbes that are associated with drug resistance
      (c) Determination of treatment efficacy (e.g., assessing viral loads in HIV and hepatitis C virus [HCV])

f. Ribonucleic acid (RNA) analysis
   (1) Not as stable as DNA-based diagnosis, but useful for the detection and quantification of RNA viruses such as HIV and HCV
   (2) Becoming an important tool for the molecular stratification of tumors

8. Referral for genetic counseling
   a. Clients who present with evidence of suspected or diagnosed genetic disorder should be referred to a genetics center for evaluation and counseling; any

genetic health condition or risk that affects one individual can affect that person's biologic and extended family

    b. Genetics professionals can be consulted through the National Society for Genetics Counselors (NSGC) website at http://www.nsgc.org

    c. Document referrals are made to a physician, a genetics professional, or both by recording:

      (1) Causes for concern

      (2) Possible diagnosis (if known)

      (3) Family history information obtained

      (4) Relevant oral examination findings, radiographs, and records

    d. Genetics consultation involves:

      (1) Confirming, diagnosing, or ruling out the genetic condition

      (2) Identifying medical management issues

      (3) Determining genetic risks

      (4) Providing psychosocial support

DIFFERENTIAL DIAGNOSIS[6]

A. Diagnostic approaches

  1. Appearance recognition—clinical manifestations of routine oral diseases can be recognized by their characteristic appearances because no other diseases produce these lesions (e.g., dental caries, gingivitis, periodontitis)

  2. Differential diagnosis—determination of which of two or more diseases with similar signs and symptoms is the one manifested in the client

    a. Requires a comparison of signs and symptoms and other pertinent details against the known features of all diseases that can produce the observed primary manifestation

    b. Reflects a conceptual process and a listing of pathologic conditions in the order of most likely to least likely

    c. Pathoses are ruled out on the basis of examinations, tests such as blood assays (see reference 5 for specific examples), urinalysis, biopsy, and so on

B. Conceptual stages of the differential diagnosis process

  1. Stage 1: classification of the abnormality by primary manifestation—describe the general nature of the lesion that makes it different from normal tissue

    a. A white mucosal discoloration without loss of mucosal integrity or enlargement

    b. A dark discoloration without loss of mucosal integrity or enlargement

    c. Loss of mucosal integrity or ulceration without enlargement

    d. Enlargement of soft tissues

    e. Radiographic manifestations of a lesion originating in bone

    f. Concurrence of several dissimilar abnormalities suggestive of a syndrome

  2. Stage 2: listing of secondary features and contributing factors—objectively describe the secondary features of

the lesion; reserve making judgments about the diagnosis based on information obtained

    a. Visual examination

      (1) Specific location of the lesion

      (2) Shape of the lesion and contours of tissue

      (3) Size of the lesion

      (4) Occurrence of the lesion as isolated, multifocal, or diffuse

      (5) Delineation of the borders of the abnormality from adjacent tissue

      (6) Consistency of appearance as homogeneous or heterogeneous

      (7) Surface color and texture

      (8) Alteration of adjacent structures, such as displacement of teeth

    b. Palpation

      (1) Degree of compressibility

      (2) Tenderness during compression

      (3) Alteration in color during compression

    c. Auscultation

      (1) Wheezing

      (2) Popping and clicking of the temporomandibular joint

      (3) Clicking of poorly fitting dentures

    d. Probing

      (1) Tissue defects

      (2) Exudates

    e. Aspiration

      (1) Pus

      (2) Cysts and nodules

    f. Evaluation of function

      (1) Tear production

      (2) Salivary glands

      (3) Tongue

      (4) Muscles of mastication

      (5) Neurologic function

    g. Client awareness

      (1) Pain, discomfort, or altered function

      (2) Duration

      (3) Course as constant, healing with recurrence, or steady progression

      (4) Response to factors such as stress and certain foods

    h. Demographics

      (1) Age

      (2) Gender

      (3) Race and ethnicity

    i. Habits

      (1) Alcohol use

      (2) Tobacco use

      (3) Oral

      (4) Other (ask client)

    j. Recent history

      (1) Injury

      (2) Infection

      (3) Surgery

k. Medical conditions
  (1) Chronic diseases
  (2) Recent acute illnesses
l. Current medical treatment
  (1) Medications
  (2) Other treatment
3. Stage 3: listing of conditions capable of causing primary manifestations
  a. Consider the variety of abnormalities that cause the condition, and compare them with the client's abnormality
  b. Create a list of plausible diagnoses
4. Stage 4: elimination of unlikely causes
  a. Identify contradictions between the features of the lesion and the known characteristics of the diagnostic possibilities
  b. The category of the lesion determines the secondary features that are most reliable; then eliminate those conditions that appear least likely

c. Elimination of malignant neoplasia as a possible cause is often more important than achieving a definitive diagnosis
5. Stage 5: ranking of possible causes by probability
  a. Rank the diseases that could explain the abnormality on the basis of the number of secondary features exhibited that correspond with the typical features of each possible diagnosis
6. Stage 6: Determination of a working diagnosis
  a. The condition considered the most likely cause of the lesion is referred to as the *working, tentative,* or *preliminary diagnosis* or the *clinical impression*
  b. Provides the basis for additional diagnostic testing and for the initial clinical management of the condition
  c. When all the diseases except one have been eliminated from the differential diagnosis, then that provides the definitive diagnosis
  d. Reevaluate to verify the correct diagnosis and that the client has responded to treatment without recurrence

Website Information and Resources

Source	Website Address	Description
National Human Genome Research Institute/ Talking Genetics Glossary	www.genome.gov/glossary.cfm	Talking glossary of genetic terms; text-only version available
Centers for Disease Control and Prevention/ Office of Genomics and Disease Prevention	www.cdc.gov/genomics	Information about human genomic discoveries and how they can be used to improve health and prevent disease
		Timely and credible information for the effective and responsible translation of genomics research into population health benefits
National Library of Medicine/Genetics Home Reference	http://ghr.nlm.nih.gov/	Allows users to search for information on diseases, tutorials about basic concepts in genetics, and educational resources
National Institutes of Health	http://stemcells.nih.gov/info/basics/ pages/basics7.aspx	Reviews stem cells; unique properties, types, and potential uses of human stem cells
International Society for Stem Cell Research	http://www.isscr.org	Provides overview of research related to stem cells; promotes professional and public education in all areas of stem cell research and application
Medline Plus	http://www.nlm.nih.gov/ medlineplus/stemcells.html	Consumer health database that includes news, health resources, and clinical trials related to stem cells

REFERENCES

1. Goljan EF: *Rapid review: pathology,* ed 4, Philadelphia, 2014, Elsevier.
2. Kumar V, Abbas AK, Fausto N, Aster JC: *Robbins and cotran pathologic basis of disease,* ed 8, Philadelphia, 2010, Saunders.
3. Rubin E, Reisner HM: *Essentials of Rubin's pathology,* ed 6, Philadelphia, 2014, Wolters Kluwer/Lippincott, Williams & Wilkins.
4. Mao JJ, Giannobile WV, Helms JA, et al: Craniofacial tissue engineering by stem cells, *J Dent Res* 85(11):966–979, 2006.
5. National Coalition for Health Professional Education in Genetics: *Genetics primer,* 2014. Available at http://www.nchpeg.org. Accessed September 5, 2014.
6. Coleman GC, Nelson JF: *Principles of oral diagnosis,* St Louis, 1993, Mosby.

SUGGESTED READINGS

Lee HN, Surh YJ: Therapeutic potential of resolvins in prevention and treatment of inflammatory disorders, *Biochem Pharmacol* 84 (10):1340–1350, 2012.
Mao JJ, Collins FM: Stem cells: sources, therapies and the dental professions, *RDH* 49–57, 2009.
Mariotti A: A primer on inflammation, *Compend Cont Educ Dent* 25(7 Suppl 1):7–15, 2004.
Nadig RR: Stem cell therapy—hype or hope? A review, *J Conserv Dent* 12(4):131–138, 2009.
National Coalition for Health Professional Education in Genetics: *Core competencies for all health professionals,* 2007, http://www.nchpeg. org. Accessed September 5, 2014.
Pagana KD, Pagana TS: *Mosby's manual of diagnostic and laboratory tests,* ed 4, Philadelphia, 2010, Mosby.

CHAPTER 7 REVIEW QUESTIONS

Answers and rationales to review questions are available on this text's accompanying Evolve site. See inside front cover for details

evolve

1. Cellular injury may be caused by all the following EXCEPT one. Which one is the *exception*?
   a. Infections
   b. Chemical agents
   c. Mitosis
   d. Tissue necrosis

2. A protective response of the body designed to rid the initial cause and consequences of cell injury explains:
   a. Inflammation
   b. Regeneration
   c. Angiogenesis
   d. Autoimmune response

3. Inflammation consists of vascular responses, migration and activation of white blood cells, and systemic reactions. It is present during cellular injury and wound repair.
   a. Both statements are TRUE.
   b. Both statements are FALSE.
   c. The first statement is TRUE; the second statement is FALSE.
   d. The first statement is FALSE; the second statement is TRUE.

4. Mr. Smith presents with generalized gingivitis with swelling, bleeding, and redness. The redness (rubor) is caused by:
   a. Vasoconstriction of blood vessels
   b. Increased vascularity
   c. Stretching of pain receptors
   d. Exudation of fluid

5. Mr. Smith's gingival swelling is caused by:
   a. Vasoconstriction of blood vessels
   b. Increased vascularity
   c. Stretching of pain receptors
   d. Exudation of fluid

6. Increased blood flow and the release of inflammatory mediators cause which cardinal sign of inflammation?
   a. Rubor
   b. Calor
   c. Dolor
   d. Functio laesa

7. Acute inflammation is characterized by a sustained inflammatory response. It is manifested by the exudation of fluid and plasma proteins and the emigration of leukocytes, most notably neutrophils.
   a. Both statements are TRUE.
   b. Both statements are FALSE.
   c. The first statement is TRUE; the second statement is FALSE.
   d. The first statement is FALSE; the second statement is TRUE.

8. What is the first white blood cell to emigrate to the site of injury?
   a. Monocyte
   b. Neutrophil
   c. Eosinophil
   d. Macrophage

9. Macrophages, lymphocytes, and eosinophils are all involved in the immune response. Neutrophils are involved in acute inflammation and not the immune response.
   a. Both statements are TRUE.
   b. Both statements are FALSE.
   c. The first statement is TRUE; the second statement is FALSE.
   d. The first statement is FALSE; the second statement is TRUE.

10. Which white blood cell produces potent vasoconstrictive mediators?
    a. Neutrophil
    b. Macrophage
    c. Lymphocyte
    d. Eosinophil

11. Which white blood cells regulate bronchial smooth muscle tone, especially in allergic hypersensitivity reactions?
    a. Neutrophils
    b. Monocytes
    c. Mast cells
    d. Lymphocytes

12. What is the term for the concentration of red blood cells in small vessels and increased viscosity of blood?
    a. Margination
    b. Pavementing
    c. Diapedesis
    d. Stasis

13. The first step in the vascular changes associated with acute inflammation is:
    a. Vasodilation
    b. Vasoconstriction
    c. Increased permeability
    d. Concentration of red cells in small vessels

14. Vasodilation results in decreased blood flow. This causes heat and redness, also known as hyperemia.
    a. Both statements are TRUE.
    b. Both statements are FALSE.
    c. The first statement is TRUE; the second statement is FALSE.
    d. The first statement is FALSE; the second statement is TRUE.

15. Endogenous chemoattractants involved in chemotaxis include all the following EXCEPT:
    a. C5a
    b. LTB_4
    c. SIRS
    d. IL-8

16. Which phase of phagocytosis involves the complete enclosure of a particle within a phagosome?
    a. Recognition and attachment
    b. Engulfment
    c. Killing and degradation
    d. Apoptosis

17. During which phase of phagocytosis does the pH drop to between 4 and 5?
    a. Recognition and attachment
    b. Engulfment
    c. Killing and degradation
    d. Apoptosis

18. The release of leukocyte products during phagocytosis may cause endothelial injury and tissue damage because neutrophils and monocytes become degranulated during this process.
    a. Both the statement and the reason are correct and are related.
    b. Both the statement and the reason are correct but are NOT related.
    c. The statement is correct, but the reason is NOT correct.
    d. The statement is NOT correct, but the reason is correct.
    e. NEITHER the statement NOR the reason is correct.

19. Examples of vasoactive amines are:
    a. Histamine and serotonin
    b. Histamine and bradykinin
    c. Serotonin and complement
    d. Serotonin and bradykinin

20. Chemical mediators perform their activities by binding to specific receptors on target cells, performing direct enzymatic activity, or mediating oxidative damage. Most mediators can last for extended periods, causing harmful effects.
    a. Both statements are TRUE.
    b. Both statements are FALSE.
    c. The first statement is TRUE; the second statement is FALSE.
    d. The first statement is FALSE; the second statement is TRUE.

21. Which chemical mediator is triggered by the activation of Hageman factor?
    a. Arachidonic acid
    b. Bradykinin
    c. Complement C3a
    d. Serotonin

22. Which mediators induce the systemic acute-phase response of infection and injury?
    a. Leukotrienes and lipoxins
    b. Tumor necrosis factor and lipoxins
    c. Tumor necrosis factor and interleukin-1
    d. Leukotrienes and interleukin-1

23. Oxygen-derived free radicals may be released from nitric oxide following a phagocytic event. These are potent mediators that can cause endothelial cell damage and increased vascular permeability.
    a. Both statements are TRUE.
    b. Both statements are FALSE.
    c. The first statement is TRUE; the second statement is FALSE.

    d. The first statement is FALSE; the second statement is TRUE.

24. Examples of acute-phase proteins seen in chronic inflammation include all the following EXCEPT:
    a. Leukocyte K
    b. C-reactive protein
    c. Fibrinogen
    d. Serum amyloid A

25. The lymphatics are a secondary line of defense in inflammation, because they help drain edema from the extravascular space.
    a. Both the statement and the reason are correct and are related.
    b. Both the statement and the reason are correct but are NOT related.
    c. The statement is correct, but the reason is NOT correct.
    d. The statement is NOT correct, but the reason is correct.
    e. NEITHER the statement NOR the reason is correct.

26. Which of the following systemic diseases is/are affected by chronic inflammation?
    a. Diabetes mellitus
    b. Cancer
    c. Gingivitis
    d. All the above

27. The first step in wound healing is:
    a. An inflammatory response
    b. Proliferation of parenchymal and connective tissue cells
    c. Formation of a thrombus
    d. Formation of new blood vessels

28. Systemic factors that influence wound healing include all the following EXCEPT:
    a. Blood supply
    b. Ionizing radiation
    c. Corticosteroids
    d. Nutritional deficiencies

29. A hallmark of healing is:
    a. Angiogenesis
    b. Granulation tissue
    c. Fibroblast proliferation
    d. Matrix metalloproteinases

30. All the following are processes of scar formation EXCEPT:
    a. Proliferation of fibroblasts in the site of injury
    b. Deposition of extracellular matrix
    c. Tissue remodeling
    d. Angiogenesis

31. During primary intention healing, granulation tissue forms within:
    a. 2 days
    b. 3 days
    c. 4 days
    d. 5 days

32. During primary intention healing, a basement membrane is formed within:
    a. 2 days
    b. 3 days
    c. 4 days
    d. 5 days

33. During primary intention healing, the inflammatory process dissipates during:
    a. Week 1
    b. Week 2
    c. Week 3
    d. Week 4

34. Delayed primary closure represents which type of healing?
    a. Primary intention
    b. Secondary intention
    c. Tertiary intention
    d. None of the above

35. What is the term for excessive scar formation?
    a. Keloid
    b. Contracture
    c. Dehiscence
    d. Ulcer

36. Autogenous stem cells are derived from the individual being treated. They may be totipotent, multipotent, or unipotent.
    a. Both statements are TRUE.
    b. Both statements are FALSE.
    c. The first statement is TRUE; the second statement is FALSE.
    d. The first statement is FALSE; the second statement is TRUE.

37. Adult stem cells are pluripotent and can generate cell tissue of the body. Embryonic stem cells have a more restricted capacity to generate different cell types.
    a. Both statements are TRUE.
    b. Both statements are FALSE.
    c. The first statement is TRUE; the second statement is FALSE.
    d. The first statement is FALSE; the second statement is TRUE.

38. All the following are types of adult stem cells EXCEPT:
    a. Amniotic fluid–derived stem cells
    b. Umbilical cord blood stem cells
    c. Adipose-derived stem cells
    d. Blastocyte-derived stem cells

39. What type of stem cell consists of both hematopoietic stem cells and mesenchymal stem cells?
    a. Amniotic fluid–derived stem cells
    b. Umbilical cord blood stem cells
    c. Bone marrow–derived stem cells
    d. Adipose-derived stem cells

40. The most common commercially available stem cells are:
    a. Embryonic stem cells
    b. Bone marrow–derived stem cells
    c. Adipose-derived stem cells
    d. Dental stem cells

41. Humans have approximately 20,000 to 25,000 chromosomes. The study of genes in the genome, their extensive DNA sequences, and their interactions define genomics.
    a. Both statements are TRUE.
    b. Both statements are FALSE.
    c. The first statement is TRUE; the second statement is FALSE.

    d. The first statement is FALSE; the second statement is TRUE.

42. Permanent changes in the DNA code is called a mutation. All mutations are harmful to the body.
    a. Both statements are TRUE.
    b. Both statements are FALSE.
    c. The first statement is TRUE; the second statement is FALSE.
    d. The first statement is FALSE; the second statement is TRUE.

43. The loss or gain of whole chromosomes resulting in monosomy or trisomy represents:
    a. Chromosome mutations
    b. Genome mutations
    c. Submicroscopic gene mutations
    d. All the above

44. The majority of mutations associated with hereditary disease are:
    a. Genome mutations
    b. Chromosome mutations
    c. Submicroscopic gene mutations
    d. Adenine gene mutations

45. Which pair of chromosomes constitutes the sex chromosomes?
    a. Twenty-first
    b. Twenty-third
    c. Thirty-eighth
    d. Forty-sixth

46. Huntington's disease exemplifies:
    a. Autosomal dominant disorder
    b. Autosomal recessive disorder
    c. X-linked recessive disorder
    d. Disorder with multifactorial inheritance

47. Cleft lip and cleft palate exemplify:
    a. Autosomal dominant disorder
    b. Autosomal recessive disorder
    c. X-linked recessive disorder
    d. Disorder with multifactorial inheritance

48. An organized graphic representation of the chromosomes of a single cell defines:
    a. Cytogenic typing
    b. Polymerase chain typing
    c. Karyotyping
    d. All the above

49. All the following are salivary DNA-PCR tests used to evaluate periodontal status EXCEPT:
    a. MyPerioPredict
    b. MyPerioPathSM
    c. MyPerioIDSM PST
    d. Perio Predict Genetic Risk Test

50. Palpating a submental node during a clinical examination represents which stage of the differential diagnosis process?
    a. Stage 1
    b. Stage 2
    c. Stage 3
    d. Stage 4

Oral Pathology

Olga A.C. Ibsen

Dental hygienists perform comprehensive extraoral and intraoral examinations, identify pathologic conditions, and communicate these findings to the dentist for diagnosis, treatment, or referral. Knowledge of oral pathology is essential for the preliminary evaluation of oral lesions. The dental hygienist differentiates between normal and abnormal findings and relates significant medical, dental, and cultural histories to clinical, radiographic, and histologic findings. Although the dental hygienist is not responsible for the dental diagnosis, skill in the use of the diagnostic process is essential for the dental hygiene diagnosis and collaborative practice.

BENIGN LESIONS OF SOFT TISSUE ORIGIN

General Characteristics

A. Etiology—unknown
B. Age and gender vary with the type of lesion
C. Clinical features
   1. Sharp line of demarcation outlines the lesion
   2. Sessile or pedunculated base
   3. Lesion is easily palpable
D. Histologic characteristics depend on the lesion (e.g., a lipoma is composed of fat cells)
E. Lesion grows slowly, or it may be encapsulated, which contributes to an evaluation of a benign state
F. Lesion is removed surgically and usually does not recur

Irritative Fibroma (or Traumatic Fibroma)

See Fig. 8-1.
A. Etiology—chronic mild irritant; chronic trauma
B. Age and gender related—40 to 60 years; more common in females (2:1)
C. Location—most common on the buccal mucosa along the area of the occlusal plane and gingiva; also found on the tongue, lips, and palate
D. Clinical features
   1. Light pink
   2. Round or semi-circular shape
   3. Less than 1 cm in size
   4. Sessile or pedunculated base
   5. Exophytic lesion
E. Histologic characteristics

1. Stratified squamous epithelium; surface may be keratinized or ulcerated (resulting from secondary trauma)
2. Contains dense connective tissue and few blood vessels
F. Treatment—complete excision

Papilloma

A. Etiology—benign lesion of squamous epithelium; long duration; slow development
B. Age and gender related—may arise at any age, but there is a 50% incidence between ages 20 and 50 years; no gender predilection
C. Location—soft palate or tongue
D. Clinical features (Fig. 8-2, *A*)
   1. Cauliflower-like appearance
   2. Usually grayish or white color; can also be pink; color depends on amount of keratin
   3. Well-delineated, exophytic nodule with a pedunculated or sessile base
   4. Under 0.5 cm in size
E. Histologic characteristics (Fig. 8-2, *B*)
   1. Composed primarily of long, finger-like projections of stratified squamous epithelium with a core of fibrous connective tissue; surface keratin
   2. Normal stratified squamous epithelium with a thick surface layer of keratin
F. Treatment and prognosis
   1. Surgical excision, including the base of the lesion to prevent recurrence
   2. Does not usually recur

Verruca Vulgaris (Wart)

A. Etiology—benign viral-induced lesion of stratified squamous epithelium; caused by human papillomavirus (HPV) (low-risk HPV)
B. Age and gender related—more common in children; but lesions have also been identified in adults; no gender predilection
C. Location—common skin lesion; lips are the most common oral site; can also be found on the tongue or mucosa
D. Clinical features (Fig. 8-3)
   1. White, papillary exophytic lesion
   2. Can spread to other areas of a person's skin
   3. Self-inoculated (finger to mouth)

FIG 8-1 Fibroma with a sessile base. (From Ibsen OAC, Phelan JA: *Oral pathology for the dental hygienist,* ed 6, St Louis, 2014, Elsevier.)

FIG 8-3 **A** and **B,** Verruca vulgaris on the tongue of a child, with a similar lesion on the thumb. (Courtesy of Dr. Edward V. Zegarelli; from Ibsen OAC, Phelan JA: *Oral pathology for the dental hygienist,* ed 6, St Louis, 2014, Elsevier.)

FIG 8-2 **A,** Clinical appearance of a papilloma on the palate showing a cauliflower-like appearance and rough surface resulting from finger-like projections. **B,** Microscopic appearance of a papilloma showing finger-like projections covered by a squamous epithelial layer and supported by thin cores of fibrous tissue. (From Ibsen OAC, Phelan JA: *Oral pathology for the dental hygienist,* ed 6, St Louis, 2014, Elsevier.)

4. Often has a sessile base
5. Differs from a papilloma in that warts grow faster, are smaller, and develop in a shorter time
E. Histologic characteristics
    1. Hyperkeratotic stratified squamous epithelium with a prominent granular cell layer in the upper spinous layer of epithelium

2. Numerous koilocytes (cells with clear cytoplasm) are located in the upper spinous layer of epithelium
3. Central cores of fibrous connective tissue
F. Treatment and prognosis
    1. Conservative surgical excision
    2. Lesions may recur because of reinoculation

Hemangioma

A. Etiology—congenital or developmental origin; when found in adults, these lesions develop as a response to trauma during the healing stages; a benign proliferation of blood capillaries
B. Age and gender related—lesions present at birth or develop shortly thereafter; more common in females (3:1); occur in adults as a response to trauma
C. Location—most common on the tongue; also found on the buccal mucosa, labial mucosa, and the vermilion border of lips
D. Clinical features (Fig. 8-4, *A*)
    1. Flat or raised, well-circumscribed lesion on tongue or mucosa
    2. Deep red or bluish purple
    3. Lesions blanch when pressure applied
    4. Two types of hemangioma:
        a. Capillary—small to moderate size; soft texture
        b. Cavernous—larger in size, more than 2 cm in diameter; exhibits a significant protrusion of tissue; deep purple; soft or semi-firm texture
E. Histologic characteristics (Fig. 8-4, *B*)
    1. Capillary—many small capillaries lined by a single layer of endothelial cells supported by a connective tissue stroma of varying density; endothelial cell proliferation
    2. Cavernous—large, dilated blood sinuses with thin walls, each having an endothelial lining; sinusoidal spaces filled with blood and lymphatic vessels

FIG 8-4 A, Clinical appearance of a hemangioma of the lower lip. **B,** Photomicrograph of a hemangioma. (From Ibsen OAC, Phelan JA: *Oral pathology for the dental hygienist,* ed 6, St Louis, 2014, Elsevier.)

F. Treatment and prognosis
   1. Treatment is variable
      a. Nonintervention for patients in whom spontaneous remission has occurred or can occur
      b. Surgical excision
      c. Sclerosing agents injected into the lesion result in its resolution
      d. Laser procedures
G. Prognosis is good

Lipoma

A. Etiology—unknown; rare; benign tumor of mature fat cells
B. Age and gender—over 40 years; no gender predilection
C. Location—most common on the buccal mucosa or in the mucobuccal fold
D. Clinical features (Fig. 8-5, *A*)
   1. Single or lobulated, well-defined, painless mass less than 3 cm in size
   2. Sessile or pedunculated base
   3. Soft to palpation
   4. Yellowish color (if aspirated, a brown-yellow fluid is withdrawn)
E. Histologic characteristics (Fig. 8-5, *B*)
   1. Circumscribed mass of mature fat cells with collagen strands and a few blood vessels
   2. Thin epithelium covers lesion
   3. If fibrous connective tissue forms a more significant part of the lesion, it is called a *fibrolipoma*
F. Treatment and prognosis
   1. Conservative surgical excision
   2. Recurrence is rare

INFLAMMATORY TUMORS (GRANULOMAS)

General Characteristics

A. Growth or enlargement of tissue composed mainly of inflammatory cells
B. Account for the major portion of all oral tumors
C. Benign tumors

Pyogenic Granuloma

A. Etiology—an exuberant tissue response to chronic irritants or trauma (i.e., plaque biofilm, calculus, poor restorative margins, hormonal levels)
B. Age and gender related—teenagers and young adults; more common in females (3:1), perhaps related to an increase in hormonal levels

FIG 8-5 A, Clinical appearance of a lipoma. **B,** Photomicrograph of a lipoma showing mature fat-cells. (**A** courtesy of Dr. Edward V. Zegarelli; from Ibsen OAC, Phelan JA: *Oral pathology for the dental hygienist,* ed 5, Philadelphia, 2009, Saunders; **B** from Regezi JA, Sciubba JJ: *Oral pathology: clinical-pathologic correlations,* ed 5, Philadelphia, 2008, Saunders.)

FIG 8-6 Pyogenic granuloma. (From Ibsen OAC, Phelan JA: *Oral pathology for the dental hygienist,* ed 6, St Louis, 2014, Elsevier.)

FIG 8-7 Papillary hyperplasia of the palate. (Courtesy of Dr. Edward V. Zegarelli; from Ibsen OAC, Phelan JA: *Oral pathology for the dental hygienist,* ed 6, St Louis, 2014, Elsevier.)

C. Location—much more common on the maxillary labial gingiva than mandibular gingiva; can occur on the lips, tongue, and buccal mucosa

D. Clinical features (Fig. 8-6)
1. Protrusive mass; pedunculated, sessile, or lobulated base
2. Deep-red to purple surface
3. Soft and spongy; freely movable; ulcerated, bleeds easily
4. Lesions are a few millimeters to several centimeters in size
5. In pregnancy, these lesions were formerly called "pregnancy tumors"

E. Histologic characteristics
1. The epithelium, if present, is thin
2. Rich in capillaries with proliferation of connective tissue; inflammatory cells
3. The lesion contains polymorphonuclear neutrophil leukocytes (PMNs), acute and chronic inflammatory cells, plasma cells, and lymphocytes

F. Treatment and prognosis
1. Removal of the irritant
2. Surgical excision of the lesion
3. These lesions can recur if the irritant remains (e.g., calculus)
4. The lesions that occur during pregnancy may resolve spontaneously, and hormonal levels return to normal

Papillary Hyperplasia of the Palate (Palatal Papillomatosis)

A. Etiology—type of denture stomatitis
1. Chronic irritation to the vault of the hard palate related to poorly fitting denture (full or partial); excessive pressure of an ill-fitting maxillary denture; and poor denture hygiene (secondary)
2. Can also be associated with poorly fitting orthodontic appliance or wearing the prosthetic device 24 hours a day

B. Age and gender related—especially individuals who wear maxillary dentures; no gender predilection

C. Location—especially in vault of the hard palate in maxillary denture wearers (suction chamber area)

D. Clinical features (Fig. 8-7)
1. Closely clustered erythematous papillary projections, 1 to 4 mm in diameter
2. Round, smooth, glistening red surface; granular appearance
3. Varying degrees of inflammation present

E. Histologic characteristics
1. Small vertical projections, each composed of stratified squamous epithelium and a central core of connective tissue
2. Epithelial proliferation
3. Infiltrated with inflammatory cells

F. Treatment
1. Surgical excision of the hyperplastic tissue before construction of a new denture or a reline
2. After surgery, emphasize denture care and removing the denture at night to rest the tissues

G. Prognosis—good

Denture-Induced Fibrous Hyperplasia (Epulis Fissuratum, Inflammatory Hyperplasia)

A. Etiology—irritation caused by poorly fitting denture, which produces a proliferation of tissue in the vestibule along the denture flange

B. Age and gender related—denture wearers; no gender predilection

C. Location—vestibule along denture border; alveolar ridge in regions along the denture border (maxillary or mandibular)

D. Clinical features (Fig. 8-8)
1. Exophytic folds of hyperplastic tissue in the vestibule under or around the denture flange
2. Pink to red color (can have ulcerated areas)
3. Firm to palpation

E. Histologic characteristics
1. Dense fibrous connective tissue covered by stratified squamous epithelium (same tissue seen in an irritation fibroma)

FIG 8-8 A, Denture-induced fibrous hyperplasia (epulis fissuratum) *(arrows)*, shown with denture in place, and **B,** denture removed. (From Ibsen OAC, Phelan JA: *Oral pathology for the dental hygienist,* ed 6, St Louis, 2014, Elsevier.)

2. Connective tissue composed of coarse bundles of collagen fibers
3. Same type of tissue as seen in irritation fibroma
F. Treatment and prognosis
1. Surgical removal of the excess tissue
2. Reline or reconstruct the denture
3. Prognosis is excellent

Peripheral Giant Cell Granuloma

A. Etiology—a reactive lesion caused by local irritants arising from the periodontal ligament
B. Age and gender related—40 to 60 years; more common in females (2:1)
C. Location—gingiva or alveolar mucosa, anterior to molars
D. Clinical features (Fig. 8-9, *A*)
1. Exophytic lesion 0.5 to 2.0 cm in diameter
2. Deep red
3. Pedunculated or sessile base
4. Arises from a deeper area in tissue than does pyogenic granuloma or fibroma
E. Radiographic appearance—peripheral giant cell granuloma
1. May cause a superficial destruction of alveolar bone
2. Radiolucent "cuffing" or erosion of bone may appear in the area
F. Histologic characteristics (Fig. 8-9, *B*)
1. Composed of a delicate reticular and fibrillar connective tissue stroma containing a large number of young, ovoid or spindle-shaped, connective tissue cells
2. Multi-nucleated giant cells

FIG 8-9 A, Peripheral giant cell granuloma. **B,** Microscopic appearance of a peripheral giant cell granuloma showing multinucleated giant cells *(M),* capillaries, and fibroblasts. (From Ibsen OAC, Phelan JA: *Oral pathology for the dental hygienist,* ed 6, St Louis, 2014, Elsevier.)

3. Proliferation of blood vessels
4. Appears to originate from the periodontal ligament or mucoperiosteum
G. Treatment and prognosis
1. Surgical removal of the entire base to eliminate recurrence

Central Giant Cell Granuloma

A. Etiology—occurs within bone; trauma caused by a fall, blow, or tooth extraction
B. Age and gender related—children and young adults; more common in females (2:1) age 10 to 30 years
C. Location—75% in the anterior segment of the mandible; also found in the maxilla
D. Clinical features
1. Appears as a swelling or bulge resulting from the expansion of cortical plates
2. No symptoms, so may be discovered on routine radiographs
3. A similar lesion, often called "brown tumor," occurs in persons with hyperparathyroidism; resolves without treatment
E. Radiographic appearance (Fig. 8-10, *A* and *B*)

FIG 8-10 Radiographs of central giant cell granulomas showing multi-locular radiolucencies. **A,** The mandible. **B,** The maxilla. (From Ibsen OAC, Phelan JA: *Oral pathology for the dental hygienist,* ed 6, St Louis, 2014, Elsevier.)

1. Usually a large radiolucent area with diffuse margins that are poorly defined with faint trabeculae
2. Displacement of teeth; divergence of the roots of teeth adjacent to the lesion is a common feature
3. Root resorption

F. Histologic characteristics
   1. Loose, fibrillar connective tissue with many fibroblasts
   2. Rich vascularity
   3. Foreign body, multi-nucleated giant cells

G. Treatment and prognosis
   1. Curettage (perhaps more than one treatment)
   2. Surgical removal
   3. Radiotherapy is contraindicated
   4. Occasionally recurs
   5. In hyperparathyroid patients, the lesion is not removed because it resolves when hyperparathyroidism is treated

Chronic Hyperplastic Pulpitis (Pulpal Granuloma, Pulp Polyp)

A. Etiology—excessive proliferation of chronically inflamed pulp tissue found in teeth with large open carious lesions; rapid caries; lesion projects from the pulp chamber

FIG 8-11 Chronic hyperplastic pulpitis (pulp polyp) *(arrow)*. (From Ibsen OAC, Phelan JA: *Oral pathology for the dental hygienist,* ed 6, St Louis, 2014, Elsevier.)

B. Age and gender related—children and young adults; no gender predilection
C. Location
   1. Usually in primary molars or permanent molars
   2. Can occur in any tooth with a large, open, carious lesion
D. Clinical features (Fig. 8-11)
   1. Red to pink outgrowth of pulp tissue protruding from the occlusal surface of the crown of a tooth that has a large, open, carious lesion
   2. Lesion is not painful because hyperplastic tissue contains few nerves
E. Histologic characteristics
   1. Originates from pulpal tissue
   2. Contains acute and chronic inflammatory cells, plasma cells, and lymphocytes
   3. Granulation tissue
F. Treatment and prognosis
   1. Extraction of the involved tooth
   2. Endodontic therapy
   3. Root canal therapy for the involved tooth plus full restorative coverage (if possible)
   4. Prognosis is good

Internal Resorption

A. Etiology—not clear; theories include:
   1. Inflammatory response in the pulp
   2. Trauma
   3. Caries-related pulpitis
B. Age and gender related—any age; no gender predilection
C. Location—usually found within a tooth in the permanent dentition
D. Clinical features
   1. Dentin immediately surrounding the pulp in the area of resorption is destroyed

FIG 8-12 Radiograph showing an area of internal resorption on the maxillary first molar *(arrow)*. (From Ibsen OAC, Phelan JA: *Oral pathology for the dental hygienist*, ed 6, St Louis, 2014, Elsevier.)

2. The crown may appear pink ("pink tooth") because of the vascularity of the lesion within (this is not easily observable on posterior teeth)
E. Radiographic appearance well defined, but radiolucent lesion in close proximity to the pulp canal (Fig. 8-12)
F. Histologic characteristics—highly vascularized, chronic inflammatory tissue; few nerves
G. Treatment—endodontic therapy if perforation of the root has not occurred; otherwise, extraction of the tooth is essential

Periapical Granuloma

A. Etiology—dental caries or deep restorations; a response to injury
B. Age and gender related—any age; no gender predilection
C. Location—apex of a nonvital tooth
D. Clinical features
  1. Nonvital tooth
  2. Fistula or parulis may be present if the condition has been chronic
  3. The affected tooth can be sensitive to percussion
  4. Many times can be asymptomatic
E. Radiographic appearance—varies from a well-defined, circular, radiolucent lesion at the apex of the involved tooth to a diffuse radiolucency or thickening of the periodontal ligament space (Fig. 8-13, *A*)
F. Histologic characteristics (Fig. 8-13, *B*)
  1. Lymphocytes, plasma cells, macrophages
  2. Dense, fibrous connective tissue
  3. Epithelial (Malassez) rests (remnants of tooth-forming tissues)
G. Treatment—endodontic therapy or extraction of the affected tooth

BENIGN INTRAOSSEOUS NEOPLASMS

General Characteristics

A. Etiology—generally unknown
B. Onset—gradual, with slow development or enlargement
C. Early stages—asymptomatic
D. With expansion of the lesion, malocclusion may occur; bone tenderness on palpation; cortical bone may become thin

Osteoma

A. Etiology—asymptomatic benign tumor of compact bone; etiology generally unknown, but the cause may be irritation or inflammation; associated with a genetic condition called Gardner syndrome
B. Age and gender related—more common in young adults but can be found at any age; no gender predilection
C. Location—most common posterior mandible; mandibular condyle; craniofacial skeleton only; exophytic or periosteal, endosteal, or central osteoma
D. Clinical features—the affected individual may be unaware of the lesion because it grows slowly; considerable growth must occur before cortical plates expand
E. Radiographic appearance
  1. Well-circumscribed radiopaque mass that is indistinguishable from scar bone

FIG 8-13 A, Radiograph of a periapical granuloma. **B,** Low-power microscopic appearance of a periapical granuloma. (From Ibsen OAC, Phelan JA: *Oral pathology for the dental hygienist,* ed 6, St Louis, 2014, Elsevier.)

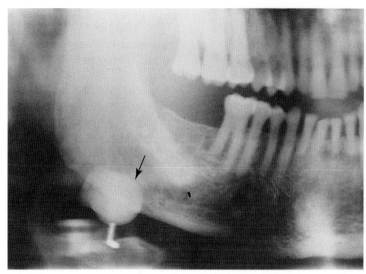

FIG 8-14 Radiograph of an osteoma showing a radiopacity *(arrow)* of the posterior mandible. (Courtesy of Dr. Sidney Eisig; from Ibsen OAC, Phelan JA: *Oral pathology for the dental hygienist,* ed 6, St Louis, 2014, Elsevier.)

2. Panoramic or lateral plate radiograph may be needed to view the lesion in its entirety (Fig. 8-14)
F. Histologic characteristics—extremely dense, compact bone or coarse, cancellous bone
   1. Compact osteomas—have minimal marrow tissue
   2. Cancellous osteomas—have fibrofatty marrow
G. Treatment and prognosis
   1. Surgical excision for large lesions
   2. Does not recur

Chondroma

A. Etiology—benign tumors of hyaline cartilage; cause unknown
B. Age and gender related—ages 30 to 40 years; no gender predilection
C. Location
   1. Maxilla—anterior area
   2. Mandible—posterior to canines
   3. May involve the body of the mandible or the coronoid or condylar process
D. Clinical features
   1. Painless
   2. Slow, progressive swelling of the jaw may loosen or malposition teeth
   3. Tendency to become malignant—potential chondrosarcoma
E. Radiographic appearance—irregular radiolucent or mottled area in bone; may displace surrounding teeth or cause root resorption
F. Histologic characteristics
   1. Mass of hyaline cartilage with areas of calcification or necrosis
   2. Cartilage cells are small, and each has one nucleus
   3. Large biopsy sample must be obtained because the lesion is similar to a malignant chondrosarcoma (more common in men)

G. Treatment and prognosis
   1. Nonconservative surgical removal; tumor may be resistant to radiation therapy
   2. Periodic follow-up evaluation is necessary to detect recurrence or possibility of a chondrosarcoma

Odontogenic Myxoma

A. Etiology—unknown; benign; originates from mesenchymal tissue of the tooth germ; odontogenic origin
B. Age and gender related—most often in young adults, ages 10 to 30 years; no gender predilection
C. Location—mandible more often than maxilla
D. Clinical features—deeply situated lesion; small lesions asymptomatic
E. Radiographic appearance (Fig. 8-15)

FIG 8-15 Radiograph of a myxoma showing multi-locular, honeycombed radiolucency. (From Ibsen OAC, Phelan JA: *Oral pathology for the dental hygienist,* ed 6, St Louis, 2014, Elsevier.)

1. May be unilocular or multi-locular
2. Several small radiolucencies occurring in groups, giving a "honeycomb" appearance
3. May show displaced teeth, mandibular canal, and antrum (may also invade the antrum)
4. Peripheral borders are irregular, diffuse, and not well defined
5. Large lesions may have a "soap bubble" radiolucent pattern similar to the ameloblastoma

F. Histologic characteristics
   1. Loosely textured tissue containing delicate reticulin fibers and mucoid material
   2. Contains stellate, spindle-shaped cells
   3. The tumor is not encapsulated and may invade surrounding tissues
   4. Does not metastasize

G. Treatment and prognosis
   1. Complete surgical excision
   2. Recurrence is common (25%)

Exostosis
Torus Palatinus

A. Etiology—inherited, autosomal dominant; some believe the cause to be genetic or environmental factors
B. Age and gender related—usually seen by the age of puberty; rarely observed in children, but peak incidence occurs before 30 years; more common in females (2:1)
C. Location—midline of the hard palate
D. Clinical features (Fig. 8-16, *A*)
   1. Bony, hard protuberance in the midline in a variety of shapes—nodular; lobulated; smooth; spindle
   2. Occurs in 20% to 35% of the U.S. population
   3. Torus may appear ulcerated because of trauma to the thin overlying mucosa

FIG 8-16 A, Clinical appearance of a lobulated torus palatinus. **B,** Clinical appearance of bilateral mandibular tori. (From Ibsen OAC, Phelan JA: *Oral pathology for the dental hygienist,* ed 6, St Louis, 2014, Elsevier.)

E. Radiographic appearance—dense radiopaque area
F. Histologic characteristics—dense cortical bone
G. Treatment—usually none, but surgical removal if the lesion interferes with a prosthodontic appliance

Torus Mandibularis

A. Etiology—inherited, autosomal dominant; possibly genetic or environmental
B. Age and gender related—first observed in early teen years; slightly more common in males
C. Location—lingual surface of the mandible above the mylohyoid line in the area of premolars; often bilateral
D. Clinical features (Fig. 8-16, *B*)
   1. Bony protuberance varying in size and shape; common exostosis—modular, lobulated, or smooth
   2. Slow growing
   3. Bilateral incidence more common (90%)
E. Radiographic appearance—dense radiopaque area
F. Histologic characteristics—dense cortical bone
G. Treatment—surgical excision if the lesion interferes with a prosthodontic appliance

Odontoma

A. Etiology—most common odontogenic tumor; composed of all tooth structure and pulp but not considered a neoplasm
B. Age and gender related—usually seen in adolescents and young adults, mean age 14 years; no gender predilection
C. Location—more frequently seen in the maxilla (especially anterior maxilla for the compound type) than in the mandible; usually between the roots of teeth or near apices; complex odontomas seen more often in posterior mandible
D. Clinical features
   1. Failure of a permanent tooth to erupt
   2. Asymptomatic
E. Radiographic appearance—irregular mass of radiopacities ("tooth-like structures") surrounded by a narrow radiolucent halo
   1. Two types
      a. Compound—tooth structures are identified radiographically (Fig. 8-17)
      b. Complex—appears as a radiopaque mass (can be confused with other lesions in bone) (Fig. 8-18)
   2. Cyst involvement may occur with an odontoma
F. Histologic characteristics—tumor in which epithelial and mesenchymal cells show differentiation, resulting in abnormal enamel and dentin formation
G. Treatment and prognosis
   1. Complete surgical removal (both forms are well encapsulated)
   2. Prognosis is good

GINGIVAL FIBROMATOSIS
General Characteristics

A. Enlargement of gingival tissue, sometimes covering teeth
B. Contains a proliferation of dense fibrous connective tissue
C. Classification includes:

FIG 8-17 Radiograph of a compound odontoma, showing a collection of numerous, small, tooth-like radiopacities *(arrows)* surrounded by a radiolucent halo. (From Ibsen OAC, Phelan JA: *Oral pathology for the dental hygienist,* ed 6, St Louis, 2014, Elsevier.)

FIG 8-18 Radiograph of a complex odontoma showing a radiopaque mass surrounded by a radiolucent halo *(arrow).* (From Ibsen OAC, Phelan JA: *Oral pathology for the dental hygienist,* ed 6, St Louis, 2014, Elsevier.)

  1. Irritative fibromatosis—localized areas associated with extraneous irritants
  2. Hereditary fibromatosis—generalized enlargement of gingival tissue
  3. Chemical fibromatosis—caused by certain medications (drug-influenced gingival enlargement)

Irritative Fibromatosis

A. Etiology—irritant such as mouth breathing, orthodontic appliances, bacterial plaque biofilm, dental calculus, debris, overhanging restorations, or poorly fitting dental appliances

B. Age and gender related—any age; no gender predilection
C. Location—localized areas on interproximal papillae; in mouth breathers, on maxillary and mandibular anterior labial gingiva
D. Clinical features—solitary round, smooth-surfaced, pink enlargement of papillae; well attached to surrounding structures
E. Histologic characteristics—proliferation of dense fibrous connective tissue with increase in number of fibroblasts
F. Treatment and prognosis
  1. Removal of the irritant
  2. Improved oral hygiene
  3. Gingivectomy in severe cases
  4. Prognosis is excellent once the cause is removed

Hereditary Gingival Fibromatosis (Gingival Lesions of Genetic Origin)

A. Etiology (see the section on "Genetics" in Chapter 7)
  1. Hereditary; believed to have genetic or developmental involvement or to be related to hormonal imbalances; a component of several syndromes (e.g., Zimmerman-Laband, Cross, Rutherfurd, Murray-Puretic-Drescher, Cowden)
  2. Contributing factors include poor oral hygiene, food impaction, calculus, and malocclusion
  3. Other conditions associated with gingival fibromatosis may include growth hormone deficiency, hypothyroidism, epilepsy, and intellectual and developmental disabilities (IDDs)
B. Age and gender related—appears during the eruption of primary or permanent teeth; slightly more common in females
C. Location—excessive enlargement of interproximal gingival tissues; can be localized
D. Clinical features
  1. Gingival enlargement may be generalized or localized
  2. Diffuse, smooth-surfaced, pink, firm tissue involving the interproximal papillae
  3. Multiple protruding pink, stippled, firm masses; labial and buccal areas are most affected; teeth may be displaced; delays eruption of teeth
E. Histologic characteristics—bundles of fibrous connective tissue with fibroblasts and fibrocytes (depending on the formative stage)
F. Treatment and prognosis
  1. Gingivectomy
  2. Rigid adherence to home care
  3. Recurrence is common

Chemical Fibromatosis (Drug-influenced Gingival Enlargement)

A. Etiology—reaction to drugs, specifically phenytoin (Dilantin); calcium channel blockers including nifedipine (Procardia), amlodipine (Norvasc), diltiazem (Cardizem), and verapamil (Calan); cyclosporin, an immunosuppressant drug given in association with organ transplants
B. Age and gender—no gender predilection

C. Location—papillae and gingivae
D. Clinical features—smooth, pink, firm enlargement of the papillae (Fig. 8-19)
E. Histologic characteristics—extensive proliferation of connective tissue
F. Treatment
   1. Change in the prescribed medication, if possible
   2. Gingivectomy
   3. Improved oral self-care; control of the biofilm

FIG 8-19 Drug-influenced gingival enlargement. **A,** Gingival enlargement caused by phenytoin (Dilantin). **B** and **C,** Gingival hyperplasia caused by nifedipine (Procardia). (**A** courtesy of Dr. Edward V. Zegarelli; **B** and **C** courtesy of Dr. Victor M. Sternberg; **A** to **C** from Ibsen OAC, Phelan JA: *Oral pathology for the dental hygienist,* ed 6, St Louis, 2014, Elsevier.)

ULCERATIVE DISEASES

General Characteristics

A. Ulcer—formed by the destruction of the epithelium and some underlying tissue
B. Factors aiding in the diagnosis of ulcers occurring in the oral cavity
   1. Number and size
   2. Location
   3. Depth
   4. Borders
   5. Patient history (personal, health, cultural, pharmacologic)
C. Etiology—not always known
D. Can be classified as an acute or chronic condition
   1. Acute ulcerative conditions include traumatic ulcers, aphthous ulcers, allergic reactions, and viral ulcerations
   2. Chronic ulcerative conditions include those caused by or associated with systemic diseases such as leukemia, colitis, malnutrition, tuberculosis, syphilis, sickle cell anemia, and drug toxicity

Traumatic Ulcer

A. Etiology—various types of trauma; history of lesion plays a significant role in the diagnosis
   1. Physical—biting the mucosa, denture irritation, toothbrush injury, sharp tooth, fractured filling (Fig. 8-20)
   2. Chemical—oral rinse, phenol, misuse of medication used to treat a toothache (e.g., misuse of aspirin causes an aspirin burn) (Fig. 8-21)
   3. Thermal—hot foods (e.g., soup) (Fig. 8-22, *A*); crack cocaine (Fig. 8-22, *B*)
   4. Electrical
B. Age and gender related—any age; no gender predilection
C. Location—lateral border of the tongue, buccal mucosa, lips, palate (especially tori)
D. Clinical features
   1. Small, single, oval, round, or irregular shape
   2. Flat or slightly depressed
   3. Covered by necrotic membrane and surrounded by an erythematous halo
   4. Painful for 2 to 5 days
   5. Heals within 7 to 14 days
E. Histologic characteristics
   1. Loss of continuity of surface epithelium
   2. Fibrinous exudate covering exposed connective tissue
   3. Infiltration of PMNs in connective tissue
   4. Fibroblastic activity can be prominent
F. Treatment and prognosis
   1. Removal of the irritant or cause
   2. Application of benzocaine (Orabase with benzocaine) to relieve symptoms
   3. Corticosteroids (recommended by some, whereas others suggest corticosteroid medications can delay healing)
   4. Topical dyclonine hydrochloride for temporary relief
   5. In severe cases, systemic antibiotics are given to prevent secondary infection (these patients may also require surgical debridement depending on the extent of tissue damage)

FIG 8-20 **A,** Traumatic ulceration caused by irritation of gingiva by fingernails. **B,** Traumatic ulcer caused by a denture. (From Ibsen OAC, Phelan JA: *Oral pathology for the dental hygienist,* ed 6, St Louis, 2014, Elsevier.)

FIG 8-22 Mucosal burns. **A,** Thermal burn of palate caused by contact with hot soup. **B,** Ulcer of midline of palate caused by heat generated during the use of crack cocaine. (**A** from Ibsen OAC, Phelan JA: *Oral pathology for the dental hygienist,* ed 6, St Louis, 2014, Elsevier; **B** from Mitchell-Lewis DA, Phelan JA, Kelly RB, Bradley JJ, Lamster IB: Identifying oral lesions associated with crack-cocaine use, *J Am Dent Assoc* 125:1104, 1994.)

FIG 8-21 Mucosal burns. **A,** Burns caused by aspirin. **B,** Chemical burn caused by contact with caustic material during endodontic treatment. (From Ibsen OAC, Phelan JA: *Oral pathology for the dental hygienist,* ed 6, St Louis, 2014, Elsevier.)

6. In patients with electrical burns, tetanus immunization is necessary
7. Prognosis is good

Necrotizing Ulcerative Gingivitis (NUG; Vincent's Infection, Trench Mouth)

A. Etiology
1. Anaerobic bacteria—fusiform bacilli (*Bacillus fusiformis*)
2. *Borrelia vincentii*, a spirochete
3. Sophisticated technology has identified the involvement of other species as well
4. Contributory factors
   a. Systemic—stress, fatigue, poor hygiene, malnutrition, suppressed immune system, recent illness
   b. Local—poor restorations, trauma, gingivitis, poor oral hygiene, heavy smoking
B. Age and gender related—any age, usually 17 to 35 years; no gender predilection
C. Location—free gingival margin, crest of gingiva, interdental papillae
D. Clinical features (Fig. 8-23)
1. Acute gingivitis with extensive necrosis
2. Blunted, "punched-out," crater-like necrosis of interdental papillae
3. Fetid mouth odor, pain, bleeding, bad taste
4. Headaches, low-grade fever
5. Regional lymphadenopathy
E. Histologic characteristics
1. Ulcerated stratified squamous epithelium
2. Thick fibrinous exudate containing PMNs
3. Significant bacterial colonization
4. Connective tissue infiltrated by dense numbers of PMNs
F. Treatment and prognosis
1. Scaling and debridement (patient may need several visits)
2. Use of ultrasonic instruments (except when contraindicated)

FIG 8-23 Necrotizing ulcerative gingivitis. (From Ibsen OAC, Phelan JA: *Oral pathology for the dental hygienist,* ed 6, St Louis, 2014, Elsevier.)

3. Topical anesthetic or even local anesthetic may be necessary for the procedure
4. Use of an oxygenating rinse four or more times daily for 1 to 2 weeks
5. 0.12% chlorhexidine rinses
6. Use of systemic antibiotics such as penicillin, tetracycline, or erythromycin, if patient has systemic symptoms such as a fever, lymphadenopathy, or both
7. Home care to improve oral hygiene status (e.g., power toothbrush, interdental cleaning)
8. Once treatment is completed, a 1-month follow-up appointment should be scheduled to evaluate therapy and reinforce oral self-care; the patient should be encouraged to have recare visits every 4 months
9. Condition can recur if the individual lacks optimal oral self-care or has associated risk factors

MINOR APHTHOUS ULCERS

Recurrent Ulcerative Stomatitis (RUS); Recurrent Aphthous Stomatitis

A. Etiology
1. Autoimmune response of oral epithelium
2. T cell–mediated immunologic response
3. Decrease of mucosal tissue barrier
4. Inherited predisposition
5. Risk factors
   a. Hormonal imbalance—premenstrual (incidence increases), pregnancy (incidence decreases)
   b. Psychological—anxiety, depression, acute emotional problems, stress
   c. Allergy—asthma, hay fever, food, drug, gluten
   d. Blood abnormalities
   e. Trauma
   f. Bacterial or viral agents (e.g., herpes simplex virus; cytomegalovirus)
6. Systemic conditions associated with aphthous stomatitis:
   a. Behçet syndrome
   b. Crohn disease
   c. Ulcerative colitis
   d. Cyclic neutropenia
   e. Sprue
   f. Intestinal lymphoma
B. Age and gender related—childhood to adolescence and young adults; more common in females
C. Location—buccal and labial mucosa, soft palate, pharynx, tongue; more common in the anterior regions
D. Clinical features (Fig. 8-24)
1. Ulcerations—oval or round in shape with distinct borders; the center of the ulcer has a yellowish white fibrous surface surrounded by an erythematous halo
2. Range from 1 to 12 in number (3 to 10 most common)
3. Size—3 to 10 mm
4. Pain, tenderness, discomfort
5. Interference with functions—speech, eating
6. Prodromal period of 1 to 2 days; characterized by a tingling or burning sensation in the area where the ulcer will appear

FIG 8-24 Example of a minor aphthous ulcer. (From Ibsen OAC, Phelan JA: *Oral pathology for the dental hygienist,* ed 6, St Louis, 2014, Elsevier.)

FIG 8-25 Example of major aphthous ulcers located on the labial mucosa. (From Ibsen OAC, Phelan JA: *Oral pathology for the dental hygienist,* ed 6, St Louis, 2014, Elsevier.)

7. Associated systemic factors can include low-grade fever and localized lymphadenopathy
E. Histologic characteristics
   1. Superficial erosion of mucosal tissue covered by a membrane
   2. Connective tissue shows increased vascularity
   3. Increase in PMNs, lymphocytes, and histiocytes
F. Treatment and prognosis
   1. Self-limiting, healing in 10 to 12 days; recurrent episodes are common
   2. Topical corticosteroids; 0.12% chlorhexidine rinse; topical tetracyclines
   3. Betamethasone syrup (rinse and expectorate)

MAJOR APHTHOUS ULCERS

Recurrent Scarifying Ulcerative Stomatitis (RSUS); Periadenitis Mucosa Necrotica Recurrens; Mikulicz Aphthae; Sutton Disease

A. Etiology
   1. Autoimmune response of oral epithelium
   2. T cell–mediated immunologic response
   3. Decrease of mucosal tissue barrier
   4. Inherited predisposition
B. Age and gender related—usually young adults, onset after puberty; more common in females
C. Location—labial mucosa, buccal mucosa, soft palate, posterior fauces
D. Clinical features (Fig. 8-25)
   1. Multiple large ulcers, 1 to 10 in number and 1 to 3 cm in diameter
   2. Crater-like formations with irregular shapes
   3. Lesions heal in 3 to 6 weeks, producing scarring
   4. Very painful
   5. Occur at frequent intervals; patient is rarely without an ulcer
E. Histologic characteristics
   1. Fibrinopurulent membrane covering the ulcerated area
   2. Necrotic epithelium

3. Intense inflammatory cell infiltration in connective tissue
4. Neutrophils and lymphocytes present
5. Granulation tissue at the base of the lesion
6. Microscopic picture is nonspecific; a conclusive diagnosis cannot be made without thorough clinical and historical data
F. Treatment and prognosis
   1. Corticosteroids
      a. Systemic
      b. Topical
   2. Inject the lesion with triamcinolone acetonide
   3. 0.05% Halobetasol propionate ointment
   4. Recurrence is common

Mucous Membrane Pemphigoid, Cicatricial Pemphigoid, Benign Mucous Membrane Pemphigoid

A. Etiology—chronic benign autoimmune disease
B. Age and gender related—ages 50 to 65 years; more common in females (2:1)
C. Location
   1. Gingiva
   2. Oral mucous membranes
   3. Eyes, nasal, esophageal, and vaginal mucosa
   4. Skin
D. Clinical features
   1. Vesicles or bullous lesions; surface is "thick" and does not rupture easily
   2. After rupture, the surface is eroded and raw (desquamated)
   3. Desquamative appearance (not descriptive of this condition alone)
E. Histologic characteristics (Fig. 8-26)
   1. Vesicles and bullae are subepithelial
   2. The epithelium appears to be detached from connective tissue

FIG 8-26 Histologic appearance of pemphigoid. (Ibsen OAC, Phelan JA: *Oral pathology for the dental hygienist,* ed 6, St Louis, 2014, Elsevier.)

3. No evidence of acantholysis—degeneration of cohesive elements of epithelial cells (as seen in pemphigus)
4. Inflammatory infiltrate in connective tissue
5. Direct immunofluorescence shows a linear pattern at the basement membrane in over 90% of cases

F. Treatment and prognosis
  1. Mild forms—topical corticosteroids
  2. With bullous eruptions or conjunctival involvement, high doses of systemic corticosteroids are needed
  3. Certain systemic antibiotics
  4. Once the diagnosis of cicatricial pemphigoid is made, the patient should be referred for an eye examination, since eye involvement can be severe but may not show any symptoms in the early stages
  5. Patients go through periods of remission; long-term disease or condition

Herpes
Primary Herpetic Gingivostomatitis
A. Etiology
  1. Virus—initial infection with herpes simplex virus (HSV)
  2. Member of the human herpesvirus (HHV) group
  3. Transmission—droplet infection; direct contact; highly contagious (the amount of virus is highest in the vesicle stage); patients can self-inoculate (especially the eyes)
B. Age and gender related—ages 6 months to 6 years; no gender predilection
C. Location—lips, gingiva, tongue, pharynx, floor of the mouth, buccal mucosa
D. Clinical features (Fig. 8-27)
  1. Systemic symptoms
    a. Abrupt onset of fever
    b. Headache, irritability
    c. Pain on swallowing
    d. Regional lymphadenopathy
  2. Oral symptoms
    a. Hypertrophic gingivitis
    b. Initially, tiny vesicles (pinhead size) that develop into ulcerations

FIG 8-27 **A,** Example of primary herpetic gingivostomatitis in a child. **B** and **C,** Primary herpetic gingivostomatitis in an adolescent. (**A** courtesy of Dr. Edward V. Zegarelli; **A** to **C** from Ibsen OAC, Phelan JA: *Oral pathology for the dental hygienist,* ed 6, St Louis, 2014, Elsevier.)

    c. Painful ulcers 1 to 3 mm in size; covered by a yellowish fibrinous surface
    d. Shallow craters covered by white or yellow plaque; bright erythematous margins ("halo")
    e. Most acute on days 3 to 7
E. Laboratory tests and findings
  1. Cytologic smear (noninvasive and inexpensive test)
  2. Blood test for HSV
  3. Viral isolation from tissue culture of intact vesicles (best diagnostic procedure but can take up to 2 weeks to obtain results)
F. Histologic characteristics
  1. Vesicle is an intraepithelial blister filled with fluid
  2. Degenerating cells show "ballooning"
  3. Displacement of chromatin around the nucleus

4. Acantholysis of epithelium (Tzanck cells)
G. Treatment and prognosis
 1. Symptomatic therapy—bed rest, fluids
 2. Antiviral medications such as acyclovir ("swish and swallow") started within the first few days
 3. Ibuprofen to reduce pain and discomfort
 4. Self-limiting; healing in 7 to 14 days
 5. Recurrence most common in the form of herpes labialis

Herpes Labialis (Cold Sore, Fever Blister)

A. Etiology
 1. Residual form of HSV type 1
 2. Recurrence of HSV from its latent stage
 3. Stimuli that can trigger the onset
  a. Exposure to sunlight
  b. Trauma
  c. Menstruation
  d. Emotional stress, anxiety, fatigue
  e. Allergic reactions
  f. Systemic diseases
B. Age and gender related—adults; no gender predilection
C. Location
 1. Lips—most common (herpes labialis)
 2. Intraorally—hard palate, attached gingiva (keratinized mucosa fixed to bone)
D. Clinical features (Fig. 8-28)
 1. Prodromal period (any time up to 24 hours before the lesion erupts)—burning sensation, feeling of tightness, tingling, or soreness where the vesicle eventually appears
 2. Several fluid-filled papules may appear in clusters (most contagious state)
 3. Vesicles rupture, and crust forms on lips
 4. Intraoral lesions can appear on keratinized mucosa
 5. Do not confuse with angular cheilitis, a fungal infection
E. Histologic characteristics
 1. Ballooning degeneration
 2. Chromatin margination around the nucleus
 3. Isolation of HSV
F. Treatment and prognosis
 1. Antiviral drugs (e.g., acyclovir, valacyclovir) especially effective if given during the prodromal period
 2. Prophylactic treatment with antivirals before encountering a risk factor, if possible
 3. Topical application of 10% n-docosanol cream has been effective
 4. Self-limiting; healing in 7 to 10 days
 5. Sunscreen to prevent the development of herpes labialis
 6. Chlorhexidine (0.12%) rinses, acyclovir suspension, or both can be helpful to treat intraoral recurrent HSV
 7. The condition does recur

Herpes Zoster (Shingles)

A. Etiology
 1. Reactivation of varicella-zoster virus (VZV, HHV-3) from its latent stage
 2. VZV also causes chickenpox, which is considered the primary infection with VZV

FIG 8-28 Herpes labialis. **A,** Twelve hours after onset. **B,** Forty-eight hours after onset. (From Ibsen OAC, Phelan JA: *Oral pathology for the dental hygienist,* ed 6, St Louis, 2014, Elsevier.)

 3. Risk factors for reactivation of VZV
  a. Systemic disease (malignancies, Hodgkin's disease, leukemia)
  b. Drug toxicity, radiation, alcohol abuse
  c. Advanced age
  d. Extreme fatigue
  e. Immunosupression
 4. Depression of cell-mediated immunity
B. Age and gender related—adults, usually over 50 years; no gender predilection
C. Location—skin or mucosa, supplied by the affected sensory nerve; any of the three branches of the trigeminal nerve (Fig. 8-29); unilateral distribution
D. Clinical features (Fig. 8-30)
 1. Three phases—prodromal, acute, chronic
 2. Prodromal period of extreme pain 1 to 3 days before eruption of the unilateral rash, which can be accompanied by systemic features such as fever, severe headaches, lymphadenopathy, and overall weakness
 3. The erythematous rash develops into vesicles; the pain becomes more intense with a burning, tingling, or stabbing sensation
 4. Clusters of these vesicles develop along the pathway of a sensory nerve

Ophthalmic branch
Maxillary branch
Mandibular branch

FIG 8-29 The divisions of the trigeminal nerve. (From Ibsen OAC, Phelan JA: *Oral pathology for the dental hygienist,* ed 6, St Louis, 2014, Elsevier.)

5. Intraoral lesions can appear as multiple vesicles with a white center, which eventually form shallow ulcerations; these lesions are also unilateral and can be on movable or attached mucosa

6. After the skin vesicles heal, a postherpetic neuralgia occurs

E. Treatment and prognosis

1. Antiviral medications (acyclovir, valacyclovir, famciclovir)

2. Postherpetic neuralgia is most difficult to control; several therapies, including analgesics, narcotics, corticosteroids, anticonvulsants; biofeedback, and nerve block

3. Cutaneous lesions should be kept clean and dry to prevent secondary infection (antibiotics may have to be prescribed if the infection does occur)

4. Antibacterial oral rinses for intraoral lesions

5. A varicella vaccine is available; Zostavax, for people 60 years and older; is 14 times more effective than Varivax, the vaccine for chickenpox

6. Prognosis is good if trigeminal nerve involvement is present (healing in 2 to 3 weeks)

7. Postherpetic neuralgia can last for extended periods

Herpangina (Aphthous Pharyngitis)

A. Etiology—coxsackievirus

B. Age and gender related—children age 6 months to 5 years; no gender predilection

C. Location—posterior hard or soft palate, fauces (pillars), uvula, tonsils; most likely seen in the summer

D. Clinical features

1. Systemic symptoms

a. Comparatively mild and of short duration

b. Sore throat; dysphagia; headaches

FIG 8-30 Herpes zoster. **A,** Unilateral distribution of vesicles along the distribution of a sensory nerve. **B,** Many vesicles coalesce to form large lesions. **C,** Unilateral facial lesions occurring along the distribution of the maxillary branch of the trigeminal nerve. (From Ibsen OAC, Phelan JA: *Oral pathology for the dental hygienist,* ed 6, St Louis, 2014, Elsevier.)

c. Fever

d. Headache; vomiting; diarrhea

e. No lymphadenopathy—differs from primary herpes, which has lymphadenopathy

f. Transmission through fecal-oral route or droplets

2. Oral symptoms (Fig. 8-31)

a. From erythematous macules to vesicles, to ulcers; ulcerations 2 to 4 mm in size

b. Vesicles are often overlooked

c. Two to six small ulcers; ulcers appear with a gray base and inflamed periphery, usually on the soft palate or tonsillar areas

FIG 8-31 Herpangina. (From Ibsen OAC, Phelan JA: *Oral pathology for the dental hygienist,* ed 6, St Louis, 2014, Elsevier.)

    d. Slightly painful; the affected person has difficulty swallowing (dysphagia)

    e. Sudden onset—mild or subclinical

    f. Erythematous pharynx

E. Laboratory tests

  1. Viral isolation (throat culture during early stage)

  2. Stool specimens

F. Treatment and prognosis

  1. Self-limiting, with few complications

  2. Nonaspirin pain relievers

  3. Usually resolves within 7 days without treatment

Infectious Mononucleosis (Glandular Fever)

A. Etiology

  1. Epstein-Barr virus (EBV)

  2. Transmission—intimate oral exchange of saliva; "kissing disease"

B. Age and gender related—children (transmission through saliva on toys) and mostly young adults; no gender predilection

C. Clinical features

  1. Systemic symptoms (depending on age)

    a. Fever, chills, prodromal fatigue, malaise

    b. Sore throat, pharyngitis

    c. Headache

    d. Nausea, vomiting

    e. Prominent lymphadenopathy—large tender nodes (however, in adults over 40, less than 30% exhibit lymphadenopathy)

    f. Enlarged spleen (rupture)

    g. Neurologic disorders, including seizures

  2. Oral symptoms

    a. Palatal petechiae

    b. Necrotizing ulcerative gingivitis

    c. Inflamed attached gingiva

    d. Ulcerations similar to those of herpes or herpangina

    e. Purpuric spots beneath the epithelium (thrombocytopenia—a decrease in the number of platelets)

    f. Edema of the soft palate and uvula

D. Laboratory tests and findings

  1. Increased white blood cells (WBCs) with atypical activated lymphocytes; presence of these atypical lymphocytes in peripheral blood is very characteristic

  2. Increased heterophil antibody titer; positive Paul-Bunnell test in young adults but not in children under 4 years old

  3. Indirect immunofluorescence test for EBV

E. Treatment and prognosis

  1. Bed rest

  2. Nonaspirin antipyretics and nonsteroidal anti-inflammatory drugs (NSAIDs)

  3. Benign and self-limiting; fatigue may last longer

  4. Mononucleosis resolves in 4 to 6 weeks

  5. Complications can include splenic, hepatic, and neurologic involvement

SKIN DISEASES

General Characteristics

A. Characterized by various forms and sizes of ulcerative eruptions

B. Lesions may appear first or during the course of the disease

C. Reaction simulates an allergic-type reaction

Erythema Multiforme

A. Etiology

  1. Etiopathogenesis, acute onset, self-limiting condition thought to be a hypersensitivity reaction

  2. May be triggered by HSV infection, tuberculosis, or histoplasmosis; drugs (e.g., barbiturates, sulfonamides); *Mycoplasma pneumoniae*

  3. Immunologic response

B. Age and gender related—young adults ages 20 to 30 years; more common in males

C. Location

  1. Extremities—hands, feet, arms, legs

  2. Skin—macular, papular, or bullous eruptions; characteristic "target" or "bull's-eye" lesions in 50% of cases.

  3. Oral findings—lips, labial and buccal mucosa, tongue, floor of the mouth, soft palate

D. Clinical features (Fig. 8-32)

  1. Systemic symptoms

    a. Abrupt onset

    b. Prodomal symptoms (e.g., fatigue, malaise, fever)

    c. Previous occurrences

    d. Has been associated with systemic conditions

    e. The characteristic skin lesion is referred to as *bull's-eye, target,* or *iris*

  2. Oral symptoms

    a. Generally lips, tongue, and buccal mucosa

    b. Red patches develop into multiple, painful ulcerations; onset is explosive

    c. Macules, papules, or vesicles ulcerate and bleed easily

    d. A raw tissue base with a grayish, necrotic slough

    e. Irregular shape; surrounded by a band of inflammation; encrustations

    f. Edema and hemorrhagic crusting of the vermilion border of lips

FIG 8-32 Skin lesions of erythema multiforme. **A,** Target lesion *(arrow).* **B,** Bullae. **C,** Crusted lip lesions with edema, ulceration, and erythema. **D,** Erythematous and ulcerated lesions of the lips and buccal mucosa. (**A** courtesy of Dr. Edward V. Zegarelli; **A** to **D** from Ibsen OAC, Phelan JA: *Oral pathology for the dental hygienist,* ed 6, St Louis, 2014, Elsevier.)

E. Laboratory tests—biopsy for differential diagnosis
F. Histologic characteristics
1. Mixed inflammatory infiltrate
2. Intraepithelial vesicle formation and thinning
3. Absence of a basement membrane
4. Dilation of capillaries and lymphatic vessels in the surface layer of connective tissue
G. Treatment and prognosis
1. Removal of the cause, if identified or even suspected
2. Topical or systemic applications of corticosteroids
3. Mild antibacterial oral rinses; antibiotics if secondary infection develops
4. If patient has significant oral pain, intravenous rehydration may be necessary
5. Condition resolves in 2 to 4 weeks
6. Recurrence is possible

Stevens-Johnson Syndrome (Erythema Multiforme Major)

A. Severe bullous form of erythema multiforme (EM)
B. Etiology—unknown; usually triggered by a drug; the most severe form of EM
C. Age and gender related—children and young adults under 25 years; more common in males; history of previous similar illness

D. Location—oral cavity, skin; lesions involving the eyes or genitalia must be present for the diagnosis to be made
E. Clinical features (Fig. 8-33)

FIG 8-33 Stevens-Johnson syndrome. (Courtesy of Dr. Sidney Eisig; from Ibsen OAC, Phelan JA: *Oral pathology for the dental hygienist,* ed 6, St Louis, 2014, Elsevier.)

1. Oral symptoms—bullae rupture, leaving ulcerations with a raw base; eating becomes impossible; lips are severely encrusted and bleed easily
2. Skin lesions—severe, numerous; cover wide areas of the body (face, chest, abdomen)
3. Eye involvement—severe conjunctivitis, photophobia, corneal ulceration, scarring, and blindness

F. Treatment and prognosis
1. Antibiotics and corticosteroids to control severity
2. Sometimes antiviral medications to reduce recurrent episodes if HSV recurs
3. Duration of 1 to 4 weeks
4. Some patients require hospitalization
5. Prognosis is usually good
6. Mortality rate is 2% to 10% with this form of EM

Behçet Syndrome

A. Etiology—chronic recurrent autoimmune disease
B. Age and gender related—young adults, no gender predilection
C. Location—although now considered a multi-system disorder, Behçet syndrome is characterized by a triad of locations: oral, occular, and genital areas are involved; two of the three areas must be involved for the diagnosis
1. Oral cavity—in most cases, the first manifestation
2. Eyes are involved in up to 85% of cases, with greater severity in men
3. Genital lesions occur in 75% of cases, with more involvement in men
D. Clinical features (Fig. 8-34)
1. Oral lesions
a. Painful ulcerations similar to minor aphthous or major aphthous ulcers, occurring in about 40% of Behçet patients, and in 3% with the herpetiform variety
b. Large ulcers with gray or yellow center surrounded by a red border

FIG 8-34 Oral lesion seen in Behçet syndrome. Aphthous-like oral mucosal ulcer. (From Ibsen OAC, Phelan JA: *Oral pathology for the dental hygienist,* ed 6, St Louis, 2014, Elsevier.)

c. Oral ulcerations involve the soft palate and oropharynx
2. Eye lesions
a. Begin with photophobia and irritation
b. Purulent conjunctivitis and uveitis
c. Healing may be followed by scarification and, consequently, blindness
d. Hypopyon (pus in anterior chamber of eye between iris and cornea) in severe cases; rare
3. Genital lesions
a. In females—painful ulcerations in the vagina, vulval folds, and labia majora
b. In males—painful ulcerations on the scrotum and base of the penis
4. Systemic symptoms
a. Occasionally fever; pallor
b. Complications can involve the central nervous system (CNS) and cardiac, vascular, and pulmonary systems
c. Arthritis involving knees, wrists, elbows, and ankles
E. Laboratory tests and findings
1. Cutaneous pathergy test is positive in many patients with Behçet syndrome
2. Specific changes involving the neutrophils
F. Histologic characteristics
1. Histopathologic features are nonspecific
2. Endothelial proliferation in lesions
3. Other characteristics similar to those of aphthous stomatitis
G. Treatment and prognosis
1. Early aggressive therapy for patients with severe clinical manifestations
2. Systemic and topical corticosteroids
3. Other immunosuppressive drugs are given for systemic and ocular involvement
4. Lesions last 2 to 4 weeks
5. Disease is long lasting with remission periods
6. Mortality is low and most often associated with CNS or pulmonary hemorrhage or bowel perforation

Pemphigus Vulgaris

A. Etiology—severe, progressive autoimmune disease that affects skin and mucous membranes
B. Age and gender related—adults, usually between ages 40 and 55 years; no gender predilection
1. More common in Ashkenazic Jews, South Asians, or persons of Mediterranean heritage
C. Location—anywhere on the oral mucosa; eyes, or skin
D. Clinical features (Fig. 8-35)
1. In over 50% of cases, the oral lesions appear first; skin lesions can erupt many months or even a year later
2. Blisters (caused by an abnormal production of autoantibodies), vesicles, or bullae collapse as soon as they are formed
a. Vary in shape and size (from several millimeters to several centimeters)
b. Ragged peripheral borders; flat or shallow; base intensely red and raw; may extend into the lips with crusting

FIG 8-35 A and **B,** Examples of oral lesions in pemphigus vulgaris. (**B** courtesy of Dr. Fariba Younai; **A** and **B** from Ibsen OAC, Phelan JA: *Oral pathology for the dental hygienist,* ed 6, St Louis, 2014, Elsevier.)

3. Filmy, necrotic slough of tissue can be detached from underlying tissue
4. Neighboring soft tissue appears normal
5. Nikolsky sign present—an intraoral bulla can form under light pressure from air syringe or tongue blade; same reaction can occur if pressure is applied to skin
6. Pain may be severe, and the person is unable to eat
7. Salivation is profuse; mouth odor
8. Gingival desquamation
E. Laboratory tests and findings
1. Biopsy and most conclusive microscopic analysis
2. Direct immunofluorescence used to identify antibodies (intercellular)
3. Indirect immunofluorescence is positive for 80% to 90% of patients with pemphigus vulgaris, showing circulating autoantibodies in the serum; also used to monitor patient's therapy
F. Histologic characteristics
1. The vesicle or bulla is entirely intraepithelial above the basal cell layer, producing a distinctive "split"; the basement layer stays attached to underlying connective tissue

2. Intercellular bridges between epithelial cells disappear, with loss of cohesiveness; epithelial cells separate (acantholysis)
3. Clumps of rounded epithelial cells, called Tzanck cells, are present
4. Some inflammatory cell infiltration in connective tissue
G. Treatment and prognosis
1. Systemic corticosteroids (prednisone)
2. Other immunosuppressive drugs such as azathioprine and methotrexate are used in addition to corticosteroids
3. Measure the titers of circulating autoantibodies using indirect immunofluorescence
4. Patient may experience periods of remission; never a "cure"
5. Mortality is under 10% and associated with complications from long-term corticosteroid therapy
6. Potential side effects associated with long-term systemic corticosteroids include diabetes mellitus, adrenal suppression, and infections

WHITE LESIONS

General Characteristics

A. Often associated with *hyperkeratosis*; clinical term for *leukoplakia*
B. Vary from simple lesions to diffuse coverage; smooth to rough surfaces; elevated to flat
C. Attached to mucous membranes
D. Color—white, grayish white, yellowish white
E. Painless
F. Associated with a variety of conditions (including variants of normal, systemic disease, and premalignant lesions)

Nicotine Stomatitis

A. Etiology—heavy tobacco smoking using cigarettes, cigars, water pipe (hookah), or pipe; often associated with pipes ("pipe smoker's palate")
B. Age and gender related—most common in male smokers over 40 years
C. Location—posterior hard and soft palates
D. Clinical features (Fig. 8-36)
1. Begins with erythema and inflammation of the palate; response to an irritant (heat)
2. Over time, the palate becomes more keratinized and grayish white; thickened nodules surround the inflamed orifices of the minor salivary ducts
3. Fissures or cracks around the nodules create an overall wrinkled appearance
E. Histologic characteristics
1. Hyperkeratosis and acanthosis
2. Thickening of the epithelium adjacent to the orifice
F. Treatment and prognosis
1. If the cause is removed—smoking—the condition may be reversible
2. The prognosis is good if the person permanently stops smoking and the tissues return to normal

FIG 8-36 Nicotine stomatitis. (From Ibsen OAC, Phelan JA: *Oral pathology for the dental hygienist,* ed 6, St Louis, 2014, Elsevier.)

3. If tissues do not return to normal after smoking irritants are removed, biopsy may be necessary

Linea Alba

A. Etiology—pattern of occlusion; pressure of teeth on buccal mucosa
B. Age and gender related—any age; no gender predilection
C. Location—buccal mucosa along the occlusal plane; usually bilateral
D. Clinical features (Fig. 8-37)
   1. "White line" on the buccal mucosa, anterior to posterior along the line of occlusion
   2. Localized, single line in thickness; usually bilateral
E. Histologic characteristics—hyperorthokeratosis; some localized intracellular edema
F. Treatment and prognosis—no treatment required

FIG 8-37 Linea alba. (From Ibsen OAC, Phelan JA: *Oral pathology for the dental hygienist,* ed 6, St Louis, 2014, Elsevier.)

Leukoedema

A. Etiology—unknown; a variant of normal
B. Age and gender related—average age 45 years; no gender predilection; African Americans are more affected (85% of incidence) than other racial groups
C. Location—bilateral buccal and labial mucosa
D. Clinical features
   1. Soft, diffuse, velvety, filmy opalescence of buccal mucosa
   2. Later becomes grayish white with a coarsely wrinkled surface
   3. When the tissue is stretched, the white opalescence disappears (this clinical characteristic can help in the differential diagnosis)
   4. Some research shows it is more prominent in smokers
E. Histologic characteristics
   1. Intracellular edema of prickle cells (spinous layer)
   2. Increased thickness of epithelium with a superficial parakeratotic layer several cells thick
   3. Broad rete pegs that appear irregularly elongated
   4. Parakeratin on epithelial surface
F. Treatment and prognosis—no treatment required; considered a variant of normal

Systemic Lupus Erythematosus (SLE)

A. Etiology—acute and chronic inflammatory autoimmune disease involving several systems
   1. Cellular and humoral immunity are impaired
   2. B lymphocytes increase function; T lymphocytes do not function properly
B. Age and gender related—much more common in females (8:1) during childbearing years; African American females more affected than white females (3:1); average age 31 years
C. Location
   1. Buccal mucosa, palate, gingiva (25% to 30% of persons with SLE)
   2. Skin—lesions occur in 85% of persons with SLE; a characteristic erythematous butterfly-shaped rash on the face (malar areas) and nose; chest, back, extremities; exposure to sunlight makes the rash worse
D. Systemic characteristics
   1. Fever, weight loss, arthritis, muscle pain
   2. Raynaud phenomenon is seen in up to 15% of persons with SLE
   3. CNS involvement, depression, and seizures
   4. Ocular involvement; retinal nerve damage
   5. Kidney involvement (complications can be fatal)
   6. Cardiac involvement (pericarditis)
   7. Warty vegetations affecting heart valves (Libman-Sacks endocarditis)
E. Clinical features (Fig. 8-38)
   1. Skin lesions—erythematous rash; scales form, scarring in the center; butterfly configuration on the malar areas of the face and nose
   2. Among those with SLE, 25% to 30% have oral manifestations
   3. Erythematous plaques with white striae; can resemble lichen planus but is less defined
   4. Burning mouth; xerostomia; candidiasis

FIG 8-38 A and **B,** Oral lesions in lupus erythematosus. (Courtesy of Dr. Edward V. Zegarelli; from Ibsen OAC, Phelan JA: *Oral pathology for the dental hygienist,* ed 6, St Louis, 2014, Elsevier.)

F. Laboratory tests and findings
   1. Direct immunofluorescence of skin lesion (95% effective for SLE)
   2. Direct immunofluorescence of normal skin showing a positive lupus band in 25% to 60% of persons with SLE
   3. Anemia; leukopenia; thrombocytopenia
   4. Positive identification of antinuclear antibodies (ANAs); not very specific
   5. Anti–double-stranded DNA antibodies, a specific finding in up to 80% of patients with SLE
   6. A combination of these test findings, multi-organ involvement, skin lesions, and possible oral lesions can all play a role in the definitive diagnosis of this very complex disease
G. Histologic characteristics
   1. Hyperkeratosis; alternating changes within the spinous layer of the epithelium
   2. Necrosis of the basal cell layer
   3. Inflammatory infiltrate around blood vessels in the connective tissue not in a subepithelial band as seen in lichen planus
   4. Deposits of a periodic acid–Schiff (PAS) stain material in the basement membrane
   5. Subepithelial edema
H. Treatment and prognosis
   1. Aspirin and NSAIDs
   2. Antimalarial and corticosteroids combined with other immunosuppressive medications
   3. Periods of remission; in mild cases, the prognosis is good; with significant organ involvement, the disease can be fatal; prognosis is worse for men
   4. Consult with patient's physician before dental treatment; prophylactic antibiotic premedication may be necessary
   5. Patients should avoid exposure to sunlight because ultraviolet light can precipitate disease activity

White Sponge Nevus (Cannon Disease, Familial White Folded Dysplasia)

A. Etiology—hereditary; autosomal dominant trait; mutation in the mucosal keratin pair K4 or K13; complete penetrance with varying degrees of expressivity
B. Age and gender related—progressive from childhood to adulthood; no gender predilection
C. Location—bilateral buccal mucosa is always affected (sometimes soft palate or ventral tongue)
D. Clinical features
   1. White, velvety, thickened, and folded tissue of the buccal mucosa
   2. Diffuse, generalized, and bilateral
   3. Early years—the white mucosa is smooth and flat; becomes corrugated over time
   4. Adolescence—tissues become increasingly folded or corrugated; appear opalescent-white when the condition peaks
E. Histologic characteristics
   1. Thickened epithelium with hyperparakeratosis and acanthosis
   2. Perinuclear condensation of keratin tonofilaments in the superficial cells of the epithelium
   3. Cells of the spinous layer toward the surface exhibit vacuolation (space filled with fluid or air)
F. Treatment and prognosis
   1. No treatment required
   2. Prognosis is excellent

Lichen Planus

A. Etiology—benign, chronic disease; immunologically mediated mucocutaneous disorder
B. Age and gender related—middle-aged adults; slight predilection for females
C. Location—skin; oral mucosa; especially buccal mucosa, dorsal tongue, gingiva, and palate
D. Clinical features—two forms: reticular and erosive
   1. Reticular lichen planus (most common) (Fig. 8-39, *B*)

FIG 8-39 Lichen planus. **A,** Erosion of the mucosa appears as erythema adjacent to white striae. **B** and **C,** Two additional examples of the oral lesions of lichen planus. (**A** courtesy of Dr. Edward V. Zegarelli; **A** to **C** from Ibsen OAC, Phelan JA: *Oral pathology for the dental hygienist,* ed 6, St Louis, 2014, Elsevier.)

    a. White, narrow, interconnecting, slightly elevated lines forming a mesh, net, or lace-like pattern (Wickham's striae); these lesions can also look like white papules; cannot be wiped off
    b. Mucous membrane between the white lines appears normal
    c. When the dorsal tongue is involved, the lesion may appear as a solid gray to white, plaque-like area
    d. Usually asymptomatic
  2. Erosive or ulcerative form
    a. Lesions are symptomatic, patient experiences pain
    b. The condition begins as an erosive, flat lesion

FIG 8-40 Lichen planus. The gingival lesions of lichen planus are described clinically as desquamative tissue. (Courtesy of Dr. Edward V. Zegarelli; from Ibsen OAC, Phelan JA: *Oral pathology for the dental hygienist,* ed 6, St Louis, 2014, Elsevier.)

    c. This erythematous area is ulcerated, painful, and surrounded by fine white borders
    d. Slightly increased risk for squamous cell carcinoma in persons with erosive lichen planus; a 3-month recare appointment with thorough extraoral and intraoral examination should be scheduled
    e. Atrophy of the gingiva is described as desquamative (Fig. 8-40); this feature can appear with other oral conditions
E. Histologic characteristics (Fig. 8-41)
  1. Hyperparakeratosis or hyperorthokeratosis on the surface epithelium
  2. Thickened spinous layer (acanthosis)
  3. Intracellular edema of cells in the spinous layer
  4. Necrosis or degeneration of the basal cell layer
  5. Band-like infiltrate of lymphocytes
F. Treatment and prognosis
  1. Treatment for symptomatic cases; no treatment for reticular lichen planus
  2. Corticosteroids to decrease ulcerations and inflammation (systemic only when absolutely necessary)

FIG 8-41 Lichen planus seen by low-power microscopy. Note the degeneration of the basal cell layer of the epithelium *(B)* and the band-like infiltrate of lymphocytes *(L)*. (From Ibsen OAC, Phelan JA: *Oral pathology for the dental hygienist,* ed 6, St Louis, 2014, Elsevier.)

3. Topical corticosteroids (e.g., fluocinonide) applied several times a day
4. Meticulous oral hygiene
5. Lesions are self-limiting; heal in a few weeks with topical corticosteroid therapy
6. The condition does recur, and corticosteroids need to be reapplied
7. Patients with erosive lichen planus should be reevaluated every 3 to 4 months

Hyperkeratosis

A. Etiology—local factors; constant, low-grade irritation (frictional keratosis; chronic tongue chewing, cheek biting, repetitive irritation); vitamin A deficiency can cause excessive keratinization of skin and mucous membranes
B. Age and gender related—usually over age 40 years; more common in males
C. Location—anywhere in the oral cavity; alveolar ridge, buccal mucosa, lateral tongue
D. Clinical features (Fig. 8-42, *A* and *B*)
    1. White, flat lesion with a diffuse boundary
    2. Three layers of epithelium affected: granular, prickle, and basal cell layers
    3. Fissures or ulcerations rare
E. Laboratory tests—incisional biopsy
F. Histologic characteristics (Fig. 8-42, *C*)
    1. Abnormal layer of keratin or parakeratosis where not normally found
    2. Increased thickness of keratin in areas where normally found (e.g., attached gingiva, palate)
    3. Normal underlying epithelial cells
    4. Scalpel biopsy necessary for microscopic evaluation
G. Treatment and prognosis
    1. Removal of the cause (irritant)
    2. Tissue should return to normal

NEOPLASIA

Squamous Cell Carcinoma (SCC)

A. Etiology—chemicals such as phenoxyacetic acids, viruses, and radiation; secondary to genetic mutation; immunosuppression
    1. Risk factors include use of all forms of tobacco, alcohol abuse, and increasing age
    2. A combination of these risks can be lethal
    3. Iron deficiency anemia, especially the severe form, Plummer-Vinson syndrome, also elevates the risk for SCC in the posterior mouth and esophagus
    4. SCC accounts for 90% to 95% of oral cancers
B. Age and gender related—young adults to adults in their 60s, 70s, and beyond
    1. Incidence increases with increasing age
    2. Sixth most common cancer in males and twelfth in females
    3. Ratio of incidence in males and females is 2:1
    4. Highest overall incidence in white males after 65 years; highest incidence in middle age found in African American males

FIG 8-42 A, Frictional keratosis *(arrow)* caused by an opposing third molar. **B,** Caused by chronic tongue chewing. **C,** Low-power microscopic appearance of hyperkeratosis showing an increase in the amount of surface keratin *(K)*. (From Ibsen OAC, Phelan JA: *Oral pathology for the dental hygienist,* ed 6, St Louis, 2014, Elsevier.)

C. Locations
    1. Tongue—37% to 50% of all oral carcinomas, excluding cancer of the pharynx
        a. Posterior third, including the lateral borders and ventral surfaces, account for most of these

b. The tongue is by far the primary location for SCC in the oral cavity

2. Floor of the mouth—30% to 35%, mostly in men

3. Lips—22%; most of these occur on lower lip; pipe, cigar smokers, patients with fair skin, and persons with an outdoor occupation who are exposed to sunlight have a definite predilection for SCC of the lower lip (Fig. 8-43)

4. Buccal mucosa—6%

5. Gingiva—6%

6. Soft palate—4%; metastasis has already occurred by the time a diagnosis is made

7. The mandible is a more common location than the maxilla and is usually the result of metastasis from other areas

D. Clinical features (Fig. 8-44, *A* to *C*)

1. Exophytic, indurated, ulcerated, firm lesion in soft tissue; feels anchored to underlying tissue

2. On lower lip, smaller crusted ulceration, indurated border; asymptomatic

3. Sores or ulcerations that do not heal

4. Stages—tumor-node-metastasis (TNM) staging system helps predict the patient's prognosis (Box 8-1)

a. Stage I—early; asymptomatic; tumor less than 2 cm in diameter

b. Stage II—intermediate; tumor 2 to 4 cm in diameter

c. Stage III—advanced; tumor greater than 4 cm

d. Stage IV—tumor metastasizes to other, adjacent areas

E. Radiographic appearance (Fig. 8-44, *D*)

1. Diffuse radiolucency with irregular borders after significant bone has been destroyed; penetration into the cortex

2. Resorption of tooth roots; expansion in between roots

F. Laboratory tests and findings

1. Biopsy—scalpel biopsy is the "gold standard"

a. Incisional—removal of a segment or piece of the lesion for microscopic analysis

b. Excisional—removal of the entire lesion in question for microscopic analysis

2. Screening tools (see the section on "Diagnostic Tools for Oral Cancer Detection" in Chapter 16)

a. Brush test—a small circular brush is rotated about 10 times on the surface cells of the lesion to obtain a transepithelial specimen from all layers of the epithelium to the basement membrane; positive and atypical results require a scalpel biopsy for complete microscopic analysis and a definitive diagnosis; research needed to establish efficacy

b. ViziLite—tissues are illuminated with a special light after patient rinses with acetic acid; areas that turn white are evaluated and, for those in question, a scalpel biopsy is performed; subtle lesions that may appear "within normal limits" during the intraoral examination can clearly be identified with ViziLite, although some variants of normal may also become more obvious; research needed to establish efficacy

c. VelScope Vx—enhanced oral assessment screening tool that uses a handheld scope and natural tissue fluorescence to discover abnormalities; used with the recommended intraoral examination; handheld device emits a fluorescent blue light into the oral cavity; normal tissue reflects green; abnormal tissue reflects brown to black; "abnormal" tissue may be linea alba; clinician needs to be experienced with variants of normal before using VelScope; research needed to establish efficacy

G. Histologic characteristics

1. Invasion of sheets of tumor cells into underlying connective tissue (neoplastic squamous cells)

2. Presence of keratin pearls (cluster of concentrically layered keratinized cells)

3. Neoplastic cells that contain large, hyperchromatic nuclei and mitotic figures

H. Treatment and prognosis

1. Surgical excision alone or excision with a combination of radiation and chemotherapy; sometimes radiation therapy alone

2. Tumor size and location both influence the treatment protocol

3. Adjunctive chemotherapeutic agents

4. When metastasis has occurred (lymph node involvement), more radical procedures are performed

5. Prognosis depends on the tumor stage

FIG 8-43 A and **B,** Clinical appearance of squamous cell carcinoma of the lower lip. (Courtesy of Dr. Edward V. Zegarelli; from Ibsen OAC, Phelan JA: *Oral pathology for the dental hygienist,* ed 6, St Louis, 2014, Elsevier.)

FIG 8-44 A, Clinical appearance of squamous cell carcinoma (SCC) of the posterolateral tongue showing an exophytic, ulcerated mass. **B,** Clinical appearance of SCC of the left side of the soft palate and fauces. **C,** Clinical appearance of SCC on the floor of the mouth. **D,** Left side of a panoramic radiograph showing destruction of the mandible by SCC. (**C** courtesy of Dr. Edward V. Zegarelli; **A** to **D** from Ibsen OAC, Phelan JA: *Oral pathology for the dental hygienist,* ed 6, St Louis, 2014, Elsevier.)

BOX 8-1 TNM Staging System for Oral Squamous Cell Carcinoma

T—Tumor
T1—Tumor <2 cm in diameter
T2—Tumor 2-4 cm in diameter
T3—Tumor >4 cm in diameter
T4—Tumor invades adjacent structures
N—Node
N0—No palpable nodes
N1—Ipsilateral (same side as primary tumor) palpable nodes (same side as tumor)
N2—Contralateral (opposite side from primary tumor) or bilateral nodes
N3—Fixed palpable nodes
M—Metastasis
M0—No distant metastasis
M1—Clinical radiographic evidence of metastasis

From Regezi JA, Sciubba JJ: *Oral pathology: clinical pathologic correlations,* ed 5, Philadelphia, 2008, Saunders.
TNM, Tumor-node-metastasis.

PLEOMORPHIC ADENOMA (BENIGN MIXED TUMOR)

A. Etiology—benign salivary gland tumor that accounts for 90% of all benign salivary gland tumors
B. Age and gender related—most common in adults ages 35 to 55 years; female predilection; can occur in children
C. Location
   1. Parotid gland
   2. Posterior hard or soft palate (most common intraoral site); unilateral
D. Clinical features (Fig. 8-45)
   1. Located on either side of the midline of the posterior palate
   2. Painless, slow growing
   3. Smooth, dome-shaped mass, not ulcerated (unless traumatized)
   4. Size from a few millimeters to a few centimeters

FIG 8-45 Benign salivary gland tumor of the palate (pleomorphic adenoma). (From Ibsen OAC, Phelan JA: *Oral pathology for the dental hygienist,* ed 6, St Louis, 2014, Elsevier.)

E. Histologic characteristics
1. An encapsulated tumor composed of epithelium and connective tissue
2. Most benign; malignant transformation in less than 5% of cases

F. Treatment and prognosis
1. Surgical excision
2. Sometimes partial or complete removal of the parotid gland in the area
3. Research reports about 5% risk of malignant transformation
4. Conservative enucleation is not recommended because it leads to high recurrence rates
5. Prognosis is excellent if proper surgical techniques are used

CYSTS

A. True cyst
1. Cavity lined by epithelium and enclosed within a capsule of connective tissue
2. Space often filled with fluid or fragments of tissues

B. Cysts are classified according to:
1. Etiology, histologic components; location
2. Odontogenic; nonodontogenic; inflammatory response

Radicular Cyst (Root-End Cyst, Periapical Cyst)

A. Etiology
1. A true cyst; develops as an inflammatory response; associated with a nonvital tooth
2. Factors could include dental caries, trauma, deep restorations causing pulpitis

B. Age and gender related—any age, but common ages 30 to 60 years; slight predilection for males

C. Location—apex of a tooth or lateral to the tooth root

D. Clinical features
1. Nonvital tooth
2. Usually asymptomatic

E. Radiographic appearance
1. Round or ovoid, well-defined radiolucent area attached to the apex or lateral to the root (Fig. 8-46, *A*)
2. Loss of lamina dura in the area; root resorption is possible
3. Same radiographic appearance as periapical granuloma

FIG 8-46 Radicular cyst. **A,** Radiograph showing a well-circumscribed radiolucency around the root of a tooth *(arrow).* **B,** Microscopic features of a radicular cyst. (From Ibsen OAC, Phelan JA: *Oral pathology for the dental hygienist,* ed 6, St Louis, 2014, Elsevier.)

F. Histologic characteristics
1. Lined by stratified squamous epithelium; developing from epithelial rest of Malassez
2. The wall is composed of well-vascularized dense fibrous connective tissue (Fig. 8-46, *B*)
3. Lumen is filled with cellular debris

G. Treatment
1. Root canal therapy
2. Extraction of the tooth and curettage of the socket and apical area to remove the cystic sac
3. If radiolucency fails to resolve the condition, retreatment endodontically; apicoectomy may be required
4. Follow-up in 1 to 2 years

Residual Cyst

A. Etiology
1. Radicular cyst that has not been removed after extraction of the involved tooth
2. Open socket with debris acting as a stimulus

FIG 8-47 **A,** Schematic of a residual cyst. **B,** Radiograph of a residual cyst showing a radiolucency at the site of a previously extracted tooth. (Courtesy of Drs. Paul Freedman and Stanley Kerpel; from Ibsen OAC, Phelan JA: *Oral pathology for the dental hygienist*, ed 6, St Louis, 2014, Elsevier.)

B. Age and gender related—usually adults who were treated for a radicular cyst
C. Location
  1. Apical area where a tooth had previously been extracted
  2. Within the socket area or on the alveolar ridge
  3. At the alveolar ridge where a tooth had previously been extracted
D. Clinical features—small and asymptomatic
E. Radiographic appearance
  1. Well-defined radiolucent area (Fig. 8-47)
  2. Round or oval in shape
  3. In time, this radiolucency can become somewhat radiopaque because of histologic changes within the lumen
F. Histologic characteristics
  1. Stratified squamous epithelium lining the lumen
  2. Dense fibrous connective tissue wall
G. Treatment—surgical removal of the cyst

DEVELOPMENTAL CYSTS

Nonodontogenic Cysts

A. Etiology
  1. Median mandibular cyst—cyst in midline of the mandible; develops from an odontogenic origin, possibly a primordial cyst; rare

  2. Globulomaxillary cyst—arises from the odontogenic epithelium between the maxillary lateral incisor and canine (not a fissural cyst)
  3. Nasolabial cyst—soft tissue cyst; develops from the inferior and anterior segments of the nasolacrimal duct; strong female predilection (4:1)
  4. Median palatine cyst—fissural cyst; posterior form of a nasopalatine canal cyst; young adults
  5. Nasopalatine canal cyst (incisive canal cyst)—develops from the epithelial remnants of embryonal nasopalatine ducts; strong male predilection
B. Age and gender related—adults; no gender predilection, unless specified
C. Location—names are based on location
  1. Median mandibular cyst—occurs at the midline of the anterior mandible; surrounding teeth are vital
  2. Globulomaxillary cyst—appears as a pear-shaped radiolucency between the roots of the maxillary lateral incisor and canine
  3. Nasolabial cyst—upper lip, lateral to midline; in the mucolabial fold in the area of the maxillary canine and the floor of the nose
  4. Median palatine cyst—arises at the midline of the hard palate
  5. Nasopalatine canal cyst—appears within the nasopalatine canal or the incisive papilla
D. Clinical features
  1. Cysts vary in size from no evidence of a lesion to a bulge or expansion of bone
  2. All teeth are vital when associated with nonodontogenic cysts
E. Radiographic appearance—well-defined radiolucent area; some have particular shapes because of the anatomical location where they develop
  1. Globulomaxillary cyst—located between the maxillary lateral incisor and canine; often pear shaped (Fig. 8-48)
  2. The nasopalatine canal (incisal canal) cyst is heart shaped
F. Histologic characteristics
  1. Median mandibular cyst—most often lined by stratified squamous epithelium; few cases of pseudostratified ciliated columnar epithelium
  2. Globulomaxillary cyst—lined by inflamed stratified squamous epithelium; can histologically resemble the components of several other cystic lesions
  3. Nasolabial cyst—lined by pseudostratified columnar epithelium; some cuboidal epithelium
  4. Median palatal cyst—lined by stratified squamous epithelium; chronic inflammation in cell wall
  5. Nasopalatine canal cyst—several types of epithelium are found in this cyst; most often, stratified squamous epithelium
G. Treatment and prognosis
  1. Enucleation of the cystic sac and curettage of surrounding bone
  2. Prognosis is excellent

FIG 8-48 Radiograph of a globulomaxillary cyst showing a characteristic pear-shaped radiolucency between the maxillary lateral incisor and canine. (From Ibsen OAC, Phelan JA: *Oral pathology for the dental hygienist,* ed 6, St Louis, 2014, Elsevier.)

FIG 8-49 A, Thyroglossal tract extends from the area of the foramen cecum, lingual to the lower part of the neck. **B,** Thyroglossal tract cyst is the cause of enlargement at the midline of the neck. (From Ibsen OAC, Phelan JA: *Oral pathology for the dental hygienist,* ed 6, St Louis, 2014, Elsevier.)

Thyroglossal Tract Cyst (Thyroglossal Duct Cyst)

A. Etiology—developmental; in the thyroglossal tract, which extends from the foramen cecum to the permanent position of the thyroid gland in the neck region; the embryonic thyroglossal tract; inflammation is the stimulus possibly associated with adjacent lymph tissue that reacts from a draining infection from the head and neck area

B. Age and gender related—usually young adults under 20 years; no gender predilection

C. Location—posterior tongue, anywhere from the foramen cecum to the suprasternal notch; 75% of these lesions are below the hyoid bone

D. Clinical features (Fig. 8-49)
1. Asymptomatic; painless; movable swelling; midline of the neck
2. Bulge is round or oval shaped; usually less than 3 cm in diameter
3. Fistulous tracts to the skin or mucosa can develop
4. Swallowing becomes difficult (dysphagia)
5. Inability to extend the tongue

E. Histologic characteristics
1. Cysts below the hyoid bone are lined with ciliated columnar epithelium; squamous epithelium or other types of epithelial tissue above the hyoid bone
2. Connective tissue wall may contain thyroid tissue

F. Treatment and prognosis
1. Complete surgical excision of the cyst (after a thyroid scan)
2. Surgical procedure will include removal of part of the hyoid bone and muscle tissue in the tract

3. Prognosis is good
4. Malignant transformation is rare

Lymphoepithelial Cyst (Branchial Cleft Cyst)

A. Etiology
1. Epithelial remnants of the embryonic brachial arches
2. About 95% develop from the second branchial arch
3. Epithelium entrapped in lymph nodes (another theory of development)

B. Age and gender related—young adults; no gender predilection

C. Location

1. Intraoral lymphoepithelial cyst—posterior floor of the mouth and lateral borders of the tongue
2. Cervical lymphoepithelial cyst—located on the lateral neck near the anterior border of the sternocleidomastoid muscle
3. Area from the clavicle to the parotid gland

D. Clinical features
1. Slow-growing, movable mass 1 to 10 cm in diameter; asymptomatic
2. Can have a pink to yellowish color when found intraorally
3. If trauma or infection is associated, pain may be present

E. Histologic characteristics (Fig. 8-50)
1. Lined by stratified squamous epithelium that may or may not be keratinized
2. Lymphoid tissue in the wall

F. Treatment and prognosis
1. Surgical removal
2. Prognosis is good

Dermoid Cyst

A. Etiology—developmental from all three germ layers: ectoderm, endoderm, mesoderm; benign cystic form of teratoma
B. Age and gender related—present at birth or in young children; no gender predilection
C. Location
1. In the oral cavity, anterior floor of the mouth; can displace tongue
2. Ovarian teratomas, or "dermoids," contain actual tooth structures

D. Clinical features
1. Semi-firm, dough-like consistency
2. Size—a few millimeters to several centimeters
3. Midline of the floor of the mouth

E. Histologic characteristics
1. Lined with orthokeratinized stratified squamous epithelium
2. Keratin within the lumen

FIG 8-50 Low-power microscopic appearance of a lymphoepithelial cyst showing lumen *(Lu),* epithelial lining *(E),* surrounding lymphocytes *(L),* and connective tissue *(CT).* (From Ibsen OAC, Phelan JA: *Oral pathology for the dental hygienist,* ed 6, St Louis, 2014, Elsevier.)

3. A fibrous connective tissue wall
4. May contain sebaceous glands, hair follicles, sweat glands, and occasionally teeth

F. Treatment and prognosis
1. Surgical removal; approach depends on the location relative to the geniohyoid muscle
2. Prognosis is good

ODONTOGENIC CYSTS

Lateral Periodontal Cyst (LPC)

A. Etiology—developmental; odontogenic cyst; develops from the rests of the dental lamina
B. Age and gender related—adults over 30 years; common ages 50 to 70 years; male predilection
C. Location—most often lateral root surface of mandibular canine or premolar teeth (occasionally seen in the maxilla in the same areas)
D. Clinical features
1. Tooth or teeth involved are vital
2. Asymptomatic, no bulge

E. Radiographic appearance
1. Small; less than 1 cm
2. Well-defined ovoid or elliptically shaped radiolucent area found lateral to a tooth root (Fig. 8-51, *A*)
3. The *botryoid odontogenic cyst* (BOC) is closely related to the LPC, and the diagnosis is used for multi-cystic or multi-locular variants; BOC is most common in the mandibular cuspid and premolar area
4. The odontogenic keratocyst and other inflammatory cysts can have the same radiographic features

F. Histologic characteristics (Fig. 8-51, *B*)
1. Stratified squamous epithelial lining only a few cells thick; focal epithelial thickening
2. Thin connective tissue wall

G. Treatment and prognosis
1. Surgical enucleation of the cyst without damage to surrounding teeth
2. Few cases of recurrence have been reported
3. BOC has greater recurrence potential than LPC

Odontogenic Keratocyst

A. Etiology—odontogenic developmental cyst with unique histologic appearance and frequent recurrence
B. Age and gender related—60% between 10 and 40 years of age; slight male predilection
C. Location—most often in posterior mandible
D. Clinical features—may be asymptomatic; does not expand bone
E. Radiographic appearance—well-defined, multi-locular radiolucent lesion; can be similar to that of an odontogenic tumor; lesion can move teeth and resorb tooth structure
F. Histologic characteristics
1. Lumen lined by epithelium 8 to 10 cell layers thick
2. Surfaced by parakeratin
3. Basal cell layer is palisaded

FIG 8-51 A, Radiograph of a lateral periodontal cyst. This biloculated, well-defined radiolucency is located lateral to the tooth root. **B,** Microscopic appearance of a lateral periodontal cyst showing a thin epithelial lining with focal epithelial thickenings. (From Ibsen OAC, Phelan JA: *Oral pathology for the dental hygienist,* ed 6, St Louis, 2014, Elsevier.)

G. Treatment and prognosis
   1. Aggressive surgical excision and osseous curettage
   2. High recurrence rate
   3. Close follow-up

Primordial Cyst

A. Etiology—neoplastic; arises from epithelium of the enamel organ or from primordial epithelium; history that a tooth was never present; the cyst develops in place of the tooth; sometimes histologically considered the same as an odontogenic keratocyst
B. Age and gender related—child to young adult; ages 10 to 40 years; slight male predilection

C. Location—posterior mandible; third molar area or posterior to an erupted third molar and up the ramus
D. Clinical features—no obvious clinical features; the affected person may be asymptomatic
E. Radiographic appearance—well-defined radiolucent oval lesion; can be multi-locular
   1. Tooth never present in the space occupied by the cyst (this history is essential to the diagnosis)
   2. An unerupted tooth can be involved in this cyst
   3. Size varies from a few millimeters to a centimeter
   4. Radiographic features not diagnostic
F. Histologic characteristics
   1. Four to eight cells of stratified squamous epithelium
   2. No rete pegs
   3. Cuboidal columnar epithelial cells are hyperchromatic and appear in the basal epithelial level
G. Treatment and prognosis
   1. Surgical removal of the cyst, biopsy, and histologic examination
   2. Recurrence depends on the histologic findings; odontogenic keratocysts recur in 30% of cases

Dentigerous Cyst (Follicular Cyst)

A. Etiology—from reduced enamel epithelium after the crown of the tooth is completely formed (unerupted or impacted tooth); accumulation of fluid between the crown and reduced enamel epithelium; cyst must be associated with a tooth; developmental or inflammatory origin
B. Age and gender related—young adults 20 to 30 years; second most common odotongenic cyst; higher predilection for white males
C. Location
   1. Mandibular third molar area—around the crown of an unerupted third molar; often extending to the ramus
   2. Maxillary canine region—compromising the maxillary sinus
D. Clinical features
   1. Always associated with the crown of an unerupted tooth; asymptomatic
   2. Can be an aggressive lesion, causing expansion of bone and extreme displacement of teeth; fracture of the mandible; or both, in which case it would be painful
E. Radiographic appearance (Fig. 8-52)
   1. Smooth, unilocular radiolucency associated with the crown of an unerupted tooth
   2. At least 4 mm of radiolucency extending from the crown to the epithelium of the reduced enamel
F. Histologic characteristics
   1. Stratified squamous epithelium lining the lumen; not keratinized
   2. Surrounded by a thin fibrous connective tissue wall
   3. In the inflamed variety, the fibrous wall has an inflammatory infiltrate
G. Treatment and prognosis
   1. Enucleation of the cystic sac, and sometimes the associated tooth

FIG 8-53 Ranula. (From Ibsen OAC, Phelan JA: *Oral pathology for the dental hygienist,* ed 6, St Louis, 2014, Elsevier.)

FIG 8-52 A, Radiographs of dentigerous cysts surrounding the crown of an unerupted premolar. **B,** Impacted third molar. (From Ibsen OAC, Phelan JA: *Oral pathology for the dental hygienist,* ed 6, St Louis, 2014, Elsevier.)

2. The tooth may be left in place, with orthodontic intervention to assist eruption
3. Rare transformation to the ameloblastoma
4. Prognosis is very good

Injuries to Oral Soft Tissue
Ranula
A. Etiology
   1. Blockage or obstruction by a salivary "stone" (sialolith) in the duct of a major salivary gland (sublingual or submandibular); unilateral
   2. Trauma to same area
   3. Term used for a mucocele that occurs in the floor of the mouth
B. Age and gender related—any age, but usually adults; no gender predilection
C. Location—unilaterally on the floor of the mouth
D. Clinical features (Fig. 8-53)
   1. Translucent, bluish, round, smooth-surfaced bulge 1 to 3 cm in diameter
   2. Semi-firm, unilateral, fluctuant mass
   3. Increases in size between meals; decreases immediately after a meal
   4. Located lateral to the midline (helpful to the differential diagnosis)

5. Small lesions can develop along the sublingual plica from the superficial ducts of Rivini
E. Radiographic appearance—radiopaque sialolith in the duct area if it is present
F. Histologic characteristics
   1. Epithelial lining is present; mucous fluid surrounded by granulation tissue
   2. Inflammatory cells
G. Treatment and prognosis
   1. Surgical excision
   2. Removal of the obstruction, if present
   3. May recur

Mucocele (Mucus Extravasation)
A. Etiology
   1. Trauma to a minor salivary gland duct; mucous secretion spills into connective tissue
   2. Mechanical trauma to the salivary duct by lip biting or pinching
B. Age and gender related—all ages but most common in children and young adults; no gender predilection
C. Location—the most common site is the lower lip mucosa
D. Clinical features
   1. Blister-like, raised, circumscribed vesicle; 1 to 4 mm in size; painless
   2. Bluish hue if the mucocele is near the surface
   3. Firm, movable on palpation
   4. Vesicle ruptures and can leave fragments of epithelial tissue
E. Histologic characteristics
   1. The lesion is not a true cyst because it is not lined with epithelium
   2. An inflammatory response occurs and granulation tissue forms
F. Treatment and prognosis
   1. Excision of the lesion and associated gland

2. Sometimes the vesicle breaks, and the lesion resolves by itself
3. Recurrence is possible (and may recur in the same place)

Necrotizing Sialometaplasia

A. Etiology
  1. Benign condition of salivary gland
  2. Lack of blood supply to the area of the lesion
  3. Trauma to the area that causes a blockage of blood supply
B. Age and gender related—adults
C. Location—most often found on the palate; however, it may be found in any site containing salivary glands
D. Clinical features (Fig. 8-54)
  1. Initial finding of tenderness and swelling in the area
  2. Well-demarcated ulcer
  3. Localized pain; can be very painful
E. Histologic characteristics
  1. Necrosis of the salivary gland tissue involved
  2. Squamous metaplasia of ductal epithelium
  3. Islands of epithelium deep in connective tissue
F. Treatment and prognosis
  1. Incisional biopsy may be performed to rule out other conditions; the ulcer may then heal by secondary intention
  2. May be self-limiting
  3. Prognosis is good

Pseudocysts

Aneurysmal Bone Cyst

A. Etiology—reactive cyst; etiologic theories include:
  1. Arteriovenous shunt—a benign fibro-osseous lesion in the area alters blood vessels
  2. Trauma—trauma ruptures a blood vessel, and blood accumulates outside the wall
B. Age and gender related—under 30 years; no gender predilection
C. Location
  1. Long bones or vertebral column
  2. When the occurrence is in the jaws, the mandible is the more common site (2:1)

FIG 8-54 Necrotizing sialometaplasia. (From Ibsen OAC, Phelan JA: *Oral pathology for the dental hygienist*, ed 6, St Louis, 2014, Elsevier.)

D. Clinical features
  1. May be asymptomatic or may appear as a slightly to moderately well-defined bulge
  2. Tenderness, pain on motion; may limit movement
  3. Mobility or migration of teeth
E. Radiographic appearance—hazy, gray, radiolucent area; appears cystic, with a "soap bubble" or honeycomb effect; multi-locular pattern can be present
F. Histologic characteristics
  1. No epithelial lining—a "pseudocyst"
  2. Walls of fibrous connective tissue
  3. Blood-filled spaces surrounded by multi-nucleated giant cells
G. Treatment and prognosis
  1. Surgical enucleation and thorough curettage (sometimes with cryosurgery—a freezing technique to help control bleeding)
  2. Follow-up treatment, if necessary
  3. May sometimes recur

Simple Bone Cyst (Traumatic Bone Cyst, Hemorrhagic Bone Cyst)

A. Etiology—theories include:
  1. Intramedullary hemorrhage following trauma; altered bone prevents fibroblasts and endothelial cells from entering the hemorrhage; clotting does not occur; blood never organizes, leaving a void within the bone
  2. Ischemic marrow necrosis
  3. Degeneration of a benign tumor
  4. Bone did not develop in the area
B. Age and gender related—ages 10 to 20 years; male predilection
C. Location
  1. More common in the mandible than in the maxilla
  2. Most common in long bones
D. Clinical features—asymptomatic (discovered through radiographic examination)
E. Radiographic appearance (Fig. 8-55)—well-defined radiolucent area 1 to 7 cm in diameter; round, oval; may be multi-locular; the radiolucent projections extend between roots of teeth, defined as "scalloping around the roots"; borders are sometimes sharp or diffuse
F. Histologic characteristics
  1. Thin vascular fibrous connective tissue lining; no epithelium so it is not a true cyst
  2. The center is a void
G. Treatment and prognosis
  1. Surgical intervention to establish bleeding and clotting is often sufficient
  2. Lesion heals 6 months to 1 year after surgical intervention
  3. Prognosis is excellent

Static Bone Cyst (Lingual Mandibular Bone Concavity, Stafne Bone Cyst)

A. Etiology—developmental; salivary gland extends laterally into the mandible
B. Age and gender related—young persons; slightly more common in males

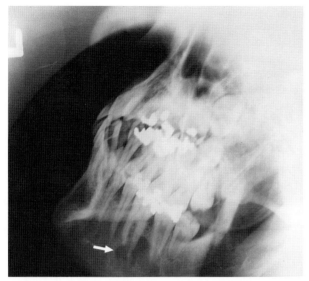

FIG 8-55 Extraoral radiograph showing a simple (traumatic) bone cyst *(arrow)* in the mandible, with its unique radiolucent characteristic scalloping around the roots. (Courtesy of Dr. Edward V. Zegarelli; from Ibsen OAC, Phelan JA: *Oral pathology for the dental hygienist,* ed 6, St Louis, 2014, Elsevier.)

C. Location—posterior of the mandible, anterior to the angle of the ramus, inferior to the mandibular canal
D. Clinical features—asymptomatic; occasionally bilateral
E. Radiographic appearance (Fig. 8-56)—sharp, well-defined ovoid radiolucency 1 to 3 cm in diameter, anterior to angle of the ramus, inferior to the mandibular canal; filled with salivary gland tissue
F. Histologic characteristics—lymphoid, fat, submaxillary salivary gland tissues; striated muscle (not a true cyst)
G. Treatment and prognosis
1. Surgical intervention to determine contents; once diagnosed, no treatment necessary
2. Prognosis is excellent; no complications

BLOOD DISORDERS

General Characteristics

A. Disease with numerous variations
B. Important to know normal blood levels and chemistries in order to make differential diagnosis
C. Anemias are categorized according to etiology
1. Blood loss
2. Excessive destruction of red blood cells (RBCs) because of a congenital or hemolytic condition
3. Decrease in production of RBCs

Sickle Cell Anemia

A. Etiology—hereditary; severe genetic disorder involving hemoglobin; abnormal hemoglobin in RBCs; decreased oxygen in RBCs
B. Age and gender related—under 30 years; female predilection; 1 in 400 African Americans in the United States are affected; also persons of Mediterranean or Asian origin
C. Clinical features
1. Systemic symptoms
   a. Weakness, easily fatigued; pallor of tissues
   b. Shortness of breath; nausea, vomiting
   c. Pain in joints
   d. Sickle cell crisis involves severe systemic complications
   e. Infections—patients are prone to infection because of early destruction of the spleen
   f. Delayed growth and development in children
   g. Cardiac, kidney, CNS, eyes, and pulmonary involvement
2. Oral symptoms
   a. Some radiographic findings
   b. Osteomyelitis of the mandible
   c. Prolonged paresthesia of the mandibular nerve
D. Radiographic appearance (Fig. 8-57)

FIG 8-56 Part of a panoramic radiograph showing a lingual mandibular bone concavity (Stafne bone cyst). Note the well-circumscribed radiolucency inferior to the mandibular canal *(arrow).* (From Ibsen OAC, Phelan JA: *Oral pathology for the dental hygienist,* ed 6, St Louis, 2014, Elsevier.)

FIG 8-57 Sickle cell anemia. The radiograph shows abnormal trabeculation. (Courtesy of Dr. Edward V. Zegarelli; from Ibsen OAC, Phelan JA: *Oral pathology for the dental hygienist,* ed 6, St Louis, 2014, Elsevier.)

1. Perpendicular trabeculations radiating outward, giving a "hair-on-end" appearance in the skull
2. Decrease in number of trabeculae in the jaws, with large marrow spaces
3. Lamina dura not affected

E. Laboratory tests and findings (Fig. 8-58)
   1. RBC count reduced to 1 million/mm^3 (normal is 4 to 6 million/mm^3)
   2. Decrease in the hemoglobin level in red blood cells (normal in males, 13.5 to 18 g/dL; in females, 12 to 16 g/dL)
   3. Blood smear showing sickle-shaped RBCs

F. Histologic characteristics
   1. Crescent-shaped erythrocytes caused by hemoglobin S
   2. Atypical chromatin distribution

G. Treatment and prognosis
   1. Symptomatic management; oxygen and intravenous fluids
   2. Bone marrow transplantation has numerous complications and is a cure for a very low percentage of patients
   3. Hydroxyurea—drug treatment for adults, but has several side effects
   4. Prognosis is unpredictable and depends on various aspects of disease activity

Pernicious Anemia (Primary Anemia, Addison Anemia, Biermer Anemia)

A. Etiology
   1. Autoimmune destruction of the parietal cells of the stomach
   2. Deficiency of intrinsic factor (produced by the parietal cells of the stomach lining) necessary to absorb vitamin B$_{12}$ (cobalamin)
   3. Deficiency of vitamin B$_{12}$ (extrinsic factor) necessary for deoxyribonucleic acid (DNA) synthesis

B. Age and gender related—older adults; rarely before age 30; no gender predilection

C. Clinical features
   1. Systemic symptoms
      a. General weakness, dizziness, pallor, anemia (caused by low oxygen in the blood)
      b. Numbness or tingling of extremities

      c. Gastrointestinal manifestations—nausea, vomiting, diarrhea, abdominal pain
      d. Loss of appetite and weight loss
      e. Shortness of breath
      f. Neurologic changes—severe paresthesias
   2. Oral symptoms
      a. Sore, painful, burning tongue; angular cheilitis
      b. Shallow ulcers on the mucosa
      c. Atrophy of papillae; distorted perception of taste
      d. Pallor of the oral mucosa with focal patches of erythema

D. Laboratory tests and findings
   1. Diagnosis of pernicious anemia is made by laboratory testing; the Schilling test is also used to determine the body's inability to absorb an oral dose of vitamin B$_{12}$ (cyanocobalamin)
   2. Achlorhydria—lack of gastric hydrochloric acid secretion
   3. Megaloblastic anemia—immature, large RBCs

E. Histologic characteristics
   1. Epithelial atrophy; no rete ridges
   2. Pale-staining nuclei

F. Treatment and prognosis
   1. Injections of vitamin B$_{12}$
   2. Increased dietary intake of folic acid (leafy green vegetables, organ meats, wheat cereals)
   3. From 1% to 2% of persons with pernicious anemia develop gastric carcinoma

Iron Deficiency Anemia (Plummer-Vinson Syndrome)

A. Etiology—iron deficiency caused by:
   1. Chronic blood loss
   2. Inadequate dietary intake of iron
   3. Decreased iron absorption
   4. Increased iron requirements (e.g., infancy, pregnancy)
   5. Longstanding iron deficiency anemia (Plummer-Vinson syndrome); symptoms include dysphagia and an increased predilection for esophageal and oral cancer

B. Age and gender related—ages 40 to 50 years; more common in females (5% to 30% female incidence in the United States)

C. Clinical features
   1. Systemic symptoms
      a. Pallor of skin, weakness; fatigue
      b. Difficulty swallowing (dysphagia)
      c. Shortness of breath
      d. Enlarged spleen (splenomegaly) (20% to 30% of cases)
      e. Absence of free hydrochloric acid in the stomach
      f. Predisposition to development of oral cancer
   2. Oral symptoms (Fig. 8-59)
      a. Angular cheilitis; pallor and atrophy of oral tissues
      b. Depapillated, smooth, burning, painful tongue
      c. Risk for oral candidiasis

D. Histologic characteristics
   1. Altered exfoliated squamous epithelial cells of the tongue and soft tissues
   2. Deficiency of keratinized cells
   3. Abnormal cell maturation; enlarged nuclei

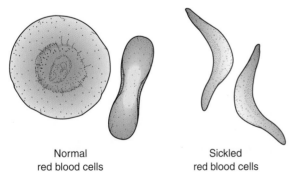

Normal red blood cells   Sickled red blood cells

FIG 8-58 Normal red blood cells compared with sickled red blood cells. (From Ibsen OAC, Phelan JA: *Oral pathology for the dental hygienist,* ed 6, St Louis, 2014, Elsevier.)

FIG 8-59 Iron deficiency anemia. The tongue is devoid of filiform papillae. Angular cheilitis is also present. (From Ibsen OAC, Phelan JA: *Oral pathology for the dental hygienist,* ed 6, St Louis, 2014, Elsevier.)

E. Laboratory findings
   1. Complete blood count (CBC) with RBC indices
   2. Hypochromatic microcytic RBCs
   3. Low number of erythrocytes (RBCs)
   4. Low hemoglobin and hematocrit
   5. In Plummer-Vinson syndrome the esophagus is evaluated for mucosal tissue growths that may inhibit swallowing
F. Treatment
   1. Increased iron intake
   2. Dietary supplement
   3. Parenteral iron occasionally

Aplastic Anemia
Primary Aplastic Anemia
A. Etiology—unknown; severe depression in bone marrow activity; rare, life-threatening disease
B. Age and gender related—young adults; no gender predilection
C. Clinical features
   1. Oral symptoms
      a. Spontaneous bleeding
      b. Petechiae
      c. Purpuric spots
      d. Gingival infection
      e. Pallor of oral tissues
   2. Systemic symptoms
      a. Fatigue, weakness
      b. Tachycardia, dizziness
      c. Retinal and cerebral hemorrhages in most severe cases
      d. Significant bruising
      e. Predisposition to infection
D. Laboratory tests and findings establish the diagnosis
   1. Reduction in the number of all blood cells (pancytopenia)
   2. Reduction in the number of RBCs (anemia)
   3. Reduction in the number of WBCs (leukopenia)
   4. Reduction in the number of platelets (thrombocytopenia)
   5. Bone marrow changes

E. Treatment and prognosis
   1. Blood transfusions
   2. Antibiotic drugs to try to control infection
   3. Bone marrow transplantation
   4. Guarded prognosis, depending on the severity of the condition
   5. Rapid decrease in various blood cells usually fatal

Secondary Aplastic Anemia
A. Etiology
   1. Result of a drug or chemical substance; chemotherapy
   2. Exposure to radiant energy—x-rays, radium, or radioactive isotopes
B. Age and gender related—any age; no gender predilection
C. Clinical features—same as in primary aplastic anemia
D. Treatment and prognosis
   1. Remove the cause
   2. Supportive therapy
   3. Prognosis is good

Thalassemia (Cooley Anemia, Mediterranean Anemia)
A. Etiology—inherited; autosomal dominant
   1. Disorder of hemoglobin synthesis
   2. Ethnic predilection—high incidence in Mediterranean and African countries and India
B. Age and gender related
   1. Thalassemia major
      a. Affects individuals within the first year of life (homozygous type)
      b. Both X and Y chromosomes are involved
      c. Is a more severe type of anemia
   2. Thalassemia minor
      a. The milder form appears in later childhood (heterozygous type)
      b. Only one gene at the locus is involved
      c. No gender predilection
C. Clinical features
   1. Systemic symptoms for thalassemia major
      a. Yellow pallor of the skin
      b. Enlarged spleen (splenomegaly); enlarged liver (hepatomegaly)
      c. Mongoloid facial features
      d. Sunken nose bridge
      e. Protruding zygoma
      f. Slanting eyes
   2. Oral symptoms for thalassemia major
      a. Malocclusion; protrusion of the anterior maxillary teeth
      b. Pallor of the mucosa
   3. No significant clinical manifestations in thalassemia minor
D. Radiographic appearance
   1. Peculiar trabecular pattern of the maxilla and the mandible—"salt and pepper" or "hair on end" of the cranial bones
   2. Mild osteoporosis of the jaws
   3. Thinning of lamina dura

E. Laboratory tests and findings
   1. Elevated white blood cell (WBC) count—10,000 to 25,000/mm^3
   2. Elevated serum bilirubin level
   3. Decreased hemoglobin level
F. Histologic characteristics—bone marrow shows cellular hyperplasia
G. Treatment and prognosis
   1. Blood transfusions (frequently administered every 2 weeks)
   2. Frequent transfusions cause a significant buildup of iron in tissues throughout the body (hemochromatosis); these toxic accumulations of iron may be fatal; treated with deferoxamine
   3. Bone marrow transplantation
   4. Prognosis is guarded; periods of remission can extend the life span to age 20

Polycythemia
General Characteristics
A. Abnormal increase in the number of circulating RBCs
B. Increased hemoglobin level
C. Three forms:
   1. Relative polycythemia—temporary increase in the number of RBCs; caused by shock, a severe burn, or excessive loss of body fluids
   2. Primary polycythemia (polycythemia vera)
   3. Secondary polycythemia

Primary Polycythemia (Polycythemia Vera)
A. Etiology—unknown; possibly familial; neoplastic proliferation of bone marrow stem cells
B. Age and gender related—ages 40 to 60 years; slightly more common in males
C. Clinical features
   1. Systemic symptoms
      a. Headache, dizziness, weakness
      b. Enlarged, painful spleen
      c. Gastric complaints; peptic ulcers
      d. Tips of fingers cyanotic
      e. Nose bleeds easily (epistaxis)
      f. Itching of skin (pruritus) without the presence of rash
   2. Oral symptoms
      a. Oral mucosa deep red to purple because of decreased hemoglobin level
      b. Gingivae edematous and spongy; bleed easily
      c. Submucosal petechiae; ecchymosis
D. Laboratory tests and findings
   1. RBC count elevated to 10 to 12 million cells/mm^3 (significant increase)
   2. Increase in:
      a. Hemoglobin content
      b. Blood viscosity
      c. WBC counts
      d. Hematocrit value
   3. Decrease in platelets
E. Treatment and prognosis
   1. Medications and procedures to control platelets
   2. Intermittent phlebotomy
   3. Chemotherapeutic drugs

Secondary Polycythemia
A. Etiology—increased number of erythrocytes caused by a physiologic response to decreased oxygen
   1. Bone marrow anoxia (lack of oxygen) caused by:
      a. Pulmonary dysfunction
      b. Heart disease
      c. High altitudes
      d. Carbon monoxide poisoning
   2. Stimulatory factors such as drugs or chemicals
B. Other characteristics and features similar to those of primary polycythemia

Relative Polycythemia
A. Etiology—decreased plasma volume (not an increase in RBCs) that may be caused by:
   1. Use of diuretics
   2. Vomiting, diarrhea
   3. Excessive sweating
B. Age and gender related—the chronic form of relative polycythemia (also called *stress polycythemia*) is more common in white, middle-aged men, who are stressed, overweight, and hypertensive and who smoke
C. Treatment—related to the type of polycythemia and risk factors; attempt to remove risk factors

Agranulocytosis
A. Etiology—significant reduction in or absence of circulating neutrophils (neutropenia)
   1. Primary form—unknown; immunologic disorder
   2. Secondary form—drug ingestion; chemotherapy; toxic effect of drugs or chemicals
B. Age and gender related—any age; more common in adults; female predilection in secondary agranulocytosis
C. Clinical features
   1. Systemic symptoms
      a. Sudden onset
      b. High fever, chills, sore throat
      c. Malaise, weakness
      d. Skin is jaundiced
      e. Regional lymphadenopathy
   2. Oral symptoms
      a. Infection (clinical signs affecting the gingiva can be similar to NUG)
      b. Ulcerations of the pharynx, palate, buccal mucosa, and tongue
D. Laboratory tests and findings—confirm the diagnosis
   1. Severe decrease in or absence of granulocytes or polymorphonuclear cells
   2. Accelerated destruction of neutrophils; bone marrow has few or no granulocytes
   3. WBC count is reduced to less than 1000 cells/mm^3
E. Histologic characteristics
   1. Necrosis of involved tissues
   2. Many bacterial microorganisms

F. Treatment
1. Removal of the causative drug or agent, if possible
2. Administration of antibiotics to control infection

Cyclic Neutropenia

A. Etiology—inherited; autosomal dominant; regular periodic episodes lasting 3 to 4 days with a significant decrease in circulating neutrophils; mutation of the neutrophil elastase (ELA2) gene.
B. Age and gender related—infants and young children; no gender predilection
C. Clinical features
1. Systemic symptoms
a. General weakness, malaise
b. Fever, sore throat, headache
c. Cervical lymphadenopathy
d. Gastrointestinal mucosal ulcerations
2. Oral symptoms (Fig. 8-60)
a. Severe gingivitis, recession, and periodontitis (gingiva severely affected)
b. Painful ulcerations on any oral mucosal tissue, especially lips, tongue, buccal mucosa, and oropharynx
c. Mild to severe loss of alveolar bone
d. Dental treatment should be performed when circulating neutrophils are normal to reduce complications and secondary infections
D. Laboratory tests and findings
1. Neutrophils may completely disappear in the acute stage
2. Cycles occur at intervals of 21 to 27 days
3. Sequential blood counts several times a week for several weeks are used to determine neutrophil cycling
E. Treatment and prognosis
1. Optimal oral hygiene practices by the patient
2. Treatment with granulocyte colony-stimulating factor (G-CSF) several times a week

FIG 8-60 Marked gingivitis, with areas of gingival recession in a patient with cyclic neutropenia. (From Ibsen OAC, Phelan JA: *Oral pathology for the dental hygienist,* ed 6, St Louis, 2014, Elsevier.)

3. Antibiotics to control significant infections
4. Premedication with antibiotics before dental hygiene or surgical procedures (which should be scheduled when neutrophils are at their highest peak)

Leukemia
General Characteristics

A. Malignant neoplastic disorder involving blood-forming cells; originates in the bone marrow
B. Excessive proliferation of WBCs in the immature state
C. Etiology—combination of genetic and environmental factors; oncogenic viruses
1. Chronic exposure to chemicals or ionizing radiation
2. Higher incidence among persons with genetic disorders, including Down syndrome and other chromosomal abnormalities, neurofibromatosis, and Klinefelter syndrome (see the section on "Genetics" in Chapter 7)
D. A number of types and subtypes of this condition exist

Acute Leukemia

A. Two types:
1. Acute myeloblastic leukemia (AML)
2. Acute lymphoblastic leukemia (ALL)
B. Age and gender related—according to cell type
1. AML generally affects adolescents and young adults but can affect children
2. ALL almost always affects children
3. Slight male predilection
C. Clinical features—onset is sudden
1. Systemic symptoms
a. Infection in lungs, urinary tract
b. Weakness, fever, headache
c. Swelling of lymph nodes
d. Bruising of the skin and mucous membranes—caused by a decrease in the number of platelets (thrombocytopenia)
e. Enlargement of organs—spleen, liver
f. Bone and joint pain
2. Oral symptoms (Fig. 8-61)
a. Purpuric spots; gingival hemorrhage
b. Severe gingival enlargement—red, soft, spongy; spontaneous bleeding
c. Gingiva sometimes similar to necrotizing ulcerative gingivitis (NUG; see earlier)—characterized by ulcerations, blunted papillae, necrosis, odor
d. Pallor of tissues; nonulcerated edema
e. Candidiasis, herpetic infection, or both
f. Toothache caused by invasion and necrosis of the pulp
g. Mobility of teeth caused by a breakdown of the periodontal membrane and supporting structures
D. Laboratory tests and findings
1. Both anemia and thrombocytopenia present
2. Prolonged bleeding and coagulation times
3. WBC count elevated to 100,000/mm^3 (many immature cells)
4. Leukemic cells in bone marrow and peripheral blood
5. Tests to identify certain enzymes can help classify the type

FIG 8-61 Generalized gingival hyperplasia in a patient with leukemia. (Courtesy of Dr. Edward V. Zegarelli; from Ibsen OAC, Phelan JA: *Oral pathology for the dental hygienist,* ed 6, St Louis, 2014, Elsevier.)

E. Treatment and prognosis
1. Chemotherapy depending on the type and form of leukemia
2. Antibiotics to control infection
3. Drug and radiation therapy to the CNS
4. Transfusions with platelets or packed RBCs
5. Optimal oral hygiene care
6. Prognosis depends on multiple factors (e.g., type of leukemia, age)

Chronic Leukemia

A. Common forms
1. Chronic myeloid leukemia (CML)—associated with the Philadelphia chromosome (first chromosomal abnormality)
2. Chronic lymphocytic leukemia (CLL)—the most common form; asymptomatic for a long time
B. Age and gender related—adults; no gender predilection; chronic leukemia affects older adults
C. Clinical features
1. Systemic symptoms
   a. Very slow onset—disease may be present for weeks or months before symptoms lead to diagnosis
   b. Weight loss, fatigue
   c. Lymph node enlargement and enlarged spleen in the CLL type, not in the CML type
   d. Petechiae on the skin with nodules of leukemic cells
   e. Destructive bone lesions—result in bone fracture
2. Oral symptoms
   a. Gingival tissues are severely affected; become tender, enlarged, and bleed easily
   b. Pallor of the gingiva and lips
   c. Purpuric spots; ecchymosis
   d. Cervical lymphadenopathy may be an early sign (underlines the importance of the extraoral clinical examination)
   e. Oral candidiasis

D. Laboratory tests and findings
1. Anemia and thrombocytopenia sometimes present
2. WBC count can increase to 500,000/mm³ (95% of the total number of blood cells)
3. Shift to the left in the maturity of cells
4. Differential count elevated in the cell type involved
E. Treatment and prognosis
1. Chemotherapy
2. Bone marrow transplantation (especially for patients with CML—better survival rates)
3. Prognosis depends on the stage of the disease; chronic leukemia—2- to 10-year survival depending on stage)

Purpura
General Characteristics
A. Purplish discoloration of the skin and mucous membranes caused by the spontaneous escape of blood into tissues
B. Caused by:
1. Defect or deficiency in blood platelets (thrombocytopenic purpura)
2. Unexplained increase in capillary fragility (vascular or nonthrombocytopenic purpura)

Thrombocytopenic Purpura
A. Etiology
1. Primary—idiopathic thrombocytopenic purpura; cause is unknown
2. Secondary—caused by a variety of conditions
   a. Drug toxicity
   b. Chemotherapy
   c. Infectious diseases
B. Age and gender related—primary form occurs in childhood before age 10 years; secondary form may appear at any age; no gender predilection
C. Clinical features
1. Systemic symptoms
   a. Spontaneous hemorrhagic skin lesions that vary in size (petechiae, ecchymosis, hematomas)
   b. Patient bruises easily
   c. Bleeding through the urinary tract (hematuria)
   d. Bleeding from the nose (epistaxis)
   e. Spleen not palpable
2. Oral symptoms
   a. Profuse gingival hemorrhage
   b. Clustered petechiae
D. Laboratory tests and findings
1. Severe reduction in the platelet count—below 50,000/mm³ (normal, 150,000 to 400,000/mm³)
2. Bleeding time prolonged to 1 hour or more
3. Positive capillary fragility test
E. Treatment
1. Discontinue causative drug, if known
2. Corticosteroid therapy
3. Blood transfusions (platelets, in particular)
4. Guarded prognosis
5. Consult patient's physician of record prior to any dental hygiene or surgical procedure

Nonthrombocytopenic Purpura

A. Etiology—results from a variety of conditions that produce capillary fragility
1. Defect in capillary walls (vitamin C deficiency, infections)
2. Disorder of platelet function (drugs, allergies, autoimmune diseases)

B. Clinical features
1. Platelet count normal
2. Other symptoms similar to those of thrombocytopenic purpura
3. Oral manifestations—spontaneous bleeding, petechial ecchymosis

C. Laboratory tests
1. Platelet count normal
2. Bleeding time prolonged

D. Treatment
1. Systemic corticosteroids
2. Splenectomy
3. Remove cause

Hemophilia

A. Etiology—a genetic deficiency of a clotting factor in the blood; prolonged clotting time; usually factor VIII or factor IX; bleeding disorder of blood coagulation
1. Inherited; X-linked disease; occurs mostly in males; occurs in females in extremely rare cases.
2. Defect carried by the X chromosome; females are carriers of the trait
3. Transmitted genetically from asymptomatic carrier mothers to sons

B. Age and gender related—usually present at birth; symptoms may not appear until later; males are most susceptible, whereas females are carriers of the trait

C. Clinical features
1. Systemic symptoms
   a. Clotting deficiency produces persistent bleeding
   b. Massive hematomas; hemorrhage
   c. Three forms—differ in the deficiency of a blood clotting factor
      (1) Type A—most common type; factor VIII; X-linked recessive
      (2) Type B—or Christmas disease; factor IX; X-linked recessive
      (3) Von Willebrand's disease—abnormal von Willebrand's factor; disorder of platelet function; autosomal dominant; both men and women
2. Oral symptoms
   a. Gingival hemorrhage
   b. Prolonged hemorrhage following tooth eruption, exfoliation, scaling, extraction, or surgery

D. Laboratory tests and findings—prolonged coagulation time (classic feature)

E. Treatment
1. Injections with clotting factor
2. Identify missing factors and replace them (complications can occur)
3. Genetic counseling

4. Optimal dental and dental hygiene care to prevent problems

HUMAN IMMUNODEFICIENCY VIRUS (HIV)

A. Etiology—infectious disease; immune deficiency resulting from HIV infection (Box 8-2)

B. Syndrome includes HIV infection, cell lymphopenia, and reduced CD4 helper T lymphocyte function

C. Age—usually adults age 20 to 40 years; infants of infected mothers; anyone to whom the virus is transmitted

D. Gender and ethnic characteristics
1. Male predilection; however, women are fastest-growing group of infected persons
2. Homosexual or bisexual men
3. Overall increased incidence among intravenous (IV) drug users
4. Others at risk include sex workers, prison inmates, and children of infected mothers

E. Transmission
1. Sexual contact
2. Infected blood serum; in infected patients, the virus has been found in blood and bodily fluids, including saliva and tears
3. Infected mothers to newborn (breast milk); artificial insemination
4. IV drug users
5. Cofactors (e.g., other infections) may influence transmission

F. Clinical features—oral (Box 8-3)
1. At the earliest stage of the disease, the oral findings can be subtle or totally asymptomatic
2. Oral candidiasis occurs in more than 85% of cases (pseudomembranous, erythematous, hyperplastic, angular cheilitis)
3. History of herpes simplex; herpes zoster; aphthous ulcers, HPV
4. NUG; linear gingival erythema; necrotizing ulcerative periodontitis (NUP)
5. Petechiae on attached gingiva
6. Sudden onset of inflammation
7. A creamy white patch covering a raw, red base, as seen in pemphigus
8. Distinct odor
9. Hairy leukoplakia
10. Kaposi's sarcoma

G. Clinical features—general
1. Opportunistic infections—candidiasis; infection by cytomegalovirus (CMV), HSV types 1 and 2; pneumocystic pneumonia; herpes zoster
2. Susceptible to forms of cancer—squamous cell carcinoma, Kaposi's sarcoma, and non-Hodgkin's lymphoma
3. Constitutional signs include sudden, unexplained weight loss, lymphadenopathy involving cervical and submandibular nodes
4. Health history—past and present history of long-term illness, slow healing, vital signs (fever is especially significant), and patient profile

---

BOX 8-2   Definition and Diagnosis of Acquired Immunodeficiency Syndrome (AIDS)

AIDS is an illness characterized by one or more of the following diseases or conditions:

HIV Laboratory Tests Not Performed or Results Inconclusive and the Patient Has No Other Cause of Immunodeficiency

1. Candidiasis of the esophagus, trachea, bronchi, or lungs
2. Cryptococcosis, extrapulmonary
3. Cryptosporidiosis with diarrhea persisting longer than 1 month
4. Cytomegalovirus disease of an organ other than liver, spleen, or lymph nodes in a patient older than 1 month of age
5. Herpes simplex virus infection causing a mucocutaneous ulcer that persists longer than 1 month, or bronchitis, pneumonitis, or esophagitis for any duration affecting a patient older than 1 month of age
6. Kaposi's sarcoma affecting a patient <60 years of age
7. Lymphoid interstitial pneumonia or pulmonary hyperplasia, or both; affecting a child <13 years of age
8. *Mycobacterium avium* or *Mycobacterium kansasii* disease, disseminated
9. *Pneumocystis jiroveci* (formerly *P. carinii*) pneumonia
10. Progressive multifocal leukoencephalopathy
11. Toxoplasmosis of the brain affecting a patient older than 1 month

With Laboratory Evidence for Human Immunodeficiency Virus (HIV) Infection

Less than 200 CD4+ T lymphocytes/mL, or a CD4+ T lymphocyte percentage of total lymphocytes of <14

Any of the diseases previously listed or those that follow:

1. Multiple bacterial infections of certain types affecting a child <13 years of age
2. Coccidioidomycosis, disseminated
3. HIV encephalopathy (HIV dementia)
4. Histoplasmosis, disseminated
5. Isosporiasis with diarrhea persisting longer than 1 month
6. Lymphoma of the brain at any age
7. Kaposi's sarcoma at any age
8. Certain types of lymphoma
9. Mycobacterial disease, other than tuberculosis, disseminated
10. Extrapulmonary tuberculosis
11. *Salmonella* septicemia, recurrent
12. HIV wasting syndrome
13. Pulmonary tuberculosis
14. Recurrent pneumonia
15. Invasive cervical cancer

Even if HIV laboratory test results are negative, if other causes of immunodeficiency are not ruled out, a diagnosis of AIDS can be made if certain of these diseases are diagnosed.

Modifed from Centers for Disease Control and Prevention: 1993 Revised classifications system for HIV infection and expanded surveillance case definition for AIDS among adolescents and adults, *MMWR* 41(RR-17), 1992.

BOX 8-3   Oral Lesions Associated with Human Immunodeficiency Virus (HIV) Infection

Candidiasis
Herpes simplex infection
Herpes zoster
Hairy leukoplakia
Human papillomavirus (HPV) lesions
Atypical gingivitis and periodontitis
Other opportunistic infections reported
  Mycobacterium avium
  Cytomegalovirus
  Cryptococcus neoformans
  Klebsiella pneumoniae
  Enterobacter cloacae
  Histoplasma capsulatum
Kaposi's sarcoma
Non-Hodgkin's lymphoma
Aphthous ulcers
Mucosal pigmentation
Bilateral salivary gland enlargement and xerostomia
Spontaneous gingival bleeding resulting from thrombocytopenia

From Ibsen OAC, Phelan JA: *Oral pathology for the dental hygienist*, ed 6, St Louis, 2014, Elsevier.

5. Other characteristics—lymphadenopathy, fatigue, diarrhea, fever, gastrointestinal involvement, weight loss; oral lesions usually manifest last
6. Epstein-Barr virus (EBV; hairy leukoplakia involving corrugated white areas, especially on the lateral tongue)

H. Laboratory
   1. Serologic testing for HIV infection using the enzyme-linked immunosorbent assay (ELISA) test twice
   2. Western blot test is performed after two positive ELISA tests
   3. The polymerase chain reaction (PCR) identifies the virus and the viral load rather than antibodies
I. Histologic findings—can be extremely variable, depending on the pathologic conditions involved and the opportunistic disease
J. Treatment—symptomatic
   1. Antiretroviral drugs; nucleoside analogs, nonnucleoside reverse transcriptase inhibitors, protease inhibitors, and fusion inhibitors
   2. Drugs that prevent or treat opportunistic diseases (e.g., protease inhibitor)
   3. Prognosis—depends on early diagnosis and current therapy

FIBROUS DYSPLASIA

General Characteristics

A. Etiology—unknown; abnormal mesenchymal cell function; rare diseases affecting bones; replacement of bone with fibrous connective tissue
B. Swelling of bones with deformities in some forms of disease
C. Benign fibro-osseous lesion

Monostotic Fibrous Dysplasia

A. Etiology—unknown; theories include:
1. Local infection
2. Trauma

B. Age and gender related—children and young adults; no gender predilection

C. Location
1. Ribs—most common site
2. Maxilla more often involved than mandible
3. Can affect any bone; most common form

D. Clinical features
1. Painless swelling; enlargement of the jaw or expansion of the buccal plate of maxilla or mandible
2. Can cause malocclusion, tipping, or displacement of teeth
3. In the maxilla, lesions are not clearly outlined because they extend into the sinus or the floor of the orbit

E. Radiographic features
1. The lesion blends into surrounding bone
2. Diffuse radiopacity; "ground glass" appearance
3. Sometimes a radiolucency with areas of radiopacity (depending on the degree of calcification)

F. Histologic characteristics
1. Proliferating fibroblasts in the stroma of woven collagen fibers
2. Irregularly shaped trabeculae; some are C shaped

G. Treatment and prognosis
1. Surgical correction of the deformed bone
2. Radiation therapy contraindicated because of possible malignant transformation

Polyostotic Fibrous Dysplasia

A. Etiology—unknown; involves more than one bone

B. Age and gender related—children; female predilection

C. Location
1. Long bones (bowing); often unilateral
2. Bones of the face and skull
3. Clavicles
4. Pelvic bones

D. Clinical features (depend on the type of polyostotic fibrous dysplasia)
1. Systemic symptoms
   a. Café au lait spots: irregular, light-brown macules on the skin
   b. Painless enlargement of affected bone(s)
   c. Bowing of long bones (pathologic fracture)
   d. Females may reach premature puberty at age 2 or 3 years
   e. Dysfunction of the endocrine system—pituitary, thyroid, and parathyroid glands
2. Oral symptoms
   a. Expansion and deformity of the jaws; unilateral enlargement of maxilla or mandible
   b. Disturbed eruption pattern caused by endocrine dysfunction
3. Types
   a. Craniofacial fibrous dysplasia—the maxilla is involved, and the lesion extends into the sinus and surrounding bones
   b. Jaffe-Lichtenstein type—lesions arise in multiple bones; café au lait skin lesions appear over the involved bone
   c. McCune-Albright syndrome—most severe form of polyostotic fibrous dysplasia
      (1) Severe endocrine abnormalities
          (a) Premature puberty in females before age 2 years
          (b) Stunted growth caused by early epiphyseal closure in both genders
          (c) Café au lait skin lesions
      (2) Other systemic complications (diabetes; hyperthyroidism)

E. Radiographic appearance—irregular bone trabeculae; expansion of cortical bone; sometimes a multi-locular cystic appearance with several radiopacities; diffuse radiopacity resembling ground glass

F. Laboratory tests and findings
1. Serum alkaline phosphatase level sometimes elevated
2. Moderately elevated basal metabolic rate

G. Histologic characteristics
1. Fibrillar connective tissue
2. Many trabeculae
3. Irregularly shaped, coarse woven fibers
4. Osteocytes

H. Treatment and prognosis
1. Surgical correction; postpone surgery as long as possible
2. No treatment for minor involvement
3. Radiation treatment is contraindicated because it has been associated with malignant transformation

Cherubism

A. Etiology—inherited; autosomal dominant gene; marked penetrance; gene 4p16

B. Age and gender related—onset at birth or early childhood (ages 2 to 5 years), females less severely affected

C. Location—only in the maxilla and the mandible (more common in the mandible)

D. Clinical features
1. Painless bilateral facial swelling or enlargement of the posterior mandible; firm and hard when palpated
2. Taut facial skin; downward pull of the eyelids; "cherubic" appearance; eyes are displaced when maxilla is affected
3. Regional lymphadenopathy
4. Has been mistaken for an ameloblastoma or multi-locular cyst
5. Primary dentition may be prematurely shed at age 3 years
6. Permanent dentition often defective; absence of teeth (hypodontia); lack of eruption of the teeth or delayed eruption
7. Speech problems; distortion of alveolar ridge

E. Radiographic appearance
1. Multi-locular radiolucencies; or typical soap bubble radiolucencies in jaw
2. Bilateral thinning of cortical plates
3. Numerous unerupted or displaced teeth in cyst-like radiolucent spaces

F. Laboratory tests and findings—all blood levels normal
G. Histologic characteristics
   1. Similar to central giant cell granuloma; fibrous tissue proliferation
   2. Numerous large, multi-nucleated giant cells in a loose, delicate, fibrous connective tissue stroma
   3. Eosinophilic cuff-like deposits surround small blood vessels
H. Treatment and prognosis
   1. Self-limiting; remission at puberty
   2. Sometimes surgical intervention
   3. Radiation contraindicated because of risk of sarcoma
   4. Prognosis is good

Periapical Cemento-osseous Dysplasia (Cementoma)

A. Etiology—unknown; a common disease that affects periapical bone
B. Age and gender related—mid-30s; more common in females (15:1) and African Americans (70%); these characteristics are critical to the diagnosis
C. Location
   1. Anterior mandible; rare in the maxilla
   2. Apex of teeth near the periodontal ligament
D. Clinical features
   1. Asymptomatic and localized; teeth in the affected area are vital (this feature is critical to the diagnosis and is seen radiographically)
   2. Pulp testing must be part of the diagnostic process to determine teeth are vital
E. Radiographic appearance—depends on the stage of development
   1. Early radiolucent lesion cannot be differentiated from several other principal pathologic lesions
   2. Mature stage showing radiopacities surrounded by radiolucency
   3. Periodontal ligament remains intact
F. Histologic characteristics
   1. Increase in connective tissue cells of the periodontal ligament
   2. Normal bone replaced with a fibrous mass; varying amounts of calcified material within
G. Treatment and prognosis
   1. Self-limiting; no treatment necessary at any time
   2. Prognosis is good

Paget Disease (Osteitis Deformans)

A. Etiology—unknown; nonneoplastic disease of bone; chronic metabolic disease of bone; resorption, osteoblastic repair, and remineralization of involved bone; theories include:
   1. Viral cause
   2. Inflammatory response
   3. Endocrine imbalance
B. Age and gender related—age over 50 years; male predilection
C. Location—especially in the pelvis and spine; more common in the maxilla than the mandible
D. Clinical features
   1. Systemic symptoms
      a. Symptoms develop slowly
      b. Enlargement of bones (bowing in long bones)—spine, femur, tibia; skull (change in hat size); pain in the involved bone
      c. Affected bones are warm to the touch as a result of increased vascularity
      d. Severe headaches, deafness, dizziness, bone neuralgia
      e. Joint pain with limited mobility
   2. Oral symptoms
      a. Enlarged maxilla; spread of the dentition
      b. No change in enamel or dentin; hypercementosis of the roots of teeth makes extractions more difficult
E. Radiographic appearance
   1. Initial decreased radiodensity
   2. Irregular radiolucent and radiopaque patches, giving a classic "cotton wool" appearance
   3. Root resorption; hypercementosis; lamina dura may be missing completely
F. Laboratory tests and findings
   1. Serum alkaline phosphatase level is significantly elevated (this is significant to the diagnosis)
   2. Serum calcium and phosphorus levels are normal
G. Histologic characteristics—characterized by both bone resorption and bone deposition
   1. Areas of resorption—osteoclast activity
   2. Areas of deposition—osteoblast activity
   3. Areas of both resorption and deposition—osteoclasts and osteoblasts present
   4. Vascular fibrous connective tissue replaces bone marrow
   5. Reversed bone lines—"mosaic bone"
H. Treatment and prognosis
   1. No treatment, if asymptomatic
   2. Bone pain—analgesics
   3. Neurologic complications (eyes, ears)
   4. Systemic bisphosphonate medications

ENDOCRINE DISORDERS

General Characteristics

A. Associated with metabolic disturbances, deficiencies, or excesses
B. Excess or deficiency in hormone

Hyperparathyroidism

A. Etiology—excess secretion of parathyroid hormone (PTH, parathormone)
   1. Primary hyperparathyroidism—parathyroid gland produces excessive PTH; results from parathyroid adenoma
   2. Secondary hyperparathyroidism—accompanies other systemic diseases, such as renal disturbances, in which calcium is excreted by the kidneys in abnormal amounts; rickets; vitamin D deficiency
B. Age and gender related—age over 60 years; female predilection (3:1)
C. Clinical features
   1. Systemic symptoms

a. Joint and bone pain, joint stiffness, and resorption of bone with spontaneous fractures

b. Urinary tract stones caused by increased calcium in urine (kidney stones)

c. Weakness, fatigue, dementia

d. Duodenal ulcers

2. Oral symptoms

a. Resembles a giant cell tumor or cyst

b. Diffuse bone loss causing malocclusion and shifting or mobility of teeth

D. Radiographic appearance (Fig. 8-62, A)

1. Cyst-like radiolucencies found in posterior jaws; ground-glass appearance

2. Lamina dura lost or sketchy

3. Mottled appearance

E. Laboratory tests and findings

1. Loss of calcium replaced by fibrous tissue

2. Serum calcium level elevated (hypercalcemia)

3. Low levels of blood phosphorus (hypophosphatemia)

F. Histologic characteristics (Fig. 8-62, B)

1. Osteoclastic resorption of trabeculae of spongiosa bone

2. Fibrosis of marrow spaces

3. Fibroblasts replace resorbed bone

4. Indistinguishable from central giant cell granuloma

5. Highly vascular granulation tissue

FIG 8-62 A, Radiograph of a mandibular lesion in a patient with hyperparathyroidism. **B,** Microscopic appearance of a jaw lesion occurring in a patient with hyperparathyroidism. The histologic appearance is identical to that of a central giant cell granuloma. (**A** courtesy of Drs. Paul Freedman and Stanley Kerpel; **A** and **B** from Ibsen OAC, Phelan JA: *Oral pathology for the dental hygienist,* ed 6, St Louis, 2014, Elsevier.)

G. Treatment

1. Correct the cause of increased PTH production (tumors, renal disease, vitamin D deficiency)

2. Surgical removal of the hyperplastic functional parathyroid gland

3. Parathyroidectomy

4. Renal transplants

Osteomalacia

A. Etiology—deficiency of calcium over a long time

1. Deficiency or impaired absorption of vitamin D (produces osteomalacia in adults and rickets in children)

2. Urinary loss of calcium and phosphorus

3. Fanconi syndrome—group of diseases related to renal tubular function

B. Age and gender related—adults; female predilection

C. Clinical features

1. Loss of calcification in bone; soft bone

a. Generalized weakness

b. Bone pain and tenderness; fractures

c. Affects gait

2. Polyuria—urine output greatly increased

3. Polydipsia—severe thirst

4. No oral symptoms

D. Radiographic appearance

1. Generalized demineralization of bone; milkman's syndrome

2. Lamina dura of teeth may be absent

3. Radiopaque renal calculi in the kidney

E. Laboratory tests and findings

1. Low serum calcium and phosphorus levels

2. Serum alkaline phosphatase level elevated

F. Treatment and prognosis

1. Increased dosage of vitamin D; if malabsorption, water-soluble, synthetic vitamin D can be given

2. Calcium supplements

3. Pathologic fractures may occur in persons with osteomalacia

Rickets

A. Etiology

1. Deficiency of vitamin D, phosphorus, and calcium

2. Form of osteomalacia; failure of calcification of cartilage and bone

B. Age related—young children

C. Clinical features

1. Systemic symptoms

a. Pliable bones; bow leg, knock-knee

b. Muscle pain

c. Enlarged skull, spinal curvature

d. Enlarged liver and spleen

2. Oral symptoms

a. Retardation of tooth eruption

b. Malposition of teeth

c. Retardation of mandibular growth; class II malocclusion

D. Treatment—increase dietary intake of vitamin D, calcium, and phosphorus; supplements

Langerhans Cell Disease
General Characteristics

A. Etiology—unknown; a reactive process
B. Cells accumulate in granulomatous masses
C. Includes a group of three diseases characterized by proliferation of Langerhans cells; a combination of histiocytic cells and eosinophils
D. Three forms:
   1. Letterer-Siwe disease (acute disseminated form)
     a. Age and gender related—first 2 years of life; infants; male predilection
     b. Clinical features
       (1) Skin rash on the trunk, scalp, and extremities
       (2) Persistent low-grade fever; malaise, irritability
       (3) Splenomegaly, hepatomegaly
       (4) Anemia
       (5) Oral lesions—not common because the disease is very rapid
       (6) Most severe form of Langerhans cell disease
     c. Prognosis—invariably fatal; sometimes responds to chemotherapy
   2. Hand-Schüller-Christian disease (chronic disseminated form)
     a. Age and gender related—early life; more common in males
     b. Clinical features
       (1) Systemic symptoms—classic triad of symptoms in 25% of patients:
         (a) Skull and jaws affected—punched-out radiolucencies
         (b) Diabetes insipidus—result of pituitary dysfunction
         (c) Exophthalmos—bulging eyes caused by massive infiltration of reticulocytes
       (2) Oral symptoms
         (a) Sore mouth, ulcerations, erythema
         (b) Halitosis, unpleasant taste, gingivitis
         (c) Loose, sensitive teeth
         (d) Failure to heal after extractions
     c. Radiographic appearance—radiolucencies in the skull and jaws; punched-out radiolucencies
     d. Treatment and prognosis
       (1) Curettage of the lesion
       (2) Radiation therapy
       (3) Cytotoxic drugs and adrenocortical hormones
       (4) Prognosis is poor; high fatality rate
   3. Eosinophilic granuloma (localized)
     a. Age and gender related—older children and young adults approximately age 20 years; male predilection (2:1)
     b. Clinical features
       (1) Most benign variety of Langerhans cell disease
       (2) May be asymptomatic; local pain, swelling, tenderness
       (3) Sore mouth, fetid breath, loosening of teeth, swollen gingiva
       (4) Mandible more involved than maxilla

FIG 8-63 Radiograph of eosinophilic granuloma. (Courtesy of Drs. Paul Freedman and Stanley Kerpel; from Ibsen OAC, Phelan JA: *Oral pathology for the dental hygienist,* ed 6, St Louis, 2014, Elsevier.)

     c. Radiographic appearance—irregular radiolucencies, single or multiple; well defined, resembling a cyst (Fig. 8-63)
     d. Treatment and prognosis
       (1) Curettage and conservative surgical excision
       (2) Radiation therapy
       (3) Prognosis is good; recurrence is rare

ABNORMALITIES OF TEETH

Loss of Tooth Structure
Attrition

A. Etiology—wearing away of tooth surfaces by active, physiologic forces
   1. Mastication
   2. Bruxism and chewing of tobacco accelerate attrition of teeth
   3. Occlusion—heavy biting forces
   4. Diet—chewing of coarse foods influences attrition
B. Age and gender related—occurs in primary and permanent dentition; the rate of attrition is higher in males
C. Clinical features (Fig. 8-64)
   1. Polished facets
   2. Flat incisal edge
   3. Discolored surface
   4. Exposed dentin
   5. Muscle tenderness (more associated with bruxism)

Abrasion

A. Etiology—wearing away of tooth structure through abnormal mechanical processes
   1. Improper toothbrushing technique

FIG 8-64 **A,** Attrition. **B,** Incisal view of attrition of the adult dentition. (From Ibsen OAC, Phelan JA: *Oral pathology for the dental hygienist,* ed 6, St Louis, 2014, Elsevier.)

2. Abrasive dentifrices
3. Repetitive oral habits

B. Clinical features (Fig. 8-65)
   1. U-shaped loss of tooth structure at the cervical margin; common in the canine and premolar areas
   2. Recession of gingiva creates sensitivity

FIG 8-65 Abrasion of the cervical area of mandibular premolars caused by aggressive toothbrushing. (From Ibsen OAC, Phelan JA: *Oral pathology for the dental hygienist,* ed 6, St Louis, 2014, Elsevier.)

3. Pipe smoking abrades teeth where the pipe rests
4. Notching associated with carpenters and tailors who hold tacks, nails, and pins between their teeth

Abfraction

A. Etiology—related to microfracture of tooth structure in areas of concentration of stress; biomechanical forces on teeth
B. Age—adults
C. Location
   1. Cervical area of teeth
   2. Predisposes the patient to abrasion
D. Clinical features—a wedge-shaped or V-shaped loss of tooth structure at the cemento-enamel junction (CEJ); the tooth is more susceptible to toothbrushing abrasion
E. Treatment
   1. Composite
   2. Glass ionomers

Erosion

A. Etiology—loss of tooth structure resulting from chemical action; when caused by gastric acids, it is known as *perimylolysis*
   1. Acid or low-pH fluid intake
   2. Acidic foods habitually used over long periods
   3. Eating disorders (bulimia)
B. Clinical features (Fig. 8-66)
   1. Usually found on the labial or buccal surfaces; loss of enamel on the anterior maxillary lingual surfaces and mesial and distal surfaces may be indicative of bulimia
   2. "Wear" depressions or etchings on cervical or occlusal surfaces
   3. Hypersensitivity of affected teeth

Drugs Affecting Teeth
Methamphetamine Abuse and Addiction

A. Street names: meth, speed, crystal, ice, glass, fire
B. Etiology—a man-made psychostimulant that can be injected, snorted, inhaled, taken orally, or smoked
   1. Mood alterations depend on how it is taken
   2. Smoking produces a high that can last 10 to 24 hours
C. Gender related
   1. Majority are males age 18 to 34
   2. Increased incidence in females
D. Clinical symptoms of use
   1. Inability to sleep
   2. Irritability
   3. Extreme anorexia (causes a decrease in appetite)
   4. Tremors
   5. Sensitivity to noise
   6. Increased craving for sweets
   7. Possession of drug paraphernalia
E. Clinical signs—oral
   1. "Meth mouth"; snorting or inhaling has the most severe effect on teeth
   2. Xerostomia; candidiasis

FIG 8-66 Erosion caused by bulimia. **A,** Decreased tooth size. **B,** Erosion of maxillary lingual surfaces. (From Ibsen OAC, Phelan JA: *Oral pathology for the dental hygienist,* ed 6, St Louis, 2014, Elsevier.)

3. "Rampant caries" caused by the acidic nature of the drug; smooth buccal or labial surfaces of teeth and interproximal surfaces of anterior teeth are especially affected
4. Bruxism and clenching, leading to cracked teeth
5. Advanced gingival problems and periodontal disease
6. One report described the oral condition as "teeth rotted to the gumline"
7. Dangerous interactions with common local anesthetics, nitrous oxide, and pain medications

F. Clinical signs—systemic
1. Cardiovascular problems, including increased heart rate and blood pressure
2. Toxic effects on the CNS
3. Hyperthermia
4. Irreversible stroke producing damage to the blood vessels in the brain
5. Acute lead poisoning in IV drug abusers
6. During pregnancy, congenital deformities, prenatal complications, and premature birth
7. Rapid aging

Tetracycline Stain

A. Etiology—ingested medication during tooth development
B. Clinical—tooth staining that can be yellow-green or gray-brown; endogenous stain

Developmental Defects Affecting Enamel and Dentin
Amelogenesis Imperfecta

A. Etiology—inherited condition affecting the enamel of teeth resulting from a malfunction of the tooth germ
B. Produces four types
1. Type 1: enamel hypoplasia—defect in the formation of the matrix
   a. Etiology—hereditary; environmental factors, nutritional deficiency, congenital syphilis, high fever, and birth injuries also can cause a hypoplastic response
   b. Clinically (Fig. 8-67), the enamel of primary and permanent teeth appears pitted; vertical grooves, deficiency in thickness, yellow to dark-brown color, open contacts, and occlusal wear are noted; seven varieties of type 1 hypoplastic amelogenesis imperfecta; the pitted, autosomal variety is most common
   c. Radiographic appearance—enamel absent or very thin layer over tips of cusps and interproximal areas
   d. Histologic characteristics—thin, defective enamel; few enamel prisms; no lamellae
   e. Treatment—restorations; crowns; bonding; laminates
2. Type 2: enamel hypocalcification—defect in mineralization of the formed matrix; normal enamel thickness, but the enamel is poorly calcified
   a. Etiology—two varieties include autosomal dominant and autosomal recessive
   b. Clinically (Fig. 8-68), the enamel appears yellow to dark brown and chalky; easily breaks down
   c. Radiographic appearance—the tooth shape is normal; enamel and dentin have the same radiodensity, which makes them difficult to differentiate; enamel appears "moth eaten" and is less radiopaque than dentin
   d. Histologic characteristics—broadening of interprismatic substance; distinct enamel prisms; enamel low in mineral content
   e. Treatment—restorations; crowns; bonding; laminates
3. Type 3: enamel hypomaturation
   a. Etiology—X-linked recessive ("snowcapped") or autosomal dominant

FIG 8-67 Pitted autosomal dominant amelogenesis imperfecta. Note the multiple pits on the labial surface of teeth. Some of the pits have been filled with composite. (From Young WG, Sedano HO: *Atlas of oral pathology,* Minneapolis, 1981, University of Minnesota Press.)

FIG 8-68 Note the loss of enamel in the teeth of a patient with hypocalcified amelogenesis imperfecta. (From Ibsen OAC, Phelan JA: *Oral pathology for the dental hygienist,* ed 6, St Louis, 2014, Elsevier.)

FIG 8-69 Note the uniform whitening of incisal edges and occlusal cusps in a case of "snowcapped" amelogenesis imperfecta. (From Ibsen OAC, Phelan JA: *Oral pathology for the dental hygienist,* ed 6, St Louis, 2014, Elsevier.)

FIG 8-70 A, Clinical view of dentinogenesis imperfecta. **B,** Radiographic view. (Courtesy of Dr. Edward V. Zegarelli; from Ibsen OAC, Phelan JA: *Oral pathology for the dental hygienist,* ed 6, St Louis, 2014, Elsevier.)

  b. Clinical appearance (Fig. 8-69)
    (1) Enamel is of normal thickness but appears mottled with large amounts of enamel matrix and is therefore softer
    (2) Occlusal third of teeth appear "white" with normal hardness
    (3) Enamel easily chips from crowns of teeth
    (4) Four varieties of this type (snowcapped type shown in Fig. 8-69)
  4. Type 4: hypoplastic—hypomaturation of enamel
    a. Etiology—characterized by association with taurodontic teeth
    b. Clinically, the enamel is thin, pitted, and appears yellow to brown in color

Dentinogenesis Imperfecta (Hereditary Opalescent Dentin)

A. Etiology
  1. Hereditary
  2. Disturbance of dentin formation
    a. Affects the mesodermal component
    b. Enamel remains normal
B. Clinical features (Fig. 8-70, *A*)
  1. Teeth appear "opalescent," a translucent hue
  2. Gray to bluish brown color
  3. Distinct constriction at the CEJ

C. Radiographic appearance (Fig. 8-70, *B*)
  1. Partial or total obliteration of pulp chambers and root canals
  2. Roots are short, blunted, and sometimes fractured
  3. Cementum, periodontal membrane, and alveolar bone appear normal
D. Histologic characteristics
  1. Disturbance of the mesoderm
  2. Dentin composed of irregular tubules; uncalcified matrix
  3. Tubules large in width; few in number
  4. Odontoblasts degenerate easily within the matrix
  5. Decrease in inorganic content
E. Treatment—cast-metal crowns; caution needed with partial appliances because of root fractures

Developmental Defects Affecting Tooth Shape
Dilaceration

A. Sharp bend or curve in the root of a formed tooth (Fig. 8-71, *A*).
B. Etiology—trauma during tooth development
  1. Calcified area displaced
  2. Amount of tooth formed at the time of trauma will affect the angle or curve of the root; usually affects the apical third of the root
C. Radiographic appearance—sharp bend or curve in the root (Fig. 8-71, *B*)
D. Treatment—none

FIG 8-71 A, Dilaceration on the distal root of an extracted tooth. **B,** Mesial root dilaceration on a mandibular second molar. (**A** courtesy of Dr. Rudy Melfi; **A** and **B** from Ibsen OAC, Phelan JA: *Oral pathology for the dental hygienist,* ed 6, St Louis, 2014, Elsevier.)

FIG 8-72 A, Clinical view of fusion involving a permanent mandibular lateral incisor. **B,** Fusion of mandibular molars. (**A** courtesy of Dr. George Blozis; **B** courtesy of Dr. Rudy Melfi; from Ibsen OAC, Phelan JA: *Oral pathology for the dental hygienist,* ed 6, St Louis, 2014, Elsevier.)

Fusion

A. Union of two normally separated tooth germs
B. Etiology—physical force or external pressure; hereditary tendency
C. Clinical features (Fig. 8-72)
  1. If the defect occurs early in development, one large tooth results
  2. If the defect occurs later, fusion of roots only
  3. Dentin always confluent (if true fusion)
  4. Can occur in both primary and permanent dentitions
  5. Can occur between two normal teeth or between one normal tooth and one supernumerary tooth
D. Location—anterior region; incisors are most often affected
E. Radiographic appearance—can have separate or fused root canals
F. Treatment—usually none; hemisection for a crown or bridge, if necessary

Gemination

A. Division of a single tooth germ by invagination; results in incomplete formation of two teeth (gemination means paired or occurring in twos)

B. Etiology—unknown; possibly trauma; hereditary tendency
C. Location—can affect the primary or permanent dentition, although it is slightly more common in the primary dentition (e.g., in mandibular incisors or in permanent maxillary incisors)
D. Clinically teeth usually have two completely or incompletely separate crowns with one root, or with one root canal (Fig. 8-73)

Concrescence

A. Fusion that occurs after root formation is complete; roots united by cementum only
B. Etiology—traumatic injury; crowding of teeth with resorption of interdental bone
C. Location—most often seen in adjacent maxillary molars
D. Radiographic appearance—establishes diagnosis because teeth are joined at the root surfaces and cannot be observed clinically (Fig. 8-74)
E. Treatment and prognosis—usually no treatment; if extraction is necessary, all teeth joined by cementum are compromised

Dens in Dente (Dens Invaginatus)

A. Tooth within a tooth
B. Etiology—increased localized external pressure; growth retardation

C. Location—maxillary lateral incisor (Fig. 8-75)

D. Often bilateral

E. Radiographic appearance—small tooth within the pulp chamber (Fig. 8-76)

F. Treatment—none, unless the pulp becomes inflamed or necrotic

Dens Evaginatus

A. An accessory cusp found on the occlusal surface

B. Etiology—rare developmental anomaly caused by proliferation of enamel epithelium

C. Location—most often mandibular premolars (tuberculated premolars)

D. Clinical appearance—small, round nodule of enamel found on the occlusal surface (Fig. 8-77)

E. Treatment—usually none, unless the condition poses occlusal problems

FIG 8-73 Clinical **(A)** and radiographic **(B)** views of gemination seen in the right maxillary central incisor. (From Ibsen OAC, Phelan JA: *Oral pathology for the dental hygienist,* ed 6, St Louis, 2014, Elsevier.)

FIG 8-75 Clinical view of dens in dente in maxillary lateral incisor. (Courtesy of Dr. George Blozis; from Ibsen OAC, Phelan JA: *Oral pathology for the dental hygienist,* ed 6, St Louis, 2014, Elsevier.)

FIG 8-74   A and **B,** Example of concrescence seen in extracted teeth and in a corresponding radiograph. (Courtesy of Dr. George Blozis; from Ibsen OAC, Phelan JA: *Oral pathology for the dental hygienist,* ed 6, St Louis, 2014, Elsevier.)

FIG 8-76 Radiograph of dens in dente in maxillary lateral incisor. (From Ibsen OAC, Phelan JA: *Oral pathology for the dental hygienist,* ed 6, St Louis, 2014, Elsevier.)

FIG 8-77 Dens evaginatus of maxillary premolar. (Courtesy of Dr. Margot Van Dis; from Ibsen OAC, Phelan JA: *Oral pathology for the dental hygienist,* ed 6, St Louis, 2014, Elsevier.)

Natal Teeth

A. Teeth present at birth
B. Etiology
 1. Develop from part of dental lamina before the deciduous bud or from bud of accessory dental lamina
 2. Neonatal teeth are those that erupt 30 days after birth
C. Location—usually found in the mandibular incisor area
D. Histologic characteristics—keratinized epithelial structures without roots (therefore not true teeth)
E. Treatment and prognosis
 1. Removal (after determining they are not prematurely erupted primary teeth)
 2. Prognosis is excellent; no complications

FIG 8-78 A and **B,** Hypodontia. The missing teeth were not extracted; they never developed. (**A** courtesy of Dr. George Blozis; **B** courtesy of Dr. Margot Van Dis; from Ibsen OAC, Phelan JA: *Oral pathology for the dental hygienist,* ed 6, St Louis, 2014, Elsevier.)

Developmental Defects Affecting the Number of Teeth

Anodontia

A. Missing teeth
B. Etiology—congenital lack of teeth; tooth germ did not develop
C. Two forms
 1. Total anodontia
  a. Rare condition—all teeth missing
  b. May involve both primary and permanent dentitions
  c. Usually associated with ectodermal dysplasia, a hereditary disturbance
 2. Hypodontia (partial anodontia) (Fig. 8-78)
  a. Rather common
  b. Teeth usually affected include third molars and maxillary lateral incisors
  c. Familial or hereditary tendency
  d. Odontodysplasia, "ghost teeth" (Fig. 8-79); teeth in this condition are malformed and unerupted
D. Treatment
 1. Space maintainers during childhood
 2. Crown and bridge work
 3. Prosthetic appliances
 4. Dental implants

Supernumerary Teeth

A. More than the normal number of teeth
B. Etiology—additional tooth buds arise from dental lamina; hereditary

FIG 8-79 Regional odontodysplasia. (From Ibsen OAC, Phelan JA: *Oral pathology for the dental hygienist,* ed 6, St Louis, 2014, Elsevier.)

C. Classification
1. Mesiodent (mesiodens)—most common; cone-shaped crown; short root; located between maxillary centrals (Fig. 8-80)
2. Maxillary fourth molar—distal to the third molar; a mandibular fourth molar occasionally is found
3. Maxillary paramolar—usually a small molar; located buccally or lingually in the area of the maxillary molars
D. Treatment—none; observe for cystic transition; remove when interference occurs with normal dentition

Developmental Defects Affecting Tooth Size
Macrodontia
Abnormally large tooth; rare; possibly a result of fusion

Microdontia
Abnormally small tooth; maxillary lateral incisor and third molar most frequently affected (Fig. 8-81)

FIG 8-80 A, Mesiodens seen between maxillary central incisors. **B,** Radiograph of a mesiodens. **C,** Radiograph showing a pair of inverted, impacted mesiodens. (**A** and **B** courtesy of Dr. George Blozis; **A** to **C,** from Ibsen OAC, Phelan JA: *Oral pathology for the dental hygienist,* ed 6, St Louis, 2014, Elsevier.)

FIG 8-81 Peg-shaped lateral incisor. (Courtesy of Dr. George Blozis; from Ibsen OAC, Phelan JA: *Oral pathology for the dental hygienist,* ed 6, St Louis, 2014, Elsevier.)

CONDITIONS OF ORAL SOFT TISSUES
Abnormalities Affecting Mucous Membranes or Skin
Amalgam Tattoo
A. Etiology—dust or particle of an amalgam restoration embedded in the mucosa or gingiva
B. Clinical features—blue to purplish area near an amalgam restoration (Fig. 8-82, *A*)
C. Radiographic appearance—radiopaque if amalgam particles are present (Fig. 8-82, *B*)
D. Treatment

Melanin Pigmentation
A. Dark pigmentation of the gingiva or mucosa (Fig. 8-83 and 8-84)
B. Etiology—hereditary; those with dark complexions are most often affected; can occur after inflammation from injury
C. Treatment—none, because tissue is healthy

FIG 8-83 Melanin pigmentation of the gingiva. (From Ibsen OAC, Phelan JA: *Oral pathology for the dental hygienist,* ed 6, St Louis, 2014, Elsevier.)

FIG 8-84 Posttraumatic melanin pigmentation. This area of melanin pigmentation on the gingiva occurred after the healing of an injury caused by trauma. (From Ibsen OAC, Phelan JA: *Oral pathology for the dental hygienist,* ed 6, St Louis, 2014, Elsevier.)

FIG 8-82 A, This blue-gray pigmentation on the gingiva is an amalgam tattoo. **B,** Periapical radiograph showing amalgam particles in the gingival tissue. (From Ibsen OAC, Phelan JA: *Oral pathology for the dental hygienist,* ed 6, St Louis, 2014, Elsevier.)

FIG 8-85 Angular cheilitis. (From Ibsen OAC, Phelan JA: *Oral pathology for the dental hygienist,* ed 6, St Louis, 2014, Elsevier.)

Angular Cheilitis

A. Etiology (considered a form of candidiasis)
   1. Infection caused by *Candida albicans*
   2. Nutritional deficiency
   3. Denture-associated cheilitis
B. Clinical features—inflammation and cracking at the corners of the lips; extend into facial skin (Fig. 8-85)
C. Histologic characteristics—inflammatory cells
D. Treatment—depends on the etiology: improved diet; correction of the vertical dimension of the denture; applying antifungal ointment or cream three to four times per day for 5 to 7 days

Fordyce Granules

A. Etiology—developmental; aberrant sebaceous glands
B. Clinical features (Fig. 8-86)
   1. Affects the vermilion border of the lips and the buccal mucosa
   2. Yellow, slightly raised spots a few millimeters in size
C. Location—buccal mucosa; lips
D. Histologic characteristics—glandular tissue; not pathologic
E. Treatment—none

Abnormalities Affecting the Tongue

See Table 12-4 in Chapter 12.

Geographic Tongue (Benign Migratory Glossitis, Erythema Migrans)

A. Etiology—unknown; theories include:
   1. Nutritional deficiency
   2. Heredity
   3. Stress
   4. Psoriasis
B. Age and gender related—any age, but more common in children and young adults; no gender predilection
C. Clinical features (Fig. 8-87)
   1. Fungiform papillae appear as red, mushroom-like projections
   2. Diffuse desquamation of filiform papillae
   3. Condition assumes variations in shape, giving a map-like appearance; remission in depapillated areas
   4. Discomfort occurs when the patient eats certain foods
D. Histologic characteristics—characteristic inflammatory cells; keratotic cells around the borders of the lesion
E. Treatment—none; variant of normal

FIG 8-86 Fordyce granules on the buccal mucosa. (From Ibsen OAC, Phelan JA: *Oral pathology for the dental hygienist,* ed 6, St Louis, 2014, Elsevier.)

FIG 8-87 **A,** Geographic tongue. **B,** Ectopic geographic tongue observed in the anterior mandibular mucosa. (From Ibsen OAC, Phelan JA: *Oral pathology for the dental hygienist,* ed 6, St Louis, 2014, Elsevier.)

Black Hairy Tongue

A. Etiology—irritation to filiform papillae caused by:
   1. Smoking
   2. Alcohol
   3. Hydrogen peroxide
   4. Antacid liquids
   5. Systemic antibiotic therapy
B. Clinical features—brownish to black appearance on the dorsal surface of the tongue (Fig. 8-88)
C. Histologic characteristics—elongation of filiform papillae; characteristic inflammatory cells
D. Treatment and prognosis
   1. Gentle brushing or scraping of the tongue; toothpaste should not be used
   2. Removal of the cause
   3. Prognosis is good; the condition is totally reversible, but may recur

FIG 8-88 Black hairy tongue. (From Ibsen OAC, Phelan JA: *Oral pathology for the dental hygienist,* ed 6, St Louis, 2014, Elsevier.)

Website Information and Resources

Source	Website Address	Description
Doctor's Guide	http://www.pslgroup.com	Articles on medical industry and medical news
National Institute of Dental and Craniofacial Research	http://www.nidcr.nih.gov/	News and information related to dentistry and information about the Institute's research
Mayo Clinic Medicine Center	http://www.mayohealth.org	Information and links to health conditions and diseases
Clinical trials listing service	http://www.centerwatch.com	International listing of clinical research trials and medical centers that perform clinical research and drug therapies newly approved by the U.S. Food and Drug Administration (FDA)
National Cancer Institute	http://www.nci.nih.gov	Information about types of cancer, treatments, risk factors, screening, tests, and statistics
American Cancer Society	http://cancer.org	Information about cancers and leukemias from both professional and patient points of view
American Society of Pediatric Hematology and Oncology	http://www.aspho.org	Information for both professionals and patients about pediatric hematology and oncology
Support for People with Oral and Head and Neck Cancers	http://www.spohnc.org	Information and support for those suffering from oral and head and neck cancers
Leukemia and Lymphoma Society of America	http://www.leukemia.org	Information about blood-related cancers

SUGGESTED READINGS

Ibsen OAC, Phelan JA: *Oral pathology for the dental hygienist,* ed 6, St Louis, 2014, Elsevier Saunders.

Neville BW, Damm DD, Allen CM, Bouquot JE: *Oral and maxillofacial pathology,* ed 3, St Louis, 2009, Elsevier Saunders.
Regezi J, Sciubba J, Jordan RCK: *Oral pathology: clinical pathologic correlations,* ed 5, St Louis, 2008, Elsevier Saunders.

▍CHAPTER 8 REVIEW QUESTIONS

Answers and rationales to review questions are available on this text's accompanying Evolve site. See inside front cover for details.

evolve

CASE A

Synopsis of Patient History	Vital Signs
Age: 30	Blood pressure: 120/80
Sex: M	Pulse rate: 60
Height: 6'3"	Respiration: 16
Weight: 200 lbs	

1. Under the care of a physician: _____ YES x NO
2. Hospitalization within the last 5 years: _____ YES x NO
3. Has or had the following conditions:
   Rheumatic fever or rheumatic heart disease _____ YES x NO
   Congenital heart disease (bicuspid aortic valve) _____ YES x NO
   Heart attack _____ YES x NO
   Angina pectoris _____ YES x NO
   Hypertension _____ YES x NO
   Diabetes mellitus _____ YES x NO
   Hepatitis _____ YES x NO
   Bleeding disorder _____ YES x NO
   Fainting spells, seizures, or epilepsy _____ YES x NO
   Asthma _____ YES x NO
   Allergies (medication, food) _____ YES x NO
4. Current medications
   Anticoagulants _____ YES x NO
   Insulin _____ YES x NO
   Antibiotics _____ YES x NO
   Aspirin _____ YES x NO
   Nitroglycerin _____ YES x NO
   High blood pressure _____ YES x NO
   Corticosteroids _____ YES x NO
   Oral contraceptives _____ YES x NO
   Other:
5. Smokes or uses tobacco products _____ YES x NO

Medical History

Patient is African American and in good health.

Dental History
Patient is meticulous with his oral hygiene, but has a tendency to brush vigorously.

Social History
Patient lives with his wife and 3-year-old son.

Chief Complaint
"I don't like the appearance of my gums pulling away from my teeth, and my teeth are sensitive around my upper canines."

Supplemental Oral Examination Findings
Patient has a generalized opalescent appearance of the buccal mucosa. Patient has generalized melanin pigmentation of the gingiva. A mucocele is noted.
   The gingiva is firm and stippled with no bleeding evident on probing. There is gingival recession on teeth #6 and #11 and mandibular anterior facials, with a 1-mm zone of attached gingiva.

Use Case A and Fig. 8-89 to answer questions 1 to 11.
1. **The generalized opalescence of the buccal mucosa is most likely:**
   a. Linea alba
   b. Leukoedema
   c. Lichen planus
   d. Leukoplakia
2. **In which layer of the stratified epithelium is the generalized opalescent condition in question 1 caused by significant intercellular edema?**
   a. Corneum
   b. Basal
   c. Prickle
   d. Granular
3. **What treatment does this condition require?**
   a. Nonsteroidal anti-inflammatory drugs
   b. Excision
   c. Antifungal drugs
   d. No treatment
4. **The patient has a 2-mm probing depth on the facial aspect of tooth #6, and he has 3 mm of recession. What is the attachment loss in this area?**
   a. 5 mm
   b. 2 mm
   c. 3 mm
   d. 1 mm
5. **The patient's sensitivity in this area is most likely related to fluid entering the:**
   a. Sulcular epithelium
   b. Rodless enamel
   c. Dentinal tubules
   d. Lacuna of cementum
6. **The tooth itself is capable of experiencing painful nerve sensation from all the following EXCEPT:**
   a. Pressure
   b. Heat
   c. Cold
   d. Olfaction

FIG 8-89 Leukoedema. (From Regezi JA, Sciubba JA, Jordan CK: *Oral pathology: clinical pathologic correlations*, ed 7, St Louis, 2017, Elsevier.)

The patient wants the areas of gingival recession treated to resolve issues of sensitivity and esthetic problems. The dental care plan includes covering the areas around the canines with soft tissue grafts. The periodontist states that she will perform connective tissue grafts. She explains that the connective tissue taken from an area (donor site) will produce the same type of epithelium at the canine area (recipient site) as the tissue that exists at that donor site.

7. **The type of tissue normally present around the canine area is:**
   a. Keratinized, stratified squamous epithelium
   b. Nonkeratinized, stratified squamous epithelium
   c. Keratinized, simple squamous epithelium
   d. Pseudo-stratified columnar epithelium

8. **The most appropriate connective tissue donor site would be the:**
   a. Buccal mucosa
   b. Soft palate
   c. Hard palate
   d. Sublingual area

9. **With this procedure, the ideal outcome would be for some of this tissue to form a fibrous attachment to the tooth cementum. From which type of tissue would the cells come to remodel the cementum in this area in which root surfaces previously were exposed?**
   a. Cellular cementum
   b. Bone
   c. Sulcular epithelium
   d. Periodontal ligament

10. **This patient also has a mucocele that is the result of trauma to a minor salivary duct. A mucocele is usually found on the:**
    a. Gingiva
    b. Lower lip mucosa
    c. Hard palate
    d. Dorsum of the tongue

11. **To prevent further recession, what changes should this patient make in his oral self-care regimen?**
    a. More frequent recare appointments
    b. Modifying flossing technique
    c. More frequent toothbrushing
    d. Modifying toothbrushing technique

12. **The radiographs in Fig. 8-90 indicate congenital absence of the:**
    a. Maxillary right first premolar and the maxillary left first premolars
    b. Mandibular right first premolar and the mandibular left first premolar
    c. Mandibular left first premolar and the mandibular right second premolar
    d. Mandibular right second premolar and the mandibular left second premolar

13. **A bony, developmental, benign asymptomatic area found on the midline of the hard palate that appears radiopaque on a radiograph is most likely a:**
    a. Odontogenic myxoma
    b. Median palatal cyst
    c. Compound odontoma
    d. Torus palatinus
    Use Fig. 8-91 to answer questions 14 to 16.

14. **On the panoramic radiograph in Fig. 8-91, the bilateral radiolucent areas apical to the mandibular molars and identified by *A* are:**
    a. Stafne bone cysts
    b. Periapical abscesses
    c. Submandibular fossae
    d. Traumatic bone cysts

15. **The horizontal radiopaque structure identified by *B* in Fig. 8-91 is the:**
    a. Anterior coronoid process
    b. Maxillary tuberosity

FIG 8-90 Radiographs.

FIG 8-91 Panoramic radiograph.

c. Mandibular condyle
d. Zygomatic arch

16. **The bilateral radiolucent areas identified by C in Fig. 8-91 are:**
   a. Nasal fossae
   b. Orbits
   c. Frontal sinuses
   d. Maxillary sinuses

17. **The Pleomorphic adenoma is most often found in the:**
   a. Palate
   b. Mandible
   c. Buccal mucosa
   d. Lymph nodes

18. **Which of the following cysts would create difficulty swallowing?**
   a. Branchial cleft
   b. Thyroglossal
   c. Nasopalatine
   d. Stafne bone

19. **Which disease may have oral characteristics similar to those found in necrotizing ulcerative gingivitis (NUG)?**
   a. Primary herpes
   b. Mononucleosis
   c. Leukemia
   d. Nonthrombocytopenic purpura

20. **A ranula usually is found on the:**
   a. Palate
   b. Lower lip mucosa
   c. Buccal mucosa
   d. Floor of the mouth

21. **A definitive dental diagnosis of soft tissue oral cancer is made by:**
   a. A complete radiographic survey
   b. Exfoliative cytology
   c. Scalpel biopsy
   d. Brush test

22. **Fig. 8-92 shows a periapical radiograph of the mandibular right quadrant, which was taken as part of a full-** mouth radiographic series. The patient was 14 years of age and asymptomatic. The periapical radiolucency indicated by the arrow on tooth #31 is most likely:
   a. Resorption caused by a traumatic injury
   b. Periapical abscesses
   c. Incomplete root formation
   d. Hypercementosis

23. **Primordial cysts are most often found radiographically:**
   a. In the anterior maxillary regions
   b. Around a supernumerary tooth
   c. Posterior to erupted third molars or in place of a tooth that was never present
   d. In the mandibular canine and first premolar areas

24. **The usual location of periapical cemento-osseous dysplasia (cementoma) is:**
   a. Mandibular anteriors
   b. Maxillary anteriors
   c. The mandibular ramus
   d. Maxillary premolars

25. **Which of the following is a rickettsial infection?**
   a. Malaria
   b. Psittacosis

FIG 8-92 Periapical radiograph.

    c. Rocky Mountain spotted fever

    d. Tularemia

26. A slightly raised, noncoated, red rectangular area in the midline of the tongue has been present as long as the patient can remember. Once thought to be developmental, it is associated with *Candida albicans*. This condition is most likely:

    a. Geographic tongue

    b. Pathologic tongue

    c. Median rhomboid glossitis

    d. Fissured tongue

27. Which of the following provides the most conclusive diagnostic evidence in distinguishing pemphigus from pemphigoid?

    a. Clinical picture

    b. History of the disease

    c. Biopsy and histology report

    d. Nikolsky's sign

28. An isolated radiopaque area in the periodontal ligament space is observed on a patient's radiographs. This radiopaque structure may be a(n):

    a. Epithelial rest

    b. Cementum spur

    c. Exostosis of alveolar bone

    d. Cementicle

29. A 30-year-old patient calls and complains of sudden swelling in both sides of his neck, which seems to be enlarging. His record indicates that he recently has canceled two appointments. He needs to have restorative care completed on the mandibular second molars, which have extensive decay. The patient may have:

    a. Actinomycosis

    b. Mumps

    c. Syphilis

    d. Ludwig angina

30. Which of the following two diseases represent different forms of infection resulting from the same virus?

    a. Measles and German measles

    b. Chickenpox and smallpox

    c. Bacterial pneumonia and croup

    d. Shingles and chickenpox

31. A lesion is noted on the lips of a 40-year-old female patient. The lesion appears as several discrete vesicles; some have ulcerated. When questioned, the patient says she "always gets a sore like that" before she develops a cold. The patient most likely has:

    a. A chancre

    b. Perlèche

    c. An aphthous ulcer

    d. Herpes labialis

32. Which of the following statements most accurately describes the most common effect of pregnancy on the health of the mother's oral tissues?

    a. Pregnancy-associated gingivitis is caused by hormonal changes, and nothing can be done about it.

    b. Pregnant women can often experience the growth of tumors in the mouth that relate to hormonal changes.

    c. Hormonal changes during pregnancy result in increased bacteria and increased gingival response to plaque biofilm.

    d. Pregnancy results in hormonal changes, but these changes do not affect the mother's oral tissues.

33. The gingival enlargement shown in Fig. 8-93 was caused by a calcium channel blocker drug. The condition was most likely caused by:

    a. Phenytoin (Dilantin)

    b. Enalapril (Vasotec)

    c. Fluoxetine (Prozac)

    d. Nifedipine (Procardia)

34. In Fig. 8-94, the soft tissue lesion on the mandibular mucosa erupted suddenly, was filled with a clear fluid, and broke easily. The condition most likely described here is:

    a. Ranula

    b. Mucocele

    c. Fibroma

    d. Fistula

35. Which of the following produce(s) no radiographic image?

    a. Dental caries

    b. Supernumerary teeth

    c. Odontoma

    d. Fibroma

FIG 8-93 Gingival enlargement. (Courtesy of Dr. Victor M. Sternberg; from Ibsen OAC, Phelan JA: *Oral pathology for the dental hygienist,* ed 6, St Louis, 2014, Elsevier.)

FIG 8-94 Soft tissue lesion.

36. Which of the following diagnostic methods is most reliable and ensures the highest degree of accuracy when evaluating squamous cell carcinoma?
    a. Surgical
    b. Microscopic
    c. Therapeutic
    d. Clinical

37. Which of the following does NOT define the term *pathogenesis*?
    a. How the lesion begins
    b. Behavior of the lesion
    c. Clinical picture of the lesion
    d. Development of the lesion

38. A pyogenic granuloma is known to scar down to a(n):
    a. Pregnancy tumor
    b. Fibrogranuloma
    c. Lipoma
    d. Osteoma

39. The patient is a 28-year-old woman who is pregnant. A gingival lesion involving the interproximal papillae between teeth #7 and #8 on the labial surface is bright red, soft, and spongy; it bleeds easily. The histology report shows proliferation of inflammatory cells and thin epithelium. The lesion described is most likely:
    a. Fibroma
    b. Pyogenic granuloma
    c. Redundant tissue
    d. Papilloma

40. Which one of the following cysts has the potential for developing into an ameloblastoma?
    a. Lateral periodontal cyst
    b. Primordial cyst
    c. Stafne bone cyst
    d. Residual cyst

41. The clinical oral examination of the patient reveals a possible leukoplakia. The first course of action should be to:
    a. Perform a scalpel biopsy
    b. Perform a cytologic smear
    c. Give the patient vitamin A therapy
    d. Have the patient return in 2 months to evaluate the growth

42. Which one of the following tests is NOT used for pemphigus?
    a. Pels-Macht
    b. Tzanck
    c. Enzyme-linked immunosorbent assay (ELISA)
    d. Nikolsky sign

43. A palatal condition of an elderly patient that is primarily caused by chronic irritation from the suction chamber of a denture is clinically observed as:
    a. Fibroma
    b. Papilloma
    c. Papillary hyperplasia
    d. Median palatal cyst

44. A lesion found on the buccal mucosa of a 30-year-old white woman is pink, well defined, and soft to palpation. It has been slow growing and histologically consists of collagenous fibers, fibroblasts, and fibrocytes, but with no fat cells or bone. It has a pedunculated base. The lesion is most likely a:
    a. Sarcoma
    b. Fibroma
    c. Fibrolipoma
    d. Fibro-osteoma

45. A radiolucent lesion in the posterior part of the mandible anterior to the angle has the radiographic features of a cyst. After surgical intervention, the histology report shows submaxillary salivary gland tissue; also, the lesion is not lined with epithelium. One may conclude that the lesion is most likely a(n):
    a. Residual cyst
    b. Traumatic bone cyst
    c. Lingual mandibular bone concavity
    d. Ameloblastoma

46. A cyst typically found unilaterally in the floor of the mouth changes size between meals. Clinically, it has a bluish hue. It may be caused by:
    a. Decayed tooth
    b. Blockage or trauma to a major salivary duct
    c. Failure of developmental fusion of the branchial arches
    d. Medications

47. The onset of this chronic, recurring autoimmune disease is at 30 years, with no gender predilection. A triad of symptomatic locations (oral, eye, and genital) is involved, and two of the three areas must be present to make the diagnosis of:
    a. Erythema multiforme
    b. Stevens-Johnson syndrome
    c. Behçet syndrome
    d. Minor aphthous ulcers

48. For which one of the following is the etiology definitely known to be an irritant?
    a. Papilloma
    b. Torus
    c. Granuloma
    d. Lipoma

49. An intraoral examination of the gingiva reveals a clinical picture of punched-out papillae. The patient complains of pain and a bad taste. The history indicates that the patient's diet is poor, that he has been under stress, and that he has had little rest. What is the best course of action for the condition you suspect?
    a. Perform culture and laboratory studies
    b. Apply a therapeutic course, debride the mouth, and recommend hydrogen peroxide oral rinse and possibly systemic antibiotics
    c. Immediately refer the patient to a periodontist
    d. Perform periodontal therapy, including extensive root planing and stain removal

50. Which one of the following is MOST important to the pathologist when a chondroma is suspected?
    a. Complete personal history of the patient
    b. Remove a very small part of the tumor in question
    c. Submission of a "large enough" sample of tissue for histologic study because a chondroma resembles a malignant chondrosarcoma
    d. Radiographs of all large bones

51. The clinical assessment of a patient's lesion is best described as a well-defined, yellowish, blister-like eruption. Straw fluid may be aspirated. It is a rare, benign neoplasm. The histology report shows a predominance of fat cells. The lesion is a(n):
    a. Papilloma
    b. Osteoma
    c. Lipoma
    d. Fibroma

52. A tooth involved in a cyst is discovered to be nonvital on pulp testing. The cyst is probably a:
    a. Residual cyst
    b. Lateral periodontal cyst
    c. Radicular cyst
    d. Dentigerous cyst

53. Which one of the following can be a characteristic of pemphigus vulgaris?
    a. Nikolsky sign
    b. Occurs predominantly in African American females
    c. Is caused by a drug reaction
    d. Occurs predominantly in white males

54. The clinical assessment reveals an inflamed, palpable benign tumor in the anterior of the palate, lingual to the maxillary incisors. The tumor arises from deeper tissue and appears to originate from the periodontal ligament. The radiograph shows the lesion infiltrating bone but no metastasis. The patient is a 35-year-old woman. A possible diagnosis is:
    a. Peripheral giant cell granuloma
    b. Lipoma
    c. Torus palatinus
    d. Pleomorphic adenoma

55. Clinical assessment of a lesion reveals a severe hypersensitivity reaction, with the lips and tongue especially affected. Additionally, "bull's-eye" or "target" skin lesions are present, and the onset of all lesions was abrupt or "explosive." The condition is most likely:
    a. Lichen planus
    b. Herpes
    c. Erythema multiforme
    d. Mononucleosis

56. Which one of the following cysts is the result of extracting a tooth without the cystic sac?
    a. Radicular cyst
    b. Residual cyst
    c. Lateral periodontal cyst
    d. Primordial cyst

57. The dental hygienist observes an adult patient with the following clinical feature and medical history; gingival enlargement resulting from a history of Zimmerman-Laband syndrome and phenytoin (Dilantin) therapy. Which one of the following statements is CORRECT?
    a. The patient should stop taking the drug.
    b. An overgrowth of the connective tissue is present.
    c. The epithelium remains the same.
    d. A gingivectomy would "cure" the condition.

58. Which one of the following diagnostic processes should be applied to establish the diagnosis of nicotine stomatitis?
    a. Surgical and microscopic
    b. Radiographic
    c. Laboratory
    d. Clinical and historical

59. Clinically, this benign white, cauliflower-like lesion usually on the palate is similar to a wart. The histology report indicates long, finger-like projections of stratified squamous epithelium. The etiology is human papillomavirus (HPV) types 6 and 11. What is the most likely condition?
    a. Verruca vulgaris
    b. Papilloma
    c. Aspirin burn
    d. Linea alba

60. In which of the following locations is a lateral periodontal cyst usually found?
    a. Between the roots of mandibular canines and premolars
    b. Between the roots of maxillary central incisors
    c. On the maxillary canine
    d. In the mandibular third molar area

61. A platelet count of 150,000 to 400,000 cells/mm^3 of blood and a normal bleeding time are NOT indicative of:
    a. Thrombocytopenia
    b. Anemia
    c. Leukemia
    d. Nonthrombocytopenic purpura

62. All the following are characteristic of necrotizing ulcerative gingivitis EXCEPT:
    a. Punched-out papillae and craters
    b. Hyperkeratinization
    c. Odor
    d. Pain and bleeding

63. Which of the following makes Behçet's syndrome different from recurrent ulcerative stomatitis?
    a. Bull's-eye skin lesions
    b. Triad of locations of lesions (oral, eye, and genital)
    c. Exudate from lesions
    d. Mesenchymal proliferations

64. What is the causative agent of herpangina?
    a. Chickenpox virus
    b. Coxsackievirus
    c. Epstein-Barr virus
    d. Varicella-zoster virus

65. In treating fibrous dysplasia, which one of the following would NOT be advised, because it can trigger a malignancy?
    a. Radiation
    b. Surgery
    c. Chemotherapy
    d. Bone marrow depressants

66. Precocious puberty is most characteristic of:
    a. Jaffe syndrome
    b. Monostotic fibrous dysplasia
    c. Cherubism
    d. McCune-Albright syndrome

67. Achlorhydria, inability to absorb vitamin B$_{12}$, and burning, painful tongue are characteristics of:
   a. Thrombocytopenia
   b. Hypervitaminosis
   c. Pernicious anemia
   d. Hyperkeratosis

68. Bone marrow anoxia occurs in:
   a. Secondary polycythemia
   b. Pernicious anemia
   c. Thalassemia
   d. Aplastic anemia

69. Which one of the following is referred to as "Cooley anemia"?
   a. Acute anemia
   b. Thalassemia
   c. Primary aplastic anemia
   d. Thrombocytopenia

70. In which of the following cysts are nonvital teeth involved?
   a. Nasoalveolar cyst
   b. Lateral periodontal cyst
   c. Radicular cyst
   d. Cyst of the incisive papilla

71. Which of the following cysts could develop into an ameloblastoma?
   a. Residual cyst
   b. Primordial cyst
   c. Median mandibular cyst
   d. Lateral periodontal cyst

72. A radicular cyst is most often caused by:
   a. Deep restorations
   b. Trauma
   c. Primary occlusal traumatism
   d. Dental caries

73. Epulis fissuratum is caused by:
   a. Denture flange
   b. Suction chamber of a denture
   c. Allergic reaction to acrylic material
   d. Denture cleaners

74. Sickle cell anemia is of hereditary origin and occurs primarily in:
   a. Whites
   b. Native Americans
   c. Eskimo population
   d. African Americans

75. Which one of the following is found in a person with achlorhydria?
   a. Low blood glucose level
   b. Lack of hydrochloric acid
   c. Too much hydrochloric acid
   d. Xerostomia

76. Which one of the following is found in a person with leukopenia?
   a. Decrease in the number of white blood cells
   b. Increase in the number of white blood cells
   c. Decrease in the number of red blood cells
   d. Decrease in the number of platelets

77. Which clinical feature is most associated with bulimia?
   a. Abrasion
   b. Abfraction
   c. Erosion
   d. Attrition

78. Aspirin burn is caused by the misuse of aspirin. It will appear on the buccal mucosa as:
   a. A white lesion with sudden onset
   b. An erythematous lesion with chronic history
   c. A lesion requiring microscopic analysis
   d. An allergic reaction

79. On which location do you normally see thermal burns?
   a. Hard palate
   b. Soft palate
   c. Buccal mucosa
   d. Floor of the mouth

80. Necrotizing sialometaplasia is observed clinically on the:
   a. Palate
   b. Buccal mucosa
   c. Lower lip
   d. Floor of the mouth

81. Which one of the following does not cause gingival enlargement?
   a. Dilantin
   b. Cyclosporine
   c. Acyclovir
   d. Norvasc

82. Pulp polyps are seen clinically:
   a. Within the open crown of a carious tooth
   b. At the apex of a tooth
   c. Between the roots of teeth
   d. On the buccal aspect of alveolar bone

83. Which one of the recurrent aphthous ulcers occurs most often?
   a. Minor aphthous ulcers
   b. Major aphthous ulcers
   c. Sutton Disease
   d. Herpetiform

84. Wickham Striae and desquamative gingivitis are characteristic features of which one of the following:
   a. Erythema multiforme
   b. Cannon disease
   c. Pemphigus
   d. Lichen Planus

85. Which one of the following is not part of the triad of symptoms associated with Reactive Arthritis?
   a. Arthritis
   b. Urethritis
   c. Conjunctivitis
   d. Appendicitis

86. The varicella zoster virus causes which one of the following:
   a. Measles
   b. Mononucleosis
   c. Verruca Vulgaris
   d. Shingles

Microbiology and Immunology

Jessica Peek Scott*

Basic concepts of microbiology and immunology relate to transmissible diseases encountered in client care. Using standard precautions in the dental setting greatly reduces the transmission of pathogens. Dental hygienists must prevent and manage potential occupational exposures from infectious diseases.

GENERAL MICROBIOLOGY

MICROORGANISMS

General Considerations

A. Ubiquitous—found virtually everywhere
B. Only 3% are pathogenic (disease causing); 97% are non-pathogenic
C. Exhibit characteristics common to all biologic systems: reproduction, metabolism, growth, response to stimuli, adaptability, mutation, and organization
D. Medically important microorganisms
  1. Eukaryotes
    a. Protozoa—unicellular, nonphotosynthetic, heterotrophic
    b. Fungi—molds (multi-cellular) or yeast (unicellular)
      (1) Nonphotosynthetic, heterotrophic
      (2) Classified by type of spores produced, presence or absence of mycelia (singular, mycelium), and mechanisms of sexual and asexual spore formation
      (3) Part of the fungi kingdom
      (4) Identification of infection is accomplished clinically and microbiologically
    c. Helminths
      (1) Multi-cellular, nonphotosynthetic, heterotrophic
      (2) Generally, macroparasites of the human alimentary tract or hemolymphatic system
      (3) Part of the animal kingdom
      (4) Identification of infection is accomplished on microbiologic and clinical grounds
  2. Prokaryotes (aerobic or anaerobic unicellular bacteria)
    a. Classified by shape
      (1) Cocci (round)
      (2) Bacilli (rod shaped)
      (3) Vibrio (comma shaped)
      (4) Spirochete (corkscrew shaped)
    b. Classified by Gram staining
      (1) Gram-positive (violet on Gram stain)
      (2) Gram-negative (pink on Gram stain)
    c. Classified into two taxa (singular, taxon):
      (1) Eubacteria—"true" bacteria; most important bacteria in medicine
      (2) Archeobacteria—primitive bacteria; can occupy and inhabit extreme environments
  3. Viruses; classification based on:
    a. Type and properties of nucleic acid
    b. Morphology of nucleoproteins
    c. Presence and properties of envelopes—the *envelope* is the protein coat that protects the capsid and nucleic acid of the virus
  4. Prion
    a. Type of protein found in brain neurons; contains no genetic material
    b. Not bacterial, viral, or fungal
    c. Improper folding and inability to be degraded allows for accumulation and damage to the nervous system
    d. Transmissible (spongiform encephalopathies)
      (1) Creutzfeldt-Jakob disease
      (2) Mad cow disease
    e. Highly resistant to traditional sterilization methods because of the extreme stability of prion proteins
E. Nomenclature—the binomial system
  1. Two-word designation
    a. Genus and species
    b. First word capitalized and both words italicized (e.g., *Escherichia coli*)
  2. Devised by Carolus Linnaeus

Methods of Measurement and Observation

A. Types
  1. Macroscopic—measurable and observable by the naked eye
  2. Microsocopic—too small to be measured or observed by the naked eye; requires a microscope or lens to see

---

*Jessica Peek Scott and the publisher acknowledge the past contributions of Marie Collins to this chapter.

B. Most commonly used units of measurement
   1. Centimeter ($cm = 10^{-2}$ m)
   2. Millimeter ($mm = 10^{-3}$ m)
   3. Micrometer or micron ($\mu m = 10^{-6}$ m)
   4. Nanometer ($nm = 10^{-9}$ m)
   5. Angstrom unit ($\mathring{A} = 10^{-10}$ m)
C. Light microscopes illuminate objects by visible light
   1. Bright-field microscopy
      a. Used to observe the morphology of microorganisms
      b. Used with stained smears
      c. Cannot be used to observe microorganisms less than 0.2 μm, such as viruses and spirochetes
      d. Compound microscopes have at least two lens systems:
         (1) Objective
            (a) Magnifies the specimen and is close to it
            (b) Four powers— $\times 4$, $\times 10$, $\times 40$, and oil immersion ($\times 100$)
         (2) Ocular
            (a) Eyepiece
            (b) Magnifies the image produced by the objective lens
   2. Darkfield microscopy
      a. Specimens seen as bright objects against a dark background
      b. Used for the examination of unstained microorganisms and spirochetes and hanging-drop preparations
      c. Advantage—allows a view of living bacteria not visible by Gram stain; undisturbed in size or shape by fixing and staining techniques
   3. Phase-contrast microscopy
      a. Useful in examining transparent, living cells, including their internal structure, and in determining motility in a fluid medium; can show dense structures
      b. Variations in density between the microbes and the surrounding medium are capitalized on to increase the contrast between the two
   4. Fluorescence microscopy
      a. Used to visualize objects that fluoresce or emit light when exposed to light of different wavelengths
      b. Ultraviolet light, fluorescent chemicals, and special filter systems required
      c. Typically used in the medical field to track antigen-antibody reactions and as a diagnostic technique (immunofluorescence)
   5. Confocal-scanning laser microscopy
      a. A conventional light microscope uses a laser light source to illuminate planes of a fluorochrome-stained specimen
      b. Confocal images combine fluorescent and reflected images
      c. Successive planes are scanned until the entire specimen is scanned
      d. Useful in creating three-dimensional pictures of biofilms
   6. Specimen preparation
      a. Viewing living organisms

(1) Methods
   (a) Hanging drop
   (b) Temporary wet mount
(2) Advantages
   (a) Maintains the shape of organisms
   (b) Is useful to determine organisms' size, shape, motility, and reactions to chemicals or immune sera
b. Staining
   (1) Procedure
      (a) Thin films of microorganisms are spread on a glass slide and allowed to dry (smear)
      (b) Films are fixed, either by a chemical fixative or by passing through a flame; this denatures the proteins and kills the cell
      (c) Dyes or stains are applied to the smear to allow for greater visualization; allows for some differentiation of species
      (d) Fixation process tends to reduce the sizes of cells; dye addition tends to increase the sizes of cells
   (2) Types of dyes
      (a) Acidic, or negative, dye is used to stain basic components of the cell (e.g., glycoproteins, matrix)
      (b) Basic, or positive, dye is used to stain acidic components of the cell (e.g., nucleic acid and polysaccharides)
   (3) Simple staining procedures
      (a) Use a single dye (e.g., carbolfuchsin, crystal violet, methylene blue, or safranin)
      (b) Are used to show shapes, sizes, and arrangements of bacterial cells
   (4) Differential staining procedures (Table 9-1)
      (a) More than one dye preparation used
      (b) Used for initial bacterial grouping
      (c) Most common methods
         [1] Gram stain—differentiates microorganisms based on color as gram-positive (blue to purple) or gram-negative (pink to red); certain characteristics of microorganisms appear correlated with their staining reactions: cell wall thickness, chemical composition, and sensitivity to

TABLE 9-1   **Comparison of Gram-Positive and Gram-Negative Bacteria**

	Gram-Positive Bacteria	Gram-Negative Bacteria
Color after Gram stain procedure	Blue to purple	Pink to red
Peptidoglycan layer in cell walls	Thick	Thin
Teichoic acid in cell walls	Present	Absent
Lipopolysaccharide in cell walls	Absent	Present

penicillin; useful in the diagnosis of infectious diseases

[2] Acid-fast stain—differentiates between acid-fast and non–acid-fast bacteria; differentiates mycobacteria (e.g., *Mycobacterium leprae, M. tuberculosis*) from other bacteria by indicating the presence or absence of special lipids in the cell wall; organisms resist decolorization with an acidic solution of alcohol after being stained with a basic dye

(5) Special staining procedures—used to color and isolate specific parts of microorganisms

    (a) Negative staining for capsules—determines if organism is encapsulated

    (b) Schaeffer-Fulton spore stain (e.g., *Bacillus, Clostridium*)—determines if organism is a spore former

    (c) Flagellar staining—determines if organism has flagella

    (d) Toluidine blue-O staining—determines prions, proteoglycans, and glycosaminoglycans in tissues

D. Electron microscopy

  1. Electrons used as a source of illumination

  2. Higher magnification and better resolving power available than with a light microscope, but because specimens must be dead, dynamic processes cannot be examined

  3. Types

    a. Transmission electron microscope—used to visualize the ultrastructures of cells and viruses

    b. Scanning electron microscope—used to visualize three-dimensional images of surface features of cells and viruses

Prokaryotic (Bacterial) Cell Structure and Function

A. Bacterial morphology

  1. Cocci (singular, coccus)

    a. Spherical or ovoid shape

    b. Occur in pairs (diplococci), chains (streptococci), four-in-a-square arrangement (tetrad), eight cells in a cubic arrangement (sarcinae), and irregular clusters (staphylococci)

  2. Bacilli (singular, bacillus)

    a. Cylindrical or rod-like

    b. Occur in pairs (diplobacilli); chains (streptobacilli); small, rounded rods (coccobacilli); and with tapered ends (fusiform bacilli)

  3. Spirilla (singular, spirillum)

    a. Spiral or curved

    b. Vary in number and fullness of turns

    c. Vibrios are portions of a spiral

  4. Palisade arrangement (bacterial cells form weird angles to one another)

    a. "Fence post" appearance

    b. *Cornynebacterium diphtheriae*

  5. Pleomorphic (no defined cell shape)

    a. Variable in shape

    b. *Mycoplasma pneumoniae*

B. External cell structures

  1. Appendages

    a. Provide motility

      (1) Flagella (singular, flagellum)

        (a) Threads of protein that extend from the cell surface and move in a whip-like motion

        (b) Vectored motility must be distinguished from brownian movement, which is caused by bacteria randomly hitting molecules in the surrounding medium; flagella enable bacteria to move toward favorable environments and away from adverse ones (chemotaxis)

      (2) Axial filaments

    b. Allow for movement—spirochetes (e.g., *Treponema pallidum, Borrelia burgdorferi*) move by this method

    c. Provide attachments

      (1) Pili (singular, pilus)

        (a) Hair-like structures often found on gram-negative bacteria; not associated with motility

        (b) Longer and fewer in number

        (c) Sex pili join bacterial cells in preparation for deoxyribonucleic acid (DNA) transfer (conjugation)

      (2) Fimbriae (singular, fimbria)

        (a) Shorter and numerous

        (b) Enable a cell to adhere to surfaces (e.g., *Neisseria gonorrhoeae, E. coli*)

  2. Surface coating (glycocalyx)

    a. Capsules

      (1) Condensed and well-defined masses of polysaccharides or polypeptides firmly attached to the cell wall

      (2) Encapsulation protects pathogenic organisms from drugs, phagocytosis, and bactericidal factors

      (3) Some bacteria need capsules to maintain virulence (e.g., *Streptococcus pneumoniae, Streptococcus mutans*)

    b. Slime layer (glycocalyx)

      (1) Unorganized, soluble mass of polysaccharides or polypeptides loosely attached to the cell wall; polymeric material (glycoprotein)

      (2) Protects microorganisms; aids in adherence and gliding motility of organism

  3. Cell wall

    a. Functions

      (1) Determines and maintains the shape of the microorganism

      (2) Provides support for flagella

      (3) Prevents rupture of the cell resulting from osmotic pressure differences on either side of the cell wall

    b. Composed of the macromolecule peptidoglycan

    c. Comparison of gram-negative and gram-positive cell walls

      (1) Gram-positive cell walls consist of many layers of peptidoglycan and contain teichoic acids

(2) Gram-negative bacteria have a lipoprotein-lipopolysaccharide-phospholipid outer membrane surrounding a thin, peptidoglycan layer

(3) Outer membrane protects gram-negative cells from phagocytosis, penicillin, lysozymes, and other chemicals

(4) Gram-negative cell walls are more easily broken by mechanical forces; susceptible to lysis by antibody, complement, and streptomycin

4. Cytoplasmic (plasma) membrane
   a. Structure—consists of a phospholipid bilayer interspersed with proteins in a mosaic pattern (fluid mosaic)
   b. Functions
      (1) Barrier that regulates movement of materials in and out of the cell
      (2) Active transport
      (3) Excretion of hydrolytic exoenzymes
      (4) Bears enzymes and carrier molecules
      (5) Bears receptors and other proteins of the chemotactic and other sensory transduction systems
   c. Lies adjacent to and beneath the cell wall and encloses the cytoplasm of the cell

5. Cell envelope
   a. Includes all external structures and appendages, including the capsule, pili, flagella, cell wall, and cytoplasmic membrane
   b. May play a role in protection from degradation, maintenance of cell shape, and cell adhesion
   c. Properties confer staining characteristics
   d. Organization and structure different in gram-positive and gram-negative bacteria

C. Internal cell structure
1. Cytoplasm (protoplasm)
   a. Fluid compartment inside the cytoplasmic membrane
   b. Prominent site for many of the cell's biochemical and synthetic activities
   c. Contains chromatin body, ribosomes, and granules
2. Mesosomes—irregular folds of the cytoplasmic membrane resulting from dehydration of cells in preparation for electron microscopy; considered artifacts
3. Genetic material or genome (nucleoid)
   a. Prokaryotes lack the distinct nucleus of eukaryotes
   b. Single chromosome is composed of a single molecule of DNA, existing as a closed loop not enclosed by the nuclear membrane; located in the nucleoplasm of the cell
   c. Additional genetic material is found in plasmids, which are extrachromosomal DNA molecules; they often carry information that determines drug resistance or sensitivity
4. Ribosomes
   a. Function in protein synthesis
   b. Composed of ribosomal protein and ribosomal ribonucleic acid (RNA)
   c. Distributed throughout the cytoplasm
5. Photosynthetic apparatus
6. Inclusions
   a. Accumulations of reserve storage materials

b. Include polysaccharide granules, metachromatic granules, sulfur granules, lipid inclusions, carboxysomes, and gas vacuoles

D. Endospores (spores)
1. Dormant structures formed within gram-positive bacterial cells as a means of survival
2. Formed during a process called *sporulation*—disintegration of parent cell releases endospore; then called *exposure* or *free spore*
3. Can remain in a spore state for years; exhibit unusual resistance to heat, drying, chemical disinfection, and radiation
4. Can transform back into a vegetative cell through a process called *germination*
5. Ability of bacteria to produce endospores restricted mainly to the genera *Bacillus* and *Clostridium*

Eukaryotic Cell Structure and Function

See Tables 9-2 and 9-3.
A. More complex than a prokaryotic cell; has a distinct nucleus bounded by a nuclear membrane, a nucleolus, and membrane-bound organelles
B. Animal cells
1. Cell membrane
   a. Surrounds the cell and interconnects with the cell's internal membrane systems
   b. Functions
      (1) Regulates the passage of substances in and out of the cell through active and passive transport
      (2) Involved in phagocytosis, tumor formation, drug sensitivity, and immune response
2. Nucleus
   a. Controls the cell's physiologic and reproductive processes
   b. Composition
      (1) Nuclear membrane
      (2) Nucleoli (involved in RNA synthesis)
      (3) Chromosomes (composed of DNA)
      (4) Nucleoprotein (chromatin)
3. Internal structures
   a. Mitochondria are sites of adenosine triphosphate (ATP), or energy, production
   b. Endoplasmic reticulum
      (1) Network of membranes involved in chemical reactions, storage, and transportation
      (2) Rough endoplasmic reticulum has ribosomes attached
   c. Golgi complex—storage and packaging structure for cellular components
   d. Lysosomes—contain digestive enzymes
   e. Microtubules
   f. Vacuoles

Microbial Growth and Cultivation

See Fig. 9-1.
A. Definitions
1. Culture media—nutrient preparations used to cultivate microorganisms

TABLE 9-2 Eukaryotic Organelles and Their Functions

Cell Part or Organelle	Associated Functions and Activities
Cell membrane	Transport of substances into and out of cells (selective permeability)
	In some cells, engulfment of foreign material (phagocytosis)
	Pinocytosis
Cell wall	Found only in plants and certain bacteria; imparts shape and strength to the cell
	Protection against certain osmotic imbalances
Centrioles	Involved in cell division
Chloroplast	Photosynthesis
Cilium	Motion, or movement of substances, past the ciliated cell
Endoplasmic reticulum	Protein synthesis
	Transport of nutrients to the nucleus
Flagellum and cilium	Propulsion
Golgi complex	Transfer of proteins and other cellular components to exterior of a secretory cell
	Storage and packing structure for cellular products
Lysosomes	Contain lysozymes and other digestive enzymes
	Break down foreign material and worn out cell parts
Microbody, or peroxisome	Enzymatic activities
Microtubule	Cell transport
	Development and maintenance of cell shape
	Cell division
	Ciliary and flagellar movement
Mitochondrion	Synthesis of the energy-rich compound adenosine triphosphate (ATP)
Nucleolus	Major site for the formation of ribosomal components
Nucleus	Control of cellular physiologic process
	Contains chromosomes
	Transfer of hereditary factors to subsequent generations
Plastids	Contain photosynthetic pigments
	Sites of photosynthesis
	Found in plant cells
Ribosome	Protein synthesis
	Attach to outer surface of rough endoplasmic reticulum
Vacuoles	Locations of water
	Storage site for certain amino acids, carbohydrates, and proteins
	Dumping ground for cellular wastes

TABLE 9-3 Major Characteristics of Eukaryotes and Prokaryotes

	EUKARYOTES		
Characteristic	Plants	Animals	Prokaryotes
Major groups	Plants, algae, fungi	Animals, protozoa	Bacteria
Size (approximate)	>5 μm	>5 μm	1 to 3 μm
Nuclear structures			
Nucleus	Classic membrane	Classic membrane	No nuclear membrane
Chromosomes	Strands of deoxyribonucleic acid (DNA) and protein	Strands of DNA and protein	Single, closed strand of DNA
Cytoplasmic structures			
Mitochondria	Present	Present	Absent
Golgi complex	Present	Present	Absent
Endoplasmic reticulum	Present	Present	Absent
Ribosomes (sedimentation coefficient)	80S	80S	70S
Cytoplasmic membrane	Contains sterols	Contains sterols	Does not contain sterols
Cell wall	Composed of cellulose or chitin	Absent	Complex structure containing protein, lipids, and peptidoglycans
Reproduction movement	Sexual or asexual	Sexual or asexual	Asexual (binary fission)
	Flagella or cilia (complex and similar to centrioles)	Flagella or cilia (complex and similar to centrioles)	Flagella, if present, are simple twisted proteins (no cilia)
Respiration	Via mitochondria	Via mitochondria	Via cytoplasmic membrane
Photosynthesis	Present (absent in fungi)	Absent	Present in cyanobacteria and some others

FIG 9-1 Bacterial production.

2. In vitro techniques—procedures using nonliving materials in a culture vessel
3. In vivo techniques—procedures using living cells or entire animals or plants
4. Colony—accumulation of bacteria on a medium

B. Conditions that affect growth
1. Physical
   a. Thermal conditions
      (1) Most bacteria grow best over a range of temperatures
         (a) Psychrophiles—0°C to 15°C
         (b) Mesophiles—20°C to 40°C
         (c) Thermophiles—45°C to 60°C
      (2) 30°C is the optimal temperature for many free-living organisms
   b. Acidity or alkalinity (pH)—most bacteria prefer a neutral pH, between 7.0 and 7.4
      (1) Acidophiles—pH 0 to 4
      (2) Neutrophiles—pH 5 to 9
      (3) Alkalinophiles—pH greater than 9
   c. Osmotic pressure
      (1) Most microorganisms must be grown in an aquatic medium
      (2) Halophilic organisms require high salt concentration
      (3) Osmophilic organisms require high osmotic pressure
2. Chemical
   a. Gaseous requirements
      (1) Aerobes require oxygen
      (2) Micro-aerophilic organisms require low concentrations of oxygen
      (3) Anaerobes do not require oxygen
      (4) Obligate (strict) anaerobes cannot tolerate any free oxygen
      (5) Facultative anaerobes can metabolize aerobically if oxygen is present or anaerobically if it is absent
      (6) Aerotolerant anaerobes metabolize substances anaerobically but are not harmed by oxygen
   b. Nutrition available

      (1) Heterotrophic organisms
         (a) Require organic compounds for growth; obtain carbon from glucose
         (b) Most often cultured on a medium of glucose
      (2) Autotrophic organisms
         (a) Do not require organic nutrients for growth
         (b) Use inorganic compounds such as carbon dioxide
         (c) Thrive in soils and bodies of water
      (3) Hypotrophic organisms
         (a) Obligate intracellular parasites; grow only within a living host cell
         (b) Include viruses and rickettsiae
      (4) Phototrophic organisms
         (a) Use light for energy
      (5) Chemotrophic organisms
         (a) Oxidize chemical compounds for energy
      (6) Nutrients needed include sulfur and phosphorus
      (7) Nitrogen is derived from proteins and their products
      (8) Certain vitamins and growth factors required

C. Types of culture media
1. Synthetic defined media—exact chemical composition is known
2. Rich complex media—exact chemical composition varies slightly from batch to batch (e.g., addition of blood or beef extract); contain digested extracts from animal organs, meats, fish, yeasts, and plants
3. Differential media
   a. Contain combinations of nutrients and pH indicators to produce visual differentiation between several microorganisms
   b. Examples
      (1) Blood agar is an enriched medium that allows streptococci to leave different signs on the medium; green discoloration around colonies indicates α-hemolytic streptococci, clear zone signifies β-hemolysis, and no effect denotes γ-hemolysis
      (2) Chocolate agar is even more enriched than blood agar
4. Selective media
   a. Allow interference with or prevention of the growth of certain microorganisms while permitting others to grow
   b. Dyes and antibiotics make the media selective
   c. Examples
      (1) Sabouraud dextrose agar is selective for fungi
      (2) Thayer-Martin agar is selective for *Neisseria gonorrhoeae*
5. Selective and differential media
   a. Combine properties of the preceding two types of media
   b. Examples—mannitol, salt agar, and MacConkey agar
6. Enriched media—similar to selective media but designed to increase the numbers of particular microbes to detectable levels

7. Reducing media
   a. Contain ingredients that chemically combine with and deplete oxygen in the culture medium
   b. Used for anaerobes
D. Pure culture techniques
   1. Used to isolate and identify a bacterial species
   2. Methods
      a. Pour-plate technique
         (1) Cool the melted agar-containing medium
         (2) Inoculate the medium
            (a) Use the loop or needle to transfer the organism
            (b) Pass the loop through the flame and heat to redness
            (c) Flame the edges of tubes from which cultures are taken before and after removal of the organism
         (3) Pour the inoculated medium into a sterile Petri dish
         (4) Allow the medium to solidify
         (5) Incubate at the desired temperature
      b. Streak-plate technique
         (1) Spread a loopful of material containing organisms over the surface of the solidified agar
         (2) Various streaking directions or patterns are possible
E. Bacterial growth
   1. Most bacteria reproduce through binary fission (i.e., two new cells are produced by one parent cell)
   2. Growth on the culture medium
      a. Typical growth curve results
      b. Phases
         (1) Lag phase—period of intense metabolic activity but no increase in cell number
         (2) Log phase or exponential growth phase—cell number increases in an exponential manner; generation time is the average time for the cell to divide; phase when cells are most metabolically active
         (3) Stationary phase—total number of viable cells is constant; metabolic activity slows
         (4) Phase of decline (death phase)—number of viable cells decreases
   3. Measurement of growth
      a. Population growth curve—made by observing an increase in mass or numbers over time
      b. Cell mass can be measured by dry weight, chemical analysis, and turbidity
      c. Population counts—cell numbers can be measured by viable platelet counts; estimates are expressed as colony-forming units (CFU) for bacteria or plaque-forming units (PFU) for viruses

Microbial Metabolism and Cell Regulation

A. Metabolism
   1. Definition—set of chemical reactions by which cells maintain life

2. Phases
   a. Anabolism—biosynthetic reactions that use energy (ATP)
      (1) Energy-consuming phase in which macromolecules such as nucleic acids, proteins, lipids, and polysaccharides are synthesized
   b. Catabolism—degradative reactions that release energy (ATP)
      (1) Energy-releasing phase in which complex compounds are broken down, creating energy in the form of ATP
3. Energy storage and transfer
   a. Chemical energy is stored as ATP
   b. May be generated through the transport of electrons (electron transport system)
   c. Energy produced through oxidation-reduction reactions
      (1) Aerobic oxidation (respiration)
      (2) Anaerobic oxidation (fermentation)
4. Metabolic pathways
   a. Series of steps to complete biochemical process
   b. Glycolytic pathway (glycolysis)
      (1) Most important way carbohydrates are metabolized
      (2) Converts glucose to pyruvic acid
      (3) Anaerobic fermentation process
      (4) Tricarboxylic acid (Krebs) cycle
   c. Occurs inside mitochondria
      (1) Follows the glycolytic pathway
      (2) Responsible for further oxidation of glucose and the production of other biochemically important intermediates
      (3) Important to aerobic bacteria
5. Protein synthesis
   a. DNA directs the formation of proteins aided by various types of RNA
   b. Transcription—synthesis of messenger RNA (mRNA) from a DNA template
   c. Translation—synthesis of protein from an mRNA template
   d. Three stages of protein synthesis occurring at the ribosome:
      (1) Initiation
      (2) Elongation
      (3) Termination
B. Metabolic control
   1. Largely by enzymatic control
   2. Types of regulation
      a. Feedback inhibition
         (1) Allosteric enzymes—end product binds to the enzyme and lowers its affinity for its substrate, thus preventing further product formation
         (2) When more end product is needed, the enzyme is released
      b. Genetic regulation—regulated by a specific unit of DNA called an *operon*
         (1) Enzyme repression—when the level of end product is sufficient, the genetic synthesis of the enzyme is suppressed

(2) Enzyme induction—enzymes are genetically synthesized only when substrates are present

Microbial Genetics

A. Eukaryotic genome
   1. Almost all the eukaryotic genome is diploid
   2. Gene expression can be recessive or dominant
   3. Mitochondria and chloroplasts have a single, circular DNA; function of DNA is related to that organelle
B. Prokaryotic genome
   1. Most prokaryotes have a single, circular chromosome
   2. Additional genes are present on plasmids (small circles of DNA)
C. Some viruses (phage) multiply in bacteria
D. Genetic recombination (see the section on "Genetics" in Chapter 7)
   1. Conjugation
      a. Transfer of genetic material between two living bacteria that are in physical contact
      b. Plasmids are most frequently transferred
   2. Transduction—a bacterial virus (bacteriophage) transfers genetic material
   3. Transformation—the direct uptake of donor DNA by a recipient cell
E. Genetic rearrangement—*transposons* are small segments of DNA that can move from one region of a chromosome to another region of the genome
F. Mutations
   1. Result in changes in DNA sequence
   2. Can be caused by agents such as ultraviolet light, radiation, nitrous acid, and carcinogens

Microbial Relationships

A. Syntrophism
   1. Organisms are not intimately associated with each other but benefit from each other
   2. Examples—yogurt production, organisms feeding in soil where decaying plant material is found
B. Competition
   1. Interaction between organisms resulting from a demand for a finite supply of nutrients and other resources
   2. Example—molds such as *Penicillium* compete by secreting substances toxic to other organisms
C. Predation—interaction that controls the population by predators feeding on another species, the prey
D. Symbiosis—interaction in which two different species live in a mutually beneficial coexistence
E. Commensalism—interaction in which only one organism benefits and the other neither benefits nor is harmed
F. Parasitism—interaction in which one organism benefits at the expense of the other

Bacteria

A. Firmicutes—gram-positive eubacteria
B. Gracilicutes
   1. Gram-negative eubacteria
   2. Largest group of bacteria
   3. Contain many medically significant microorganisms
C. Tenericutes (mycoplasmas)
   1. Eubacteria lacking cell walls—because they lack cell walls, they are highly pleomorphic
   2. Enclosed by the plasma membrane—plasma membranes have lipids called *sterols* that aid in resisting lysis
   3. Mycoplasmas are the smallest self-replicating microorganisms
D. Mendosicutes (archaeobacteria)
   1. Conventional peptidoglycan in the cell wall is replaced with pseudomurein
   2. Often live in extreme environments
   3. Carry out atypical metabolic processes
   4. No known medically significant species

Fungi

A. Description
   1. Eukaryotic
   2. Nonphotosynthetic
   3. Heterotrophic saprophytes—use preexisting organic products, either living or dead
   4. Grow well in dark, moist environments
   5. Few species are pathogenic to humans
B. Forms
   1. Molds (mycelial forms)
      a. Long filaments are structural units called *hyphae*; multi-cellular hyphae result in a cobweb-like growth called a *mycelium*
      b. Reproduce by sexual or asexual spores
   2. Yeasts
      a. Oval or spherical single cells
      b. Produce moist, shiny colonies
      c. Reproduce asexually by producing new buds or daughter cells
   3. Dimorphic fungi—some fungi exhibit characteristics of both molds and yeasts, depending on growth conditions
C. Classification of medically important fungi
   1. Zygomycota (the phycomyces)—include the common bread molds *Rhizopus* and *Mucor*
   2. Ascomycota (sac fungi)—include *Histoplasma, Microsporum, Aspergillus, Trichophyton, Penicillium* (a source of antibiotics), and *Saccharomyces* (leavened bread and fermented beer and wine)
   3. Basidiomycota—include *Cryptococcus neoformans*
   4. Deuteromycota (the imperfect fungi)—include *Candida, Pneumocystis, Coccidioides, Sporothrix,* and *Epidermophyton*; do not produce sexual spores
D. Fungal diseases (mycoses)
   1. Generally long-lasting infections
   2. Classification
      a. Systemic—involving a number of tissues and organs
      b. Subcutaneous—beneath the skin
      c. Cutaneous (superficial)—involving only the epidermis, hair, and nails
         (1) Tinea infections caused by *Microsporum, Trichophyton,* and *Epidermophyton*

d. Opportunistic—generally harmless; can become pathogenic in a debilitated host

Protozoa

A. Description
1. Unicellular
2. Eukaryotic
3. Heterotrophic
4. Most have a motile feeding stage called *trophozoite*
5. Many can form cysts
   a. Protective resting stage
   b. Can serve as a site for division or spreading of pathogenic protozoans (e.g., *Entamoeba histolytica,* which causes amoebic dysentery)
6. Reproduce asexually by fission, budding, or schizogony (multiple fission); reproduce sexually by conjugation

B. Four phyla (Sarcomastigophora, Mastigophora, Ciliophora, Microspora)

Viruses

A. Properties of a mature virus particle, or virion
1. Has a single type of nucleic acid, RNA or DNA, that contains genetic material, or a genome
2. Nucleic acid is surrounded by an outer protein coat, the capsid; nucleic acid and capsid compose the nucleocapsid
3. Capsids may or may not be covered by an envelope
4. Viral nucleic acid contains the necessary information for programming an infected host cell
5. Absence of cellular structures
6. Lack components for energy production and protein synthesis
7. Obligate intracellular parasites

B. Bacteriophages (bacterial viruses)
1. Contain either RNA or DNA
2. Life cycles: lytic and lysogenic
   a. Lytic cycle—virus enters a host cell, takes over cell replication mechanism, makes viral DNA and protein, then lyses (breaks open) the cell; this allows newly produced viruses to leave host cell and infect other cells (destroys host cell)
   b. Lysogenic cycle—virus attaches to host cell's DNA and replicates when host cell divides; once integrated, the virus is referred to as a *prophage,* and a stable association is established between the host cell and the virus (no harm done to host cell)

C. Plant viruses (most contain RNA)—viroids
1. Small, single-stranded, circular RNA molecules
2. Found mainly in plants

D. Human viruses (Table 9-4)
1. Classified by structure and type of nucleic acid, mode of replication, and morphology
2. Destructive effects on cells are termed *cytopathic*
3. Prions

TABLE 9-4   Selected Important Groups of Viruses and Viral Diseases

Virus Type	Viral Characteristics	Virus	Disease
Poxviruses	Large brick shape with envelope, double-stranded (ds) segment of deoxyribonucleic acid (DNA)	Variola	Smallpox
		Vaccinia	Cowpox
Polyoma-papilloma	Polyhedral, ds DNA	Papillomavirus	Warts
		Polyomavirus	Some tumors, some cancers
Herpesvirus	Polyhedral with envelope, ds DNA	Herpes simplex 1	Cold sores or fever blisters
		Herpes simplex 2	Genital herpes
		Herpes zoster	Shingles
		Varicella	Chickenpox
Adenovirus	Icosahedral, with envelope, ds DNA		Respiratory infections, pneumonia, conjunctivitis, some tumors
Picornaviruses (means "small ribonucleic acid [RNA] viruses")	Tiny icosahedral, with envelope, single-stranded (ss) RNA	Rhinovirus	Colds
		Poliovirus	Poliomyelitis
		Hepatitis types A and B	Hepatitis
		Coxsackievirus	Respiratory infections, meningitis
Reoviruses	Icosahedral, with envelope, ds RNA	Enterovirus	Intestinal infections
Myxoviruses	Helical with envelope, RNA	Orthomyxoviruses types A and B	Influenza
		Myxovirus parotidis	Mumps
		Paramyxovirus	Measles (rubeola)
		Rhabdovirus	Rabies
Arbovirus	Cubic, arthropod-borne RNA	Mosquito-borne type B	Yellow fever
		Mosquito-borne type A and B	Encephalitis (many types)
		Tick-borne coronavirus	Colorado tick fever
Retrovirus	Helical with envelope, ds RNA	RNA tumor virus	Tumors
		Human T lymphotropic virus (HTLV)	Leukemia
		Human immunodeficiency virus (HIV)	Acquired immunodeficiency syndrome (AIDS)

From Burton GRW, Engelkirk PG: *Microbiology for the health sciences,* ed 7, Philadelphia, 2004, Lippincott, Williams & Wilkins.

a. Proteinaceous infectious particles believed to cause kuru and Creutzfeldt-Jakob disease (CJD)

b. Organization, replication, and how they cause disease are unknown

E. Viral replication

1. Uses biosynthetic mechanisms of the host cell

2. Phases

   a. Attachment, penetration, and uncoating

   b. Synthesis of viral components

   c. Morphogenesis and release

F. Modes of viral transmission

1. Direct transmission from person to person

2. Transmission from animal to animal

3. Transmission by an arthropod vector

G. Role of virus in cancer

1. Oncogenous viruses can induce various types of cancers (RNA-type or DNA-type viruses)

2. Proto-oncogenes are highly conserved, "friendly" transforming genes

3. Mechanisms of oncogene activation

   a. Transduction by a virus

   b. Insertional mutagenesis

   c. Translocation

   d. Gene amplification

   e. Mutation

4. Role oncogenes play in the development of cancer is unclear

MICROBIAL VIRULENCE AND DISEASE TRANSFER

A. Bacteria that produce disease or pathologic changes in humans (Table 9-5)

B. Definitions

1. Pathogen—agent producing disease or pathologic changes

2. Opportunist—commensal bacterium that invades the host under favorable conditions

3. Virulence—the degree of pathogenicity; properties that determine pathogenicity of an organism include invasiveness (transmissibility), ability to multiply in the host, and toxin production

4. Infection—invasion of the tissue by a pathogenic microorganism and multiplication of the organism

   a. Localized—organism remains in a particular area of the body

   b. Generalized or systemic—microorganism invades the bloodstream and the lymphatic system

   c. Acute—runs a rapid course; terminates abruptly (less than 6 months)

   d. Chronic—slow onset; infection of long duration

   e. Primary—original infection

   f. Secondary—infection that follows a primary infection and is often caused by an opportunistic organism

   g. Toxemia—presence of toxin in the blood

   h. Subclinical—lacking recognizable symptoms

   i. Focal—localized in one area and spreading elsewhere in the body from that point

   j. Bacteremia—presence of bacteria in the bloodstream

   k. Latent—causative agent remains inactive for a time but then becomes active to produce symptoms of the disease

   l. Sequelae—long-term or permanent damage to diseased tissues or organs

   m. Nosocomial—acquired during a hospital stay

   n. Sign—objective changes that a health care provider can observe and measure

   o. Symptom—subjective changes in body experienced by the patient or client

5. Infectious disease—interference with the normal functioning of the host; proof by Koch's postulates:

   a. Microorganisms are present in every case of disease

   b. Microorganisms grow in pure culture from the diseased host

   c. Same disease is reproduced when pure culture is inoculated into a healthy host

   d. Microorganism is recovered from the inoculated host

C. Transmission of disease

1. Reservoir of infection—contains potential sources of the disease-causing agent

   a. Human

      (1) Active cases of infectious disease

      (2) Carriers—persons (asymptomatic) harboring infectious agents potentially pathogenic for other members of the population

      (3) Endogenous infection—the causative organism is derived from the host's own microflora

   b. Animal—zoonosis; disease transmitted from animal to human

   c. Insects and arthropods—flies, mosquitoes, fleas, lice, ticks, and mites

   d. Nonliving—water, food, soil, and dust

2. Portals of exit are sources of infectious body fluids

   a. Gastrointestinal (GI) tract

   b. Genitourinary system

   c. Oral region

   d. Respiratory tract

   e. Blood and blood derivatives

   f. Skin lesions

   g. Conjunctiva

3. Routes of transmission

   a. Contact

      (1) Direct

      (2) Indirect—involves nonliving reservoir (fomite)

      (3) Droplet transmission (short distance)

   b. Vehicles

      (1) Waterborne transmission

      (2) Foodborne transmission

      (3) Airborne transmission

   c. Vectors—insects and arthropods

4. Basic path of an infectious disease

   a. Exposure to the pathogen

   b. Incubation period

   c. Prodromal period

TABLE 9-5 Bacteria of Human Importance

Organism	Diseases	Other Features
Gram-Positive Cocci		
Staphylococcus aureus	Boils, carbuncles, septicemia, food poisoning, pneumonia	Common skin commensal; phage typing identifies virulent strains; enterotoxin causes food poisoning
Streptococcus pyogenes	Tonsillitis, scarlet fever, erysipelas, septicemia, strep throat, rheumatic fever	Also causes glomerulonephritis and rheumatic fever, with immunopathologic basis
Streptococcus viridans group (Streptococcus sanguis, etc.)	Infective endocarditis	Oral commensals settle on abnormal heart valves during bacteremia
Streptococcus mutans	Dental caries	Regular inhabitant of mouth; initiates plaque on tooth surface
Streptococcus pneumoniae	Pneumonia, otitis, meningitis	Normal upper respiratory tract commensal; can spread to infected or damaged lungs
Gram-Negative Cocci		
Neisseria gonorrhoeae	Gonorrhea	Obligate human parasite
Neisseria meningitidis	Meningitis, nasopharyngitis	Obligate human parasite; increased upper respiratory carriage in epidemics
Gram-Positive Bacilli		
Corynebacterium diphtheriae	Diphtheria	Natural host humans; noninvasive disease caused by toxin
Bacillus anthracis	Anthrax	Pathogen of herbivorous animals that ingest spores; occasional human infection
Clostridium spp.	Tetanus, gas gangrene, botulism	Widely distributed in soil and intestines
Gram-Negative Bacilli		
Escherichia coli	Urinary tract infections, infantile gastroenteritis	Normal intestinal inhabitant (humans and animals); many antigenic types
Salmonella spp.	Enteric fever, food poisoning, gastroenteritis	Salmonella typhi—natural host is humans; invasive Other Salmonella—1000 species, mainly animal pathogens
Shigella spp.	Bacillary dysentery (shigellosis)	Obligate parasites of humans; local invasion only
Proteus spp.	Urinary tract infection, gastroenteritis, wound infection	Common in soil, feces; occasionally pathogenic
Klebsiella spp.	Urinary tract and wound infection, otitis, meningitis, pneumonia	Present in vegetation, soil, sometimes feces; pathogenic when host resistance lowered
Pseudomonas aeruginosa	Urinary tract, respiratory and wound infection	Common human intestinal bacteria; resists many antibiotics
Haemophilus influenzae	Pneumonia, meningitis	Human commensal; invades damaged lung
Bordetella pertussis	Whooping cough	Specialized human respiratory parasite
Yersinia pestis	Plague	Flea-borne pathogen of rodents; transfer to humans as greatest infection in history
Brucella spp.	Undulant fever, brucellosis	Pathogens of goats, cattle, and pigs with secondary human infection
Acid-Fast Bacilli		
Mycobacterium tuberculosis	Tuberculosis	Chronic respiratory infection in humans; 10 to 15 million active cases in the world; enteric infection with bovine type via milk
Mycobacterium leprae	Leprosy (Hansen's disease)	Obligate parasite of humans; attacks skin, nasal mucosa, and nerves; 15 million people with leprosy in the world
Miscellaneous		
Vibrio cholerae	Cholera	Obligate parasite of humans; noninvasive intestinal infection
Treponema pallidum	Syphilis	Obligate human parasite; sexual transmission; related nonvenereal human bacteria
Actinomyces israelii	Actinomycosis	Normal inhabitant of the human mouth
Leptospira spp.	Leptospirosis (Weil's disease, etc.)	Mostly pathogens of animals; human infection from urine of rats, etc.
Legionella pneumophila	Legionnaires disease	Respiratory pathogen of humans, often acquired from contaminated air-conditioning units

d. Appearance of the signs and symptoms of the disease

e. Outcome of the disease (e.g., convalescence, disability, or death)

Microbial Virulence Factors

A. Capsules (Streptococcus pneumoniae)—resist the host's defenses by impairing phagocytosis

B. Enzyme production—includes coagulases, kinases, hyaluronidases, collagenases, mucinases, lecithinases, leukocidins, and hemolysins

C. Toxin production

1. Exotoxins

a. Soluble substances secreted by gram-positive bacteria

b. Clinically significant exotoxins are associated with botulism, tetanus, diphtheria, gas gangrene, scarlet fever, staphylococcal food poisoning, toxic shock syndrome, and traveler's diarrhea

2. Endotoxins
   a. Heat-stable lipopolysaccharides—toxic component associated with cell wall
   b. From gram-negative bacteria
   c. Pathologic effects
      (1) Fever
      (2) Interference with hemostatic mechanisms of blood
      (3) Activation of the complement system
      (4) Leukopenia
      (5) Hypotension and shock
      (6) Organ dysfunction
      (7) Activation of complement system
      (8) Death

Disease Barriers

A. Normal or indigenous flora
   1. Most highly specialized bacteria; highly adapted to commensal life; cause minimal damage under normal conditions
   2. Includes beneficial microorganisms and pathogens
   3. When ecologic balance is disturbed, infection can occur (e.g., antibiotic therapy may result in *Candida albicans* infection)
B. Nonspecific immunity
   1. Physical and chemical barriers
      a. Intact skin
      b. Mucous membranes and their secretions
      c. Gastric acid barrier
   2. Blood and lymphatics
      a. Leukocytes—proportionate number changes in response to infection
         (1) Granulocytes (basophils, eosinophils, and neutrophils [polymorphonuclear leukocytes])
         (2) Agranulocytes (lymphocytes and monocytes)
      b. Lymphatic system transports white blood cells and removes foreign cells and tissue debris
         (1) Consists of lymphatic vessels, lymph fluid, nodes, and lymphocytes
         (2) Mononuclear phagocyte system—mononuclear phagocytic cells that remove particulate matter from bloodstream and lymph (e.g., Kupffer cells in the liver)
   3. Phagocytosis
      a. Digestion of the invading matter
      b. Accomplished by neutrophils and mature monocytes, or macrophages
   4. Inflammation
      a. Produced by disease agents or irritants such as chemicals, heat, or mechanical injury
      b. Cardinal signs include heat, pain, redness, swelling, and loss of function
      c. Pus formation possible
   5. Fever
      a. Bacterial endotoxins and interleukin-1 (IL-1) can induce fever

b. Intensifies the effect of interferon (IFN)
c. Inhibits the growth of some microorganisms

6. Antimicrobial substances
   a. Complement system—a defense system consisting of serum proteins that participate in lysis of foreign cells, inflammation, and phagocytosis
   b. Interferons (IFN-α, -β, and -γ)—interfere with viral replication

C. Specific immunity—the immune system (Fig. 9-2 and Box 9-1)
   1. Humoral immunity—B lymphocyte production and release of specific antibodies into the circulating blood or body fluids; antibodies then interact with foreign antigens; defends primarily against bacteria, toxins, and viruses; antibodies protect the host as follows:
      a. Recognize an organism or its toxin by binding to it
      b. Opsonize or coat bacteria, which enhances ingestion by macrophages or natural killer (NK) cells
      c. Cause antigens to clump or agglutinate, which enhances phagocytosis
      d. Activate complement system, resulting in cell lysis
   2. Cell-mediated (cellular) immunity—stimulation of T lymphocytes to activate a variety of effector T cells in response to foreign organisms or tissues (antigens); defends primarily against bacteria, viruses, fungi, protozoa, helminths, foreign tissue, and cancerous cells
   3. Acquired immunity
      a. Natural
         (1) Active—person is exposed to an antigen and the body produces antibodies
         (2) Passive—antibodies of a mother are passed to her infant
      b. Artificial
         (1) Active—vaccination with killed, inactivated, or attenuated microorganisms or toxoid
         (2) Passive—injection of immune serum or γ-globulin
D. Hypersensitivity or allergy is an exaggerated response to specific substances; the inciting agent is the allergen (Fig. 9-3; see Box 9-1)

Immunodeficiency

See the section on "Human Immunodeficiency Virus" in Chapter 8.
A. Inability of the immune system to perform normally; properly functioning system recognizes and destroys all that is foreign or "non-self"
B. Results in increased susceptibility to infection
C. Autoimmune disease (autoallergic)
   1. "Self" antigens stimulate the production of antibodies or sensitized lymphocytes; antigen-antibody complex
   2. Mechanisms
      a. May be caused by the release of sequestered antigens; escape of tolerance to the "self" antigen at the T cell level; diminished suppressor T cell function
      b. Intolerance of self antigen because of cross-reactions
      c. Decreased function of suppressor T cells
   3. Includes systemic lupus erythematosus, rheumatoid arthritis, myasthenia gravis, and Graves disease

FIG 9-2 The duality of the immune system. *Left,* Humoral immunity mediated by soluble antibody proteins produced by B lymphocytes. *Right,* Cellular immunity mediated by T lymphocytes. (Modified from Kumar V, Cotran R, Robbins S: *Basic pathology,* ed 7, Philadelphia, 2005, Saunders.)

D. Immunodeficiencies in B cells or T cells
  1. Hypergammaglobulinemias—overabundance of immunoglobulin
  2. Hypogammaglobulinemias—decreased catabolism, or loss of immunoglobulins
  3. Thymic aplasia (DiGeorge syndrome)—congenital absence of thymus gland
E. Drug-induced immunosuppression
  1. Used as an adjunct to organ transplantation and other organ grafts; also used for the treatment of immunologically mediated disease
  2. Examples of drugs used include corticosteroids, rapamycin (now sirolimus), 15-deoxy- spergualin trihydrochloride (now gusperimus trihydrochloride), and cyclosporine; common complication is infection
F. Acquired immunodeficiency syndrome (AIDS)
  1. Definition
    a. Disease that occurs because of a defect in cell-mediated immunity
    b. Cellular immunity is profoundly suppressed, allowing development of opportunistic infections and cancers
    c. U.S. Centers for Disease Control and Prevention (CDC) surveillance case definition includes all human immunodeficiency virus (HIV)–infected persons with a CD4+ T lymphocyte count of less than 200 cells/mm^3 of blood
    d. AIDS diagnosis can also be established by the development of one or more opportunistic infections regardless of CD4+ count[1]
  2. Irreversible acquired defect
  3. Etiology
    a. Lentivirus subfamily of human retroviruses
    b. Infects lymphocytes, macrophages, promyelocytes, and epidermal Langerhans cells
  4. High fatality rate
  5. Virus isolated from blood, semen, vaginal secretions, saliva, tears, breast milk, cerebrospinal fluid, amniotic fluid, and urine
  6. Transmission
    a. Susceptible exposure to infected blood (e.g., intravenous [IV] drug use, blood transfusion)
    b. Sexual contact
    c. Mother to newborn (perinatal)
    d. Cofactors (e.g., genital herpes) may influence transmission

BOX 9-1 Immunology Terms

Anaphylatoxin: a substance produced by complement activation (especially C3a, C5a) that results in increased vascular permeability through release of pharmacologically active mediators from mast cells

Antibody (Ab): a protein that is produced as a result of the introduction of an antigen and has the ability to combine with the antigen that stimulated its production

Antigen (Ag): a substance that can induce a detectable immune response when introduced into an animal

B cell (B lymphocyte): strictly, a bursa-derived cell in avian species and, by analogy, a cell derived from the equivalent of the bursa in nonavian species; B cells are the precursors of plasma cells that produce antibody

Chemotaxis: a process whereby phagocytic cells are attracted to the vicinity of invading pathogens

Complement: a system of serum proteins that is the primary mediator of antigen-antibody reactions

Cytokine: a factor such as a lymphokine or monokine produced by cells that affect other cells (e.g., lymphocytes and macrophages) and have multiple immunomodulating functions; cytokines include interleukins and interferons

Cytolysis: the lysis of bacteria or of cells such as tumor cells or red blood cells by the insertion of the membrane attack complex derived from complement activation

Hapten: a molecule that is not immunogenic by itself but can react with a specific antibody

Histocompatible: sharing transplantation antigens

Hypersensitivity reactions: these occur in four types:

Antibody-mediated hypersensitivity

Type I. Anaphylactic ("immediate"): immunoglobulin E (IgE) antibody is induced by allergen and binds via its Fc receptor to mast cells and basophils; after encountering the antigen again, the fixed IgE becomes cross-linked, inducing degranulation and release of mediators, especially histamine (e.g., in asthma, hay fever, hives, anaphylactic shock)

Type II. Cytotoxic: antigens on a cell surface combine with antibody, which leads to complement-mediated lysis (e.g., transfusion or Rh reactions) or other cytotoxic membrane damage (e.g., in autoimmune hemolytic anemia)

Type III. Immune complex: antigen-antibody immune complexes are deposited in tissues, complement is activated, and polymorphonuclear cells are attracted to the site, causing tissue damage (e.g., in serum sickness, Arthus reactions)

Cell-mediated hypersensitivity

Type IV. Delayed: T lymphocytes, sensitized by an antigen, release lymphokines on second contact with the same antigen; the lymphokines induce inflammation and activate macrophages (e.g., in contact dermatitis, poison ivy, graft rejection, tuberculin skin reaction)

Immune response: development of resistance (immunity) to a foreign substance (e.g., infectious agent); it can be antibody mediated (humoral), cell mediated (cellular), or both

Immunoglobulin: a glycoprotein composed of H and L chains that functions as an antibody; all antibodies are immunoglobulins, but not all immunoglobulins have an antibody function

Immunoglobulin class: a subdivision of immunoglobulin molecules based on unique antigenic determinants in the Fc region of the H chains; five immunoglobulin classes in humans
1. IgG: principal immunoglobulin of the secondary immune response; the only immunoglobulin capable of crossing placental barriers
2. IgM: first immunoglobulin to appear in a given immune response
3. IgA: principal immunoglobulin in external secretions of mucosal surfaces, tears, saliva, bile, urine, and colostrum
4. IgD: thought to activate the B cell
5. IgE: plays important role in immediate hypersensitivity reactions and parasitic infections

Interferon: one of a heterogeneous group of low-molecular-weight proteins elaborated by infected host cells that protect noninfected cells from viral infection; interferons, which are cytokines, also have immunomodulating functions

Interleukin (IL): a cytokine that stimulates or otherwise affects the function of lymphocytes and some other cells
IL-1: induces T helper cell synthesis of IL-2; activates T cells; induces chemotaxis for neutrophils
IL-2: stimulates antibody synthesis, T cytotoxic cells, and natural killer cells
IL-3: stimulates hematopoiesis
IL-4: induces isotype switching
IL-5: promotes the growth and differentiation of B cells
IL-6: stimulates B cell differentiation; activates T cells
IL-7: promotes pre–B cell growth and pre–T cell growth
IL-8: stimulates chemotaxis of neutrophils
IL-9: promotes T cell growth; enhances mast cell
IL-10: inhibits T helper cell 1 (TH1) and cytokine release; stimulates mast cell growth
IL-11: stimulates development of B cells; stimulates hematopoiesis
IL-12: activates T cells; stimulates TH1 cell development
IL-13: anti-inflammatory activity; B cell growth and differentiation
IL-14: induces proliferation of activated B cells
IL-15: stimulates growth of intestinal epithelium, T cells, and natural killer cells
IL-16: lymphocyte chemoattractant factor

Lymphocyte: a mononuclear cell 7 to 12 μm in diameter containing a nucleus with densely packed chromatin and a small rim of cytoplasm; lymphocytes include T cells and B cells, which have primary roles in immunity

Lymphokine: a cytokine that is a soluble product of a lymphocyte; lymphokines are responsible for multiple effects in a cellular immune reaction

Macrophage: a phagocytic mononuclear cell derived from bone marrow monocytes and found in tissues and at the site of inflammation; macrophages serve accessory roles in cellular immunity

Major histocompatibility complex (MHC): a cluster of genes located close to each other; this determines the histocompatibility antigens of the members of a species

Membrane attack complex (MAC): the end product of activation of the complement cascade, which contains C5, C6, C7, and C8 (and C9); the MAC makes holes in the membranes of gram-negative bacteria, killing them and, in red blood cells or other cells, resulting in lysis

Monocyte: a circulating phagocytic blood cell that develops into tissue macrophages

Opsonin: a substance capable of enhancing phagocytosis; antibodies and complement are the two main opsonins

Opsonization: the coating of an antigen or particle (e.g., infectious agent) by substances such as antibodies, complement components, fibronectin, and so on, that facilitate uptake of the foreign particle into a phagocytic cell

Polymorphonuclear cell (leukocyte, PMN): also known as a neutrophil or granulocyte; a PMN is derived from a hematopoietic cell of bone marrow and is characterized by a multi-lobed nucleus; PMNs migrate from the circulation to a site of inflammation by chemotaxis and are phagocytic for bacteria and other particles

T cell (T lymphocyte): a thymus-derived cell that participates in a variety of cell-mediated immune reactions
TH1 (helper) or CD4 cell: activates macrophages and cytotoxic and other T cells
TH2 (helper) or CD4 cell: activates B cells to secrete immunoglobulin
TC (cytotoxic) or CD8 cell: destroys target cells
TD (delayed hypersensitivity) cell: causes inflammation associated with allergic reactions and tissue transplant rejection
TS (suppressor) or CD8 cell: regulates the immune response

Modified from Stites DP, Stobo JD, Wells JV, editors: *Basic and clinical immunology,* ed 8, East Norwalk, Conn, 1994, Appleton & Lange.

FIG 9-3 Hypersensitivity reactions are secondary responses to antigens that occur in an exaggerated or inappropriate form. These reactions have been classified into four major types. **A,** Type I reaction (antibody mediated). **B,** Type II reaction (antibody mediated). *(Continued)*

7. CDC classification system for HIV-infected adolescents and adults categorizes persons based on CD4+ T lymphocyte counts and clinical conditions associated with HIV infection
   a. CD4+ T lymphocyte categories
      (1) Three CD4+ T lymphocyte categories:
         (a) Category 1—500 or more cells/μL
         (b) Category 2—200 to 499 cells/μL
         (c) Category 3—less than 200 cells/μL
      (2) These categories correspond to CD4+ T lymphocyte counts per microliter of blood and

guide clinical and therapeutic actions in the management of HIV-infected adolescents and adults; the revised HIV classification system also allows for the use of the percentage of CD4+ T cells
      (3) Classification of HIV-infected persons should be based on existing guidelines for the medical management of HIV-infected persons; thus, the lowest accurate but not necessarily the most recent CD4+ T-lymphocyte count should be used for classification purposes

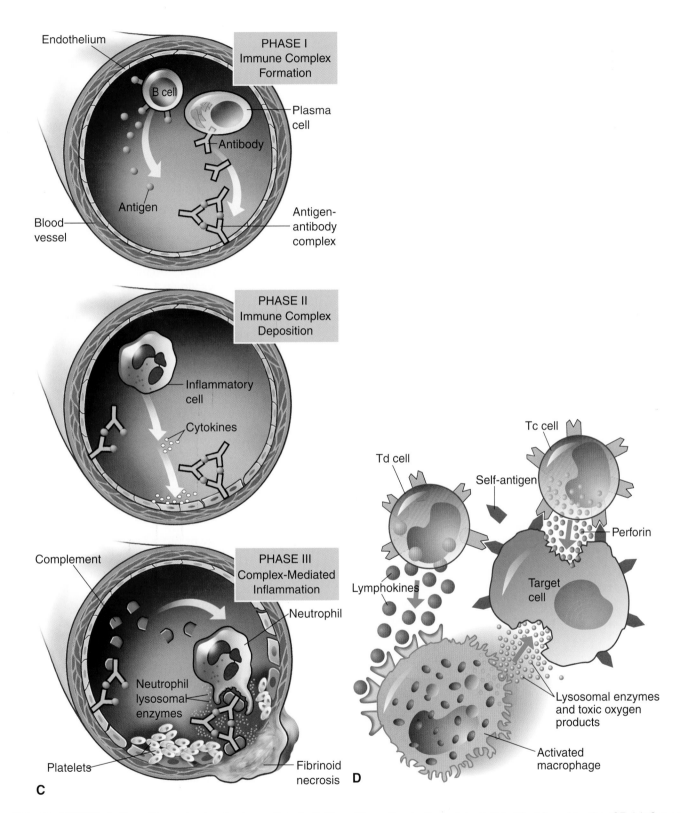

FIG 9-3, CONT'D C, Type III reaction (antibody mediated). **D,** Type IV reaction (cell mediated). (Modified from Huether SE, McCance KL: *Understanding pathophysiology,* ed 6, St Louis, 2017, Elsevier.)

b. Clinical categories of HIV infection
  (1) Category A—consists of one or more of the conditions listed below in an adolescent or adult (at least 13 years old) with documented HIV infection; conditions listed in categories B and C must not have occurred
    (a) Asymptomatic HIV infection
    (b) Persistent generalized lymphadenopathy
    (c) Acute (primary) HIV infection with accompanying illness or history of acute HIV infection
  (2) Category B—consists of symptomatic conditions in an HIV-infected adolescent or adult that are not included among conditions listed in clinical category C and that meet at least one of two criteria: the conditions are attributed to HIV infection or are indicative of a defect in cell-mediated immunity, or the conditions are considered by physicians to have a clinical course or to require management that is complicated by HIV infection; examples of conditions in clinical category B include, but are not limited to:
    (a) Bacillary angiomatosis
    (b) Candidiasis, oropharyngeal (thrush)
    (c) Candidiasis, vulvovaginal; persistent, frequent, or poorly responsive to therapy
    (d) Cervical dysplasia (moderate or severe) or cervical carcinoma in situ
    (e) Constitutional symptoms such as fever (38.5°C) or diarrhea lasting longer than 1 month
    (f) Hairy leukoplakia, oral (Fig. 9-4)
    (g) Herpes zoster (shingles), involving at least two distinct episodes or more than one dermatome
    (h) Idiopathic thrombocytopenic purpura
    (i) Listeriosis
    (j) Pelvic inflammatory disease, particularly if complicated by tubo-ovarian abscess
    (k) Peripheral neuropathy
  (3) For classification purposes, category B conditions take precedence over those in category A; for example, someone previously treated for oral or persistent vaginal candidiasis (and in whom a category C disease has not developed) but who is now asymptomatic should be classified in category B
  (4) Category C—includes the clinical conditions listed in the AIDS surveillance case definition; for classification purposes, once a category C condition has occurred, the person will remain in category C
8. Secondary neoplasms
  a. Kaposi's sarcoma—skin lesions; may be oral; multiple small, reddish blue, purple, or hyperpigmented brown papules, plaques, or nodules; associated with human herpesvirus 8 (HHV-8) (Fig. 9-5)
  b. B cell lymphomas
9. Opportunistic infections
  a. Cytomegalovirus—frequently involves the eye, causing retinal lesions
  b. Tuberculosis
  c. *Pneumocystis jiroveci (P. carinii)*
  d. Oral and esophageal infection from *Candida albicans*
  e. Herpes simplex viruses 1 and 2
10. Incidence and prevalence
  a. Approximately 1.1 million people live with AIDS in the United States
  b. Leading cause of death among men (25 to 44 years) and the fifth leading cause of death among women (15 to 44 years) in the United States
  c. Risk factors
    (1) Unsafe sexual practices
    (2) Exposure to blood or blood products
    (3) IV drug use
    (4) Infant of infected individual
  d. Transmission to health care personnel providing care to infected individuals is rare
11. Treatment (see the section on "Antiviral Agents" in Chapter 11)
  a. No known cure or vaccine yet available
  b. Vaccine will have to be targeted both to free virus in bloodstream and to virus present in infected host cells
  c. Food and Drug Administration (FDA)–approved antiretroviral drugs used for the treatment of HIV:
    (1) Multi-class combination products (e.g., Atripila)
    (2) Nucleoside reverse transcriptase inhibitors (NRTIs) (e.g., zidovudine [AZT], didanosine [ddI], stavudine [d4T], lamivudine [3TC])
    (3) Nonnucleoside reverse transcriptase inhibitors (NNRTIs) (e.g., nevirapine [NVP], efavirenz [EFV])
    (4) Protease inhibitors (PIs) (e.g., amprenavir [AP], indinavir [IDV], darunavir, atazanavir sufate [ATV])
    (5) Fusion inhibitors (e.g., enfuvirtide [T-20])
    (6) Entry inhibitors (e.g., maraviroc [Selzentry, Celsentri])
    (7) HIV integrase strand transfer inhibitor (e.g., raltegravir)
12. Oral manifestations
  a. Hairy leukoplakia

FIG 9-4 Hairy leukoplakia.

FIG 9-5 Kaposi's sarcoma of the neck *(top)*; presenting as a dark macule in the right posterior palate *(bottom)*. (From Regezi JA, Sciubba JA, Jordan CK: *Oral pathology: clinical pathologic correlations,* ed 7, St Louis, 2017, Elsevier.)

b. Herpetic lesions

c. Oral and esophageal candidiasis

d. Kaposi's sarcoma

e. Linear gingival erythema and necrotizing ulcerative periodontitis

f. Human papillomavirus

g. Lymphoma

h. Recurrent aphthous ulcers

Infections of the Skin, Nails, and Hair

A. Bacterial infections

1. Tetanus
   a. Etiology—*Clostridium tetani*
   b. Pathogenesis and transmission—by spores that germinated in the wound and produce tetanus-causing toxin
   c. Clinical findings and symptoms
      (1) Trismus (stiff jaw); eventually, locked jaw
      (2) Spasms of facial muscles
      (3) Dysphagia
      (4) Difficulty breathing
2. Leprosy
   a. Etiology—*Mycobacterium leprae*
   b. Pathogenesis and transmission—transmitted via prolonged direct contact or inhalation of organisms
   c. Clinical findings and symptoms
      (1) Skin lesions
      (2) Oral lesions are tumor-like masses of tissue that involve the oral lining, tongue, lips, or palate
3. *Pseudomonas aeruginosa* infections
   a. Pathogenesis
      (1) Low pathogenicity for humans, except in debilitated persons (e.g., burn victims or those taking antibiotics or immunosuppressive drugs)
      (2) Ubiquitous in nature
   b. Clinical findings and symptoms
      (1) *Pseudomonas* dermatitis—self-limiting rash associated with swimming pools, hot tubs, and saunas
      (2) Otitis externa—infection of the external ear canal

4. Staphylococcal infections
   a. Etiology—*Staphylococcus aureus* and *Staphylococcus epidermidis*
   b. Pathogenesis—determined by extracellular factors and invasive properties of the strain
   c. Clinical findings and symptoms
      (1) Most *S. aureus* strains are resistant to penicillin
      (2) Causes furuncles (boils), carbuncles, impetigo, and cellulitis
5. Streptococcal infections
   a. Etiology—*Streptococcus pyogenes* (group A β-hemolytic)
   b. Pathogenesis
      (1) Determined by portal of entry
      (2) Diffuse and rapidly spreading infection
   c. Clinical findings and symptoms
      (1) Scarlet fever
         (a) Acute inflammation of the upper respiratory tract
         (b) Generalized rash caused by erythrogenic exotoxin
         (c) Oral mucosa is red; "strawberry tongue"
         (d) Sequelae from group A streptococcal infection include rheumatic fever and hemorrhagic glomerulonephritis
      (2) Erysipelas
6. Lyme disease
   a. Etiology—*Borrelia burgdorferi* (spirochetes)
   b. Pathogenesis
      (1) Transmitted by ticks (zoonotic)
      (2) Antigen-antibody complexes may be responsible for arthritic or neurologic difficulties
   c. Clinical findings and symptoms
      (1) Initial phase—rash, headache, fever, and myalgia
      (2) Secondary phase—possible cardiac involvement
      (3) Recurring neurologic symptoms, arthritis, or both
B. Fungal infections
1. Ringworm infections (tinea)
   a. Etiology—dermatophytes most important; *Microsporum, Trichophyton, Epidermophyton*
   b. Pathogenesis—grow only within dead keratinized tissue

c. Clinical findings and symptoms—inflammatory response, especially at the border of lesions; patching; scaling

2. Candidiasis
   a. Etiology—*Candida albicans*
   b. Pathogenesis
      (1) Dissemination and sepsis in compromised patients (opportunistic infection)
      (2) Normal inhabitant of the skin and mucosal surfaces
      (3) Predisposing factors include diabetes mellitus, pregnancy, obesity, vitamin deficiency, use of broad-spectrum antibiotics, and immunologic defects
   c. Clinical findings and symptoms—vary with site

C. Viral infections
   1. Herpes simplex
      a. Etiology—herpes simplex virus (HSV)
      b. Pathogenesis
         (1) Transmission through oral and ocular secretions
         (2) Virus is present in saliva, even in apparent good health
         (3) Indirect contact (e.g., fomites)
         (4) Infects epithelial cells
         (5) Establishes a latent infection from retroviruses
      c. Clinical findings and symptoms
         (1) Types
            (a) HSV-1—generally above the waist; usually found in and around the mouth
            (b) HSV-2—herpes genitalis
         (2) Frequently asymptomatic
         (3) Most often, acute gingivostomatitis; usually in children—fever, malaise, irritability, local lymphadenopathy, and anorexia; red, edematous gingiva and adjacent mucosa; lesions are vesicles with yellowish contents that rupture and ulcerate; bright margin of erythema; sharply defined; pain may be severe; duration of about 7 days; self-limiting

      (4) Herpetic whitlow infection of fingers; can be caused by HSV-1 or HSV-2; abrupt onset; local irritation; tenderness, edema, erythema, and vesicles; difficult to differentiate from bacterial pyoderma caused by staphylococci
      (5) Recurrent secondary infections by HSV-1
         (a) Virus now latent but permanently established in nerve ganglia (carrier)
         (b) Infections may be induced by stress, sun, or colds
      (6) Herpes labialis is the most common clinical manifestation of recurrent infection
         (a) Cold sores, fever blisters
         (b) Vesicles on an erythematous base
         (c) Prodromal burning and hyperesthesia
         (d) Swollen lymph nodes
      (7) Intraoral lesions
         (a) Usually found on the mucosa or hard palate overlying bone
         (b) Small, discrete lesions; vesicles of clear fluid; ulcerate with a red base

   2. Chickenpox
      a. Etiology—varicella-zoster virus (VZV)
      b. Pathogenesis
         (1) Route of infection through the mucosa of the upper respiratory tract
         (2) Highly infectious
         (3) Virus probably circulates in the blood and localizes on the skin
         (4) Incubation period 2 weeks
         (5) Vaccine available
      c. Clinical findings and symptoms
         (1) Earliest symptoms are malaise and fever, followed by a rash and formation of vesicles
         (2) Oral lesions may occur throughout the mouth and appear as small canker sores or aphthae; vesicles rupture quickly (Fig. 9-6)

FIG 9-6 Herpes labialis.

3. Shingles
   a. Etiology—VZV
   b. Pathogenesis
      (1) Reactivation of latent virus in dorsal root ganglion
      (2) Closely follows area of innervation
      (3) Chickenpox and shingles represent different forms of infection by the same agent
      (4) Virus resides in ganglia; usually affects sensory nerves (thoracic area most often involved; ophthalmic division of trigeminal nerve next most involved)
      (5) Vaccine available
   c. Clinical findings and symptoms
      (1) Mostly found in adults
      (2) Malaise, fever, followed by severe pain in area
      (3) Rash and vesicles along the nerve trunk
4. Warts
   a. Etiology—papillomaviruses
   b. Pathogenesis—affects epithelial cells of skin and mucous membranes
   c. Clinical findings and symptoms
      (1) Skin warts, plantar warts, flat warts, genital condylomas, laryngeal papillomas
      (2) Oral warts are papular or nodular lesions covered with papilliferous projections; also may look like common warts
5. Measles
   a. Etiology—rubeola virus
   b. Pathogenesis
      (1) Transmission through the respiratory tract
      (2) Spreads to regional lymphoid tissue
      (3) Primary viremia disseminates the virus
      (4) Secondary viremia seeds the epithelial surfaces of the body
   c. Clinical findings and symptoms
      (1) Koplik's spots
         (a) Small, bluish white spots with a red surrounding zone; cannot be wiped off
         (b) Occur on the buccal mucosa opposite the molars
      (2) Followed by a diffuse skin rash and fever
      (3) Bacterial secondary infections occur, such as middle ear infections or pneumonia
6. German measles
   a. Etiology—rubella virus
   b. Pathogenesis
      (1) Occurs through the upper respiratory tract
      (2) Incubation period 2 to 3 weeks
   c. Clinical findings and symptoms
      (1) Malaise, low-grade fever, rash, and lymphadenopathy
      (2) Rash starts on face; extends to trunk and extremities
7. Erythema infectiosum (also called fifth disease)
   a. Etiology—human parvovirus B19
   b. Pathogenesis

(1) Children most affected by the virus
(2) Virus transmitted through the upper respiratory tract
   c. Clinical findings and symptoms
      (1) Low-grade fever, malaise, and bright-red rash on cheeks spreading to the rest of the body
      (2) Sequelae include arthritis in adulthood

Infections of the Respiratory Tract
Upper Respiratory System Infections
A. Bacterial infections
   1. Diphtheria
      a. Etiology—*Corynebacterium diphtheriae*
      b. Pathogenesis
         (1) Droplets or by contact with susceptible individuals
         (2) Bacilli grow on mucous membranes or in skin abrasions
         (3) Damage caused by the systemic distribution of toxin
      c. Clinical findings and symptoms
         (1) Enlarged lymphadenopathy of the neck; possibly edema
         (2) Pseudomembrane forms on tonsils
   2. Streptococcal pharyngitis ("strep throat")
      a. Etiology—*Streptococcus pyogenes* (group A)
      b. Pathogenesis—transmitted by the respiratory route and contaminated food, water, and milk
      c. Clinical findings and symptoms: severe inflammation of the throat and tonsils; fever
B. Viral infections—common cold (Table 9-6)

Lower Respiratory System Infections
A. Bacterial infections
   1. Pneumococcal pneumonia
      a. Etiology—most common agent is *Streptococcus pneumoniae*
      b. Pathogenesis
         (1) Spread by droplets from nasal or pharyngeal secretion
         (2) Person may contract the disease or become an asymptomatic carrier
         (3) Predisposing factors include age, impaired resistance, and bacteremia
      c. Clinical findings and symptoms: symptoms include sudden onset of high fever, chills, chest pain, dry cough, and rust-colored sputum
   2. Bacterial pneumonia
      a. Etiology—several species—*Streptococcus pyogenes, Staphylococcus aureus, Klebsiella pneumoniae, Haemophilus influenzae*
      b. Pathogenesis is similar to that caused by *S. pneumoniae*
      c. Inflammation of the lungs
   3. Legionnaires disease
      a. Etiology—*Legionella pneumophila*
      b. Pathogenesis

TABLE 9-6 Viral Infections of the Respiratory Tract

Syndrome	Main Symptoms	MOST COMMON VIRAL CAUSES		
		Infants	Children	Adults
Common cold	Nasal obstruction, nasal discharge	Rhinovirus Adenovirus	Rhinovirus Adenovirus	Rhinovirus Coronavirus
Pharyngitis	Sore throat	Adenovirus Herpes simplex virus	Adenovirus Coxsackievirus	Adenovirus Coxsackievirus
Laryngitis/croup	Hoarseness, "barking" cough	Parainfluenza virus Influenza virus	Parainfluenza virus Influenza virus	Parainfluenza virus Influenza virus
Tracheobronchitis	Cough	Parainfluenza virus Influenza virus	Parainfluenza virus Influenza virus	Influenza virus Adenovirus
Bronchiolitis	Cough, dyspnea	Respiratory syncytial virus Parainfluenza virus	Rare virus	Rare virus
Pneumonia	Cough, chest pain	Respiratory syncytial virus Influenza virus	Influenza virus Parainfluenza virus	Influenza virus Adenovirus

From Brooks GF, Butel JS, Morse SA: *Jawetz, Melnick & Adelberg's medical microbiology*, ed 23, Columbus, Ohio, 2004, McGraw-Hill.

(1) Inhalation of bacteria from aerosols
(2) Bacteria multiply in lungs and produce pneumonia
c. Clinical findings and symptoms
  (1) Influenza-like illness with pneumonia
  (2) Complications include renal failure, GI hemorrhage, and respiratory failure
4. Tuberculosis
  a. Etiology—*Mycobacterium tuberculosis*
  b. Pathogenesis
    (1) Transmitted by inhalation of droplets, ingestion, or direct inoculation; disseminated by coughing, sneezing, or contaminated dust
    (2) Predisposing factors include advanced age, chronic alcoholism, poor nutrition, diabetes mellitus, and prolonged stress
    (3) Incubation period is generally 28 to 47 days; can be as long as 6 months
  c. Clinical findings and symptoms
    (1) Symptoms vary but include fever, general discomfort, weight loss, tubercle formation (nodule in lung tissue), night sweats, and persistent cough
    (2) Oral lesions may appear as an ulcerated lesion on the tongue or mucosa (rare)
    (3) Diagnosis by a skin test and a radiograph
5. Whooping cough (pertussis)
  a. Etiology—*Bordetella pertussis*
  b. Pathogenesis—transmitted by inhalation of droplets; produce toxins
  c. Clinical findings and symptoms—spasmodic coughing and gasping noise with inhalation
6. Mycoplasmal pneumonia
  a. Etiology—*Mycoplasma pneumoniae*
  b. Pathogenesis—transmitted in airborne droplets; binds respiratory epithelium and inhibits ciliary action
  c. Clinical findings and symptoms—mild symptoms of low fever, cough, and headache that persist for 3 weeks or longer

B. Fungal infections
1. Histoplasmosis
  a. Etiology—*Histoplasma capsulatum*
  b. Pathogenesis—transmitted by inhalation of spores, especially in excreta of wild birds, poultry, and bats
  c. Clinical findings and symptoms
    (1) Skin lesions are common
    (2) Meningitis
2. Pneumocystis pneumonia
  a. Etiology—*Pneumocystis jiroveci*
  b. Pathogenesis—inhalation of spores; disease more common among immunosuppressed persons, especially those with AIDS
  c. Clinical findings and symptoms—nonspecific; fever; dry, nonproductive cough
3. Coccidioidomycosis
  a. Etiology—*Coccidioides immitis*
  b. Spores in desert soils are inhaled along with dust (common in the southwestern United States)
  c. Clinical findings and symptoms—chest pain, fever, cough, weight loss
C. Viral infections
1. Influenza virus infection
  a. Etiology—orthomyxoviruses
  b. Pathogenesis
    (1) The genome can undergo sudden genetic reassortment
    (2) Spread by airborne droplets or contact with contaminated objects
    (3) Virus attaches to the respiratory epithelium
  c. Clinical findings and symptoms
    (1) Chills, headache, dry cough, fever, malaise, muscular ache, and inflammation of the soft palate
    (2) Secondary infection by *S. aureus, H. influenzae, S. pyogenes,* and *S. pneumoniae*; may result in bronchitis and pneumonia
    (3) Reye syndrome may be a complication

2. Hantavirus pulmonary syndrome
   a. Etiology—hantavirus
   b. Pathogenesis—inhalation of excreta of deer mice
   c. Clinical findings and symptoms—severe cold followed by an internal hemorrhage of blood plasma in the lungs

Infections of the Gastrointestinal Tract

A. Bacterial infections
   1. Cholera
      a. Etiology—*Vibrio cholerae*
      b. Pathogenesis
         (1) Transmitted as a result of unsanitary living conditions and through ingestion of the organisms
         (2) Organisms attach to microvilli of epithelial cells; produce toxin
      c. Clinical findings and symptoms—dehydration, nausea, vomiting, profuse diarrhea, and abdominal and leg cramps
   2. Salmonellosis
      a. Etiology—several species of *Salmonella*
      b. Pathogenesis—organisms enter by the oral route usually through contaminated food or drink
      c. Clinical findings and symptoms—organisms cause enteric fevers, bacteremia, followed by focal lesions or endocarditis
   3. Shigellosis (bacillary dysentery)
      a. Etiology—*Shigella dysenteriae, S. flexneri, S. boydii,* and *S. sonnei*
      b. Pathogenesis
         (1) Transmitted through contaminated food or water
         (2) The organism invades the mucosal epithelium
      c. Clinical findings and symptoms—abdominal pain, fever, and watery or bloody diarrhea
   4. Enteric infections caused by *Escherichia coli*
      a. Etiology
         (1) Enterotoxigenic *E. coli* (ETEC)—traveler's diarrhea
         (2) Enteroinvasive *E. coli* (EIEC)
         (3) Enteropathogenic *E. coli* (EPEC)
         (4) Enterohemorrhagic *E. coli* (EHEC)—serotype O157: H7
         (5) Enteroaggregative *E. coli* (EaggEC)
      b. Pathogenesis
         (1) Acquired by ingestion of contaminated food or water or through contact with contaminated persons
         (2) Factors responsible for the different ways in which *E. coli* produces disease vary with strain
      c. Clinical findings and symptoms—abdominal pain, malaise, loss of appetite, diarrhea, and dehydration; diarrhea may be watery or bloody, depending on the strain of *E. coli*
   5. Typhoid fever
      a. Etiology—*Salmonella typhi*
      b. Pathogenesis—transmitted through contaminated food or water
      c. Clinical findings and symptoms
         (1) Fever, severe headache, abdominal pain, and abdominal rash
         (2) Complications include carrier state, relapses, inflammation of the gallbladder, and intestinal bleeding
   6. *Helicobacter* peptic disease syndrome
      a. Etiology—*Helicobacter pylori*
      b. Pathogenesis—*H. pylori* produces ammonia, which neutralizes stomach acid, allowing the bacteria to colonize the stomach mucosa
      c. Clinical findings and symptoms—peptic ulcers
   7. Food poisoning
      a. Botulism
         (1) Etiology—*Clostridium botulinum*
         (2) Pathogenesis
            (a) Regularly contaminates human, plant, and animal food products
            (b) Produces a deadly toxin that acts on nerves
            (c) Transmitted through improperly preserved foods and uncooked fish and meats; foods do not appear contaminated
         (3) Clinical findings and symptoms
            (a) Difficulty speaking, blurred vision, inability to swallow, heart failure, and respiratory paralysis
            (b) Infant botulism may be one of the causes of sudden infant death syndrome
      b. Staphylococcal food poisoning
         (1) Etiology—toxin produced by staphylococci (usually *S. aureus*) in unrefrigerated foods such as dairy products, custard, cream-filled products, fish, or processed meats
         (2) Pathogenesis
            (a) Caused by ingestion of preformed enterotoxin
            (b) Incubation period is from 1 to 8 hours
            (c) Symptoms include nausea, violent vomiting, diarrhea; no fever
            (d) Rapid convalescence; self-limiting
      c. *Perfringens* poisoning
         (1) Etiology—*Clostridium perfringens*
         (2) Pathogenesis
            (a) Precise mechanism is unknown
            (b) Organism produces an enterotoxin
            (c) Incubation period is 8 to 16 hours
         (3) Clinical findings and symptoms
            (a) Symptoms are similar to those of staphylococcal food poisoning
            (b) Usually self-limiting
B. Viral infections
   1. Hepatitis A (Tables 9-7 and 9-8)
      a. Etiology—hepatitis A virus (HAV)
      b. Pathogenesis
         (1) Oral-fecal route in unsanitary conditions; contaminated food and water; close, intimate contact with infected person
         (2) Rarely through the blood

TABLE 9-7 Characteristics of the Various Types of Viral Hepatitis

Characteristic	Hepatitis A	Hepatitis B	Hepatitis C	Hepatitis D	Hepatitis E	Hepatitis G*
Transmission	Fecal-oral (ingestion of contaminated food, ice, and water)	Parenteral (injection of contaminated blood or other body fluids)	Parenteral	Percutaneous, permucosal, or parenteral (host must be co-infected with hepatitis B or as a superinfection in persons with chronic HBV infection)	Fecal-oral (contaminated drinking water most common)	Bloodborne and co-infection with HCV
Agent	Hepatitis A virus (HAV); single-stranded (ss) ribonucleic acid (RNA); no envelope	Hepatitis B virus (HBV); double-stranded deoxyribonucleic acid (DNA); envelope	Hepatitis C virus (HCV); ss RNA; envelope	Hepatitis D virus (HDV); defective ss RNA, envelope from HBV	Hepatitis E virus (HEV); ss RNA; no envelope	Hepatitis G virus, although causal association remains to be confirmed
Incubation period	15 to 50 days	45 to 160 days	2 to 26 weeks	Uncertain	15 to 60 days	Acute disease spectrum unknown
Manifestations or symptoms	Children under age 6 years may not have signs of illness; severe cases: fever, headache, malaise, jaundice, fatigue, loss of appetite, nausea, dark urine	Clinical manifestations are age dependent; anorexia, nausea, malaise, vomiting, jaundice, dark urine, clay-colored stools, abdominal pain, and more likely to progress to severe liver damage	Similar to HBV	Severe liver damage; high mortality rate	Similar to HAV, but pregnant women may have high mortality rate; less common symptoms include arthralgia, diarrhea, pruritus, and urticaria	
Chronic liver disease	No	Yes	Yes	Yes	No	No
Vaccines	A sterile suspension of inactivated virus	Genetically engineered	None	HBV vaccine is protective because co-infection is required	None	None

*Information on hepatitis G, from the Centers for Disease Control and Prevention: *Guidelines for viral hepatitis surveillance and case management,* Atlanta, 2005. Available at http://www.cdc.gov/ncidod/diseases/hepatitis/resource/PDFs/revised_GUIDELINES_formatted5.pdf.
From Tortora GJ, Funke BR. Case DL: *Microbiology: an introduction,* ed. 8, Menlo Park, Calif, 2003, Benjamin/Cummings.

(3) The incubation period is 15 to 50 days
(4) Usually occurs in children and young adults
c. Clinical findings and symptoms
(1) Preicteric (before jaundice appears)—similar to influenza; fever, headache, nausea, vomiting, fatigue, abdominal pain, loss of appetite, dark urine
(2) Icteric—jaundice (rare in children); other symptoms continue
(3) Anicteric—without jaundice; two or three times more prevalent than the icteric state; symptoms resemble those of influenza
(4) Recovery and immunity
  (a) Antibody to HAV (anti-HAV) is usually in the blood 2 weeks after onset
  (b) Most individuals recover completely in 4 to 6 weeks
  (c) Immunity develops after recovery
  (d) No carrier state develops
  (e) Usually self-limiting
d. Active immunization
(1) Hepatitis A vaccine (Havrix) at least 2 weeks before expected exposure; booster dose recommended 6 to 12 months later for adults

(2) The vaccine may be administered concomitantly with immunoglobulin in persons exposed to HAV
2. Hepatitis B (see Tables 9-7 and 9-8)
a. Etiology—hepatitis B virus (HBV)
b. Pathogenesis
(1) Infected blood or serum through parenteral inoculation (e.g., blood transfusions, contaminated dental or medical instruments, needles and syringes used by IV drug abusers, accidental self-inoculation by health care professionals)
(2) Other body fluids, including saliva, semen, tears, urine, sweat, and nasopharyngeal secretions
(3) Oral or sexual contact or other close, personal contact
(4) Coughing, sneezing, and aerosols
(5) Salivary transmission by way of hands, instruments, and other equipment is an important consideration in the practice of dental hygiene
c. Incubation
(1) Between 45 and 160 days
(2) Presence of hepatitis B surface antigen (HBsAg) indicates potential to be infective

TABLE 9-8   Viral Hepatitis: Significance of Key Terms

Abbreviations	Term	Significance
Hepatitis A		
HAV	Hepatitis A virus	Causative agent for hepatitis A
Anti-HAV	Antibody to hepatitis A virus	Acute or resolved infection
		Protective immune response to infection
		Passively acquired antibody
		Response to vaccination
IgM anti-HAV	Immunoglobulin M (IgM) antibody to hepatitis A virus	Recent HAV infection
HAV-RNA	Ribonucleic acid (RNA) of HAV	Detected by nucleic acid amplification, hybridization, or both
Hepatitis B		
HBV	Hepatitis B virus (Dane particle)	Causative agent for hepatitis B
		Current HBV infection
HBsAg	Hepatitis B surface antigen	Surface marker in acute disease and carrier state
		Antigen used in hepatitis B vaccine
Anti-HBs	Antibody to hepatitis B surface antigen	Indicates:
		(1) Active immunity to HBV (past infection)
		(2) Passive immunity from HBIg
		(3) Immune response from HB vaccine
HBeAg	Hepatitis B e antigen	High-titer HBV in serum indicates high infectivity
		Persists into carrier state
Anti-HBe	Antibody to hepatitis B e antigen	Low-titer HBV
		Low-degree infectivity
HBcAg	Hepatitis B core antigen	Indicates acute, chronic, or resolved HBV infection
		Not elicited by vaccination
Anti-HBc	Antibody to hepatitis B core antigen	Indicates prior HBV infection
IgM anti-HBc	IgM class antibody to hepatitis B core antigen	Indicates recent HBC infection
HBV-DNA	Deoxyribonucleic acid (DNA) of HBV	Detected by nucleic acid amplification, hybridization, or both
Hepatitis C		
HCV	Hepatitis C virus (formerly parenterally transmitted non-A, non-B)	Causative agent for hepatitis C
Anti-HCV	Antibody to hepatitis C virus	Indicates acute disease and chronic state
		Resembles hepatitis B
HCV-RNA	RNA of HCV	Defines viremia; detected by nucleic acid amplification
Hepatitis D		
HDV	Hepatitis delta virus	Causative agent for hepatitis D
		Only infectious in presence of acute or chronic HBV infection
HDV-Ag	Delta antigen	Detectable during early acute HDV infection
Anti-HDV	Antibody to hepatitis D virus	Indicates acute, resolved, or chronic infection
IgM anti-HDV	IgM-class antibody to HDV	Indicates either acute or chronic infection with active viral replication
HDV-RNA	RNA of HDV	Detected by nucleic acid amplification, hybridization, or both
Hepatitis E		
HEV	Hepatitis E virus (formerly enterically transmitted non-A, non-B)	Causative agent for hepatitis E
Anti-HEV	Antibody to hepatitis E virus	Indicates acute or resolved infection
IgM anti-HEV	IgM-class antibody to hepatitis E virus	Indicates acute infection
Non-ABCDE		
Parenterally transmitted (HSG)	Diagnosis of exclusion	Epidemiologic evidence of parenteral or sexual transmission
Enterically transmitted (HSF)	Diagnosis of exclusion	Epidemiologic evidence of fecal-oral transmission
Immunoglobulins		
Ig	Immunoglobulin	Contains antibodies to HAV and low-titer HBV antibodies
HBIg	Hepatitis B immunoglobulin	Contains high-titer antibodies to HBV

From Wilkins EM: *Clinical practice of the dental hygienist,* ed 10, Philadelphia, 2009, Lippincott, Williams & Wilkins.

d. Symptoms
  (1) Similar to hepatitis A
  (2) Slower onset; longer duration
  (3) Asymptomatic to severe and debilitating
  (4) Patient may have subclinical disease and remain undiagnosed
  (5) May result in chronic liver disease; strong evidence for link between chronic HBV infection and hepatocellular carcinoma (liver cancer)
e. Recovery
  (1) Development of antibody to HBsAg (anti-HBs) indicates immunity
  (2) Approximately 5% to 10% of those infected develop a chronic carrier state; HBsAg still present after 6 months; carriers are usually asymptomatic and often remain undetected
f. Risk factors
  (1) Exposure to virus at birth (e.g., infants born to mothers infected with HBV)
  (2) Exchange of blood or blood products (e.g., during hemodialysis, blood transfusions, or IV drug use)
  (3) Exposure to blood or blood products (e.g., in the case of health care workers)
  (4) Close, intimate contact with infected person
  (5) Unsafe sexual practices
  (6) Institutionalization (e.g., in the case of some individuals with Down syndrome and prisoners)
  (7) Immunosuppressive therapy
g. Immunization
  (1) Two types of HBsAg vaccines
    (a) Obtained from HBsAg-positive carriers (Heptavax)
    (b) Obtained from recombinant DNA in yeast cells (Recombivax)
  (2) Passive immunization results from hepatitis B immune globulin (HBIg); used for postexposure prophylaxis; preferably within 24 to 48 hours; partially effective
  (3) Given as a series of 3 or 4 shots
3. Hepatitis type C (see Tables 9-7 and 9-8)
  a. Etiology—hepatitis C virus
  b. Pathogenesis
    (1) Originally named "non-A, non-B" hepatitis virus
    (2) Risk factors include blood transfusion, IV drug use, and heterosexual transmission
  c. Clinical findings and symptoms
    (1) Mild symptoms; most asymptomatic
    (2) Development of chronic hepatitis in 50%; may develop into cirrhosis and hepatocellular carcinoma
4. Hepatitis D (formerly delta hepatitis) (see Tables 9-7 and 9-8)
  a. Etiology—hepatitis D virus
  b. Pathogenesis
    (1) Similar to HBV
    (2) Infection dependent on HBV replication
  c. Clinical findings—may produce acute exacerbations of chronic HBV and fulminant hepatitis

5. Hepatitis type E (see Tables 9-7 and 9-8)
  a. Etiology—hepatitis E virus
  b. Pathogenesis
    (1) Originally named "non-A, non-B" hepatitis virus
    (2) Enteric transmission
    (3) Epidemic outbreaks occurring in developing countries
6. Hepatitis G (see Table 9-7)
  a. Etiology—hepatitis G virus
  b. Pathogenesis
    (1) Bloodborne transmission and co-infection with HCV
    (2) Acute disease spectrum unknown
7. Rotavirus
  a. Pathogenesis—disease spread via the fecal-oral route; the virus replicates in the epithelial cells on the tips of villi in the small intestine
  b. Clinical findings and symptoms—acute onset of vomiting, watery diarrhea, fever, and abdominal pain in children younger than 2 years
8. Norwalk virus and Norwalk-like virus
  a. Pathogenesis—disease spread via the fecal-oral route
  b. Clinical findings and symptoms—nausea, vomiting, abdominal cramps, lethargy, and diarrhea in older children and adults

Infections of the Circulatory System
Diseases of the Heart
A. Rheumatic fever
  1. Etiology—β-hemolytic group A streptococcal infection
  2. Pathogenesis
    a. Rheumatic fever—hypersensitivity state developing after streptococcal infection; associated with β-hemolytic group A streptococci
    b. Heart valves become inflamed; subsequent abnormal growths of connective tissue; scarring of valves occurs, resulting in rheumatic heart disease
  3. Clinical findings and symptoms
    a. Fever, malaise, polyarthritis, inflammation of the heart
    b. Defective heart valves are a result of carditis
    c. Heart valve damage
      (1) Stenosis—narrowing of the valve opening
      (2) Valvular insufficiency—failure of the valve to close completely
  4. Prophylactic antibiotic premedication is necessary before dental and dental hygiene treatments
B. Infective endocarditis
  1. Etiology—most often associated with the normal flora of the respiratory or intestinal tract
  2. Pathogenesis
    a. Inflammatory condition of the heart; microbial colonization of the endothelial membrane that covers the inner surface of the heart and the heart valves
    b. Predisposing factors
      (1) Artificial heart valves
      (2) Congenital heart defects
      (3) History of endocarditis

(4) Damaged heart valves

(5) History of IV drug use

c. Dental and dental hygiene procedures may allow bacteria to enter the bloodstream (bacteremia) and lodge in the heart valves

3. Clinical findings and symptoms

a. Fever, anemia, weakness, and heart murmur

b. Inflammation of the heart

c. May result in death

Other Microbial Diseases of the Circulatory System

A. Bacterial infections

1. Rickettsial infections

a. Etiology—obligate intracellular parasites

b. Pathogenesis

(1) Transmitted by arthropods such as fleas, lice, mites, and ticks

(2) Rocky Mountain spotted fever (tick vector)

(3) Typhus (flea-borne, common in rats)

(4) Rickettsialpox (mouse-mite vector)—usually involves fever, rash, and vasculitis

B. Protozoan infections

1. Malaria—*Plasmodium* species (spp.)

a. Spread by mosquitoes

b. Symptoms—shaking, chills, fever, headache, and nausea, which appear at 2- to 3-day intervals

C. Viral infections

1. Infectious mononucleosis

a. Etiology—Epstein-Barr virus (EBV)

b. Pathogenesis

(1) Transmitted by kissing or sharing drinking glasses with an infected person

(2) Involves lymph nodes and the spleen; increase in lymphocytes

c. Clinical findings and symptoms

(1) Acute leukemia-like infection

(2) Primarily found in young adults

(3) Symptoms include mild jaundice, fever, enlarged and tender lymph nodes, sore throat, bleeding gingiva, and general weakness

2. Cytomegalovirus (CMV) infections

a. Etiology—cytomegalovirus

b. Pathogenesis

(1) Cytomegalic inclusion disease is caused by intrauterine or perinatal infection

(2) Virus may persist in organs in a latent state or as a chronic infection

(3) CMV mononucleosis occurs spontaneously or through blood transfusions

(4) The route of infection in older infants, children, and adults is unknown

c. Clinical findings and symptoms

(1) May result in death in infants

(2) Prematurity, jaundice, pneumonitis, central nervous system (CNS) damage, and mental or motor retardation can occur in infants

(3) Acquired infection in children results in hepatitis, pneumonitis, and anemia

(4) CMV mononucleosis produces a mononucleosis-like disease

Infections of the Reproductive and Urinary Systems
Reproductive System Infections

A. Bacterial infections

1. Gonorrhea

a. Etiology—*Neisseria gonorrhoeae*, a gram-negative aerobic bacterium; often co-infection with *Chlamydia trachomatis*

b. Pathogenesis

(1) Risk of infection is 20% to 30% from a single exposure for men; higher percentage for women

(2) Grows primarily in the genitourinary tract; possesses pili that allow attachment to mucosal cells and resist phagocytosis; can infect the eye, rectum, and throat

c. Clinical findings and symptoms

(1) Sometimes found in the pharynx; localized yellow or gray-white raised patches or generalized lesions with a gray membrane; the membrane sloughs, leaving a bright area; seen on the gingiva, tongue, and soft palate; may have itching or burning

(2) Gonococcal glossitis (Fig. 9-7)

(3) The newborn's eyes may be infected while the baby is passing through the birth canal (ophthalmia neonatorum); use of silver nitrate or antibiotic after birth alleviates the condition

(4) Men experience painful and frequent urination and discharge containing mucus and pus

(5) Women often do not have symptoms; may have urethral or vaginal discharge, backache, or abdominal pain (pelvic inflammatory disease)

(6) Oral infection results in pharyngitis, glossitis, or stomatitis, including some areas of ulceration

(7) Complications include sterility, disseminated infection, and meningitis

FIG 9-7 Gonococcal glossitis. (Courtesy of Beverly Entwistle Isman, formerly with the Department of Applied Dentistry, University of Colorado School of Dentistry, Denver.)

FIG 9-8 Primary, secondary, and tertiary stages of syphilis.

2. Syphilis (Fig. 9-8)
   a. Etiology—*Treponema pallidum*; spirochete, anaerobic
   b. Pathogenesis
      (1) Usually transmitted by sexual contact with skin or mucous membrane lesions of an infected person
      (2) Infection limited to the human host
      (3) Congenital syphilis occurs when the organism crosses the placenta
      (4) *T. pallidum* can pass through abraded skin and can probably pass through intact mucous membranes
      (5) If the organisms gain access to the circulatory system, they can affect all organs and spread rapidly to the lymphatic system and bloodstream
   c. Clinical findings and symptoms (Fig. 9-9)
      (1) Primary stage—chancre, a single granulomatous lesion; often asymptomatic; common on the lips; may involve the tongue and oral mucosa; highly contagious; occurs 2 to 3 weeks after exposure and lasts 3 to 5 weeks; red, small, elevated nodule; heals spontaneously; no scarring
      (2) Secondary stage

FIG 9-9 Chancre lesion of primary syphilis. (From Sapp JP, Eversole LR, Wysocki GP: *Contemporary oral and maxillofacial pathology,* ed 2, St Louis, 2004, Mosby.)

    (a) Appears 6 to 8 weeks after exposure; patient can be asymptomatic for 2 to 6 months, and then secondary lesions appear

    (b) Flu-like symptoms

    (c) Skin rashes—maculopapular rash on the face, hands, and feet

    (d) Mucous patches on the lips, soft palate, and tongue—painless shallow ulcers; grayish white areas may be removed, leaving red areas of erosion; highly contagious

    (e) Swollen lymph nodes

  (3) Tertiary stage

    (a) Gumma—inflammatory granulomatous lesion with a central zone of necrosis; may be on the tongue, palate (perforation), or facial bones; soft, swollen areas or tumors; not contagious and usually asymptomatic

    (b) Often takes 5 to 20 years to develop

    (c) Involvement of the CNS and spinal cord leads to paresis, loss of fine muscle coordination, and personality changes

    (d) Involvement of the cardiovascular system—major cause of death

  (4) Congenital syphilis

    (a) Hutchinson's incisors—notched, bell shaped (Fig. 9-10)

    (b) "Mulberry molars"—first molars are irregular with poorly developed cusps (Fig. 9-11)

    (c) Skin, mucous membrane lesions

    (d) High mortality

3. Toxic shock syndrome (TSS)

  a. Etiology—*Staphylococcus aureus*

  b. Pathogenesis

    (1) Short incubation period of 1 to 8 hours

    (2) The toxin is produced by the microorganism

  c. Clinical findings and symptoms

FIG 9-10 Congenital syphilis. The patient exhibits anomalously shaped teeth, consisting of incisors with screwdriver-shaped crowns and notched incisal edges and molars with constricted crowns and a lack of cuspal development (mulberry molars). (From Sapp JP, Eversole LR, Wysocki GP: *Contemporary oral and maxillofacial pathology,* ed 2, St Louis, 2004, Mosby.)

FIG 9-11 "Mulberry molars" of congenital syphilis. (Courtesy of Beverly Entwistle Isman, formerly with the Department of Applied Dentistry, University of Colorado School of Dentistry, Denver.)

(1) Rash, nausea, violent vomiting, and diarrhea, but no fever
(2) Rapid convalescence
(3) Often occurs within 5 days of the onset of menses
(4) Can recur

B. Viral infections (Fig. 9-12)
  1. Genital herpes
    a. Etiology

FIG 9-12 Primary herpetic gingivostomatitis.

(1) Herpesvirus
(2) HSV-2—herpes genitalis (genital herpes)
  b. Pathogenesis—transmitted by sexual contact
  c. Clinical findings and symptoms
    (1) Lesions appear 2 to 7 days after exposure
    (2) Lesions appear in or on the genitalia and skin
    (3) Lesions may ulcerate early and be painful or crust over
    (4) Fever, lymphadenopathy, malaise, anorexia
    (5) Initial lesions subside and heal in 2 to 3 weeks
    (6) Recurrent lesions have a milder course
    (7) Highly infectious
    (8) Primary and recurrent infections
      (a) Most (90%) primary infections are subclinical
      (b) Recurrent infections in women often serve as a source of neonatal herpes

Urinary Tract Infections

A. Etiology—primarily caused by *E. coli*
B. Pathogenesis—predisposing conditions
  1. Diabetes mellitus
  2. Neurologic diseases (e.g., polio and spinal cord injury)
  3. Lesions (e.g., kidney stones) interfering with urine flow
  4. Eclampsia of pregnancy
C. Clinical findings and symptoms
  1. Blood in urine
  2. Accumulation of fluid in tissue
  3. Pain

Infections of the Central Nervous System

A. Bacterial infections
  1. Meningitis
    a. Etiology
      (1) Aseptic meningitis—caused by a variety of agents, including viruses, spirochetes, bacteria, mycoplasmas, and chlamydiae
      (2) Meningococcal meningitis—caused by *Neisseria meningitidis*
    b. Pathogenesis—meningococcal meningitis is transmitted by droplet inhalation
    c. Clinical findings and symptoms
      (1) Aseptic meningitis produces an acute onset, fever, headache, and stiff neck
      (2) Meningococcal meningitis produces headache, vomiting, stiff neck, and coma within a few hours
B. Viral infections
  1. Poliomyelitis
    a. Etiology—poliomyelitis virus
    b. Pathogenesis—virus transmitted through the mouth and intestines
    c. Clinical findings and symptoms
      (1) Flaccid paralysis; destruction of motor neurons in the spinal cord
      (2) Acute inflammation of the meninges
      (3) May range from mild illness to paralysis
  2. Rabies
    a. Etiology—rabies virus

b. Pathogenesis
   (1) Transmitted to humans through the bite of a rabid animal
   (2) Incubation period is 4 to 6 weeks or longer
c. Clinical findings and symptoms—include visual difficulties, painful throat spasms, convulsions, and respiratory paralysis
3. Viral encephalitis
   a. Etiology—usually caused by arboviruses
   b. Pathogenesis—virus replicates in, and is spread by, arthropods, usually mosquitoes or ticks
   c. Clinical findings and symptoms
      (1) Causes extensive nervous tissue damage and encephalitis
      (2) Symptoms—include fever, chills, nausea, fatigue, drowsiness, pain, stiff neck, general disorientation, blindness, deafness, and paralysis
C. Protozoan infection—toxoplasmosis
   1. Etiology
      a. *Toxoplasma gondii*
      b. Sources include infected cat feces, contaminated raw meat and soil, and rodents (cats may eat infected mice)
   2. Pathogenesis
      a. Inhaling or ingesting cysts when handling cat litter or sandboxes frequented by the infected cat
      b. Eating raw meat
      c. Through the placenta (pregnant women must not eat raw or undercooked meat and handle litter boxes)
   3. Clinical findings and symptoms
      a. Resembles infectious mononucleosis in adults
      b. Congenital infection can lead to stillbirth, psychomotor dysfunction, blindness, and other congenital defects
D. Fungal infection—cryptococcosis
   1. Etiology—*Cryptococcus neoformans*
   2. Pathogenesis
      a. The organism tends to reside in pigeon droppings
      b. Transmitted by inhalation of dehydrated yeasts
   3. Clinical findings and symptoms
      a. Meningitis most common; often associated with immunocompromised patients
      b. Disseminated disease can affect skin, lungs, or other organs

Infections of the Eye

A. Bacterial infections
   1. Conjunctivitis
      a. Etiology—*Haemophilus aegyptius*
      b. Clinical findings
         (1) Purulent conjunctivitis
         (2) Epidemic in warmer climates
   2. Trachoma-inclusion conjunctivitis
      a. Etiology—*Chlamydia trachomatis*
      b. Pathogenesis—transmitted through person-to-person contact; associated with poor sanitation and poor personal hygiene
      c. Clinical findings and symptoms
         (1) Inflammation of conjunctiva; scarring of eyelids or cornea; can lead to secondary infection; can lead to partial or complete blindness
         (2) "Swimming pool conjunctivitis," which results in conjunctival inflammation; is usually self-limiting
B. Viral infections
   1. Adenovirus infection
      a. Etiology—adenoviruses
      b. Pathogenesis
         (1) Hand-to-eye contact is the most significant factor
         (2) Swimming pool conjunctivitis most likely transmitted by the waterborne route
      c. Clinical findings and symptoms—inflammation of the conjunctiva, excessive lacrimation, periorbital edema
   2. Enterovirus type 70 is one of the causes of acute hemorrhagic conjunctivitis
   3. Herpetic keratitis
      a. Etiology—primarily caused by HSV-1; occasionally by HSV-2
      b. Pathogenesis—cytolytic, herpetic infection of the cornea
      c. Clinical findings and symptoms
         (1) Severe keratoconjunctivitis; corneal ulcers or vesicles on the eyelids
         (2) May recur
         (3) May cause blindness

Chemotherapeutic Agents

See Tables 9-9 and 9-10.

TABLE 9-9   Choice of Antibacterial Agents for Therapy

Causative Organism	Disease	Agent(s) of First Choice
Gram-Negative Cocci		
Neisseria gonorrhoeae	Gonorrhea	Ceftriaxone
Neisseria meningitides	Meningitis	Penicillin
Gram-Positive Cocci		
Enterococcus spp.	Endocarditis	Ampicillin or vancomycin ± gentamicin
	Urinary tract infection	Ampicillin, amoxicillin
Staphylococcus aureus	Furuncles, abscesses, pneumonia, meningitis, osteomyelitis, bacteremia, endocarditis	
Non–penicillinase producing		Penicillin

(Continued)

TABLE 9-9 Choice of Antibacterial Agents for Therapy—cont'd

Causative Organism	Disease	Agent(s) of First Choice
Penicillinase producing		Methicillin, oxacillin
Methicillin resistant		Vancomycin
Streptococcus pneumonia	Pneumonia	Penicillin*
Streptococcus		
Group A	Strep throat, scarlet fever, postpartum fever, erysipelas	Penicillin
Group B	Neonatal meningitis, bacteremia	Penicillin, ampicillin
Vrindans group	Endocarditis	Penicillin ± gentamicin
Other (including anaerobic) streptococci		Penicillin
Gram-Positive Bacilli		
Actinomyces spp.	Actinomycosis	Penicillin
Bacillus anthracis	Anthrax	Ciprofloxacin, doxycycline
Clostridium perfringens	Gas gangrene	Penicillin ± clindamycin
Clostridium tetani	Tetanus	Metronidazole
Corynebacterium diphtheria	Diphtheria	Erythromycin
Listeria monocytogenes	Meningitis, bacteremia	Ampicillin
Nocardia spp.	Nocardiosis	Trimethoprim-sulfamethoxazole
Gram-Negative Bacilli		
Prevotella	Anaerobic infections	
– Mouth strains		Penicillin
– Gastrointestinal strains		Metronidazole
Brucella spp.	Brucellosis	Doxycycline ± rifampin or gentamicin
Enterobacter spp.	Urinary tract infection	Imipenem
Escherichia coli	Urinary tract infection	A cephalosporin
Francisella tularensis	Tularemia	Streptomycin, gentamicin
Haemophilus influenza	Meningitis, epiglottitis	Cefotaxime, ceftriaxone
Klebsiella spp.	Pneumonia, urinary tract infection	A cephalosporin
Legionella spp.	Pneumonia	Erythromycin ± rifampin
Proteus mirabilis	Urinary tract infection	Ampicillin
Proteus, Providencia spp.	Urinary tract infection	Cefotaxime, ceftizoxime, ceftriaxone
Pseudomonas aeruginosa	Urinary tract infection	A fluoroquinolone
	Other infections	Ticarcillin, mezlocillin ± an aminoglycoside
Salmonella spp.	Typhoid, paratyphoid, enteritis	Ceftriaxone, a fluoroquinolone
Shigella	Dysentery	A fluoroquinolone
Vibrio cholera	Cholera	Tetracycline
Yersinia pestis	Plague	Streptomycin, gentamicin
Acid-Fast Bacilli		
Mycobacterium tuberculosis	Tuberculosis	Isoniazid ± rifampin ± pyrazinamide
Mycobacterium leprae	Hansen's disease (leprosy)	Dapsone ± rifampin ± clofazimine
Spirochetes		
Borrelia burgdorferi	Lyme disease	Ceftriaxone, doxycycline, amoxicillin
Borrelia recurrentis	Relapsing fever	Tetracycline
Leptospira interrogans	Leptospirosis	Penicillin
Treponema pallidum	Syphilis	Penicillin
Other Bacteria		
Mycoplasma pneumonia	Pneumonia	Erythromycin, azithromycin, clarithromycin, tetracycline
Rickettsia spp.	Rocky Mountain spotted fever, typhus, and other fevers	Tetracycline
Chlamydia psittaci	Psittacosis	Erythromycin
Chlamydia trachomatis	Inclusion conjunctivitis, pneumonia	Doxycycline or azithromycin
	Urethritis, cervicitis	Tetracycline
	Lymphogranuloma venereum	
Chlamydia pneumonia	Pneumonia	Doxycycline

*Penicillin-allergic patients are often treated with erythromycin or clarithromycin. Resistant strains are treated with vancomycin ± rifampin.

Modified from Morello JA, Mizer HE, Granato PA: *Microbiology in patient care,* ed 6, Boston, 1998, WCB/McGraw-Hill.

TABLE 9-10   Antimicrobial Agents for Fungi, Parasites, and Viruses

Agent	Mechanism of Action	Susceptible Microorganisms	Comments
Antifungal Agents			
Amphotericin B	Binds to sterols in fungal cell membranes, increasing their permeability and causing leakage of cellular constituents	Systemic fungi, including *Paracoccidioides brasiliensis, Coccidioides immitis, Cryptococcus neoformans, Histoplasma capsulatum, Sporothrix schenckii, Blastomyces dermatitidis, Candida* spp., *Aspergillus fumigatus*	Toxic for mammalian cells that contain sterols, such as certain kidney cells and erythrocytes; used only for severe systemic fungal infections; may have activity against some protozoa *(Leishmania, Naegleria)*
Flucytosine	Degrades in cell to an antimetabolite; also inhibits deoxyribonucleic acid (DNA) synthesis	Some *Cryptococcus, Candida* spp.	Used only for serious infections caused by susceptible strains of *Cryptococcus* and *Candida*, or topically in ophthalmic preparations
Griseofulvin	Interrupts fungal cell mitosis; causes defective DNA production	Ringworm fungi, including species of *Trichophyton, Microsporum,* and *Epidermophyton*	Used to treat ringworm infections of the hair, skin, and nails only; may need treatment for a year or longer for fungal nail infections
Ketoconazole*	Alters cellular membranes and increases cell permeability	Active against a wide range of systemic and ringworm fungi (see above) and *Candida* spp.	Given orally for systemic and superficial fungal infections; not recommended for fungal meningitis; topical preparation available; may cause liver toxicity
Miconazole	Alters cellular membranes and interferes with intracellular enzymes	Same as ketoconazole	Given orally or intravenously for severe systemic fungal infections and intravenously for fungal meningitis; may be effective for eye infections caused by the parasite *Acanthamoeba*
Nystatin	Binds to sterols in fungal cell membranes and alters their permeability	*Candida* spp.	Used orally or topically for local, but not systemic, *Candida* infections
Terbinafine	Kills fungal cells by inhibiting an enzyme important for synthesis of the fungal cell wall and membrane	Ringworm fungi, yeasts	Used to treat ringworm infections, especially of the nails; requires 6 weeks of therapy for fingernail infections and 12 weeks for toenail infections; may cause liver dysfunction and skin reactions
Antiparasitic Agents			
Albendazole	Kills worms and their larvae by interfering with adenosine triphosphate (ATP) production and thus causing depletion of energy	Larval forms of *Taenia solium* and *Echinococcus granulosus*	The first drug approved in the United States for treating neurocysticercosis and hydatid cyst disease, the infections caused by these organisms; effective in 70% to 80% of patients
Chloroquine	Binds to nucleoproteins and interferes with protein synthesis	*Plasmodium* spp.	Effective against circulating forms of malarial parasites, but not *P. falciparum* gametocytes; many *P. falciparum* strains now resistant
Emetine	Causes nuclear degeneration; interferes with trophozoite multiplication	*Entamoeba histolytica* trophozoites	Used in severe amebic dysentery only; used in combination with iodoquinol to eradicate disease completely
Iodoquinol	Unknown	*Entamoeba histolytica*	Used alone for treating mild or asymptomatic intestinal disease; or in combination with emetine for severe disease
Mebendazole	Inhibits uptake of glucose by helminths, depleting glycogen stores and interfering with absorptive and secretory functions	Pathogenic roundworms, including hookworm, pinworm, whipworm, threadworm; some tapeworms (beef, pork, dwarf), *Echinococcus* larvae (hydatid cyst)	Highly effective in curing infection caused by susceptible worms
Niclosamide	Inhibits mitochondrial oxidative phosphorylation in worms	Most tapeworms, pinworm	Does not act on larval or tissue stage of tapeworm infection (cysticercosis)
Piperazine	Causes paralysis of the worm by inhibiting nerve transmissions at neuromuscular junctions	*Ascaris lumbricoides* (roundworm), *Enterobius vermicularis* (pinworm)	Effective only when given in multiple doses
Praziquantel	Unknown, but result is paralysis of the worm's suckers, causing the worm to dislodge from the intestine	*Schistosoma* spp., flukes, some tapeworms, larval stage of *T. solium*	Highly effective against susceptible worms
Primaquine	Interferes with DNA function of malarial parasites	*Plasmodium* spp.	Active against tissue forms of malarial parasites and *P. falciparum* gametocytes; not active against other erythrocytic forms, therefore must be used in conjunction with chloroquine to eradicate all parasite forms

(Continued)

TABLE 9-10   Antimicrobial Agents for Fungi, Parasites, and Viruses—cont'd

Agent	Mechanism of Action	Susceptible Microorganisms	Comments
Pyrimethamine	Folic acid inhibitor similar to the antibacterial trimethoprim	*Toxoplasma gondii, Plasmodium* spp.	Used with a sulfonamide to treat toxoplasmosis; less effective against malarial parasites than other drugs
Quinacrine	Unclear, but may inhibit nucleic acid synthesis in *Giardia lamblia*	*G. lamblia*, tapeworms, blood forms of malarial parasites (*Plasmodium* spp.)	Drug of choice for giardiasis; used for chemoprophylaxis against malaria; not effective for circulating gametocytes of *P. falciparum*
Thiabendazole	Unclear, but may deprive worm of energy source by decreasing formation of ATP	Most intestinal roundworms	Drug of choice for *Strongyloides* infections; variable results against other roundworms
Antiviral Agents			
Acyclovir	Interferes with DNA synthesis and inhibits viral replication of herpes simplex and varicella-zoster viruses; others unknown	Herpesvirus family (including herpes simplex virus, varicella-zoster virus, Epstein-Barr virus, cytomegalovirus)	Used for treating initial and recurring herpes simplex infections in immunocompromised children and adults; in the immunocompetent host, used only against severe genital herpes; some herpesviruses now resistant
Amantadine[†]	Prevents the virus from penetrating the host cell or inhibits uncoating so that the virus cannot replicate	Influenza A virus only	Virustatic drug; effective primarily for prophylaxis or symptomatic treatment of early influenza A; most effective when given on exposure before symptoms develop
Didanosine	Competitively inhibits reverse transcriptase enzyme; causes premature termination of viral replication	Retroviruses, including human immunodeficiency virus (HIV)	Used for the treatment of patients with advanced HIV infection (acquired immunodeficiency syndrome, AIDS) who cannot tolerate zidovudine therapy or who deteriorate clinically and immunologically during zidovudine therapy
Ganciclovir	Competes with guanosine compound for uptake into viral DNA, interferes with DNA synthesis	Herpesvirus family	Used almost exclusively to treat human cytomegalovirus infections, especially in immunosuppressed organ or bone marrow transplant patients; some viruses already resistant
Lamivudine	Interferes with viral DNA synthesis by acting as a competitive inhibitor of the viral reverse transcriptase enzyme	HIV	Approved for use in combination with zidovudine; may delay viral development of resistance to zidovudine or improve its effectiveness
Ribavirin	Interferes with ribonucleic acid (RNA) and DNA synthesis, inhibiting protein synthesis and replication	In vitro, many RNA and DNA viruses	Available in the United States only for aerosol therapy; used in infants to treat severe lower respiratory infections caused by respiratory syncytial virus
Saquinavir	Blocks the action of a protease vital to the final stages of viral replication; the first of a type of drug known as a protease inhibitor to gain the U.S. Food and Drug Administration (FDA) approval	HIV	Approved for use in combination with zidovudine; does not work well alone; ritonavir and indinavir are newer such drugs now in use in combination with zidovudine and other anti-HIV drugs
Zalcitabine	Same as didanosine	HIV	Approved for use only in combination with zidovudine for adults with full-blown AIDS
Zidovudine	Inhibits reverse transcriptase enzyme in retroviruses	Retroviruses, including HIV	An "orphan" drug used only to treat symptomatic HIV infections (AIDS)

*A number of antifungal imidazole drugs that are similar to ketoconazole in mechanisms of action and spectra of antifungal activity are available as topical preparations. These agents, which include clotrimazole, econazole, and terconazole, are *not* used to treat serious systemic disease.
†Rimantadine, a similar agent for prophylaxis of influenza A, may produce fewer side effects than does amantadine.
Modified from Morello JA, Mizer HE, Granato PA: *Microbiology in patient care*, ed 6, Boston, 1998, WCB/McGraw-Hill.

MICROBIOLOGY OF THE ORAL CAVITY

NORMAL ORAL FLORA

A. Composition and distribution—different types of surfaces create distinct habitats within the mouth, so the distribution of microflora is not uniform throughout the mouth (Table 9-11)

1. Lips—predominantly facultatively anaerobic streptococci; *Streptococcus vestibularis* found in the vestibule

2. Palate—predominantly *Actinomyces* spp. and *Streptococcus* spp.

3. Cheek—predominantly *Streptococcus* spp. and *Haemophilus* spp.; 5 to 25 bacteria per epithelial cell

    a. Majority of streptococci are *Streptococcus oralis* and *S. mitis*, and fewer are *S. sanguis*

    b. *Simonsiella* spp. isolated primarily from human cheek cells

TABLE 9-11   Bacterial Genera Found in the Oral Cavity

	Gram-Positive	Gram-Negative
Cocci	Abiotrophia	Moraxella
	Enterococcus	Neisseria
	Peptostreptococcus	Veillonella
	Staphylococcus	
	Stomatococcus	
	Streptococcus	
Rods	Actinomyces	Aggregatibacter
	Bifidobacterium	Campylobacter
	Corynebacterium	Cantonella
	Eubacterium	Capnocytophaga
	Lactobacillus	Centipeda
	Propionibacterium	Desulfovibrio
	Pseudoramibacter	Desulfobacter
	Rothia	Eikenella
		Fusobacterium
		Haemophilus
		Johnsonii
		Leptotrichia
		Porphyromonas
		Prevotella
		Selenomonas
		Simonsiella
		Tannerella
		Treponema
		Wolinella

4. Tongue (100 bacteria per tongue epithelial cell)—papillae allow for a large surface area for colonization, resulting in higher bacterial density and diverse microflora
   a. Predominantly *S. oralis*, *S. mitis*, and *Streptococcus salivarius*
   b. *Stomatococcus mucilagenosus* is found exclusively on the tongue
   c. *Veillonella* spp., *Actinomyces naeslundii*, *Actinomyces odontolyticus*, and *Haemophilus* spp. also isolated
   d. Increased numbers of *Porphyromonas*, *Prevotella*, *Fusobacterium*, and *Treponema* spp. lead to halitosis resulting from an increase in volatile sulfur compound production
5. Saliva—108 to 109 bacteria/mL of saliva; normal salivary flow ensures that bacteria do not multiply in saliva; so saliva does not contain resident flora but rather bacteria from other surfaces—primarily from the dorsum of the tongue and dental plaque
6. Tooth surfaces (plaque)
   a. Pits and fissures
      (1) Morphologic condition allows for proliferation
      (2) Predominantly *Streptococcus mutans* and *A. naeslundii*
      (3) Common sites for caries
   b. Interproximal surfaces
      (1) Inaccessible to routine oral hygiene care
      (2) Bacteria in biofilm can proliferate in microcolonies undisturbed
      (3) Predominantly *A. naeslundii*, *Actinomyces israelii*, and *Streptococcus*, *Veillonella*, and *Prevotella* spp.
      (4) Majority of streptococci are *S. sanguis*
      (5) Common site for caries
   c. Smooth coronal surfaces
      (1) Can be covered with plaque if oral hygiene is not practiced
      (2) Plaque formation limited by the cleaning action of saliva, the movement of soft tissue, and the action of food particles
      (3) Oral bacteria colonize in a predictable succession
B. Factors that influence microbial composition
   1. Temperature 35°C to 36°C (95°F to 96.8°F)
      a. Temperature may influence proportions of bacterial species
      b. Periodontal pockets with active disease have higher temperatures—up to 39°C (102.2°F)
   2. Nutrient sources
      a. Exogenous sources include the host's diet, especially dietary sugar, which is needed for acid and polysaccharide production
      b. Endogenous sources
         (1) Saliva
         (2) Gingival exudate
         (3) Epithelial cells and leukocytes
         (4) Continuing existence of flora even when humans and animals are fed by a stomach tube
         (5) Certain bacteria use metabolic byproducts from other bacteria
   3. pH requirements
      a. The pH of most surfaces regulated by saliva (pH 6.75 to 7.25)
      b. Dietary sugars provide a selective force favoring predominance of certain organisms that tolerate an acidic medium (pH 5)
      c. Strains of *S. mutans*, related streptococci, and lactobacilli are both acidogenic (produce acid) and aciduric (tolerate low pH values)
      d. Dairy products can elevate pH
      e. The pH of the gingival sulcus becomes alkaline during the host inflammatory response in periodontal disease (pH 7.2 to 7.8)
      f. Alkaline pockets favor the growth of the pathogen *Porphyromonas gingivalis*
   4. Oxygen concentration
      a. Distribution of microorganisms in the mouth is related to the redox potential at a particular site
      b. The majority of organisms are micro-aerophilic, facultative, or obligate anaerobes
   5. Microbial interactions
      a. Microbial aggregation
         (1) Certain species undergo reactions between host cell surfaces (adhesion receptor)
         (2) Bacterial cells can attach to each other (co-aggregation)
         (3) Some bacteria produce extracellular polysaccharides (glucans, fructans, heteropolysaccharides) that provide structural and energy sources for plaque

b. Interspecies antagonisms
   (1) Competition for host receptors
   (2) Competition for endogenous nutrients
   (3) Production of inhibitory substances (e.g., hydrogen peroxide by *S. mitis* and *S. sanguis*; bacteriocin by streptococci; formation of acid by *S. mutans, S. salivarius,* and lactobacilli)

6. Saliva
   a. Nonspecific factors
      (1) Flow of saliva removes planktonic bacteria from oral surfaces
      (2) Flow rate bears some relationship to caries susceptibility
      (3) Rate of secretion is correlated to buffering capacity
      (4) Proteins and glycoproteins form acquired pellicles on teeth; bacteria can attach to the pellicle
      (5) Proteins and glycoproteins act as nutrient source for microflora
      (6) Proteins and glycoproteins can aid in co-aggregation of bacteria, thus facilitating their clearance
      (7) Antibacterial components include lysozymes, lactoperoxidase, lactoferrin, salivary thiocyanate, and peptides
   b. Specific factors—secretory immunoglobulin A inhibits microbial attachment

7. Host factors that affect microflora
   a. Oral hygiene—antimicrobial agents in toothpaste and mouth rinses; mechanical force of toothbrush and interdental care
   b. Gender and race
   c. Age
   d. Alterations in the food web
   e. Long-term use of antibiotics and development of antimicrobial resistance
   f. Scratches and grooves on tooth surfaces or restorations, or margins between dental restorations and tooth surface that enhance biofilm formation
   g. Genetics

Development of Oral Microflora

A. The oral cavity is usually sterile at birth
B. Initial colonization of the infant's mouth by the microflora of the mother, milk, water, and saliva of those in close contact
   1. Oral microflora consist of aerobic and facultatively anaerobic gram-positive species
   2. *S. salivarius, S. oralis,* and *S. mitis* predominate by the first month of the infant's life
C. The microflora diversify in the next few months with several gram-negative anaerobes—*Prevotella melaninogenica, Fusobacterium nucleatum,* and *Veillonella* spp.
D. At 12 months, most children have the following organisms:
   1. Streptococci
      a. *S. salivarius, S. oralis,* and *S. mitis* predominate
      b. *S. mutans* and *S. sanguis* are not established until tooth eruption
      c. *S. mutans* disappears when full-mouth extractions occur; reappears with dentures

2. Staphylococci
3. *Veillonella* spp.
4. *Neisseria* spp.
5. *Actinomyces* spp.
6. Lactobacilli
7. *Nocardia* spp.
8. *Fusobacterium* spp.

E. Preschool-age child
   1. Adult-like microflora
   2. *P. melaninogenica* and spirochetes not common at age 5 years, but increase in numbers by age 13 years
F. Relatively stable oral microflora in healthy adults
G. Age-related changes in oral microflora
   1. Increase in numbers of yeast (*C. albicans*) may be associated with increased denture wear, changes in the oral mucosa, blood glucose level, and malnutrition
   2. Increased use of medications common with aging; may decrease salivary flow

BACTERIAL PLAQUE

See the section on "Bacterial Dental Biofilm" in Chapter 14.
A. Definition
   1. Deposit formed by the colonization of teeth by members of the normal oral flora
   2. Complex of bacteria in the matrix mainly of bacterial polysaccharides; biofilm
   3. Bacteria embedded in an exopolymeric matrix that provides a protective environment for bacteria
B. Stages of formation
   1. Cell-free pellicle
      a. High-molecular-weight salivary glycoproteins
      b. Quickly colonized by bacteria
   2. Supragingival plaque formation
      a. Phase I—initiation
         (1) Begins in 1 to 2 days of plaque accumulation
         (2) Gram-positive cocci and short rods show early dominance
         (3) Streptococci (aerobe)
      b. Phase II
         (1) From 2 to 4 days of plaque accumulation
         (2) Cocci still dominate, but gram-positive rods and gram-negative cocci begin to appear
         (3) *Streptococcus sanguis, S. oralis,* or *S. mitis* usually first colonizer, but *Haemophilus* and *Neisseria* spp. may also be early colonizers
      c. Phase III
         (1) From 4 to 7 days of plaque accumulation
         (2) After 7 days, streptococci remain the dominant organism, but by day 8, their numbers decrease
         (3) Filamentous bacteria (*Veillonella* and *Actinomyces* spp.) appear in 7 to 14 days
         (4) Respiration becomes increasingly anaerobic; rods and filaments predominate (increase in *Tannerella, Actinomyces, Capnocytophaga, Treponema, P. melaninogenica,* and *Fusobacterium*)

(5) Composition of mature plaque biofilm varies with site, oxygen and nutrient sources, and level of protection

3. Subgingival plaque formation
  a. Microbiota
    (1) Vibrios and spirochetes prevalent
    (2) Anaerobic, gram-negative, motile, asaccharolytic
  b. Types
    (1) Tooth associated (attached)
    (2) Tissue associated
    (3) Unattached subgingival

C. Factors that affect adherence and retention
  1. Salivary glycoprotein
    a. Affinity for hydroxyapatite
    b. Causes bacteria to aggregate
  2. Specific bacterial attachment mechanisms
    a. Electrostatic forces
    b. Bacterial surface components (adhesions) bind specific sites of the pellicle (receptors)
    c. Hydrophobic interactions
  3. Bacterial competition
    a. Relative numbers of a species may affect colonization patterns
    b. *Streptococcus sanguis* has a stronger affinity for enamel than does *S. mutans;* fewer numbers of *S. mutans* are in saliva to compete for tooth sites
  4. Bacterial interactions—some evidence that *S. mutans* and *S. sanguis* are antagonistic
  5. Natural local cleansing activity and retentive areas
  6. Diet

D. Plaque polysaccharides
  1. Extracellular glucans—structural component of plaque
    a. Synthesized from sucrose
    b. Properties
      (1) Insoluble
      (2) May mediate attachment of bacteria to dental tissues
      (3) May entrap bacterial enzymes or metabolic products
      (4) Ability of *S. mutans* to produce glucans appears essential for cariogenicity
  2. Levans (fructans and heteropolysaccharides)—produced by *S. mutans, S. sanguis, S. salivarius, Lactobacillus* spp., *Rothia* spp., *Eubacterium* spp., and *A. naeslundii*
    a. Soluble
    b. Reserve nutrients
    c. Can be used as sources of energy in bacterial metabolism

E. Microbial composition of plaque
  1. Bacterial composition of supragingival (supramarginal) plaque
    a. Thin layer; 1 to 20 cells thick
    b. Mostly gram-positive facultative anaerobic organisms
    c. Most predominant organisms are *S. sanguis* and *A. naeslundii*
    d. Other species found include *A. israelii, S. mutans, Veillonella* and *Fusobacterium* spp., *Treponema* spp., and *Capnocytophaga* spp.

2. Bacterial composition of normal gingival crevicular plaque
  a. Gingival crevice—an area of stagnation and bacterial proliferation—environmental influences include an increase in crevicular fluid, desquamation of epithelial cells, and bacterial acid products
  b. Quantity of species relatively constant; proportions of species vary among people and even within the same mouth
  c. Predominant organisms are *S. mitis, S. sanguis, A. naeslundii, A. odontolyticus, A. meyeri, A. georgiae, Rothia dentocariosus,* and *Eubacterium, Fusobacterium,* and *Treponema* spp.

3. Calculus
  a. Inorganic salts, 70% to 90%
  b. Microbes similar to those of the gingival crevicular area
  c. Main role in periodontal disease is to serve as a collection site for more bacteria

DENTAL CARIES

See Fig. 9-13.
A. Prerequisites for caries development
  1. Cariogenic bacteria
  2. Supply of substrate for acid production
  3. Susceptible host
B. Cariogenic bacteria
  1. Essential properties
    a. Acidogenic and aciduric; acid must be produced and a low pH maintained for a long period
    b. Ability to attach to tooth surfaces
    c. Formation of a protective matrix

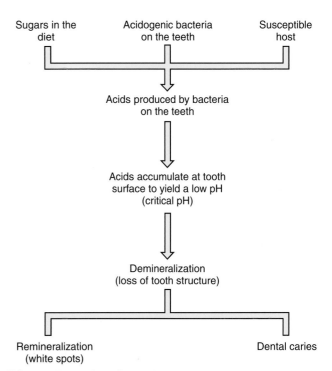

FIG 9-13 Formation of dental caries.

2. Streptococci
   a. *Streptococcus mutans*
      (1) Most strongly cariogenic bacteria in animals
      (2) Hard surfaces are a prerequisite for its presence; the organisms disappear if teeth are extracted and reappear with dentures
      (3) Homofermentive lactic acid former
      (4) Produces insoluble and soluble glucans
      (5) A high-sucrose diet is generally associated with an increase in the *S. mutans* population
      (6) Usually found in the early stages of plaque formation
   b. *Streptococcus sobrinus*
      (1) A *mutans* streptococcus
      (2) Possible roles in caries are still evolving
   c. *Streptococcus sanguis*
      (1) Produces glucans
      (2) Some strains cariogenic in animals
      (3) Colonizes tooth enamel
      (4) Is present in plaque and sometimes cheek
   d. *Streptococcus mitis*
      (1) Cariogenic in animals
      (2) Found on oral soft tissues
   e. *Streptococcus salivarius*
      (1) Produces fructans
      (2) Usually has a strong affinity for oral soft tissues, especially the tongue
      (3) Some strains cariogenic in animals
3. Lactobacilli
   a. Present in small numbers in plaque
   b. Increase in number in the mouth when the sugar content in the diet is high
      (1) Present in the mouth where sugar is retained
      (2) Carious lesions act as retention sites
   d. Strongly acidogenic and aciduric
   e. May have important role in the progression of caries
2. *Actinomyces*
   a. *Actinomyces naeslundii* primary cause of root-surface caries
   b. Plaque-forming organisms
   c. Ferment glucose to produce mostly lactic acid
   d. *A. naeslundii* present on tongue, tooth surfaces, and plaque
C. Acid production in plaque
   1. Decalcification of teeth caused by acids produced through bacterial fermentation
   2. Cariogenic plaque, when exposed to sugar, shows a decrease in pH that is low enough to decalcify enamel within minutes; pH returns to resting levels after approximately 40 minutes; even though sugar is washed away by saliva, pH can remain at a low level for 20 minutes
   3. Important features of the acid production process
      a. Amount of plaque
      b. Predominant microflora
      c. Rate of salivary flow
      d. Substrate characteristics
      e. Location of plaque
   4. More lactic acid present than any other acid

D. Bacterial substrates and diet
   1. Sucrose
      a. Main substrate for cariogenic bacteria
      b. Important in the formation of smooth-surface caries
      c. Metabolized to form acids and glucans
      d. Essential for caries production in animals
      e. Epidemiologic evidence has established its role in human caries
      f. Increase in the frequency of sucrose consumption is associated with an increase in caries
      g. High cariogenic effect when retained on teeth for a long period
   2. Starches
      a. Low cariogenicity
      b. Probably influences plaque microflora
E. Host factors
   1. Tooth surface
      a. Caries formation influenced by tooth morphology and arch form
      b. Enamel surfaces are probably more caries resistant than the subsurface
   2. Saliva
      a. Functions that affect the carious process
         (1) Clearance of food
         (2) Buffer activity
         (3) Bacterial aggregation
         (4) Antibacterial function (e.g., immunoglobulin A, lysozymes, salivary peroxidase)
      b. Amount of ambient calcium, phosphate, and fluoride ions in the saliva for remineralization of tooth structure
      c. Rate of flow and buffering abilities
         (1) As flow rate increases, pH rises
         (2) High salivary flow rates and buffering are associated with low caries activity

PERIODONTAL DISEASES

See the section on "Diseases of the Periodontium" in Chapter 14.
A. Classification of periodontal diseases
   1. Gingival diseases
      a. Dental plaque–induced gingival diseases
         (1) Early gingivitis
            (a) Plaque is thicker (100 to 300 cells thick) and more complex than in healthy tissue
            (b) Proliferation of *Fusobacterium nucleatum* and *Actinomyces* organisms
            (c) Mostly gram-positive organisms
         (2) Chronic gingivitis (Box 9-2)
            (a) Anaerobic, gram-negative organisms increase; rods form 75% of the subgingival flora
            (b) Presence of *Actinomyces naeslundii, Fusobacterium nucleatum, Prevotella intermedia,* and *Veillonella parvula*
            (c) Spirochetes are elevated at affected sites

BOX 9-2   Predominant Bacteria of Experimental Gingivitis in Young Adults

Gram-Positive Bacteria	Gram-Negative Bacteria
Actinomyces israelii	Prevotella oris
Actinomyces naeslundii	Prevotella intermedia
Actinomyces odontolyticus	Campylobacter spp.
Propionibacterium acnes	Veillonella parvula
Lactobacillus spp.	Fusobacterium nucleatum
Streptococcus anginosus	Treponema spp.
Streptococcus mitis	Wolinella spp.
Peptostreptococcus micros	
Eubacterium spp.	

From Marsh P, Martin MV: *Oral microbiology,* ed 4, Boston, 1999, Wright.

BOX 9-3   Some Bacterial Species That Have Been Commonly Implicated in Chronic Periodontitis

Gram-Positive Bacteria	Gram-Negative Bacteria
Eubacterium brachy	Tannerella forsythensis
Eubacterium nodatum	Dialister pneumosintes
Eubacterium timidium	Fusobacterium nucleatum
Peptostreptococcus anaerobius	Porphyromonas gingivalis
Peptostreptococcus micros	Prevotella intermedia
	Prevotella loescheii
	Prevotella oralis
	Campylobacter rectus
	Treponema spp.
	Aggregatibacter actinomycetemcomitans

---

b. Plaque-induced gingival disease is modified by systemic factors
  (1) Endogenous sex-steroid–hormone gingival disease (pubertal-associated gingivitis, pregnancy-associated gingivitis, menstrual gingivitis)
  (2) Diabetes mellitus–associated gingivitis
  (3) Hematologic (leukemic) gingival disease
  (4) Drug-influenced gingival enlargement
  (5) Gingival disease associated with nutrition
c. Non–plaque-induced gingival disease
  (1) Gingival disease of specific bacterial, viral, fungal, or genetic origin
  (2) Gingival manifestations of systemic conditions
  (3) Traumatic lesions, foreign-body reactions, and nonspecific gingival lesions
2. Periodontal diseases
a. Necrotizing periodontal diseases
  (1) Necrotizing ulcerative gingivitis (NUG)
    (a) Anaerobic infection of gingival margins causes ulceration; if allowed to progress, destruction of gingivae and underlying bone occurs; onset is sudden and acute
    (b) The interproximal areas are affected first
    (c) Appears to be an opportunistic infection based on predisposing factors (e.g., plaque formation, depression of polymorphonuclear leukocyte [PMN] function, stress, poor diet, immunocompromise)
    (d) Predominant microflora include *P. intermedia,* spirochetes, and fusiform bacteria
  (2) Necrotizing ulcerative periodontitis (NUP)
    (a) Appearance—necrosis of gingival tissues, periodontal ligaments, and alveolar bone
    (b) Indications—client presents with pain and excessive necrosis
    (c) Severe and rapid periodontal destruction; lack of deep-pocket formation
    (d) Occurs in persons infected with HIV and those undergoing immunosuppressive therapies
    (e) Predominant microflora include *C. albicans, Haemophilus actinomycetemcomitans, F. nucleatum,* and *Porphyromonas gingivalis*

b. Chronic periodontitis (slight or early; moderate; severe or advanced) (Box 9-3)
  (1) Extension of inflammatory changes into deeper periodontal structures, with resulting bone loss
  (2) May indicate multiple diseases that share similar characteristics
  (3) Pockets provide a favorable environment for bacterial growth
  (4) Different bacterial populations associated with destructive periodontitis have been described (Boxes 9-4 and 9-5)
  (5) Periodontitis can be a manifestation of systemic diseases such as hematologic or genetic disorders
  (6) Associated with abscesses of the periodontium and endodontic lesions

---

BOX 9-4   Species of Bacteria for Which Proportions in Plaque Rise with Increasing Severity of Periodontal Disease

Gram-Positive Bacteria	Gram-Negative Bacteria
Eubacterium alactolyticum	Aggregatibacter actinomycetemcomitans
Eubacterium brachy	Bacteroides gracilis
Eubacterium nodatum	Campylobacter concisus
Eubacterium saphenum	Campylobacter rectus
Eubacterium timidium	Campylobacter curvus
Eubacterium spp.	Filifactor alocis
Atopobium rimae	Fusobacterium nucleatum
Peptostreptococcus anaerobius	Prevotella denticola
	Prevotella intermedia
	Prevotella nigrescens
	Prevotella melaninogenica
	Prevotella oris
	Prevotella tannerae
	Prevotella veroralis
	Porphyromonas gingivalis
	Selenomonas flueggei
	Selenomonas infelix
	Selenomonas noxia
	Selenomonas sputigena

BOX 9-5   Principal Bacteria Associated with Periodontal Disease

Chronic periodontitis	*Porphyromonas gingivalis, Prevotella intermedia, Campylobacter rectus, Fusobacterium nucleatum, Tannerella forsythensis*
Aggressive periodontitis	*Aggregatibacter actinomycetemcomitans, P. intermedia, Eikenella corrodens, Capnocytophaga sputigena*
Necrotizing periodontal diseases	*P. gingivalis, A. actinomycetemcomitans, F. nucleatum, P. intermedia, Streptococcus* spp., *Candida albicans, Treponema, Selenomonas*

BOX 9-6   Identification of the Bacterial Cause in Periodontal Diseases

1. Large numbers of the bacteria are associated with the disease state, and absence or reduced numbers are associated with health.
2. Elimination or suppression of the organism reverses or reduces the disease.
3. Elevated host responses are associated with the disease.
4. Animal pathogenicity similar to periodontal disease occurs on implantation of the organism(s) into germ-free animals.
5. Bacteria possess potentially pathogenic mediators that could contribute to the disease process.

From Newman MG, Nisengard R: *Oral microbiology and immunology,* ed 2, Philadelphia, 1994, Saunders.

---

(7) Causative organisms include *P. intermedia, Aggregatibacter actinomycetemcomitans, P. gingivalis, Eubacterium* spp., *F. nucleatum,* spirochetes, *Tannerella forsythensis,* and *Campylobacter rectus*

   c. Aggressive periodontitis
   (1) Onset occurs before age 35 years and is associated with a rapid rate of progression of tissue destruction, host defense defects, and composition of subgingival flora
   (2) Subclassifications are identified as:
      (a) Prepubertal periodontitis
      (b) Juvenile periodontitis—localized and generalized forms
   (3) Primary organism—*Aggregatibacter actinomycetemcomitans*
   (4) Clinical findings and symptoms
      (a) Periodontitis as a manifestation of systemic diseases such as hematologic or genetic disorders
      (b) Abscesses of the periodontium
      (c) Periodontitis associated with endodontic lesions
      (d) Developmental or acquired deformities and conditions

B. Bacterial plaque (dental) biofilm and periodontal disease
   1. Factors that determine the severity of periodontal disease
      a. Level of oral hygiene
      b. Type of bacteria in plaque biofilm
      c. Host resistance and immunity
   2. Evidence supports microbial cause of periodontal disease (Box 9-6)
      a. Gram-negative microorganisms are the principal bacteria associated with disease
      b. Plaque associated with gingivitis and periodontitis has different bacterial populations
   3. Pathogenic mechanisms of plaque bacteria
      a. Attachment mechanisms—attachment to the tooth surface may depend on early colonizers of tooth surface and pellicle (e.g., *Streptococcus* and *Actinomyces,* which are gram-positive organisms)
      b. Products of bacteria
      (1) Bacteria themselves may invade tissue
      (2) Products may cause tissue destruction
         (a) Endotoxins
         (b) Enzymes (collagenase, lysozyme, and hyaluronidase)
      c. Survival mechanism—slime layer and biofilm formation
   4. Immunologic aspects of periodontal disease
      a. Bacteria in biofilm are antigenic in varying degrees; present a challenge to the immune system
      b. Immune responses are just as likely to be protective as they are injurious to tissue
      c. Mechanisms of tissue destruction may involve anaphylactic, cytotoxic, immune complex, and cell-mediated or delayed hypersensitivity reactions
      d. Participation of the humoral immune system
      (1) Lymphocytes and plasma cells are the predominant cells in the gingiva in the vicinity of plaque
      (2) Antibody production is stimulated
      (3) Complement system is activated
         (a) Mediates inflammatory response and immunologic reactions
         (b) Complement is activated by plaque bacteria, either by endotoxin (lipopolysaccharide) or by bacterial antigen-antibody complexes
         (c) Involved in chemotaxis (directed migration of inflammatory cells)
      e. Participation of the cell-mediated immune system
      (1) Cell-mediated immunity leads to release of lymphokines (e.g., osteoclast-activating factor)
      (2) Reports on the relationship between cell-mediated reactivity and the severity of periodontal disease are conflicting
      (3) Clinically not possible to distinguish between cell-mediated immunity (resistance) and delayed hypersensitivity (damaging) reactions in humans; both reactions depend on the same cellular participants

PERIAPICAL INFECTIONS AND ORAL-FACIAL TISSUE INFECTIONS

A. Infections
   1. Abscesses (periodontal and periapical)
   2. Postsurgical and postextraction wound infections

3. Endodontically involved infections
4. Sinus tract infections
5. Cellulitis
6. Traumatic injuries
7. Osteomyelitis
8. Postextraction alveolar osteitis (dry socket)
9. Pericoronitis
10. Periodontally involved infections

B. Bacteria cultivated from such infections
   1. Polymicrobial and opportunistic in nature
   2. Obligate anaerobic bacteria predominate in acute endodontic infections

C. Ludwig's angina
   1. Mixed infection
      a. *Fusobacterium* spp., *Prevotella* spp., *Porphyromonas* spp., and streptococci
      b. Often caused by the normal oral flora gaining access through the infected tooth
   2. Symptoms
      a. Rapidly spreading, diffuse bilateral cellulitis of the floor of the mouth and neck
      b. Swelling that may block air passages
      c. Fever and malaise
   3. Predisposing factors
      a. Infected mandibular molars
      b. Thin lingual cortical plate of the mandible

OPPORTUNISTIC INFECTIONS OF THE ORAL CAVITY

A. Definition—opportunistic organisms take advantage of a compromised situation in the host and subsequently invade and cause infections of the oral cavity

B. Actinomycosis
   1. Etiology
      a. *Actinomyces israelii* most common
      b. *A. naeslundii* and *Arachnia propionica* found in some lesions
   2. Pathogenesis
      a. Gram-positive bacteria; member of the normal oral flora
      b. Infection may follow injury with introduction of contaminated debris into tissue
   3. Clinical findings and symptoms
      a. Facial swelling, most frequently in soft tissue below the angle of the jaw
      b. Small, chronic, superficial mass
      c. Abscess with sinus and chronic discharge develops

C. Oral candidiasis—four clinically distinct forms:
   1. Pseudomembranous candidiasis
      a. A removable soft, creamy, white plaque; red or bleeding base
      b. Predominantly found on the buccal and labial mucosa, tongue, hard and soft palates

   2. Erythematous candidiasis
      a. A smooth, flat, red lesion on the dorsum of the tongue; associated with loss of papillae
      b. Can also be found on the hard palate
   3. Angular cheilitis—cracking or redness around the corners of the mouth
   4. Hyperplastic candidiasis
      a. A raised, white, nonremovable plaque
      b. Appears on the buccal mucosa, hard palate, or dorsum of the tongue

D. Staphylococci
   1. Etiology—*S. aureus* and *S. epidermidis*
   2. Pathogenesis—normal flora of the skin, oral cavity, and anterior nares
   3. Clinical manifestations
      a. Mandibular osteomyelitis
      b. Acute suppurative parotitis

E. Other oral diseases
   1. Mumps
      a. Etiology—mumps virus
      b. Clinical findings and symptoms
         (1) Painful, swollen parotid or submaxillary glands
         (2) Fever and malaise
         (3) Red and swollen papilla of Stensen's duct
      c. Prevention through vaccine
   2. Herpangina (vesicular pharyngitis)
      a. Etiology—coxsackievirus A
      b. Pathogenesis
         (1) Transmitted by ingestion of contaminated materials
         (2) Primarily occurs in children
      c. Clinical findings and symptoms—fever and vomiting; vesicles and later ulcers on the mucous membrane of the throat, palate, or tongue
      d. Recovery in 7 to 10 days; complications rare
   3. Recurrent aphthous ulcers
      a. Etiology—unknown; evidence suggests immunologic etiology
      b. Clinical findings and symptoms
         (1) Canker sore, small ulcer
         (2) Covered by pseudomembrane
         (3) Surrounding erythematous halo
         (4) Occur on nonkeratinized mucosa
   4. Hand-foot-and-mouth disease
      a. Etiology—coxsackievirus A
      b. Pathogenesis
         (1) Highly infectious
         (2) Typically affects many children, particularly in schools
      c. Clinical findings and symptoms
         (1) Vesicular stomatitis and rash
         (2) Affects the buccal mucosa, tongue, gingiva, lips, hands, and feet
         (3) Pain

Source	Website Address	Description
Bergey's Taxonomic Outline	http://www.bergeys.org/outlines.html	Online publication, updated approximately six times per year and is free to registered users
Centers for Disease Control and Prevention (CDC)	http://www.cdc.gov/	One of the 13 major operating components of the Department of Health and Human Services (HHS), which is the principal U.S. government agency for protecting the health and safety of all Americans and for providing essential human services, especially for persons who are least able to help themselves
Organization for Asepsis and Safety Procedures (OSAP)	http://www.osap.org/	Promotes infection control and related science-based health and safety policies and practices through quality education and information dissemination
Morbidity and Mortality Weekly Report (MMWR)	http://www.cdc.gov/mmwr/	The MMWR series is prepared by the CDC and provides data regarding a variety of health and safety concerns

Website Information And Resources

REFERENCE

1. Centers for Disease Control and Prevention: *About HIV/AIDS,* 2014, http://www.cdc.gov/hiv/statistics/basics.html.

CHAPTER 9 REVIEW QUESTIONS

Answers and rationales to review questions are available on this text's accompanying Evolve site. See inside front cover for details.

evolve

1. **What cellular structure is involved in energy synthesis (ATP production)?**
   a. Golgi complex
   b. Ribosome
   c. Mitochondrion
   d. Nucleus

2. **The type of microscopic technique used to examine unstained microorganisms, spirochetes, and hanging drop preparations.**
   a. Phase-contrast microscopy
   b. Darkfield microscopy
   c. Bright-field microscopy
   d. Scanning electron microscopy

3. **Identify the type of staining procedure used to distinguish between gram-positive and gram negative bacteria.**
   a. Flagellar stain
   b. Acid-fast stain
   c. Gram staining
   d. Schaefer-Fulton stain

4. **What is the CORRECT morphologic name for bacteria that do not have a defined shape?**
   a. Staphylococci
   b. Diplococci
   c. Sarcinae
   d. Pleomorphic

5. **Heterotropic organisms do NOT require organic compounds for growth. Autotrophic organisms do require organic compounds for growth.**
   a. Both statements are TRUE.
   b. Both statements are FALSE.
   c. The first statement is TRUE; the second statement is FALSE.

   d. The first statement is FALSE; the second statement is TRUE.

6. **The type of microbial relationship in which one organism benefits at the expense of another organism is called:**
   a. Symbiosis
   b. Predation
   c. Commensalism
   d. Parasitism

7. **In which phase of metabolism is energy released?**
   a. Catabolism
   b. Anabolism
   c. Glycolysis
   d. Protein synthesis

8. **Which immunoglobulin plays an important role in hypersensitivity reactions?**
   a. IgG
   b. IgM
   c. IgA
   d. IgE

9. **Infection acquired during a hospital stay is called:**
   a. Latent
   b. Primary
   c. Toxemia
   d. Nosocomial

10. **A gumma is present during which stage of a syphilis infection?**
    a. Primary
    b. Secondary
    c. Tertiary
    d. Quaternary

11. **The incubation period for hepatitis B is:**
    a. 28 to 47 days

b. 45 to 160 days

c. 8 to 16 hours

d. 15 to 50 days

12. The structure that functions as storage site for amino acids, carbohydrates, and proteins is:

a. Ribosome

b. Plastid

c. Cytoplasmic membrane

d. Vacuole

13. In eukaryotes, respiration occurs through what cellular structure?

a. Cytoplasmic membrane

b. Mitochondria

c. Ribosomes

d. Lysosomes

14. The type of media used to produce visual differentiation between several microorganisms is called:

a. Reducing media

b. Enriched media

c. Selective media

d. Differential media

15. Exotoxins are soluble microbial virulence factors secreted by gram-positive bacteria. Endotoxins are heat-stable polysaccharide microbial virulence factors secreted by gram-negative bacteria.

a. Both statements are TRUE.

b. Both statements are FALSE.

c. The first statement is TRUE; the second statement is FALSE.

d. The first statement is FALSE; the second statement is TRUE.

16. All the following are clinical signs and symptoms associated with a tetanus infection EXCEPT one. Which one is the *exception*?

a. Trismus

b. Spasms of facial muscles

c. Infection of the external ear canal

d. Dysphagia

17. The type of bacteria associated with rheumatic fever is:

a. Streptococcal species

b. *Plasmodium* spp.

c. *Salmonella* spp.

d. None of the above

18. Warts are caused by this virus:

a. Rubella virus

b. Human parvovirus B19

c. Varicella-zoster virus

d. Papillomavirus

19. The cardinal signs of inflammation include heat, pain, redness, swelling, and loss of function. Pus formation is NOT possible in the inflammatory process.

a. Both statements are TRUE.

b. Both statements are FALSE.

c. The first statement is TRUE; the second statement is FALSE.

d. The first statement is FALSE; the second statement is TRUE.

20. The bacterial species primarily responsible for root caries is:

a. *Streptococcus mitis*

b. *Streptococcus sanguis*

c. *Streptococcus salivarius*

d. *Actinomyces naeslundii*

21. An infection caused by a pathogen that does not normally cause disease in a healthy individual is indicative of which type of infection?

a. Latent

b. Systemic

c. Local

d. Opportunistic

22. The type of immunity acquired by injection of immune serum is called:

a. Natural active

b. Artificial active

c. Natural passive

d. Artificial passive

23. Direct uptake of donor DNA by a recipient cell is called:

a. Transformation

b. Mutation

c. Transduction

d. Conjugation

24. Kaposi's sarcoma is associated with the herpesvirus. B cell lymphomas are associated with the AIDS virus.

a. Both statements are TRUE.

b. Both statements are FALSE.

c. The first statement is TRUE; the second statement is FALSE.

d. The first statement is FALSE; the second statement is TRUE.

25. Gingival inflammation without the presence of periodontal pocketing and bone loss is indicative of:

a. Chronic periodontitis

b. Necrotizing ulcerative periodontitis

c. Gingivitis

d. Aggressive periodontitis

26. Varicella-zoster viruses are responsible for the formation of:

a. Cold sores

b. Warts

c. Chickenpox

d. Measles

27. The causative agent of infectious mononucleosis is:

a. *Neisseria gonorrhoeae*

b. Epstein-Barr virus

c. *Treponema pallidum*

d. Rubella virus

28. The primary organism in necrotizing ulcerative gingivitis is:

a. *Streptococcus mutans*

b. *Aggregatibacter actinomycetemcomitans*

c. *Candida albicans*

d. *Prevotella intermedia*

29. All the following are prerequisites for caries development EXCEPT:

a. Cariogenic bacteria

b. Supply of substrate for acid production

c. Susceptible host

d. Calculus

30. **The causative agent of syphilis is:**
    a. *Chlamydia psittaci*
    b. *Treponema pallidum*
    c. *Borrelia burgdorferi*
    d. *Mycobacterium tuberculosis*

31. **Transmission of hepatitis A occurs through the fecal-oral route. Transmission of hepatitis B occurs through the parenteral route.**
    a. Both statements are TRUE.
    b. Both statements are FALSE.
    c. The first statement is TRUE; the second statement is FALSE.
    d. The first statement is FALSE; the second statement is TRUE.

32. **Skin and oral lesions are clinical symptoms of what disease?**
    a. Trismus
    b. Leprosy
    c. Lyme
    d. Ringworm

33. **Escherichia coli is a gram-positive bacillus. Escherichia coli is the causative agent of urinary tract infections.**
    a. Both statements are TRUE.
    b. Both statements are FALSE.
    c. The first statement is TRUE; the second statement is FALSE.
    d. The first statement is FALSE; the second statement is TRUE.

34. **Endospores are formed during a process called:**
    a. Sporulation
    b. Germination
    c. Binary fission
    d. None of the above

35. **The causative agent of urinary tract infections is:**
    a. *Yersenia pestis*
    b. *Bacillis anthracis*
    c. *Escherichia coli*
    d. *Bordetella pertussis*

36. **In which phase of bacterial growth is there a decrease in the number of cells?**
    a. Lag phase
    b. Log phase
    c. Stationary phase
    d. Phase of decline

37. **Necrotizing ulcerative gingivitis is an anaerobic infection. Predominant microflora present include *Prevotella intermedia*, spirochetes, and fusiform bacteria.**
    a. Both statements are TRUE.
    b. Both statements are FALSE.
    c. The first statement is TRUE; the second statement is FALSE.
    d. The first statement is FALSE; the second statement is TRUE.

38. **The antibacterial agent used to treat tetanus is:**
    a. Doxycycline
    b. Erythromycin
    c. Penicillin
    d. Metronidazole

39. **Coxsackievirus A is responsible for causing:**
    a. Herpangina
    b. Mumps
    c. Recurrent apthous ulcers
    d. Orthomyxovirus

40. **Hand-foot-and-mouth disease is frequently seen in the elderly population. The causative agent in hand-foot-and-mouth disease is coxsackievirus A.**
    a. Both statements are TRUE.
    b. Both statements are FALSE.
    c. The first statement is TRUE; the second statement is FALSE.
    d. The first statement is FALSE; the second statement is TRUE.

41. **Acidophiles prefer a pH of:**
    a. 0 to 4
    b. 5 to 9
    c. Greater than 9
    d. None of the above

42. **Prokaryotes reproduce via binary fission. Binary fission is a form of asexual reproduction.**
    a. Both statements are TRUE.
    b. Both statements are FALSE.
    c. The first statement is TRUE; the second statement is FALSE.
    d. The first statement is FALSE; the second statement is TRUE.

43. **A person presents with raised, white, nonremovable plaques on the buccal mucosa, hard palate, and dorsum of tongue. This condition is most likely:**
    a. Herpetic whitlow
    b. Recurrent apthous ulcer
    c. Hyperplastic candidiasis
    d. Ludwig's angina

44. **All the following are functions of the cell wall EXCEPT:**
    a. Determines and maintains the shape of the microorganism
    b. Provides support for flagella
    c. Prevents rupture of the cell resulting from differing osmotic pressures
    d. Protein synthesis

45. **During the initiation phase of plaque formation, the predominant bacteria present are:**
    a. Gram-positive cocci and rods
    b. Gram-negative cocci
    c. Filamentous organisms
    d. None of the above

Use the following case study to answer questions 46-50.

A 50-year-old woman with a full dentition presents for a continued dental hygiene care appointment. Her chief complaint is that her lower-right mandibular molar is hurting her. Extraoral examination reveals a bilateral swelling of her neck and floor of the mouth and a cold sore on her right lip near the commissure. Intraoral examination reveals a cavitated lesion on tooth #30 occlusal; a raised, white, nonremovable plaque on her hard palate; and generalized probing depths of 5 to 6 mm.

46. **The bilateral swelling is MOST likely indicative of what disease?**
    a. Syphilis
    b. AIDS
    c. Ludwig's angina
    d. Shingles
47. **Which of the following infections is the MOST likely cause of the cold sore?**
    a. Herpesvirus
    b. Candida
    c. Influenza
    d. Cytomegalovirus
48. **The raised, white, nonremovable plaque on the hard palate is MOST likely:**
    a. Angular cheilitis
    b. Hyperplastic candidiasis
    c. Erythematous candidiasis
    d. Pseudomembranous candidiasis
49. **The bacteria primarily responsible for the lesion on #30 occlusal is:**
    a. *S. mutans*
    b. *A. actinomycetemcomitans*
    c. *C. albicans*
    d. *P. intermedia*
50. **The cause of the bilateral swelling in the neck and floor of the mouth is MOST likely a result of:**
    a. Infected tooth #30
    b. Immunocompromised health history
    c. *Candida* infection
    d. None of the above

10 CHAPTER

Infection Control and Prevention of Disease Transmission in Oral Health Care

Darnyl M. Palmer

Preventing disease transmission in dental hygiene practice requires an understanding of microbial transfer, infection, and disease in the oral health care environment. Implementing and practicing the elements of standard precautions is essential.

DISEASE TRANSMISSION

See the section on "Microbial Virulence and Disease Transfer" in Chapter 9.

A. Development of an infectious disease
   1. Source of microorganism or pathogen (microorganism capable of causing infectious disease)
      a. Primarily originating from a person's mouth
      b. May originate from a dental team member (this mode less likely than from a client's mouth)
      c. Microbes may be present in saliva, blood, respiratory secretions, and other bodily fluids
   2. Portal of exit—escape of microorganism from a person
      a. Coughing, sneezing, and talking
      b. Contaminated dental equipment, instruments, and supplies used in a client's mouth
      c. Spatter droplets and aerosol particles generated by using power instrumentation, low-speed and high-speed handpieces, and air/water syringe
         (1) Spatter droplets—large, visible particles that settle quickly, contaminating the clinician and the surfaces of the treatment area
         (2) Aerosol particles—small, invisible particles that may be inhaled or remain airborne for an extended period
   3. Transfer of microorganisms to another person
      a. Direct contact with microorganisms in a client's mouth that penetrate through nonintact skin
      b. Indirect contact with items contaminated by a client's microorganisms, including sharps (all items that can puncture skin), instruments, surfaces, hands, and equipment
      c. Droplet infection from spatter that contacts nonintact skin or mucous membranes (oral, nasal, ocular)
      d. Airborne infection from inhaling aerosols
   4. Portal of entry—entry of microorganisms into a person
      a. Inhalation—breathing aerosol particles
      b. Ingestion—swallowing droplets of saliva or blood spattered into the mouth
      c. Through mucous membranes—droplets of saliva or blood spattered into the eyes, nose, or mouth
      d. Through breaks in the skin—by touching contaminated objects, spattering of microorganisms onto nonintact skin, or punctures with contaminated sharps
         (1) Percutaneous injury—injury that penetrates the skin
         (2) Parenteral—piercing mucous membranes or skin
   5. Infection
      a. The infectious agent has a portal of entry into a susceptible (not immune) host
      b. Establishment and survival of microorganism in the body
   6. Damage to the body—the disease occurs when microorganisms multiply to a harmful level
   7. Pathogenic agents and diseases associated with oral health care (Table 10-1)

B. Infection control
   1. Goal—to prevent oral health care–related infections, injuries, and illnesses among clients and dental health care personnel (DHCP)
   2. Reducing the numbers of microorganisms that may be transmitted from person to person or from persons to the oral health care environment, and vice versa
   3. Infection control protocols seek to reduce or eliminate the likelihood of disease transmission by eliminating one or more factors required for disease transfer (Fig. 10-1)
      a. Asepsis—absence of infectious materials; achieved by removing or killing microorganisms
      b. Disinfection—reducing the number of pathogenic organisms in or on an object, thereby minimizing the potential for disease transmission
         (1) Disinfectants are applied to inanimate objects
         (2) Antiseptics are applied to living tissues
      c. Engineering controls—devices that reduce the risk of exposure to potentially infectious materials (e.g., self-sheathing needles and instrument cassettes)
      d. Personal protective equipment—items designed to protect DHCP from exposure to bloodborne and other pathogens (e.g., gloves, masks, safety glasses, face shields, barrier gowns)

TABLE 10-1   Pathogenic Agents Important in Oral Health Care

Disease	Pathogen
Bloodborne Diseases	
Viral	
Hepatitis B	Hepatitis B virus (HBV)
Hepatitis C	Hepatitis C virus (HCV)
Hepatitis D	Hepatitis D virus (HDV)
Acquired immunodeficiency syndrome (AIDS)	Human immunodeficiency virus (HIV)
Oral Diseases	
Bacterial	
Gonococcal pharyngitis	*Neisseria gonorrhoeae*
Streptococcal pharyngitis and scarlet fever	*Streptococcus pyogenes*
Syphilis	*Treponema pallidum*
Viral	
Primary herpetic gingivostomatitis	Human herpesvirus 1 or 2
Recurrent herpes (e.g., herpes labialis)	Human herpesvirus 1 or 2
Hand-foot-and-mouth disease	Coxsackievirus
Herpangina	Coxsackievirus
Hairy leukoplakia	Human herpesvirus 4
Fungal	
Candidiasis (thrush)	*Candida albicans*
Denture stomatitis	*Candida albicans*
Systemic Diseases with Oral Lesions	
Bacterial	
Secondary syphilis	*Treponema pallidum*
Viral	
Chickenpox	Human herpesvirus 3 (varicella-zoster virus)
Infectious mononucleosis	Human herpesvirus 4 (Epstein-Barr virus)
Other Diseases Spread by Respiratory or Oral Fluids	
Bacterial	
Tuberculosis	*Mycobacterium tuberculosis*
Diphtheria	*Corynebacterium diphtheriae*
Pneumonia	*Streptococcus pneumoniae, Staphylococcus aureus, Mycoplasma pneumoniae, Chlamydia pneumoniae, Moraxella catarrhalis, Haemophilus influenzae*
Meningitis, sinusitis, conjunctivitis	*Haemophilus influenzae* type B
Meningitis	*Neisseria meningitidis*
Bronchitis	*Haemophilus influenzae, Moraxella catarrhalis*
Viral	
Common cold	Rhinoviruses and several others
Influenza	Influenza viruses
Bronchitis	Influenza A, parainfluenza virus, coronavirus
Pneumonia	Influenza virus, adenovirus, respiratory syncytial virus
Cytomegalovirus (CMV) disease	Cytomegalovirus
Infectious mononucleosis	Human herpesvirus 4 (Epstein-Barr virus)
Erythema infectiosum (fifth disease)	Human parvovirus B19
Measles	Rubeola (measles) virus
Rubella	Rubella virus
Mumps	Mumps virus

Modified from Miller CH: *Infection control and management of hazardous materials for the dental team,* ed 5, St Louis, 2014, Mosby.

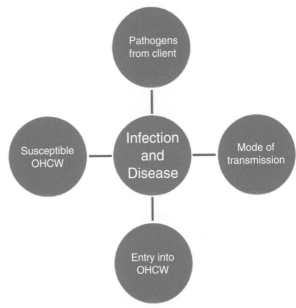

FIG 10-1 Factors related to infection and disease transfer. *OHCW,* Oral health care worker.

e. Standard precautions—treating all blood and bodily fluids (including secretions and excretions, except sweat), nonintact skin, and mucous membranes as potentially infectious in all clients
   (1) In the oral health care setting, saliva is an important source of contamination; although invisible, it is capable of containing infectious agents that can survive on surfaces for a long period
f. Transmission-based precautions—additional measures beyond standard precautions provided during urgent care to clients with certain diseases having multiple modes of transmission (e.g., tuberculosis); in this situation, care would be provided in a facility equipped with a respiratory protection program including an airborne infection isolation room (AIIR)
g. Sterilization—the destruction or removal of all microorganisms in or on an object
h. Work practice controls—procedures that reduce the chance of exposure to potentially infectious materials (e.g., using a one-handed technique to recap needles; maintaining a 14-inch to 18-inch working distance to reduce exposure to droplets; fulcruming one to four teeth away from tooth being treated)
i. DHCP-related controls
   (1) Maintaining a healthy lifestyle and immune status
   (2) Receiving recommended vaccinations
   (3) Obtain a baseline tuberculin skin test
   (4) Abiding by the recommended U.S. Public Health Service (PHS) work restrictions for DHCP in the case of certain infections and after exposure to some diseases
j. Client-related controls
   (1) Prophylactic antibiotic premedication to reduce the possibility of infection in immunocompromised individuals and others with various conditions

(2) Preprocedural rinse to decrease the microbial load in spatter and aerosols and to help protect against autogenous (self-derived) infection

(3) Avoiding treatment of clients with known communicable illnesses (e.g., influenza) or contagious lesions (e.g., herpes)

4. Infection control protocols are designed to reduce or prevent the spread of pathogens from:
   a. Client to DHCP
   b. DHCP to client
   c. Client to client
   d. Dental office to community, including families of DHCP
   e. Community to client

5. Table 10-2 outlines the mechanisms of the spread and the prevention of diseases

INFECTION CONTROL PROCEDURES FOR DENTAL HEALTH CARE PERSONNEL

A. Health history
   1. Obtain, review, and update clients' health histories at all visits
   2. Address specific questions related to present health status, physician care, hospitalizations, surgery, diseases, medications, allergies, current or chronic illness, review of major organ systems, and recent overseas travel
   3. Be aware that obtaining health histories will not identify all infectious clients; clients may suppress information purposely or unknowingly (many persons with hepatitis B virus [HBV], hepatitis C virus [HCV], and human immunodeficiency virus [HIV] are asymptomatic)

TABLE 10-2 Mechanisms of Disease Spread and Prevention

Pathway of Cross-Contamination	Source of Microorganism	Mode of Disease Spread	Mechanism or Site of Entry into Body	Infection-Control Procedure
Client to DHCP	Client's mouth	Direct contact	Through breaks in skin of dental team	Gloves or handwashing
				Immunizations
		Droplet infection	Inhalation by DHCP	Facemask
				Rubber dam
				Mouth rinsing
			Through breaks in skin of DHCP	Gloves or handwashing
				Protective clothing
				Face shield
				Rubber dam
				Mouth rinsing
			Through mucosal surfaces of DHCP	Facemask
				Eyewear
				Face shield
				Rubber dam
				Mouth rinsing
				Immunizations
		Indirect contact	Cuts, punctures, or needlesticks in DHCP	Needle safety and waste management
				Heavy gloves for cleanup
				Ultrasonic cleaning rather than hand scrubbing
				Instrument cassettes to reduce direct handling during cleaning
				Antimicrobial holding solution
				Antimicrobial cleaning solution
			Through breaks in skin of DHCP	Heavy gloves for cleanup
				Protective clothing
				Immunizations
	Client's skin lesions	Direct contact	Through breaks in skin of DHCP	Gloves or handwashing
				Immunizations
DHCP to client	DHCP hands (lesions or bleeding)	Direct contact	Through mucosal surfaces of client	Gloves or handwashing
				Care in handling sharp objects
				Immunizations
		Indirect contact	Bleeding on items used in client's mouth	Gloves or handwashing
				Instrument sterilization
				Surface disinfection
				Immunizations

TABLE 10-2   Mechanisms of Disease Spread and Prevention—cont'd

Pathway of Cross-Contamination	Source of Microorganism	Mode of Disease Spread	Mechanism or Site of Entry into Body	Infection-Control Procedure
	DHCP mouth (oral or respiratory fluids)	Droplet infection	Inhalation by client	Facemask Face shield
			Through oral mucosal surfaces of client	Facemask Face shield
Client to client	Client's mouth	Indirect contact (instruments, surfaces, hands)	Through oral mucosal surfaces of client	Instrument and handpiece sterilization Sterilization monitoring Surface covers Surface disinfection Handwashing and proper gloving Changing mask Decontaminating protective eyewear Changing protective clothing when needed Use of sterile or clean supplies Flushing dental unit water lines Monitoring water line antiretraction valves Use of disposable items
OHC setting to community	Patient's mouth	Indirect contact	Cuts, punctures, breaks in skin of dental laboratory worker, waste disposal, or laundry personnel	Waste management Disinfection of impressions and appliances Proper management of contaminated laundry Handwashing
DHCP to DHCP's family	DHCP bodily fluids	Direct or indirect contact	Intimate contact	Immunization
Community to client	Municipal water	Direct contact or airborne	Client's mouth or lungs	Use of new and separate water source Periodically disinfecting inside of dental unit water lines Use of water containing an approved antimicrobial agent Filtering the water

DHCP, Dental health care personnel; *OHC*, oral health care.
Modified from data from US Department of Labor, Occupational Safety and Health Administration: *Controlling occupational exposure to bloodborne pathogens*, Washington, DC, 1996, 2001, OSHA 3127 (revised).

4. Health history may identify conditions requiring:
   a. Diagnostic evaluation and laboratory testing
   b. Medical consultations
   c. Prophylactic antibiotic premedication to reduce the incidence of autogenous infections, that is, conditions caused by introducing the microflora of clients into injured tissues (e.g., bacteremia, abscess)
5. The U.S. Centers for Disease Control and Prevention (CDC) recommends conducting a tuberculosis risk assessment for an oral health care setting and then formulating a prevention program appropriate for its designated risk category; most dental settings will be low or very low risk
B. Immunizations are recommended for DHCP
1. Essential component of an infection control program
2. Most effective method to prevent contracting a vaccine-preventable disease
3. Immunizations are recommended for the following diseases, unless evidence of past infection and immunity: hepatitis B, varicella, influenza, measles, mumps, rubella, tetanus, diphtheria, pertussis, and

meningococcal disease; consult with a primary care physician before vaccination because some vaccines are contraindicated for immunocompromised and pregnant persons
4. The U.S. Occupational Safety and Health Administration (OSHA) policies regarding hepatitis B vaccination
   a. OSHA requires employers to make hepatitis B vaccine available at no cost to employees who are or may be exposed by occupation to bloodborne pathogens and within 10 working days
   b. Employers must provide information about the vaccine and ensure that all medical records concerning the vaccination are kept confidential
   c. Employees have the right to refuse vaccination but must read and sign an OSHA declination statement
   d. Employers cannot demand that employees be serologically prescreened before vaccination
5. Hepatitis B vaccine
   a. Two single-antigen vaccines available:
      (1) Recombivax HB (Merck & Co., Inc.)
      (2) Engerix-B (GlaxoSmithKline)

b. Process
   (1) Serologic screening for antibodies to hepatitis B surface antigen (HBsAg) before vaccination is not recommended, unless infection is suspected
   (2) Pregnancy is not a contraindication for vaccination
   (3) A series of three injections in the deltoid muscle given at 0, 1, and 6 months
   (4) Seroconversion rates are 95% to 97% in healthy younger adults; lower rates (approximately 70%) in persons over 40 years old, smokers, overweight persons, and those receiving injections in the buttocks
   (5) Genetic factors may influence seroconversion rates
   (6) Testing for antibody (anti-HBsAg) is recommended after vaccination to ensure protection against HBV; testing should be conducted 1 to 2 months after the final injection
   (7) With successful seroconversion, protective antibodies have been sustained for at least 20 years
   (8) Failure to seroconvert requires a second series of three injections
   (9) Continued failure to seroconvert could signal chronic HBV infection in a person who is unable to produce antibodies; nonresponders should be evaluated by a medical provider
   (10) The CDC currently does not recommend a booster injection
   (11) Minimal side effects of vaccine include injection site soreness, headache, and fever
   (12) Individuals with allergies to yeast or iodine (vaccine preservatives) must consult a physician before the vaccination

6. Recommended screenings for DHCP
   a. DHCP should know their HBV status
   b. Tuberculin skin test (TST), also known as the Mantoux test for tuberculosis (TB), should be administered annually according to the CDC risk level of dental setting
      (1) In the majority of cases, a positive test indicates previous infection with *Mycobacterium tuberculosis* but not active disease; in some persons, 6 months of preventive chemotherapy is advised
      (2) Only 10% of individuals infected will eventually develop disease
      (3) Drug-resistant TB does not respond to medication, which ultimately leads to death

C. Hand hygiene
   1. Extremely important disease prevention practice
   2. Hands are a primary source of microorganisms capable of disease transmission
   3. Rationale
      a. Handwashing reduces both resident and transient flora on skin
         (1) *Resident flora* are permanent residents that colonize several skin layers and cannot be completely removed; this type is less important and less likely to transmit disease than transient flora
         (2) *Transient flora* contaminate hands when hands touch contaminated surfaces; this type colonizes the outer layers of skin, only survive for a limited time, and can be easily removed by routine handwashing
      b. Protects clients and DHCP by reducing the spread of microorganisms and subsequent infections by the hands
      c. Unwashed, contaminated hands can transfer microbes to sterile instruments, dental equipment, and environmental surfaces
   4. Use of gloves is *not* a substitute for routine handwashing
   5. Hands must be washed before gloves are put on to minimize organisms that can multiply rapidly when enclosed in a moist, warm environment; bacteria and yeast growth can cause skin irritation
   6. Hands must be washed after removal of gloves because defects, tears, and punctures may occur in gloves, permitting microorganisms to be transferred to hands; this also helps remove glove powder, which contains latex protein and other glove chemicals that can elicit irritant contact dermatitis or an allergic reaction in sensitized individuals
   7. Watches, bracelets, and rings must be removed to prevent harboring of microorganisms; also, rings may perforate glove materials
   8. Nails must be kept short and clean and the cuticles well maintained; artificial nails and nail jewelry should not be worn, since current research has implicated them in disease transmission in hospitals
   9. Intact skin is the best protection against infection; this can be achieved by:
      a. Minimizing trauma to hands (e.g., cuts, scrapes) while outside the dental setting
      b. Protecting hands from drying and chapping during cold weather
      c. Frequent use of lubricating hand lotions
         (1) When at work, use hand lotion containing petroleum or oil emollients at the end of the day, because these ingredients can negatively affect the integrity of latex gloves
   10. DHCP who have open or weeping lesions or dermatitis on hands should not provide client care until the condition resolves, since dermatitis reduces the effectiveness of handwashing, and nonintact skin provides a portal of entry for microorganisms
   11. Hand hygiene procedures for routine dental hygiene care include:
      a. Vigorous lathering of hands using an interlacing finger motion with either antimicrobial or plain soap for 15 seconds
         (1) Plain soap will remove soil and transient microorganisms
         (2) Antimicrobial soap will remove or destroy transient microorganisms and reduce resident flora

(3) Disposable soap containers should not be refilled, and when empty should be discarded and replaced

(4) Soap dishes accumulate microorganisms and are not recommended

(5) Sinks and soap dispensers should be electronically operated or have foot controls; if not, paper towels should be used to turn off sink faucet

b. Rinsing with cool to lukewarm water while rubbing hands together for 10 seconds

c. Drying hands with single-use paper towels

d. Using alcohol-based hand sanitizers as an alternative to handwashing

(1) Used when no visible soil appears on the hands

(2) Have been shown to be effective, sometimes reducing bacterial counts more effectively than soap and water

(3) Most effective at inactivating microorganisms at 60% to 95% alcohol concentrations

(4) May increase the frequency of hand hygiene because of ease of use

(5) According to manufacturer's directions, place an adequate amount of alcohol-based hand sanitizer in hand and then vigorously rub hands until dry

(6) Alcohol-based hand sanitizers may cause dry skin (choose ones that contain emollients)

e. Washing hands between clients, before and after lunch, before and after restroom visits, or any time hands become contaminated

f. Maintaining asepsis by touching only sterile instruments or disinfected surfaces

12. For surgical procedures, use an antimicrobial soap with persistent or residual activity (inhibits growth and survival of microorganisms); chlorhexidine digluconate or triclosan

D. Personal protective equipment (PPE)

1. Protective barriers used to reduce exposure of mucous membranes, hands, and body of DHCP to microorganisms and also to prevent injury from chemicals and particles of debris

2. Used during client care, laboratory, disinfection, and sterilization procedures

3. PPE includes gloves, masks, protective eyewear, and protective clothing

4. Sequence for donning PPE: protective clothing, then mask and eyewear, and finally, after handwashing, gloves

5. The employer is responsible for providing and maintaining appropriate PPE for employees

6. Gloves

a. The use of gloves provides a high level of protection for both DHCP and clients

(1) Prevents direct contact with microorganisms in the client's mouth and on contaminated surfaces (bare hands often will have areas of nonintact skin providing portals of entry for pathogenic microorganisms)

(2) Prevents saliva and blood from being retained under fingernails; saliva and blood have been shown to persist for several days even with handwashing

(3) Protects against contact with disinfecting and cleaning chemicals and x-ray solutions

(4) Protects clients from the microorganisms on the hands of DHCP

(5) Examination gloves provide minimal protection against sharps injuries; utility gloves provide more protection; however, injuries still can occur

b. Risks associated with not routinely wearing gloves

(1) DHCP exposure to potentially infectious client tissues and contaminated surfaces—most likely route by which DHCP have acquired HBV from clients

(2) Client exposure to infectious agents originating from the DHCP

(a) Documented source of transmission of HBV from ungloved dentist to clients

(b) Documented case in which an ungloved hygienist transmitted herpes to 20 of her clients

(3) Skin irritation from contact with disinfecting chemicals

(4) Burns resulting from contact with hot items from sterilizer

c. Protocol for glove use

(1) Wear during intraoral procedures and when in contact with contaminated items or surfaces (e.g., contaminated laundry or waste)

(2) If it is necessary to leave the chairside during client care, remove gloves, and after hand hygiene, don a new pair on returning (prevents contamination of additional surfaces one may touch and also prevents contamination of the client with microorganisms that already may be present on those surfaces)

(3) Ensure that gloves cover the cuff of a long-sleeved gown

(4) Change gloves between clients and during long appointments because defects in gloves increase with use beyond 60 minutes

(5) Do not wash or disinfect gloves; may cause "wicking" or enhanced penetration of liquids through undetected defects in gloves

(6) Remove torn or punctured gloves as soon as possible; wash hands and don new gloves

(7) If using latex gloves, do not use petroleum or oil-based hand lotion or apply petroleum-based lubricants to client's lips

d. Types of gloves—Table 10-3 outlines glove materials

(1) Nonsterile, ambidextrous gloves in sizes extra-small, small, medium, and large are adequate for most procedures; proper glove fit is important to ensure efficient instrumentation and to prevent hand fatigue and possibly carpal tunnel syndrome

TABLE 10-3   Types of Gloves Used in Oral Health Care

Type	Material
Nonsterile (examination) gloves	Latex
	Nitrile
	Neoprene
	Vinyl
	Polyurethane
	Styrene-based co-polymer
	Butadiene methyl methacrylate
Sterile (surgical) gloves	Latex
	Nitrile
	Neoprene
	Polyurethane
	Styrene-based co-polymer
	Synthetic polyisoprene
Utility gloves	Latex
	Nitrile
	Neoprene
	Butyl rubber
	Fluoroelastomer
	Polyethylene and ethylene vinyl
	Alcohol co-polymer
Overgloves	Thin co-polymer
	Thin plastic ("food handlers")

(2) Sterile gloves are recommended for surgical procedures

(3) Use puncture-resistant and chemical-resistant utility gloves to prepare chemicals, handle contaminated instruments, and clean and disinfect surfaces

(a) Utility gloves are reusable and can be disinfected or sterilized in an autoclave

(b) Replace utility gloves when they show any signs of wear (e.g., cracks, punctures, discoloration)

(4) Overgloves are worn over treatment gloves to prevent cross-contamination of items and surfaces such as pens, charts, and drawers

(5) Heat-resistant gloves are worn when handling hot items (e.g., unloading sterilizers)

e. Dermatitis and latex allergy

(1) Irritant contact dermatitis

(a) Nonimmunologic (nonallergic) reaction of skin to chemicals used in glove manufacturing

(b) Skin on hands becomes dry, red, itchy, and cracked

(c) The condition is aggravated by soaps, not rinsing or drying hands completely, perspiration, or cornstarch powder

(d) Most skin reactions from wearing gloves are caused by irritant contact dermatitis and are not true allergic reactions

(2) Allergic contact dermatitis

(a) Type IV, or delayed, hypersensitivity occurring within hours or days because of allergy to glove chemicals

(b) Limited to area of contact, causing itching, redness, and vesicles to appear within 24 to 48 hours, followed by dry skin, fissures, and sores

(c) Patch test identifies sensitivity to specific chemical

(3) Latex allergy

(a) Type I, or immediate, hypersensitivity within minutes or hours

(b) Allergy to naturally occurring latex proteins

(c) Symptoms: skin (hives, swelling, burning, tightness, itching, redness, tingling), lungs (asthma, wheezing, constriction, coughing, sneezing, rhinitis, angioedema), and other (nausea, vomiting, diarrhea, cramps, hypertension, tachycardia, shock)

(d) Anaphylactic shock and death can occur with subsequent exposures to latex

(e) High-risk individuals for latex allergy include: persons who have had multiple surgeries and persons with spina bifida, urogenital anomalies, spinal cord injuries, and allergies to bananas, kiwis, chestnuts, or avocados

(f) Reductions in exposure to latex proteins are known to decrease sensitivity (important for DHCP to reduce their daily exposure to airborne latex proteins by wearing powder-free, reduced-protein latex or latex-free gloves)

(g) The CDC indicates that DHCP need to be educated about skin problems that can occur with frequent hand hygiene and the use of gloves

(h) Latex-free environment should be provided to clients and DHCP with a latex allergy

(4) Procedures for management of persons with latex allergy

(a) Include questions in health history appropriate for identifying possible latex allergy

(b) Document latex allergy in health history record in a way that will ensure observation by DHCP

(c) Schedule allergic clients for the first appointment of the day, when airborne latex proteins are at their lowest levels (still risky)

(d) Ensure that DHCP uses latex-free gloves for treatment area preparation and for touching all items that will come in contact with the client

(e) Use latex-free gloves and dental materials during client care

7. Masks

a. Purpose

(1) Worn to protect the mucous membranes of the nose and mouth from spatter of oral fluids

(2) Provide a lesser degree of protection from inhalation of aerosol particles

(a) Surgical masks will not provide protection from airborne infections (e.g., SARS)

(b) The N-95 respirator is needed to protect against airborne infections

(3) May provide some protection to client from nasal or oral secretions of DHCP

b. Composed of synthetic material that should filter at least 95% of small particles

c. Types of masks
  (1) Dome mask with elastic band
  (2) Tie-on or ear-loop mask

d. Should have a seal against the face to minimize leakage around the margins

e. Maximizing effectiveness and minimizing cross-contamination
  (1) Use a new mask for each client
  (2) Change the mask if it becomes moist; moistness compromises its effectiveness by increasing the passage of unfiltered air around the edges of the mask and may wick contaminants through the mask
  (3) Don a new mask every 20 to 30 minutes to maintain high filterability
  (4) Adjust the mask so that it fits snugly against the face, covering nose and mouth
  (5) Avoid touching the mask during the appointment
  (6) Keep the mask on after completing the procedure to reduce inhalation of aerosols
  (7) When removing the mask, handle it by its strings or elastic
  (8) Do not leave the mask on the head, dangling around neck, or in your pocket

8. Protective eyewear
  a. Purpose—protect the eye from microbial invasion, chemicals, physical projectiles, ultraviolet (UV) light, and lasers
  b. Risks for unprotected eyes
    (1) Conjunctivitis
    (2) Ocular herpes (can cause blindness)
    (3) Hepatitis B (eye as portal of entry)
    (4) Eye injury (physical or chemical)
  c. Types of eyewear
    (1) Regular glasses offer limited side or top protection and are not recommended
    (2) Safety glasses, goggles, or loupes
      (a) Cover entire eye orbit (providing protection on all sides)
      (b) Some may be worn over prescription glasses
      (c) Are more shatter resistant than regular glasses
      (d) Provide minimal visual distortion
      (e) Are able to withstand disinfection (should be cleaned and disinfected between clients)
      (f) Should meet American National Standards Institute (ANSI) guidelines for spatter and impact protection
    (3) Face shields
      (a) An alternative to safety glasses
      (b) Should be chin-length and provide top and side protection

(c) Masks should still be worn to reduce inhalation of aerosols

(d) Provide maximum coverage of face for high-spatter procedures (e.g., air polishing, power scaling)

(e) Face shields made of thin plastic may have limited impact resistance

(4) Protective eyewear should be provided to clients
  (a) Protection against damage from UV (curing) light and lasers
  (b) Protection against physical and chemical injury to the client's eyes during treatment

9. Protective (barrier) clothing
  a. Purpose
    (1) Protects nonintact skin from contamination by microorganisms
    (2) Reduces the risk of bringing contaminants on unprotected clothing beyond dental setting
    (3) May protect client from microorganisms on street clothing or may provide protection against disease transmission when soiled protective clothing is changed between clients (*fomites*—clothing and paper that can absorb and transmit infectious agents)
    (4) Microorganisms adhere to clothing; however, lack of evidence exists to support the extent to which barrier clothing protects against disease transmission
  b. Characteristics of protective clothing
    (1) Reusable or disposable
    (2) Gowns, aprons, laboratory coats, or uniforms used as a covering for street clothing or scrub uniforms
    (3) High collar that fits closely around the neck
    (4) Long-sleeved garments with fitted cuffs allow gloves to extend over them for complete coverage
  c. To maximize effectiveness and minimize cross-contamination
    (1) Use fabric made of synthetic material, which is more fluid resistant
    (2) Do not wear protective clothing outside treatment area (remove before going out [e.g., to lunch] or leaving the dental setting)
    (3) Change protective clothing daily or when visibly soiled
    (4) Avoid touching clothing during client care and throughout the day
    (5) Roll protective clothing inside out to minimize contact with exposed surface

10. Additional barrier protection used when cleaning or performing surgery
  a. Plastic aprons or other fluid-proof garments
  b. Head covers
  c. Shoe covers

11. Laundering of reusable clothing
  a. Laundered in the office following the manufacturer's instructions

b. Sent to a laundry service in a leak-proof bag labeled with the biohazard symbol

c. It is against OSHA regulations for DHCP to take contaminated protective clothing home for laundering

ORAL HEALTH CARE ENVIRONMENT AND PROMOTION OF INFECTION CONTROL

A. Design and equipment selection emphasizes:
1. Smooth construction—eliminates knobs, hooks, and crevices
2. Design of client chairs and operator stools that:
   a. Minimize buttons and seams
   b. Use vinyl upholstery instead of cloth
   c. Provide foot-control operation
3. Avoidance of fabric-covered, coiled, or mechanically retracted tubings
4. Sink faucets and soap dispensers with foot or electronic controls
5. Paper towel dispenser designed to avoid touching hardware or electronically controlled
6. Plastic-lined waste containers recessed under cabinet, with opening on countertop
7. Surfaces that are compatible with disinfectants and detergents
8. Plastic laminate instead of wood for cabinets and countertops
9. Vinyl flooring and walls that are smooth and seamless
10. Carpeting or wallpaper not recommended
11. Dental unit water lines (DUWLs) that provide:
    a. Antiretraction valves to prevent the aspiration of microorganisms into water lines
    b. Equipment, devices, and treatments for DUWLs
       (1) Filtration unit
       (2) Sterile-water delivery system
       (3) Flushing the lines with antimicrobial agents
       (4) Independent water reservoirs
12. Reduction of airborne microbes
    a. Air circulation exchange system or single-room filtration units
    b. Ventilation systems to control noxious sterilization and laboratory vapors
    c. Prevention of recirculation of contaminated air or transport of microbes
    d. Cooling and heating system filters that prevent transfer of microbes
13. Housekeeping surfaces are surfaces that are not contaminated by hands or equipment (e.g., walls, floors) and should be cleaned and disinfected routinely or when visibly soiled with detergents or low-level hospital disinfectants
    a. Clean mops and cloths after use and allow to dry before reuse, or use single-use items
    b. Clean walls, blinds, and window treatments in client care areas
    c. Perform cleaning with a wet cloth or mop to prevent distribution of microorganism-laden dust particles
14. Keep treatment area free of unnecessary or seldom-used equipment and items

Maintaining Asepsis in the Oral Health Care Environment

A. Items associated with oral health care are classified as:
1. Critical—instruments that penetrate oral soft tissue or bone, enter the bloodstream, or enter other sterile tissues of the mouth (e.g., curette); must be heat-sterilized or a single-use (disposable) device (SUD)
2. Semi-critical—items that come in contact with mucous membranes (used in the mouth) but will not penetrate soft tissue, contact bone, enter the bloodstream, or enter other sterile tissues of the mouth (e.g., radiographic positioning devices)
   a. Preferably heat-sterilized or an SUD (disposable)
   b. If heat sensitive, decontaminate using a chemical sterilant or cover the device with a Food and Drug Administration (FDA)–approved barrier to prevent contamination (e.g., digital radiography sensors)
3. Noncritical—items that contact intact skin (e.g., blood pressure cuff)
   a. If contamination is possible, cover the device to prevent contamination
   b. If the device is contaminated, clean and disinfect
      (1) If contaminated by blood, use intermediate-level disinfectant
      (2) If not contaminated by blood, use low-level disinfectant
B. Maintaining asepsis with the use of chemicals and surface covers
1. Categories of disinfecting or sterilizing chemicals (Table 10-4)
   a. Sterilant—destroys all microorganisms, including high numbers of bacterial spores
   b. High-level disinfectant—destroys all microorganisms but may not destroy bacterial spores (depending on contact time, can be either a disinfectant or sterilant)
   c. Intermediate-level disinfectant—destroys vegetative bacteria, most fungi, and most viruses; inactivates *Mycobacterium tuberculosis* var. *bovis*
   d. Low-level disinfectant—destroys vegetative bacteria, some fungi and viruses; does *not* inactivate *M. tuberculosis* var. *bovis* (Fig. 10-2)
C. Surface disinfection of clinical contact surfaces
1. Any surface that is touched by contaminated hands, instruments, devices, or other items during the provision of oral health care (e.g., light handles, dental equipment)
2. Identify and list surfaces that will be contaminated during treatment
3. Post the list in the treatment area to increase effectiveness and efficiency of decontamination procedures
4. Approaches to clinical contact surface asepsis
   a. Avoid unnecessarily contaminating surfaces during treatment by:
      (1) Using unit doses of materials to avoid contamination of multiple-use containers

TABLE 10-4	Categories of Disinfecting or Sterilizing Chemicals		
Category	**Definition**	**Examples**	**Use**
Sterilant*	Destroys all microorganisms, including high numbers of bacterial spores	Glutaraldehyde, glutaraldehydephenate, hydrogen peroxide, hydrogen peroxide with peracetic acid, peracetic acid	Heat-sensitive reusable items: immersion only
High-level disinfectant*	Destroys all microorganisms, but not necessarily high numbers of bacterial spores	Glutaraldehyde, glutaraldehydephenate, hydrogen peroxide, hydrogen peroxide with peracetic acid, peracetic acid, orthophthaldehyde	Heat-sensitive reusable items: immersion only
Intermediate-level disinfectant	Destroys vegetative bacteria, most fungi, and most viruses; inactivates *Mycobacterium tuberculosis* var. *bovis* (is tuberculocidal)	Environmental Protection Agency (EPA)–registered hospital disinfectant[†] with label claim of tuberculocidal activity (e.g., chlorine-based products, phenolics, iodophors, quaternary ammonium compounds with alcohol, bromides)	Clinical contact surfaces, noncritical surfaces with visible blood
Low-level disinfectant	Destroys vegetative bacteria, some fungi, and some viruses; does not inactivate *M. tuberculosis* var. *bovis* (is *not* tuberculocidal)	EPA-registered hospital disinfectant with no label claim of tuberculocidal activity (e.g., quaternary ammonium compounds)	Housekeeping surfaces (e.g., floors, walls); noncritical surfaces without visible blood; clinical contact surfaces[‡]

*Some, but not all, of these products can serve as high-level disinfectants and sterilants, depending on the immersion time used.
[†]A hospital disinfectant is one that has been shown to kill *Staphylococcus aureus*, *Pseudomonas aeruginosa*, and *Salmonella choleraesuis*.
[‡]The Centers for Disease Control and Prevention (CDC) indicates that low-level disinfectants can be used on clinical contact surfaces if the product has a label claim of killing human immunodeficiency virus (HIV) and hepatitis B virus (HBV) in addition to being an EPA-registered hospital disinfectant.
Modified from Centers for Disease Control and Prevention: Guidelines for infection control in dental health-care settings, *MMWR* 52(RR-17):1-66, 2003.

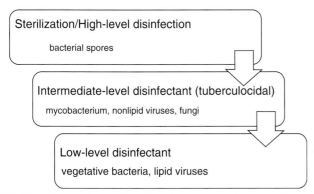

FIG 10-2 Decreasing order of resistance of microorganisms to germicidal chemicals. (Modified from Centers for Disease Control and Prevention: Guidelines for infection control in dental health-care settings, *MMWR* 52(RR-17):1-68, 2003.)

   (2) Using prearranged tray setups and cassettes containing a complete selection of instruments needed for a particular procedure
   (3) Gathering the needed supplies and equipment at the beginning of treatment to eliminate the need to open drawers and cabinets or to leave the treatment area to retrieve supplies during client care
   (4) Having sterile pliers, overgloves, gauze, and paper towels available for use as barriers between contaminated gloved hands and uncontaminated objects (e.g., drawer handle, dental record)
  b. Prevent contamination by using a surface cover or barrier protection
   (1) Surface covers protect surfaces that are difficult to preclean adequately
   (2) May be less time-consuming than precleaning or disinfecting surfaces before and after client care

   (3) Surface covers include clear plastic wrap, bags, and tubing
   (4) May be placed using bare hands on cleaned and disinfected surfaces
   (5) Should be placed to protect the entire surface and to ensure that the barrier protection will not come off when the surface is touched
   (6) Reduce the use of chemicals that may stain or corrode and are hazardous to DHCP and the environment
  c. Disinfection of surfaces not covered by barriers
   (1) Requires purchase and proper use of disinfecting chemicals
   (2) Chemical use requires that Safety Data Sheets (SDSs) be filed on site and that DHCP be provided information and training on the hazards and proper use of chemicals
   (3) Disinfection is best reserved for surfaces that are difficult to cover, smooth surfaces, and those not involving electricity
  d. A dual approach consisting of both barrier protection and disinfection with chemicals is most often used in oral health care settings
 5. Clinical contact surfaces to be covered or disinfected
  a. Mobile cart, master control unit, countertop, and radiographic equipment
  b. Air/water syringe, high-volume and low-volume evacuators (parts of these may be sterilized or disposable, which is preferred because these items come in contact with mucous membranes)
  c. Hoses, tubing, and controls attached to handpieces
  d. Supports for handpieces, air/water syringe, and suction devices
  e. Chairs, including switches and levers

f. Control switches

g. Light handles

h. Faucet handles and soap dispenser (if manually operated)

i. Instrument tray (if it cannot be sterilized)

j. Stethoscope earpieces

k. Floss dispenser, hand mirror, pens, pencils

l. Chairside computers and keyboards

m. Phones, intercoms

6. Factors influencing effectiveness of surface disinfection with chemicals

a. Numbers and types of organisms present; some organisms have a higher resistance to destruction by chemicals (e.g., *Mycobacterium* species)

b. Amount of *bioburden* (blood, saliva, and microorganisms)

(1) Organic materials in blood and saliva insulate microorganisms from chemicals

(2) May partially inhibit the active ingredient in the disinfectant

c. Selection of an Environmental Protection Agency (EPA)–registered disinfectant that is tuberculocidal (sterilant or high-level disinfectant should *not* be used for clinical contact surfaces)

d. Use of a water-based disinfectant is reported to clean organic material better than alcohol-based disinfectants

e. Performing procedures carefully and following manufacturer's instructions by using appropriate disinfectant concentration, use life, and contact time

(1) Do not store gauze squares or other materials moistened in disinfectant; instead, wet material before use

(2) If using container of disinfectant towelettes, keep lid closed to prevent drying

f. Clean surfaces with a combination of a detergent and a disinfectant to maximize the removal of bioburden before the disinfection step

(1) The detergent or disinfectant used for the cleaning step must contain a surfactant

(a) Surfactant—an agent that loosens, emulsifies, and holds soil in suspension, allowing for easier removal of debris and for more thorough cleaning

(2) An advantage to using a combination agent is that a chemical disinfectant starts the killing process during the cleaning step and reduces the opportunity for contaminants to spread to other surfaces

7. Cleaning or disinfection technique for clinical contact surfaces

a. Exercise care when using disinfectants, and wear PPE, including utility gloves

(1) To prevent irritation or injury to eyes, mucous membranes, and skin

(2) To avoid breathing in noxious vapors

b. Step 1—clean; spray the detergent or disinfectant, or apply with a premoistened cloth

TABLE 10-5 Chemical Agents for Surface Disinfection

Chemical Classification	Advantages	Disadvantages
Chlorines	Rapid acting Broad spectrum Economical	Prepare solution daily Diminished activity by organic matter Corrosive Strong odor
Iodophors	Broad spectrum Few reactions Residual biocidal activity	Unstable at high temperatures Dilution and contact time critical Prepare solution daily Discoloration of some surfaces Inactivated by hard water
Synthetic phenolics	Broad spectrum Residual biocidal activity Compatible with most metals	Degrades certain types of plastic over time Difficult to rinse Film accumulation Alcohol-based products are only fair to poor in cleaning ability
Dual or synergized quaternaries	Broad spectrum Contains detergent for cleaning	Easily inactivated by anionic detergents and organic matter Damaging to some materials

c. Step 2—wipe; vigorously wipe surfaces with a paper towel to remove stuck-on debris

d. Step 3—reapply the disinfectant

(1) Leave surfaces undisturbed for a specified contact time, usually 10 minutes

(2) Wipe any remaining wet areas with a paper towel

8. Chemical disinfectants for surface disinfection (Table 10-5)—selection criteria

a. EPA-registered intermediate-level disinfectant that is tuberculocidal (kills *M. tuberculosis* var. *bovis*)

b. Effective within 10 minutes or less

c. Does not have an offensive odor

d. Reasonable cost

e. Provides persistent or residual effect on treated surfaces

f. Retains stability and effectiveness in the presence of bioburden, preferably water-based

g. Good penetrating and cleaning ability

h. Compatible with and innocuous to equipment and clinical surfaces (consult product manufacturer for recommendations)

i. The CDC does not recommend alcohol, household bleach, or early-generation quaternary ammonium compounds as surface disinfectants

D. Dental unit water line asepsis

1. High concentrations of bacteria have been found in untreated DUWLs (e.g., power instrumentation, air-polishing units, high-speed handpieces, air/water syringes)

a. Municipal water entering the dental unit is not sterile and contains 0 to 500 colony-forming units per milliliter (CFU/mL) of heterotrophic bacteria

b. Water exiting untreated DUWLs may contain more than 100,000 CFU/mL
   (1) Consists of waterborne bacteria of low pathogenicity or opportunistic pathogens, which pose the greatest risk to immunocompromised individuals
   (2) Organisms of greatest concern are *Pseudomonas, Legionella,* and *Mycobacterium* species
2. Microorganisms attach to and accumulate on the inside of the water line tubing, creating biofilm colonies (an organized, protected, and highly resistant colony of live microorganisms attached to a surface) (see the section on "Bacterial Dental Biofilm" in Chapter 14); formation of biofilm:
   a. Biofilm includes naturally occurring waterborne bacteria and may include microorganisms from the oral cavities of clients treated before the current client
   b. Stagnation of water and small-diameter tubing in DUWLs encourages biofilm formation
   c. Incoming water brings a continuous source of nutrients to bacteria
   d. As water flows past the biofilm in the water line, it picks up detached bacteria before exiting through dental equipment
3. Dental unit water and infection control
   a. No epidemiologic evidence of a widespread public health problem caused by dental unit water
      (1) In 2011, one confirmed case of an 82-year-old woman in Italy who died after contracting legionnaires disease from aspirating *Legionella*-contaminated dental unit water at her dental office
   b. Using water that does not meet the standards for drinking water increases client and DHCP exposure to microorganisms (immunocompromised individuals most at risk)
   c. Oral health care facilities should use water that meets the American Dental Association (ADA) recommendation of no more than 200 CFU/mL of aerobic mesophilic heterotrophic bacteria for routine dental care
   d. Dental unit water from a municipal supply should not be used for oral surgery or in the treatment of immunocompromised persons (sterile water delivery systems must be used)
   e. Boil water notices in the community
      (1) Do not use dental unit or faucet water until the notice is lifted
      (2) After the notice is lifted, flush all water lines for 1 to 5 minutes, and disinfect them following manufacturer's recommendations
4. Improving the quality of dental unit water
   a. Routinely check antiretraction valves (valves can become stuck in the open position with age)
   b. Flush water lines for 3 to 5 minutes at the beginning of each day; flush for 30 seconds between clients
      (1) Flushing does not remove biofilm but may temporarily reduce planktonic (free-floating) microbes

   (2) Flushing may help remove client materials that have entered the turbine, air, and water lines
   c. Use an independent water reservoir—a bottle that supplies nonmunicipal water to dental unit
   d. Chemical treatment of DUWLs is still necessary to control biofilm formation, even when an independent water reservoir is used

Maintaining the Treatment Area During Client Care

A. Spatter and aerosol management to reduce the number of microorganisms escaping from the source
   1. Use a preprocedural, antimicrobial rinse containing chlorhexidine, essential oils, or iodophor to reduce microbial counts in spatter and aerosols
   2. Use air and water separately instead of a combination spray
   3. Use high-volume evacuation, whenever possible
      a. When using the saliva ejector, do not allow the client to close the lips around the tip, creating a seal
      b. Research has shown that in one in five cases, previously suctioned fluids might enter a client's mouth by way of a reverse flow in the vacuum line
   4. Use of a rubber dam will not only reduce spatter and aerosols but also will lessen the chance of a client's saliva retracting into the dental handpiece and the air/water syringe
B. Reducing the risk of contamination and disease transmission
   1. Limit the areas of contamination; use overgloves when touching clinical contact surfaces
   2. Disinfect anything not covered with barriers when touched by contaminated hands
   3. Avoid accessing drawers, cabinets, and other storage areas with contaminated gloves; ask for assistance if additional supplies are needed
   4. Protect dental records from contamination
      a. Ask for the help of a hygiene assistant or other personnel to record
      b. Use overgloves
      c. Record data on audio, and make manual entries in client record after glove removal
      d. Generate client record with voice-activated computer software
   5. Eating, drinking, smoking, applying of cosmetics or lip balm, and handling of contact lenses are prohibited in client care areas
   6. Food and drink cannot be stored in refrigerators, freezers, or cabinets or on shelves and countertops where blood or saliva is present
C. Waste disposal during treatment
   1. Immediately discard blood-soaked items in a small biohazard bag taped to the mobile cart or the cabinet
   2. Do not allow contaminated waste to accumulate on trays
D. Precautions and care in handling syringes or sharp instruments
   1. Needlestick injuries are a major cause of disease transmission to health care personnel
      a. Never permit "sharps" to be directed toward the body

b. Do not allow uncovered needles to remain on tray
c. Never recap a needle using a two-handed technique
   (1) Using one hand, the cap is scooped up from the tray
   (2) Use the sheath holder
   (3) Use self-sheathing disposable needles
d. Never bend, break, or otherwise manipulate a needle
e. DHCP giving an injection should appropriately recap the needle to eliminate the danger of passing an uncovered needle to another worker for recapping
f. Sharps containers should be located in each treatment area

2. Instrument sharpening
   a. Sharpening contaminated instruments poses risk of disease transmission
      (1) Avoid sharpening during a procedure
      (2) Instead, include duplicates of most-used instruments in the cassette for difficult cases
   b. The ideal method involves sharpening sterile instruments and then sterilizing again before use

3. Avoid injury with contaminated instruments during client care (i.e., curettes and scalers)
   a. Avoid fulcruming on the same tooth being treated
   b. Never wipe instruments on gauze held in your hand or wrapped around your finger
   c. Instruments should be organized and lying flat (instruments should not be on top of each other, sticking up, or balancing crosswise on the edges of cassettes)
   d. Never grab instruments by the working end
   e. Avoid holding more than one instrument in each hand
   f. Do not adjust dental light while holding an instrument

E. Exposure incident protocol (Box 10-1)
   1. Includes all needlesticks, puncture wounds, cuts, and scrapes with contaminated instruments and all nonintact skin and mucous membrane exposure to blood and saliva

---

BOX 10-1 Recommendations for Contents of the Occupational Exposure Report

Date and time of exposure

Details of the procedure being performed, including when and how the exposure occurred

   If related to a sharps device, the type and brand of device and how and when in the course of handling the device the exposure occurred

Details of the exposure, including the type and amount of fluid or material and the severity of exposure; for example:

   For a percutaneous exposure, depth of injury and whether fluid was injected

   For a skin or mucous membrane exposure, the estimated volume of material and the condition of the skin (e.g., chapped, abraded, intact)

Details about the exposure source; for example:

   Whether the source material contained hepatitis B virus (HBV), hepatitis C virus (HCV), or human immunodeficiency virus (HIV)

   If the source is HIV infected, the stage of disease, history of antiretroviral theapy, viral load, and anitiretroviral resistance information, if known

Details about the exposed person (e.g., hepatitis B vaccination and vaccine response status)

Details about counseling, postexposure management, and follow-up

---

a. In DHCP, 90% of exposures result from sharps penetrating the hands and fingers
2. Immediately wash the injured area with antimicrobial soap and water or flush with water for a mucous membrane exposure (eye)
3. Inform the employer about the incident
4. If the source individual can be identified, request his or her consent for blood testing for HBV, HCV, and HIV as soon as possible (if the source individual's disease status is not already known)
5. Results of the source individual's tests are confidential and are revealed only to the exposed employee, not to the employer
6. The employer is responsible for providing to the exposed employee laboratory testing for HBV, HCV, and HIV (30-minute rapid test available), medical evaluation, and counseling by a preselected, qualified, licensed health care provider (HCP)
7. HCP should be familiar with most current PHS recommendations for testing and postexposure prophylaxis (PEP)
8. Within 2 hours of exposure, the employee should seek medical care allowing PEP, if indicated, which offers the greatest chance of success in preventing disease transmission (seroconversion)
   a. Seroconversion depends on dose of blood transferred, titer of virus (viral load), resistant viral strain, depth of injury, and host factors
   b. PEP may reduce the risk of infection by 80%
9. If the employee declines testing, a blood sample from the employee may be preserved for 90 days in case the employee later consents to testing
10. The HCP informs the employee about both his or her own test results and the source client's test results and of any conditions that require further evaluation and treatment
11. The employer receives a written report from the HCP confirming that the employee was tested, informed of results, and counseled if further evaluation or treatment was needed
    a. Report notes if hepatitis B vaccine was administered
    b. Report does *not* include test results, diagnoses, or treatment because this information is confidential and protected employee health information

F. Prevention of disease transmission during radiographic procedures (see the section on "Infection Control" in Chapter 6)
   1. Although radiographic procedures are generally noninvasive, the potential for disease transmission does exist
   2. The use of barriers on equipment will prevent contamination and promote efficiency
      a. Plastic bag to cover position-indicating device (PID), tubehead, and swivel arms
      b. Plastic cover for exposure control switch
      c. Cover for headrest and chair controls
      d. FDA-approved plastic barrier for digital sensor
      e. Plastic barrier underneath exposed films and on countertop

3. If contamination occurs, disinfect
    a. Use EPA-registered intermediate-level disinfectant
    b. Disinfect all touched surfaces that are unprotected by barriers
    c. Do not directly spray disinfectant on the control panel because it has electrical components
    d. Follow manufacturer's directions for digital sensors (most cannot be disinfected)
4. Radiographic film holders—use reusable film holders that can be heat-sterilized, or use disposable items (SUDs)
5. Radiographic film options
    a. Digital radiographs (no film processing necessary for some methods)
    b. Film in plastic covering or pouch (best option when using film)
    c. Film without plastic covering (during processing, special handling is necessary when removing the film from the packet to avoid contaminating the film)
6. Aseptic procedure for imaging and processing dental radiographs in plastic pouches
    a. Drape the client with lead apron and thyroid shield, and position the client's bib to act as a barrier; if shields become contaminated, disinfect with an intermediate-level disinfectant
    b. Wear PPE
    c. After exposing the film, drop it into a disposable cup
    d. Remove the plastic pouches, and drop the film packet into a new cup without contaminating the film packet or the outside of the cup
    e. Remove gloves, and wash hands before transporting the film to the processing area
    f. With ungloved hands, unwrap the film and put it into the automatic processor
7. Aseptic procedure for processing dental radiographs without plastic covering
    a. After exposure, contaminated film should be placed in a plastic cup without contaminating the outside of the cup
    b. Don a new pair of gloves before transporting the film to the darkroom
    c. Open the film packet, and drop the film on a paper towel (proceed carefully to avoid contaminating the film)
    d. Remove gloves, wash hands, and with bare hands, feed the film into the automatic processor
G. Infection control for the dental laboratory
    1. Prevention of disease transmission between the treatment area and the dental laboratory
    2. OSHA regulations include measures for the protection of dental laboratory personnel from bloodborne pathogens
    3. Impression materials, prostheses, and appliances are exposed to oral microflora
    4. Protective attire and barrier techniques
        a. When performing laboratory procedures, PPE should be worn; use caution with lathes because gloves can become caught and cause injury
        b. Masks and eyewear protect against chemicals, aerosols, spatter, and projectiles

5. Preparation of materials and transport to laboratory
    a. Clean and disinfect impressions, prostheses, and casts before transport
    b. Always disinfect prostheses before sending them to another location or returning to the client
    c. Use new packing material every time the prosthesis is transported between the laboratory and the oral health care facility to prevent contamination of shipping materials
    d. Communicate the infection control protocol to the laboratory and DHCP
6. Minimizing contamination of common areas in laboratory
    a. Use paper covers on countertops
    b. Place plastic barriers on frequently touched areas
    c. Procedures for using the lathe
        (1) Use fresh pumice each time
        (2) Use disposable trays
        (3) Use sterile or disposable ragwheels (polishing devise made of cloth)
7. Use a shielding device and air-suction motor with the polishing lathe, model trimmer, or grinding bench to minimize aerosol spray
8. An EPA-registered intermediate-level disinfectant should be used to disinfect contaminated laboratory materials (e.g., impressions, fixed and removable prostheses, retainers, crowns)
    a. Spray the chemical or, preferably, immerse the material in the chemical using minimal effective exposure time (at least 15 minutes) to prevent damage to the material
    b. Consult with the manufacturer to determine which chemicals are compatible with the item to be disinfected and the immersion time required
9. Professional cleaning of removable prostheses
    a. Use of denture-cleaning solutions is *not* a substitute for disinfection
    b. To prevent microbial contamination:
        (1) Use resealable plastic bags
        (2) Do not reuse the denture-cleaning solution or plastic bags
        (3) Place sealed bags in a disinfected beaker in the ultrasonic unit
        (4) Sterilize or dispose of the equipment used in cleaning (e.g., brushes)
    c. Rinse the prosthesis with water to remove any residual chemical, and place it in a mouthwash solution to ensure a pleasant taste for the client

Maintaining the Oral Health Care Environment After Client Care

A. Decontamination of the treatment area
    1. Wear PPE, including utility gloves
    2. Seal and transport the biohazard bag (that is taped to the mobile cart) containing blood-soaked gauze to the biohazard waste container
    3. Deliver instruments in a closed, puncture-proof container (cassette) to the instrument-processing area

4. Remove surface barriers carefully to avoid contamination of the surfaces underneath, and dispose of in a trash receptacle

5. Remove and dispose of SUDs (air/water syringe tip, saliva ejector)

6. Using air/water syringe, flush low-volume and high-volume (if used) evacuator tubing for 30 seconds

7. Flush all other water lines for 30 seconds between clients (ultrasonic unit)

8. If instrument sterilization is delayed, place the instruments in a holding solution to prevent bioburden from drying on the instruments

9. At the end of the workday, flush high-volume and low-volume evacuator tubing with a cleaning and disinfecting solution; at least weekly, clean the trap of the evacuation system, or preferably, replace with a disposable trap

B. Regulated infectious waste

1. Medical waste that has the potential for disease transmission and requires special handling and disposal

2. OSHA regulates the handling of infectious waste; EPA regulates the disposal of infectious waste for three categories:
   a. Sharps (e.g., needles, scalpel blades, instruments)
   b. Tissue and extracted teeth; CDC allows extracted teeth to be returned to the client
   c. Blood, items soaked or caked with blood, or items that could release potentially infectious materials when compressed; CDC considers saliva as infectious material but not as regulated medical waste

3. Unregulated medical waste—solid waste that is generated, including all disposable items other than sharps, tissues, extracted teeth, and blood-soaked items (e.g., gloves, saliva ejectors, cups, surface barriers); unregulated medical waste may be potentially infectious; however, it is unregulated and may be disposed of as common trash unless restricted by state and local laws

4. Contact state and local governments for regulations on the disposal of regulated and unregulated medical waste

C. Waste management

1. Line trash receptacles with plastic bags

2. Sharps containers should be placed in each treatment area

D. Waste disposal

1. Regulated infectious waste must be separated from other waste, put in a color-coded ("red bagged") container, and labeled with the biohazard symbol (Fig. 10-3)
   a. Sharps must be in a closed, leakproof, and puncture-resistant sharps container
   b. Nonsharp items must be placed in a leakproof container (e.g., biohazard bag)

2. Disposal options
   a. Sterilization on-site and disposal according to local and state regulations
      (1) Do not process instruments and waste in same load

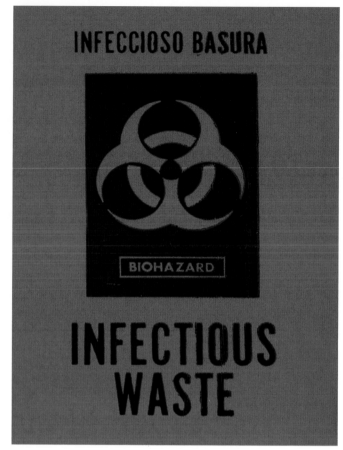

FIG 10-3 Biohazard symbol: (Sorrentino SA, Gorek B: *Mosby's textbook for long-term care nursing assistants*, ed 6, St Louis, 2011, Mosby.)

      (2) Properly perform biologic monitoring during sterilization
      (3) Extracted teeth, to be used for educational purposes, with amalgam restorations must not be heat-sterilized because this will generate toxic vapors; use a chemical sterilant instead; teeth without restorations must be heat-sterilized
   b. Hazardous waste removal service by an EPA-approved waste hauler
      (1) The oral health care facility is ultimately responsible for the proper disposal of infectious waste; therefore the waste hauler's credentials should be checked carefully
      (2) A manifest should be provided by the waste hauler indicating the method by which the waste was treated and its final disposal site

E. Instrument processing

1. Organization of sterilization area
   a. For efficiency, the instrument-processing area should be centrally located
   b. The area is designed to allow for linear progression of instrument processing and for the separation of contaminated and clean or sterile items
   c. The area should be divided into three designated areas:

(1) Decontamination area—receiving area for contaminated instruments (soaking and waste disposal), ultrasonic cleaning, rinsing, and drying

(2) Packaging area—instruments are arranged in sets; chemical and biologic indicators are added; instruments are wrapped or bagged, sealed, and labeled

(3) Sterilization and storage area—instruments are processed and stored

2. Decontamination area procedures

   a. Use PPE, including utility gloves

   b. If a delay occurs before decontamination, soak instruments in a holding solution to prevent the drying of saliva and blood

   (1) Extended soaking is not recommended because it can damage the instruments

   (2) The holding solution can be water, enzyme solution, heparin solution (dissolves blood), or detergent

   c. Cleaning instruments in an ultrasonic unit or instrument washer is an important step; otherwise, stuck-on blood or other organic material will remain on the instruments even after sterilization (instruments with adhered debris are not sterile)

   d. Ultrasonic cleaning

   (1) Vibrations dislodge and dissolve organic material

   (2) The safest and most efficacious method of cleaning

   (3) Eliminates the need for hand scrubbing and potential for injury with contaminated instruments

   (4) Procedure for using ultrasonic instrument cleaner

   (a) Use solution specifically designed for ultrasonic cleaners; may contain antimicrobial properties

   (b) Time—4 to 16 minutes, depending on the unit, the instruments, and the amount of material on the instruments (instruments in cassettes require longer exposure time)

   (c) Keep the unit covered to prevent exposure to aerosols

   (d) Rinse the instruments, and let excess water drain from the cassettes

   (e) Open cassette and inspect instruments to ensure absence of debris

   (f) Replenish the ultrasonic solution, and disinfect the unit daily

   (g) Periodically test the unit (aluminum foil test)

   e. Manual scrubbing technique—used rarely when bioburden remains on instruments or when ultrasonic exposure would cause damage to instruments or devices (ultrasonic inserts, some handpieces)

   (1) Scrub with a long-handled, stiff brush; wear utility gloves

   (2) Scrub the item, holding it low in the sink to minimize spatter

   (3) Manual scrubbing is not advised because it poses an increased risk for injury

f. Asepsis for high-speed and low-speed dental handpieces

   (1) Refer to the manufacturer's instructions for cleaning, lubrication, and sterilization

   (2) Some handpieces can be cleaned ultrasonically; all handpieces must be able to withstand heat sterilization

   (3) Flush the water lines of high-speed handpieces for 30 seconds after use

g. Prophylaxis angles; should be heat-sterilized or SUDs (disposable); consult the manufacturer's instructions for cleaning, lubrication, and sterilization

3. Packaging area procedures

   a. Surgical and hinged instruments

   (1) Instruments can be dipped in surgical milk to prevent rusting and to lubricate hinged instruments (rusted instruments should be discarded and never used because sterility of these instruments cannot be ensured)

   (2) Hinged instruments should be opened before packaging

   b. The instruments to be bagged should be dry to avoid penetrating the packaging, and excess moisture can interfere with sterilization

   c. Packaging materials vary according to the type of sterilization method (Table 10-6)

   d. Packaging materials include plastic or paper pouches, plastic tubing, cassettes, or trays to be wrapped with paper or cloth, sealed with appropriate tape, dated, and labeled with the type of instrument setup and sterilizer used (in the case of more than one sterilizer)

   (1) With more than one sterilizer in use, if one was to malfunction, it would be important to identify the packages that had been processed in that sterilizer

   e. To maintain package integrity, do not seal the package using staples, pins, or paper clips

   f. Packages should be tightly sealed, eliminating gaps

   g. Autoclave bags are designed for single use because of pores in the paper that open during sterilization, allowing steam to penetrate, and then close on cooling to inhibit microbes from entering into package

   h. The packaging materials used must NOT:

   (1) Melt or char

   (2) Prevent the sterilizing agent from penetrating

   (3) Be easily torn by sharp instruments

   i. Instruments should be packaged loosely to allow for maximum contact with steam or chemical vapors; overloaded packages can lead to incomplete sterilization

   j. Biologic and chemical indicators are added during packaging procedures

4. Sterilization area procedures

5. Sterilization methods (see Table 10-6)

   a. Steam (moist heat under pressure) sterilization—autoclave

   (1) Types based on how air is removed the chamber

   (a) Gravity displacement

TABLE 10-6   Comparison of Heat Sterilization Methods

Method	Sterilizing Conditions*	Packaging Materials	Advantages	Precautions
Steam Autoclave		Paper wrap	Time-efficient	No closed containers
		Nylon "plastic" tubing	Good penetration	Damage to plastic and rubber
Standard cycles	20 to 30 minutes at 250°F	Paper or plastic peel pouches		Non–stainless steel items corrode
		Thin cloth		Use of hard water may leave deposits
		Wrapped, perforated cassettes		Items may be wet after cycle
Flash cycles	3 to 10 minutes at 273°F	No packaging (unwrapped)		Unwrapped items quickly contaminated after processing
Unsaturated Chemical Vapor	20 minutes at 270°F	Paper wrap	Time-efficient	No closed containers
		Paper or plastic peel pouches	No corrosion	Damage to plastic and rubber
		Wrapped, perforated cassettes	Items dry quickly after cycle	Must use special solution
				Pre-dry instruments
				Provide adequate ventilation
				Cannot sterilize liquids
				No cloth wrap (absorbs too much chemical vapor)
Dry Heat	60 to 120 minutes at 320°F	Paper wrap	No corrosion	Some paper may get charred
				Pre-dry instruments
Oven type (static-air)		Appropriate nylon "plastic" tubing	Can use closed containers†	Long sterilization time (oven type)
				Damage to plastic and rubber
		Closed containers	Low cost	Door cannot be opened during cycle
		Wrapped, perforated cassettes	Items are dry after cycle	Cannot sterilize liquids
Rapid heat transfer (forced air)	12 minutes at 375°F (wrapped)	Aluminum foil‡	No corrosion	Unwrapped items quickly contaminated after processing
	6 minutes at 375°F (unwrapped)		Short cycle	
			Items are dry after cycle	

*These conditions do not include warm-up or cool-down time, and they may vary, depending on the contents and volume of the load and brand of the sterilizer.
†Biologic indicator must be used to ensure sterility.
‡Tears or punctures easily.
Modified from Miller CH: *Infection control and the management of hazardous materials for the dental team,* ed 5, St Louis, 2014, Mosby.

(b) Vacuum pump (type B sterilizer)—perform air removal test (Bowie-Dick) at the beginning of each day to ensure complete air removal from the chamber
(c) Pressure pulse
(2) Moist heat denatures and coagulates microbial proteins; pressure serves to elevate temperature
(3) Periodically check gasket on door to ensure a tight fit
(4) Steam must be able to penetrate the instrument package; pack loosely to allow for free passage of steam
(5) Packages and cassettes should be placed on their edges, not laid flat
(6) Avoid the package coming in contact with chamber walls
(7) Use distilled or deionized water to prevent deposits on instruments
b. Dry-heat sterilization
(1) Sterilizes by oxidizing cell parts
(2) Keeps air spaces between packages
(3) If the sterilizer is opened, timer must be restarted
c. Unsaturated chemical vapor sterilization

(1) Alcohols, formaldehyde, ketone, acetone, and water are heated under pressure to produce the gas that permeates and destroys microbes
d. Ethylene oxide gas sterilization
(1) Used mostly in hospitals and large clinics
(2) Operation
(a) Sterilize at room temperature, 75°F (25°C), for 10 to 16 hours
(b) Alternatively, sterilize at 120°F (49°C) for 2 to 3 hours
(c) Aerate plastic and rubber materials for at least 16 hours after sterilization to remove gas molecules
(d) *Warning:* Residual gas can cause tissue burns
e. Liquid chemical sterilants
(1) Used for heat-sensitive, semi-critical items when ethylene oxide gas is not available
(a) Should not be used as a substitute for heat sterilization of semi-critical items that are not heat sensitive
(b) Should be avoided because mostly heat tolerant, or SUDs are available

      (c) Biologic monitoring is not possible, so this method cannot ensure sterility

    (2) Follow the manufacturer's instructions for dilution, temperature, and contact time

    (3) Ensure that the instruments are dry to avoid diluting the solution

    (4) Remove the instruments with sterile forceps, rinse with sterile water, and package or cover with sterile towel

    (5) Chemicals used for sterilization (see Table 10-4); the disadvantages of chemicals are:

      (a) They produce toxic fumes and are irritating to tissues

      (b) Biologic indicators (BIs) are not available with the use of chemical sterilants; therefore, the sterility of items cannot be verified

      (c) When removed from chemicals, items are exposed to the environment and can easily become contaminated because of lack of packaging

      (d) Chemical sterilization requires an extended contact time of 3 to 12 hours, depending on the chemical

6. Verification of sterilization
  a. Failure of sterilization can occur as a result of operator or mechanical failure
    (1) Overloading—the reason for failure in the majority of cases
    (2) Improper packaging
    (3) Improper timing
    (4) Improper unit operation
    (5) Unit malfunction
    (6) Improper maintenance of equipment
  b. The CDC recommends routine use of BIs (spore tests) for verification of sterility
    (1) Biologic monitoring is a process in which highly resistant spores are passed through the sterilizer and then cultured to determine whether they have been killed
      (a) If spores have been killed, all the less-resistant microorganisms exposed to the same conditions will also have been destroyed
      (b) Primary method to ascertain sterility
      (c) Biologic monitoring with BIs can be done in the dental setting or in a processing facility
    (2) Types of BIs
      (a) Spore strips—paper strips containing one or two types of spores enclosed in a glassine envelope
        [1] After sterilization, remove the spore strip aseptically, place it in a culture medium, and incubate for 7 days
        [2] If spores are present, they will grow and change the color of the growth medium, indicating sterilization failure
        [3] Strips can be used for all methods of heat sterilization

      (b) Self-contained vial—contains spore strip with an ampule of growth medium in a plastic vial
        [1] After sterilization, squeeze the vial to break the internal ampule, which would mix the growth medium with the spores
        [2] Incubate the vial; if spores are present, they will multiply and change the color of the growth medium, indicating sterilization failure
        [3] Vials can only be used in a steam autoclave
      (c) Specific bacterial endospores used in BIs
        [1] Steam autoclave and chemical vapor sterilizer—spores of *Geobacillus stearothermophilus*
        [2] Dry heat and ethylene oxide gas sterilizer—spores of *Bacillus atrophaeus*
    (3) Use of BIs
      (a) Place a strip inside one of each type of package (e.g., autoclave bag, cassette)
      (b) Incubate a control BI that has not been sterilized, along with the test BI
      (c) Growth of spores from the control BI confirms that live spores were present
      (d) No growth from the test BI indicates that sterilization has been achieved
    (4) Use BIs once a week to test sterilization equipment and when:
      (a) The equipment has been repaired
      (b) New packaging material is used
      (c) A new sterilizer is operated
      (d) Training new staff
      (e) The loading procedure is changed
      (f) Sterilizing an item to be implanted
    (5) Sterilization failure (growth on the BI test, or positive spore test)
      (a) Review the procedures to determine any operator error
      (b) Take the sterilizer out of operation, and retest with mechanical, chemical, and biologic monitors
      (c) If the repeat BI test is negative, put the sterilizer back in service
      (d) If the repeat BI test is positive, determine the cause of failure, and repeat the BI test three times before putting the sterilizer back into service
      (e) Withdraw the instruments, and repeat the process
    (6) Documentation
      (a) Record the results of biologic monitoring in a log book
      (b) Necessary for compliance with federal regulations
      (c) Serves quality assurance and risk management purposes

c. Chemical monitoring
  (1) Chemical indicators—items containing heat-sensitive chemicals that change color when exposed to certain temperatures to assess conditions during the sterilization process (e.g., autoclave tape, special markings on autoclave bags, chemical indicator strips)
  (2) Chemical monitoring does not provide proof of sterilization
  (3) Types of chemical indicators
    (a) Integrated indicator (class V)—changes color slowly when exposed to a combination of time, temperature, and steam; placed inside each instrument package to confirm whether instruments have been exposed to sterilizing conditions
    (b) External chemical indicator—changes color after a certain temperature has been reached (e.g., autoclave tape)
      [1] Distinguishes those instruments that have been in the sterilizer from those that have not, preventing accidental use of unprocessed items
      [2] Should be present on packaging material or applied on the outside of every instrument package and cassette
d. Mechanical monitoring
  (1) Observation of sterilizer gauges, including temperature, pressure, and exposure time
  (2) Incorrect reading indicates a functional problem
7. Storage area procedures
  a. After sterilization, allow the instrument packages to cool and dry before storage
    (1) Microorganisms and instrument tips can penetrate wet packaging material and compromise sterility
    (2) Microorganisms on contaminated surfaces can wick through wet packaging
  b. Instruments must not be stored unwrapped or unpackaged (unpackaged instruments are immediately contaminated when exposed to the environment)
  c. Packaged instruments should not be stored above the sterilizers and should be stored away from treatment areas to lessen chances of contamination
  d. Sealed packages should be kept on shelves protected by doors for dry, low-dust storage
  e. Sealed instrument packages have been shown to maintain sterility for up to 6 months; however, to err on the side of caution, repackage and sterilize after 30 days
  f. Instrument packages should be rotated so that the oldest dated instrument pack is used first
  g. Packages that are dropped on the floor, punctured, torn, or wet are considered contaminated and must be reprocessed
  h. Wrapped cassettes are ideal for storing and then serving as sterile instrument trays

GOVERNMENTAL AGENCIES AND INFECTION CONTROL

A. U.S. Food and Drug Administration (FDA)
  1. Regulates all medical devices
    a. Examples in oral health care include liquid sterilants, biologic and chemical indicators, ultrasonic cleaners, PPE, dental instruments, and sterilizers
  2. Ensures products are safe and effective
  3. Ensure devices fulfill performance standards before marketing
B. U.S. Environmental Protection Agency (EPA)
  1. Mission to protect human health and the environment
  2. Ensures the safety and effectiveness of chemical disinfectants (EPA registration number displayed on container)
  3. Regulates medical and chemical waste after leaving the OHC setting
C. Centers for Disease Control and Prevention (CDC)
  1. Under the auspices of the U.S. Department of Health and Human Services
  2. Health and quality-of-life promotion mitigating injury, disability, and disease
  3. Infection control guidelines and recommendations for dentistry (infection procedures used in oral health care settings are based on 2003 recommendations)
  4. Regulatory agency only; does not have authority to enforce guidelines
D. Occupational Safety and Health Administration (OSHA)
  1. Within the U.S. Department of Labor (federal and state divisions)
  2. Ensuring a safe and healthy working environment for employees
    a. Instrument sterilization is *not* covered by OSHA regulations because it is considered a procedure involved in client protection instead of DHCP (employee) protection
  3. OSHA formulates and has the authority to enforce regulations related to occupational safety and health
  4. Protection of DHCP against exposure to bloodborne pathogens
  5. OSHA Bloodborne Pathogens Standard
    a. The most important infection control regulation in dentistry for the protection of DHCP
    b. The final Bloodborne Pathogens Standard was published in 1991 and became effective in 1992
    c. The Needlestick Safety and Prevention Act was added to the Standard in 2001
      (1) On an annual basis, employers must solicit input from DHCP to identify, evaluate, and select safer medical devices to minimize or eliminate occupational exposures (e.g., self-sheathing needles)
    d. Employers are responsible for staff compliance with the Standard; this includes:
      (1) Review of the Standard and ensuring that a copy is available on-site
      (2) Formulation of a written exposure control plan that contains:

(a) Clarification of which employees face a potential risk for occupational exposure and will be covered under the Standard

(b) Description of how and when provisions will be implemented (i.e., communication of the hazards to employees, hepatitis B vaccination, postexposure evaluation and follow- up, record keeping, use of PPE, engineering and work practice controls, and housekeeping)

(c) Prevention and evaluation of exposure incidents (sharps injuries)

(d) In 2005, OSHA determined that oral health care settings are of low hazard and are exempt from keeping an injury and illness log unless the government requires it

(e) Employers still must report any workplace incident that results in the hospitalization of three or more employees or a fatality

(3) Training of employees

(a) Training that provides information about the hazards and preventive measures related to occupational exposure to bloodborne pathogens

(b) Training to be completed at the initial time of assignment and annually thereafter

(c) Person conducting the training must be qualified and knowledgeable

(d) Training must provide an opportunity for interactive questions and answers with the person conducting the training

(4) Providing employees with necessary materials to comply with the Standard

(a) Offer and pay for hepatitis B vaccination

(b) Provide, maintain, and ensure use of PPE and engineering controls

(c) Establish appropriate work practices and decontamination procedures in the oral health care setting to ensure the safety of DHCP (appropriate decontamination, laundry handling, and infectious waste disposal)

(d) Establish and provide postexposure medical evaluation and follow-up without any cost to employees

(e) Provide appropriate biohazard communication by posting signs, biohazard waste labels, and red containers that indicate infectious waste on-site

(5) Maintain appropriate records

(a) Training sessions (participants, trainers, summary of content, evaluations)

(b) Employee medical records (HBV immunization status, postexposure evaluation and follow-up)

6. Inspections conducted by OSHA

a. Initiated by employee complaints or other interested parties

b. Programmed inspections of randomly selected worksites employing 11 or more people

c. Noncompliance with any provision in the Standard can result in the imposition of fines

Evaluation of Infection Control Programs

Table 10-7 lists program elements with corresponding activities in the evaluation of infection control programs. The websites listed in the Website Information and Resources table provide the oral health care professional with immediate access to current recommendations and regulations concerning infection control.

TABLE 10-7 Evaluating Infection Control Programs	
Program Element	**Evaluation Activity**
Appropriate immunization of dental health care personnel (DHCP)	Conduct annual review of personnel records to ensure up-to-date immunization.
Assessment of occupational exposures to infectious agents	Report occupational exposures to infectious agents. Document the steps that occurred around the exposure, and plan how such exposure can be prevented in the future.
Comprehensive postexposure management plan and medical follow-up program after occupational exposures to infectious agents	Ensure the postexposure management plan is clear, complete, and available at all times to all DHCP. All staff should understand the plan, which should include toll-free phone numbers for access to additional information.
Adherence to hand hygiene before and after patient care	Observe and document circumstances of appropriate or inappropriate handwashing. Review findings in a staff meeting.
Proper use of personal protective equipment (PPE) to prevent occupational exposures to infectious agents	Observe and document the use of barrier precautions and careful handling of sharps. Review findings in a staff meeting.
Routine and appropriate sterilization of instruments using a biologic monitoring system	Monitor paper log of steam cycle and temperature strip with each sterilization load, and examine results of weekly biologic monitoring. Take appropriate action when failure of sterilization process is noted.
Evaluation and implementation of safer medical devices	Conduct an annual review of the exposure control plan, and consider new developments in safer medical devices.

(Continued)

TABLE 10-7   Evaluating Infection Control Programs—cont'd

Program Element	Evaluation Activity
Compliance of water in routine dental procedures with current drinking U.S. Environmental Protection Agency water standards (fewer than 500 colony-forming units [CFU] of heterotrophic water bacteria)	Monitor dental water quality as recommended by the equipment manufacturer, using commercial self-contained test kits or commercial water-testing laboratories.
Proper handling and disposal of medical waste	Observe the safe disposal of regulated and nonregulated medical waste, and take preventive measures if hazardous situations occur.
Health care–associated infections	Assess the unscheduled return of patients after procedures, and evaluate them for an infectious process. A trend might require formal evaluation.

From Centers for Disease Control and Prevention: Guidelines for infection control in dental health-care settings, *MMWR* 52(RR-17):1-68, 2003.

BOX 10-2   Legal and Ethical Guidelines in Disease Prevention

Treat all clients regardless of disease status
Practice infection control according to the standard of care
   Adhere to the Centers for Disease Control and Prevention (CDC) and the Occupational Safety and Health Administration (OSHA) guidelines
   Adhere to state and federal laws
   Use evidence-based protocols

Follow state board of dentistry laws and regulations
Follow expert opinion related to infection control
Stay current of new protocols and guidelines
Abide by U.S. Public Health Service (PHS) guidelines for employee work restrictions

Legal and Ethical Issues in Disease Prevention

Box 10-2 lists recommendations to address legal and ethical considerations in infection control measures.

SUGGESTED READINGS

Centers for Disease Control and Prevention: Guidelines for infection control in dental health-care settings, *MMWR* 57, 2003.

Centers for Disease Control and Prevention: Guidelines for disinfection and sterilization in healthcare facilities, *MMWR* 57:2008.

Miller CH: *Infection control and management of hazardous materials for the dental team,* ed 5, St Louis, 2014, Mosby.

US Department of Labor, Occupational Safety and Health Administration: *Controlling occupational exposure to bloodborne pathogens,* 2001, Washington, DC, 1996, OSHA. 3127 (revised).

Website Information And Resources

Source	Website Address	Description
Association for Professionals in Infection Control and Epidemiology (APIC)	http://www.apic.org	Infection control organization for health care
Centers for Disease Control and Prevention (CDC)	http://www.cdc.gov	U.S. government agency that provides resources and recommendations for numerous health and safety topics
Organization for Safety, Asepsis, and Prevention (OSAP)	http://www.osap.org	Organization that promotes infection control and safety policies to the dental community
Occupational Safety and Health Administration (OSHA)	http://www.osha.gov	U.S. government agency responsible for ensuring the health and safety of employees at workplaces
National Institutes for Occupational Safety and Health (NIOSH)	http://www.cdc.gov/niosh	U.S. government agency that provides national and world leadership to prevent illness and injury

CHAPTER 10 REVIEW QUESTIONS

Answers and rationales to review questions are available on this text's accompanying Evolve site. See inside front cover for details.

evolve

CASE A

Isabelle Sanchez, RDH, has been practicing dental hygiene for 7 years and has decided to return to college to pursue her master's degree in dental hygiene. She has moved to another state and is currently working during the summer as a temporary hygienist to earn money for living expenses. For the last two consecutive Mondays, she has been working in the same practice, substituting for a hygienist who is on maternity leave. Today, when she reports to work, Isabelle is told by the dental assistant that the elderly man whom Isabelle treated last Monday is in the hospital and has been diagnosed with legionnaires disease. During the last week, he had only left his house to go to his dental visit, and the water tested in his house was negative for *Legionella*. In hindsight, Isabelle realizes that in her treatment room, she did not see a water bottle attached to the master control unit that would have indicated use of an independent water system. She just assumed that the dental unit water lines were being treated with another method.

Use Case A to answer questions 1 to 6.

1. **Which of the following pathways of cross-contamination is depicted in this case?**
   a. Client to DHCP
   b. DHCP to client
   c. Client to client
   d. Community to client

2. **Which of the following modes of disease spread is depicted in this case?**
   a. Direct contact
   b. Indirect contact
   c. Droplet infection
   d. Airborne infection

3. **What is the source of the microbes in this case?**
   a. Client's oral cavity
   b. Hygienist's hands
   c. Contaminated instrument
   d. Dental unit water

4. **In this case, which of the following infection control procedures likely would have prevented disease transmission?**
   a. Using barriers
   b. Cleaning the housekeeping surfaces
   c. Treating dental unit water lines
   d. Wearing proper PPE

5. **Which of the following microorganism types is responsible for legionnaires disease?**
   a. Bacterium
   b. Prion
   c. Virus
   d. Fungus

6. **What was the portal of entry of *Legionella* into the elderly client's body?**
   a. Breathing in contaminated water vapor
   b. Swallowing contaminated water
   c. Infiltrating microbes into nonintact mucosa
   d. Splashing of droplets on mucous membranes

CASE B

After dismissing his last client of the day, Preston Miller, RDH, returns to his treatment room. He is in a rush because his son's baseball team has a game tonight and he is the coach. Preston hurriedly closes his instrument cassette, not taking care to arrange the instruments beforehand. In the instrument-processing area, he lifts the cassette off the metal tray to place it into the ultrasonic unit. Unknowingly, an explorer is protruding from a hole in the cassette and penetrates his finger through the exam glove. He removes his gloves and sees a small amount of blood forming on his index finger.

Use Case B to answer questions 7 to 13.

7. **What should Preston the dental hygienist do next?**
   a. Scrub the finger using a stiff brush
   b. Squeeze the finger to let out the contaminants
   c. Wash the finger with antimicrobial soap
   d. Immerse the finger in bleach for 1 minute

8. **Preston, the employee, has sustained a percutaneous injury and may have been exposed to a bloodborne pathogen. In this situation, what is the responsibility of the employer (dentist) according to OSHA?**
   a. None; an employee works at his own risk
   b. Pay for the treatment of any acquired disease
   c. Give the employee the following day off with pay
   d. Arrange for a consultation with a qualified HCP

9. **Which of the following modes of disease spread is depicted in this case?**
   a. Direct contact
   b. Indirect contact
   c. Droplet infection
   d. Airborne infection

10. **What is the source of the microbes in this case?**
    a. Contaminated droplets
    b. Hygienist's hands
    c. Contaminated instrument
    d. Dental unit water

11. **The dental hygienist elects to be tested for bloodborne pathogens (HCV and HIV), and he is informed of the**

results. Which of the following actions is he then required to take?

a. Inform his employer of the results
b. Document the results in his employee file
c. Inform the CDC and OSHA
d. None of the above is required

12. **According to OSHA, which of the following does NOT need to be included in a dental office's record keeping?**
   a. Employee vaccine declination statements
   b. Records of annual staff trainings on infection control
   c. Log of employee injuries and illnesses
   d. Employees' Social Security numbers

13. **What is the level of risk related to the transmission of HCV or HIV from this exposure?**
   a. High
   b. Moderate
   c. Low
   d. Very low

14. **All the following viruses are bloodborne pathogens EXCEPT:**
   a. Human immunodeficiency virus
   b. Hepatitis B virus
   c. Hepatitis C virus
   d. Varicella-zoster virus

15. **Which term is used for the practice of treating a client's blood, body fluids, nonintact skin, and mucous membranes as potentially infectious?**
   a. Standard precautions
   b. Pervasive precautions
   c. Universal precautions
   d. Protective precautions

16. **Glutaraldehyde is a high-level disinfectant; therefore it can be used to sterilize critical items.**
   a. Both statements are TRUE.
   b. Both statements are FALSE.
   c. The first statement is TRUE; the second statement is FALSE.
   d. The first statement is FALSE; the second statement is TRUE.

17. **A dental health care employee has occupationally acquired tuberculosis. Which of the following modes of disease spread would be implicated in this case?**
   a. Direct contact
   b. Indirect contact
   c. Droplet infection
   d. Airborne infection

18. **Which of the following methods will achieve sterilization?**
   a. Dry heat at 320°F for 50 minutes
   b. Steam autoclave at 200°F for 30 minutes
   c. Chemical vapor at 270°F for 20 minutes
   d. Ethylene oxide gas for 5 hours

19. **The CDC recommends disinfecting clinical contact surfaces with an intermediate-level disinfectant that is tuberculocidal, because *Mycobacterium tuberculosis* var. *bovis* is a resistant microbe and all other, less resistant microbes would also be killed.**

a. Both the statement and the reason are TRUE.
b. Both the statement and the reason are FALSE.
c. The statement is TRUE, but the reason is FALSE.
d. The statement is FALSE, but the reason is TRUE.

20. **What is the ultimate goal of disease prevention in the oral health care (OHC) setting?**
   a. Prevent pathogens from entering the OHC setting
   b. Sterilize clinical contact surfaces between clients
   c. Prevent OHC-related infections and diseases
   d. Eliminate all microbes in the OHC setting

21. **Alcohol-based sanitizers may be used instead of handwashing when no visible soil is present, because the sanitizers have been found to be as effective as handwashing.**
   a. Both the statement and the reason are TRUE.
   b. Both the statement and the reason are FALSE.
   c. The statement is TRUE, but the reason is FALSE.
   d. The statement is FALSE, but the reason is TRUE.

22. **All the following are TRUE related to using instrument cassettes EXCEPT:**
   a. Unwrap the cassette in view of the client.
   b. Sterilized cassettes are used as instrument trays.
   c. Exposure to sharps is decreased.
   d. Using cassettes is less time-efficient.

23. **Many DHCP experience skin problems on their hands related to the use of gloves. In most cases, these problems are caused by an allergic response to latex proteins in gloves.**
   a. Both statements are TRUE.
   b. Both statements are FALSE.
   c. The first statement is TRUE; the second statement is FALSE.
   d. The first statement is FALSE; the second statement is TRUE.

24. **Which of the following indicators is used to determine sterility?**
   a. External indicator
   b. Integrated indicator
   c. Biologic indicator
   d. Chemical indicator

25. **Which of the following is OSHA primarily concerned with protecting?**
   a. Employee
   b. Employer
   c. Client
   d. Community

26. **Which of the following characteristics is an advantage of chemical-vapor sterilization?**
   a. A ventilation system is not required.
   b. It can sterilize closed containers.
   c. Extra drying time is not needed.
   d. It is the least costly method of sterilization.

27. **All the following are vaccine-preventable illnesses EXCEPT:**
   a. Hepatitis B virus (HBV)
   b. Hepatitis A virus (HAV)
   c. Hepatitis C virus (HCV)
   d. Varicella-zoster virus (VZV)

28. **Which of the following statements BEST characterizes the resident flora on hands?**
    a. They colonize the deeper layers of the skin.
    b. They are less resistant to removal by handwashing.
    c. They are the primary source of disease transmission.
    d. They are associated with allergic contact dermatitis.

29. **Which of the following statements is TRUE regarding the handling of regulated infectious waste?**
    a. Containers of infectious waste must be identified with the biohazard symbol.
    b. Infectious waste can be disinfected and then combined with the regular trash.
    c. Infectious waste must be sterilized before leaving the oral health care setting.
    d. Infectious waste does not require any special handling in some states.

30. **Examination gloves to be used intraorally should be donned *before*:**
    a. Operatory setup
    b. Unwrapping the cassette
    c. Taking the blood pressure
    d. Entering the client's mouth

31. **Which of the following packaging materials should NOT be used with chemical vapor sterilization?**
    a. Paper wrap
    b. Paper pouches
    c. Plastic pouches
    d. Cloth wrap

32. **Which of the following characteristics BEST describes the use of protective barriers for clinical contact surfaces?**
    a. They need to be changed only when visibly soiled.
    b. They should be used after sterilization of the surface.
    c. They are ideally used for surfaces that are difficult to disinfect.
    d. They decrease the cost of maintaining asepsis.

33. **All following characteristics describe EPA-registered intermediate-level disinfectants EXCEPT:**
    a. Must inactivate *Mycobacterium tuberculosis* var. *bovis*
    b. Will kill vegetative bacteria and most viruses
    c. Must be used on surfaces with visible blood
    d. Will achieve sterilization if long contact time is used

34. **All DHCP who are vaccinated for hepatitis B will become immune to the virus. Therefore, the CDC does not recommend booster injections.**
    a. Both statements are TRUE.
    b. Both statements are FALSE.
    c. The first statement is TRUE; the second statement is FALSE.
    d. The first statement is FALSE; the second statement is TRUE.

35. **Face shields provide maximum coverage for the face and protection from spatter during oral health care procedures. Therefore, wearing a facemask is not required when using a face shield.**
    a. Both statements are TRUE.
    b. Both statements are FALSE.

    c. The first statement is TRUE; the second statement is FALSE.
    d. The first statement is FALSE; the second statement is TRUE.

36. **Which of the following pathogens has been identified in the biofilm that accumulates inside dental unit water lines?**
    a. *Pseudomonas aeruginosa*
    b. *Neisseria meningitidis*
    c. *Candida albicans*
    d. *Treponema pallidum*

37. **Which of the following governmental agencies is responsible for approving the safety and effectiveness of small office sterilizers and ultrasonic units?**
    a. EPA
    b. FDA
    c. CDC
    d. OSHA

38. **An individual should be tested for antibodies to HBV 1 to 2 months after receiving the last dose of the hepatitis B vaccine. The reason for this testing is that not all individuals will seroconvert.**
    a. Both statements are TRUE.
    b. Both statements are FALSE.
    c. The first statement is TRUE; the second statement is FALSE.
    d. The first statement is FALSE; the second statement is TRUE.

39. **In which of the following methods are biologic monitors containing spores of *Geobacillus stearothermophilus* used to verify sterilization?**
    a. Steam autoclave
    b. Dry-heat oven
    c. Ethylene oxide gas
    d. Rapid heat transfer

40. **Which of the following is NOT considered a safe work practice control?**
    a. Using an instrument cassette instead of autoclave bags
    b. Hand scrubbing instruments using exam gloves
    c. Using a one-handed technique to recap needles
    d. Fulcruming a couple of teeth away from instrumented tooth

41. **Sterilization failure is most often caused by:**
    a. The autoclave not working properly
    b. Improper packaging materials used
    c. Overloading the office sterilizer
    d. Inadequate sterilization time

42. **A chemical indicator is used on the outside of packaging to identify the items that have been processed through the sterilizer. The chemical indicator changes color when the packages are sterile.**
    a. Both statements are TRUE.
    b. Both statements are FALSE.
    c. The first statement is TRUE; the second statement is FALSE.
    d. The first statement is FALSE; the second statement is TRUE.

43. **Dental handpieces are considered semi-critical items, and therefore they can be disinfected by wiping with an intermediate-level disinfectant.**
    a. Both statements are TRUE.
    b. Both statements are FALSE.
    c. The first statement is TRUE; the second statement is FALSE.
    d. The first statement is FALSE; the second statement is TRUE.

44. **What is the maximum level of bacteria that the ADA has recommended in dental unit water?**
    a. 100 CFU/mL
    b. 200 CFU/mL
    c. 300 CFU/mL
    d. 400 CFU/mL

45. **In most cases, what is the number of bacteria in the water exiting from an untreated dental unit water line?**
    a. Lower than in drinking water
    b. The same as in drinking water
    c. Slightly higher than in drinking water
    d. Much higher than in drinking water

46. **All the following materials are considered regulated infectious waste EXCEPT:**
    a. Extracted tooth
    b. Blood-soaked gauze
    c. Anesthetic needle
    d. Contaminated exam gloves

47. **The primary reason for clients to perform a preprocedural rinse before undergoing oral health care is to:**
    a. Remove malodorous breath
    b. Remove adherent food debris
    c. Reduce the microbes in aerosols
    d. Eliminate oral infections

48. **Using biologic indicators to test sterilizing equipment, biologic monitors should be used once every:**
    a. Day
    b. Week
    c. Month
    d. Quarter

49. **All the following methods inhibit the formation of bio-film in dental unit water lines EXCEPT:**
    a. Flushing water lines for 2 minutes
    b. Independent water reservoir
    c. Chemical disinfection of water lines
    d. Sterile water delivery systems

50. **To prevent cross-contamination, the practice of using a cotton roll taped to the bracket tray for wiping debridement instruments, instead of a gauze square wrapped around the finger, is considered:**
    a. Standard bioburden control
    b. Safe practice control
    c. Engineering control
    d. Work practice control

Pharmacology

Elena Bablenis Haveles

As a health care provider responsible for client assessment and care, a dental hygienist must understand drugs, the conditions for which these drugs are used, and the actions, range of effects, and interactions of the drugs. The health, dental, and pharmacologic histories are the foundation on which decisions regarding client care rest. For example, some clients may need prophylactic antibiotic premedication before dental and dental hygiene care. Therefore, before care is planned, the client's medical conditions and medications used to manage them are assessed and recorded in the client's permanent record. Contraindications or cautions to professional care concerning these drugs are determined using appropriate references and consultations. Through this knowledge, medical emergencies may be prevented; and, if an emergency occurs, the oral health care team can act within the standard of care.

GENERAL CONSIDERATIONS

Definitions

A. Pharmacology—the study of drugs and their effects on living organisms
B. Pharmacotherapy—the use of medications to treat different disease states
C. Pharmacodynamics—the action of drugs on living organisms
D. Pharmacokinetics—what the body does in response to the drugs (e.g., absorption, distribution, metabolism, excretion)
E. Pharmacy—the practice of compounding, preparing, and dispensing drugs and of counseling clients about their medications
F. Toxicology—the study of the harmful effects of drugs on living organisms
   1. Drugs—biologically active substances that can modify cellular function; used in the prevention, diagnosis, treatment, and cure of disease or in the prevention of pregnancy
   2. Nomenclature—each drug has several names
      a. Chemical name—based on the drug's chemical formula (e.g., *N*-acetyl para-amino phenol)
      b. Trade (proprietary) name—each drug company makes up its own product trade name (e.g., Tylenol, Peridex, Atridox, Arestin)
      c. Brand name—technically, the name of the drug company itself, but often used interchangeably with the

trade name (e.g., either Astra [company that makes Xylocaine] or Xylocaine can be considered the brand name)
      d. Generic name—official name of the drug determined by the U.S. Adopted Names Council that is used by all manufacturers of a particular drug (e.g., acetaminophen, chlorhexidine gluconate)
G. Table 11-1 lists the Latin abbreviations used in prescription writing

Agencies and Legislation

A. U.S. Food and Drug Administration (FDA)—determines drugs to be marketed in the United States; after considering safety, efficacy, and physical and chemical data, the FDA requires quality control of manufacturing facilities, determines what drugs are sold by prescription, and regulates the advertising and labeling of prescription drugs
B. U.S. Drug Enforcement Administration (DEA)—branch of the Department of Justice; determines the degree of control for substances with abuse potential; controlled substances used in dentistry are classified under schedules I to V (Table 11-2)

Drug Action

A. Log dose–response curve—as the dose of a drug increases (*x* axis), the percentage of maximum response increases (*y* axis) until increasing the dose further produces no increase in the percentage of response (the effect of the drug reaches a plateau) (Fig. 11-1)
B. Definitions
   1. Effective dose (ED) 50—dose that produces 50% of the maximum response, or the dose of a drug that produces a specific response in 50% of the subjects
   2. Lethal dose (LD) 50—dose that is lethal to (kills) 50% of the subjects; laboratory animals are used to derive LD
   3. Therapeutic index (TI)—LD_{50} divided by ED_{50}; a measure of the safety of a drug
   4. Onset—time required for a drug's effect to begin; onset is short if the drug is given intravenously, longer if administered orally
   5. Duration—length of time a drug's effect lasts; related to a drug's half-life

TABLE 11–1 Common Latin Abbreviations Used in Prescription Writing

Abbreviation*	Interpretation
a., ante	Before
a.c., ante cibum	Before meals
A.D., aurisdextra	Right ear
A.L., aurislaeva	Left ear
b.i.d., bis in die	Twice per day or twice daily
gt., gutta	Drop (plural gtt.)
h., hora	Hour
h.s., hora somni	At bedtime
o.d., oculus dexter	Right eye
o.s., oculus sinister	Left eye
o.u., oculus uterque	Each eye
p.c., post cibum	After meals
p.o., per os	By mouth
p.r.	By rectum
p.r.n., pro re nata	As needed
q.d., quaque die	Once per day or once daily
q.i.d., quater in die	Four times per day
q.o.d.	Every other day
q.h.	Every 6 hours
sl.	Sublingual
supp.	Suppository
t.i.d., ter in die	Three times per day
u.d.	As directed

*Periods usually omitted (e.g., bid, po) when abbreviations used (as with dosages).

TABLE 11–2 Drug Enforcement Administration Schedules Used in Dentistry (I Through V)

Schedule	Abuse Potential	Examples	Handling
I	High	Heroin, phencyclidine (PCP)	Prescriptions may not be sent by telephone
II	High	Morphine, meperidine, oxycodone mixtures (Percodan, Percocet), hydrocodone mixtures (Vicodin)	Prescriptions must be signed by the prescriber; may not be telephoned to pharmacist; emergency prescriptions may be phoned; however, signed original prescription order must be delivered to the pharmacy within 72 hours of the phone order; no refills
III	Some	Codeine mixtures (Tylenol and codeine), "weaker" stimulants and sedatives	Prescriptions may be telephoned to pharmacy; may be refilled five times within 6 months
IV	Low	Dextropropoxyphene (Darvon), diazepam (Valium)	Same as schedule III
V	Very low	Some cough syrups containing codeine	Same as schedule III

6. Half-life (t½)—time required for a drug's serum concentration to decrease by 50%; five half-lives are required for a drug to be eliminated from the body
7. Potency—amount of drug (e.g., in milligrams) needed to produce an effect; the more potent an agent is, the lower is the dose needed to produce an effect (Fig. 11–2)
8. Efficacy—the desired effect elicited by a drug, independent of dose (see Fig. 11–2)
9. Tolerance—physiologic response to the same dose produces less effect, or a higher dose is required to achieve the same effect
10. Therapeutic effect—desired pharmacologic effect
C. Routes of administration
   1. Oral (PO)—by mouth; easiest to use; good client acceptance; however, a latency period exists
   2. Rectal—administration by suppository or enema; produces either local or systemic effect
   3. Parenteral—a route other than an oral route; usually refers to an injection
   4. Intravenous (IV)—administration into a vein; shortest onset of action and higher risk of adverse events compared with other routes of administration
   5. Intramuscular (IM)—administration into the muscle; sometimes painful
   6. Subcutaneous (SC, SQ)—injected beneath the skin (e.g., insulin)
   7. Oral or nasal—particles, volatile liquids, or gasses that are inhaled (e.g., nitrous oxide–oxygen [N_2O-O_2] analgesia;

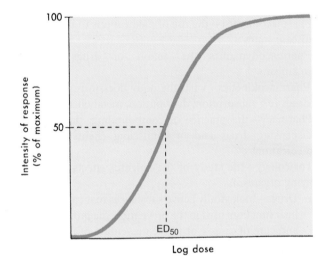

FIG 11–1 Log dose-effect curve. *ED*, Effective dose.

as are some medications used to treat allergies and asthma)
8. Topical—ointments or creams applied to the skin or mucous membranes (e.g., hydrocortisone)

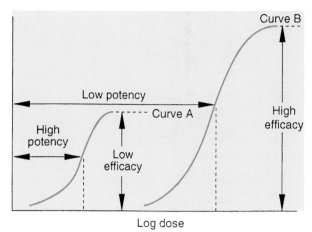

FIG 11–2 Potency and efficacy of a drug. *Curve A* has high potency and low efficacy; *Curve B* has low potency and high efficacy.

9. Sublingual—a tablet that dissolves or a solution that is sprayed under the tongue (for systemic effect)
D. Dosage forms
1. Capsule—gelatin shell
2. Tablet—compressed or molded dosage form
3. Ointment or cream—semi-solid for topical application
4. Suppository—penile, rectal, or vaginal; systemic or local
5. Solution—single-phase system consisting of more than one constituent
6. Suspension—insoluble particles in liquid (e.g., milk of magnesia)
E. Dosage
1. Varies depending on the client's:
a. Age—older adults may require lower doses because they may metabolize and excrete drugs more slowly
b. Weight—total body weight, muscle-to-fat ratio, and body size can affect drug absorption
c. Condition (disease)—many different disease states can affect drug absorption, metabolism, or excretion (e.g., congestive heart failure slows down metabolism; hyperthyroidism speeds up metabolism)
d. Route of administration
2. Pediatric dose
a. Less than the adult's dose
b. Based on:
(1) Manufacturer's recommendations—best method
(2) Surface area—good method
(3) Weight—adequate method
(4) Age—very poor method

Adverse Reactions
Side Effect
A. Side effect on a nontarget organ—effect on an organ other than that intended to be altered (e.g., insomnia resulting from a β_2-agonist or theophylline); dose related and often predictable
B. Toxic reaction—predictable and dose-related effect on a target organ (e.g., insulin can lower blood glucose levels to the point of hypoglycemia)

C. Allergic reaction—varies from mild rash to anaphylaxis; involves an antigen-antibody reaction (e.g., rash from penicillin); can include urticaria, soft tissue swelling, and difficulty breathing; not predictable and not dose related
D. Idiosyncrasy—abnormal drug response that is genetically related
E. Interference with natural defense mechanisms—body is less able to fight infection (e.g., steroids weaken the immune system)
F. Teratogenic effect—adverse effect on a fetus (e.g., alcohol intake during pregnancy produces fetal alcohol syndrome)

Pharmacokinetics
Pharmacokinetics is the way in which the body responds to drugs through the four processes of absorption, distribution, metabolism, and excretion (ADME).
A. Absorption depends on:
1. Degree of ionization—the more ionized (charged) the drug, the less it will be absorbed; conversely, the less ionized the drug, the more it will be absorbed; with weak acids or bases, this is a function of pH
2. Lipid solubility—the more lipid soluble the drug, the more readily it will be absorbed; the less lipid soluble it is, the less readily it will be absorbed
3. Factors that affect absorption
a. Client compliance
b. Age
c. Gender
d. Other disease states
e. Genetic variations
f. Placebo effect
B. Distribution of the drug (Fig. 11–3)[1]
1. Drugs are transported to the site of action
2. Only the free, or unbound, drug can cross cell membranes (indicated by arrows between boxes in Fig. 11–3)
3. In each cellular compartment, equilibrium is reached between the bound and unbound (free) drug
4. Redistribution—the drug moves from one tissue (where it exerts an effect) to another tissue (where it is inactive); this is one method of terminating a drug's effect
5. Protein binding—drugs bind to protein receptors to varying degrees; once the drug binds to a protein receptor, it cannot exert its pharmacologic effect; when more than one drug is present in the system, the drugs may compete for the same receptor site; the drug with the stronger affinity will bind to the receptor site, and the drug with the weaker affinity will then exert its pharmacologic effect
6. Tissue binding—some drugs can also bind to body tissues and cause significant chemical effects (e.g., tetracycline has an impact on developing bones and teeth of the fetus and of a young child)
C. Metabolism (biotransformation)—takes place mainly in the liver by hepatic microsomal enzymes; metabolites are more polar, less protein bound, and more easily excreted; drugs metabolized by microsomal enzymes can affect their own metabolism or that of other drugs (e.g., either increasing [as with barbiturates] or decreasing [as with cimetidine,

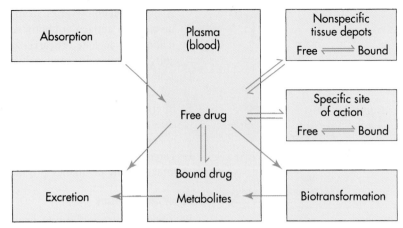

FIG 11–3 Absorption and outcome of a drug. (Modified from Holroyd SV, Wynn RL, Requa-Clark B: *Clinical pharmacology in dental practice,* ed 4, St Louis, 1989, Mosby.)

erythromycin] the rate of metabolism); biotransformation is a source of drug interactions

D. Excretion—usually by way of kidneys (urine); can also occur through feces (enterohepatic circulation), sweat, tears, or lungs (e.g., N_2O is exhaled)

Receptors

A receptor site is an area in the body to which a drug binds.

A. Agonist—a drug that has an affinity for a receptor site and binds to it, producing an effect (e.g., opioid [narcotic] analgesic agent)

B. Antagonist—a drug has an affinity for a receptor site and binds to it but produces no effect; competitively blocks the effect of an agonist (e.g., naloxone, an opioid [narcotic] antagonist blocks the effect of the agonist, an opioid)

AUTONOMIC NERVOUS SYSTEM AGENTS

Agents affecting the autonomic nervous system (ANS) are divided into four groups: parasympathetic (P) nervous system stimulation (P+) and inhibition (P−), and sympathetic (S) nervous system stimulation (S+) and inhibition (S−).

Sympathetic (Adrenergic) Agents

Mimic the action of the sympathetic autonomic nervous system (SANS); act like norepinephrine (NE) in the SANS, producing stimulation of the SANS; epinephrine produces the same effect (Fig. 11–4)

A. Adrenergic agonists

1. The SANS is activated by fear (the "fight-or-flight" response)

2. Catecholamine—chemical structure of some adrenergic agents

3. Receptors in the SANS include alpha (α) and beta (β) types:

a. α_1-Receptors—produce constriction of smooth muscles and blood vessels (vasoconstriction)

b. β-Receptors

(1) β_1-Receptors—stimulate the heart, increase heart rate (HR), increase the contractility and

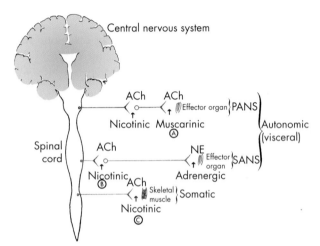

FIG 11–4 Typical neurons with neurotransmitters (*ACh*, acetylcholine; *NE*, norepinephrine), and the typical parasympathetic nervous system *(PANS)*; the sympathetic nervous system *(SANS)*; somatic nerves; and muscarinic *(A)* and nicotinic *(B and C)* receptors.

conduction velocity of the heart, and cause bronchodilation

(2) β_2-Receptors—relax smooth muscles, causing dilation of the blood vessels of skeletal muscle (vasodilation) and bronchodilation

B. Pharmacologic effects and adverse reactions

1. The central nervous system (CNS)—stimulation produces increased alertness; may also cause anxiety, anorexia

2. Stimulation of the heart—S+, produces

a. Positive chronotropic effect (increased HR)

b. Positive inotropic effect (increased strength of contraction of the heart)

c. Arrhythmias, with higher doses

d. α-Receptor stimulation—decreases HR because of the indirect (reflex vagal) effect

3. Vascular effects (on the arterial tree) result from

a. α-Receptors—causing vasoconstriction of blood vessels

   b. β-Receptors—causing vasodilation of skeletal muscle blood vessels
   c. Total peripheral resistance (TPR)—force against which the heart works to circulate blood
      (1) α-Receptors—increased TPR
      (2) β-Receptors—decreased TPR
4. Mydriasis (pupil dilation) and reduced intraocular pressure; useful in treating glaucoma
5. Bronchodilation (by action of β2-agonist); useful in treating clients with asthma
6. Production of thick, viscous saliva
C. Drug interactions—examples of interactions caused by adrenergic agents:
   1. Tricyclic antidepressants (TCAs; e.g., amitriptyline [Elavil], imipramine [Tofranil])—interaction increases blood pressure; produces dysrhythmias
   2. β-Blockers (e.g., propranolol [Inderal])—produce hypertension and bradycardia (slowed HR)
   3. Antidiabetic agents (e.g., insulin, glipizide [Glucotrol], glyburide (DiaBeta)—increase the blood glucose level
   4. Monoamine oxidase inhibitors (MAOIs)— no problem with epinephrine; indirect-acting amines (e.g., pseudoephedrine) must be avoided
   5. General anesthetics—halogenated hydrocarbons (e.g., halothane [Fluothane]) sensitize the myocardium to catecholamines; epinephrine is a catecholamine; increase the risk of arrhythmia/dysrhythmias
D. Dental hygiene considerations—the client's pulse and blood pressure (BP) must be checked; all these medications can increase HR and BP
E. Therapeutic uses (Table 11–3)
   1. Medical purposes—treatment of:
      a. Anaphylaxis
      b. Cardiac arrest
      c. Nasal congestion—decongestant
      d. Asthma (β2-agonist)
      e. Attention deficit hyperactivity disorder (ADD or ADHD)
      f. Glaucoma

2. Dental purposes
   a. Local anesthetic additive (vasoconstrictor)
   b. Hemostatic additive to reduce bleeding; provides adequate tissue retraction (cord)
F. Adrenergics as vasoconstrictors are contained in local anesthetic solutions
   1. Examples
      a. Epinephrine (Adrenalin)
      b. Levonordefrin (Neo-Cobefrin)
   2. Advantages of adrenergic vasoconstriction
      a. Prolongs duration of anesthesia
      b. Reduces systemic toxicity
      c. Provides hemostasis
      d. Reduces absorption (vasoconstriction)
      e. Increases concentration of anesthetic at the nerve membrane
   3. Disadvantages of adrenergic vasoconstriction
      a. Excessive amount produces systemic toxicity
      b. In persons with cardiovascular disease:
         (1) Reasonable amounts can be used in local anesthetic additives for clients whose cardiovascular conditions are stable
         (2) Avoid using epinephrine-impregnated retraction cords
         (3) Maximum (safe) dose (MD) varies for normal and clients with cardiovascular disease
            (a) Epinephrine—dose for normal clients, 0.2 mg; for clients with cardiovascular disease, 0.04 mg
            (b) Levonordefrin (Neo-Cobefrin)—dose for normal clients, 1 mg; for clients with cardiovascular disease, 0.2 mg (some sources state 1.0 mg)
      c. Hyperthyroidism—vasoconstrictors may produce a thyroid storm in clients who have not received treatment and in those receiving drug therapy
         (1) *Thyroid storm* or *thyroid crisis* is characterized by an acceleration of all body processes (e.g., increases in HR, BP, respiration, body temperature, and pulse)
         (2) Pulmonary edema and congestive heart failure can occur
   4. Minimize toxicity by:
      a. Injecting slowly
      b. Aspirating before injecting
      c. Calming the client
      d. Using the lowest effective dose
   5. Dental hygiene considerations
      a. Use is contraindicated in clients with uncontrolled cardiovascular disease
      b. Check blood pressure and pulse

α-Adrenergic Blockers (α-Blockers)

See the section on "Cardiovascular Agents" for a more detailed discussion.
A. Mechanism of action—block α-receptors, which block action of the SANS
B. Used to treat hypertension (e.g., Raynaud disease)

TABLE 11–3 Adrenergic Agents and Their Use		
Adrenergic Agent	Receptor Stimulated	Comments
Epinephrine (Adrenalin)	αβ	Endogenous catecholamine; local anesthetic additive
Methylphenidate (Ritalin)	α	Attention deficit hyperactivity disorder (ADHD)
Phenylephrine (Neo-Synephrine)	α	Nasal decongestant
Levonordefrin (Neo-Cobefrin)	α > β	Local anesthetic additive
Amphetamine	αβ	Diet pill (abused)
Pseudoephedrine (Sudafed)	αβ	Orally active nasal decongestant

C. Examples (note generic names ending with "-sin")
 1. Prazosin (Minipress)
 2. Terazosin (Hytrin)
 3. Doxazosin (Cardura)

β-Adrenergic Blocker (β-Blocker) Antagonists

See the section on "Cardiovascular Agents" for more information.

A. Mechanism of action—drug blocks SANS action (β-receptors); some β-blockers are more selective for the β_1-receptor than β_2-receptor; some drugs are formulated to target β_1-receptors, others to β_2-receptors; other drugs target both β_1- and β_2-receptors
B. Used to treat hypertension, angina, arrhythmias; also congestive heart failure, anxiety, and glaucoma; used to prevent myocardial infarction (MI, heart attack)
C. Examples (note generic names ending with "-olol")
 1. Propranolol (Inderal)—nonselective β_1- and β_2-blocker
 2. Metoprolol (Lopressor)—selective β_1-blocker
 3. Atenolol (Tenormin)—selective β_1-blocker
D. Dental hygiene considerations
 1. Check the client's BP and pulse—these medications can increase or decrease HR
 2. Raise the dental chair slowly, and allow the client to remain seated for a few minutes to minimize the risk of orthostatic hypotension

Adrenergic Neuronal Agonists and Antagonists

A. Pharmacologic effects—affect the release of norepinephrine from nerve endings and the level of adrenergic activity; influence α-receptor and β-receptor activities
B. Therapeutic use—treatment of hypertension; use is limited by adverse effects (e.g., can cause xerostomia and sedation)
C. Examples
 1. Reserpine (Serpasil)
 2. Methyldopa (Aldomet)
 3. Clonidine (Catapres)

Parasympathomimetic (Cholinergic) Agents

A. Cholinergic agonists—mimic the action of the parasympathetic autonomic nervous system (PANS); stimulation of the PANS
 1. Receptors—see Fig. 11–4 for an illustration of a typical cholinergic nerve
  a. Muscarinic—receptor stimulated by the compound found in the poisonous mushroom *Amanita muscaria* (Fig. 11–4, *A*)
   (1) Areas affected (*A*)
    (a) Smooth muscle
    (b) Cardiac muscle
    (c) Gland cells
   (2) Neurotransmitter—acetylcholine (ACh)
   (3) Location—the synapse between the postganglionic fiber and the neuroeffector organ in the PANS
   (4) Stimulated by muscarine

   (5) Blocked by atropine
  b. Nicotinic—receptor stimulated by nicotine; found in cigarettes (Fig. 11–4, *B* and *C*)
   (1) Areas affected
    (a) Postganglionic neurons (*B*)
    (b) Skeletal muscle end plates (*C*)
   (2) Neurotransmitter—acetylcholine (ACh)
   (3) Location—autonomic ganglia (*B*) and neuromuscular junction (*C*)
   (4) Stimulated by nicotine
   (5) Blocked by hexamethonium (autonomic, *B*) and *d*-tubocurarine at the neuromuscular junction (*C*)
 2. Acetylcholine—the following diagram illustrates synthesis and inactivation of ACh

$$A \qquad Ch \qquad Choline \qquad ACh$$
$$\text{acetyltransferase}$$
$$\text{Acetyl + Choline} \rightleftharpoons \text{Acetylcholine}$$
$$\text{(CoA)} \qquad \text{Acetylcholinesterase}$$
$$\text{(AChE)}$$

 3. Classification and mechanism of action
  a. Direct-acting drugs—act just as ACh at the receptor site, such as:
   (1) Choline derivatives
   (2) Pilocarpine (Salagen)
  b. Indirect-acting drugs—increase the amount of ACh indirectly; block ACh inactivation by inhibiting acetylcholinesterase (AChE), the enzyme that normally destroys ACh
   (1) "Reversible" cholinesterase inhibitors—drugs that block action of AChE, but whose action is terminated (ACh is then destroyed)
    (a) Edrophonium (Tensilon)
    (b) Physostigmine (Eserine)
    (c) Neostigmine (Prostigmin)
   (2) "Irreversible" cholinesterase inhibitors—drugs that attach to and inactivate AChE (e.g., organophosphates used as insecticides [malathion, parathion])
 4. Pharmacologic effects—similar to stimulation of the PANS
  a. Smooth muscle stimulation
   (1) Increase in gastrointestinal (GI) motility—diarrhea may result; advantageously used to treat postoperative GI and genitourinary (GU) retention
   (2) Bronchoconstriction—causes constriction of bronchial smooth muscle, an adverse reaction
  b. Glands—increased secretion of saliva; used to treat dry mouth (xerostomia)
  c. Eye—decreased intraocular pressure; used to treat glaucoma
 5. Toxic reactions—symptoms of overdose are extensions of the pharmacologic effects; the "too much" effect
  a. SLUD—excessive salivation, lacrimation (tearing), urination, and defecation

b. Treatment of overdose
   (1) Pralidoxime (2-PAM, Protopam)—regenerates AChE
   (2) Atropine—antimuscarinic; blocks the muscarinic effects of ACh excess (not nicotinic effects)
6. Dental hygiene considerations
   a. Oral forms can cause increased salivation and may cause hypotension and bradycardia
   b. Clients should maintain good oral hygiene
   c. Have client rise slowly from the dental chair to minimize orthostatic hypotension
7. Dental use—treatment of xerostomia; pilocarpine tablets may increase salivary flow

B. Anticholinergic agents—block muscarinic actions of the PANS
1. Basic principles
   a. Decreased salivary flow; used advantageously to dry up saliva
   b. Many drugs can have an anticholinergic, atropinic, or atropine-like effect
   c. Anticholinergic agents block the muscarinic receptors
2. Pharmacologic effects on the:
   a. Heart—tachycardia (increased HR; useful during general anesthesia when HR may fall too low)
   b. Eye—produces:
      (1) Mydriasis—dilation of pupils; results in photophobia
      (2) Cycloplegia—paralysis for distant vision; client cannot focus or read up close
      (3) Avoid repeated doses in clients who have narrow-angle glaucoma (this is the only autonomic drug group relatively contraindicated in certain forms of glaucoma)
   c. Salivary secretions—salivary flow reduced; useful in dentistry (Table 11–4 lists several drug groups that produce xerostomia)
   d. CNS—can cause sedation or excitation
3. Adverse reactions and toxicity—contraindications to use
   a. Xerostomia, dry skin, and dry eyes—caution in persons wearing contact lenses; reduces lactation in nursing mothers
   b. Eyes—blurred vision; avoid use in clients with narrow-angle glaucoma; careful use of eyedrops in persons with wide-angle glaucoma is usually acceptable
   c. Urinary retention—avoid use in persons with prostatic hypertrophy (enlarged prostate)
   d. Dizziness and fatigue—toxic levels can cause delirium, hallucinations, coma, and convulsions
   e. Tachycardia—monitor persons with cardiovascular disease
   f. Reduced GI motility—avoid in persons with gastric retention or intestinal obstruction
4. Clinical uses—effects offer advantageous treatment in:
   a. GI activity—has antispasmodic properties (reduced GI overactivity) and reduces secretions (e.g., stomach acid)

TABLE 11–4 Xerostomia-Producing Drug Groups with Examples

Drug Group	Examples
Antiacne	Isotretinoin
Anticholinergics* (P-)	Atropine
Anticonvulsants	Carbamazepine, felbamate, gabapentin, lamotrigine
Antidepressants	Amitriptyline, imipramine, fluoxetine, fluvoxamine
Antihistamines	Astemizole, brompheniramine, chlorpheniramine, loratadine
Antihypertensives*	Clonidine, guanethidine, methyldopa, captopril
Antinauseants	Cyclizine, diphenhydramine, meclizine
Antiparkinson drugs	Benztropine mesylate, biperiden, carbidopa, levodopa, trihexyphenidyl
Antipsychotics	Chlorpromazine, clozapine, fluphenazine, haloperidol, thioridazine
Antispasmodics	Dicyclomine, propantheline
Antidiarrheal	Diphenoxylate, loperamide
Benzodiazepines	Diazepam, alprazolam, lorazepam
Decongestants	Pseudoephedrine
Diuretics	Hydrochlorothiazide, furosemide
Muscle relaxants	Baclofen, orphenadrine
Nonsteroidal anti-inflammatory drugs (NSAIDs)	Diflunisal, ibuprofen, naproxen

*More likely to produce xerostomia; effect still dose related.

b. Ophthalmology—dilates eyes and paralyzes the muscles of accommodation (the person can see only distant objects); used for eye examinations
c. Parkinson's disease
d. Drug-induced Parkinson's disease
e. Dental
   (1) Used before general anesthesia to dry up saliva and to prevent vagal slowing of the heart
   (2) Used to prepare the mouth for procedures that require a drier field
5. Dental hygiene considerations
   a. Xerostomia—instruct the client to drink plenty of water, suck on tart sugarless gum or candy with xylitol or ice chips, avoid products containing alcohol and caffeine, and avoid juices and soft drinks to reduce the risk of dental caries; saliva substitutes (Xero-lube, Salivart) can also be recommended
   b. Tachycardia—check the client's BP and pulse
   c. Sedation—an increased risk of sedation exists if combined with other sedating agents; client should be instructed to avoid driving or operating heavy machinery or any task that requires thinking or concentration
6. Examples of anticholinergic agents
   a. Atropine
   b. Benztropine mesylate (Cogentin)
   c. Dicyclomine (Bentyl)

d. Methantheline (Banthine)

e. Propantheline (Pro-Banthine)

f. Trihexyphenidyl hydrochloride (Artane)

Local Anesthetic Agents

See the section on "Management of Pain and Anxiety" in Chapter 18.

A. Chemistry

1. Three components common to local anesthetics (LAs)

   a. Aromatic lipophilic group—contains a benzene ring

   b. Intermediate chain—either ester or amide

   c. Hydrophilic amino group—secondary or tertiary amine

2. Intermediate chain

   a. Composed of esters

   (1) Tetracaine (Pontocaine)

   (2) Procaine (Novocain)

   (3) Propoxycaine (in Ravocaine)

   b. Composed of amides

   (1) Articaine (Septocaine)

   (2) Lidocaine (Xylocaine)

   (3) Mepivacaine (Carbocaine)

   (4) Prilocaine (Citanest)

   (5) Bupivacaine (Marcaine)

B. Mechanism of action by:

1. Nerve fiber susceptibility—nerves and sensations generally are affected in this order: autonomic, cold and warmth, pain, touch pressure, vibration, proprioception, and motor; sensations and nerve functions are regained in reverse order

2. Specific receptor theory—the anesthetic agent binds to receptors on the sodium channel; permeability to sodium ions is decreased, and nerve conduction is interrupted

3. Base and salt forms of LAs (Fig. 11–5)—both forms are needed; the base penetrates the lipid membranes, and the salt traverses the cellular fluid

$$R_3N + H^{\oplus} \rightleftharpoons R_3N^{\oplus} - H$$

Free base

Uncharged, un-ionized

Fat soluble (lipophilic)

Penetrates nerve tissue

Salt

Charged, cation (ionized)

Water soluble (hydrophilic)

Form present in dental cartridge (pH 4.5-6.0)

Infection, doesn't penetrate

FIG 11–5 Base and salt forms of local anesthetics. The pH determines the amounts on each side (in equilibrium).

4. Inflammation—reduces LA effect

   a. Acid environment (pH 5.5) of inflammation increases the ionized form and reduces the anesthetic effect

   b. Edema—dilutes the LA because of an increase in fluids

   c. Increased tissue vasculature—increased blood supply carries away the LA; duration of action is shortened

C. Pharmacokinetics

1. Absorption

   a. Effect on the vasculature—LAs produce vasodilation (except cocaine); vasoconstrictors are added to counteract dilation

   b. Absorption and distribution of LAs are determined by the pH of the environment, as shown in the following reaction:

Inflammation $\rightarrow \downarrow$ pH $\rightarrow \uparrow$ [H$^+$] $\rightarrow \uparrow$ charged form (more acide)(more hydrogen ions)

S $\rightarrow \downarrow$ un-ionized form B $\rightarrow \updownarrow$; charged distribution

   c. Solubility

   (1) Lipid-soluble—the nonionized form penetrates membranes

   (2) Water-soluble—the ionized form crosses the cell membrane and exerts its effect at the nerve

   d. Rate of absorption

   (1) The faster the rate of absorption, the greater the chance of systemic toxicity and the shorter the duration of action

   (2) Route of administration alters the rate of absorption; the topical anesthetic agent can be absorbed quickly

2. Distribution—the level of the LA in the blood is determined by movement of the LA around the body; side effects occur if the LA reaches a high enough level in other organs (e.g., CNS, heart); blood level is determined by:

   a. Rate of injection

   b. Speed of absorption (depends on proximity to blood vessels)

   c. Speed of distribution to other tissues

   d. Speed of metabolism and excretion

3. Metabolism (biotransformation)

   a. Esters—hydrolyzed by plasma pseudo-cholinesterases

   (1) Procaine—metabolized to para-aminobenzoic acid (PABA)—allergenic

   (2) Congenital cholinesterase deficiency—LAs containing esters are absolutely contraindicated

   b. Amides—metabolized in the liver

   (1) Liver dysfunction—LAs containing amides should be given cautiously; they may be metabolized more slowly; toxic levels can build up if repeated doses are administered

   (2) Prilocaine—metabolized to orthotoluidine, which can produce methemoglobinemia, a condition in which excess methemoglobin in the blood results in lowered oxygen-carrying capacity; not usually a problem in healthy clients

4. Excretion capacity
   a. Esters are almost completely metabolized before they are excreted
   b. Amides are mostly metabolized before they are excreted
   c. The presence of significant renal disease can cause all LA metabolites to accumulate
D. Adverse reactions
   1. Factors influencing toxicity
      a. Drug
      b. Concentration
      c. Route
      d. Tissue inflammation
      e. Vasoconstriction
      f. Body weight
      g. Rate of metabolism and excretion
   2. Symptoms of LA toxicity—the CNS and the cardiovascular system (CVS) are affected most; the severity of effects is related directly to the amount of the LA in blood
      a. CNS response—stimulation followed by depression
         (1) CNS stimulation (excitatory)—produces restlessness, shivering, tremors, convulsions
         (2) CNS depression—results in sedation, drowsiness, respiratory and cardiovascular depression, coma; can occur without previous excitation
      b. CVS response
         (1) Antidysrhythmic action—lidocaine used intravenously to treat dysrhythmias
         (2) Vasodilation produces hypotension; releases vascular smooth muscle; lowers resistance
   3. Malignant hyperthermia—life-threatening complication associated with the administration of general anesthesia, characterized by tachycardia, tachypnea, cardiac dysrhythmia, muscle rigidity, and extreme increase in body temperature; LA agents containing amide administered in standard doses in oral health care appear to be safe for individuals susceptible to malignant hyperthermia
   4. Allergic reactions
      a. Range of reactions—mild rash to anaphylaxis
      b. Esters—much more allergenic than amides; note that the presence of true allergic reactions to amides is still debated; it is unclear whether people are actually allergic to amides
      c. Other ingredients may produce allergic reactions (preservatives, antioxidants); see H. Composition of LA solutions
      d. Administer LAs containing amides to clients allergic to esters, and vice versa
E. Drug interactions
   1. Esters administered in the presence of sulfonamides—esters may interfere locally with the sulfonamides' anti-infective action
   2. Lidocaine administered in the presence of cimetidine (Tagamet)—cimetidine prolongs the metabolism of lidocaine in the liver; levels of lidocaine in blood may increase with repeated doses; not important to dentistry

F. Dental hygiene considerations
   1. CNS stimulation—calm client with a soothing voice and manner
      a. Administer a lower dose of the LA
      b. Switch to another LA
   2. Sedation
      a. Have someone drive the client home
      b. Have the client sit in the reception area until he or she no longer feels tired
      c. Use caution while using opioid analgesics, antianxiety drugs, or other sedating drugs if sedation persists
   3. Have the client refrain from imbibing very hot and very cold foods or drinks
   4. Advise patient to be conscious of accidentally biting the cheek until all feeling has returned after LA
G. Vasoconstrictors and cardiovascular disease
   1. Clients with controlled cardiovascular disease (e.g., hypertension, angina, arrhythmias) can receive LAs
   2. Do not exceed the maximum dose of a vasoconstrictor in clients with cardiovascular disease; use caution
   3. Check the client's pulse rate and BP before administering an LA that contains a vasoconstrictor
H. Composition of LA solutions
   1. Other ingredients
      a. Vasoconstrictors—epinephrine (Adrenalin), levonordefrin (Neo-Cobefrin)
      b. Preservatives (antiseptics)—methylparabens and propylparabens are no longer present in dental anesthetic cartridges
      c. Antioxidant (preservative)—sodium bisulfite, acetone sodium bisulfite, or sodium metabisulfite; the antioxidant is present if the LA contains a vasoconstrictor
         (1) May precipitate asthma attacks in susceptible persons
         (2) Sulfite, sulfa, and sulfur are not cross-allergenic
      d. Alkalinizing agent—sodium hydroxide; adjusts pH; maintains the LA in salt form so that it will be soluble in water
      e. Sodium chloride—makes the solution isotonic
   2. LAs in dental cartridges (Table 11–5)
I. Topical LAs and injection-free local anesthesia
   1. Benzocaine—ester-based anesthetic; used topically because it cannot be used systemically; some sensitization occurs; use gloves to avoid skin contact with the drug, rash, and sensitization
   2. Lidocaine—topically effective
   3. Tetracaine—avoid use because of toxicity and slow onset
   4. Lidocaine and prilocaine (injection-free local anesthesia)
      a. Used in adults who require limited pain control during root debridement or in those who fear injections
      b. Gel applied into the periodontal pocket to provide pain relief during scaling and root-planing procedures (e.g., Oraqix)
      c. Amide-type topical anesthetic agent

TABLE 11-5 Local Anesthetic Agents in Dental Cartridges*

Local Anesthetic	Concentration (%)	Vasoconstrictor	
Amides			
Lidocaine	2	Epinephrine	1:100,000
(Xylocaine,	2	Epinephrine	1:50,000
Octocaine)			
Mepivacaine	2	Levonordefrin	1:20,000
(Carbocaine,	3	(Neo-Cobefrin)	
Isocaine)		None	
Prilocaine (Citanest,	4	Epinephrine	1:200,000
Forte Citanest)	4	None	
Bupivacaine	0.5	Epinephrine	1:200,000
(Marcaine,			
Sensorcaine)			
Articaine	4	Epinephrine	1:100,000
(Septocaine)			1:200,000

*Cartridge = 1.8 mL.

5. Dental hygiene considerations
   a. Use the smallest volume and the lowest concentration to avoid adverse effects
   b. Limit area of application
   c. Instruct the client not to swallow the topical LA
   d. Instruct the client to avoid very hot and very cold foods; client may not be able to sense temperature changes because of the topical LA

LOCAL ANESTHETIC REVERSAL AGENT

General Considerations

A. Dental use—for reversal of soft tissue anesthesia (lip, tongue) and functional deficits resulting from an intraoral submucosal injection of an LA with a vasoconstrictor; reduces recovery time of normal sensation
B. Contraindications—not recommended for use in children less than 6 years of age or weighing under 15 kg (33 lb)
C. Mechanism of action—expands blood vessels and increases blood flow, thereby accelerates the reversal of soft tissue numbness
D. Adverse effects
   1. Transient pain at injection site
   2. Tachycardia and arrhythmia may occur with parenteral administration but are uncommon after submucosal administration
E. Example—phentolamine mesylate (OraVerse)

GENERAL ANESTHETICS

General Considerations

A. Dental use—in extensive oral surgery and in an anxious client, a mentally challenged client who cannot cooperate, and any client who cannot control behavior during dental care
B. Stages and planes of anesthesia
   1. Stage I—analgesia
   2. Stage II—excitement and delirium; avoid, if possible

3. Stage III—surgical anesthesia; divided into four planes
4. Stage IV—respiratory paralysis (medullary paralysis); death ensues without intervention
C. Routes of administration
   1. Intravenous anesthetics—fixed anesthetics (cannot be removed by respiration)
      a. Barbiturates (e.g., thiopental [Pentothal])
      b. Dissociative—ketamine (Ketalar, Ketaject)
      c. Neuroleptanalgesic—fentanyl (Sublimaze) plus droperidol (Inapsine, Innovar)
   2. Inhalation gases
      a. Nitrous oxide combined with oxygen
   3. Inhalation volatile liquids
      a. Halogenated hydrocarbons (e.g., halothane [Fluothane])

Specific Agents

A. Nitrous oxide–oxygen (N_2O-O_2) analgesia
   1. Incomplete anesthetic; if used alone, the client cannot reach stage III
   2. Usual concentration maintained at 30% to 50% to prevent O_2 deprivation
   3. Administration
      a. Begin with 100% O_2 for 2 to 3 minutes
      b. Then add N_2O in 5% to 10% increments until the desired state of sedation is reached (usually 3 to 5 minutes)
      c. Once the procedure is terminated, the client should receive O_2 for 5 minutes
   4. Advantages
      a. Rapid onset and recovery
      b. Least toxic; safe when used appropriately
      c. May be used in children
      d. Nonflammable
      e. Nonirritating to the GI tract
      f. Good analgesic properties; anxiolytic (antianxiety) effect
   5. Disadvantages
      a. "Misuse" potential exists with both clients and oral health care professionals
      b. Reduces fertility
      c. Associated with high rate of miscarriages
      d. Improper use (without concomitant LA block injection) gives N_2O a "bad name"; analgesia from N_2O-O_2 still requires the use of an LA agent
      e. Nausea—most common complaint; caused by rapid changes in N_2O concentration of inspired air, change levels slowly
      f. Diffusion hypoxia—low level of O_2 in lungs because of diffusion of O_2 into the blood supply rarely occurs; administer 100% oxygen at the end of the procedure to prevent this
   6. Adverse effects
      a. Misuse or faulty installation of equipment
      b. Nausea, vomiting
      c. Headache, if oxygen is not given at the end of the procedure
      d. N_2O abuse

7. Drug interactions—occur with any drug that can cause CNS depression or sedation
8. Contraindications
   a. Respiratory problems
      (1) Upper respiratory tract infection (URI)—difficult to administer N_2O-O_2 analgesia when nasal passages are congested
      (2) Chronic obstructive pulmonary disease (COPD), such as emphysema or bronchitis
         (a) Administering O_2 at the usual concentration with N_2O could produce apnea (cessation of respiration)
         (b) The client's respiration is driven by carbon dioxide (CO_2) levels
   b. Pregnancy—the first trimester is the most critical; the greatest number of spontaneous abortions occur at this stage (especially in oral health care personnel); teratogenic effect unknown, but not probable
   c. Epilepsy
   d. Emotional instability
   e. Multiple sclerosis
   f. Previous negative experience
9. Dental hygiene considerations
   a. The client's emotional and psychiatric history
   b. Clients may have fanciful dreams while under the effects of N_2O-O_2; male dental personnel should ensure that female dental personnel are always present with female clients to avoid unfounded accusations
B. Halogenated hydrocarbons
   1. Examples
      a. Halothane (Fluothane)
      b. Enflurane (Ethrane)
      c. Isoflurane (Forane)
      d. Desflurane
      e. Sevoflurane
   2. Does not cause irritation of the mucosal membrane; not explosive; poor muscle relaxation; no analgesia; little nausea or vomiting
   3. The myocardium is sensitized to catecholamines (epinephrine)—can produce dysrhythmias
   4. Hepatotoxic—greater with more exposures
   5. Drug interaction—can occur if administered with drugs that cause CNS depression or sedation (e.g., opioid analgesics, barbiturates, benzodiazepines, antipsychotic drugs, antidepressants, antihistamines)
   6. Dental hygiene considerations
      a. Sedation and amnesia—clients should have someone to drive them home after the procedure
      b. Clients should be instructed to avoid driving or operating heavy machinery or any task that requires thinking or concentration
C. Ultrashort-acting barbiturates
   1. Examples
      a. Thiopental (Pentothal); also known as "truth serum"
      b. Methohexital (Brevital)
      c. Thiamylal (Surital)

2. Rapid onset; short duration secondary to redistribution to brain, muscles, and adipose tissue
3. Used to induce general anesthesia; the client advances rapidly to stage III
4. Adverse reaction—laryngospasm
5. Contraindicated in porphyria and status asthmaticus
D. Ketamine (Ketalar, Ketaject) produces dissociative anesthesia
   1. Not a complete anesthetic
   2. The client is not asleep and does not respond to stimuli in the environment (trance-like state)
   3. Reactions—bad dreams, may be described by the client as "bad trip"; more likely to occur in adults
   4. Can produce hyperactive reflexes such as coughing, gagging, or tongue movements
E. Neuroleptanalgesia—anesthetic, analgesic (Innovar)
   1. Fentanyl (opioid) plus droperidol (tranquilizer)
   2. Adverse reaction—produces "board-like" chest, which requires ventilatory action; performing cardiopulmonary resuscitation (CPR) is difficult

SEDATIVE-HYPNOTIC MEDICATIONS

General Considerations

A. Used to treat anxiety disorder, situational anxiety, and insomnia
B. Other drugs, in addition to sedative-hypnotics, can cause sedation; all can increase a client's risk for sedation when used together (Box 11–1)
C. Dental concerns
   1. Additive CNS depressant effects when taken with alcohol, opioid analgesics, or other CNS depressants
   2. The client should be instructed to avoid driving or operating heavy machinery or any task that requires thinking or concentration

Benzodiazepines

A. Mechanism of action—potentiates the inhibitory neurotransmitter γ-aminobutyric acid (GABA); GABA-ergic neurotransmission increases sedation
B. Wide therapeutic index when ingested alone; much safer than barbiturates

---

BOX 11–1 Select Pharmacologic Groups Producing Sedation

Alcohol, ethyl
Antihistamines
Antipsychotics (phenothiazines)
Barbiturates
Benzodiazepines
Centrally acting muscle relaxants
Nonbarbiturate sedative-hypnotics
Nonsteroidal anti-inflammatory drugs (NSAIDs)
Opioid (narcotic) analgesic agents
Tricyclic antidepressants

C. Adverse reactions
 1. Sedation—the client should be instructed to avoid driving or operating heavy machinery or any task that requires thinking or concentration
 2. Addiction potential—some potential exists but less than that for barbiturates
 3. Teratogenicity—increased incidence of birth defects if taken during the first trimester; this is an FDA (U.S. Food and Drug Administration) category D or X drug
 4. Thrombophlebitis—when administered intravenously; local irritation may occur with diazepam because of the use of propylene glycol as diluent; midazolam (Versed) is soluble in water, so no propylene glycol is used
 5. Overdose—treated with flumazenil (Mazicon), a benzodiazepine antagonist

D. Specific agents
 1. Examples of benzodiazepines and typical doses are provided in Table 11–6 (see also Table 11–3)
 2. Differences between benzodiazepines
  a. Equivalent dose—usual dose varies with agent
  b. Duration—varies from a few hours to a few days
  c. Metabolism
   (1) Most benzodiazepines are metabolized by oxidation to active metabolites
   (2) Oxazepam, lorazepam, and temazepam are inactivated by glucuronidation
   (3) The client's age is a factor that can reduce the metabolism of oxidized benzodiazepines
 3. Drug interactions—the presence of cimetidine reduces the metabolism of oxidized benzodiazepines; clients who smoke experience less sedation (smoking induces liver enzymes)

E. Dental hygiene considerations
 1. Can cause anterograde amnesia (limited to events occurring after drug administration); clients should be cautioned about making life-changing decisions after taking a benzodiazepine
 2. All other dental hygiene considerations are the same as the general considerations

Barbiturates

A. Pharmacologic effects
 1. Continuum with increasing doses—from sedation and anxiety relief, to sleep, and then anesthesia

 2. Anticonvulsant—long-acting agents are usually the most useful
 3. Muscle relaxation—this action is inseparable from CNS sedation effects
 4. No analgesic action—in the presence of pain, agitation may result if an analgesic is not given concurrently

B. Adverse reactions
 1. CNS depression—drowsiness and impaired performance and judgment; the client should be instructed to avoid driving or operating heavy machinery, or anything that requires thinking or concentration (see Box 11–1 for drugs that produce sedation)
 2. Abuse—euphoria, habituation, withdrawal, increased tolerance
 3. Acute overdose—causes depression of respiratory system and respiratory arrest
 4. Barbiturates—contraindicated in porphyria; stimulate liver microsomal enzymes (drugs metabolized by the liver disappear more quickly)

C. Therapeutic uses
 1. Medical uses—treatment of epilepsy, sedation, or anxiety
 2. Dental uses
  a. Preoperative anxiety reduction—oral or intramuscular administration
  b. Induction of general anesthesia—intravenous barbiturates
  d. Dental hygiene considerations—same as earlier "General Considerations" under "Sedative-Hypnotic Medications"

E. Examples—barbiturates
 1. Ultrashort-acting—for induction of general anesthesia
  a. Thiopental (Pentothal)
  b. Methohexital (Brevital)
 2. Short-acting—for insomnia; most abused form
  a. Pentobarbital (Nembutal)
  b. Secobarbital (Seconal)
 3. Intermediate-acting—for insomnia or daytime sedation; frequently abused
  a. Amobarbital (Amytal)
  b. Butabarbital (Butisol)
 4. Long-acting—treatment of seizure disorders, anticonvulsant; seldom abused
  a. Phenobarbital (Luminal)
  b. Primidone (Mysoline)

Nonbarbiturate Nonbenzodiazepines

A. Nonbenzodiazepine—benzodiazepine receptor agonists
 1. Zolpidem (Ambien)
 2. Zaleplon (Sonata)
 3. Eszopiclone (Lunesta)
B. Melatonin receptor agonist—ramelteon (Rozerem); used to treat insomnia characterized by difficulty falling asleep
 1. Centrally acting muscle relaxants
  a. Carisoprodol (Soma)—Class 2 (CII) drug
  b. Chlorzoxazone (Paraflex)
  c. Methocarbamol (Robaxin)
  d. Orphenadrine (Norflex)

TABLE 11–6 Examples of Benzodiazepines	
Drug	Usual Dose (oral) (mg/day)
Alprazolam (Xanax)	0.5-4.0
Chlordiazepoxide (Librium)	15.0-100.0
Diazepam (Valium)	2-10
Flurazepam (Dalmane)	15-30
Lorazepam (Ativan)	2-6
Midazolam (Versed)	Intravenous
Oxazepam (Serax)	15-30
Temazepam (Restoril)	15-30
Triazolam (Halcion)	0.125-0.5

2. Miscellaneous
    a. Baclofen (Lioresal)
    b. Tizanidine (Zanaflex)
    c. Dantrolene (Dantrium)
C. Dental hygiene considerations—same as earlier "General Considerations"

Analgesics

See Table 11–7.

General Considerations

A. Pain is characterized by:
    1. Perception—experienced uniformly through the nerve (signal from the site of pain to the CNS)
    2. Reaction—varies greatly from person to person (interpretation of the signal within the CNS)
B. Variables—client's age, gender, race, ethnic group, fatigue, and pain threshold

Salicylates (Aspirin)

A. Mechanism of action—primarily peripheral; prostaglandin synthesis inhibitor functions by inhibiting the enzyme cyclooxygenase (COX) or prostaglandin synthetase
B. Pharmacologic effects—"the three As"
    1. Analgesic—reduces pain
    2. Antipyretic—therapeutic dose reduces elevated body temperature
    3. Anti-inflammatory—higher dose reduces inflammation
C. Adverse reactions
    1. GI upset—minimized by ingesting the drug with food, water, or antacids
    2. Alteration in bleeding
        a. Platelet adhesiveness—reduced platelet adhesion for the life of the platelet (4 to 7 days); normal clotting reappears 72 hours after ingestion; reduced clotting

effect requires only a low single dose; useful in low doses to prevent clotting
        b. Hypoprothrombinemia—reduced prothrombin levels; requires several consecutive doses to reduce prothrombin levels
    3. Salicylate toxicity ("salicylism")—symptoms include tinnitus, hyperthermia (increased body temperature), electrolyte and glucose problems, and altered sensorium
    4. Allergic reactions—true allergy is uncommon; if person is allergic, some cross-reactivity exists with other agents (e.g., nonsteroidal anti-inflammatory drugs [NSAIDs]); can produce an acute asthma attack; persons with asthma and nasal polyps are more susceptible
    5. Reye syndrome—children with chickenpox or influenza should not be given aspirin; avoid aspirin in children and adolescents up to 18 years of age
D. Drug interactions—adverse reactions occur with aspirin used in conjunction with:
    1. Warfarin (Coumadin)—used as an anticoagulant; bleeding or hemorrhage
    2. Probenecid (Benemid)—used to treat gout; acute attack of gout
    3. Tolbutamide (Orinase)—used to control diabetes; altered blood glucose level
    4. Methotrexate (MTX)—used to treat cancer or control arthritis; MTX toxicity in bone marrow
    5. Alcohol—can increase bleeding or hemorrhage
    6. Other anti-inflammatory drugs—can increase bleeding or hemorrhage
E. Dental hygiene considerations
    1. Avoid drugs that can cause GI upset or prolong bleeding time
    2. Check for aspirin allergies
    3. If taken before procedure, client may experience more bleeding than normal

TABLE 11–7 Analgesic Summary

Pharmacologic Effects and Adverse Reactions	Aspirin	NSAIDs	Acetaminophen	Opioids (Narcotics)
Analgesic	+	++	+	++++
Antipyretic	+	+/0	+	0
Anti-inflammatory	+	++	0	0
Central nervous system (CNS) effects (drowsiness)	++[a]	++	0[b]	++
Gastrointestinal (GI) effects	++[c]	+[c]	0	+[d]
Bleeding	++	+[e]	0	0
Hepatotoxic	+[f]	+	+[g]	0
Nephrotoxic	+[e]	+[e]	+[e]	0
Addicting effects	0	0	0	++++

+, Very low; ++, low; +++, moderate; ++++, high; 0, no effect.
[a]Poisoning—salicylism.
[b]Very high doses.
[c]Upset stomach, ulcers, pain.
[d]Nausea, constipation.
[e]Aspirin or nonsteroidal anti-inflammatory drugs (NSAIDs) and acetaminophen.
[f]Hepatitis in persons with systemic lupus erythematosus or rheumatoid arthritis.
[g]With acute overdose.

Nonsteroidal Anti-Inflammatory Agents (NSAIAs) and Drugs (NSAIDs)

A. Mechanism—similar to that of aspirin, drug inhibits prostaglandin synthesis (COX)
B. Pharmacologic effects—"the three As" (similar to aspirin)
   1. Analgesic
   2. Antipyretic
   3. Anti-inflammatory
C. Adverse reactions
   1. GI—more severe than aspirin; abdominal problems range from discomfort to ulcers; treated or managed with prostaglandin—misoprostol (Cytotec); increased risk for severe GI events, including bleeding and ulcers
   2. CVS—may increase the risk for serious cardiovascular thrombotic events, stroke, and MI
   3. CNS—dizziness, sedation; the client should be instructed to avoid driving or operating heavy machinery, or any task that requires thinking or concentration
   4. Blood coagulation—reduction in platelet aggregation and possible prolongation of bleeding time; alteration is reversible, unlike the effect of aspirin, which is not reversible
   5. Oral—can produce stomatic gingival ulceration and xerostomia
   6. Renal—can result in renal failure or cystitis
   7. Hypersensitivity—ranges from mild rash to anaphylaxis
D. Drug interactions
   1. Lithium—can increase lithium levels
   2. Digoxin—can increase the effects of digoxin
   3. Methotrexate—can increase the effects of MTX
   4. Antihypertensives—can reduce the antihypertensive effects of diuretics, angiotensin-converting enzyme (ACE) inhibitors, and β-blockers
   5. Other inflammatory drugs—can increase bleeding and hemorrhage
   6. Alcohol—can increase bleeding or hemorrhage
E. Contraindications
   1. Contraindicated in patients that have experienced asthma or allergic reaction to aspirin therapy
   2. Fluid-retention problems
   3. Coagulation problems
   4. Peptic ulcer disease
   5. Ulcerative colitis
   6. Renal disease; especially in patients at risk for renal disease or for patients taking ACE inhibitors or angiotensin receptor blockers (ARBs)
F. Dental hygiene considerations
   1. Same as for aspirin
   2. CNS sedation—the client should be instructed to avoid driving or operating heavy machinery or any task that requires thinking or concentration
G. Therapeutic uses
   1. Pain control—analgesic; stronger than aspirin, equal to or stronger than some opioids; strength of effect is dose dependent; anti-inflammatory effect makes NSAIDs especially useful in dentistry

   2. Arthritis—anti-inflammatory action
   3. Dysmenorrhea (painful menstruation)—effective because the mechanism of action is specific for the problem of excess prostaglandins caused by excessive uterine contractions
H. Examples
   1. Ibuprofen (Motrin-IB, Rufen, Nuprin, Advil); naproxen sodium (Anaprox; Aleve); available without a prescription
   2. Naproxen (Naprosyn)
   3. Indomethacin (Indocin)—prescription only
   4. Celecoxib (Celebrex)—prescription only
      a. Caution should be exercised because COX-2 inhibitors can increase the risk of a heart attack
      b. Caution should be exercised because of an increased risk for significant GI bleeding

Acetaminophen (N-Acetyl-p-Aminophenol [NAPAP]; Tylenol [Available Over the Counter; OTC])

A. Pharmacologic effects—"the two As"
   1. Analgesic
   2. Antipyretic
   3. Not an anti-inflammatory
B. Adverse reactions
   1. Analgesic nephropathy—adversely affects the kidneys; more likely to occur if used chronically in combination with aspirin or NSAIDs
   2. Hepatotoxicity—may occur with acute overdose or chronic use; delayed reaction; treated with N-acetylcysteine; may be fatal without liver transplantation
C. Drug interactions—alcohol increases the risk of acetaminophen toxicity
D. Contraindications
   1. Hepatotoxicity
   2. Renal toxicity
   3. Clients with alcohol-abuse problems
E. Dental hygiene considerations—avoid use in clients with hepatotoxicity, renal toxicity, or alcohol abuse problems

Opioid (Narcotic) Analgesic Agents

A. Pharmacologic effects—proportional to the "strength" of the opioid
   1. Analgesia
   2. Sedation (anxiety relief)
   3. Euphoria
   4. Dysphoria
   5. Cough suppressant
   6. GI effects
   7. Respiratory effects
B. Examples of agonists (combine with opioid receptor and produce an effect) are provided in Table 11–8)
   1. Agonist–antagonist agents
      a. Example—pentazocine (Talwin-NX)
      b. Principle
         (1) Maintain analgesic properties
         (2) Have lower abuse potential
      c. Can precipitate withdrawal in opiate addicts

TABLE 11-8 Examples of Agonists

Drug	Usual Dose (Oral) (mg/day)	"Strength"
Morphine	10-30 po q4h	Stronger
Hydromorphone (Dilaudid)	1-6 q4-6 h	
Meperidine (Demerol)	50-150 po q4h	
Oxycodone (in Percodan)	5 q6h	
Hydrocodone (in Vicodin)	5-10 po q4-6 h	
Codeine (in Tylenol No. 3, Empirin No. 3)	30-60 q4-6 h	Weaker

po, By mouth; *q4h,* every 4 hours; *q4-6 h,* every 4 to 6 hours; *q6h,* every 6 hours.

2. Antagonists
   a. Example—Naloxone (Narcan), Naltrexone (Vivitrol), Nalmefene (Revex)
   b. Combine with opioid receptor; produces no effect; reverses opioid overdose
   c. Therapeutic uses
      (1) Treat opioid overdose
      (2) Counteract respiratory depression
      (3) Include in any dental emergency kit
C. Adverse reactions—proportional to the "strength" of the opioid
   1. CNS effects—sedation, euphoria, dysphoria
   2. Respiratory depression—dose related; overdose can result in death; reversed with naloxone
   3. GI—nausea, vomiting, constipation; diphenoxylate can be useful therapeutically
   4. Abuse—can occur with all opioid analgesics; tolerance develops to all pharmacologic effects except miosis (pupillary constriction) and constipation; withdrawal produced if the drug is abruptly stopped
   5. Miosis
   6. Urinary retention
   7. Cardiovascular effects—orthostatic hypotension
D. Therapeutic uses
   1. Pain relief—this is the central mechanism; agent affects a person's perception of pain; some opioids can relieve severe pain
   2. Sedation and anxiety relief—not the main use of opioids; used preoperatively
   3. Cough suppression—antitussive action (cough suppressant); low dose needed (e.g., codeine-containing cough syrups)
   4. Diarrhea—symptomatic relief only; reduce GI motility by increasing tone and spasm; diphenoxylate (in Lomotil)
E. Drug interactions
   1. Increase sedation when used with other CNS depressant drugs
   2. Increase constipation when combined with anticholinergic drugs
F. Dental hygiene considerations
   1. Decrease the dose in hypertensive clients because of associated urinary retention caused by opioids

2. Increased risk for sedation—as with other CNS depressant drugs
3. Increased risk for xerostomia—as with anticholinergic drugs

Drugs Used for Gout

A. Disease—gout is a metabolic condition involving increased serum uric acid, with episodes of acute attacks of pain in joints (big toe, knee) and severe inflammation caused by deposition of monosodium urate
B. Prevention
   1. Probenecid (Benemid)—uricosuric (promotes uric acid excretion); aspirin interferes with this effect of probenecid
   2. Allopurinol (Zyloprim)—xanthine oxidase inhibitor (inhibits uric acid synthesis); also used in clients with cancer before chemotherapy or radiation therapy when many cells are killed and release their amino acids, which leads to accumulation of uric acid and attacks of gout
C. Treatment
   1. Colchicine—binds to microtubular protein tubulin (prevents leukocyte migration and phagocytosis); inhibits formation of leukotrienes; GI toxicity—nausea, vomiting, diarrhea are end points of treatment and adverse reactions
   2. NSAIDs—anti-inflammatory action ameliorates symptoms (e.g., indomethacin)

ANTI-INFECTIVES (ANTIBIOTICS)

General Considerations

A. Prevention of infection (see the section on "Disease Transmission" in Chapter 10)
   1. Sterilization measures prevent infection
   2. Many infections—treat with local measures (e.g., incision and drainage), antibiotics are often not needed; the client's resistance and the development of resistant strains of bacteria must be considered
   3. Antibiotic administration carries risks
   4. Prophylaxis is rarely indicated except for decreasing the likelihood of infective endocarditis in persons who have the highest risk, prosthetic joint infection, or when client is immunosuppressed[2] (see Chapter 15, Table 15-2).
B. Definitions
   1. Antimicrobial—agent that acts against microbes
   2. Anti-infective—agent that acts against the organisms that cause infections
   3. Antibacterial—agent that acts against bacteria
      a. Bactericidal—kills bacteria
      b. Bacteriostatic—retards or incapacitates bacteria (reversible)
   4. Antiviral—agent that acts against viruses
   5. Antifungal—agent that acts against fungi
   6. Antibiotic—agent that is effective in low concentrations; produced by microorganisms; kills or suppresses growth of other organisms
   7. Spectrum—range of an antibiotic's anti-infective properties; can be narrow (acting on few organisms) to wide

or broad (acting on many organisms); may include effectiveness against gram-positive and gram-negative bacteria

8. Resistance—the organism is unaffected by an anti-infective; the resistance may be natural (always has been resistant) or acquired (resistance has developed); prolonged exposure to antibiotics allows for the organism to develop resistance towards the antibiotic.

9. Suprainfection (superinfection)—onset of a new infection from an organism other than the original organism; occurs after taking an antimicrobial agent; the new infection is usually more difficult to treat, and commonly occurs when the spectrum is the widest; for example, Candida infection may arise in person taking tetracycline

10. Synergism—agent's effect is more than additive $(1+1>2)$

11. Antagonism—agent's effect is less than additive $(1+1<2)$

C. General side effects
1. GI side effects—variable, depending on antibiotic; includes nausea, vomiting, diarrhea, dyspepsia
2. Suprainfection from antibiotic-resistant bacteria is possible, usually in the form of a vaginal yeast infection
3. Drug interactions
   a. Oral contraceptives—some antibiotics may reduce effectiveness; inform the client that alternative forms of birth control should be used for the duration of the prescription, plus an additional 7 days or until the end of their menstrual cycle
   b. Warfarin (Coumadin)—antibiotics alter the GI flora that make vitamin K, which then can potentiate warfarin's effect

D. Treatment versus prophylaxis
1. Treatment—the anti-infective is used to treat an infection that is present
2. Prophylaxis—used to prevent some potential future infection; only proven beneficial in a few instances

E. General dental concerns for all antibiotics—make sure that the client:
1. Knows the name of the antibiotic and how to take it
2. Understands the need to complete the full course of therapy
3. Understands the rationale for prophylactic antibiotic medication
4. Takes all antibiotics with a full glass of water
5. Takes antibiotics on an empty stomach; if the medicine causes nausea, it should be taken with food

Penicillins

A. Mechanism—inhibit cell wall synthesis; bactericidal
B. Spectrum—three penicillin subgroups:
1. Penicillin G, penicillin V
2. Penicillinase-resistant penicillin
3. Extended-spectrum penicillins
   a. Ampicillin-like
   b. Carbenicillin-like

C. Stability
1. Acid labile—degrades in stomach acid; therefore administered parenterally (e.g., penicillin G, methicillin, carbenicillin)
2. Acid stable—may be used orally (e.g., penicillin VK, amoxicillin)

D. Pharmacokinetics
1. Peak—penicillin blood levels peak between 30 minutes and 1 hour when administered by the oral or intramuscular route; peak immediately when administered intravenously
2. Half-life ($t\frac{1}{2}$)—between 30 minutes and 1 hour
3. Excretion very rapid, actively secreted; duration prolonged by concomitant probenecid (Benemid) administration

E. Adverse effects
1. GI—mild GI upset to nausea and vomiting
2. Allergic reactions—range from mild rash to anaphylaxis
3. Nephrotoxicity—occurs occasionally; kidney damage more likely with broader-spectrum penicillins

Penicillin G and Penicillin V

A. Examples
1. Penicillin G potassium
2. Penicillin G procaine (Wycillin, Crysticillin)
3. Penicillin G benzathine (Bicillin)
4. Penicillin VK (V-Cillin K, Pen-Vee K)

B. Spectrum—potent against many gram-positive aerobic organisms, such as *Streptococcus* and *Staphylococcus*, certain gram-negative aerobic cocci, such as *Neisseria gonorrhoeae*, and some anaerobic organisms; not resistant to penicillinase

C. Penicillin G—parenteral administration
1. Dose specified in units (e.g., 5 million units [MU])
2. Intramuscular salts (procaine and benzathine) provide longer duration of action than do sodium and potassium salts

D. Penicillin V—more acid stable than penicillin G, thus, can be used orally; potassium salt better absorbed; therefore, penicillin VK is the most frequently used antibiotic in dentistry; 400,000 units (U) = 250 mg

Penicillinase (β-Lactamase)–Resistant Penicillins

A. Examples
1. Methicillin (Staphcillin)
2. Nafcillin (Unipen, Nafcil)
3. Oxacillin (Prostaphlin, Bactocill)

B. Therapeutic use—limited; used against penicillinase-producing staphylococci

Extended-Spectrum ("Broader-Spectrum" or "Wider-Spectrum") Penicillins

A. Ampicillin-like
1. Examples
   a. Ampicillin (Omnipen, Totacillin, Polycillin)
   b. Amoxicillin (Amoxil, Larotid, Polymox)
2. Spectrum—effective against many gram-positive and some gram-negative bacteria such as *Haemophilus influenzae*, *Escherichia coli*, and *Proteus mirabilis*

3. Not penicillinase resistant
4. Augmentin—amoxicillin combined with clavulanic acid, which binds with penicillinase, so amoxicillin is not inactivated; can be used with penicillinase-producing organisms

B. Extended-spectrum penicillins
1. Examples
   a. Ticarcillin (Ticar)
   b. Carbenicillin (Geopen, Pyopen)
   c. Piperacillin (Pipracil)
2. Spectrum—provides coverage against gram-negative bacteria such as *Pseudomonas aeruginosa, Proteus,* and organisms resistant to ampicillin-like drugs
3. Administered parenterally (in hospitalized clients) for systemic action

Macrolides

A. Mechanism—interfere with protein synthesis by binding to the 50S ribosomal subunit; provide bacteriostatic action
B. Spectrum
1. Erythromycin
   a. Effective primarily against gram-positive microorganisms; ineffective against anaerobes
   b. Used against certain strains of *Rickettsia, Chlamydia,* and *Actinomyces*; drug of choice for treating infections caused by *Mycoplasma pneumoniae* and *Legionella pneumophila*
2. Azithromycin (Zithromax)
   a. Recommended by the American Heart Association (AHA) for use in the prevention of bacterial endocarditis before certain dental procedures, in persons who are allergic to penicillin[2]
   b. Adverse effects—stomatitis, candidiasis, angioedema (allergic reaction), heart palpitations, chest pain, nausea, vomiting, diarrhea, abdominal pain, hepatotoxicity, heartburn, flatulence
   c. Alternative drug of choice for mild infection caused by susceptible organisms in persons allergic to penicillin
3. Clarithromycin (Biaxin)
   a. Recommended by the AHA for use in the prevention of bacterial endocarditis prior to certain dental procedures in persons who are allergic to penicillin[2]
   b. Adverse effects—abnormal taste, candidiasis, stomatitis, nausea, abdominal pain, diarrhea, hepatotoxicity, heartburn, anorexia, vomiting, vaginitis, moniliasis, urticaria, rash, pruritus
   c. Alternative drug of choice for mild infection caused by susceptible organisms in persons allergic to penicillin
C. Pharmacokinetics of erythromycin
1. Erythromycin—high acid lability (instability) requires enteric coating (does not dissolve in the stomach; dissolves in the intestine) or formulation as an ester to protect against stomach acid (e.g., ethylsuccinate, erythromycin ethylsuccinate [EES])
2. Effect peaks in 2 to 4 hours
D. Adverse effects
1. GI upset is very common; must be taken with food to decrease

2. Cholestatic jaundice is primarily associated with the estolate ester
E. Drug interactions—theophylline and erythromycin; increase theophylline levels
F. Examples—erythromycin
1. Erythromycin base (E-mycin)
2. Erythromycin estolate (Ilosone)
3. Erythromycin ethylsuccinate (EES, Pedia-mycin)
4. Erythromycin stearate (Erythrocin)
G. Therapeutic uses
1. Treatment of dental infections in persons allergic to penicillin
2. Specific suspected infections (see earlier B. Spectrum)

Cephalosporins

A. Mechanism—similar to penicillins; inhibits cell wall synthesis; bactericidal
B. Chemistry similar to penicillins
C. Spectrum—effective against many gram-positive and gram-negative bacteria; the third-generation cephalosporins and the newest fourth-generation cephalosporins have the widest spectrum of action
D. Adverse reactions
1. GI upset common (33%)
2. Other—similar to those of the broader-spectrum penicillins (e.g., nephrotoxicity, suprainfection)
3. Allergy—some cross-hypersensitivity (10%) with penicillin allergy (possess a similar chemical structure)
E. Examples
1. Cefuroxime (Ceftin)
2. Cephalexin (Keflex)
3. Cephradine (Velosef, Anspor)
F. Suggested oral antibiotic regimen for the client with joint prosthesis less than 2 years after surgery[2]

Clindamycin (Cleocin)

A. Mechanism—inhibits protein synthesis (binds to the 50S ribosomal subunit); bacteriostatic protection
B. Spectrum—effective against gram-positive organisms and many anaerobes such as *Bacteroides*
C. Adverse reactions
1. GI—diarrhea; pseudomembranous colitis (PMC) or antibiotic-associated colitis (AAC, incidence up to 10%); drug must be discontinued if bloody stools with mucus occur
2. The FDA states that this agent should be "reserved for serious anaerobic infections"
D. Dental use—used against certain anaerobic infections thought to be caused by *Bacteroides* species (spp.), jaw infections, and periodontal infections; and for the prophylaxis of infective endocarditis[2]

Tetracyclines

A. Mechanism—inhibit protein synthesis by binding to the 30S ribosome; provide bacteriostatic action
B. Spectrum—truly broad spectrum; effective against many gram-positive and gram-negative bacteria

C. Pharmacokinetics
   1. Tetracyclines—divalent and trivalent cations (e.g., calcium [Ca^{+2}; in dairy products], magnesium [Mg^{+2}] and aluminum [Al^{+3}] in antacids, iron [Fe^{+2}]); inhibit the absorption of tetracycline by chelation
   2. Doxycycline (Vibramycin) and minocycline (Minocin)—less affected by food or dairy products than is tetracycline; avoid taking antacids or Ca^{+2} supplementation concomitantly
D. Resistance—cross-transference can occur; organisms can become resistant without being exposed to drug
E. Adverse effects
   1. GI upset—relatively common
   2. Suprainfection—very common because of the wide spectrum of action; drug alters normal flora (e.g., may result in vaginal candidiasis)
   3. Photosensitivity—exaggerated sunburn with exposure to ultraviolet (UV) light
   4. Teeth—both hypoplasia and intrinsic stain can occur if the drug is taken during enamel development; primary teeth affected from the last half of the pregnancy to age 4 to 6 months; permanent teeth are affected from age 2 months to 7 to 12 years
F. Examples
   1. Doxycycline (Vibramycin, Atridox)
   2. Minocycline (Minocin, Arestin)
   3. Tetracycline (Achromycin-V)
   4. Tetracycline fibers (Actisite)
G. Therapeutic uses
   1. Medical—treatment of acne, respiratory tract infections in clients with COPD (emphysema or bronchitis), certain sexually transmitted diseases (STDs)
   2. Dental—management of periodontal diseases; drug placed in periodontal pocket (e.g., tetracycline fibers [Atridox, Actisite, Arestin])
H. Dental hygiene considerations
   1. Must be taken 1 hour before or 2 hours after eating
   2. Should be taken with crackers if stomach upset occurs
   3. Should not be taken with antacids or dairy products
   4. Clients must be counseled about photosensitivity

Quinolones

A. Mechanism—inhibition of bacterial gyrase so that the daughter segment of deoxyribonucleic acid (DNA) cannot acquire the proper configuration to divide
B. Spectrum—effective against gram-negative bacteria, including *Enterobacter* spp., *Escherichia coli*, and *Morganella morganii*
C. Adverse reactions—abdominal pain, nausea, vomiting, diarrhea, rash, urticaria, angioedema
D. Dental concerns—the client must avoid direct light (e.g., dental light); offer the client dark glasses to be worn during dental procedures; the client must also avoid direct sun exposure
E. Examples
   1. Ciprofloxacin (Cipro)
   2. Enoxacin (Penetrex)
   3. Ofloxacin (Floxin)

Aminoglycosides

A. Mechanism—inhibit protein synthesis by binding to the 30S ribosomal subunit; provide bactericidal action (the only group that combines the inhibition of protein synthesis with "cidal" action)
B. Spectrum—effective against some gram-positive and many gram-negative bacteria
C. Pharmacokinetics—not effective systemically when administered orally; must be administered parenterally, intravenously, or by intramuscular injection
D. Adverse reactions—toxicity usually results from excessive levels in blood
   1. Ototoxicity—adverse effect on cranial nerve VIII; both vestibular (balance) and auditory functions are affected
   2. Nephrotoxicity—adverse effect on kidney
E. Examples
   1. Gentamicin (Garamycin)
   2. Kanamycin (Kantrex)
   3. Neomycin (Mycifradin)
   4. Tobramycin (Tobrex)

Sulfonamides ("Sulfa" Drugs)

A. Mechanism—competitive antagonist of para-aminobenzoic acid (PABA); prevents the use of PABA to make the folic acid needed in an organism
B. Adverse reactions
   1. Allergic reactions—rash
   2. Photosensitivity
C. Examples
   1. Sulfisoxazole (Gantrisin)
   2. Trimethoprim-sulfamethoxazole (TMP-SMX; Bactrim, Septra)
D. Therapeutic uses
   1. Urinary tract infections (UTIs)
   2. Otitis media (children's ear infections)
   3. Respiratory infections
   4. Dental use unclear; probably not useful

Metronidazole (Flagyl)

A. Mechanism—breaks DNA structure, which inhibits protein synthesis; provides bactericidal action
B. Spectrum
   1. Trichomonicidal (effective against *Trichomonas vaginalis*)
   2. Bactericidal (effective against anaerobes such as *Bacteroides* spp.)
C. Adverse reactions
   1. GI—anorexia, nausea, vomiting, headache, dizziness
   2. CNS—disulfiram (Antabuse)–like reaction; concurrent alcohol ingestion produces nausea and vomiting
   3. Carcinogenic in animals; mutagenic in bacterial organisms; however, significance with regard to cancer is unknown
D. Dental use—management of periodontal clients with anaerobic infections; effective against organisms; inexpensive
E. Dental hygiene considerations
   1. Clients must avoid alcohol-containing products, including beverages, foods cooked with alcohol, colognes, aftershaves, perfumes

2. Clients must avoid mouth rinses with alcohol; recommend alcohol-free mouth rinses

Antituberculosis Agents

A. Tuberculosis (TB)—a chronic disease
   1. Resistant organisms develop easily
   2. Treatment is difficult, so drug combinations are frequently required; multidrug-resistant (MDR) organisms are common
   3. Requires drug treatment regimen of 6 to 9 months
B. Drugs
   1. Isoniazid (INH)—used alone as prophylaxis; used in combination with other agents; hepatitis is an adverse side effect
   2. Rifampin (Rifadin, Rimactane)
   3. Pyrazinamide
   4. Ethambutol (Myambutol)
C. Dental implications—use standard precautions; affected persons are treated for 6 weeks to 2 months; the client is generally not contagious if compliant with TB treatment regimen; direct observation and monitoring of the client are needed

Antifungal Agents

A. Disease—candidiasis (*Candida albicans*), called *thrush* in infants
B. Nystatin (Mycostatin, Nilstat)—dosage forms: oral suspension or pastille (rubbery lozenge)
C. Clotrimazole (Mycelex)—lozenges available
D. Ketoconazole (Nizoral)
   1. Tablets—dose: once per day
   2. An acid stomach environment is required for adequate absorption—be alert to histamine (H_2)-blockers
   3. Adverse reactions
      a. Nausea and vomiting
      b. Hepatocellular dysfunction
      c. Teratogenic potential
      d. Drug interactions
E. Fluconazole (Diflucan)
   1. Tablets, oral suspension, and intravenous administration
   2. Therapeutic use—systemic fungal infections
   3. Adverse reactions—headache, abdominal pain, nausea, diarrhea, hepatic toxicity
F. Itraconazole (Sporanox)
   1. Capsules
   2. Therapeutic use—indicated for the treatment of certain fungal infections in both immunocompromised clients and those who are not
   3. Adverse reactions—nausea, vomiting, diarrhea, abdominal pain, anorexia, edema, rash, fatigue, fever, malaise

Antiviral Agents

A. Acyclovir (Zovirax)
   1. Topical, oral, and intravenous forms available
   2. Therapeutic uses
      a. Treatment of initial genital herpes in clients who are not immunocompromised
      b. Treatment of recurrent genital herpes in immunocompromised clients
      c. Oral administration is recommended with continuous use as a prophylactic
B. Docosanol (Abreva)
   a. Treatment of oral herpes simplex labialis (cold sores)
   b. Available without a prescription
   c. Adverse effects—stinging at the site of application
   d. L-lysine (an amino acid) is often recommended with docosanol to aid in tissue repair and growth
C. Ganciclovir (Cytovene)
   1. Inhibits replication of most herpesviruses
   2. Therapeutic use—prevention and treatment of cytomegalovirus (CMV) in persons with acquired immunodeficiency syndrome (AIDS)
   3. Adverse effects—fever, coma, chills, confusion, abnormal thoughts, dizziness, bizarre dreams, headaches, psychosis, tremors, paresthesia, dysrhythmia, hypertension, hypotension, hemorrhage, anorexia, blood dyscrasia
D. Antiretroviral drugs—indications: HIV-positive clients and those with AIDS
   1. Zidovudine (AZT, Retrovir)
   2. Didanosine (ddI, Videx)
   3. Zalcitabine (ddC, Hivid)
E. Dental hygiene considerations—use standard precautions

CARDIOVASCULAR AGENTS

See Chapters 8 and 19 for contraindications and cautions involving dental treatment in persons with cardiovascular disease.[3]

Digitalis Glycosides

A. Pharmacologic effects—heartbeats are stronger (positive chronotropic effect) but usually slower (bradycardia); therefore, efficiency is increased
B. Adverse reactions
   1. GI disturbances—nausea, vomiting
   2. CVS—arrhythmias/dysrhythmias
   3. CNS—yellow-green vision; halos around lights
C. Therapeutic uses—heart failure, certain arrhythmias
D. Dental hygiene considerations
   1. Hypokalemia—decreased potassium levels because of diuretics; digitalis toxicity may exacerbate dysrhythmias; epinephrine exacerbates dysrhythmias
   2. Epinephrine—use of epinephrine may increase the risk for arrhythmias (dysrhythmias)
   3. Pulse rate must be monitored
   4. Tetracycline and erythromycin can increase the levels of digoxin in blood, causing digoxin toxicity (signaled by nausea, vomiting, and copious salivation)
E. Example—digoxin (Lanoxin)

ANTIARRHYTHMICS

A. Pharmacologic effects—suppress arrhythmias
B. Dental considerations—in clients with cardiac problems, use caution when administering local anesthetics with epinephrine
C. Examples
   1. Lidocaine (Xylocaine)—local anesthetic agent can be used parenterally as an antidysrhythmic agent
   2. Procainamide
   3. Propranolol (Inderal)
   4. Quinidine
D. Dental hygiene considerations
   1. Review health history to determine the client's state of health
   2. Check BP and pulse

Antianginal Agents

A. Pharmacologic effects—reduce the "work" of the heart because these agents function as nonspecific vasodilators, thereby reducing the amount of blood returning to the heart
B. Adverse reactions—hypotension and severe headache are common; client should be in the sitting position to take nitroglycerin (NTG)
C. Drug interactions – phosphodiesterase-5 inhibitors (sildenafil, tadalafil, vardenafil)
D. Therapeutic use—angina pectoris
E. Dental hygiene considerations
   1. Storage—unstable products; must be stored properly; heat, light, and moisture cause further degradation; discard opened containers after 2 months or on the basis of the expiration date on the original vial, whichever comes first
   2. Acute anginal attack—administer NTG sublingually
   3. Routes of NTG administration
      a. Sublingual (SL)—tablets or spray
      b. Transdermal—patches applied to chest or arm
      c. Ointment—in ointment applied to skin
   4. Anxiety about the dental appointment may cause the angina attack; the client can take tablet prophylactically
F. Examples
   1. Nitroglycerin (Nitrostat), SL tablet or spray (Nitrolingual SL spray)
   2. Isosorbide dinitrate (Isordil) or mononitrates

Antihypertensives

See Table 11–9.
A. Pharmacologic effects—reduce elevated BP
B. Adverse reaction—CNS depression, fatigue, xerostomia, orthostatic hypotension, constipation and diarrhea, sexual dysfunction, upset stomach
C. Therapeutic use—treatment of hypertension
D. Dental hygiene considerations
   1. Take BP reading to ensure it is normal
   2. Xerostomia—instruct the client to drink plenty of water; suck on tart sugarless gum or candy that contains xylitol, or ice chips; avoid products containing alcohol and caffeine; and avoid juices and soft drinks to reduce the risk of dental caries; saliva substitutes (Xero-lube, Salivart) can also be recommended
   3. Have the client rise slowly from the dental chair
   4. Some calcium channel blockers can cause drug-influenced gingival enlargement; clients should perform meticulous oral hygiene and obtain frequent periodontal maintenance care
   5. CNS sedation—several antihypertensive medications can cause sedation; the client is at an increased risk for sedation if an opioid analgesic or benzodiazepine is prescribed; the client should be instructed to avoid driving or operating heavy machinery, or any task that requires thinking or concentration
   6. GI effects—several antihypertensives can cause GI irritation; NSAIDs may increase the risk of GI irritation; these agents must be taken with food, milk, or an antacid
   7. Constipation—may be further aggravated by the addition of an opioid analgesic; have the client drink plenty of water and eat fruits, vegetables, and other high-fiber foods

Diuretics

A. Pharmacologic effects—remove excess water and sodium by way of the kidneys; direct vasodilating action on blood vessels lowers total peripheral resistance and BP
B. Adverse reactions
   1. Hypokalemia (low potassium)—the client may need to take a potassium replacement
   2. Hyperglycemia, hyperuricemia
   3. The client may urinate more frequently after taking the medicine (usually in the morning)
C. Therapeutic uses—treatment of hypertension, edema
D. Dental hygiene considerations—hypokalemia (reduced potassium level) potentiates epinephrine-induced arrhythmias; pulse rate must be monitored
E. Examples
   1. Thiazide diuretics—hydrochlorothiazide (HCTZ, HydroDiuril)
   2. Loop diuretics—furosemide (Lasix)
   3. Combinations of thiazide diuretics with potassium-sparing diuretics—Dyazide, Max-zide; reduce the side effect of hypokalemia

Anticoagulants
Warfarin (Coumadin)

A. Mechanism—interfere with vitamin K–dependent clotting factors (II, VII, IX, X)
B. Pharmacologic effects—reduce the ability of blood to clot; latent time required before full effect is seen (several days); a certain amount of time is required for the effect to subside after discontinuation of treatment
C. Adverse reactions—bleeding, hemorrhage
D. Therapeutic uses—used after MI, thrombophlebitis, atrial fibrillation, emboli, valve replacement (any condition in which too much blood clotting occurs)
E. Dental hygiene considerations

TABLE 11–9 Selected Antihypertensives

Examples, Mechanisms, and Adverse Reactions

Drug Group	Examples	Mechanism	Adverse Reactions
Diuretics–thiazides	Hydrochlorothiazide (HCTZ)	Inhibits sodium (Na) resorption, direct vasodilator, moderate potency	Hypokalemia Hyperuricemia Hyperglycemia NSAIDs ↓ effect
Loop diuretic	Furosemide (Lasix)	Loop of Henle, high potency	Similar to thiazides
Thiazides combined with potassium (K^{+2}) sparing	Maxzide Dyazide	K-sparing, low potency	Hyperkalemia
α-Adrenergic selective blockers	Terazosin (Hytrin) Doxazosin (Cardura) Prazosin (Minipress)	Blocks α_1-receptor in arterioles/venules	Sedation D/C gradually Also used for benign prostatic hypertrophy
β-Adrenergic blockers (select drugs)	Propranolol (Inderal) Atenolol (Tenormin) Metoprolol (Lopressor)	Blocks sympathetic effect on heart (↓ CO); ↓ PVR, inhibits stimulation of rennin	NSAIDs ↓ effect
Angiotensin-converting enzyme (ACE) inhibitor	Captopril (Capoten) Lisinopril (Zestril) Enalapril (Vasotec) Quinapril (Accupril)	Inhibits ACE, angiotensin II (vasoconstriction; aldosterone secretion) production inhibited	Neutropenia Bone marrow depression Cough Dysgeusia (altered taste) NSAIDs ↓ effect
Angiotensin receptor blocker	Irbesartan (Avapro) Losartan (Cozaar) Valsartan (Diovan)	Blocks the binding of angiotensin I to angiotensin II receptors; blocks vasoconstriction and aldosterone-secreting effects of angiotensin II	Oral lesions, nausea, vomiting, dyspepsia
Calcium channel blocking agents	Verapamil (Isoptin, Calan) Diltiazem (Cardizem) Nifedipine (Procardia) Nisoldipine (Sular) Isradipine (Dynacire)	Blocks calcium channel: relaxes vascular smooth muscle, decreases myocardial contractility (force)	Gingival enlargement Hyperkalemia Renal failure Dysgeusia
Adrenergic blockers Centrally acting antiadrenergic agents	Clonidine (Catapres) Methyldopa (Aldomet)	Stimulates arteriolar and the central nervous system (CNS; medulla) α-receptors	Transdermal patch Xerostomia
Postganglionic sympathetic blockers	Guanethidine (Ismelin) Reserpine (Serpasil)	Inhibits release of NE, replaces NE (false neurotransmitter) Blocks uptake and storage of amines	Postural hypotension Diarrhea Impaired ejaculation Mental depression Sedation
Vasodilators	Hydralazine (Apresoline) Minoxidil (Loniten)	Relaxes smooth muscles of arterioles	Combined with sympathetic blockers, β-blockers, and diuretics Hirsutism

CO, Cardiac output; *D/C*, discontinue; *NE*, norepinephrine. *NSAIDs*, nonsteroidal anti-inflammatory drugs; *PVR*, peripheral vascular resistance.

1. Excessive bleeding may result; assess health history at every appointment
2. Monitoring—performed using international normalized ratio (INR);[3,4] older test is prothrombin time (PT)—clients with INR of 3 or less can safely receive periodontal debridement

F. Examples—warfarin (Coumadin)
G. Drug interactions—occur with warfarin given with:
1. Aspirin or NSAID—potentiates bleeding problems; do not use concomitantly; alternative is acetaminophen

2. Vitamin K—helps blood clot; used to treat overdose or to reduce the latent period for improving the clotting status; antibiotics may reduce vitamin K levels by altering the intestinal flora that would potentiate the anticoagulant's effect

H. New oral anticoagulants
1. Factor XA inhibitors—Rivaroxaban (Xarelto); apixaban (Eliquis)
2. Direct thrombin inhibitor—Dabigatran (Pradaxa)

I. Others—Ticlopidine (Ticlid); clopidogrel (Plavix)

TABLE 11–10 Antiepileptic Drugs of Choice for Seizures

Seizure Type	First-Choice Agent—FDA Approved	Alternatives—FDA Approved
Generalized Seizures		
Absence (petit mal)	Ethosuximide (Zarontin) Valproate (Depakote)	Clonazepam (Clonopin)
Tonic-clonic (grand mal)	Carbamazepine (Tegretol) Phenytoin (Dilantin) Valproate (Depakote)	Phenobarbital (Luminal) Primidone (Mysoline) Lamotrigine (Lamactil) Topiramate (Topamax)
Status epilepticus	Diazepam (Valium) Phenytoin (Dilantin) Phenobarbital (Luminal)	
Partial Seizures		
Simple Complex Secondarily generalized	Carbamazepine (Tegretol) or Phenytoin (Dilantin) or Lamotrigine (Lamactil) or Oxcarbazepine (Trileptal)	Valproate (Depakote) Gabapentin (Neurontin) Topiramate (Topamax) Tiagabine (Gabitril) Zonisamide (Zonegran) Levetiracetam (Keppra) Primidone (Mysoline) Phenobarbital (Luminal) Pregabalin (Lyrica) Felbamate (Felbatol)

FDA, U.S. Food and Drug Administration.

Anticonvulsants

A. General properties of anticonvulsants (Table 11–10)
   1. Pharmacologic effects—reduction of frequency or elimination of seizures (see Table 11–10)
   2. GI upset—common side effect
   3. Teratogenicity—variable teratogenic potential (pregnant women with epilepsy need to be treated)
   4. Sedation—tolerance to sedative effect occurs without tolerance to anticonvulsant effect
   5. Blood dyscrasias—sudden and drastic drops in either white blood cell (WBC) count or red blood cell (RBC) count, or both, which can be serious; laboratory monitoring is important
   6. Dental hygiene considerations
      a. Sedation—client should be instructed to avoid driving or operating heavy machinery, or any task that requires thinking or concentration
      b. GI upset—need to avoid NSAIDs and aspirin because they increase the risk of GI upset
      c. Increased risk for sedation with CNS depressants or sedating drugs
      d. CNS stimulant effects—may be difficult to treat a client who cannot sit still
      e. Xerostomia—instruct the client to drink plenty of water; suck on tart sugarless gum or candy containing xylitol, or ice chips; avoid products containing alcohol and caffeine; and avoid juices and soft drinks to reduce the risk of dental caries; saliva substitutes (Xero-lube, Salivart) can also be recommended

B. Barbiturates—CNS adverse effects: sedation, hyperactivity in children, confusion, excitation, or depression in older adults
C. Phenytoin (Dilantin)—adverse effects
   1. Drug-influenced gingival enlargement—meticulous oral hygiene reduces the enlargement
      a. Wait 1 year after medication change before performing surgical interventions
   2. Vitamin deficiencies—may induce deficiency in vitamins D and folate
   3. Fetal hydantoin syndrome—associated with teratogenic conditions
D. Valproic acid (Depakene, Depakote)—adverse effects
   1. Hepatic failure—liver function tests are required to monitor the client's liver status
   2. Thrombocytopenia—bleeding; use caution when combining with aspirin, NSAIDs, or warfarin
   3. GI—nausea, vomiting
   4. CNS—sedation, drowsiness; hyperactivity, aggressiveness in children
E. Carbamazepine (Tegretol)—adverse effects
   1. Induces metabolism of itself and other drugs
   2. CNS—drowsiness, dizziness
   3. GI—nausea and vomiting
   4. Hematologic—can cause agranulocytosis; frequent monitoring of WBC count is necessary; signs and symptoms of a low count include fever, chills, aches, and pains
   5. Hepatic—liver function tests are necessary
   6. Indications—various seizures and trigeminal neuralgia
   7. Drug interactions—carbamazepine increases the metabolism of warfarin, theophylline, and doxycycline; the drug's metabolism is inhibited by erythromycin, verapamil, and diltiazem; increases the effect of lithium
F. Benzodiazepines
   1. Diazepam (Valium)—used for status epilepticus and emergency treatment of seizures; usually administered through an IM injection (adults) or rectally (children)
   2. Clonazepam (Clonopin)—taken orally for absence seizures (nonconvulsive seizures characterized by "staring off") and psychiatric conditions; oral adverse effects include coated tongue, xerostomia, encopresis, abnormal thirst, tender gums
G. Ethosuximide
   1. Used to treat absence seizures
   2. GI—anorexia, GI upset, nausea, vomiting
   3. CNS—drowsiness, dizziness, lethargy, hyperactivity
   4. Oral adverse drug reactions—drug-influenced gingival enlargement, swollen tongue
H. Newer agents
   1. Gabapentin—no reported drug interactions
   2. Felbamate—increased risk for developing aplastic anemia, severe liver disease
   3. Lamotrigine
   4. Topiramate
   5. Tiagabine
   6. Fosphenytoin—parenteral use only
   7. Levetiracetam
   8. Oxcarbazepine

9. Pregabalin—a schedule V drug, because of reported euphoria in some clinical trials
10. Zonisamide

PSYCHOTHERAPEUTIC AGENTS

Antipsychotics

A. Pharmacologic effects
1. Antipsychotics—used in the management of psychoses; the client may perceive comments as threats (paranoia)
2. Sedation and drowsiness—additive CNS depression with other CNS depressants
3. Antiemetics—depress the chemoreceptor trigger zone (CTZ); reduce nausea and vomiting

B. Adverse reactions
1. Orthostatic hypotension—dizziness or fainting on rising from a supine position
2. Extrapyramidal effects—areas in the brain affecting body movements
   a. Dyskinesia—uncontrollable movements of the tongue or face
   b. Tardive dyskinesia—abnormal involuntary movements that occur with prolonged use of conventional antipsychotic agents
   c. Parkinsonian symptoms—tremors and rigidity resembling Parkinson's disease
   d. Akathisia—motor restlessness (e.g., swinging legs)
   e. Acute dystonic reaction—difficulty in opening the mouth; jaw muscles are contracted; dislocation of the jaw might occur
3. Anticholinergic—xerostomia increases the risk of dental caries

C. Drug interactions—occur with antipsychotic agent given with:
1. CNS depressants—additive CNS depression
2. Anticholinergic—additive anticholinergic toxicity

D. Dental hygiene considerations
1. Dyskinesia, akathisia, and tardive dyskinesia—the client may not be able to perform self-care
2. Acute dystonic reaction—can occur during a procedure; the client needs to be treated with an anticholinergic drug
3. Orthostatic hypotension—raise the dental chair slowly; have the client remain seated for a few minutes before standing to prevent a fall
4. Xerostomia—instruct the client to drink plenty of water; suck on tart sugarless gum or candy containing xylitol, or ice chips; avoid products containing alcohol and caffeine; and avoid juices and soft drinks to reduce the risk of dental caries; saliva substitutes (Xero-lube, Salivart) can also be recommended

E. Therapeutic uses
1. Treatment of psychosis (e.g., schizophrenia) and bipolar disorder
2. Antiemetic—for nausea or vomiting
3. Opioid potentiation—combined with an opioid to potentiate analgesia and sedation; reduce the dose of the opioid if an antipsychotic is added

TABLE 11-11	Selected Antipsychotic Drugs
Group	**Drug**
First Generation	
High potency	Haloperidol (Haldol)
Medium potency	Trifluoperazine (Stelazine)
	Thiothixene (Navane)
Low potency	Chlorpromazine (Thorazine)
	Thioridazine (Mellaril)
Second Generation	
	Clozapine (Clozaril)
	Risperidone (Risperdal)
	Olanzapine (Zyprexa)

F. Table 11-11 provides examples of select antipsychotic agents

Antidepressants

A. Pharmacologic effects
1. Affect norepinephrine and serotonin levels in the brain (require 4 to 6 weeks to be effective)
2. Adverse reactions
   a. Cardiotoxic in overdose— arrhythmias (mainly with TCAs); usual cause of death when used in a suicide attempt
   b. Xerostomia (anticholinergic action)
   c. Sedation
   d. GI—nausea resulting from selective serotonin reuptake inhibitors (SSRIs)
   e. Orthostatic hypotension

B. Drug interactions—occur with TCAs given with:
1. Epinephrine—results in hypertension (increased vasopressor response); low doses contained in local anesthetic solutions can be used safely in normotensive persons (those with normal BP)
2. Anticholinergic—results in additive anticholinergic action and excessive xerostomia

C. Therapeutic uses
1. Treatment of depression
2. Migraine headache prophylaxis
3. Treatment of nocturnal enuresis (bedwetting) in children
4. Chronic pain treatment adjuvant

D. Drugs
1. Select tricyclic antidepressants (TCAs)
   a. Amitriptyline (Elavil)
   b. Imipramine (Tofranil)
2. MAOIs—phenelzine (Nardil); tranylcypromine (Parnate)
   a. Infrequently used for depression
   b. Potential for numerous severe drug-food interactions (e.g., wine, sausage, cheese; indirect-acting adrenergic agents, meperidine)
3. Dopamine-norepinephrine reuptake inhibitors
   a. Bupropion (Wellbutrin, Zyban)
   b. Bupropion, sustained release (Wellbutrin SR)
   c. Bupropion, extended release (Wellbutrin ER)

4. Select SSRIs
   a. Fluoxetine (Prozac)
   b. Sertraline (Zoloft)
   c. Paroxetine (Paxil)
   d. Citalopram (Celexa)
5. Serotonin and norepinephrine reuptake inhibitors
   a. Venlafaxine (Effexor)
   b. Venlafaxine, extended release (Effexor XR)
6. Serotonin modulators
   a. Nefazodone (Serzone)
   b. Trazodone (Desyrel)
7. Norepinephrine-serotonin modulator—mirtazapine (Remeron)

Other Psychotherapeutic Agents

A. Lithium—for treating bipolar-affective disorder (manic depression); blood level is difficult to maintain; NSAIDs increase serum lithium levels
B. Carbamazepine, valproate—these drugs are also used to treat seizure disorders; drug interactions and dental concerns are the same as those in the treatment of seizure disorders

ENDOCRINE AGENTS

Adrenocorticosteroids (Steroids)

A. Classification
   1. Glucocorticoids—regulate glucose metabolism and have an anti-inflammatory effect
   2. Mineralocorticoids—regulate sodium (minerals) and water
B. Pharmacologic effect—anti-inflammatory, antiallergenic, involved in carbohydrate metabolism, and have catabolic effects
C. Adverse reactions
   1. Cushing syndrome—long-term, high-dose steroids produce symptoms including:
      a. Metabolic effects—"moon face," "buffalo hump," truncal obesity
      b. Peptic ulcers—exacerbation or stimulation of stomach acid secretion
      c. Skin conditions—bruising, striae, delayed healing
      d. Mental changes—euphoria, depression, psychosis, mood swings
      e. Infection—caused by suppression of immunity, symptoms may be masked; close observation and aggressive treatment are necessary
      f. Osteoporosis—bones break more easily
      g. Hypertension—elevated water and sodium retention (mineralocorticoid action)
      h. Hyperglycemia—exacerbation of diabetes
   2. Adrenal crisis (thyroid storm)—abrupt withdrawal or stress (e.g., a dental appointment) can precipitate a crisis; can be prevented by premedicating with additional steroids; potentially serious situation
D. Contraindications and cautions
   1. Ulcers—ulcerogenic

2. Cardiovascular disease—can precipitate congestive heart failure, edema (result of mineralocorticoid effect)
3. Acute psychoses
4. Infection—increased susceptibility to bacterial, fungal, or viral infections
5. Diabetes—hyperglycemia is induced
E. Dental hygiene considerations
   1. Check BP before procedure or administration of a vasoconstrictor
   2. Avoid NSAIDs, aspirin, and opioid analgesics because of the increased risk of GI upset
   3. Steroids can delay wound healing and mask the symptoms of infection; consider administration of prophylactic antibiotic before procedure
   4. Osteoporosis may be evident on dental radiographs
   5. The steroid-dependent client may need short-term increase in steroid dose before a dental procedure to avoid an adrenal crisis
F. Therapeutic uses
   1. Medical—treatment of many inflammatory conditions (e.g., arthritis, asthma, dermatitis)
   2. Dental—treatment of:
      a. Aphthous lesions—palliative treatment; topical or intralesional therapy
      b. Oral lesions secondary to collagen vascular diseases—respond to topical, intralesional, or systemic therapy
      c. Temporomandibular joint disease—intra-articular injection (into the joint) if the patient has arthritis
G. Table 11–12 provides examples of steroid agents

Agents for Diabetes Mellitus

See also the section on "Diabetes Mellitus" in Chapter 19.
A. Definition
   1. Symptoms
      a. Polyuria—increased urination
      b. Polydipsia—increased thirst
      c. Polyphagia—increased hunger
      d. Weight loss
      e. Xerostomia
   2. Classifications
      a. Type 1 diabetes (insulin-dependent diabetes mellitus)—circulating insulin is absent; usually is a result of autoimmune destruction of pancreatic beta (β-) cells; requires insulin therapy

TABLE 11–12 Common Steroids

Steroid	Comments	Equivalent Dose (mg/day)
Hydrocortisone	Some mineralocorticoid action	20-240
Prednisone	Most commonly used orally	5-60
Triamcinolone (Kenalog)	Used topically and injected into joints	2-20
Dexamethasone (Decadron)	Very potent, thus lower dose used	0.75-9.0

b. Type 2 diabetes (non–insulin-dependent diabetes mellitus)—decreased tissue sensitivity to insulin and impaired β-cell response to glucose; controlled by diet, oral hypoglycemic agents, and insulin, alone or in combination

3. Microvascular and macrovascular complications
   a. Cardiovascular problems—circulation and heart problems, MI, stroke
   b. Retinopathy—vision problems, cataracts, blindness
   c. Neuropathy—reduced sensations in the extremities
   d. Renal failure—nephropathy (kidney problems)
   e. Immunity—reduced ability to fight infections
   f. Healing—slower or delayed
   g. Oral manifestations—reduced immunity caused by WBC dysfunction; reduced vascular supply (small-vessel disease), and other alterations in immune system function; predisposes a client to periodontal disease; loss of alveolar bone is characteristic

B. Dental hygiene considerations
   1. Reinforce the importance of good oral hygiene to minimize the risk of xerostomia, candidiasis, and dental caries
   2. Keep at hand a source of glucose that will act quickly (e.g., tube of cake frosting or orange juice) in case the client experiences hypoglycemia
   3. Clients with diabetes are at increased risk for periodontal disease and disease progression
   4. These clients are at a higher risk for delayed wound healing and infection; those with poorly controlled diabetes may require prophylactic antibiotic premedication
   5. Epinephrine, steroids, and opioid analgesics can decrease insulin release or increase insulin requirements; therefore must be used with caution in clients with diabetes

C. Adverse reactions
   1. Hypoglycemia—too much drug or too little food (intakes are not balanced)
      a. Symptoms—nervousness, sweating, tremulousness, compulsive talking, mental confusion, nausea, convulsions, coma
      b. Treatment—administer glucose orally if the client is conscious and able to swallow; if the client is unconscious, administer glucose intravenously, or administer glucagon subcutaneously or intramuscularly
   2. Hyperglycemia—less common cause of problems in the person with diabetes; treated in the emergency room with insulin and fluids
   3. Lipodystrophy—occurs when insulin is injected into the same site for a prolonged period

D. Examples of hypoglycemic agents
   1. Insulin
      a. Rapid-acting—insulin lispro, insulin aspart
      b. Short-acting—regular insulin (Humulin R, Novolin R) and prompt insulin zinc suspension (Semilente, Semilente Insulin, Semitard)
      c. Intermediate-acting—insulin time suspension (Lente, Humulin L); isophane insulin suspension (Humulin, WPH, Novolin N)

d. Long-acting—extended insulin zinc suspension (Ultralente, Humulin U Ultralente)
      e. Mixed preparations—isophane insulin suspension and regular insulin injection (Humulin 70/30)
   2. Use and sources
      a. Combined regular and neutral protamine Hagedorn (NPH) insulin—given one to two times per day
      b. Human insulin—from gene splicing (made from *E.coli*) or altered pork insulin
   3. Oral hypoglycemic agents (sulfonylureas)
      a. First-generation agents
         (1) Chlorpropamide (Diabinese)
      b. Second-generation agents
         (1) Glyburide (DiaBeta, Micronase)
         (2) Glipizide (Glucotrol)
         (3) Glimepiride (Amaryl)
   4. Other, newer agents
      a. Biguanides—metformin (Glucophage)
      b. α-Glucosidase inhibitors—acarbose (Pre-cose); miglitol (Glyset)
      c. Thiazolidinediones—pioglitazone (Actos); rosiglitazone (Avandia)
      d. Meglitinides—nateglinide (Starlix); repaglinide (Prandin)
      e. GLP-1 receptor agonist—exenatide (Byetta)
      f. Bile acid sequestrant—colesevelam (Welchol)
      g. DPP-4 inhibitors—alogliptin (Nesina); linagliptin (Tradjenta); saxagliptin (Onglyza); sitagliptin (Januvia)

Thyroid Agents

A. Hypothyroidism—also hypothyroidosis, athyroidosis, hypothyrosis, thyroid insufficiency; deficient thyroid activity results in lowered metabolism, fatigue, lethargy; more common in women than in men; can lead to cretinism in infants
   1. Thyroid replacements used; leads to a euthyroid condition (normal thyroid)
   2. Examples of hypothyroidism agents
      a. Levothyroxine (Synthroid, Levothroid)
      b. Liotrix (Euthroid, Thyrolar)
   3. The client requires no special handling if the dose is adequate
   4. Dental hygiene considerations
      a. Carefully examine children suspected of having hypothyroidism and children diagnosed with hypothyroidism; the client with hypothyroidism must maintain good oral health
      b. Clients with hypothyroidism are more sensitive to medications that depress the CNS; lower doses may therefore be necessary; counsel the client about the CNS side effects

B. Hyperthyroidism—also Graves disease; various causes lead to the excessive production of thyroid hormones; produces goiter, cardiopulmonary dysfunction (atrial fibrillation, palpitations, widened pulse rate), skin and behavioral conditions (tremor, excessive sweating, heat intolerance, nervousness, fatigue), and ocular symptoms (exophthalmos)

1. Partial thyroidectomy (treated surgically or with radioactive iodine [^{131}I]) ablates part of the thyroid gland—the client requires supplemental thyroid hormone therapy; no unusual dental considerations if the client is taking drug treatment
2. Clients awaiting surgery or those who are poor surgical candidates are maintained on a regimen of thyroid suppressants
   a. Drugs suppress thyroid function—propylthiouracil (PTU)
   b. β-Blockers are given to bring down elevated HR (e.g., propranolol)
   c. Dental hygiene considerations—avoid epinephrine because it can trigger a thyroid storm; clients have a lower pain threshold and may require higher doses of local anesthetic agents or higher doses of CNS-depressing medications

Estrogens and Progesterone

Estrogen

A. Responsible for female sex characteristics, reproduction development, and preparing for conception
B. Adverse reactions
   1. Nausea, vomiting
   2. Uterine bleeding, vaginal discharge
   3. Edema
   4. Thrombophlebitis
   5. Weight gain
   6. Headache
   7. Hypertension
C. Dose forms
   1. Oral tablets
   2. Creams
   3. Transdermal patches
D. Clinical uses include treatments for:
   1. Symptoms of menopause
   2. Menstrual disturbances
   3. Osteoporosis

Progesterone

A. Responsible for preparing the uterus for implantation of the fertilized egg
B. Adverse reactions
   1. Abnormal menstrual bleeding
   2. Breakthrough bleeding
   3. Spotting between menstrual periods
   4. Change in amount of menstrual blood flow
   5. Amenorrhea
C. Dose forms
   1. Oral
   2. Parenteral
D. Clinical uses include treatments for:
   1. Dysfunctional uterine bleeding
   2. Endometriosis
   3. Dysmenorrhea
   4. Premenstrual tension

Oral Contraceptives

A. Pharmacologic activity—inhibits the release of follicle-stimulating hormone (FSH) and luteinizing hormone (LH), which prevent ovulation and pregnancy
B. Contain either progesterone alone or a combination of estrogen and progesterone; both come in varying doses
C. Adverse reactions
   1. Nausea, dizziness, weight gain, headache, breast tenderness
   2. Hypertension, liver damage, thrombophlebitis, thromboembolism
   3. Oral—increased gingival fluid, susceptibility to gingivitis, gingival inflammation, increased risk of dry socket after extraction (newer formulations contain less hormone and therefore are less likely to cause these conditions)
D. Dental hygiene considerations
   1. Review with the client the importance of good oral hygiene because of the potential for gingivitis
   2. Extractions should be performed on days 23 to 28 of the oral contraceptive cycle to reduce the risk of dry socket
   3. Check BP at each appointment because of the risk of hypertension
   4. During long procedures, have scheduled breaks to minimize risk of thrombophlebitis; have the client stretch the legs and walk around, if possible
   5. Instruct clients to use a contingent method of birth control if they require antibiotic therapy

RESPIRATORY SYSTEM AGENTS

Agents for Asthma

A. Disease—dyspnea, cough, and wheezing, secondary to bronchospasm (hyperirritable bronchioles), inflammation of bronchioles with secretions
B. Drugs
   1. Adrenergic agonists (sympathomimetics)—see the earlier section on "Autonomic Nervous System"
      a. Dose forms—oral inhalers, tablets, liquid
      b. Inhalers—β$_2$-adrenergic agonists
         (1) Short-acting β$_2$-agonists
            (a) Albuterol (Proventil, Ventolin)
            (b) Metaproterenol (Alupent, Metaprel)
         (2) Long-acting β$_2$-agonists
            (a) Salmeterol (Serevent)
            (b) Formoterol (Foradil Aerolizer)
      c. Epinephrine—administered intravenously for an acute attack
      d. Used for maintenance and prophylactic therapy
      e. Adverse reactions—nervousness, tachycardia, insomnia, xerostomia with oral inhalers
      f. Dental hygiene considerations for short-acting and long-acting β$_2$-agonists
         (1) Measure the client's BP and pulse rate before the procedure because of the potential for tachycardia
         (2) Have the client "rinse, swish, and expectorate" after each inhaler use to reduce xerostomia

(3) Instruct the client to maintain good oral hygiene, especially with the use of oral inhalers
2. Methylxanthines
   a. Examples
      (1) Theophylline (Theo-dur, Slo-bid)
   b. Pharmacologic effects
      (1) Bronchodilation (smooth muscle relaxation) helps reduce the symptoms of asthma
      (2) CNS stimulation—alertness, insomnia
      (3) Diuresis—increased urination
3. Cromolyn sodium (Intal, Nasalcrom)
   a. Used for asthma prophylaxis by inhalation, for allergic rhinitis, and for maintenance therapy for asthma
   b. Adverse reactions—nausea, vomiting, restlessness, anxiety
   c. Dental concerns—same as with β_2-adrenergic agonists
4. Ipratropium bromide (Atrovent); tiotropium bromide (Spiriva)
   a. Anticholinergic bronchodilator; used mainly to treat emphysema
   b. Adverse reactions—xerostomia and bad taste
   c. Dental concerns
      (1) Counsel the client to rinse well and expectorate after each use
      (2) Counsel the client about the importance of good oral hygiene
5. Adrenocorticosteroids
   a. Used for acute and maintenance therapy
   b. Dose forms—oral, parenteral, metered-dose inhaler (MDI), tablets
   c. Adverse reactions with MDI—dysphonia (hoarseness), xerostomia, cough, and candidiasis
   d. Dental hygiene considerations
      (1) MDI—same as with other oral inhalers
   e. Examples
      (1) Flunisolide (Aerobid)
      (2) Fluticasone (Flovent)
C. Dental hygiene considerations
1. Disease considerations
   a. Degree of control—avoid elective treatment if the asthma is poorly controlled
   b. The client's anxiety may precipitate an acute attack; an antianxiety agent may be useful (e.g., benzodiazepine)
2. Analgesic choice—sometimes difficult to make
   a. Aspirin-containing compounds—may precipitate an attack
   b. NSAIDs—if aspirin causes bronchospasm, NSAIDs are contraindicated
   c. Acetaminophen—best choice; may be used in combination with a weak opioid (e.g., Tylenol No. 3)

GASTROINTESTINAL AGENTS

Agents Affecting Gastrointestinal Motility

A. Laxatives—increase GI motility; symptomatically used to treat constipation (e.g., milk of magnesia)

B. Antidiarrheals—reduce GI motility; symptomatically used to treat diarrhea (e.g., Lomotil, Imodium, any opioid)
C. Dental hygiene considerations
1. CNS sedation—the client should be instructed to avoid driving or operating heavy machinery, or anything that requires thinking or concentration
2. Xerostomia—instruct the client to drink plenty of water; suck on tart sugarless gum or candy containing xylitol, or ice chips; avoid products containing alcohol and caffeine; and avoid juices and soft drinks to reduce the risk of dental caries; saliva substitutes (Xero-lube, Salivart) can also be recommended

Agents for Gastroesophageal Reflux Disease—Histamine (H_2-) Blockers

A. Mechanism of action—block stomach acid secretion; pain subsides and no further damage occurs from esophageal exposure to stomach acid
B. Examples (all available OTC [over the counter])
1. Cimetidine (Tagamet HB)
2. Famotidine (Pepcid AC)
3. Nizatidine (Axid AR)
4. Ranitidine (Zantac 75)
C. Dental hygiene considerations
1. These agents interfere with the absorption of drugs that need acid for absorption (e.g., ketoconazole [Nizoral])
2. Avoid ulcerogenic medications unless absolutely necessary (e.g., aspirin, NSAIDs, glucocorticoids)
3. Cimetidine
   a. Reduces hepatic blood flow
   b. Inhibits the metabolism of certain drugs (diazepam, warfarin)

Proton Pump Inhibitors

A. Mechanism—irreversibly bind to the proton pump, resulting in acid suppression lasting more than 24 hours
B. Examples
1. Omeprazole (Prilosec)
2. Lansoprazole (Prevacid)
3. Esomeprazole (Nexium)
C. Adverse reactions
1. Esophageal candidiasis
2. Mucosal atrophy of the tongue
3. Xerostomia
D. Dental hygiene considerations
1. Evaluate for adverse oral reactions
2. Xerostomia—instruct the client to drink plenty of water; suck on tart sugarless gum or candy that contains xylitol, or ice chips; avoid products containing alcohol and caffeine; and avoid juices and soft drinks to reduce the risk of dental caries; saliva substitutes (Xero-lube, Salivart) can also be recommended

Emetics and Antiemetics

A. Emetics—induce vomiting; used to treat most poisonings (e.g., syrup of ipecac, which is available without a prescription); abused by persons with bulimia

B. Antiemetics
1. Reduce nausea or vomiting
2. Examples
   a. Benzquinamide (Emete-Con)
   b. Prochlorperazine (Compazine)
   c. Trimethobenzamide (Tigan)
C. Dental hygiene considerations
1. CNS sedation—the client should be instructed to avoid driving or operating heavy machinery or performing any task that requires thinking or concentration
2. Xerostomia—instruct the client to drink plenty of water; suck on tart sugarless gum or candy containing xylitol, or ice chips; avoid products containing alcohol and caffeine; and avoid juices or soft drinks to reduce the risk of dental caries; saliva substitutes (Xero-lube, Salivart) can also be recommended

ANTINEOPLASTIC AGENTS

A. Mechanism—interfere with the metabolism or reproductive cycle of malignant cells; also affect normal cells
B. Drugs
1. Alkylating agents
   a. Nitrogen mustards
      (1) Cyclophosphamide (Cytoxan)
      (2) Chlorambucil (Leukeran)
      (3) Melphalan (Alkeran)
   b. Nitrosureas—carmustine (BiCNU)
   c. Busulfan (Myleran)
2. Antimetabolites
   a. Folic acid analog—methotrexate (MTX)
   b. Purine antagonists
      (1) Mercaptopurine (6-MP)
      (2) Thioguanine (6-TG)
   c. Pyrimidine antagonists
      (1) 5-Fluorouracil (5-FU)
      (2) Cytarabine (Cytosar-U, ara-C)
3. Other antineoplastics
   a. Plant alkaloids
      (1) Vinblastine (Velban)
      (2) Vincristine (Oncovin)
   b. Antibiotics
      (1) Dactinomycin (actinomycin D, Cos-megen)
      (2) Daunorubicin (Cerubidine)
      (3) Doxorubicin (Adriamycin)
      (4) Mitomycin (Mitocin-C)
   c. Hormones
      (1) Adrenocorticosteroids
      (2) Androgens
      (3) Estrogens
      (4) Progestin
      (5) Tamoxifen (Nolvadex)—antiestrogen
   d. Aminobisphosphonates
      (1) Alendronate (Fosamax)
      (2) Ibandronate (Boniva)
      (3) Pamidronate (Aredia)
      (4) Risedronate (Actonel)
      (5) Zoledronic acid (Zometa)
   e. Miscellaneous
      (1) Asparaginase (Elspar)
      (2) Bleomycin (Blenoxane)
      (3) Cisplatin (Platinol)
      (4) Hydroxyurea (Hydrea)
C. Adverse reactions
1. Lack of specificity against tumor cells because normal cells are also destroyed; cells with the fastest life cycle are affected first
2. Bone marrow activity suppression
   a. Leukopenia—lowered WBC count; infections are more likely
   b. Thrombocytopenia—lowered platelets; risk of bleeding is increased
   c. Anemia
3. GI—stomatitis, mucosal sloughing
4. Infection—reduced immunity and ability to fight infection
5. Skin and hair—rash, alopecia (baldness)
6. Oral effects
   a. Symptoms—pain, ulcers, dryness, impaired taste, gingival hemorrhage, sensitivity of teeth and gingivae
   b. Treatment—avoid mouth rinses with alcohol; substitute saline or sodium bicarbonate; avoid alcohol
   c. Candidiasis—use antifungal agents (e.g., Nystatin)
   d. Xerostomia—instruct the client to drink plenty of water; suck on tart sugarless gum or candy with xylitol, or ice chips; avoid products containing alcohol and caffeine; and avoid juices and soft drinks to reduce the risk of dental caries; saliva substitutes (Xero-lube, Salivart) can also be recommended
7. Osteonecrosis of the jaw (ONJ)
   a. In cancer, primarily breast cancer, patients receiving intravenous bisphosphonates, 94% of cases with ONJ have been reported; the incidence is much lower in patients taking oral bisphosphonates for osteoporosis
   b. Prolonged use may suppress bone turnover—leads to microdamage
   c. Most cases of ONJ occur after tooth extractions or other procedures that cause trauma to the jawbone
   d. Very difficult to treat once it occurs
   e. Oral health examinations and other dental procedures should be performed before starting bisphosphonate therapy and continued every 3 months thereafter
   f. Any dental procedures that are performed should involve minimal trauma to the jaw and adjacent tissue
   g. ONJ treatment by oral and maxillofacial surgeons; treatment varies according to size of the lesion
   h. If clinically necessary, 0.12% chlorhexidine gluconate rinses, systemic antibiotics, and analgesics can be used
D. Dental hygiene considerations
1. Have clients improve their oral hygiene before chemotherapy, if possible
2. Avoid elective procedures during chemotherapy; timing is important; the best time for procedures is the day on

which chemotherapy begins (period of highest blood counts)

3. Check the coagulation status before any emergency surgery

4. Use of prophylactic antibiotic premedication is controversial

5. If xerostomia is a problem, client will need custom-fitted mouth trays for at-home, self-administered fluoride therapy

SUBSTANCE ABUSE

See the section on "Chemical Dependency" in Chapter 19.

Definitions

A. Tolerance—increasingly higher doses are required to produce the same effect; the same dose produces less effect; occurs with repeated administration

B. Physical dependence—symptoms of withdrawal occur if the drug is abruptly discontinued

C. Psychological dependence—craving occurs if the drug is stopped; no physical withdrawal syndrome; however, psychological dependence is just as likely to result in relapse (e.g., cocaine)

D. Abuse—improper or excessive self-administration of a drug that results in an adverse outcome

E. Addiction—pattern of abuse that continues despite medical or social complications

F. Withdrawal—a physical reaction attributable to physical dependence

G. Abstinence—drug-free state

H. Enabling—a pattern of coping methods (e.g., making excuses for absences) used by the associates of those addicted, which allows the addicted person to continue the drug use

Drugs of Abuse

A. Depressants

1. Alcohol—impaired judgment, slurred speech, ataxia, seizures, coma, death; withdrawal produces autonomic hyperactivity, hallucinations, or seizures; cirrhosis with chronic use

2. Opioids (hydrocodone, heroin, codeine, morphine)—euphoria, abscesses, constipation, respiratory depression; withdrawal produces "cold turkey" syndrome; methadone maintenance and naltrexone (acts similar to orally active naloxone) used to suppress a "high"

3. Barbiturates—secobarbital, pentobarbital

4. Volatile solvents—glue sniffing and paint solvent inhaling; called "huffing"

5. Benzodiazepines—diazepam

6. Anesthetics—N_2O-O_2 analgesia

B. Stimulants

1. Amphetamines—methamphetamine; highly addictive; street name "ice"

2. Cocaine—most psychologically addicting drug; produces euphoria, hyperactivity, paranoia; risk of acute MI; street names include coke and crack

3. Nicotine—in cigarettes, chewing tobacco, and cigars

4. Caffeine—in soft drinks, coffee, and tea

C. Psychedelics

1. Lysergic acid diethylamide (LSD)—flashbacks occur (without the drug); called "bad trip"

2. Psilocybin—hallucinogen derived from mushrooms of the genus Psilocybe

3. Phencyclidine (PCP)—disorientation, seizures; treatment consists of "talking down"

4. Marijuana (cannabis)—active ingredient is tetrahydrocannabinol (THC); causes silliness, relaxation, euphoria, paranoia, confusion, chronic amotivational syndrome; entrance drug (used first before trying other addictive drugs)

D. Dental hygiene considerations

1. Cocaine—cardiac stimulant effect; causes addictive effect on heart with local anesthetic agents with vasoconstrictors

2. Nitrous oxide (N_2O)—sense of euphoria; incidence of dental personnel abuse (unsupervised use); abuse produces neuropathy (sometimes irreversible); without adequate O_2, hypoxia is produced

3. Addicts—"shopper" clients attempt to obtain prescriptions for controlled substances from several dental offices; feign dental pain but refuse definitive treatment; suspicion is warranted

4. Caffeine—increased HR and BP with excessive caffeine intake

5. Nicotine—check for oral manifestations of tobacco use (e.g., nicotine stomatitis, periodontal disease, oral leukoplakia, precancerous lesions, hairy tongue, halitosis)

DRUG USE DURING PREGNANCY

A. General—pregnant women must:

1. Avoid any unnecessary drugs

2. Consult with an obstetrician

B. Pregnancy and professional oral health care

1. First trimester—period of highest risk for drug effects on the fetus; negative organogenic effects possible

2. Second trimester—best for elective dental treatment

3. Third trimester—use of any unnecessary drugs must be avoided because of client comfort and proximity to delivery

C. Drugs used in dental practice that are probably safe

1. Amoxicillin

2. Penicillin

3. Erythromycin

4. Lidocaine

5. Epinephrine (limit dose)

D. Drugs used in dental practice that must be avoided

1. Aspirin

2. NSAIDs

3. Metronidazole

4. N_2O—dental personnel who are pregnant should be especially careful

a. Women exposed to high levels of N_2O (more than 5 hours per week) were significantly less fertile than

unexposed women; levels of allowable exposure vary from state to state
  b. Dental practices should improve room air circulation and cleaning procedures and use an air evacuation system to reduce adverse outcomes[5,6]
  c. More information is available at http://www.osha.gov/dts/osta/anestheticgases/index.html#C1

Smoking Cessation

A. Nicotine reduction systems
  1. Nicotine is a ganglionic cholinergic receptor agonist
  2. Nicotine reduction (also known as *replacement*) therapies reduce the withdrawal symptoms associated with smoking cessation
  3. Smoking cessation reduces the risk of oral and lung cancers, heart disease, and other lung diseases
B. Types of nicotine reduction systems
  1. Chewing gum—Nicorette 2 or 4 mg; available without a prescription
  2. Transdermal systems—all available without a prescription
    a. Habitrol
    b. Nicoderm
    c. Nicotrol
    d. Prostep
  3. Nasal spray—Nicotrol NS
  4. Adverse effects
    a. Chewing gum—sore mouth, hiccups, dyspepsia, jaw ache, nausea
    b. Chewing gum can stick to dentures and dental work
    c. Transdermal systems—nausea, hypersalivation, abdominal pain, vomiting, diarrhea, perspiration, headache, dizziness, hearing and visual disturbances, confusion, weakness
    d. Nasal spray—runny nose, throat irritation, watery eyes, sneezing, cough
  5. Dental hygiene considerations
    a. Evaluate the client who smokes for oral benign and malignant changes
    b. Stress the importance of tobacco cessation
    c. Evaluate clients using the chewing gum for any problems(e.g., gum sticking to dentures or dental work); recommend using another form of smoking cessation aid
C. Bupropion (Zyban)
  1. Antidepressant used to reduce nicotine cravings
  2. Also called Wellbutrin; the pills are identical and made by the same manufacturer, but coded differently for insurance purposes
  3. Concomitant treatment modalities are encouraged (behavior modification)
  4. Recommended dosing—150 mg once daily for 3 days, followed by 150 mg twice daily for 2 to 3 months if the client is experiencing success
D. Varenicline (Chantix)
  1. Nicotine receptor blocker; amount of dopamine released into the brain is reduced; thereby blocking the feelings of pleasure associated with tobacco use
  2. Dosing—once daily for the first 3 days, twice daily thereafter for the full course of therapy (usually 12 weeks)
  3. Taken after meals and with a full glass of water
  4. Adverse effects include nausea, sleep problems, constipation, gas, vomiting, and changes in mood and behavior
  5. Cannot be used in conjunction with other smoking cessation products

Website Information And Resources

Source	Website Address	Description
RxList, The Internet Drug Index	http://www.rxlist.com	A HealthCentral.com Network site providing information about medications, indications, contraindications, dosages, and client information
Drug Topics	http://www.drugtopics.modernmedicine.com	Current news on drug-related topics
FDA - Drugs	http://www.fda.gov/Drugs/	Information on new drug development and regulatory issues
Med Watch	http://www.fda.gov/medwatch/safety.htm	Safety information
American Herbal Products Association	http://www.ahpa.org	Current information on herbal remedies
Malignant Hyperthermia Association of the United States	http://www.mhaus.org	Online brochures, including an explanation of malignant hyperthermia as a concern in dentistry and oral and maxillofacial surgery

REFERENCES

1. Holroyd SV: *Clinical pharmacology in dental practice*, ed 4, St Louis, 1989, Mosby.
2. Wilson W, Taubert KA, Gewitz M, et al: Prevention of infective endocarditis: guidelines from the American Heart Association, *Circulation* 116:1736.11, 2007.
3. Hirsh J, Dalen J, Guyatt G, editors: The sixth (2000) ACCP guidelines for antithrombotic therapy for prevention and treatment of thrombosis. American College of Chest Physicians. In *Chest* 119(I suppl):1S–2S.
4. American Hospital Formulary Service: *Drug information*, Bethesda, Md, 2013, American Society of Hospital Pharmacists.
5. Crawford JS, Lewis M: Nitrous oxide in early pregnancy, *Anaesthesia* 41:900–905, 1986.
6. Little JW, Falace DA, Miller CS, Rhodus NL: *Dental management of the medically compromised patient*, St Louis, 2008, Mosby.

CHAPTER 11 REVIEW QUESTIONS

Answers and rationales to review questions are available on this text's accompanying Evolve site. See inside front cover for details.

evolve

CASE A

Synopsis of Patient History
Age:16
Sex: M
Height: 5'9"
Weight: 162 lbs (73.6 kg)

Vital Signs
Blood pressure: 102/60 mm Hg
Pulse rate: 70 bpm
Respiration rate: 22 rpm

1. Under care of physician: x YES   ___ NO
    Condition: Asthma
2. Hospitalized within the last 3 years: ___ YES   x NO

Current Medications
Albuterol inhaler: as needed
Montelukast (Singulair) 10 mg: one tablet daily
Fluticasone/salmeterol (Advair HFA) inhaler: one inhalation twice daily

Multivitamin: once daily
Doxycycline
Cetirizine (Zyrtec) 10 mg daily

Medical History
Patient has a history of asthma and is under the care of his pediatrician. Patient also has acne, which is being treated by his pediatrician.

Dental History
Visits the dental office for regular examination and cleaning.

Social History
He lives with his mother, father, and brother.
He enjoys golf, soccer, movies, and traveling.
He is a junior at a local high school.

Chief Complaint
Sore and dry throat

Use Case A to answer questions 1 to 10.

1. **Which of the following drugs could be causing the sore throat and dry mouth?**
    a. Albuterol
    b. Montelukast
    c. Multivitamins
    d. Doxycycline
2. **Albuterol is a bronchodilator that can be administered via a metered-dose inhaler. It is recommended for treating an acute asthma attack.**
    a. Both statements are TRUE.
    b. Both statements are FALSE.
    c. The first statement is TRUE; the second statement is FALSE
    d. The first statement is FALSE; the second is TRUE
3. **Which one of the following drugs can result in oral candidiasis?**
    a. Cetirizine
    b. Ibuprofen
    c. Acetaminophen
    d. Fluticasone
4. **All the following are recommendations that you should make to patients with asthma EXCEPT one. Which one is the *exception*?**
    a. Bring your inhaler (albuterol) to the dental appointment.
    b. Rinse after using corticosteroid inhaler.
    c. Avoid erythromycin.
    d. Avoid aspirin.
    e. Avoid acetaminophen.
5. **Although this teenager with asthma does not have emphysema, several of the drugs used to treat asthma**

are also used to treat emphysema. Which of the following is the drug of choice for treating emphysema?
    a. Albuterol
    b. Zileuton
    c. Ipratropium
    d. Cetirizine
6. **Which of the following orally inhaled drugs should the patient bring with him to each appointment in case of an acute asthma attack?**
    a. Salmeterol
    b. Albuterol
    c. Flunisolide
    d. Ipratropium bromide
7. **Which of the following is the BEST recommendation you could make to your patient if he required oral prednisone (steroid therapy)?**
    a. Continue to rinse, swish, and spit after taking your oral tablet.
    b. Rinse, swish, and swallow after taking your oral tablet.
    c. Check for any signs of infection, since this medication can mask the signs of infection and can delay wound healing.
    d. Be careful, since this drug can cause significant dry mouth.
8. **Patients using the fluticasone/salmeterol inhaler should be instructed about all the following EXCEPT:**
    a. Rinse, swish, and spit after each use of the inhaler.
    b. The inhaler must be discarded 1 month from the date of first use.
    c. It is a good idea to brush your teeth after each inhaler use.
    d. This inhaler can be used for acute attacks.

9. Patients taking doxycycline should be counseled about all the following EXCEPT:
   a. Esophageal irritation
   b. Photosensitivity
   c. Gastrointestinal upset
   d. Sedation

10. Histamine-1 (H$_1$)–blocking drugs such as cetirizine are preferred over drugs such as diphenhydramine because

they are less sedating. Cetirizine is a nonsedating H$_1$-blocking drug.
   a. Both statements are TRUE.
   b. The first statement is TRUE; the second statement is FALSE.
   c. The first statement is FALSE; the second statement is TRUE.
   d. Both statements are FALSE.

CASE B

Synopsis of Patient History
Age: 55
Sex: M
Height: 5'10"
Weight: 220 lbs (100 kg)

Vital Signs
Blood pressure: 145/85 mm Hg
Pulse rate: 75 bpm
Respiration rate: 25 rpm

1. Under care of physician: x YES   ___ NO
   Condition: Hypertension, high cholesterol, type 2 diabetes, coronary artery disease, depression
2. Hospitalized within the last 3 years: x YES   ___ NO
   Rule out MI

Current Medications
Lisinopril (Zestril)
Hydrochlorothiazide
Baby aspirin

Atorvastatin (Lipitor)
Glipizide (Glucotrol) 10 mg bid
Metformin (Glucophage)
Citalopram (Celexa) 40 mg qd
Sublingual nitroglycerin as needed

Medical History
Client has a history of cardiovascular disease, type 2 diabetes, depression, and high cholesterol. Patient being treated by a cardiologist and his general physician.

Dental History
Visits the dental office for regular examination and cleaning.

Social History
Married with three children
Enjoys golf, football, television, and good meals
Currently employed as a government contractor

Chief Complaint
Presents for routine oral health examination

Use Case B to answer questions 11 to 25.

11. **What is meant by the term essential hypertension?**
   a. Hypertension of unknown cause
   b. Iatrogenic hypertension
   c. Hypertension precipitated by another disorder
   d. A rapidly developing form of hypertension, requiring aggressive therapy

12. **Eating a banana or drinking a glass of orange juice when taking a thiazide diuretic will:**
   a. Deplete calcium
   b. Prevent diuresis
   c. Replenish potassium
   d. Inhibit the drug's metabolism

13. **Patients who have experienced a myocardial infarction 9 months prior to an office visit would be considered a CONTRAINDICATION to dental treatment. After 9 months, if treatment is provided, the patient should receive prophylactic antibiotic premedication.**
   a. Both statements are TRUE.
   b. The first statement is TRUE; the second statement is FALSE.
   c. The first statement is FALSE; the second statement is TRUE.
   d. Both statements are FALSE.

14. **One of the main differences between angiotensin-converting enzyme (ACE) inhibitors and angiotensin receptor blockers (ARBs) is that ACE inhibitors cause a dry, nonproductive cough. ARBs do not cause a dry, nonproductive cough.**
   a. Both statements are TRUE.
   b. The first statement is TRUE; the second statement is FALSE.
   c. The first statement is FALSE; the second statement is TRUE.
   d. Both statements are FALSE.

15. **Clients taking antihypertensive agents who have been supine for some time should rise from that position slowly. They should dangle their legs over the side of the chair and wiggle them before rising to the standing position.**
   a. Both statements are TRUE.
   b. Both statements are FALSE.
   c. The first statement is TRUE; the second statement is false.
   d. The first statement is FALSE; the second statement is true.

16. **Which of the following drugs inhibits hydroxymethyl-glutaryl coenzyme A (HMG-CoA) reductase?**

a. Pravastatin
b. Ramipril
c. Nifedipine
d. Ezetimibe

17. Which agent reduces serum cholesterol by increasing its use for bile acid synthesis?
    a. Niacin
    b. Atorvastatin
    c. Gemfibrozil
    d. Cholestyramine

18. Which class of drugs is recommended in persons with diabetes?
    a. β-Adrenergic blockers
    b. Ca^{+2} channel blocker
    c. Angiotensin-converting enzyme (ACE) inhibitors
    d. Anticholinergic agents

19. All the following drugs inhibit platelet function EXCEPT:
    a. Clopidogrel
    b. Dipyridamole
    c. Ticlopidine
    d. Aspirin

20. Patients taking nitroglycerine (NTG) sublingual tablets should be instructed to:
    a. Store their NTG in plastic
    b. Keep their NTG in the refrigerator
    c. Use NTG once every 5 minutes until the anginal attack has stopped
    d. Bring their NTG to the dental appointment and make it available to the practitioner in the event that the patient experiences an acute anginal attack

21. Your patient complains of chest pain while sitting in the dental chair. Even though the information is not recorded on his health history or pharmacologic history form, it is a good idea for you to ask if he has taken sildenafil (Viagra) within the last 24 hours. The use of nitroglycerine is contraindicated if sildenafil has been taken within 24 hours because the nitroglycerine-sildenafil combination can precipitate a hypertensive crisis.
    a. Both statements are TRUE.
    b. Both statements are FALSE.
    c. The first statement is TRUE; the second statement is FALSE.
    d. The first statement is FALSE; the second statement is TRUE.

22. Which oral antidiabetic agent produces lactic acidosis as a significant adverse effect?
    a. Tolbutamide
    b. Metformin
    c. Repaglinide
    d. Acarbose

23. Patients taking glipizide should be instructed to:
    a. Schedule their dental appointments after mealtimes and take their medicine on time
    b. Schedule their dental appointments around the time they take their medicine
    c. Schedule their dental appointments around mealtimes only
    d. Schedule their dental appointment any time, as the timing of the appointment is not a significant factor

24. Which antidepressant is LEAST likely to cause xerostomia?
    a. Bupropion
    b. Citalopram
    c. Chlorpromazine
    d. Amitriptyline

25. Selective serotonin reuptake inhibitors (SSRIs) tend to produce central nervous system (CNS) stimulation rather than CNS depression. Therefore, SSRIs are less sedating.
    a. Both statements are TRUE.
    b. The first statement is TRUE; the second statement is FALSE.
    c. The first statement is FALSE; the second statement is TRUE.
    d. Both statements are FALSE.

CASE C

Synopsis of Patient History
Age: 49
Sex: F
Height: 5'2"
Weight: 125 lbs (57 kg)

Vital Signs
Blood pressure: 95/68 mm Hg
Pulse rate: 65 bpm
Respiration rate: 20 rpm

1. Hospitalized within the last 3 years: ___ YES   x NO

Current Medications
LoEstrin 24
Occasional over-the-counter ibuprofen and acetaminophen

Medical History
Menopausal; otherwise healthy

Dental History
Visits the dental office for regular examination and cleaning.
Predental anxiety, requires pretreatment with a benzodiazepine

Social History
Married with two children
She enjoys golf, gardening. scrapbooking, reading, and traveling.
She is a pharmacist.

Chief Complaint
Requires a crown

Anticipated Medications
Lorazepam 2 mg the night before the appointment
N_2O-O_2 conscious sedation during procedure
Acetaminophen with codeine post procedure

Use Case C to answer questions 26 to 40.

26. **Patients should be warned that an acute overdose with acetaminophen can result in damage to the:**
    a. Eyes
    b. Liver
    c. Spleen
    d. Kidney

27. **Alcohol consumption in combination with acetaminophen stimulates the breakdown of acetaminophen, thereby increasing the toxic potential of acetaminophen use.**
    a. Both statements are TRUE.
    b. Both statements are FALSE.
    c. The first statement is TRUE; the second statement is FALSE.
    d. The first statement is FALSE; the second statement is TRUE.

28. **Approximately 90% of dental pain is BEST managed with:**
    a. Codeine 60 mg
    b. Ibuprofen 400 mg
    c. Acetaminophen 650 mg
    d. Aspirin 650 mg

29. **Which of the following drugs should you avoid recommending to a person taking lithium?**
    a. Aspirin
    b. Ibuprofen
    c. Acetaminophen
    d. Oxycodone

30. **Patients taking ibuprofen should be counseled about all the following EXCEPT:**
    a. Gastrointestinal upset
    b. Heartburn
    c. Sedation
    d. Increased risk for bleeding

31. **Both opioid and nonopioid analgesics relieve pain by raising the pain threshold. Raising the pain threshold increases one's reaction to pain.**
    a. Both statements are TRUE.
    b. The first statement is TRUE; the second statement is FALSE.
    c. The first statement is FALSE; the second statement is TRUE.
    d. Both statements are FALSE.

32. **Following the dental procedure, the patient developed itching and urticaria after taking her acetaminophen with codeine. This response MOST likely represents a:**
    a. Pharmacologic action of codeine
    b. Hypersensitivity reaction to codeine
    c. Placebo effect from receiving codeine
    d. Reaction unrelated to codeine administration

33. **Which of the following is the major symptom of opioid overdose?**
    a. Miosis

b. Respiratory depression
c. Urticaria
d. Mydriasis

34. **For pain control, often an opioid analgesic is combined with a nonopioid analgesic. This combination produces an additive analgesic effect with fewer adverse reactions.**
    a. Both statements are TRUE.
    b. The first statement is TRUE; the second statement is FALSE.
    c. The first statement is FALSE; the second statement is TRUE.
    d. Both statements are FALSE.

35. **Which of the following is an adverse reaction to codeine?**
    a. Diarrhea
    b. Miosis
    c. CNS excitation
    d. Hepatotoxicity

36. **Antianxiety agents are most frequently administered as the oral dose form. This is because the blood levels achieved from the oral administration of the antianxiety agent are very predictable.**
    a. Both statements are TRUE.
    b. Both statements are FALSE.
    c. The first statement is TRUE; the second statement is FALSE.
    d. The first statement is FALSE; the second statement is TRUE.

37. **Once a benzodiazepine is absorbed into the systemic circulation, all the following contribute to the rate at which it reaches its site of action EXCEPT:**
    a. Lipid solubility
    b. Protein binding
    c. Ionization
    d. Client's gender

38. **The patient has begun to inhale nitrous oxide and oxygen (N_2O-O_2) as part of conscious sedation. The BEST way to determine her level of sedation under N_2O-O_2 is:**
    a. Response to a painful stimulus
    b. Percent N_2O being delivered
    c. Response to questions
    d. Muscle tone

39. **Conscious sedation with N_2O-O_2 is CONTRAINDICATED in a patient with:**
    a. Diabetes
    b. Emotional instability
    c. Hypertension
    d. Glaucoma

40. **Nitrous oxide and oxygen (N_2O-O_2) is often combined with a halogenated inhalational anesthetic because it:**
    a. Increases the minimum alveolar concentration (MAC)
    b. Decreases the MAC
    c. Typically precipitates a toxic reaction
    d. Inhibits the metabolism of the halogenated anesthetic

CASE D

Synopsis of Patient History
Age: 76
Sex: F
Height: 5'3"
Weight: 140 lbs (63.6 kg)

Vital Signs
Blood pressure: 115/75 mm Hg
Pulse rate: 70 bpm
Respiration rate: 22 rpm

1. Under care of physician: x YES   ___ NO
   Condition: Arthritis
2. Hospitalized within the last 3 years: ___ YES   x NO

Current Medications
Ibuprofen 400 mg tid
Hydrochlorothiazide 25 g qd
Phenytoin (Dilantin)

Medical History
Patient has a history of arthritis, seizure disorders, and hypertension. She is being treated by a general physician for all three. She often complains of GI upset after taking ibuprofen. She is also 1 year post–joint replacement surgery on her right knee.

Dental History
Visits the dental office for regular examination and cleaning.

Social History
She is widowed and lives alone.
She enjoys volunteering, reading, gardening and traveling

Chief Complaint
Routine visit
Requires antibiotic prophylaxis: amoxicillin 2 g 1 hour before procedure

---

Use Case D to answer questions 41 to 50.

41. **The distribution of a drug across biologic membranes is determined by all the following EXCEPT:**
    a. Blood flow to the organ
    b. Presence of certain barriers
    c. Plasma-protein binding capacity
    d. Half-life

42. **A drug effect that is NEITHER predictable NOR dose related is called a:**
    a. Therapeutic effect
    b. Toxic reaction
    c. Side effect
    d. Allergic reaction

43. **Infective endocarditis prophylaxis with an anti-infective agent is indicated for patients who have had:**
    a. Mitral valve prolapse
    b. Prosthetic cardiac valve
    c. Rheumatic heart disease
    d. Atrial septal defect

44. **Which drug should be used as an antibiotic premedication before invasive dental or dental hygiene care for a patient who has a history of congenital heart disease, artificial heart valves, and an allergy to penicillin?**
    a. Amoxicillin
    b. Tetracycline
    c. Clindamycin
    d. Cephalexin

45. **Which of the following drugs can result in a severe drug interaction with alcohol?**
    a. Erythromycin
    b. Tetracycline
    c. Metronidazole
    d. Aminoglycosides (e.g., streptomycin)

46. **Which organ is involved in the "first-pass" effect after oral administration of a drug?**
    a. Kidney
    b. Lungs
    c. Liver
    d. Spleen

47. **All the following are TRUE with regard to cytochromes P450 EXCEPT for which one?**
    a. Cytochromes P450 are located in the endoplasmic reticulum.
    b. Cytochromes P450 exist as numerous isozymes.
    c. Cytochromes P450 are involved in the first-pass effect.
    d. Cytochromes P450 inactivate drugs through conjugation reactions.

48. **NSAIDs, such as ibuprofen, can antagonize the effects of which of the following antihypertensive medications?**
    a. ACE inhibitors
    b. β-Adrenergic antagonists
    c. Calcium channel blockers
    d. Diuretics

49. **Which anticonvulsant medication has been documented to cause osteomalacia?**
    a. Carbamazepine
    b. Phenytoin
    c. Ethosuximide
    d. Gabapentin

50. **Alopecia may be an adverse effect of phenytoin. Carbamazepine can cause hirsutism.**
    a. Both statements are TRUE.
    b. Both statements are FALSE.
    c. The first statement is TRUE; the second statement is FALSE.
    d. The first statement is FALSE; the second statement is TRUE.

Biochemistry, Nutrition, and Nutritional Counseling

Lisa F. Harper Mallonee

Humans require specific chemicals or nutrients from food to grow, maintain homeostasis, and achieve optimal health. An understanding of cellular biochemistry and nutrition is essential for preventing and treating disease and for promoting health. Nutrition science includes the intake of food and the processes involved in digestion, absorption, transportation, metabolism of nutrients, and excretion. As an applied science, it involves counseling people to adapt food patterns to nutritional needs within the cultural, economic, and psychosocial environment. Nutrition assessment counseling, when performed effectively, motivates individuals to modify eating behaviors so that optimal health can be achieved.

This chapter reviews the six major nutrient groups and their metabolic activities in mammalian cells, dietary modifications for diseases, nutritional diseases and disorders, and oral manifestations of nutritional deficiencies and toxicities. The effects of nutrients on oral tissues and the dietary assessment tools and techniques available for counseling individuals with various types of oral diseases are also described. Because nutritional problems in the developed countries are a result of overeating and undereating, a review of energy balance and weight control is included. Cellular biochemistry is fundamental to the study of nutrition; therefore the reader is referred to the section on "General Histology" in Chapter 2 for a review of structural and functional similarities in cells.

SIX MAJOR CLASSES OF ESSENTIAL NUTRIENTS

Carbohydrates

A. Definition—polyhydroxy aldehydes or ketones that serve as the body's primary sources of quick energy; carbohydrates (CHO) are composed of monosaccharides, basic units that contain carbon, hydrogen, and oxygen
B. Basic chemical structure
   1. The ratio of carbon, hydrogen, and oxygen is 1:2:1
   2. The reactive portion of the molecule may be in a ketose form or an aldose form

3. The position of the hydroxyl (–OH) groups determines properties such as sweetness and absorbability
C. Classification
   1. Simple carbohydrates
      a. Monosaccharides
         (1) Trioses (C3) and tetroses (C4)—usually formed during intermediary metabolism and are not important dietary components
         (2) Pentoses (C5)—important in nucleic acids and coenzymes; do not occur in free form (uncombined); not important dietary components (e.g., ribose)
         (3) Hexoses (C6)—most important group physiologically
            (a) Glucose—blood sugar; primary energy source
            (b) Galactose—seldom found free; but found in lactose
            (c) Fructose—fruit sugar; sweetest tasting sugar; found in honey and fruits
      b. Disaccharides—composed of two monosaccharide units
         (1) Sucrose—glucose plus fructose (e.g., cane and beet sugar)
         (2) Lactose—glucose plus galactose (e.g., milk sugar)
         (3) Maltose—glucose plus glucose (intermediate of starch hydrolysis [digestion])
D. Oligosaccharides—composed of two to six monosaccharide units
   1. Complex carbohydrates
      a. Homopolysaccharides—made up of more than six identical monosaccharide units
         (1) Starch—plant storage form of glucose; source of half of dietary carbohydrates
            (a) Amylose—straight chain
            (b) Amylopectin—branched chain
         (2) Glycogen—animal storage form of glucose; found in the liver and muscle of living animals; insignificant source of dietary carbohydrates
         (3) Cellulose—chief constituent of the framework of plants; glucose units are in β-linkages, not capable of being hydrolyzed by human digestive enzymes; provides bulk and fiber in the diet

b. Heteropolysaccharides—carbohydrates associated with noncarbohydrates or carbohydrate derivatives
   (1) Pectin, lignin—important contributors to fiber in the diet
   (2) Glycoproteins—carbohydrate and protein in a specific, functional arrangement (e.g., blood group substances and many hormones)
   (3) Glycolipids—carbohydrate and lipid, as in gangliosides
   (4) Mucopolysaccharides—protein and carbohydrate in a loose binding
      (a) Hyaluronic acid—vitreous humor and joint lubricant
      (b) Heparin—anticoagulant
      (c) Chondroitin sulfate—cartilage, skin, bone, and teeth
      (d) Keratin sulfate—nails and teeth

E. Digestion, absorption, and transport
   1. Digestion (Table 12-1)
      a. Mouth
         (1) Teeth and tongue—mechanical breakdown and mixing of food
         (2) Saliva—hydration and lubrication of food
         (3) Salivary amylase (ptyalin)—initial enzymatic hydrolysis of starch
      b. Stomach—no digestive enzymes for carbohydrates; initial enzymatic hydrolysis of starch by salivary amylase may continue
      c. Small intestine
         (1) Pancreatic juices—pancreatic amylases
         (2) Intestinal villi (brush border) enzymes—disaccharidases
            (a) Sucrase—converts sucrose to glucose and fructose
            (b) Lactase—converts lactose to glucose and galactose
            (c) Maltase—converts maltose to glucose

d. Large intestine—bacterial "fermentation" of some undigested carbohydrates
   (1) No significant contribution to absorbable carbohydrates
   (2) May be the cause of gas production and bloating during primary or secondary disaccharidase deficiency (e.g., "lactose intolerance")

2. Absorption (Fig. 12-1)
   a. Factors affecting absorption
      (1) Intestinal motility
      (2) Type of food mixture
      (3) Integrity of intestinal mucosa
      (4) Endocrine activity
   b. Mechanism
      (1) Passive diffusion along the osmotic gradient—when the intestinal concentration of carbohydrates is greater than the level of carbohydrate in the blood
      (2) Facilitated diffusion—only certain molecules allowed to pass across a membrane using an ion channel or a carrier protein
      (3) Active transport—requires energy and allows molecules to pass against a concentration gradient with the aid of an ion channel or a carrier protein at the brush border
   c. Route
      (1) Carbohydrates are water soluble and are absorbed directly into the capillaries of the intestinal mucosa
      (2) Carried by the portal circulation to the liver

F. Metabolism—glucose is the main immediate source of energy for the body; a glucose level of 70 to 120 mg/100 mL blood is maintained by most healthy persons (Fig. 12-2)
   1. Sources of blood glucose
      a. Dietary carbohydrates—sugars, starches
      b. Stored liver glycogen breakdown—glycogenolysis

TABLE 12-1	**Digestive Action at Various Points Along the Gastrointestinal Tract**		
	Carbohydrates	**Proteins**	**Fats**
Mouth	Salivary amylase: starch → maltose	No enzymatic action	No enzymatic action
Stomach	No enzymatic action	Hydrochloric acid (HCl): denatures proteins → activates pepsinogen → pepsin → hydrolysis of peptide bonds → peptides + proteoses	Gastric lipase*: → short- and medium-chain triglycerides → fatty acids + monoglycerides
Small intestine Pancreatic enzymes	Pancreatic amylase: starch → dextrin dextrin → maltose	Trypsin → chymotrypsin + aminopeptidase + carboxypeptidase → hydrolysis of peptide bonds	Pancreatic lipase: fatty acids → triglycerides → diglycerides + monoglycerides
Bile salts	No action	No action	Bile salts: emulsification of fats
Brush-border enzymes	Disaccharidases → monosaccharides: Sucrose → glucose → fructose Lactase → lactose → glucose + galactose Maltaste → maltose → glucose	Dipeptidases → dipeptides → amino acids	Lecithinase: lecithin → monoglyceride + fatty acid + PO_4 + choline
Large intestine	Some fermentation of undigested nutrients but with negligible absorption of the fermentation products		

*A minor role in total fat digestion.

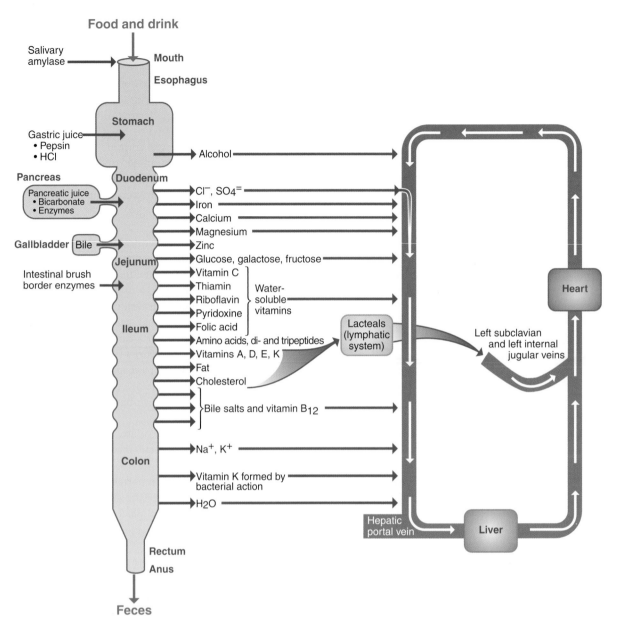

FIG 12-1 Absorption of major nutrients, vitamins, and minerals. (From Mahan LK, Escott-Stump S: *Krause's food and nutrition therapy*, ed 13, St Louis, 2012, Saunders.)

c. Synthesis from intermediary metabolites such as pyruvic acid—glyconeogenesis
d. Synthesis from noncarbohydrate sources— gluconeogenesis
   (1) Deaminated (glucogenic) amino acids
   (2) Glycerol portion of lipids
2. Reactions of blood glucose—"burned" (oxidized) for energy
a. Glycolysis—end product is pyruvate or lactic acid in the absence of oxygen (anaerobic conditions) or acetyl–coenzyme A (acetyl-CoA) in the presence of oxygen (aerobic conditions)
b. Tricarboxylic acid cycle (TCA) or Krebs cycle—oxidation of acetyl-CoA with the release of carbon dioxide (CO_2)

c. Oxidative phosphorylation and electron transport—production of adenosine triphosphate (ATP, a high-energy molecule) and water
3. Storage for reserve use
a. Glycogenesis—glycogen is the short-term storage form of glucose in the liver and muscle (6 to 18 hours)
b. Lipogenesis—excess carbohydrate in the diet is converted to fat to be stored in adipose tissue as a long-term energy storage form
4. Conversion to other molecules, such as:
a. Other carbohydrates needed for structural or functional roles
b. Keto acids to be used in protein synthesis
G. Metabolic regulators

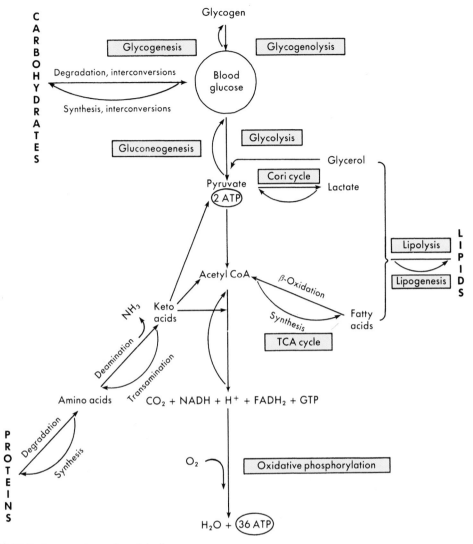

FIG 12-2 An overview of metabolism.

1. Anabolic hormones—lower the blood glucose level (e.g., insulin)
   a. Increase the entry of glucose into cells
   b. Increase glycogenesis
   c. Increase lipogenesis
2. Catabolic hormones—raise the blood glucose level
   a. Glucagon—stimulates glycogenolysis
   b. Steroid hormones—stimulate gluconeogenesis
   c. Epinephrine—stimulates glycogenolysis
   d. Growth hormone and adrenocorticotropic hormone (ACTH)—act as insulin antagonists
   e. Thyroxine—increases insulin breakdown, intestinal absorption of glucose, and epinephrine release
3. Coenzymes—B-complex vitamins are important precursors of the coenzymes involved in the catabolism of carbohydrates

H. Fiber
1. Definition—substance, usually nonstarch polysaccharide, found in plants; not broken down by human digestive enzymes; some of it is digested by bacteria in the gastrointestinal (GI) tract

   a. Insoluble fiber—substance (e.g., cellulose, hemicellulose, lignin) that gives structure to plant cell walls; adds bulk and softness to stools; reduces contact with possible carcinogens by decreasing transit time through the colon; foods high in insoluble fiber include wheat bran, raw fruits, and vegetables
   b. Soluble fibers—substances (e.g., gums, mucilages, pectin, oat bran) that dissolve to become gummy or viscous; lower blood cholesterol; regulate the use of sugars and slow down gastric emptying; foods high in soluble fiber include legumes, raw apples, and whole oats
2. Epidemiologic studies indicate that individuals whose diets include a significant amount of fiber have a low incidence of chronic "Western" diseases, such as coronary heart disease, diabetes, atherosclerosis
3. Specific fibers are believed to play roles in decreasing the incidence of obesity, irregularity, hemorrhoids, appendicitis, diverticulosis, colon cancer, hyperlipidemia, and fluctuations in blood glucose

4. Excessive dietary fiber
   a. For persons with a limited intake, diets high in fiber bulk may cause nutritional deficiency
   b. Use of large doses of purified fiber may inhibit absorption of calcium, potassium, zinc, and iron
   c. Phytic acid, often found in high-fiber foods such as cereal grains, can bind and prevent absorption of minerals such as iron, calcium, and zinc
5. Recommended fiber intake—for adults, 21 to 38 grams per day (g/day), depending on age and gender

I. Biologic role and functions of carbohydrates
1. Provide precursors of structural and functional molecules (e.g., gangliosides)
2. Energy source (4 kilocalories per gram [kcal/g])
3. Spare protein
4. Provide bulk and palatability to the diet

J. Role in oral biology
1. Preeruptive effect on teeth
   a. Energy source for growth and development
   b. Protein-sparing nutrient
2. Posteruptive effect on teeth
   a. Energy source for oral cariogenic bacteria (e.g., *Streptococcus mutans*)
   b. Acidogenic bacteria metabolize monosaccharides and disaccharides, particularly sucrose, for the production of energy through glycolysis that results in the formation of lactic acid, pyruvate, and other acetyl-CoA, dependent on the conditions
   c. *S. mutans* synthesizes polysaccharides (glucans, levans, and glycogen) from sucrose
      (1) Polysaccharides are used for energy when sucrose is unavailable
      (2) Glucans form insoluble complexes with *S. mutans* and have a strong affinity for enamel, thus enhancing bacterial plaque formation
      (3) The organic acids are liberated into the interface between the bacterial plaque and surface enamel
      (4) At pH 5.5, decalcification and demineralization begin
   d. The firm texture of some complex carbohydrates, as found in raw fruits and vegetables, can help to remove food debris retained between teeth; the chewing action can also stimulate salivary flow
3. Dietary sweeteners (Table 12-2)
   a. Nutritive sweeteners are used by the body as an energy source; they provide calories

TABLE 12-2 Dietary Sweeteners

Common Category	Chemical Structure and Category	Examples	Caries Promoting Potential	Relative Sweetness in Comparison to Sucrose*	Food Sources
Sugars	Monosaccharide	Glucose, dextrose	Yes	0.7	Most foods
		Fructose, high fructose corn syrup	Yes	1.4-1.8	Fruits, honey, condiments, soft drinks
		Galactose	Yes	0.6	_____
	Disaccharide	Sucrose, granulated, powdered or brown sugar, turbinado, molasses	Yes	1.0	Fruits, vegetables, table sugar
		Lactose	Yes	0.2	Milk
		Maltose	Yes	0.4	Beer
Other carbohydrates	Polysaccharide	Starch	Yes	N/A	Potatoes, grains, rice, legumes, bananas, cornstarch
	Fiber	Cellulose, pectin, gums, β-glucans, fructans	No	N/A	_____
Sugar alcohols	Polyol-monosaccharide	Sorbitol, mannitol, xylitol, erythritol	No	0.5-1.0	Grains, fruits, vegetables
	Polyol-disaccharide	Lactitol, isomalt, maltitol	No	0.3-0.9	Fruit, seaweed, exudates of plants or trees
	Polyol-polysaccharide	Hydrogenated starch, hydrolysates (HSH) or maltitol syrup	No	0.7	Derived from lactose, maltose, or starch
Nonnutritive sweeteners	Aspartame	Nutrasweet, Equal	No	200	
	Saccharin	Sweet' n Low	No	300	Derived from monosaccharides
	Acesulfame-K	Sunett	No	200	_____
	Sucralose	Splenda	No	600	_____
	Lu han guo	Monk fruit	No	200	_____
	Rebaudioside A	Truvia, Stevia	No	250-300	_____

N/A, Not applicable.
*Sucrose = 1.0

Modified from Hubrich B, Nabors LO. Glycemic response. In *Formulating glycemic strategies,* a supplement to Food Product Design. July 2006, pp 1-9. Adapted from Davis JR, Stegeman CA: *The dental hygienist's guide to nutritional care,* ed 4, Philadelphia, 2015, Saunders; and Palmer C: *Diet and nutrition in oral health,* ed 2, Upper Saddle River, NJ, 2007, Pearson Prentice Hall, p 68.

(1) Sugar alcohols (xylitol, sorbitol, and mannitol) are noncariogenic nutritive sweeteners that are slowly fermented through anaerobic metabolism by oral bacteria; excessive intake of these polyols can cause diarrhea because of the osmotic transfer of water into the bowel

(2) Xylitol is found naturally in plants and is equal to or sweeter than sucrose; consumption of xylitol-containing products after eating food has been shown to interfere with the metabolism of *S. mutans* and decrease the demineralization of enamel

b. Nonnutritive sweeteners are calorie free and have no nutritive value; aspartame, saccharin, and acesulfame-K are nonnutritive sweeteners approved by the United States Food and Drug Administration (FDA); are noncariogenic

c. Aspartame should be avoided by patients who have phenylketonuria, a genetic disorder characterized by an inability to metabolize the amino acid phenylalanine

d. Food labels often list sugar content in its various forms (e.g., invert sugars, dextrose, fructose, corn sweeteners) to give an appearance of lower sugar content

4. Cariogenicity factors of diet habits (from *most* important to *least* important)

a. Intake frequency of simple sugars—the more frequent the exposure to sugar, the more cariogenic is the diet; six candy bars eaten at six different times during the day are more harmful in terms of acid and bacterial plaque formation than six candy bars consumed at the same time

b. Form of simple sugars (liquid or retentive)—liquid sweets clear the oral cavity faster than solid or retentive sweets do and therefore are less cariogenic

c. Time of ingestion of simple sugars—combining sweets with liquids and other noncariogenic foods during a meal is less cariogenic than a concentrated exposure to sweets between meals as a snack

d. Total intake of simple sugars—average daily intake of sugar is 22 teaspoons (tsp); the majority of our simple sugar intake comes from soft drinks, fruit drinks, desserts, candies, and ready-to-eat cereals; the American Heart Association (AHA) recommends 6 tsp/day for women and 9 tsp/day for men[1]

e. Starch-rich foods that are retained on the teeth for prolonged periods are ultimately degraded to organic acids and can contribute to the production of dental caries

f. Combining cariogenic foods with noncariogenic foods—recent studies indicate that certain cariogenic foods (e.g., canned pears in syrup) are less cariogenic when combined with a particular noncariogenic food (e.g., cheese)

5. Importance of carbohydrates in periodontal health

a. Energy source for the growth and repair of periodontal tissues

b. Protein-sparing nutrient

c. Firm texture of complex carbohydrates can promote circulation in gingival tissue

d. Dietary monosaccharides and disaccharides enhance supragingival bacterial growth and plaque formation; these bacteria set the stage for the growth and development of subgingival bacteria and plaque, which are responsible for the destructive effects of periodontitis

K. Requirements

1. The recommended daily allowance (RDA) of digestible carbohydrate is 130 g/day for adults and children

a. Minimum adult intake (50 to 100 g) prevents use of body protein as an energy source

b. Pregnant and lactating women need additional carbohydrates to prevent ketosis

2. Recommendations

a. The Food and Nutrition Board recommends that 45% to 65% of calories should come from carbohydrates[2]

b. Calories from simple carbohydrates (monosaccharides and disaccharides)—10% or less of the total caloric intake

c. The majority of calories should come from complex carbohydrates (including fiber)

L. Dietary modifications for persons with disease conditions

1. Obesity—reduce total calories and percentage of simple carbohydrates (concentrated sweets) to increase the nutrient density of a lower-calorie diet

2. Genetic defects

a. Lactose intolerance (inability to hydrolyze lactose)—eat fewer milk products, use fermented products, or add a commercial lactose enzyme (lactase) to milk

(1) Yogurt with active-bacteria culture is recommended because the lactose is digested by the yogurt

(2) The main concern for oral and systemic health is an inadequate intake of calcium and vitamin D; a hydrogen breath test can be used for diagnosis

(3) Types of lactose intolerance

(a) Primary—congenital absence of lactase (a brush-border enzyme)

(b) Secondary—temporary or permanent loss of lactase activity resulting from intestinal injury, diseases (e.g., Crohn), or infections which cause injury to the GI mucosa

b. Galactosemia—congenital inability to metabolize galactose; lactose and milk products should be removed from the diet

c. Fructose intolerance—congenital inability to metabolize fructose; fructose and sucrose should be removed from the diet; individuals with fructose intolerance have significantly fewer dental caries

3. Dental caries and periodontal disease—a protective diet should be implemented

a. A diet that is low in retentive carbohydrates

b. Avoidance of cariogenic snacks

c. A diet that is adequate in all nutrients (Table 12-3)

d. Inclusion of foods of firm or hard texture

TABLE 12-3   Dietary Reference Intake, Adequate Intake, and Tolerable Upper Limits of Nutrients Specific to Bone Health

Nutrient	Dietary Reference Intake (DRI)/ Recommended Dietary Allowance (RDA)*	Adequate Intake (AI) (Therapeutic Range)†	Tolerable Upper Limit (UL)‡
Calcium (mg/d)	—	200-1300 mg/d	1000-2500 mg/d
Phosphorus (g/d)	460-1250 g/d for most healthy adults and children	100-275 g/d for infants	3-4 g/d for most healthy adults and children; no determined tolerable UL for infants
Magnesium (mg/d)	80-420 mg/d for most healthy adults and children	30-75 mg/d for infants	65-350 mg/d for most healthy adults and children; No determined tolerable UL for infants.
Vitamin D (µg/d)	13-15 µg/d	—	25-100 µg/d
Fluoride (mg/d)	—	0.01-3 mg/d	0.7-10 mg/d

*Recommended dietary allowance values meet the needs of 97% of individuals in a group. Daily reference intake values are groups of values that provide quantitative estimates of nutrient intake for planning and assessing diets for all healthy individuals.
†Adequate intake (AI), also known as a therapeutic range, is the mean intake for healthy individuals that is used when an RDA value cannot be determined. The lower number represents the adequate intake for infants and children, and the higher range of numbers will vary depending on life stage and gender group. Refer to the National Academies Press website (http://nap.edu/) for more in-depth information. The therapeutic range (AI) is the dose at which physiologic benefits for healthy individuals and decreased risk for toxicity may exist.
‡The lower number represents the upper limits for infants and children, and the higher number represents upper limits for males and females (pregnant and lactating). The tolerable upper limit is the highest level of daily nutrient intake that is likely to pose no risk of adverse health effects.

4. Diabetes (inability to regulate glucose because of insufficiency or relative ineffectiveness of insulin)—dietary treatment (see the section on "Diabetes Mellitus" in Chapter 19)
   a. Two major forms
      (1) Type 1 diabetes—persons with type 1 diabetes require:
         (a) Daily injections of insulin
         (b) Routine blood testing to monitor blood sugar levels
         (c) Routine urine testing to monitor ketone levels
      (2) Type 2 diabetes—persons with type 2 diabetes require:
         (a) Medication to facilitate glucose metabolism
         (b) Specialized diet to help control the disease
         (c) Routine blood testing to monitor blood sugar levels
   b. Signs and symptoms of diabetes mellitus
      (1) Frequent urination (polyuria)
      (2) Excessive thirst (polydipsia)
      (3) Recurring gingival infections
      (4) Extreme hunger (polyphagia)
   c. Dietary recommendations
      (1) Type 1 diabetes
         (a) Is managed primarily with insulin therapy
         (b) A regular pattern of three meals per day, with one or more snacks between meals
         (c) A diet that is rich in complex carbohydrates and dietary fiber
         (d) A diet high in carbohydrates replaced with unsaturated fat and dietary fiber, if elevated triglycerides are present
      (2) Type 2 diabetes
         (a) Regular meal patterns
         (b) Regular physical activity
         (c) Monitoring carbohydrate intake and increasing the consumption of unsaturated fat and dietary fiber, if elevated triglycerides are present

5. Reactive hypoglycemia—rare; symptoms of dizziness, hunger, and heart palpitations are lessened with a low-carbohydrate diet
6. Dumping syndrome—occurs after gastric surgery; postprandial symptoms of nausea, dizziness, cramping, and diarrhea are lessened by a low-monosaccharide, low-disaccharide diet
7. Alcoholism—overconsumption of alcohol may cause malnutrition (see the section on "Chronic Alcohol Abuse and Dependence" in Chapter 19)
   a. Depresses the appetite
   b. Empty-calorie food—provides energy but few other nutrients (e.g., concentrated sweets, alcohol, and fats)
   c. Causes vitamin B depletion because the liver needs niacin and thiamine to metabolize alcohol
   d. Causes folate and iron deficiency
   e. Depresses antidiuretic hormone, causing loss of magnesium, potassium, and zinc in urine
8. Alcohol consumption during pregnancy—has a direct teratogenic effect on the developing fetus: fetal alcohol syndrome (see the section on "Fetal Alcohol Spectrum Disorders" in Chapter 19)
9. Carbohydrate regulation in some hyperlipoproteinemias—total carbohydrate and alcohol intake is controlled; concentrated sweets are restricted

Proteins

A. Definition—complex biologic compounds of high molecular weight that contain nitrogen, hydrogen, oxygen, carbon, and small amounts of sulfur; each protein has a specific size and is made up of amino acid building blocks linked through peptide bonds in a specific arrangement
B. Classifications
   1. Chemical
      a. Simple proteins—contain amino acids only
      b. Compound (conjugated) proteins—contain simple proteins and a nonprotein group

(1) Nucleoproteins
(2) Metalloproteins
(3) Phosphoproteins
(4) Lipoproteins

c. Derived proteins—fragments produced during digestion or hydrolysis (e.g., peptides, peptones, proteases)

2. Biologic

a. Complete proteins contain sufficient amounts of the essential amino acids for normal metabolic reactions; found in foods of animal origin

(1) A total of 20 essential amino acids that cannot be synthesized by humans and must be provided in the diet in sufficient amounts to meet the body's needs

(a) Adult—histidine, isoleucine, leucine, lysine, methionine, phenylalanine, threonine, tryptophan, and valine

(b) Infant—all the above plus histidine and probably taurine

(c) Premature infant—all the above plus cysteine

(2) Nonessential amino acids can be synthesized by the body and need not be provided by the diet but are necessary for normal metabolic reactions; include alanine, arginine, aparagine, aspartic acid, cysteine, glutamic acid, glutamine, glycine, proline, serine, and tyrosine

b. Incomplete proteins have insufficient quantities of one or more essential amino acids to support protein synthesis in humans; plant proteins are often incomplete (e.g., corn protein is low in lysine; legume protein is low in methionine)

c. Complementary proteins are proteins that are incomplete when ingested singly but, when combined, provide sufficient essential amino acids

(1) In a "vegan" (or strict vegetarian) diet, the complementing of plant proteins can be accomplished by combining appropriate incomplete proteins

(a) The amino acids in different foods can complement one another, even when eaten at different meals

(b) Persons on a strict vegetarian diet are at the greatest risk for developing deficiencies in calcium, iron, zinc, and vitamin B_{12} because the major food sources of these nutrients come from animal products

(2) In an "ovolacto"-vegetarian diet, milk and egg proteins can provide the essential amino acids that are inadequate in incomplete plant proteins; however, this diet still may be deficient in iron

d. Protein quality is a measure of a protein's ability to support protein synthesis; it is measured by comparing the test protein with a reference protein, usually egg protein

(1) Amino acid or protein chemical score (CS)—compares the essential amino acid content in a dietary protein to that of a reference protein

(2) Protein efficiency ratio (PER)—measures a protein's ability to support growth

(3) Biologic value (BV)—expression of the percentage of nitrogen retained for maintenance and growth compared with the amount absorbed

(4) Net protein utilization (NPU)—expression of the percentage of retained nitrogen compared with the amount ingested; differs from BV because it takes into account the protein's digestibility

(5) Protein digestibility–corrected amino acid score (PDCAAS)—compares the amino acid balance of a food protein with the amino acid requirements of preschool-aged children and then corrects for digestibility; used by the FDA for labeling

C. Structure

1. Primary—linear sequence of the component amino acids

2. Secondary—steric interaction of amino acids that are close to one another in the linear sequence (e.g., the α-helix and β-sheet)

3. Tertiary—steric interaction between amino acids that are far apart in the linear sequence, which causes folding and the ultimate functional structure of the protein (e.g., disulfide bonds)

4. Quaternary—steric interaction between subunits of proteins with more than one polypeptide chain (e.g., hemoglobin)

D. Digestion, absorption, and transport (see Table 12-1 and Fig. 12-1)

1. Mouth—mechanical breakdown and moistening

2. Stomach

a. Hydrochloric acid from parietal cells denatures or unfolds proteins and activates pepsinogen to give pepsin

b. Pepsin begins the hydrolysis of the peptide bonds of proteins to form peptides and proteoses

3. Small intestine

a. The pancreas secretes bicarbonate into the duodenum to neutralize the acidic products from the stomach and proteolytic enzymes into an inactive form; enzymes activated by trypsin through a hormonal feedback mechanism are chymotrypsin, aminopeptidase, and carboxypeptidase; each hydrolyzes peptide bonds formed by different classes of amino acids

b. Enzymes of the brush border are dipeptidases that hydrolyze dipeptides to amino acids

4. Absorption—at the brush border of the microvilli of the small intestine, absorption occurs both by simple diffusion along a concentration gradient and by active transport at specific amino acid sites involving carrier enzymes, a sodium-ATP pump, and vitamin B_6

5. Transport—absorbed amino acids collected by the portal blood system and transported to the liver

E. Metabolism (see Fig. 12-2)

1. Amino acid pool—a collection of amino acids in a dynamic equilibrium in the liver, blood, and other cells that provides the raw material for the body's protein and amino acid needs

a. Input into the pool comes from proteins in the diet, breakdown of body proteins, and synthesis of nonessential amino acids

b. Output from the pool is for synthesizing body structures, specialized substances (e.g., melanin from tyrosine), and energy, as needed

2. Anabolism
   a. De novo synthesis—requires deoxyribonucleic acid (DNA), messenger ribonucleic acid (mRNA), and ribosomal ribonucleic acid (rRNA)
      (1) In the nucleus, DNA carries the genetic information in groups of three bases that provide the code for the individual amino acids comprising a specific protein
      (2) mRNA transports a copy of the code from DNA into the cytoplasm
      (3) mRNA attaches to a ribosome and acts as a template for the alignment of amino acids that are attached to transfer RNA (tRNA)
      (4) If the proper amino acids are in the correct proportions and the synthetic enzymes and energy are available, the polypeptide chain is synthesized
   b. Transamination
      (1) Nonessential amino acids can be synthesized from the corresponding α-keto acids, an α-amino acid (as the NH_3^+ donor), a specific transaminase enzyme, and the coenzyme pyridoxal phosphate (vitamin B_6)
      (2) The intermediate complex formed in this reaction is called a *Schiff base*

3. Catabolism—amino acids in excess of those needed for the synthesis of proteins and other biomolecules cannot be stored or excreted; they may, however, be deaminated and the α-keto acid used as a metabolic fuel for immediate energy needs or for long-term energy storage as fat
   a. Amino group
      (1) Deamination—loss of the α-amino group, usually in the liver, through transfer to α-ketoglutarate to form glutamate; glutamate is then oxidatively deaminated to yield ammonia (NH_3)
      (2) Urea cycle—series of steps whereby the ammonia produced during deamination is converted to urea for excretion
   b. α-Keto acid
      (1) Ketogenic amino acids are those whose carbon skeleton, after deamination, yields acetyl-CoA or acetoacetyl-CoA, which then yields ketone bodies; high concentrations of ketone bodies lead to some of the undesirable side effects of high-protein, low-carbohydrate diets (e.g., ketoacidosis)
      (2) Glucogenic amino acids are those that yield pyruvate, α-ketoglutarate, and other intermediates of the citric acid cycle that, if needed, can be converted to glucose

4. Nitrogen balance—comparison measurement of the amount of nitrogen ingested with the amount excreted (e.g., urinary nitrogen plus approximately 1 g/day for nail, hair, skin, and perspiration losses) made to determine whether net protein catabolism, anabolism, or equilibrium exists
   a. Positive balance—intake is greater than output; indicates net protein synthesis and is the normal situation for anyone building protein-containing tissue, such as during childhood, pregnancy, and recovery from undernutrition, surgery, or illness
   b. Negative balance—intake is less than output; indicates net protein breakdown, when the body must break down its own protein to meet energy or metabolic needs; can result from insufficient protein (or essential amino acids) or energy intake or from fever, infection, anxiety, or prolonged stress

F. Metabolic regulation
   1. Hormones
      a. Anabolic—growth hormone, insulin, normal thyroid hormone, and sex hormones
      b. Catabolic—adrenocortical hormones and large amounts of thyroid hormone
   2. Vitamins—pyridoxine and riboflavin are necessary for protein synthesis; when they are deficient in the diet, synthesis may be limited

G. Functions
   1. Structural—formation of:
      a. Collagen and elastin
      b. Bone and tooth matrix
      c. Myosin fibrils
      d. Keratin
   2. Dynamic
      a. Transport of nutrients by:
         (1) Lipid-soluble and fat-soluble vitamins
         (2) Iron—transferrin
         (3) Hemoglobin and myoglobin—oxygen
         (4) Protein-bound molecules
         (5) Membrane transport
      b. Regulation and control by:
         (1) Immunoglobulins
         (2) Buffers
         (3) Hormones
         (4) Enzymes
         (5) Blood coagulation—fibrin
         (6) Muscle contraction—actin and myosin
   3. Energy source (4 kcal/g)
   4. Role of proteins in oral biology
      a. Preeruptive effects on teeth—essential for all cells and therefore necessary for normal tooth bud and pulp formation and synthesis of protein matrix for enamel and dentin
      b. Posteruptive effects on teeth
         (1) Essential for maintaining the integrity of pulpal tissue throughout life
         (2) Chemical nature of protein foods can neutralize acids produced by oral bacteria
      c. Periodontal health and disease
         (1) Essential for all cells in the growth, development, and maintenance of the periodontium
         (2) Essential for the normal function of cellular defenses against subgingival bacteria and toxins
         (3) Necessary in the healing and repair of injured tissues from periodontitis or periodontal surgery

H. Requirements
  1. Determination and estimates of protein requirements
    a. Studies of nitrogen balance are used to determine the lowest protein intake that will support homeostasis or equilibrium
    b. Average requirement for reference proteins of 0.8 g/kg/day for young adult males; other groups by extrapolation or interpolation
    c. Estimates for growth needs in infants are based on the amount of protein provided by that quantity of human milk that ensures a satisfactory growth rate
  2. Recommended dietary allowances—developed by the National Research Council; based on 1985 World Health Organization (WHO) recommendations, which use nitrogen balance data; these allowances assume ingestion of good-quality protein in a mixed diet; adjustments are made for growth, pregnancy, and lactation
  3. Food sources—protein needs of an average adult can be met by choosing two or more servings per day of meats, poultry, fish, eggs, dried beans, and nuts
I. Dietary modifications for disease
  1. Genetic disorders
    a. Phenylketonuria (PKU)—inherited enzyme defect in which individuals cannot metabolize the phenylalanine found in almost all proteins; the prescribed diet provides only enough phenylalanine to meet growth and maintenance needs; dietary protein is restricted, but amino acids are provided by a synthetic formula from which the phenylalanine has been removed
    b. Other genetic disorders—maple syrup urine disease, homocystinuria, tyrosinemia, methylmalonic aciduria, propionic acidemia, and isovaleric acidemia are genetic disorders in which amino acid metabolism is altered; treated with low-protein diets and synthetic amino acid formulas
    c. Gout—characterized by excessive uric acid production leading to the formation of urate crystals deposited in the joints; treatment often includes restriction of protein to limit purine and uric acid production
  2. Protein needs are increased during fever, after severe injury and surgery, and by intestinal malabsorption, increased protein loss from the kidneys, or diminished protein synthesis by the liver
  3. Dietary protein must be restricted when the kidneys can no longer remove nitrogenous wastes from the body or in severe liver disease when the nitrogenous byproducts of protein catabolism can no longer be synthesized
  4. Protein-energy (or protein-calorie) malnutrition (PEM or PCM)
    a. Kwashiorkor (classic)—failure of the young child to grow because of insufficient protein intake (usually following weaning from mother's milk); edema often masks muscle wasting
    b. Marasmus (classic)—failure of the infant or young child to grow because of partial starvation; total caloric and protein intakes are insufficient

    c. Adult PEM or PCM—seen even in the developed countries among alcoholic persons and long-term hospitalized patients with acquired immunodeficiency syndrome (AIDS), tuberculosis, or anorexia nervosa

Lipids (Fats)

A. Definition—biochemical compounds composed of carbon, hydrogen, oxygen, and small amounts of phosphorus; insoluble in water and soluble in fatty substances and organic solvents
B. Classification
  1. Simple lipids
    a. True fats—contain fatty acids attached to glycerol (a trihydroxy alcohol) through an ester linkage; these may be monoglycerides, diglycerides, or triglycerides, depending on the number of glycerol-hydroxyl groups esterified; chemical and biochemical characteristics of glycerides depend on the number, order, and types of fatty acids attached
      (1) Saturated fatty acids—contain no double bonds and are found in lipids from animal sources; are solids at room temperature (high melting point)
      (2) Unsaturated fatty acids—contain one or more double bonds and come from plant sources; are usually liquids at room temperature (low melting point)
      (3) Hydrogenation—addition of hydrogen to some or all of the double bonds; used in the manufacture of margarine or butter substitutes from vegetable oils; in partial hydrogenation, some trans bonds are formed and may present a health risk
      (4) Rancidity—addition of oxygen to some of the double bonds of fatty acids that contributes to spoilage; occurs spontaneously in foods and can be reduced by the addition of antioxidants, such as butylated hydroxytoluene (BHT)
      (5) Iodine number—chemical indication of the degree of unsaturation of a fatty acid; the more molecules of iodine bound by the fatty acid, the more unsaturated and the higher the iodine number
    b. Waxes—esters of a fatty acid and an alcohol other than glycerol; the body is unable to use waxes because digestive enzymes do not hydrolyze their ester linkage
  2. Compound lipids contain compounds added to the glycerol and fatty acids
    a. Phospholipids (glycerol + 2 fatty acids + phosphate group = R group)
      (1) Water-soluble emulsifiers (e.g., lecithin, with choline as the R group)
      (2) Membrane constituents (e.g., sphingomyelin)
      (3) Active intermediates in metabolism of lipid compound (e.g., CoA)
    b. Glycolipids—contain a carbohydrate component and are found in the brain and nervous tissue (e.g., cerebrosides)
    c. Lipoproteins—are water soluble and responsible for carrying lipids throughout the body

(1) Chylomicrons—approximately 2% protein; carry exogenous (absorbed from the diet) triglycerides throughout the body

(2) Very-low-density lipoproteins (VLDLs)—9% protein; carry endogenous triglycerides around the body

(3) Low-density lipoproteins (LDLs)—21% protein; carry mostly cholesterol from the liver to peripheral sites

(4) High-density lipoproteins (HDLs)—50% protein; carry cholesterol back to the liver; can be elevated by exercise

3. Derived lipids are compounds whose synthesis begins like fatty acid synthesis, with acetyl groups added on one at a time

a. Sterols—all have a polycyclic nucleus

b. Cholesterol is a precursor for the synthesis of many steroid compounds and a constituent of cell membranes

(1) Sources

(a) Exogenous—average dietary intake is 400 to 600 milligrams (mg) from foods of animal origin

(b) Endogenous—average synthesis in the body is 1 to 2 g/day

(2) Regulation of cholesterol—dietary cholesterol, percentage of fat, ratio of polysaturated to monosaturated to unsaturated fat, and amount of certain fibers in the diet

c. Steroids—similar to sterols but with side-chain modification (e.g., bile acids, sex hormones, adrenocortical hormones, vitamin D)

4. Artificial fats—substances developed for use in foods; have the flavor, appearance, and feel of dietary fats without their physiologic effects

a. Olestra—a zero-kilocalorie (0-kcal) artificial fat made from an indigestible combination of sucrose and fatty acids; may help serum cholesterol levels by directly interfering with cholesterol absorption; may increase the requirement for vitamin E; approved for use in snack foods

b. Simplesse—has approximately 15% of the kilocalorie of the fat it replaces; made by microparticulation of protein; the small protein particles have the feel of fat; not suitable for use in cooking but used in fat-free dairy products and salad dressings

c. Oatrim and maltodextrim—carbohydrate-based fat replacements; mimic the texture and feel of fat by forming gels; are digestible and contribute some calories

C. Digestion, absorption, and transportation (see Table 12-1 and Fig. 12-1)

1. Digestion

a. Mouth—no enzymatic action; mechanical and moistening action only

b. Stomach—gastric lipase hydrolyzes some short-chain and medium-chain fatty acids from triglycerides

c. Small intestine

(1) Gallbladder—bile salts emulsify fats before digestion

(2) Pancreas—pancreatic lipase hydrolyzes fatty acids from triglycerides to form diglycerides and monoglycerides

(3) Intestinal mucosa—lecithinase converts lecithin to fatty acids, monoglyceride, phosphate, and choline

2. Absorption and transport

a. Short-chain fatty acids can be absorbed into the portal system

b. Medium-chain and long-chain fatty acids are water insoluble, require bile as a carrier (emulsifier), and are absorbed in stages

(1) Bile separated out at the intestinal wall and recirculated

(2) Complete breakdown of triglycerides within the mucosal cells by mucosal lipase

(3) Resynthesis of new triglycerides that combine with protein carriers to form chylomicrons

(4) Passage into the lymph system (lacteals) and blood through the thoracic duct

(5) At its destination, lipoprotein lipase hydrolyzes the triglycerides, clearing chylomicrons from blood

(6) Lipoprotein carriers (VLDLs, LDLs, and HDLs) carry endogenous lipids and cholesterol

D. Metabolism (see Fig. 12-2)

1. Anabolism

a. Lipogenesis—synthesis of triglycerides for long-term storage of energy; starting material is acetyl-CoA, which can come from glucogenic amino acids, carbohydrates, or breakdown of dietary lipids; lipogenesis takes place in almost all cells but is most active in adipose cells

b. Synthesis of steroids occurs in all cells

c. Synthesis of lipoproteins occurs mainly in the liver

2. Catabolism

a. β-Oxidation—fatty acids are broken down in a stepwise manner to yield one molecule of acetyl-CoA for every two carbon atoms; acetyl-CoA can be catabolized further by means of the TCA and oxidative phosphorylation

b. Ketone production—when the body's supply of carbohydrates is low, the TCA is depressed and acetyl-CoA from β-oxidation accumulates; alternative route for acetyl-CoA is ketone production; acetoacetone, acetone, and β-hydroxybutyrate are the ketone bodies; excess ketone production can cause ketosis, ketonuria, and ketoacidosis (which is sometimes fatal)

E. Metabolic regulators

1. Vitamins as coenzyme precursors

a. Anabolism—biotin, riboflavin (in flavin adenine dinucleotide [FAD]), niacin (in nicotinamide adenine dinucleotide [NAD]), and pantothenic acid (in CoA) (see Fig. 12-2)

b. Catabolism—riboflavin, niacin, and pantothenic acid
2. Hormones
   a. Anabolism—insulin
   b. Catabolism—ACTH, thyroid-stimulating hormone (TSH), epinephrine, and glucagon
3. Enzymes necessary for the metabolism of lipids are synthesized or inhibited in response to the relative amounts of substrates and products available
F. Biologic role and functions of lipids
   1. Structural components of cell membrane
   2. Energy source
      a. Provide 9 kcal/g (compared with 4 kcal/g for protein or carbohydrates)
      b. Long-term storage of energy
   3. Carrier medium of fat-soluble vitamins
   4. Protective padding for body organs
   5. Insulation for the maintenance of body temperature
   6. Role of lipids in oral biology
      a. Cariostatic properties
         (1) Lipids provide a coating on the tooth's surface and form a protective pellicle on the tooth
         (2) Lipids act by neutralizing the acids produced by bacterial metabolism of the plaque biofilm; they raise the pH and decrease risk of the demineralization of enamel
      b. No relationship between dietary fat and periodontal disease
      c. A review of the literature on obesity and periodontal disease suggests that they both confound each other, and obesity itself has been recognized as a major risk factor for periodontal disease; adverse effects of obesity on periodontium may be mediated through proinflammatory cytokines and various other bioactive substances
G. Nutritional requirements
   1. Essential fatty acids (EFAs)—cannot be synthesized in sufficient amounts to meet the body's needs; must be supplied in the diet; for humans the only EFAs are linoleic (ω-6) and linolenic (ω-3) (omega fatty acids); requirement is approximately 3% of total kilocalories
      a. Function—necessary for the synthesis of membranes and prostaglandins (local hormone)
      b. Deficiency symptoms—seen in infants on low polyunsaturated fatty acid (PUFA) diets and in adults receiving total parenteral nutrition feedings without lipids; the deficiency is characterized by slow growth, reproductive failure, and skin lesions
   2. Recommendations (dietary goals as recommended by the AHA)
      a. Total fats: 30% or less of total kilocalories; majority of calories should come from monounsaturated and polyunsaturated fatty acids
      b. Cholesterol: 300 mg/day or less; 200 mg/day for high-risk individuals
      c. Saturated fats—avoid saturated and *trans* fatty acids (found in processed foods); less than 10% of total kilocuries should come from saturated fatty acids
      d. Two weekly servings of fatty fish such as tuna or salmon

3. The seventh edition of *Dietary Guidelines for Americans* (2010) makes similar recommendations for healthy persons age 2 years and older
H. Dietary modifications for disease
   1. Cardiovascular disease (CVD)—blood vessel lumens become narrower and sometimes completely blocked because of the plaques caused by the accumulation of fatty substances, cellular debris, and calcium; blood pressure and the work required of the heart increase; formation of clots increase, and the result may be a heart attack (myocardial infarction) or stroke (cerebrovascular accident)
      a. Hyperlipoproteinemias—for diagnosis, elevation of serum VLDL, LDL, and chylomicron levels indicates that a client is at risk for CVD; a genetic predisposition for certain hyperlipoproteinemias exists; elevated HDL levels may exert a protective effect against CVD; routine exercise elevates HDL levels in most people
      b. Dietary factors that may increase serum lipids—high intake of cholesterol, saturated fats, total fats, sucrose, fructose, and ethanol (alcohol)
      c. Dietary factors that may decrease serum lipids—monounsaturated and polyunsaturated fatty acids, omega fatty acids (fish oils), and pectin; ethanol in moderate amounts may have a protective effect by increasing HDL levels; unidentified substances in garlic, yeast, onions, and some wines may also have a protective effect
   2. Obesity—because fats are a concentrated source of calories (9 kcal/g), most reducing diets recommend a decrease in fat intake; fat should not be too severely restricted because it adds to the palatability and satiety of the diet
   3. Gallbladder disease and chronic pancreatitis—often cause pain after lipid ingestion; diet may have to be restricted in fats until the conditions are corrected
   4. Cystic fibrosis and malabsorption disorders—often treated with synthetic medium-chain triglyceride formulas that are more easily absorbed
   5. Dumping syndrome and gastric ulcers—often treatment involves increasing fat in the diet to delay gastric emptying
   6. Epilepsy—children with some types of epilepsy may be effectively treated with a ketogenic diet that is high in fats, is low in carbohydrates, and causes a ketotic condition

Vitamins

A. Definition—organic substances that are essential to life and are needed in very small amounts; serve in regulatory functions and often act as coenzymes or precursors of coenzymes; some vitamins can be produced in precursor form or activated in the body
B. Classification
   1. Water-soluble vitamins
      a. Vitamin C
      b. B-complex vitamins
   2. Fat-soluble vitamins
      a. Vitamin A

b. Vitamin D
c. Vitamin E
d. Vitamin K

C. Chemistry and general properties
1. Water-soluble vitamins
   a. Soluble in water
   b. Sensitive to heat, light, and oxygen
   c. Contain the elements carbon, hydrogen, oxygen, and nitrogen, and, in some cases, other elements such as cobalt or sulfur
   d. Absorbed into blood by both active and passive transport from the upper portion of the digestive tract (see Fig. 12-1); vitamin B_{12} requires the intrinsic factor for absorption
   e. Transported free and unbound to cells by blood
   f. Minimal storage of excess dietary vitamins except for:
      (1) Vitamin C—stores may last 30 to 90 days
      (2) Vitamin B_{12}—stores may last many years in those without pernicious anemia
      (3) Folic acid—stores may last 4 to 5 months
   g. Are excreted in urine
   h. Should be supplied in the diet almost every day
   i. Deficiency symptoms often develop rapidly
   j. Are relatively nontoxic with excessive dietary intake, although the increased use of over-the-counter (OTC) "megavitamin" preparations has caused the appearance of toxic symptoms
2. Fat-soluble vitamins
   a. Soluble in fat and fat solvents (some water-soluble derivatives are available)
   b. More stable than water-soluble vitamins in light, heat, and oxygen
   c. Contain only elements of carbon, hydrogen, and oxygen
   d. Must be emulsified and carried across the membranes of the intestinal cells in the presence of fat and bile (see Fig. 12-1); any conditions that decrease the digestion, absorption, or transport of lipids will lower the usable amount of fat-soluble vitamins
   e. Absorbed into the lymphatic system and transported by attachment to protein carriers
   f. Not readily excreted
   g. Not absolutely necessary in the diet every day
   h. Amount ingested in excess of the daily need is stored in the liver and fatty tissues
   i. Deficiency symptoms slow to develop
   j. Toxic with chronic excessive intake
D. General functions
1. Water-soluble vitamins
   a. Form coenzymes for energy metabolism
   b. Synthesis of red blood cells and DNA
2. Fat-soluble vitamins—play a role in:
   a. Vision
   b. Maintenance of the body's mucosal linings and epithelial cells
   c. Integrity of mineralized tissues of bone and teeth by regulating the calcium biond phosphorus levels in the body

d. Cellular antioxidant
e. Normal blood clotting

E. Nutritional requirements—dietary reference intake (DRI) and RDA are based on vitamin and mineral intake from food, not supplements; for an elaboration of DRI and RDA, see the section on "Methods for Assessment of Dietary Intake" later in this chapter. Refer to "Food and Nutrition" at the National Academies Press website of the National Academy of Science, available at http://nap.edu/; also see Website Information and Resources table at the end of this chapter
F. Dietary sources, specific body functions, and symptoms of deficiencies and toxicities (Table 12-4)
G. Role of vitamins in oral biology
1. Functions
   a. Tooth formation (Table 12-5)
   b. Periodontium (Table 12-5)
2. Oral manifestations of deficiencies and toxicities (see Table 12-4)

Minerals

A. Definition—inorganic elements that are essential to life; serve both structural and regulatory functions
B. Classification (see Table 12-4)
1. Macrominerals—present in relatively high amounts in body tissues
2. Trace elements—present at less than 0.005% of body weight
C. Chemistry and general functions
1. Exist as inorganic ions
2. Chemical identity not altered in the body or in food
3. Indestructible
4. Soluble in water and tend to form acidic or basic solutions
5. Vary in amounts absorbed and in pathways of excretion (see Fig. 12-1)
6. Some readily absorbed into blood and transported freely
7. Some require carriers for absorption and transportation
8. Excessive intake can be toxic
D. General functions
1. Maintenance of acid-base balance
2. Coenzymes or catalysts for biologic reactions
3. Components of essential body compounds
4. Maintenance of water balance
5. Transmission of nerve impulses
6. Regulation of muscle contraction
7. Growth of oral and other body tissues
E. Nutritional requirements (see information on the National Academies Press website)
F. Dietary sources, specific body functions, and symptoms of deficiencies and toxicities (see Table 12-4)
G. Role of minerals in oral biology
1. Function (see Table 12-5)
   a. Tooth formation
   b. Periodontium
2. Oral manifestations of deficiencies and toxicities (see Table 12-4)

TABLE 12-4 Nutrients and Their Related Effects on the Oral Cavity

Nutrient	Dietary Sources	Major Body Functions	Oral Manifestations of Nutrient Deficiency	Oral Manifestations of Nutrient Excess
Vitamins				
Vitamin A	Provitamin A, orange, yellow, and green vegetables and fruit Retinol: milk, cheese, butter, fortified margarine, egg yolk	Antioxidant Constituent of rhodopsin Maintains epithelial tissue involved in bone growth and remodeling	Ameloblast atrophy Faulty bone and tooth formation Enamel hypoplasia Xerostomia Cleft lip Increased risk of candidiasis Decreased taste sensitivity	Hypertrophy of bone Cracking and bleeding lips Cheilosis Erythemic gingivae
Vitamin D	Sunlight, oily fish, eggs, dairy, fortified milk, margarine	Promotes growth and mineralization of bones and teeth Increases absorption of calcium at intestine	Loss of alveolar and mandibular bone Delayed dentition Increased caries rate Loss of lamina dura around roots of tooth Failure of bones to heal	Pulp calcification Enamel hypoplasia
Vitamin E	Vegetable oils, seeds, green leafy vegetables, margarine and whole-grain or fortified cereals, wheat germ, nuts	Antioxidant Involved in cellular respiration and synthesis of body compounds Prevents hemolysis of red blood cells (RBCs)	Loss of resistance to inflammation in peridontium	No effect noted
Vitamin K	Green and yellow vegetables, meats, microflora in the gut	Important in blood clotting Involved in the formation of active prothrombin	Gingival hemorrhage Increased risk of candidiasis	No effect noted
Vitamin C	Citrus fruits, tomatoes, green peppers, broccoli, strawberries, melons	Important in collagen synthesis Important in the body's use of iron, B_{12}, and folic acid	Odontoblast atrophy Porotic dentin formation Gingival inflammation Cyanotic gingival tissues Ulceration and necrosis Slow wound healing Defects in collagen formation	No effect noted
Thiamin	Pork, whole grains, nuts, legumes	Coenzyme in reactions involving removal of carbon dioxide in carbohydrate metabolism Synthesized by intestinal bacteria in large intestine	Increased sensitivity and burning sensation of oral mucosa Loss of taste and appetite	No effect noted
Riboflavin	Dairy products, grains	Functions as a coenzyme in the metabolism of carbohydrate, protein, and fat Synthesized by intestinal bacteria in the large intestine	Angular cheilosis Atrophy of filiform papillae Enlarged fungiform papillae Shiny, red lips Painful tongue Glossitis	No effect noted
Niacin	Liver, meat, fish, poultry, cereals, legumes, peanuts	Coenzyme in energy (ATP) production	Loss of filiform and fungiform papillae Mucositis Stomatitis Glossitis Ulcerative gingivitis Glossodynia	No effect noted
Pyridoxine	Meat, poultry, fish, vegetables, whole-grain cereals, egg yolk	Coenzyme involved in amino acid metabolism Converts tryptophan to niacin Role in hemoglobin synthesis	Angular cheilosis Sore, burning mouth Glossitis Glossodynia Stomatitis Deficiency usually occurs in combination with other B vitamins	No effect noted
Pantothenic acid	Organ meats, whole-grain cereals, broccoli, avocados	Constituent of coenzyme A, which plays a central role in energy metabolism	No effect noted	No effect noted

(Continued)

TABLE 12-4   Nutrients and Their Related Effects on the Oral Cavity—cont'd

Nutrient	Dietary Sources	Major Body Functions	Oral Manifestations of Nutrient Deficiency	Oral Manifestations of Nutrient Excess
Cobalamin	Meat, poultry, eggs, fish, shellfish, dairy products	Coenzyme involved in synthesis of single carbon units in nucleic acid metabolism Important in RBC formation and myelin synthesis	Stomatitis Hemorrhagic gingiva Pale to yellow mucosa Glossopyrosis Glossitis Atrophy and burning tongue Altered taste Halitosis Oral paresthesia Detachment of periodontal fibers Bone loss Xerostomia Aphthous ulcers	No effect noted
Folate	Fortified grain products, liver, kidney, yeast, mushrooms, leafy green vegetables, legumes	Coenzyme involved in RNA and DNA synthesis Important in the proper formation of neural tubes during fetal development	Glossitis Enlargement of fungiform papillae Ulcerations along edge of tongue Gingivitis Neural tube defects: cleft palate and lip	Excess can mask cobalamin deficiency Pale mucosa Angular cheilosis
Biotin	Liver, kidney, milk, egg yolk, cereals	Coenzyme required for the synthesis and oxidation of fats and carbohydrates and for deamination of proteins	Glossitis Gray mucosa Atrophy of lingual papillae	No effect noted
Minerals				
Calcium	Milk, cheese, dark-green vegetables, fortified breads, juices and cereals, canned salmon	Bone and tooth formation Blood clotting Nerve transmission Muscle contraction	Incomplete calcification of teeth Risk of hemorrhage Increased susceptibility to caries and periodontal disease	No effect noted
Phosphorus	Milk, cheese, meat, poultry, grains, eggs	Bone and tooth formation Acid-base balance Release of energy: adenosine triphosphate (ATP), adenosine diphosphate (ADP)	Incomplete calcification of teeth Failure of dentin formation Increased susceptibility to caries during tooth development Increased susceptibility to periodontal disease	No effect noted
Sulfur	Meat, fish, poultry, legumes	Important in oxidation reduction reactions Body water balance	No effect noted	No effect noted
Potassium	Meats, milk, many fruits, fish, eggs	Acid-base balance Body water balance Nerve function Affects heart muscle contraction	No effect noted	No effect noted
Chlorine	Table salt, cured and pickled foods, water	Formation of gastric juice Body water balance Acid-base balance	No effect noted	No effect noted
Sodium	Table salt; cured, processed, canned, and pickled foods; broth	Acid-base balance Body water balance Nerve function	Decrease in salivary flow	Dry, sticky tongue and oral mucous membranes
Magnesium	Whole grains, green leafy vegetables, nuts, beans, bananas	Activates enzymes involved in energy metabolism Maintains calcium homeostasis	Alveolar bone fragility Gingival hyperplasia Enamel hypoplasia Widening of periodontal ligament	No effect noted
Iron	Egg yolk, meats, liver, whole grains, dark-green vegetables, dried fruits	Constituent of hemoglobin and enzymes involved in energy metabolism	Angular cheilosis Pallor of lips or oral mucosa Atrophy of filiform papillae Decreased resistance to infection Glossitis Increased risk of candidiasis	No effect noted

TABLE 12-4 Nutrients and Their Related Effects on the Oral Cavity—cont'd

Nutrient	Dietary Sources	Major Body Functions	Oral Manifestations of Nutrient Deficiency	Oral Manifestations of Nutrient Excess
Fluoride	Drinking water, tea, seafood	Important in the maintenance of bone structure. Forms strong apatite crystals during tooth formation	Decreased resistance to dental caries	Enamel fluorosis
Zinc	Lamb, beef, oysters, eggs, peanuts, whole grains	Required for synthesis of DNA, RNA, and protein. Bone growth and metabolism	Impaired taste. Loss of tongue sensation. Delayed wound healing. Impaired keratinization of epithelial cells. Increased susceptibility to periodontal disease. Flattened filiform papillae	No effect noted
Copper	Shellfish, oysters, crabs, liver, nuts, soy products, legumes	Important catalyst in hemoglobin synthesis	Decreased trabecular pattern. Decreased tissue vascularity. Fragility of tissue	No effect noted
Selenium	Seafood, kidney, liver, dairy products, whole grains, nuts	Antioxidant	No effect noted	Associated with increased dental caries
Manganese	Whole grains, legumes, nuts, tea, green leafy vegetables	Normal skeletal development. Involved in fat synthesis, urea formation, and energy release	No effect noted	Associated with increased dental caries
Iodine	Marine fish and shellfish, table salt, eggs	Constituent of thyroid hormones. Regulates energy metabolism	No effect noted	No effect noted
Molybdenum	Legumes, whole grain cereals, organ meats	Constituent of enzymes involved in uric acid formation and oxidation of aldehydes	No effect noted	No effect noted
Chromium	Vegetables, whole grains, wheat germ, nuts, mushrooms, beer and wine	Involved in carbohydrate and lipid metabolism	No effect noted	No effect noted
Cobalt	Liver, kidney, fish, poultry eggs, tempeh	Important in RBC formation as a component of B_{12}	No effect noted	No effect noted
Other Nutrients				
Carbohydrates	Breads, cereals and grains, starchy vegetables, fruits	Source of energy	Decrease in caries rate as carbohydrate intake decreases in population and individuals	Cariogenic; causative risk factor for dental caries. Form, frequency, and total contact time influence cariogenicity
Fats	Cooking oils, butter, fats found in meat, fish, poultry with skin, dairy products, etc.	Source of energy. Cariostatic; antimicrobial action that produces an oily film on enamel and protects against cariogenic challenges	Difficult to develop a deficiency	Cariostatic: antimicrobial action that produces an oily film on enamel and protects against cariogenic challenges
Protein	Meat, lean meat, fish, poultry, eggs, legumes, tofu, dairy products, peanut butter	Source of energy. Cariostatic	Defects in composition, eruption pattern, and resistance to decay during periods of tooth development. Increased susceptibility to soft tissue infection, poor healing, and tissue regeneration	No effect noted
Water	Tap water, bottled water, water used in coffee and tea; some fruits and vegetables contain water	Source of hydration	Dehydration. Fragility of epithelial tissues. Decreased muscle strength for chewing. Xerostomia. Fissured tongue	No effect noted

Data from DePaola DP, Touger-Decker R, Rigassio-Radler D, Faine MP: Nutrition and dental medicine. In Shils ME et al, editors: *Modern nutrition in health and disease,* ed 11, Baltimore, 2012, Williams & Wilkins; Davis JR, Stegeman CA: *The dental hygienist's guide to nutritional care,* ed 4, Philadelphia, 2015, Saunders; and Palmer C: *Diet and nutrition in oral health,* ed 2, Upper Saddle River, NJ, 2007, Pearson Prentice Hall.

TABLE 12-5 Effects of Nutrients on Oral Tissues and Their Role in Tooth Formation

Nutrients	Effects on Oral Soft and Hard Tissue	Role in Tooth Formation
Vitamin A	Synthesis and function of epithelial cells Maintenance of the integrity of the sulcus Normal growth and function of salivary glands Essential for activity of epiphyseal cartilage cells and normal endochondral bone growth	Normal growth of dentin and enamel Normal growth of periodontal tissues and maintenance of epithelium
Vitamin D	No effects noted	Controls calcification of dentin and enamel by regulating calcium absorption in the intestines
Vitamin C	Synthesis of connective tissue Essential for integrity of capillaries and oral mucosa Needed for normal bone matrix formation Needed for normal phagocytic function and antibody synthesis in host defense system	Integrity of blood vessels in gingival and pulpal tissues Hydroxylation of proline and lysine in collagen synthesis Normal formation of dentin
B-Complex Vitamins		
Niacin	Integrity of oral tissues	No effects noted
Folacin	Normal synthesis of protein compounds in oral tissues (e.g., hemoglobin and enzymes)	No effects noted
Thiamin	Normal energy metabolism during development and maintenance of oral tissue	No effects noted
Riboflavin	Energy metabolism of oral tissues	No effects noted
Pyridoxine	Normal carbohydrate metabolism and hemoglobin synthesis in oral tissues	No effects noted
Cobalamin	Integrity of nerve tissue and normal red blood cell formation in oral tissues	No effects noted
Other Nutrients		
Calcium/phosphorus ratio	No effects noted	Normal tooth and bone mineralization
Fluoride	No effects noted	Forms dentin and enamel
Iron	Normal hemoglobin formation and carbon dioxide transport to tissue	No effects noted
Fiber	Stimulates salivary flow and integrity of periodontal tissues	No effects noted
Protein	Synthesis of antibodies and leukocytes Synthesis of epithelial and connective tissues in the healing process Maintains integrity of periodontal tissues	Formation of matrix of dentin and enamel Collagen formation

Data from DePaola DP, Touger-Decker R, Rigassio-Radler D, Faine M: Nutrition and oral medicine. In Shils ME et al, editors: *Modern nutrition in health and disease,* ed 12, Baltimore, 2012, Williams & Wilkins.

Water

A. Definition—essential nutrient abundantly found in foods and beverages; makes up 50% to 60% of total body weight; survival without water is possible only up to 2 or 3 days

B. Total body water
   1. Body water, as a percentage of body weight, decreases with age, ranging from 69% in newborn infants to 49% in women
   2. Distribution—majority is intracellular, with the remainder being extracellular in serum, cerebrospinal fluid, tissue spaces, and saliva
      a. Intracellular
         (1) Enclosed within the cell membrane
         (2) Accounts for two thirds of the total
         (3) Increases with increased body cell mass
      b. Extracellular compartment
         (1) Intravascular
            (a) Approximately 3 liters (L)
            (b) Includes water in blood vessels

         (2) Intercellular (interstitial)
            (a) Approximately 12 L
            (b) Fluids that leave blood vessels
            (c) Fluids present in spaces between and surrounding each cell

C. Biologic role and functions
   1. Is the medium in which most of the body's reactions take place
   2. Is the means for transporting vital materials to cells and waste products away from cells
   3. Regulates a constant body temperature
   4. Maintains a constant composition of elements in body fluids (e.g., calcium, sodium, fluoride)
   5. Is part of the chemical structure of compounds that form cells (e.g., proteins)
   6. Is active in many chemical reactions (e.g., digestion of a disaccharide)
   7. Serves as a solvent (e.g., amino acids dissolve in water); this permits their transport to body cells

8. Lubricates and protects sensitive tissue around joints and mucosal linings
D. Water balance
 1. Intake—controlled by thirst sensations; total daily intake need ranges from 1 to 3 L at a minimum to replace daily water losses; sources of water intake are:
  a. Ingested liquids and foods—1200 to 2000 milliliters (mL) per day
  b. Metabolic water from the oxidation of foods—300 to 350 mL/day
 2. Elimination—total water output is 1500 to 3000 mL/day
  a. Sensible or measurable losses—occur through the kidneys as urine and through the bowel as feces; constant daily losses amount to 500 to 800 mL
  b. Insensible or unmeasurable losses—occur through the lungs with expired air and through the skin as perspiration; daily losses vary considerably, with an average of 850 to 1200 mL
E. Regulation
 1. Potassium and sodium concentrations are responsible for maintaining water balance; when extracellular sodium equals intracellular potassium, water will not move into or out of the cell
 2. Mechanisms of regulation
  a. Thirst response—when sodium increases, it stimulates the hypothalamus and increases the urge to drink
  b. Excretion regulation
   (1) Increased sodium stimulates the hypothalamus to signal the pituitary to release antidiuretic hormone (ADH), and water is resorbed in the kidney tubules
   (2) Decreased sodium causes the release of aldosterone, which causes resorption of sodium at the kidney tubules
F. Requirements—include water from liquids and food
 1. For men, the adequate intake (AI) is 15 to 16 cups (3.7 L) per day
 2. For women, the adequate intake (AI) is 11 to 12 cups (2.7 L) per day
G. Causes of water deficiency and conditions of toxicity
 1. Dehydration
  a. Malfunction of kidneys
  b. Blood loss
  c. Vomiting
  d. Diarrhea
  e. Inadequate fluid intake
 2. Water intoxication
  a. Edema
  b. Hypertension
  c. Sodium retention

SPECIALIZED CELLS OF ORAL TISSUES: EFFECTS OF NUTRIENTS

A. Epithelial cells
 1. Important in tooth formation during the embryonic period
 2. Make up the outer layers of tissue in the oral mucosa

  a. Rapid cell renewal, especially in the sulcular area
  b. Cell renewal more frequent with increasing age
 3. Important in the normal development of salivary glands
 4. Vitamin A and protein are essential for the normal proliferation of epithelial cells
B. Fibroblasts
 1. Synthesize collagen fibrils in connective tissues of the gingiva, periodontal ligament, and pulp
 2. Throughout life, fibroblasts maintain a rate of collagen synthesis equal to that of collagen breakdown; nutrient deficiencies can interfere with this equilibrium and cause a net loss of collagen tissue
 3. Vitamin C, zinc, copper, and protein are important in collagen formation
C. Cementoblasts and cementocytes
 1. Synthesize the protein matrix for cementum; vitamin C, zinc, copper, and protein are essential
 2. Calcify the protein matrix; protein, calcium, phosphorus, and vitamin D are essential
 3. Cementum is avascular and part acellular
 4. Cellular cementum consists of cementocytes that depend on diffusion from the periodontal ligament for their nutrient supply
D. Ameloblasts
 1. Synthesize the protein matrix for enamel; vitamins A and C, zinc, copper, and protein are essential
 2. Calcify the protein matrix; protein, calcium, phosphorus, and vitamin D are essential; fluoride improves the quality of the apatite crystals formed
 3. Once enamel is formed, no metabolic cells are present
E. Odontoblasts
 1. Synthesize the protein matrix for dentin; vitamins A and C, zinc, copper, and protein are essential
 2. Calcify the protein matrix; protein, calcium, phosphorus, and vitamin D are essential; fluoride improves the quality of the apatite crystals formed
 3. Once dentin is formed, no metabolic cells are present, except in reaction to trauma; with trauma, new odontoblasts can form (possibly from pulpal tissue), and secondary dentin can be laid down
F. Osteocytes—osteoblasts and osteoclasts
 1. Function in the synthesis of the alveolus
 2. Function in the lifelong process of bone apposition (osteoblasts) and resorption (osteoclasts) in the alveolus
 3. Nutrients important in the formation and maintenance of the alveolus are protein; vitamins A, C, and D; zinc; copper; calcium; and phosphorus

ENERGY BALANCES AND WEIGHT CONTROL

A. Definition—energy balance is a dynamic state in which the calories from food are equal to the caloric needs of the body; changes in energy balance result in a relative gain or loss in body weight
 1. Lean body mass is highly metabolically active; basal metabolism is generally higher in people with greater amounts of lean body mass

2. In older adults, increases in body weight and body fat are not attributed to increased intake but are related to decrease in energy expenditure from loss of lean body mass

B. Measurement of energy
   1. By calorimetry—food sample is burned in oxygen in an enclosed vessel surrounded by water; 1 kcal is the amount of heat produced sufficient to raise the temperature of 1 kg of water to 1°C; the commonly used term *calorie* has the same definition
   2. In the body—carbon, hydrogen, and oxygen (from protein, carbohydrates, alcohol, or fats) are converted to carbon dioxide, water, and energy; energy is produced in the form of ATP; when needed, each ATP molecule loses a high-energy phosphate bond and becomes adenosine diphosphate (ADP) with a release of approximately 7.3 kcal/mole

C. Energy-producing systems
   1. Blood glucose—immediate and preferred source of energy for cellular metabolism; glycogen stores provide glucose through glycogenolysis during the short periods of fasting between meals and in response to hormonal signals during sudden movement or intense exercise
      a. Protein—can be used as an energy source when the blood glucose level falls; glucogenic amino acids are converted to glucose after deamination by gluconeogenesis; in a starvation state, body proteins are used for energy, which may cause irreversible damage if the essential protein components of the body are catabolized
      b. Fat—mobilized from adipose tissue; triglycerides are broken down into glycerol and fatty acids in the liver; fatty acids are catabolized by β-oxidation to acetyl-CoA
      c. Ethanol (alcohol)—can be oxidized to acetaldehyde, which is then converted into acetyl-CoA
   2. Acetyl-CoA—enters the TCA from many sources
   3. ATP—made during the process of oxidative phosphorylation in the mitochondria; proteins, carbohydrates, and fats do not yield the same number of ATP molecules per molecule of starting material because of their difference in molecular structure; to estimate the stored energy of foods, use these approximations: protein, 4 kcal/g; carbohydrate, 4 kcal/g; fat, 9 kcal/g; and ethanol, 7 kcal/g

D. Energy-using systems—ATP produced during catabolism is used by the body for biosynthetic activities, muscle contraction, ion transport, nerve conduction, and maintenance of body temperature
   1. Energy for basal metabolism—*basal metabolic rate* (BMR) is a measure of the energy required to maintain a living state while at rest and without food; includes respiration, circulation, maintenance of body temperature, muscle tone, glandular activities, and cellular metabolism
      a. Conditions for BMR measurement—postabsorptive state; muscles totally relaxed; awake; environmental temperature between 20°C and 25°C (68°F and 77°F); free of emotional stress; not during ovulation

   b. Factors influencing the BMR—age, genetics, gender, body size, nutritional state, muscular training, pathologic conditions, thyroid gland activity, climate, and altitude
   2. Energy for activity—the activity component of the energy requirement is for voluntary physical activity and varies from 20% of the BMR for sedentary activity to 50% or more of the BMR for heavy activity; factors influencing energy needs for the activity component include the size of the individual and the intensity and duration of the activity
   3. Thermic effect of food (TEF)—energy required to digest, absorb, and metabolize food; also called *nonshivering thermogenesis* because a slight elevation in body temperature occurs after a meal; not a clearly defined phenomenon; believed to include the energy needed to increase muscular contractions of the digestive tract, increases the synthesis of digestive enzymes and transports molecules; amounts to about 5% to 10% of the BMR and activity energy components

E. Nutritional requirements: determined by intake of food energy that allows the maintenance of ideal weight; data have been gathered from animal studies, balance studies, and intake surveys
   1. Recommendations represent the average needs of people in each age group and within a given activity category
   2. Recommendations are influenced by body size, gender, climate, age, and activity level

F. Weight management and control
   1. Calculating caloric intake needs—body mass index (BMI) and ideal body weight (IBW); see the section on "Complete Nutritional Assessment" later in this chapter
      a. BMI—approximate positive correlation of height and weight with body fat ($r = +0.7 - 0.8$); used to assess obesity and as an indicator of optimal weight for health (Table 12-6); for example, overweight adults with a BMI greater than 25 are at risk for comorbid diseases
      (1) Calculate BMI by dividing body weight in kilograms (kg) by the height in square meters (m^2); for example, a man weighing 270 pounds (122.7 kg) who is 6 feet (3.34 m^2) tall has a BMI of approximately 37

TABLE 12-6   Body Mass Index Classification Chart

	Obesity Class	Body Mass Index (BMI) (1 kg/m²)
Underweight	—	<18.5
Normal	—	18.5-24.9
Overweight	—	25.0-29.9
Obesity	I	30.0-34.9
	II	35.0-39.9
Extreme obesity	III	≥40

Modified from National Institutes of Health: *Clinical guidelines on the identification, evaluation, and treatment of overweight and obesity in adults: The Evidence Report.* Washington, DC, 1998, NIH.

(2) BMI does not differentiate between lean body mass and fat mass; thus could inaccurately label an individual as "obese"

b. Waist circumference is a more accurate method of determining central obesity, also known as *abdominal obesity* in an individual; puts an individual at greater risk of CVD

   (1) Women with waist measurements greater than 35 inches are at risk for comorbid conditions

   (2) Men with waist measurements greater than 40 inches are at risk for comorbid conditions

   (3) Waist circumference standards used for the general population may not apply to individuals under 5 feet in height or with a BMI of 35 or greater

c. Determining ideal body weight (IBW)

   (1) Male IBW $= 106 + (6 \times$ inches over 5 feet tall)

   (2) Female IBW $= 100 + (5 \times$ inches over 5 feet tall)

   (3) For individuals under 5 feet, subtract 2 lb for each inch below 5 feet

d. Alternative method—decreasing usual caloric intake by 500 kcal/day usually allows a weight loss of 1 lb per week; this loss may reach a plateau as the body adjusts to a new BMR

e. Refer to www.choosemyplate.gov to determine individual caloric needs

2. Types of diet modifications

a. Balanced, low-calorie diet—the safest and healthiest reducing diet (e.g., Weight Watchers diet), if calories are approximately 1200 kcal/day and the intake is balanced and varied

b. Low-carbohydrate, high-protein diet—risk of development of ketosis (e.g., Atkins diet, the Zone diet, South Beach diet) exists

c. Low-fat diet—may deprive the individual of essential fatty acids and fat-soluble vitamins; causes rapid emptying of the stomach (low satiety) and may make food seem flavorless; most individuals can decrease their usual fat intake without any harmful effects

d. High-fiber diet—increases fiber and bulk in the diet and allows a more rapid transit time for food in the GI tract; fiber also binds other nutrients, so they are not completely absorbed; moderate increases in the fiber content of the diet (e.g., in well-designed vegetarian diets) appear to be helpful in treating diabetes, diverticulosis, and hypercholesterolemia as well as in decreasing the total caloric intake of reducing diets; very-high-fiber diets cause GI discomfort and may induce mineral deficiencies

e. Single-food (monotonous) diet—no one food by itself can provide a balance of nutrients; diets that promote a single food with unrealistic claims are not recommended (e.g., the grapefruit diet, the cabbage soup diet)

f. Liquid formulas (protein)—very-low-calorie diets; have been successfully used in treating morbidly obese persons in carefully monitored hospital settings but are not recommended for the individual (e.g., Optifast)

3. Prescription drugs used for weight loss are recommended for individuals with a BMI of 30 or greater with no obesity-related risk factors or for those with a BMI of 27 to 29.9 with obesity-related risk factors; adverse side effects have been observed in long-term use of such drugs; prescription drugs include:

a. Noradrenergic drugs for short-term weight loss

   (1) Diethylpropion

   (2) Phentermine (e.g., Zantry, Adipex-P, Fastin)

   (3) Mazindol

b. Serotonergic drugs

   (1) Fenfluramine (also phentermine plus fenfluramine, or Phen-Fen) and dexfen-fluramine (Redux) were removed from the U.S. market because of reports of primary pulmonary hypertension, heart valve abnormalities, and death associated with their use

   (2) Fluoxetine (not FDA approved for treating obesity)

c. Sibutramine (Meridia) is an approved combination of serotonin and adrenergic drugs; centrally acting agent that increases satiety but has little effect on hunger

d. Orlistat (Xenical prescription or alli OTC) is a lipase inhibitor; interferes with fat digestion; taking the drugs with meals inhibits fat absorption by 30%

4. Activity in weight management—even moderate activity such as walking will increase caloric expenditure and should be considered in every weight loss program; moderate exercise also improves muscle tone, stimulates circulation, increases BMR, and often creates a sense of well-being

5. Behavior modification—eating habits and attitudes often must be changed to prevent weight regain; many successful diet programs combine decreased food intake and increased activity with an analysis and modification of eating behaviors; group programs such as Weight Watchers help make behavioral changes

6. Dietary aids—represent a multimillion-dollar business, and although they may help cause an initial rapid weight loss, they are no more effective than mere calorie cutting in long-term weight maintenance; moreover, most diet drugs have the potential for serious side effects if used habitually over a long period or by persons with certain medical conditions; types most often used are appetite suppressants, stimulants, laxatives, diuretics, and bulk-producing agents

7. Surgical therapy—gastric bypass surgery may be recommended to individuals with BMI of 40 or greater and for those with BMI greater than 35 and comorbid conditions

a. This surgical approach is used to reduce the size of the stomach to decrease its reserve capacity

b. Bloating, nausea, vomiting, dumping syndrome, anemia, and nutrient deficiencies may result if diet instructions are not followed after surgery

c. Fluids are consumed separately from meals; more frequent small meals throughout the day are recommended

d. Increased risk of caries because of alterations in eating habits

G. Eating disorders
1. Treatment
   a. Correction of any underlying physiologic causes of weight loss
   b. Increased caloric intake with foods that are concentrated sources of energy; several small meals per day
   c. Limiting weight gain goals to 1 to 2 lb per week
   d. Team approach; physician, registered dietitian, psychotherapist, or all should be involved in the treatment
2. Signs and symptoms of disordered eating
   a. Erosion of tooth enamel (perimylolysis)
   b. Halitosis
   c. Severe weight loss
   d. Dental caries
   e. Lanugo
   f. Enlarged tongue
   g. Angular cheilosis
   h. Enlarged parotid glands
   i. Xerostomia
   j. Goosebumps on skin
   k. Glossitis
3. *Anorexia nervosa*—state of protein-energy malnutrition brought on by voluntary starvation (and often with the use of diet aids, intense exercise, and self-induced vomiting)
   a. Seen most often in middle-income and upper-income adolescent females, who are typically described as perfectionists, overachievers, and models of good behavior; they begin dieting because they have a distorted perception of body shape and weight
   b. Death may occur from failure of multiple organ systems
   c. Treatment usually includes specially tailored counseling and hospitalization before voluntary weight gain is possible; treatment encourages regular mealtimes, varied and moderate intake, and gradual introduction of feared foods
   d. The client should be referred to a physician, a registered dietitian, or a psychologist for treatment
4. *Bulimia*—condition of alternate food gorging and purging by vomiting; occasional use of laxatives to maintain weight
   a. Most often found in adolescent females who appear to be of normal weight
   b. Is more prevalent than anorexia nervosa
   c. Treatment involves counseling; self-induced vomiting can cause swelling of the salivary glands and esophagus and the destruction of tooth enamel by acid that results in sensitive teeth
   d. The client should be referred to a physician, a registered dietitian, or a psychologist for treatment
5. *Eating disorders not otherwise specified* (EDNOS)—a broad category in which individuals do not meet the strict criteria for anorexia nervosa or anorexia bulimia; binge-eating disorder falls into this category

NUTRITIONAL ASSESSMENT AND COUNSELING

Malnutrition

A. Overconsumption of nutrients such as:
1. Fat—can result in excess weight gain; associated with coronary heart disease (CHD), obesity, and certain types of cancers
2. Sugar—can result in excess weight gain; associated with obesity, dental caries, and plaque-induced gingivitis
3. Salt or sodium—can result in retention of excess body fluid; associated with high blood pressure; increased sodium may also decrease calcium levels
4. Excess calories—can result in obesity; associated with CHD, hypertension, and diabetes mellitus type 2
5. Vitamin and mineral supplements—"megadoses" may result in toxicity of one or many nutrients and inhibition of others

B. Nutrient deficiencies—the health of a person is at risk because of the unavailability of nutrients for cellular activities; end result of deficiencies is the same, but the multiple causes can be classified as primary or secondary
1. *Primary deficiency* is a result of an inadequate food intake and can result from the following conditions:
   a. Fad diets—low-calorie or imbalanced diet plans
   b. Economics—inadequate resources to obtain a healthy diet
   c. Illness—loss of appetite
   d. Improper food preparation—destruction of nutrients because of delayed storage and overcooking of foods
   e. Accessibility to food—nutritious foods unavailable because of problems with transportation or market supplies encountered by individuals
   f. Ignorance—lack of nutritional knowledge
   g. Flavor preferences—palatability of sweets and fats can lead to a diet high in empty-calorie foods
   h. Time constraints—inadequate time for food preparation can lead to the use of highly processed convenience foods, which tend to have low nutrient density
   i. Poor oral health—inability to masticate food because of edentulism or oral disease; altered taste perceptions result from oral disease
2. *Secondary deficiency* is the result of inability to digest, absorb, and use foods consumed; an individual may eat a balanced diet, but other factors interfere with the body's use of nutrients in foods; examples of these conditioning factors include:
   a. Disease—any GI or metabolic disease can interfere with the digestion and use of foods and nutrients (e.g., ulcers, lactase deficiency, partial obstruction of the GI tract, inborn errors of metabolism)
   b. Drug-nutrient interactions—certain drugs can interfere with and reduce the absorption, transportation, and metabolism of nutrients (e.g., grapefruit juice with high blood pressure medication)
   c. Nutrient-nutrient interactions—excess or deficiency of certain nutrients can affect the absorption of other nutrients (e.g., vitamin C and iron)

d. Allergies—sensitivity to certain foods or chemicals in foods can lead to malabsorption syndromes (e.g., gluten sensitivity, as in celiac disease)

3. Manifestations of primary and secondary deficiencies
   a. Gradual decreases in the tissue level of nutrients
      (1) Earliest sign of malnutrition
      (2) Determined by blood and urine analyses for each nutrient
   b. Biochemical disturbances
      (1) Occur if duration of deficiency is long enough to deplete the body's stores and interfere with cellular metabolism
      (2) Determined by blood and urine analyses for alterations in cellular levels of enzymes and metabolites
   c. Anatomical lesions
      (1) Signs of chronic and severe malnutrition, leading to destruction of body tissues
      (2) Determined by clinical examination of body tissues

Complete Nutritional Assessment

A. Health and pharmacologic history
   1. Factors that influence food intake
      a. Socioeconomic conditions—food-purchasing power
      b. Home environment—culture, family values, and eating practices
      c. Client motivation and education—interest and awareness of the principles of a nutritious diet
      d. Prescriptive drugs that may suppress appetite, alter taste perception, or negatively interact with foods
   2. Factors that influence food use
      a. Oral health—ability to masticate, saliva production, and presence of oral disease
      b. Systemic health—ability to digest, absorb, and metabolize nutrients in food; therapeutic diets for disease control
      c. Mental health—desire to eat
      d. Drug use—alcohol abuse and illegal drugs
B. Assessment of dietary intake
   1. Collection of objective data on what a person eats
      a. Assessment tools—screening questionnaire for food intake frequency, 24-hour recall method, and food record or diary
         (1) Food-frequency questionnaires—ask how often food items are consumed; elicit specific details; work better with large groups in the community setting
         (2) A 24-hour recall method—mental recall of everything eaten in the previous 24 hours; useful for individual counseling in a clinical setting; does not represent "usual" diet
         (3) Food record diary—exact record of everything eaten in a specific period; more accurate account
         (4) Combining 3- to 7-day food record with a 24-hour recall method presents a more accurate measure of intake
      b. Specific amounts or quantities of foods eaten must be recorded to use assessment tools effectively

2. Analysis and evaluation of food intake
   a. Methods of analysis—the USDA MyPlate (Fig. 12-3)
   b. Methods of evaluation—comparing results of diet analysis with standards of adequacy
3. Diet modifications
   a. Adding foods to the diet to correct for nutrient deficiencies
   b. Eliminating or reducing excessive nutrient intake for disease control and prevention (e.g., sugar, fat, oils, sodium)
   c. Collaborate with a registered dietitian for in-depth analysis and modification of dietary intake
C. Biochemical analysis and immune function
   1. Blood and urine analyses
      a. Most objective and precise assessment data
      b. Determine marginal nutritional deficiencies before overt clinical signs appear by measuring either the concentration of a nutrient or the functional activity of the nutrient
   2. Delayed cutaneous hypersensitivity skin tests
      a. Assessment of host defense mechanisms by evaluating the client's reaction to common skin test antigens as a nonspecific indicator of malnutrition
      b. Most useful for evaluating the critically ill client's ability to withstand the stresses of surgery
D. Clinical examination of body tissues—indicator of systemic health and nutritional status (see Table 12-4)
   1. Oral tissues
      a. Dental caries—excessive sugar or acid exposure (supports *S. mutans* and *Lactobacillus acidophilus*)
      b. Gingivitis and periodontal disease—excessive sugar intake (supports growth of plaque biofilm and nutritional deficiencies)
      c. Glossitis—nutritional deficiencies affecting the papillae and color of the tongue
      d. Stomatitis—nutritional deficiencies affecting oral soft tissues
      e. Cheilosis—nutritional deficiencies affecting the lips and the corners of the mouth
      f. Necrotizing ulcerative gingivitis (NUG)—excessive sugar and caffeine intake, smoking, stress, and poor oral hygiene combined with nutritional deficiencies result in lowered host resistance to bacterial plaque (dental) biofilm and bacterial challenges
   2. Anthropometric analysis—determines the body structure, form, and composition (e.g., content of lean body mass and fat tissue); the following tools are useful, but each has its limitations:
      a. BMI, IBW, and waist circumference (see the earlier section on "Energy Balances and Weight Control")
      b. Skinfold thickness measurements
         (1) Obtained by using skinfold calipers to measure subcutaneous fat in millimeters in selected areas (e.g., triceps and subscapular regions)
         (2) Measurements are compared with standards to estimate total body fat composition
      c. Arm muscle circumference

FIG 12-3 Anatomy of USDA MyPlate. (From www.choosemyplate.gov. Accessed October 27, 2014.)

(1) Sensitive indicator of the muscle mass that reflects protein stores

(2) Determined by measuring the arm circumference at the midpoint of the upper arm and by measuring triceps skinfold

d. Bioelectrical impedance and ultrasound methods

(1) Potential predictors of total body fat

(2) Lean body mass conducts electricity better than fat mass

e. Underwater weighing

(1) Measures body weight when the person is under water

(2) One of the most accurate methods used to determine body volume

f. Dual-energy x-ray absorptiometry (DEXA)—can distinguish fat mass, fat-free mass, and bone mineral loss; most accurate method to determine body fat

Methods for Assessment of Dietary Intake

A. Dietary intake standards

1. *Dietary Reference Intake* (DRI) and *Recommended Dietary Allowance* (RDA)

a. Published by the Panel on Micronutrients of the Food and Nutrition Board, Institute of Medicine, National Academy of Sciences; principally used as measurement tools by nutrition professionals who plan and evaluate food supplies for groups; to establish guidelines for new food products; used as the basis for regulatory standards in determining nutritional quality; and used to set standards for nutritional labeling (e.g., percentage of daily value)

b. DRI is the updated version of the RDA established by the National Academy of Sciences, Food and Nutrition Board; DRI values are based on the observed average or experimentally set intake by individuals that appear to sustain a defined nutritional status

(1) Unlike RDA values, DRI values aim to prevent nutrient deficiency as well as reduce the likelihood of chronic disease

(2) DRI includes five sets of standards:

(a) RDA—intake level sufficient to meet nutrient requirements of almost all healthy individuals

(b) AI (adequate intake)—value based on approximation of nutrient intake by a group of healthy people, used when an RDA value cannot be determined

(c) UL (upper limit)—highest level of daily nutrient intake that is likely to pose no risk of adverse health effects to almost all individuals in the general population; risk of adverse effects increases as intake increases above the UL

(d) EAR (estimated average requirement)—nutrient intake value that is estimated to meet the requirements of half the healthy individuals in a group

(e) EER (estimated energy requirement)—average calorie need estimates for various life stage groups and genders

2. *Dietary Guidelines for Americans* are issued by the U.S. Department of Agriculture (USDA) and the U.S. Department of Health and Human Services (HHS) and are revised every 5 years

a. The seventh edition of the *Dietary Guidelines for Americans* (2010) includes 23 key recommendations for the general population and six additional key recommendations for special populations[3]

b. Special populations include children and adolescents, women capable of becoming pregnant, pregnant women, women who are breastfeeding, older adults and adults at high risk of chronic disease

c. The updated guidelines are intended for Americans ages 2 years and older, including those with chronic disease

d. Two common themes are weaved throughout the updated guidelines: encouragement of balanced caloric intake to manage body weight and the consumption of nutrient-dense foods and beverages

e. The key recommendations within these chapters include the following[3]:

(1) Men ages 19 and older should eat between 2000 and 3000 calories a day depending on degree of activity; women should eat 1600 and 2400 calories daily; individuals should aim for the lower caloric levels if inactive

(2) SoFAS (solid fats and added sugars) should make up no more than 13% of your daily caloric intake based on a 2000-calorie diet

(3) Reduce consumption of refined grains; half of grain consumption should come from whole grains; based on a minimum consumption of 6 ounces, 3 ounces should come from whole-grain foods

(4) Limit sodium intake to 2300 mg/day; African Americans and individuals 51 and older or who have hypertension, diabetes, or chronic kidney disease should decrease their intake to 1500 mg/day

(5) Increase intake of fruits and vegetables; consume 2 cups of fruit and 2.5 cups of vegetables (including beans and peas) each day

(6) Aim for 3 cups of low-fat or fat-free dairy foods each day

(7) Consume at least 8 oz of seafood a week

(8) Limit protein foods; consume no more than 5.5 oz daily.

(9) Consume a variety of food sources to ensure optimum intake of potassium, calcium, and vitamin D; choose whole-food sources of nutrients; limit use of supplements

3. Dietary guidelines for oral health

a. Eat a balanced diet representing moderation and variety as shown by MyPlate, and follow the recommendations of the *Dietary Guidelines for Americans* (2010)[3]

b. Combine and eat foods in sequence to enhance mastication, saliva production, and oral clearance; for example, combine dairy foods with sweet or starchy foods, or combine protein-rich foods with cooked or processed starches

c. Plan eating intervals that allow time for the pH of the plaque to return to neutral; for example, up to 120 minutes may be needed for the plaque pH to return to neutral after exposure to a fermentable carbohydrate

d. Take care not to replace other foods needed to maintain optimum health with sweets and soft drinks; obtain most calories from whole grains, fruits and vegetables, low-fat or nonfat dairy products, and lean meats or meat alternatives

e. Drink water often; consume sweetened and acidic beverages *with* meals to allow for a buffering action, rather than consuming soft drinks *between* meals

f. Limit the consumption of sugar-free beverages and sports drinks; demineralization of tooth structure can still occur as a result of the low pH of these beverages; consume these with meals

4. The Food and Nutrition Board's recommendations for healthy adult Americans

a. Maintain a healthy weight by balancing energy intake and energy expenditure

b. If the requirement for energy is low (e.g., weight-reducing diet), reduce the consumption of foods such as alcohol, sugars, fats, and oils that provide calories but few other essential nutrients

c. Use salt in moderation; recommended intake is no more than 2300 mg (1 teaspoon) per day; 1500 mg/day for those with hypertension

d. Select a nutritionally adequate diet from the foods available by each day consuming appropriate servings

TABLE 12-7   Daily Guide to Food Choices

Dietary Component	Source of	DAILY RECOMMENDED SERVINGS		
		1600 kcal	2200 kcal	2800 kcal
Water	Fluids to maintain water balance and hydration	64 oz	64 oz	64 oz
Breads, cereals, grains	Riboflavin, thiamin, niacin, iron, protein, fiber, magnesium	5 oz	7 oz	10 oz
Vegetables	Vitamins A and C, folate, potassium, magnesium, iron, fiber, phytochemicals	2 cups	3 cups	3.5 cups
Fruits	Vitamins A and C, potassium, iron phytochemicals, fiber	1.5 cups	2 cups	2.5 cups
Milk, yogurt, cheese	Calcium, protein, riboflavin, vitamins A and D, phosphorus	3 cups	3 cups	3 cups
Meat and meat alternatives	Protein, zinc, iron, vitamin B_{12}, niacin, thiamin, vitamin A, folacin, pyroxidine, magnesium, phosphorus, vitamin B_6	5 oz	6 oz	7 oz
Fats and oils	Essential fatty acids, energy	5 teaspoon (tsp)	6 tsp	8 tsp
Added sugar	Energy	Women:6 tsp	Women: 6 tsp	Women: 6 tsp
		Men: 9 tsp	Men: 9 tsp	Men: 9 tsp
Alcohol	Energy	—	—	—

Courtesy of Connie Mobley, RD, PhD, University of Nevada Las Vegas, School of Dental Medicine, Las Vegas, Nevada.
Data from My Pyramid Food Intake Patterns, US Department of Agriculture, Center for Nutrition Policy and Promotion, MyPyramid Food Guidance System, April 2005, www.choosemyplate.gov/food-groups/downloads/MyPyramid_Food_Intake_Patterns.pdf, accessed October 30, 2014; and Johnson RK, Appel LJ, Brands M, et al: Dietary sugars intake and cardiovascular health: a scientific statement from the American Heart Association, *Circulation* 120:1011-1020, 2009.

of low-fat dairy products, lean meats or legumes, vegetables, fruits, cereals, grains, and breads (Table 12-7)
  e. Select as wide a variety of foods in each of the major food groups, as practical, to ensure a high probability of adequate quantities of all essential nutrients
5. The USDA MyPlate (see Fig. 12-3)
  a. Graphic design is similar to a pie chart; organizes foods into four colorful sections with a side portion for dairy.
    (1) Red represents fruits; green is for vegetables; orange is for grains; purple is for protein (a separate blue section for dairy is on the side of the plate)
    (2) Encourages healthier eating habits and the consumption of a more plant-based diet
    (3) Promotes balanced proportions of each food group to be consumed at meals
      (a) Half of your plate should be fruits and vegetables
      (b) At least half of your grains should be whole grains
      (c) Make the switch to fat-free or low-fat milk
      (d) Balance calories
      (e) Avoid oversized portions
    (4) Recommends reduced intake of those foods high in sodium; read labels to compare
    (5) Supports the consumption of water over sugary drinks
B. Methods for collecting data on food intakes
  1. Nutritional Screening and Assessment of Dietary Intake Questionnaire (Fig. 12-4)
    a. Description—interviewer collects data from the client about all food consumed in the previous 24-hour period; additional questions help determine frequency of sugar and food group intake
    b. Nutrition tools used to guide recommendations
      (1) USDA MyPlate
      (2) *Dietary Guidelines*

    (3) Dietary Reference Intake (DRI) based on life stage
  c. Advantages
    (1) Can be filled out by the client while waiting in the oral health care setting
    (2) Requires only 15 to 20 minutes to complete
    (3) Allows analysis of food group consumption
    (4) Allows evaluation of sugar intake
  d. Limitations
    (1) No nutrient analysis
    (2) Relies on the client's memory
2. The 24-hour dietary recall
  a. Description—interviewer collects data from the client about all food consumed in the previous 24-hour period
  b. Advantages
    (1) Requires 20 minutes or less for the interview
    (2) Allows nutrient analysis
    (3) Allows analysis of food group consumption
    (4) Allows evaluation of sugar intake
  c. Limitations
    (1) Requires a trained interviewer
    (2) Relies on the client's memory
    (3) Represents only 1 day of food consumption
    (4) Requires a nutrient data file on foods to analyze nutrients
3. A 3- to 7-day food record or diary
  a. Description—client keeps a record of food and eating times for 3 to 7 days
  b. Advantages
    (1) No interviewer required except to give directions on how to fill out the record
    (2) Allows for analyses of both nutrients and food groups
    (3) Allows for evaluation of sugar intake
    (4) An average intake of several days may be more representative of client's food intake than that of just 1 day

Nutritional Screening and Assessment of Dietary Intake Questionnaire

Client's Name _____   Gender: M   F   Age: _____

Height _____   Weight _____   # IBW _____   Occupation/Activity Level _____

FOR THE EDENTULOUS CLIENT, COMPLETE ONLY THOSE ITEMS WITH AN ASTERISK (*).

* _____ Complete Oral Health Evaluation   CRA Score†:   low   moderate   high   very high

*Review client chart and Oral Health Evaluation Form for the following:

____ Does client have a chronic disease (diabetes, hypertension, etc.)?
____ Is client taking medication or a dietary supplement with nutritional implications?
____ Does client have periodontal disease or xerostomia?
____ Does client have a dietary screening score greater than 3?

*Obtain typical dietary intake information: (record 24-hour recall of dietary intake)
*Use nutritional tools as a guide to making recommendations (USDA MyPlate, Dietary Guidelines, DRIs/RDIs)

Determine if diet is caries promoting, using the following criteria:	If YES, circle:
a. Do the total number of servings from the combined sugars and sweet beverages group exceed the number of servings from the grains group?	**4 points**
b. Are food and beverage sources of sugars consumed alone?	**2 points**
c. Are foods from the grains group consumed alone? Are foods from the grains group consumed in combination with foods that are sources of sugars? Are these combined foods eaten alone?	**2 points**
d. Is diet lacking foods and/or adequate servings of foods from 1 or more food groups? Do number of servings for food groups exceed recommendations?	**2 points**

e.   Does the client have an unusual meal pattern?
  –Eating snacks or drinking beverages in place of meals
  –Spacing meals/snacks more than 6 hours apart
  –Eating or drinking every 1–2 hours
	1 point

f. Does the client eat or drink late in the evening or immediately prior to bedtime?	**1 point**
g. Does the client report chewing gum that is not sugar free?	**1 point**
Total Score (6=caries promoting diet)	

*Chart findings using SOAP format.

*Educate client, using appropriate nutrition education handouts and models. Refer client to other healthcare professionals, as appropriate.

FIG 12-4 Nutritional Screening and Assessment of Dietary Intake Questionnaire. *The caries risk assessment (CRA) score is determined from an oral health evaluation tool that is used to determine the level of caries risk on an individual basis. (Modified from Connie Mobley, RD, PhD, University of Nevada Las Vegas, School of Dental Medicine, Las Vegas, Nevada.)

c. Limitations
   (1) Represents the food consumption of only the days included in the record
   (2) Relies on the cooperation and ability of the client to keep the record
   (3) Requires a nutrient data file for nutrient analysis
B. Methods for evaluating food intake
   1. USDA MyPlate
      a. Nutrient contributions (see Table 12-7)
         (1) Role in general health
         (2) Role in oral health
      b. Advantages for use in counseling
         (1) Client participation
         (2) Simple
         (3) Inexpensive
         (4) Fairly accurate
         (5) Detailed nutrient analysis
      c. Limitations
         (1) No provisions made for combination foods (e.g., pizza, casseroles); need to break down into ingredients that correspond to the six groups
         (2) Website can be difficult to navigate
   2. Computerized analysis of diet
      a. Definition—food nutrient data are individually entered into a computer program, and the specific amounts of each nutrient for each food consumed are calculated
      b. Nutrient data file (software)—lists foods and their nutrients;[4,5] the USDA has a nutrient database website: http://fnic.nal.usda.gov/; MyPlate has an online dietary assessment tool MyPyramid Tracker that can be accessed at https://www.supertracker.usda.gov/ (see Website Information and Resources table at the end of this chapter)
      c. DRI and RDA values—used as a standard for comparison with the client's daily nutrient intake
      d. Advantages
         (1) Accurate
         (2) Specific
         (3) Cost-efficient when technology is available
            (a) Computers in oral health care settings with Internet access
            (b) Services available for a fee outside the oral health care setting
      e. Limitations
         (1) Limited client participation and home use
         (2) Hardware and software availability
         (3) Expense
         (4) Requires training for accurate interpretation of output
   3. Sugar analysis and evaluation
      a. Dental caries and periodontal disease are multifactorial infectious diseases that result from the interaction of the resistance of oral tissues (host factor) with the destructive effects of bacterial plaque and acids (agent factor) produced from the metabolism of dietary sugars (diet or environment factor); dental disease occurs when all three factors exist simultaneously; often called the "triad" of dental disease; nutritional assessment of exposure to sugar is an essential part of nutritional counseling in disease prevention programs and can be conducted by using precise or simplified methods
         (1) Precise analysis—computer analysis of the diet for carbohydrate content: total carbohydrate in grams, monosaccharides and disaccharides in grams (e.g., grams of sucrose), and fiber in grams; percentage of the total daily calorie intake from simple and complex carbohydrates can be calculated and compared with the recommendations; added sugars should contain no more than 25% of total calories consumed; fiber needs range from 21 to 38 g, depending on age and gender[2]
         (2) Simplified analysis—dietary sugars (sweets and foods processed with sugars; see Table 12-3) are circled on the food record or recall; cariogenicity of the diet is assessed on the basis of frequency and form of sugar exposure; frequent exposure to retentive solid sugars, especially between meals, is harmful; acid production potential of the diet can be calculated by using the following formula:

Total daily *solid* sugar exposures $\times 40\,\text{min}$
$+$
Total daily *liquid* sugar exposures $\times 20\,\text{min}$
$=$ Total min acid exposure to otal tissues from *all* dietary sugars
Total should not exceed 100 min of exposure

The formula is based on research that shows glucose-rich food products (either liquid or sugar) result in a decrease of oral pH below the critical level (pH 5.5, the point at which acids decalcify enamel) and that it takes 20 minutes after consumption of liquid sugars for healthy saliva to neutralize acids and raise the pH to a safe level; solid sugars adhere to teeth and have approximately double the potential for acid production
      b. Caries activity tests—often involve counting the number of acidogenic bacteria or measuring the acids produced by these bacteria; provide information about the current oral environment and help to detect dental caries risk; are valuable adjuncts in plaque control programs and can be used to monitor a client's progress in oral home care and diet modifications

Nutritional Counseling Techniques

A. Direct approach—counseling technique that focuses on the dietary problem
   1. Role of the client—the client provides information about his or her diet; is passive and listens to the counselor
   2. Role of the counselor—the counselor controls the session; analyzes and evaluates the client's diet and makes recommendations for improvement

3. Advantages—easier for the counselor and often requires less time than a more client-oriented approach
4. Limitations—fosters client dependence; little chance of success if the client is not committed to dietary changes; client is not involved in decision making

B. Nondirect or behavior modification approach—counseling technique that focuses on the client
   1. Role of the client—the client actively participates in the diet analysis, evaluation, and modification program
   2. Role of the counselor—the counselor provides information on the causes of dental disease, the role of the diet, and the use of dietary assessment tools
   3. Method
      a. Assumption—dietary habits are learned behaviors and can be "unlearned" and replaced with new behaviors
      b. Collection of baseline data
      c. Client takes ownership of his or her dietary problems and is committed to change
      d. Client determines his or her behavioral changes and goals; develops own reward system to use when goals are met
      e. Changes are gradually made in small steps; appropriate changes are rewarded and failures ignored
      f. Close monitoring of progress until new behaviors become self-reinforcing
   4. Advantages—fosters client independence; success is more likely because the client is in control of the change process
   5. Limitations—more time and effort needed to arrive at appropriate solutions to dietary problems and rewards for behavior modification

B. Factors that influence the client's food intake—any combination of the following influences affects food choices and needs to be addressed in a modification program:
   1. Environmental influences—economics, lifestyle, geography, seasons, markets
   2. Social influences—family, culture, religion, social pressures, marketing strategies
   3. Psychological influences—self-image, emotions, stresses, values, priorities

C. Determinants for dental client selection
   1. High-risk clients—those with conditions that would benefit most from nutritional counseling
      a. Pregnancy—nutrient needs are high; hormonal changes may lead to exaggerated responses to plaque and bacterial toxins; maternal diet affects the formation of fetal oral tissues
      b. Adolescence—nutrient needs are high; vulnerable to nutritional problems from "fad" diets for weight loss and muscle building; frequent snacking on empty-calorie foods; problems of anorexia and bulimia can lead to enamel erosion, irritation of oral mucosa, and infected or enlarged salivary glands, with possible xerostomia
      c. Rampant caries—high bacterial plaque and calculus and a positive caries activity test may indicate a problem of frequent exposure to sugar

      d. Periodontal disease or NUG—frequent exposure to sugar and nutritional deficiencies can contribute to the development and progression of these conditions
      e. Oral and maxillofacial surgery—nutritional counseling before and after surgery is important for optimal surgical recovery; postsurgical nutrient needs are high because of blood loss, tissue repair, and host defense activities; modifications in food texture (e.g., soft foods) are made according to the client's ability to masticate
      f. Edentulism—inability to masticate can result in nutrient deficiencies because of the limited nutrient content in soft and liquid foods
         (1) Food choices are altered because of difficulties with chewing or fear of choking; reduced intake of meats, fresh fruits, and vegetables; softer foods are usually eaten
         (2) Lowered intake of magnesium, folic acid, fluoride, zinc, and calcium
      g. Oral cancer—nutrient needs are high because of host defense activities and tissue repair from cancer and its treatment; cancer or treatment may result in inadequate food intake because of decreased appetite, altered taste perceptions, irritated oral tissues, and xerostomia
   2. Dental office resources—availability of trained personnel, time, and facilities to conduct nutrition counseling services
   3. Client factors—level of client motivation to use and benefit from nutritional counseling and financial and intellectual capabilities for using nutritional counseling services

Dietary Modifications for Specific Dental Conditions

A. Dental caries (see Tables 12-4 and 12-5)
   1. Role of nutrients in tooth formation
      a. Preeruptive effects—nutrients are used systemically for enamel, dentin, and pulp formation; tooth bud formation begins at 6 weeks in utero, and calcification is completed at 13 years
      b. Posteruptive effects—fluoride aids in the remineralization of small enamel lesions; evidence indicates that specific minerals or combinations of minerals and fats have local cariostatic properties
   2. Local effect of dietary carbohydrates on bacteria growth and plaque formation
   3. Role of diet and nutrients in salivary gland function
      a. Nutrients are used systemically for the normal development and secretory function of salivary glands
      b. Foods of firm texture (e.g., raw vegetables) enhance mastication, stimulate the salivary flow rate, and modify the concentration of constituents in saliva, possibly improving antibacterial properties and the buffering capacity to neutralize decalcifying acids

B. Periodontal disease (see Table 12-5)
   1. Role of nutrients in the formation of periodontal tissues

a. Nutrients are used systemically for the normal development of the gingiva, periodontal ligament, cementum, and alveolus
b. Periodontal tissues are metabolically active throughout a person's life, and nutrients are constantly needed for maintenance (e.g., the cell population of the sulcal epithelium completely renews itself within 3 to 6 days)
2. Local effect of dietary carbohydrates on bacteria growth and plaque formation
3. Role of nutrients in the host defense system
   a. During the initial stages of periodontitis, the nutritional status of the client is important in cellular immunocompetence for combating bacterial insults to the periodontium
   b. After periodontal surgery, cellular immunocompetence is important for optimal healing and prevention of infection
C. Oral and maxillofacial surgery
1. Presurgical nutritional counseling
   a. Adequate nutrient intake is needed to build up nutrient reserves in tissues to cope with postsurgical nutrient demands and complications
   b. Counseling is helpful for advising the client to plan and purchase appropriate foods before surgery in anticipation of convalescence
   c. Need for referral to registered dietitian prior to surgery should be evaluated
2. Postsurgical nutritional counseling
   a. Nutrient requirements are high because of blood loss, increased catabolism, tissue repair, and host defense activities
   b. Dietary intake is influenced by surgical complications of anorexia, dysphagia, and oral discomfort; a liquid diet should be used initially for the first few days, followed by a soft diet until the client can eat normally; during convalescence, high-protein liquid products fortified with vitamins and minerals (e.g., Ensure, Sustacal, Instant Breakfast) are helpful but contain cariogenic sweeteners; safe levels of vitamin and mineral supplements (100% to 200% of DRI or RDA values) may be recommended
D. Prosthodontics
1. Nutritional counseling in the preparation of the mouth for a prosthesis
   a. Nutrients—systemically important for the health of oral soft tissues and the alveolar ridge
      (1) Surgery—if surgery is necessary, nutrient requirements will be higher for postsurgical healing
      (2) Tissue state—if any inflamed or soft tissue injuries and bone resorption conditions exist, nutrient requirements will be higher for repair and host defense activities
   b. Dietary sugars—condition of the remaining dentition is important for maintaining the use of a new prosthesis; cariogenic sugars need to be restricted to control bacterial growth, acid production, and bacterial plaque formation

c. Texture of foods—partial or fully edentulous clients will often need to eat chopped, soft foods; if nutrient intake is compromised, fortified liquid products or nutrient supplements are helpful
2. Nutritional counseling after prosthesis insertion
   a. Food texture—liquid foods for the first 24 hours, followed by soft foods and chopped or cut-up foods; this minimizes biting and chewing and allows time for the muscles and tongue to adjust to the new prosthesis
   b. Counter-dislodgement forces—for every bite of food, food should be evenly divided in the right and left sides of the mouth before chewing to equalize occlusal forces
   c. Nutrients—adequate intake for the integrity of the oral mucosa and alveolar ridge
   d. Dietary sugars—should be restricted to prevent bacterial growth, acid production, and bacterial plaque formation on the remaining dentition and prosthesis
   e. Food flavors—initially, flavors of foods will be altered because of the new prosthesis, but this side effect will eventually disappear with continued denture use
E. Orthodontics
1. Role of nutrients—systemically important for the integrity of periodontal tissues; requirements are higher as stresses of tooth movement result in more bone apposition and the synthesis of a new periodontal ligament; nutrients are needed for the healing and repair of gingival injuries and irritations from orthodontic bands
2. Role of sugars—to prevent enamel erosion and decay, dietary sugars (especially retentive sweets) must be restricted during the wearing of appliances
3. Role of food textures—when appliances or bands are tightened, chewing hard-textured foods may be painful, and liquid and soft foods should be eaten temporarily; retentive and sticky foods should be avoided because they become trapped in the appliance and are difficult to remove

Dietary Considerations for Immunocompromised Clients and Those with Special Needs

A. Oral cancer
1. Nutritional support for healing and cellular immunocompetence
   a. Compromised nutritional status—weight loss and nutrient deficiencies increase the risk of not withstanding the physiologic stresses of cancer and anticancer therapies
   b. Surgical treatment—primary method in treating cancer; nutrient requirements are higher as a result of the increased catabolic activities, tissue repair, and host defense activities
   c. Chemotherapy and radiation treatment—nutrient needs are higher because of the destruction of healthy cells and tissues that occurs during these types of treatments
   d. Possible need for referral to registered dietitian to monitor client's dietary intake during the compromised state

2. Diet modifications useful in treating complications from cancer or cancer treatments
   a. Client unable to ingest or digest food
      (1) Home enteral feedings can provide nutrients (e.g., nasogastric tube feedings)
      (2) Home parenteral feedings can provide nutrients (e.g., intravenous feedings)
   b. Eating problems arising from complications or side effects of anticancer therapies
      (1) Nausea and vomiting—client should suck on ice chips; eat frequently; eat dry, bland foods; eat and drink slowly; avoid highly spiced and fatty foods; new antinausea medications are effective
      (2) Loss of appetite—client should eat foods that are appealing; make up nutrient requirements at times when the appetite is good; eat foods with a high nutrient density
      (3) Food aversions and alterations in taste and smell—client should eliminate offending foods; include highly spiced and distinctive textures to improve taste perceptions; cook and serve food with plastic utensils rather than metal utensils
      (4) Dry mouth (xerostomia)—client should use xylitol-containing gum, mints, and sprays; suck on ice chips or use synthetic saliva; drink liquids with meals; eat cold-temperature foods rather than hot-temperature foods; concentrate on highly nutritious liquids
      (5) Radiation-induced caries—client should restrict cariogenic foods; because of changes in both the quality and the quantity of saliva after cancer treatment, rapid demineralization of the tooth surface can occur
      (6) Glossitis and stomatitis—client should eat a variety of soft, easy-to-chew foods; eat stewed foods rather than broiled and fried foods; avoid highly spiced or acidic foods; eat moderate-temperature foods; use straws if swallowing is difficult

B. Human immunodeficiency virus (HIV)
   1. Causes of malnutrition in HIV-infected persons
      a. Reduced food intake
         (1) Drug treatments cause vomiting, nausea, and food aversions
         (2) Fatigue, depression, and fear cause anorexia
         (3) Oral infections alter taste, cause pain, and reduce saliva flow
         (4) Esophageal infections and respiratory complications hamper swallowing
      b. Increased nutrient loss
         (1) Cancers of the GI tract cause malabsorption
         (2) Drugs cause diarrhea and malabsorption
         (3) PEM leads to malabsorption
      c. Altered metabolism
         (1) Cancer, infections, and fevers increase BMR
         (2) Drug therapy alters nutrient utilization
   2. Nutrient support

      a. Any subclinical nutrient deficiencies and weight loss should be corrected at the time of a positive HIV test
      b. At least 100% of the DRI or RDA values of all vitamins and minerals must be provided
      c. Client must avoid all foodborne illnesses
      d. The nutrition plan should be designed on the basis of individual complications, with emphasis on controlling weight loss by eating nutrient-dense foods throughout the day
      e. Dietary recommendations should be regulated only by a medical physician (MD) or a registered dietitian (RD), or both

C. Clients with special needs (see Chapter 19)
   1. Dental problems—unmet oral health care needs in this population significantly exceed those in the general population
      a. The oral caries rate may be higher than that of the general population because of poor oral hygiene and cariogenic food habits
      b. Increased periodontal disease compared with the general population because of:
         (1) Poor oral hygiene; limited self-care
         (2) Diets consisting of soft-textured foods
         (3) Frequent exposures to fermentable carbohydrates
         (4) Metabolic disturbances affecting disease resistance and the reparative process
         (5) Nutritional deficiencies associated with diet or metabolic disturbance
         (6) Malocclusion and developmental defects
      c. Barriers to health care
   2. Nutritional problems—slow growth, excessive weight loss or gain, and nutrient deficiencies can occur in the following situations:
      a. Inability to consume an adequate diet
         (1) Absence or weak sucking response (e.g., cleft lip and palate)
         (2) Poor control of arm and head (e.g., cerebral palsy)
         (3) Inadequate control of jaw, lip, and tongue (e.g., tongue thrust and tonic bite)
         (4) Attention deficit (e.g., intellectual disability and hyperactivity)
      b. Impaired nutrient use
         (1) Malabsorption conditions (e.g., cystic fibrosis)
         (2) Inborn errors of metabolism (e.g., phenylketonuria)
         (3) Drug-nutrient interactions (e.g., anticonvulsant medications can interfere with calcium and phosphorus use)
         (4) Poor muscle control (e.g., constipation)
      c. Excessive intake of foods, calories, and sweets
         (1) Food, especially sweets, often used to reinforce good behavior
         (2) Overfeeding because of parental guilt
         (3) Overemphasis on feeding because mealtime is perceived as the most important time for parent-child interaction
         (4) Excessive calorie intake resulting from inactivity and the pleasurable aspects of eating

Web Site Information And Resources

Source	Web Site Address	Description
Food and Nutrition Center: US Department of Agriculture National Agricultural Library	http://fnic.nal.usda.gov/	Resource for *Dietary Nutrient* database, *Dietary Guidelines for Americans,* and the Food Guide Pyramid
Healthy People 2020	http://www.healthypeople.gov	Information on *Healthy People 2020;* includes tips for speakers. Oral health objectives provide a valuable resource for community-based activities.
American Dental Association	http://www.mouthhealthy.org/en/nutrition	Provides a nutrition link for food tips, nutrition concerns, and nutrition during pregnancy
National Academy of Science	http://www.nasonline.org/	Information available for purchase by the public about food and nutrition. Specific subtopics include diet and health and dietary reference intakes.
Choose My Plate	http://www.choosemyplate.gov	Provides guidance on balance, moderation, and adequate consumption of essential food groups; interactive resource for individual groups Provides specific dietary requirement based on age, gender, and level of physical activity

REFERENCES

1. Johnson RD, Lawrence LJ, Brands M, et al: Dietary sugars intake and cardiovascular health scientific statement from the American Heart Association, *Circulation* 120:1011–1020, 2009.
2. Institute of Medicine (IOM): National Academy of Sciences, Food and Nutrition Board: *Dietary Reference Intakes for energy, carbohydrates, fiber, fat, fatty acids, cholesterol, protein, and amino acids.* Washington, DC, 2010, The National Academy Press. http://www.nap.edu/openbook.php?record_id=10490. Accessed October 26, 2014.
3. U.S. Department of Agriculture and U.S. Department of Health and Human Services: *Dietary guidelines for Americans,* ed 7, Washington, DC, 2010, US Government Printing Office.
4. Axxya Systems: Nutritionist Pro Diet analysis software, PO Box 3157, Redmond, WA 98073. http://www.axxya.com. Accessed October 30, 2014.
5. ESHA Research: Food processor nutrition and fitness analysis software, PO Box 13028, Salem, OR 97309-1028. http://www.esha.com. Accessed October 30, 2014.

SUGGESTED READINGS

Harper Mallonee LF: Nutrition counseling. In Darby M, editor: *Dental hygiene: theory and practice,* ed 4, St Louis, 2015, Elsevier Saunders.

Harper Mallonee L, Boyd L, Stegeman C: Practice paper of the Academy of Nutrition and Dietetics (AND). Oral health and nutrition, *J Acad Nutr Diet* 114:958, 2014. Full article available for purchase to the public at http://www.sciencedirect.com/science/article/pii/S2212267214003670. Accessed October 2, 2015.

Lamster I: *Primary health care in the dental office,* Dental clinics of North America 2012, Elsevier Saunders.

Stegeman CA, Davis JR: *The dental hygienist's guide to nutritional care,* ed 4, St Louis, 2015, Elsevier Saunders.

Touger Decker R, Mobley C: Position paper of the Academy of Nutrition and Dietetics (AND). Oral health and nutrition, *J Acad Nutr Diet* 113(5):693–701, 2013. http://www.eatright.org/About/Content.aspx?id=8384. Accessed September 22, 2014.

Touger -Decker R, Mobley C, Epstein JB: *Nutrition and oral medicine,* ed 2, Totowa, NJ, 2014, Humana Press.

■ CHAPTER 12 REVIEW QUESTIONS

Answers and rationales to the review questions are available on this text's accompanying Evolve site. See inside front cover for details.

evolve

1. **All the following are disaccharides EXCEPT one. Which one is the *exception*?**
   a. Glucose
   b. Sucrose
   c. Lactose
   d. Maltose

2. **Oligosaccharides are composed of how many monosaccharide units?**
   a. More than six identical monosaccharide units
   b. Two to six monosaccharide units
   c. Two monosaccharide units
   d. One monosaccharide unit

3. **In the mouth, salivary amylase initiates the enzymatic hydrolysis of starch. Salivary amylase also activates pepsin and denatures proteins in the mouth.**
   a. Both statements are TRUE.
   b. Both statements are FALSE.
   c. The first statement is TRUE; the second statement is FALSE.
   d. The first statement is FALSE; the second statement is TRUE.

4. **Which of the following emulsifies fat during the digestive process?**
   a. Pancreatic enzymes

b. Bile salts
c. Brush-border enzymes
d. Salivary enxymes

5. **All the following are monosaccharides EXCEPT:**
   a. Galactose
   b. Sucrose
   c. Glucose
   d. Fructose

6. **Endocrine activity can affect the absorption process. Type of food mixture would not have an influence.**
   a. Both statements are TRUE.
   b. Both statements are FALSE.
   c. The first statement is TRUE; the second statement is FALSE.
   d. The first statement is FALSE; the second statement is TRUE.

7. **One of the end products of glycolysis is**
   a. Carbon dioxide
   b. Adenosine triphosphate
   c. Lactic acid
   d. Water

8. **What is the process called in which glycogen is the short-term storage form of glucose in the liver and muscle?**
   a. Glycogenolysis
   b. Gluconeogenesis
   c. Glycogenesis
   d. Glyconeogenesis

9. **Anabolic hormones raise the blood glucose levels. Catabolic hormones lower the blood glucose level.**
   a. Both statements are TRUE.
   b. Both statements are FALSE.
   c. The first statement is TRUE; the second statement is FALSE.
   d. The first statement is FALSE; the second statement is TRUE.

10. **Anabolic hormones are metabolic regulators of all the following EXCEPT:**
    a. Lower blood glucose level
    b. Stimulate gluconeogenesis
    c. Increase glycogenesis
    d. Increase lipogenesis

11. **Which of the following is an example of a soluble fiber?**
    a. Oat bran
    b. Cellulose
    c. Hemicellulose
    d. Lignin

12. **All the following are biologic roles of carbohydrates EXCEPT:**
    a. Provides an energy source of 4 kcal/g
    b. Protein sparing
    c. Structural component of cell membrane
    d. Precursors of structural and functional molecules

13. **The congenital absence of lactase enzyme is considered a primary lactose intolerance. Temporary or permanent loss of lactase enzyme activity as a result of injury or illness is considered a secondary lactose intolerance.**
    a. Both statements are TRUE.

b. Both statements are FALSE.
c. The first statement is TRUE; the second statement is FALSE.
d. The first statement is FALSE; the second statement is TRUE.

14. **Which of the following nonnutritive sweeteners should be avoided by patients who have phenylketonuria?**
    a. Saccharin
    b. Acesulfame-K
    c. Sucralose
    d. Aspartame

Questions 15 to 20: Order the following cariogenicity factors of the diet (a to f) from MOST important (15) to LEAST important (20).

____15. a. Total intake of sugars (liquid or retentive)
____16. b. Form of simple sugars
____17. c. Frequency of intake
____18. d. Consumption of starch-rich foods
____19. e. Timing of ingestion
____20. f. Combining cariogenic foods with noncariogenic foods

21. **What is the recommended daily allowance (RDA) for digestible carbohydrate for adults and children?**
    a. 50 g
    b. 65 g
    c. 100 g
    d. 130 g

22. **All the following are TRUE about patients with type 2 diabetes EXCEPT:**
    a. A specialized diet is recommended to maintain blood glucose control.
    b. Daily injections of insulin are needed.
    c. Routine blood testing to monitor blood sugar levels is recommended.
    d. Medication is often prescribed to facilitate glucose metabolism.

23. **All the following signs and symptoms of diabetes mellitus EXCEPT:**
    a. Recurring gingival infections
    b. Excessive thirst
    c. Poor appetite
    d. Frequent urination

24. **Alcoholism can cause B-vitamin depletion. It can also depress antidiuretic hormone, resulting in a loss of magnesium, potassium, and zinc in urine.**
    a. Both statements are TRUE.
    b. Both statements are FALSE.
    c. The first statement is TRUE; the second statement is FALSE.
    d. The first statement is FALSE; the second statement is TRUE.

25. **Essential amino acids can be synthesized by the body and do not need to be provided by the diet. Nonessential amino acids are found in food of animal origin.**
    a. Both statements are TRUE.
    b. Both statements are FALSE.
    c. The first statement is TRUE; the second statement is FALSE.

    d. The first statement is FALSE; the second statement is TRUE.

26. Although an ovolactovegetarian diet can provide essential amino acids that are inadequate in incomplete plant proteins, which of the following nutrients might an ovolactovegetarian be deficient?
    a. Iron
    b. Vitamin B_{12}
    c. Calcium
    d. Zinc

27. The linear sequence of the components of amino acids is referred to as which type of structure?
    a. Primary
    b. Secondary
    c. Tertiary
    d. Quaternary

28. Absorption of proteins occurs at the brush border of the microvilli of the small intestine. Absorption occurs only by active transport at specific amino acid sites.
    a. Both statements are TRUE.
    b. Both statements are FALSE.
    c. The first statement is TRUE; the second statement is FALSE.
    d. The first statement is FALSE; the second statement is TRUE.

29. All the following are used for de novo synthesis of proteins EXCEPT:
    a. Deoxyribonucleic acid
    b. Alpha keto acid
    c. Messenger ribonucleic acid
    d. Ribosomal ribonucleic acid

30. Positive nitrogen balance is the normal situation for building protein-containing tissue. Negative nitrogen balance indicates net protein breakdown.
    a. Both statements are TRUE.
    b. Both statements are FALSE.
    c. The first statement is TRUE; the second statement is FALSE.
    d. The first statement is FALSE; the second statement is TRUE.

31. All the following are examples of anabolic hormones EXCEPT:
    a. Growth hormone
    b. Adrenocortical hormones
    c. Insulin
    d. Thyroid hormone

32. The cariogenic potential of foods:
    a. Can be affected by the amount of sugar in food
    b. Is related to the retentive quality of the food
    c. Is related to the time foods are beverages are in the mouth
    d. All the above
    e. Both b and c

Questions 33 to 35: For each nutrient listed below, select the physiologic fuel value (kilocalories) associated with each.
___**33.** Carbohydrates   a. 9 kcal/g
___**34.** Lipids (fats)   b. 4 kcal/g
___**35.** Proteins

___**36.** The recommended daily allowance of digestible carbohydrate is:
    a. 90 g/day
    b. 100 g/day
    c. 110 g/day
    d. 130 g/day

37. All the following are TRUE about water-soluble vitamins EXCEPT:
    a. They are sensitive to heat, light, and oxygen.
    b. They are absorbed into the blood by both active and passive transport.
    c. Deficiency symptoms are slow to develop.
    d. They are transported free and unbound.

38. Vitamins are inorganic substrates that are essential to life. Minerals are organic substrates that are essential to life.
    a. Both statements are TRUE.
    b. Both statements are FALSE.
    c. The first statement is TRUE; the second statement is FALSE.
    d. The first statement is FALSE; the second statement is TRUE.

39. Which of the following have cariostatic properties, providing a coating on the tooth's surface and forming a protective pellicle on the tooth?
    a. Proteins
    b. Carbohydrates
    c. Lipids (fats)
    d. Vitamins

40. All the following are examples of fat-soluble vitamins EXCEPT:
    a. Vitamin A
    b. Vitamin C
    c. Vitamin D
    d. Vitamin K

41. The energy required to digest, absorb and metabolize food is known as which of the following?
    a. Basal metabolic rate
    b. Kilocalories
    c. Thermic effect of food
    d. Adenosine triphosphate

42. What is a more accurate method of determining central or abdominal obesity?
    a. Body mass index
    b. Ideal body weight
    c. Waist circumference
    d. Weighing on a scale

43. Which of the following statements is TRUE regarding the diet of individuals who are edentulous or who have limited mastication due to loss of teeth?
    a. There is a reduced intake of dairy products.
    b. There is a reduced intake of grain products.
    c. There is reduced intake of meats.
    d. More fruits and vegetables are consumed.

44. All the following are important posteruptive effects of carbohydrate on the teeth EXCEPT:
    a. *Streptococcus mutans* synthesizes polysaccharides from sucrose, which enhances bacterial plaque formation.

b. Carbohydrates provide an energy source for oral bacteria.

c. Lactic acid, pyruvic acid, or acetyl–coenzyme A are the end products of glycolysis for acidogenic bacteria.

d. Carbohydrates contribute to enamel remineralization.

45. **Increased caries rate is attributed to a deficiency of vitamin D. Pulp calcification can occur if there is an excess of vitamin D.**

a. The first statement is TRUE; the second statement is FALSE.

b. The first statement is FALSE; the second statement is TRUE.

c. Both statements are TRUE.

d. Both statements are FALSE.

CASE A

Margaret is a 56-year-old patient who presents to the dental clinic for her 4-month recare appointment. As a divorced mother, she has been struggling to support her three children in college. She is currently self-employed and cleans homes and babysits for a living. Her chief complaint is sensitivity to hot and cold when eating. She also complains of dry mouth and states she sips on citrus-flavored water throughout the day.

Margaret's medical history reveals she is currently being treated by a physician for type 2 diabetes, hyperlipidemia, hypertension, and gastroesophageal reflux disease (GERD). Her medications include 1000-mg metformin, 15-mg atorvastatin, 30-mg atenolol, 20-mg Prilosec, 81-mg aspirin tablet, 600 mg of calcium twice daily, and a multivitamin. Her height is 5 feet, 2 inches, and she weighs 150 pounds. Her BMI is 27.43. She reports brushing her teeth morning and night, and she tries to floss but is not very compliant. Her plaque score is 43%. She has several "watches" that are noted on previous dental charting. New bitewing radiographs were taken at this appointment. Secondary decay was identified on the distal of tooth #19 and mesial of tooth #30. Her periodontal assessment reveals isolated probing depths of 4 to 5 mm on the maxillary and mandibular posterior teeth.

The dental hygienist questions Margaret about her diet. She reports she eats small meals throughout the day and states that she "would rather snack than eat full meals." She is also lactose intolerant, so she avoids dairy products. She likes fruits and vegetables but thinks it is time-intensive to have to prepare them, so she has developed a new habit of juicing fruits and vegetables and having a morning "smoothie." Margaret states she also consumes energy drinks each day because she believes they give her "an extra boost" to get through her day.

Answer questions 46 to 50 based on Case A.

46. **The secondary decay is most likely caused by all the following EXCEPT:**

a. GERD

b. Lactose intolerance

c. Energy drink consumption

d. Flavored-water consumption

e. Juicing with fresh fruits and vegetables

47. **Based on her calculated body mass index (BMI) of 27.43, Margaret would be classified in which of the following categories?**

a. Obesity

b. Oveweight

c. Underweight

d. Normal weight

e. Extreme obesity

48. **The direct-approach counseling technique would be best used to address Margaret's dietary concerns in relation to her oral disease risk. The counselor (dental hygienist) should provide information on the causes of the dental disease, the role of the diet, and the use of dietary assessment tools, with the client (Margaret) as an active participant.**

a. Both statements are TRUE.

b. Both statements are FALSE.

c. The first statement is TRUE; the second statement is FALSE.

d. The first statement is FALSE; the second statement is TRUE.

49. **During nutrition counseling, it is important for the dental hygienist to:**

a. Assess patient knowledge of information provided

b. Tell the patient which diet to follow

c. Include the patient in the diet planning

d. All the above

e. Both a and c

50. **Margaret has a 43% plaque score. Supragingival biofilm or plaque formation is influenced by frequent intake of which of the following in the diet?**

a. Dietary monosaccharides and disaccharides

b. Fiber-rich foods

c. Protein-rich foods

d. Fat-rich foods

13 CHAPTER

Biomaterials

Stephen C. Bayne, John M. Powers

Biomaterials, restorative materials, and tissue engineering are fundamental to dental hygiene practice and are used in a variety of dental hygiene roles. This chapter provides an overview of general applications, terminology, and classification for specific biomaterials, including preventive and restorative materials. Structure and the properties of materials, including physical, chemical, mechanical, and biologic characteristics, are also reviewed.

Direct applications of materials include dental amalgams; dental composites; pit-and-fissure sealants; infiltrants for lesions; bonding agents; cement liners and bases and luting cements; fluoride-releasing restorative materials, topical fluorides and fluoride varnishes; dentifrices and prophylactic pastes; and bleaching agents. Indirect applications include impression materials, provisional materials, models, casts, dies, waxes, investment materials, casting alloys, dental solders, chromium alloys for partial dentures, porcelain-fused-to-metal (PFM) alloys, dental ceramics, crown-and-bridge cements, acrylic appliances, acrylic denture bases, denture teeth, denture liners, denture cleansers, mouth protectors, veneers, digital scanning, computer-assisted design and computer-assisted machining (CAD/CAM), three-dimensional (3-D) printing, and dental implants. Indirect applications continue to move toward digital workflow in which all fabrication operations use computer operations to replace all traditional fabrication stages. Originally, these depended on subtractive processes (e.g., CAD/CAM machining from blocks of ceramic or composite), but many newer applications (e.g., stereolithography, inkjet printing, selective layer sintering) are additive processes.

INTRODUCTION

General Considerations

A. Applications for dental biomaterials
   1. Direct preventive and restorative dental procedures
   2. Indirect preventive and restorative dental procedures
B. Definitions and terminology
   1. Materials science terminology
   2. Biomaterials terminology for classification
C. Classification of materials for applications by:
   1. Key parts of composition-influencing properties
   2. Extent of cavity preparation

Structure

A. Composition
   1. Generally, two components in a specific ratio
      a. Powder and liquid (P/L)
      b. Powder and powder (P/P)
      c. Water and powder (W/P)
      d. Paste and paste (p/p)
      e. Paste and light
   2. Generally, the liquid part is the major reactant
B. Reaction during use
   1. Physical reaction—solidification by drying or cooling with no chemical reaction
   2. Chemical reaction—solidification by creating new primary bonds within the composition
C. Manipulation
   1. Proportioning variables
      a. Ratio of parts
      b. Temperature
      c. Relative humidity
   2. Mixing variables
      a. Manual mixing
         (1) Method of combining components (e.g., stirring and stropping)
         (2) Rate of mixing (e.g., fast and slow)
      b. Auto-mixing and machine mixing
   3. Stages of manipulation
      a. Definitions of times
         (1) Mixing time—time elapsed from onset to completion of mixing
         (2) Working time—time elapsed from onset of mixing to onset of initial setting time
         (3) Initial setting time—time at which sufficient reaction has occurred to cause the materials to be resistant to further manipulation
         (4) Final setting time—time at which the material is practically set, as defined by its resistance to indentation
      b. Definitions of intervals
         (1) Mixing interval—length of time of mixing stage
         (2) Working interval—length of time of working stage
         (3) Setting interval—length of time of setting stage
      c. All water-based materials lose their gloss at the time of setting

Properties

A. Physical properties—events that do not involve changes in composition or primary bonds
1. Descriptive properties
   a. Weight—gravitational force that attracts a body
   b. Mass—resistance of a body to acceleration (or being moved)
   c. Volume—a defined region in three-dimensional space
   d. Density—a body's weight per unit of volume
2. Thermal properties
   a. Linear coefficient of thermal expansion (LCTE, α)
      (1) Rate of expansion or contraction of one dimension of a material with temperature change (Fig. 13-1)
      (2) LCTE $= [(L_2 - L_1)/(L_1)]/(T_2 - T_1)$, where
         (a) L_1 = original length
         (b) L_2 = new length
         (c) T_1 = original temperature
         (d) T_2 = new temperature
      (3) Values reported as: in/in/°F (inch per inch per degree Fahrenheit), 10^{-6}/°F; cm/cm/°C, (centimeter per centimeter per degree Celsius), 10^{-6}/°C; ppm/°C (parts per million per degree C)
      (4) LCTE values—tooth, 9 to 11 ppm/°C; amalgam, 25 ppm/°C; composite, 35 to 45 ppm/°C; inlay wax, 300 ppm/°C
      (5) When the thermal expansion of restorative material does not match the tooth structure, percolation of fluids occurs at the margins during cyclic heating and cooling
   b. Thermal conductivity
      (1) Insulators transmit heat poorly (e.g., dental enamel, dental cements, acrylic polymers, dental porcelain, ceramic restorations)
      (2) Conductors transmit heat easily (e.g., dental amalgam, cast-gold alloys)
      (3) Teeth with metal restorations may be sensitive to hot and cold foods because of their good thermal conduction
      (4) Individuals wearing dentures may not sense normal temperature differences attributable to the thermal insulation of the acrylic denture base

FIG 13-1 Linear coefficient of thermal expansion.

$$\text{LCTE} = \alpha = \frac{\text{Fractional change in length}}{\text{Change in temperature}} = \frac{(L_2-L_1)/(L_1)}{(\Delta T)}$$

      (5) To be an effective insulator, the material must be at least 0.5 mm thick
3. Electrical properties—electrical conductivity
   a. Conductors transmit electrons easily (e.g., metals)
   b. Semiconductors transmit electrons sometimes, including ceramics and often composites
   c. Insulators transmit electrons poorly (e.g., ceramics, polymers)
4. Surface properties
   a. Contact angle—internal angle of liquid droplet with solid surface
      (1) Good wetting (angle = 0 degrees)
      (2) Spreading (angle < 90 degrees)
      (3) Poor wetting (angle ≥ 90 degrees)
   b. Reflection—degree of surface backscattering
5. Color properties
   a. Perception—physiologic response to physical stimulus by the eye, which can distinguish three parameters
      (1) Dominant wavelength—blue, green, yellow, orange, and red
      (2) Luminance—lightness of color from black to white
      (3) Excitation purity—saturation of light
   b. Measurement
      (1) Munsell Color System (e.g., 5R 6/4)
         (a) Hue—color family (R, YR, Y, GY, G, BG, B, PB, P, RP)
         (b) Value—lightness from black to white (0/ to 10/)
         (c) Chroma—saturation from gray upward (/0 to /18)
      (2) Instrumentation techniques—record the spectral reflectance versus wavelength curves (405 to 700 nm)
      (3) L*a*b* color system
         (a) L* is value
         (b) a* is red, −a* is green
         (c) b* is yellow, −b* is blue
      (4) Dental manufacturer shade guides
         (a) Custom product shades guides
         (b) VITA Classical
         (c) VITA Linearguide 3D-Master
         (d) VITA Bleachguide 3D-Master
   c. Definitions
      (1) Metamerism—colors with different spectral energy distributions that look the same under certain lighting conditions but look different with different light sources
      (2) Fluorescence—emission of light by a material when a beam of light is shined on it
      (3) Opacity—degree of light absorption by a material
      (4) Translucency—degree of internal light reflection
      (5) Transparency—degree of light transmission through a material
B. Chemical properties
1. Primary chemical bonding types
   a. Types

(1) Metallic (e.g., metals)

(2) Ionic (e.g., ceramics)

(3) Covalent (e.g., polymers)

b. Events related to changes in primary chemical bonding

  (1) Contraction attributable to chemical reaction

    (a) Rate of contraction of size of material during chemical reaction or phase change at constant temperature

    (b) Linear change (percent) $= [(L_1 - L_0)/(L_0)] \times 100\%$, where

      [1] $L_0 =$ original length

      [2] $L_1 =$ final length (after 24 hours)

    (c) Values reported as percentage changes

  (2) Corrosion of surfaces

2. Secondary chemical bonds

a. Types

  (1) Hydrogen bonding—where hydrogen is attracted to an electronegative element; found in most water-based liquids

  (2) Van der Waals forces—dispersion forces caused by fluctuating dipoles; found in dental composites and acrylics

b. Events related to changes in secondary chemical bonding

  (1) Adsorption—uptake "onto" the surface of the solid

  (2) Absorption—uptake "into" the solid

    (a) Example—water absorbed by denture

    (b) Example—moisture absorbed by alginate (imbibition)

  (3) Desorption—fluid lost from the solid; for example, water lost from alginate (syneresis)

  (4) Solubility—material loss by dissolution of surface

  (5) Disintegration—material loss by disruption of solid, usually by absorbed water

3. Corrosion

a. Chemical corrosion—chemical reaction at surface

  (1) Products may be soluble

  (2) Products may be insoluble and form layers (tarnish)

b. Electrochemical corrosion—chemical reaction that requires an anode (e.g., dental amalgam), a cathode (e.g., gold crown), an electrolyte (e.g., saliva), and an electrical circuit (e.g., contact) for electron flow (Fig. 13-2)

  (1) Galvanic corrosion—dissimilar metals in contact (previous examples)

  (2) Local galvanic corrosion (structure selective corrosion)—dissimilar phases in the same metal in contact

  (3) Crevice corrosion—corrosion in the crack under plaque, between a restoration and the tooth structure, or in the scratch on the surface of a restoration, where the metals may be the same but the electrolytes are different locally

c. Corrosion potential

  (1) Immune—does not corrode (i.e., cathodic)

  (2) Active—corrodes readily (i.e., anodic)

  (3) Passive—corrosion produces protective film, for example, chromium oxide film on stainless steel

C. Mechanical properties

1. Resolution of forces (Fig. 13-3)

a. Uniaxial (one-dimensional) forces—compression, tension, and shear

b. Complex forces—torsion, flexure, and diametral tension or compression

2. Normalization of forces and deformations

a. Stress

  (1) Applied force (or material's resistance to force) per unit area

  (2) Stress $=$ force/area

FIG 13-2 Electrochemical corrosion.

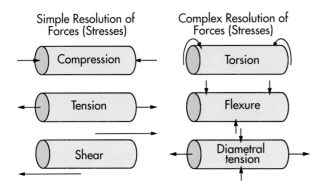

FIG 13-3 Resolution of forces.

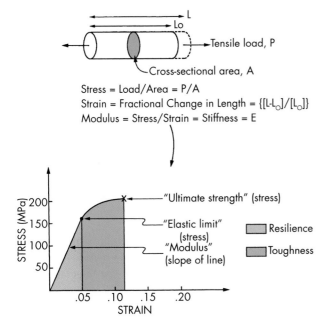

Stress = Load/Area = P/A
Strain = Fractional Change in Length = {[L-L$_0$]/[L$_0$]}
Modulus = Stress/Strain = Stiffness = E

FIG 13-4 Stress-strain curve.

    (a) lb/in^2 (pounds per square inch, psi)
    (b) kg/cm^2 (kilograms per square centimeter)
    (c) N/m^2 (megapascals, MPa)
  b. Strain (Fig. 13-4)
    (1) Change in length per unit of length because of force
    (2) Strain = $(L - l_0)/(l_0)$; dimensionless units
3. Stress-strain diagrams
  a. Plot of stress (vertical) versus strain (horizontal)
    (1) Allows convenient comparison of materials
    (2) Different curves for compression, tension, and shear
    (3) Curves depend on rate of testing and temperature
  b. Analysis of curves (see Fig. 13-4)
    (1) Elastic behavior
      (a) Elastic strain—initial response to stress (*elastic*—when the stress is removed, the strain returns to zero and the material returns to its original length)

      (b) Elastic modulus—slope of first part of curve; represents the stiffness of the material, or the resistance to elastic deformation under force
      (c) Elastic limit (proportional limit)—stress above which the material no longer behaves totally elastically
      (d) Yield strength—stress that is an estimate of the elastic limit at 0.002 permanent strain
      (e) Hardness—value on a relative scale that estimates the elastic limit in terms of a material's resistance to indentation
        [1] Examples—Knoop hardness scale, Diamond pyramid hardness scale, Brinnell hardness scale, Rockwell hardness scale, Barcol scale, Shore A hardness scale, Mohs hardness scale (Table 13-1)
        [2] Hardness values are used to determine the ability of abrasives to alter the substrates they contact
      (f) Resilience—area under the stress-strain curve up to the elastic limit; estimates the total elastic energy that can be absorbed before the onset of plastic deformation
  (2) Elastic and plastic behavior
    (a) Beyond the stress level of the elastic limit, a combination of both elastic and plastic strain exists
    (b) Ultimate strength—highest stress reached before fracture; the ultimate compressive strength is greater than the ultimate shear strength and the ultimate tensile strength
    (c) Elongation (percent elongation)—percent change in length up to the point of fracture = strain × 100%
    (d) Brittle materials—less than 10% elongation at fracture
    (e) Ductile materials—greater than 10% elongation at fracture
    (f) Toughness—area under the stress-strain curve up to the point of fracture (it estimates the total energy absorbed up to fracture)

TABLE 13-1	Mohs' Scale for Hardness*
Number	**Hardness**
10	Diamond
9	Corundum
8	Topaz
7	Quartz
6	Orthoclase
5	Apatite
4	Fluorite
3	Calcite
2	Gypsum
1	Talc

*Standard for checking hardness of abrasives and substrates.

(3) Time-dependent behavior
    (a) Strain rate sensitivity—the faster a stress is applied, the more likely a material is to store the energy elastically and not plastically
    (b) Creep—strain relaxation with time in response to a constant stress, such as dental wax deforming because of built-in stresses created during cooling
    (c) Stress relaxation—with time in response to a constant strain
    (d) Fatigue—failure caused by cyclic loading

4. Principles of cutting, polishing, and surface cleaning
  a. Terminology
    (1) Cutting—gross removal of excess material from the surfaces of restorations or teeth
    (2) Finishing—fine removal of surface material in an effort to produce finer surface scratches
    (3) Polishing—smoothing of surfaces by removal of fine scratches
    (4) Debriding—removal of unwanted material attached to surfaces
    (5) Air abrasion (air polishing)—removal or polishing of hard tissue by the kinetic energy from particles sprayed against the surface
    (6) Microabrasion—removal of stains by a mixture of an abrasive and hydrochloric acid
  b. Surface mechanics for materials (Table 13-2)
    (1) Cutting—requires materials with the highest possible hardness to produce the cuts
    (2) Finishing—requires materials with the highest possible hardness for the best effect, except at the margins of restorations, where the tooth structure may be inadvertently affected
    (3) Polishing—requires materials with small particles and with a Mohs hardness that is only 1 to 2 units above that of the substrate
    (4) Debriding—requires materials with a Mohs hardness that is less than or equal to that of the substrate to prevent scratching

TABLE 13-2 Hardness Values for Dental Substrates*

Hardness Value	Number
CAD/CAM ceramic	6-7
Porcelain	6-7
Composite	5-7
Glass	5-6
Dental enamel	5-6
Dental amalgam	4-5
Dentin	3-4
Hard gold alloys	3-4
Pure gold	2-3
Acrylic	2-3
Cementum	2-3

*Based on Mohs hardness scale: diamond = 10; talc = 1 (see Table 13-1).

c. Factors affecting cutting, polishing, and surface cleaning
  (1) Applied pressure
  (2) Particle size of abrasive
  (3) Hardness of abrasive
  (4) Hardness of substrate
  (5) Speed of rotary instrument
d. Factors affecting air abrasion
  (1) Abrasive particle size: 27-μm or 50-μm aluminum oxide
  (2) Air pressure—higher air pressure cuts faster but may cause discomfort
e. Precautions
  (1) During cutting, heat will build up and change the mechanical behavior of the substrate from brittle to ductile and will encourage formation of a smear layer
  (2) Instruments may transfer debris onto the cut surface from their own surfaces during cutting, polishing, or cleaning operations (this has important implications in cleaning dental implant surfaces)

D. Biologic properties
1. Definitions of biohazards
  a. Toxicity—cell or tissue death attributable to material concentration
  b. Sensitivity—systemic reaction to a substance
    (1) Allergy—reaction to relatively small amounts of a material
    (2) Hypersensitivity—reaction to minute amounts of a material
2. Definitions of local tissue interactions with biomaterials
  a. Fibrous tissue capsule formation (tissue encapsulation)
  b. Integration at the interface (osseo-integration)
    (1) Bone ingrowth
    (2) Bone ongrowth
  c. Biodegradation (desorption or resorption)
3. Classification of biologic materials—tissue interfaces
  a. Intraoral and supragingival—in enamel or dentin
  b. Intraoral, pulpal, or periapical
  c. Transcutaneous
  d. Subcutaneous
  e. Intraosseous
4. Clinical analysis of biocompatibility
  a. Risk versus benefits
  b. Safety and efficacy
5. Agencies that oversee materials, devices, and therapeutics
  a. Regulatory agencies—U.S. Food and Drug Administration (FDA)
  b. Standards development for manufacturing practices (for physical, chemical, mechanical, and biologic properties and for clinical testing)
    (1) American Dental Association (ADA)—Council on Scientific Affairs and Standards Committee on Dental Products (SCDP)
    (2) American National Standards Institute (ANSI)
    (3) Fédération Dentaire Internationale (FDI; International Dental Association)
    (4) International Standards Organization (ISO)

DIRECT PREVENTIVE AND RESTORATIVE MATERIALS

Dental Amalgam

A. General considerations
1. Applications
    a. Load-bearing restorations for posterior teeth (class I, class II)
    b. Pin-retained restorations
    c. Buildups (foundations) or cores for cast restorations
    d. Retrograde root canal filling material
2. Terminology
    a. Amalgam alloy—powder particles of silver-tin-copper-(zinc), or Ag-Sn-Cu-(Zn) (minor elements are indicated in parentheses)
    b. Amalgam—reaction product of any material with mercury
    c. Dental amalgam—reaction product of amalgam alloy (Ag-Sn or Ag-Sn-Cu) with mercury
3. Classification of dental amalgam by:
    a. Powder particle shape
        (1) Irregular (comminuted, filing, or lathe-cut)
        (2) Spherical (spherodized)
        (3) Blends, including irregular-irregular, irregular-spherical, or spherical- spherical
    b. Total amount of copper
        (1) Low-copper alloys (conventional, traditional); less than 5% copper (Ag-Sn-Cu)
        (2) High-copper alloys (corrosion-resistant); 12% to 28% copper (Ag-Sn-Cu)
    c. Presence of zinc
    d. Other modifications
4. Examples
    a. Low-copper, irregular-particle alloy (e.g., 70Ag-26Sn-4Cu)
    b. High-copper, blended-particle alloy with irregular particles (e.g., 70Ag-26Ag-4Cu) and spherical particles (e.g., 72Ag-28Cu)
    c. High-copper, spherical-particle alloy (e.g., 60Ag-27Sn-13Cu)
B. Structure
1. Components
    a. Mercury (Hg) mixed with amalgam alloy
    b. Mercury reacts with periphery of alloy particle to produce crystalline silver-mercury, tin-mercury, and copper–tin phases
2. Reaction (Fig. 13-5)

FIG 13-5 Amalgam reaction.

a. Setting reactions
    (1) Low-copper dental amalgam

$$Hg + Ag - Sn \rightarrow Ag - Sn + Ag - Hg + Sn - Hg$$

    (2) High-copper dental amalgam

$$Hg + Ag - Sn - Cu \rightarrow Ag - Sn - Cu + Ag - Hg + Cu - Sn$$

and

$$Hg + Ag - Sn + Ag - Cu \rightarrow Ag - Sn + Ag - Cu + Ag - Hg + Cu - Sn$$

b. Phases in set amalgams
    (1) Residual alloy (Ag-Sn, Ag-Sn-Cu, or Ag-Cu)—strongest; most corrosion-resistant
    (2) Ag-Hg ($= \gamma_1$) = major matrix phase in low-copper or high-copper dental amalgams
    (3) Sn-Hg ($= \gamma_2$) = second matrix phase in low-copper dental amalgams
    (4) Cu-Sn (η or ε) = second matrix phase in high-copper dental amalgams
3. Manipulation
    a. Selection—based on clinical requirements for strength
    b. Packaging
        (1) Powder or pressed tablets; mercury
        (2) Precapsulated powder and mercury
    c. Mixing
        (1) Mercury alloy—specific to each product but generally less than 1:1 so that amalgam contains 41% to 50% mercury
        (2) Mechanical amalgamators—variable time, speed (frequency and amplitude), and amalgamator motion for different equipment; variables affect the mixing process
        (3) Each amalgamator has specific settings for each different amalgam alloy (e.g., high-copper amalgams require 5 to 10 seconds)
        (4) Amalgamator capsules are disposable
        (5) Pestle may be included in the capsule for mixing efficiency
        (6) Overmixed mass is difficult to remove from capsule
        (7) Undermixed mass is crumbly
    d. Condensation
        (1) Adaptation of amalgam to cavity walls
        (2) Removal of excess mercury-rich matrix produces a stronger and more corrosion-resistant amalgam because it minimizes the formation of the matrix phases of amalgam, which are the least desirable parts of the set material
        (3) Amalgams with spherical alloys are more fluid and require larger-tipped condensers
        (4) It is important to condense in small increments, overpack restoration, avoid delays, and avoid saliva contamination
    e. Finishing
        (1) The anatomy should be carved within a few minutes after condensing

(2) The surface should be burnished or the final finish performed at least 24 hours later

C. Properties
1. Physical
   a. Coefficient of thermal expansion = 25 ppm/°C
   b. Thermal conductivity—high (therefore the amalgam may need an insulating liner or base in very deep cavity preparations)
2. Chemical
   a. Dimensional change on setting, should be less than ±20 μm (excessive expansion can produce postoperative pain)
   b. The cavity varnish or the bonding agent electrically insulates a dental amalgam restoration, but it does not prevent corrosion
   c. Chemical corrosion produces a black or green tarnish on the surface that is aesthetically unacceptable but is not detrimental to oral health
   d. Electrochemical corrosion produces penetrating corrosion of low-copper amalgams but produces only superficial corrosion of high-copper amalgams
3. Mechanical
   a. Compressive strength—ranges from 310 to 480 MPa, comparable with enamel (410 MPa) but is not significant in preventing marginal fracture
   b. Because of low tensile strength, enamel support is needed at the margins
   c. Spherical high-copper alloys develop high tensile strength quickly and can be polished sooner than enamel
   d. Excessive creep occurs during the Ag-Hg phase of incorrectly mixed amalgams and contributes to early marginal fracture
   e. Marginal fracture is correlated with creep and electrochemical corrosion in low-copper amalgams (Fig. 13-6)
   f. Bulk fracture (isthmus fracture) occurs across the thinnest portions of amalgam restorations because of high stresses during traumatic occlusion, the accumulated effects of fatigue, or both
   g. Dental amalgam is relatively resistant to abrasion, that is, wear; similar to human enamel

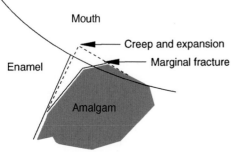

FIG 13-6 Marginal ditching in an amalgam restoration is produced by creep and expansion, which elevate the margins of the amalgam, and functional stresses produce marginal fracture.

4. Biologic
   a. Mercury hygiene
      (1) All personnel must be trained; all personnel must be made aware of mercury sources in the oral care setting
      (2) A proper work-area design is important; personnel must work in well-ventilated spaces; the treatment area atmosphere must be periodically checked for mercury vapor
      (3) Precapsulated products should be stored in tight containers
      (4) Mercury should not come into contact with the skin
      (5) Spills should be cleaned up immediately to minimize mercury vaporization
      (6) Amalgamators should be used with covers enclosing the mixing arm
      (7) High-vacuum suction should be used during amalgam alloy placement, setting, polishing, or removal when mercury may be vaporized
      (8) All scrap amalgam should be salvaged and stored in tightly closed containers and recycled in accordance with applicable laws
      (9) Mercury-contaminated items must be disposed of in sealed bags and not in medical waste containers
      (10) The dental office personnel must be aware of aerosols created by vacuuming mercury spilled on the floor or the carpet
      (11) Floor coverings should be replaced every 5 years to eliminate spilled mercury that might have accumulated in carpet pores
      (12) Professional clothing must be removed before leaving the workplace
   b. Mercury bioactivity
      (1) Depends on whether the form is metallic, inorganic, or organic mercury
      (2) Metallic mercury is the least toxic form and is absorbed primarily through the lungs rather than through the gastrointestinal (GI) tract or skin
      (3) Mercury accumulated in the body may come from air, water, food, dental sources (a low amount), or medical sources
      (4) Average half-life for mercury elimination from the body is 55 days
      (5) The U.S. Occupational Safety and Health Administration (OSHA) has set the average level for mercury toxicity by exposure as less than 50 μg/m^3 per 40-hour workweek
      (6) Incidence of mercury hypersensitivity is estimated to be less than 1 per 100 million persons
   c. Environment issues-important to:
      (1) Use best management practices (BMPs)
      (2) Use precapsulated alloys
      (3) Manage mercury through recycling—recycle used disposable amalgam capsules; salvage, store, and recycle noncontact amalgam; salvage amalgam

pieces from restorations after removal, and recycle amalgam waste
- (a) Use chairside traps to retain amalgam and recycle contents
- (b) Recycle contents retained by vacuum pump filter or other amalgam-collecting devices
- (c) Disinfect extracted teeth that contain amalgam restorations using bleach, and recycle them with chairside trap wastes

D. Amalgam alternatives
1. Direct esthetic filling materials (composites, compomers)
2. Indirect filling materials (cast gold, PFM, all-ceramic materials)

Dental Composites

A. General considerations
1. Applications
   a. Anterior restorations created for aesthetic purposes (class III, IV, and V cervical erosion, or abrasion lesions)
   b. Low-stress posterior restorations (small class I and II)
   c. High-stress posterior restorations with certain formulations
   d. Veneers
   e. Cores for cast restorations
   f. Cements for ceramic restorations
   g. Cements for resin-bonded bridges
   h. Repair systems for composites or ceramic restorations
2. Terminology (Fig. 13-7)
   a. Composite—physical mixture of materials to average the properties of the materials involved
   b. Dental composite—restorative material resulting from the mixture of ceramic reinforcing filler particles in a monomer matrix that is converted to polymer on setting
   c. Polymerization—reaction of small molecules (monomers) into very large molecules (polymers)
   d. Cross-linking—tying together of polymer molecules by chemical reaction between the molecules to produce a continuous 3-D network
3. Classification by:
   a. Amount of filler—25% to 85% by volume, 45% to 90% by weight
      (1) Very high—bulk-fill; packable or condensable composite

(2) High—universal composite
(3) Moderate—flowable composite
(4) Low—microfill
b. Filler particle size
   (1) Average sizes—minifill = 0.1 to 1.0 μm; microfill = 0.01 to 0.1 μm; nanofill = 0.001 to 0.01 μm
   (2) Mixture of sizes—hybrid (microhybrid = mini + micro)
   (3) Presence of pre-cured composite (heterogeneous)
c. Polymerization method
   (1) Auto-cured (also self-cured, SC)
   (2) Visible light–cured (VLC)
   (3) Dual-cured (VLC + SC)
d. Matrix chemistry
   (1) Bisphenol A–glycidylmethacrylate (Bis-GMA) or Bis-GMA–like monomers
   (2) Urethane dimethacrylate (UDM or UDMA) monomers
   (3) Tetraethylene glycol dimethacrylate (TEGDMA)—diluent monomer to reduce viscosity
   (4) Expanding monomers—to control overall polymerization shrinkage

B. Structure
1. Components
   a. Filler particles—colloidal silica or silicate glasses (noncrystalline) of various particle sizes (containing Ba, Li, Al, Zn, Yr, and others)
   b. Matrix—Bis-GMA (or UDMA) with lower-molecular-weight diluents (e.g., TEGDMA) that co-react during polymerization; ring-opening monomers
   c. Coupling agent—silane, which chemically bonds the surfaces of the filler particles to the polymer matrix
2. Reaction
   a. Free-radical polymerization—monomers + initiator + accelerators → polymer molecules
   b. Initiators—start polymerization by decomposing and reacting with monomer
      (1) Benzoyl peroxide typically used in SC systems
      (2) Camphorquinone typically used in VLC systems
   c. Accelerators—speed up initiator decomposition; different amines used for accelerating initiators in SC and VLC systems
   d. Retarders or inhibitors—prevent premature polymerization

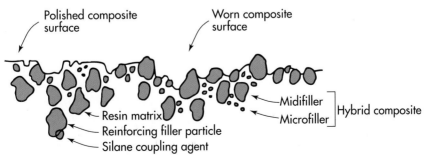

FIG 13-7 Hybrid dental composite.

3. Manipulation
    a. Selection
        (1) Microfill composites or microhybrids for anterior class III, IV, and V restorations
        (2) Microhybrids for class I, II, III, IV, and V restorations
    b. Conditioning of enamel and dentin (see later section on "Bonding Agents")
        (1) Total-etch technique:
            (a) Acid-etch with 15% to 38% phosphoric acid
            (b) Have the patient rinse for 5 to 10 seconds with water
            (c) Air-dry enamel for 5 to 10 seconds, but do not desiccate or dehydrate
            (d) Apply bonding agent and polymerize
        (2) Self-etch technique (apply bonding system)
    c. Mixing (if required)—two pastes are mixed for 20 to 30 seconds
        (1) Self-cured composite—working time is 60 to 120 seconds after mixing
        (2) Light-cured composite—working time is nearly unlimited; used for most anterior and some posterior composite restorations; natural light and dental chair lights may slowly start the reaction
        (3) Dual-cured composite—working time is 5 to 8 minutes
    d. Placement—a plastic instrument or syringe or a unidose (compule) should be used
    e. Light curing—it is important to:
        (1) Check the output of the light-curing unit
        (2) Use high-intensity quartz-tungsten-halogen (QTH) or light-emitting-diode (LED)
        (3) Cure incrementally in 1.5 to 2.0 mm–thick layers; use a matrix strip, where possible, to produce a smooth surface and to contour the composite
    f. Finishing and polishing—it is important to:
        (1) Remove the oxygen-inhibited layer (with alcohol swab)
        (2) Use stones, carbide burrs, or diamonds for gross reduction
        (3) Use multi-fluted carbide burs or special diamonds for fine reduction
        (4) Use aluminum oxide strips or discs for finishing or rubber points, cups, and discs
        (5) Use fine aluminum oxide or diamond finishing pastes
        (6) Microfill and nanofill composites develop smoothest finish because of small size of filler particles
        (7) Keep in mind that liquid polishes provide short-term smooth-surface coatings
C. Properties—generally improve with filler content
    1. Physical
        a. Radiopacity depends on the ions in silicate glass
        b. Coefficient of thermal expansion is 35 to 45 ppm/°C and decreases with increasing filler content
        c. Thermal and electrical insulators

2. Chemical
    a. Water absorption is 0.5% to 2.5% and increases with polymer content
    b. Acidulated topical fluorides (e.g., acidulated phosphate fluoride [APF]) tend to dissolve glass particles, and thus composites should be protected with a non–petroleum-based jelly during these procedures, or a different topical fluoride (e.g., neutral sodium fluoride) should be used
    c. In the past, major color changes occurred in resin matrix with time because of oxidation, which produces colored byproducts, but the modern composites are highly color stable; some composites experience a slight shade shift when light-cured
3. Mechanical
    a. The compressive strength is 310 to 410 MPa, which is adequate
    b. Wear resistance—improves with higher filler content, higher percentage of conversion in curing, use of microfiller, and closer interparticle spacing of fillers
    c. Surfaces that are rough from wear retain plaque biofilm and stain more readily
4. Biologic—the components may be cytotoxic, but the cured composite is biocompatible as restorative filling material

Pit-and-Fissure Sealants

A. General considerations—see the section on "Dental Sealants" in Chapter 16.
    1. Applications
        a. Occlusal surfaces of newly erupted posterior teeth
        b. Lingual surfaces of anterior teeth with fissures
        c. Occlusal surfaces of teeth in older persons with reduced flow of saliva (because low levels of saliva increase susceptibility to dental caries)
    2. Classification by:
        a. Polymerization method
            (1) Self-curing
            (2) Light-curing—90% of current products
        b. Filler content
            (1) Unfilled—many systems are unfilled because filler tends to interfere with and wear away from self-cleaning occlusal areas; sealants are designed to wear away, except where no self-cleaning action occurs; a common misconception is that sealants should be wear resistant
            (2) Lightly filled—10% to 30% by weight
B. Structure
    1. Components
        a. Monomer—Bis-GMA–like or UDMA monomers with TEGDMA, a diluent monomer, to facilitate flow into pits and fissures before cure
        b. Initiator—benzoyl peroxide (in self-cured) and camphorquinone (in light-cured)
        c. Accelerator—amine
        d. Opaque filler—1% titanium dioxide or other colorant to make the material detectable on tooth surfaces

e. Reinforcing filler—silicate glass (generally not added because wear resistance is not required within pits and fissures)

f. Fluoride—may be added for slow release

2. Reaction—free-radical reaction (see the previous section on "Dental Composites")

3. Manipulation

a. Preparation—this involves:

(1) Cleaning the pits and fissures of organic debris

(2) Etching the occlusal surfaces, pits, and fissures with 37% phosphoric acid

(3) Washing the occlusal surfaces for 5 to 10 seconds

(4) Drying the etched area for 5 to 10 seconds with clean air spray

(5) Applying the sealant and polymerizing

b. Mixing or dispensing

(1) Self-cured—equal amounts of liquids are mixed in a Dappen dish for 5 seconds with a brush applicator

(2) Light-cured—syringes or unidose tips are used for dispensing

c. Placement—pits, fissures, and occlusal surfaces; this involves:

(1) 60 seconds for self-cured materials to set

(2) Light-curing according to manufacturer's instructions

d. Finishing

(1) Unpolymerized (air-inhibited layer) and excess materials should be removed

(2) The hardness and marginal adaptation of the sealant should be examined

(3) Occlusal adjustments should be made, where necessary, in the sealant; most unfilled sealant materials are self-adjusting

C. Properties

1. Physical—wetting: low-viscosity sealants wet acid-etched tooth structure the best

2. Mechanical

a. Wear resistance should not be too great because the sealant should be able to wear off the self-cleaning areas of tooth

b. To prevent loss, sealants should be protected during polishing procedures with air-abrading units

3. Biologic—no apparent biologic problems

4. Clinical efficacy

a. Effectiveness is 100% if retained in pits and fissures

b. Requires routine clinical evaluation (every 1.5 to 2 years) to check the integrity and resealing of defective areas if sealant loss is attributable to poor retention

c. Sealants resist attack from topical fluorides (also applied for prevention of dental caries)

Infiltrants

A. General considerations

1. Applications—approximal and smooth-surface uncavitated lesions where sealing would not be a permanent solution to stop lesion growth and to create good esthetics

2. Definition—a resin system capable of penetrating through slightly porous enamel, embedding into an existing decalcified region of dentin, stopping lesion activity by preventing the diffusion of organic acids below plaque and restoring the esthetics of the tooth structure

3. Classification—this is a new and novel approach to minimally invasive dentistry for interproximal, uncavitated lesion repair; currently, only one system is available on the market

a. Approximal application kit

b. Smooth-surface application kit

B. Structure

1. Components—acrylic monomer infiltrant after use of a hydrochloric acid (HCl; hydrogen chloride, hydrochloride) etchant to create micropores in the enamel overlying the lesion and to allow resin penetration

2. Reaction—the resin is light-cured

3. Manipulation (approximal repair)

a. Wedging of teeth to separate interproximal contacts

b. Application of acid etchant (more than 90 seconds with 15% aqueous HCl) to create micropores through the overlying enamel by using a unique holder and a film packet to deliver materials

c. VLC materials

C. Properties

1. Physical—the tooth structure appears to have normal color and opacity after infiltration

2. Chemical—no evidence of dentin decalcification after infiltration

3. Mechanical—previously decalcified dentin is restored to approximately the same hardness

4. Biologic—no evidence of any threat to the pulp before setting

Bonding Agents

A. General considerations

1. Applications—composites, resin-modified glass ionomers, compomers, bonded ceramic restorations, veneers, orthodontic brackets, desensitizing dentin by covering exposed tubules, resin-bonded bridges, composite-repair and ceramic-repair systems, and amalgams

2. Definitions

a. Smear layer—thin layer (0.5 to 5.0 μm) of compacted debris on enamel and dentin resulting from the cavity-preparation process (Fig. 13-8) that is weakly held to the surface (5 to 6 MPa) and that limits bonding agent strength if not removed

FIG 13-8 The surface of cut dentin, with a smear layer and smear plugs occluding the dentinal tubules.

b. Etching (or conditioning)—smear layer removal and production of microspaces for micromechanical bonding by dissolving minor amounts of surface hydroxyapatite crystals
   (1) Total-etch (or etch-and-rinse) system—phosphoric acid should be used
   (2) Self-etch system—reliance on acidic monomer to dissolve smear layer, etch surface of intertubular dentin, and embed collagen fibers; no rinsing
c. Priming—micromechanical (and possibly chemical) bonding to the microspaces created by the conditioning step
d. Conditioning and priming agent (self-etching primer)—agent that accomplishes both actions
e. Bonding—formation of resin layer that connects the primed surface to the overlying restoration (e.g., composite)

3. Classification
   a. Major substrate
      (1) Enamel and dentin bonding system—for bonding to enamel and dentin composite or other restorative materials
      (2) Amalgam bonding system—for bonding amalgam to enamel and dentin to amalgam
      (3) Universal bonding system—for bonding an appliance to enamel, dentin, amalgam, ceramic, metallic alloy, or any other substrate that may be necessary for a restorative procedure using the same set of procedures and materials
   b. Number of components and type of etching (Fig. 13-9)
      (1) Three-component total-etch system—etching +priming+bonding (E+P+B) (also called *fourth-generation*; involves two layers of material)
      (2) Two-component total-etch system—etching+ priming/bonding (E+PB) (also called *fifth-generation*; involves one layer of material)
      (3) Two-component self-etch system—etching/priming+bonding (EP+B) (also called *sixth-generation type 1*; involves two layers of material)
      (4) One-component self-etch system—etching/priming/bonding) (EPB)—materials are mixed (if necessary) and scrubbed onto the surface to be bonded using the applicator tip [also called *sixth-generation type 2* or *seventh-generation* (no mixing), involves one layer of material]
      (5) Universal system—etching/priming/bonding (EPB) system is compatible with etching with phosphoric acid, system may contain components that prime zirconia-based ceramics, silica-based ceramics, and metals

B. Structure
   1. Components of bonding systems
      a. Conditioning agent—mineral (e.g., 10% to 40% phosphoric acid), organic acid (e.g., polyacrylic acid), or acidic acrylic monomer (e.g., phosphonate)
      b. Priming agent—resin and monomer in alcohol, acetone, or water
      c. Bonding agent—Bis-GMA or UDMA monomers
   2. Reaction
      a. Bonding occurs primarily by intimate micromechanical retention, with the relief created by the conditioning step
      b. Chemical bonding is possible but is not recognized as contributing significantly to the overall bond strength
   3. Manipulation (manufacturer's instructions should be followed)
      a. Conditioning

FIG 13-9 Evolution of bonding system types with fewer components.

(1) Total-etch technique—this involves:
    (a) Applying phosphoric acid solution or equivalent
    (b) Rinsing and drying without desiccation (dentin should be kept moist with "glistening" appearance)
    (c) In case of overdried dentin, remoistening surface with water or a rewetting solution for 10 to 15 seconds
(2) Self-etch technique—this involves applying an acidic primer or a bonding agent, no rinsing
  b. Priming—this involves:
    (1) Applying a priming agent, and gently drying to remove excess solvent (but air-thinning must not be done unless recommended by manufacturer)
    (2) Applying several layers until dentin is fully impregnated to surface
  c. Bonding—this involves:
    (1) Applying one to two coats of bonding agent when bonding composites
    (2) Applying multiple coats of the bonding agent or mixing it with a thickening agent in preparation for bonding with amalgam restorations

C. Properties
  1. Physical—thermal expansion and contraction may create fatigue stresses that debond the interface and permit microleakage
  2. Chemical—water absorption into the bonding agent may chemically alter the bonding
  3. Mechanical—mechanical stresses may produce fatigue that can debond the interface and permit microleakage
    a. Enamel bonding—adhesion occurs by macrotags (between enamel prisms) and microtags (into enamel prisms) to produce micromechanical retention
    b. Dentin bonding—adhesion occurs by removal of smear layer and formation of microtags within intertubular dentin to produce a hybrid zone (interpenetration or diffusion zone) that microscopically intertwines collagen bundles and bonding agent polymer; macrotags within tubules do not add much to retention because they are poorly polymerized and poorly adapted
  4. Biologic
    a. Conditioning agents may be locally irritating if they come into contact with soft tissue
    b. Uncured priming agents, particularly those based on hydroxyethyl methacrylate (HEMA), may become skin sensitizers for dental personnel after several contacts
      (1) Hands and face must be protected from inadvertent contact with unset materials and their vapors
      (2) HEMA and other priming monomers may penetrate through rubber gloves in relatively short times (60 to 90 seconds)

Cement Liners (Calcium Hydroxide; Zinc Oxide–Eugenol; Bioceramic)

A. General considerations—applications (if remaining dentin thickness is less than 0.5 mm)

1. Thermal insulation where the cavity preparation is close to the pulp
2. Delivering medications to the pulp
    a. Calcium hydroxide (CH) liners—in self-cured and light-cured versions that stimulate reparative dentin
    b. Zinc oxide–eugenol (ZOE) relieves pain by desensitizing nerves
    c. Bioceramic promotes remineralization

B. CH structure (for ZOE types; see the section on "Dental Sealants")
  1. Components
    a. Paste of CH reactant powder, ethyl toluene sulfonamide dispersant, zinc oxide filler, and zinc stearate radiopacifier
    b. Paste of glycol salicylate reactant liquid, titanium dioxide filler powder, and calcium tungstenate radiopacifier
  2. Reaction
    a. Chemical reaction of calcium ions with salicylate to form methylsalicylate salts
    b. Moisture absorbed to allow CH to dissociate into ions to react with salicylate
    c. Mixture sets from outside surface to inside as water diffuses
  3. Manipulation
    a. Dentin should not be dehydrated, or material will not set
    b. A drop each of the pastes should be mixed together for 5 seconds
    c. The material should be applied to dentin; 1 to 2 minutes should be allowed for the material to set

C. CH properties
  1. Physical—good thermal and electrical insulator
  2. Chemical—poor resistance to water solubility, so may dissolve
  3. Mechanical—low compressive strength (0.7 to 3.4 MPa)
  4. Biologic—releases constituents, which diffuse toward the pulp and stimulate reparative dentin formation

Cement Bases

A. General considerations (limited use)
  1. Applications
    a. Thermal insulation below a restoration (Fig. 13-10)
    b. Mechanical protection where dentin is inadequate to support amalgam condensation pressures

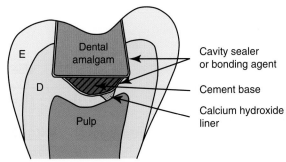

FIG 13-10 Sealer, liner, and base applications for use with dental amalgam. *E*, Enamel; *D*, dentin.

2. Classification (many materials have been used in the past)
   a. Glass ionomer (GI) cement bases
   b. Resin-modified glass ionomer (RMGI)—light-curing compositions
B. Structure (see the section on "Crown-and-Bridge Cements")
   1. Components
      a. Self-curing cements (ZP, PC, GI)—reactive powder (chemically basic) and reactive liquid (chemically acidic)
      b. Light-curing cements (RMGI)—paste
      c. Bioceramic—paste containing calcium silicate or bioactive filler and resin
   2. Reaction
      a. Self-curing cement—acid–base reaction that forms salts or cross-linked matrix; reaction may be exothermic
      b. Light-curing cements—monomer polymerization is exothermic
   3. Manipulation—consistency for basing includes more powder, which improves all of the cement properties
C. Properties
   1. Physical—excellent thermal and electrical insulation
   2. Chemical—much more resistant to dissolution than cement liners
      a. Polycarboxylate (PC) and GI cements are chemically adhesive to tooth structure
      b. Solubility of all cement bases is lower than that of cement liners if they are mixed at higher powder-to-liquid ratios
   3. Mechanical—much higher compressive strengths (80 to 210 MPa) than those of luting cements
      a. Light-cured RMGI cements are the strongest
      b. ZOE cements are the weakest
   4. Biologic (see the section on "Crown-and-Bridge Cements" for details)—PC, GI, and RMGI cements, properly handled, provide good biocompatibility with pulp

Other Cement Applications

A. Root canal sealers
   1. Applications
      a. Cementing of silver cone or guttapercha point
      b. Paste filling material
   2. Classification
      a. Zinc oxide–eugenol cement types
      b. Noneugenol cement types
      c. Therapeutic cement types
      d. Flowable composite types
   3. Important properties
      a. Physical—radiopacity
      b. Chemical—insolubility
      c. Mechanical—flow; tensile strength
      d. Biologic—inert
B. Gingival tissue packs
   1. Application—provide temporary displacement of gingival tissues
   2. Composition—slow-setting ZOE cement mixed with cotton twills for texture and strength
C. Surgical dressings
   1. Application—gingival covering after periodontal surgery
   2. Composition—modified ZOE cement (containing tannic acid, rosin, and various oils)
D. Orthodontic cements
   1. Application—cementing of orthodontic bands
   2. Composition—composite (see the sections on "Crown-and-Bridge Cements" and "Bonding Agents")
   3. Manipulation
      a. Resin (composite) cements use total-etch or self-etch bonding systems for improved bonding
      b. Band, bracket, or cement removal requires special care

Fluoride-Releasing Restorative Materials

A. General considerations
   1. Applications for glass ionomers (GIs), resin-modified glass ionomers (RMGIs), compomers, and atraumatic restorative technique (ART) materials
      a. Class V restorations—GIs and RMGIs for geriatric dentistry
      b. Class I and II restorations—RMGIs and compomers in pediatric dentistry; and ART temporary restorations in people living in the underserved regions of the world
      c. Class III restorations—RMGIs and compomers
   2. Classification by composition (Fig. 13-11)
      a. Conventional GIs—limited use
      b. Metal-modified GIs—limited use
      c. RMGIs (hybrid ionomers)—popular use
      d. Compomers—limited use
      e. Giomers—limited use
      f. RMGIs (ART materials)—extremely popular use for temporaries, ART, and permanent restorations in

FIG 13-11 Evolution of glass ionomer composites over 35 years, leading toward composites. *ART,* Atraumatic restoration technique.

pediatric dentistry applications (representing the largest use of GI restorative material)

B. Structure
1. Components
   a. Conventional glass ionomers—aluminosilicate glass powder and liquid water solution of co-polymers (or acrylic acid with maleic, tartaric, or itaconic acid)
   b. Metal-modified glass ionomers—used for cores
   c. Resin-modified glass ionomers—aluminosilicate glass powder and liquid with water solution of co-polymers (or acrylic acid with maleic, tartaric, or itaconic acids) and water-soluble monomers, for example, HEMA
   d. Compomers—hybrid of RMGI and composite
   e. Giomers—compomers with precured GI particles blended into a mixture
   f. Resin-reinforced (ART materials)—high fluoride-releasing conventional GI that may have small amounts of resin added for increased tackiness
2. Reactions (may involve several reactions and stages of setting)
   a. Glass ionomer reaction (acid-base reaction of polyacid and ions released from aluminosilicate glass particles)
      (1) Calcium, aluminum, fluoride, and other ions released by the outside of the powder particle dissolving in acidic liquid
      (2) Calcium ions initially cross-link acid-functional co-polymer molecules
      (3) Calcium cross-links are replaced in 24 to 48 hours by aluminum ion cross-links, with increased hardening of system
      (4) If no other reactants are present in the cement (e.g., resin modification), protection from saliva is required during the first 24 hours, unless otherwise indicated by manufacturer's instructions
   b. Polymerization reaction (polymerization of double bonds from water-soluble monomers or pendant groups on the co-polymer to form cross-linked matrix)
      (1) Polymerization reaction can be initiated with chemical (self-curing) or light-curing steps
      (2) Cross-linked polymer matrix ultimately interpenetrates the GI matrix
      (3) Occurs in resin-modified GI materials and compomers
3. Manipulation
   a. Self-curing materials—powder and liquid components may be manually mixed or may be precapsulated for mechanical mixing; light-curing materials—directly placed from a syringe or a unidose tip
   b. Placement—mixture is normally placed by using a syringe
   c. Finishing—can be immediate if the system is resin modified or is a compomer system (but otherwise must be delayed 24 to 72 hours until aluminum ion replacement reaction is complete)
   d. Sealing—the resin sealer is applied to smooth the surface (and to protect against moisture affecting the GI reaction)

C. Properties
1. Physical
   a. Good thermal and electrical insulation
   b. Better radiopacity than with most composites
   c. Linear coefficient of thermal expansion and contraction is closer to that of the tooth structure than that of composites (but is less well matched for resin-modified and compomer systems)
   d. The esthetics of resin-modified and compomer systems is not quite as good as those of most composites
2. Chemical
   a. Reactive acid side groups of co-polymer molecules produce chemical bonding to the tooth structure
   b. Fluoride ions are released
      (1) Rapid release at first because of excess fluoride ions in the matrix
      (2) Slow release after 7 to 30 days because of slow diffusion of fluoride ions out of aluminosilicate particles (Fig. 13-12)
      (3) Presence of fluoride in topical fluorides and fluoride-containing toothpastes may recharge the fluoride content in the cement matrix temporarily for 2 to 3 days
   c. The solubility resistance of resin-modified systems is close to that of composites
3. Mechanical
   a. Compressive strength of resin-modified systems and compomers is much better than that of conventional glass ionomers but not quite as strong as that of composites
   b. Glass ionomers are more brittle than are composites
4. Biologic
   a. Ingredients are biologically compatible with pulp
   b. Fluoride ion release may reduce the incidence and severity of secondary caries (Fig. 13-12), but no definitive clinical research studies exist

Topical Fluorides and Fluoride Varnishes

A. General considerations (see the section on "Fluoride Agents for Professional Application" in Chapter 16)
1. Applications—used to prevent smooth-surface caries
2. Classification
   a. Acidulated phosphate fluoride (APF) gels (acid pH)
   b. Neutral fluoride gels (sodium fluoride at neutral pH)
   c. Fluoride varnishes (5% sodium fluoride, 2.26% fluoride, 22,600 ppm fluoride)
B. Structure for APF
1. Composition
   a. Acidulated phosphate fluoride
      (1) Fluoride ion concentration ranges from 1.22% to 1.32%
      (2) Ingredients—2% sodium fluoride, 0.34% hydrogen fluoride, 0.98% orthophosphoric acid, thickening agent, flavoring agent, coloring agent, and aqueous gel
      (3) pH ranges from 3 to 4; may dissolve glass in restorations, thus those surfaces must be protected

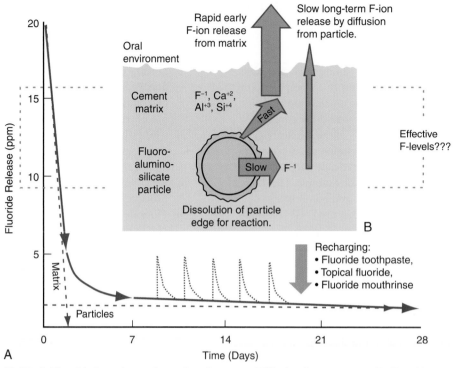

FIG 13-12 A, Fluoride ion release from glass ionomer. Diffusion from cement. **B,** Fluoride concentration released over time. (From Bayne SC, Thompson JY: Biomaterials. In Roberson TM, Heymann HO, Swift EJ, editors: *Sturdevant's art and science of operative dentistry*, ed 5, St Louis, 2006, Mosby.)

b. Neutral fluoride gels
c. Fluoride varnishes—fluoride source mixed with urethane or other resin and dissolved in solvent

2. Reactions
  a. APF—acid demineralization of the outer layer of enamel; fluoride accelerates the remineralization of demineralized enamel; fluoride ions are incorporated to produce fluoride-substituted hydroxyapatite
  b. Neutral fluoride gels—form fluoride salts on surfaces of teeth
  c. Fluoride varnishes—provide temporary film to allow longer-term fluoride diffusion from varnish into enamel

3. Manipulation
  a. Gels are applied in a soft, spongy tray after extrinsic stain removal; teeth should be free from saliva; maxillary and mandibular trays are loaded, placed in position, and squeezed to mold the trays tightly around teeth; the tray is held in position for 4 minutes (shorter applications are not effective); the client is told not to eat, smoke, or drink for 30 minutes
  b. Varnishes are painted onto all tooth surfaces; wear away after several hours

C. Properties
  1. Chemical—enamel solubility is decreased by fluoride ion incorporation
  2. Biologic—enamel is more resistant to carious dissolution

Dentifrices and Prophylactic Pastes

A. General considerations
  1. Cleansing—removal of exogenous stains, pellicle, materia alba, and other oral debris without causing undue abrasion to tooth structure
  2. Polishing—smoothing surfaces (without significant abrasion) of amalgam, composites, glass ionomers, ceramic, and other restorative materials
  3. Factors influencing cleaning and polishing
    a. Hardness of abrasive particles versus that of the substrate (see Tables 13-1 and 13-2)
    b. Particle size of abrasive particles
    c. Pressure applied during procedure
    d. Temperature of abrasive materials
    e. Speed of the rotating instrument used (easiest factor to control)

B. Structure
  1. Composition—contain abrasives, such as kaolinite, silicon dioxide, calcined magnesium silicate, diatomaceous silicon dioxide, pumice, sodium-potassium–aluminum silicate, and zirconium silicate; some pastes also may contain sodium fluoride or stannous fluoride, but they have not been shown to produce therapeutic effects
  2. Reactions—abrasion for cleansing and polishing
  3. Manipulation (see the earlier section on "Properties," B. Mechanical properties, Principles of cutting, polishing, and surface cleaning)

C. Properties
  1. Mechanical
    a. Products with pumice and quartz enable more efficient cleansing but also generate greater abrasion of enamel and dentin
    b. Coarse pumice is the most abrasive
    c. Dentin is abraded five to six times faster than enamel, regardless of the product used, and cementum is abraded even more quickly than is dentin
    d. Polymeric restorative materials such as denture bases, denture teeth, composites, and composite veneers can easily be scratched during polishing
    e. Ceramic restorations that are externally characterized should not be polished, or the surface color will be lost
  2. Biologic—no known problems

Whitening Agents

A. General considerations
  1. Lighten discolored teeth
  2. Classification by:
    a. Site of application
      (1) External—applied to the tooth surface
      (2) Internal—applied inside the pulpless (endodontically treated) tooth
    b. Method of application
      (1) In-office—applied professionally
      (2) At-home—dispensed by the dentist or obtained over the counter (OTC) and applied by the client
B. Structure
  1. In-office systems use light, heat, or both to "activate" a high concentration (up to 30% to 39%) hydrogen peroxide gel or paste, but little evidence that light or heat provides any benefit
  2. At-home systems typically use a 10% carbamide peroxide (equivalent to 3.4% hydrogen peroxide) or higher (15% to 20% carbamide peroxide) concentration that is applied in a custom-fitted, mouthguard-type, soft-plastic tray
  3. New systems use thin polyethylene strips impregnated with 5.3% hydrogen peroxide (OTC) and 14% hydrogen peroxide (office dispensed)
C. Properties
  1. The effectiveness of whitening depends on application time and dose
  2. In-office whitening can provide faster results but is more expensive than at-home bleaching
  3. Yellow-colored teeth bleach more rapidly than do gray-colored teeth
  4. Tetracycline-stained teeth whiten very slowly (several months of daily at-home treatment needed) or not at all
  5. Most common side effects are tooth sensitivity and gingival irritation; both are transient

INDIRECT PREVENTIVE AND RESTORATIVE MATERIALS

Impression Materials

A. General considerations
  1. Applications
    a. Dentulous impressions
      (1) For casts in prosthodontics
      (2) For pediatric and orthodontic appliances
      (3) For study models in orthodontics
    b. Edentulous impressions for casts in denture construction
  2. Terminology
    a. Rigid—inflexible and cannot be removed from undercut area
    b. Flexible—can be removed from undercut area
    c. Hydrocolloid—gel produced by interconnection of small particles (colloid, less than 1 μm) dispersed in water
    d. Elastomeric—based on flexible polymeric material
  3. Classification
    a. Rigid impression materials (very limited use)
      (1) Plaster
      (2) Compound
      (3) Zinc oxide–eugenol
    b. Flexible hydrocolloid impression materials
      (1) Agar-agar (reversible hydrocolloid [limited use])
      (2) Alginate (irreversible hydrocolloid)
    c. Flexible, elastomeric, general-purpose impression materials
      (1) Polysulfide elastomer (mercaptan rubber [limited use])
      (2) Silicone elastomer (condensation silicone [laboratory use])
      (3) Polyether (PE) elastomer
      (4) Polyvinyl siloxane (PVS) (addition silicone)
      (5) PE-PVS hybrid
    d. Precision impression materials used for prosthodontics
      (1) Addition silicones—contain surfactants to make surface wetting easier
      (2) Polyethers—more hydrophilic
B. Structure
  1. Components (Table 13-3)
    a. Most contain fillers to control shrinkage
    b. Matrix
  2. Reaction (Table 13-3)
    a. Physical reaction—cooling causes reversible hardening
    b. Chemical reaction—irreversible reaction during setting
  3. Manipulation
    a. Mixing
      (1) Powder-liquid (P/L) types mixed in bowl (plaster and alginate)
      (2) Thermoplastic materials not mixed (compound and agar-agar)

TABLE 13-3   Impression Materials

Materials	Type	Reaction	Composition	Manipulation	Initial Setting Time
Plaster (limited use)	Rigid	Chemical	Calcium sulfate hemihydrate, water	Mix powder and liquid (P/L) in bowl	3-5 min
Compound (limited use)	Rigid	Physical	Resins, wax, stearic acid, and fillers	Soften by heating	Variable (sets on cooling)
Zinc oxide–eugenol (limited use)	Rigid	Chemical	Zinc oxide powder, oils, eugenol, and resin	Mix pastes on pad	3-5 min
Agar-agar (limited use)	Flexible	Physical	12%-15% agar, borax, potassium sulfate, and 85% water	Conditioned in heated bath	Variable (sets on cooling)
Alginate	Flexible	Chemical	Sodium alginate, calcium sulfate, retarders, and 85% water	Mix P/L in bowl	4-5 min
Polysulfide (limited use)	Flexible	Chemical	Low-molecular-weight (LMW) mercaptan polymer, fillers, lead dioxide, copper hydroxide, or peroxides	Mix pastes on pad	5-7 min
Silicone (limited use)	Flexible	Chemical	Hydroxyl functional dimethyl siloxane, fillers, tin octoate, and orthoethyl silicate	Mix pastes on pad	4-5 min
Polyether	Flexible	Chemical	Aromatic sulfonic acid ester and polyether with ethylene imine groups	Mixing gun or mixing machine	4-6 min
Polyvinyl siloxane (addition silicone)	Flexible	Chemical	Vinyl silicone, filler, chloroplatinic acid, LMW silicone, and filler	Mixing gun or mixing machine	4-5 min

(3) Hand-mix—paste-paste (p/p) types are hand-mixed on a pad (ZOE, polysulfide rubber, silicone rubber, PE rubber, and PVS)

(4) Auto-mix—p/p types are mixed through a disposable nozzle on an auto-mixing gun (PVS, PE)

(5) Machine-mix—components mixed and extruded through a disposable nozzle using small machine (e.g., Dynamix speed, Pentamix 3)

b. Placement
   (1) Mixed material—carried in a tray to the mouth (full arch, quadrant, or triple tray)
   (2) The material sets in the mouth more quickly because of higher temperature

c. Removal—rapid removal of the impression encourages deformation to take place elastically rather than permanently (elastic recovery requires approximately 20 minutes)

d. Cleaning and disinfection of impressions (see the section on "Maintaining the Treatment Area During Client Care" in Chapter 10)

e. Problems—PVS may be inhibited from bonding at the surface of the preparation wall by the bonding agent and also may be dissolved by subsequent infection control solutions; components from latex gloves can contaminate the impression

Provisional Materials

A. General considerations
   1. Applications
      a. While waiting for laboratory fabrication of cast restoration
      b. While observing the reaction of pulp tissue
   2. Terminology
      a. Temporary—provisional or nonpermanent; range of use is 2 to 52 weeks
      b. Short-term use—2 to 6 weeks
      c. Longer-term use—6 to 52 weeks
      d. Provisional materials—usually include both provisional restoration and provisional cement
      e. Direct—set intraorally (in situ)
      f. Indirect—set out of the mouth
   3. Objectives
      a. Physiologic objectives—protection of hard and soft tissues, pulpal protection, delivery of medication, stabilization of tooth, provision of function for chewing, patient comfort
      b. Esthetic objectives—short-term resistance to staining
      c. Clinical objectives—ease of use, low cost, ease of repair, low polymerization exotherm, minimal surface reactions on curing, absence of sensitivity reactions
      d. Material performance objectives—fracture resistance, wear resistance
   4. Classification
      a. Provisional resins
      b. Temporary or provisional cements
B. Structure
   1. Components
      a. Provisional restorations
         (1) ZOE cement, with cotton fibers
         (2) Acrylic P/L products
         (3) Bis-acryl and bis-methacryl resin products
      b. Provisional cements
         (1) ZOE-based cements
         (2) Calcium hydroxide cements
         (3) Admix cements (cements mixed with petroleum jelly)
         (4) Composite cements (without bonding systems)

2. Reaction (see the sections on "Dental Composites" and "Cement Liners")
3. Manipulation (see "Dental Composites" and "Cement Liners")

C. Properties
   1. Physical
      a. Excellent thermal and electrical insulation
      b. Percolation resistance is good for cements but poor for resins
   2. Chemical—generally good resistance to dissolution
   3. Mechanical
      a. Good short-term resistance to fracture
      b. Poor resistance to abrasion
      c. Limited color stability and stain resistance
   4. Biologic—cements are biocompatible, but resins with low-molecular-weight monomers may cause pulpal inflammation if cured in situ without caution

Model, Cast, and Die Materials

A. General considerations
   1. Applications
      a. Gold casting, ceramic, and porcelain-fused-to-metal veneer fabrication procedures
      b. Orthodontic and pediatric appliance construction
      c. Study models for occlusal records
   2. Terminology
      a. Models—replicas of hard and soft tissues for study of dental symmetry
      b. Casts—working replicas of hard and soft tissues for use in the fabrication of appliances or restorations
      c. Dies—working replicas of one tooth (or a few teeth) used for the fabrication of a restoration
      d. Duplicates—second casts prepared from original casts
   3. Classification by materials
      a. Models (model plaster, orthodontic stone, or printed resin)
      b. Casts (regular stone or printed resin)
      c. Dies—may be electroplated (very limited use)
         (1) Diestone—gypsum product
         (2) Epoxy dies—epoxy polymer; abrasion-resistant dies
         (3) Printed resin—produced from digital files using 3-D printer

B. Structure of gypsum products
   1. Components (Table 13-4)
      a. Powder (calcium sulfate hemihydrate = β-$CaSO_4 \times$ ½ H_2O)
      b. Water (for mixing and reacting with powder)
   2. Reaction
      a. Calcium sulfate hemihydrate (one-half mole of water) crystals dissolve and react with water
      b. Calcium sulfate dihydrate (two moles of water) form and precipitate new crystals
      c. Unreacted (excess) water is left between crystals and slowly evaporates
   3. Manipulation of gypsum products
      a. Selection—based on strength for models, casts, or dies
      b. Mixing

TABLE 13-4 Gypsum Products

Characteristics	Plaster	Stone	Diestone
Chemical name	β-Calcium sulfate hemihydrates	α-Calcium sulfate hemihydrate	α-Calcium sulfate hemihydrate
Formula	$CaSO_4 \cdot \times$ ½ H_2O	$CaSO_4 \cdot \times$ ½ H_2O	$CaSO_4 \cdot \times$ ½ H_2O
Uses	Plaster models, impression plaster	Cast stone, investments	Improved stone, diestone
Water (W)			
Reaction water	18 mL	18 mL	18 mL
Extra water	32 mL	12 mL	6 mL
Total water	50 mL	30 mL	24 mL
Powder (P)	100 g	100 g	100 g
W/P ratio	0.50	0.30	0.24

      (1) Appropriate proportions of water and powder are dispensed (Table 13-4)
      (2) The powder is sifted into the water in a rubber mixing bowl
      (3) A stiff-bladed spatula is used to mix the mass on the side of the bowl
      (4) The mixing is completed in 60 seconds
   c. Placement
      (1) Vibration is used to remove air bubbles created through mixing
      (2) Vibration is used to keep the mixture wet and help it flow into the impression

C. Properties of gypsum products
   1. Physical
      a. Excellent thermal and electrical insulator
      b. Dense
      c. Excellent dimensional accuracy (setting expansion)
         (1) Plaster: 0.20%
         (2) Stone: 0.10%
         (3) Diestone: 0.05%
         (4) High-expansion diestone: 0.20% (for all-ceramic restoration fabrication)
      d. Good reproduction of fine detail of hard and soft tissues
   2. Chemical
      a. Heating will reverse the reaction, that is, decompose the material into calcium sulfate hemihydrate, the original dry component
      b. Models, casts, and dies should be wet during the grinding or cutting to prevent heating
   3. Mechanical
      a. Better powder packing and lower water content at mixing lead to higher compressive strengths (plaster < stone < diestone)
      b. Poor resistance to abrasion (polymer added to improve resistance)
   4. Biologic
      a. Materials are safe for contact with external epithelial tissues

b. Masks should be worn during grinding or polishing operations, which are likely to produce gypsum dust

D. Printed resin—produced from digital files using 3-D printer

Waxes

A. General considerations
   1. Applications
      a. Making impressions
      b. Registering of tooth or soft tissue position
      c. Creating restorative patterns for laboratory fabrication
      d. Aiding in laboratory procedures
   2. Terminology
      a. Inlay wax—used to create a pattern for inlay, onlay, or crown for subsequent investing and casting in a metal alloy
      b. Casting wax—used to create a pattern for metallic framework for removable partial dentures
      c. Baseplate wax—used to establish the vertical dimension, plane of occlusion, and initial arch form of a complete denture
      d. Corrective impression wax—used to form a registration pattern of soft tissues on an impression
      e. Bite registration wax—used to form a registration pattern for the occlusion of opposing models or casts
      f. Boxing wax—used to form a box around an impression before pouring a model or cast
      g. Utility wax—soft, pliable adhesive wax for modifying appliances, such as alginate impression trays
      h. Sticky wax—sticky when melted and used to temporarily adhere pieces of metal or resin in laboratory procedures
      i. Printed wax—produced from digital files using 3-D printer
   3. Classification
      a. Pattern waxes—inlay, casting, and baseplate waxes
      b. Impression waxes—corrective and bite registration waxes
      c. Processing waxes—boxing, utility, and sticky waxes

B. Structure
   1. Components
      a. Base waxes—hydrocarbon (paraffin) or ester waxes
      b. Modifier waxes—carnauba, ceresin, beeswax, rosin, gum dammar, or microcrystalline waxes
      c. Additives—colorants
   2. Reaction—waxes are thermoplastic (soften on heating, harden on cooling)

C. Properties
   1. Physical
      a. High coefficients of thermal expansion and contraction
      b. Insulators (cool unevenly); should be placed in increments to allow heat dissipation
   2. Chemical
      a. Degrade prematurely if overheated
      b. Designed to degrade into CO_2 and H_2O during burnout for inlay waxes
   3. Mechanical—stiffness, hardness, and strength depend on modifier waxes used and on temperature

Investment Materials

A. General considerations
   1. Applications
      a. Mold-making materials for casting alloys or castable ceramics to facilitate the creation of oversize mold space to compensate for shrinkage during cooling of casting alloy
      b. Mold-making materials for denture production
   2. Terminology—*investment* refers to the mold-making material
   3. Classification
      a. Gypsum-bonded investment (GBI)—based on gypsum products for matrix
      b. Phosphate-bonded investment (PBI)
      c. Silicate-bonded investment (SBI)
      d. Specialty investments—for glass ceramics, titanium alloys, and other specialized fabrication procedures

B. Structure—66% filler, 33% binder (matrix forms on setting), 1% modifiers
   1. Components
      a. Liquid—water or other reactant starts the formation of the matrix binder by reacting with the powder
      b. Powder—reactant powder, filler, or modifiers
   2. Reactions and mold expansion
      a. Setting expansion while material reacts, forming crystals that push on each other
      b. Hygroscopic expansion while setting mold placed under water
      c. Thermal expansion during heating of mold to casting temperature
      d. Filler expansion caused by the inversion of crystalline lattice during heating
   3. Manipulation
      a. P/L is mixed and placed in a container around the wax pattern
      b. After setting, the investment is heated to eliminate the wax pattern in preparation for casting

Casting Alloys

A. General considerations
   1. Applications—inlays, onlays, crowns, and bridges
   2. Terminology
      a. Precious (metals)—based primarily on valuable elements (Au, Pt, Pd, Ag, Ir, Rh, Rd)
      b. Noble or immune—corrosion-resistant element or alloy
      c. Base or active—corrosion-prone alloy
      d. Passive—corrosion resistant because of surface oxide film (*passivation* is prevention of corrosion by formation of a thin, adherent oxide film on metal surface, which acts as a barrier to further oxidation)
      e. Purity by weight (99.99% = "4 nines pure")
      f. Karat (24 karat is 100% gold; 18 karat is 75% gold)
      g. Fineness (1000 fineness is 100% gold; 500 fineness is 50% gold)
   3. Classification
      a. High-gold alloys are greater than 75% wt gold or other noble metals (= 50% atoms that are immune)

(1) ADA type I alloys are 83% wt noble metals (e.g., in simple inlays)

(2) ADA type II are $\geq$78% wt noble metals (e.g., in inlays and onlays)

(3) ADA type III are $\geq$75% wt noble metals (e.g., in crowns and bridges)

(4) ADA type IV are $\geq$75% wt noble metals (e.g., in partial dentures)

  b. Medium-gold alloys are 25% wt to 75% wt gold or other noble metals

  c. Low-gold alloys are less than 25% wt gold or other noble metals

  d. Gold-substitute alloys do not contain gold

(1) Palladium-silver alloys—passive because of mixed oxide film

(2) Cobalt-chromium or nickel-chromium alloys—passive because of Cr_2O_3 oxide film

  e. Titanium alloys are based on 90% to 100% titanium; passive because of TiO_2 oxide film

B. Structure

  1. Components of gold alloys

    a. Gold contributes to corrosion resistance

    b. Copper contributes to hardness and strength

    c. Silver counteracts orange color of copper

    d. Palladium increases melting point and hardness

    e. Platinum increases melting point

    f. Zinc acts as oxygen scavenger during casting

  2. Manipulation

    a. Heated to just beyond melting temperature for casting

    b. Cooling shrinkage causes substantial contraction

C. Properties

  1. Physical

    a. Electrical and thermal conductors

    b. Relatively low coefficient of thermal expansion

  2. Chemical

    a. Silver content affects susceptibility to tarnish

    b. Corrosion resistance is attributed to high noble metal content or passivation

  3. Mechanical

    a. High tensile and compressive strengths but relatively weak in thin sections such as margins; can be deformed relatively easily

    b. Good wear resistance except in contact with ceramic

Dental Solders

A. General considerations

  1. Applications—fabrication of cast bridges and metallic orthodontic appliances

  2. Terminology

    a. Soldering—joining using filler metal that melts below 500°C

    b. Brazing—joining using filler metal that melts above 500°C

    c. Welding—melting and alloying of pieces to be joined

    d. Fluxing

(1) Oxidative cleaning of area to be soldered

(2) Oxygen scavenging to prevent oxidation of alloy being soldered

    e. Numerical terminology: 16 to 650 = 650 fineness solder to be used with 16-karat alloys; *fineness* refers to the gold or other precious metal content

  3. Classification

    a. Gold solders—bridges

    b. Silver solders—gold-substitute bridges and orthodontic alloys

B. Structure of gold solders

  1. Composition—lower gold content than of alloys being soldered

  2. Manipulation—solder must melt below melting temperature of alloy

C. Properties

  1. Physical—similar to alloys being joined

  2. Chemical—more prone to chemical and electrochemical corrosion

  3. Mechanical—similar to alloys being joined but weaker

  4. Biologic—similar to alloys being joined

Chromium Alloys for Partial Dentures

A. General considerations

  1. Applications—casting partial denture metal frameworks

  2. Classification

    a. Cobalt-chromium

    b. Nickel-chromium

B. Structure

  1. Composition

    a. Chromium—produces a passivating oxide film for corrosion resistance

    b. Cobalt—increases the rigidity of the alloy

    c. Other elements—increase strength and castability

  2. Manipulation

    a. Require higher temperature investment materials (PBI or SBI)

    b. More difficult to cast because less dense than gold alloys; usually require special casting equipment

    c. Much more difficult to finish and polish because of higher strength and hardness

C. Properties

  1. Physical—less dense than gold alloys

  2. Chemical—passivating corrosion behavior

  3. Mechanical—stronger, stiffer, and harder than gold alloys

  4. Biologic

    a. Nickel may cause sensitivity in some individuals (approximately 6% of men, and 11% to 24% of women)

    b. Beryllium in some alloys forms oxide that is toxic, which is a significant problem for dental laboratory technicians if grinding dust is inhaled

Porcelain-Fused-to-Metal Alloys

A. General considerations

  1. Applications—substructures for porcelain-fused-to-metal (PFM) crowns and bridges

  2. Classification

a. High-gold alloys
b. Palladium-silver alloys
c. Cobalt-chromium alloys
B. Structure
1. Composition
   a. High-gold alloys are 98% gold, platinum, palladium, or both
   b. Palladium-silver alloys are 50% to 60% palladium and 30% to 40% silver
   c. Chromium-cobalt alloys are 60% to 65% chromium and 25% to 30% cobalt, with other metals
2. Manipulation
   a. Must have melting temperatures above that of porcelains (low-fusing porcelains) that will be fabricated onto their surfaces
   b. More difficult to cast (see the previous section on "Chromium Alloys for Partial Dentures")
C. Properties
1. Physical
   a. Except for high-gold alloys; others are less dense alloys
   b. Alloys are designed to have low thermal expansion coefficients that must be matched to the veneering porcelain
2. Chemical—high-gold alloys are immune to corrosion; others passivate
3. Mechanical—high modulus and hardness
4. Biologic—biologically acceptable if they do not corrode

Dental Ceramics

A. General considerations
1. Applications
   a. Veneering material for PFM crowns and bridges
   b. All-ceramic, high-strength inlays, onlays, crowns, and bridges
   c. Denture teeth
2. Terminology
   a. Ceramic—any inorganic material containing metallic and nonmetallic elements, generally formed at a high temperature
   b. Porcelain—ceramic composition based primarily on silica, alumina, and potassium oxide; created by mixing clay, feldspar, and quartz, and then heating
   c. PFM restoration—metal-based coping (substructure) coated with a porcelain veneer
   d. All-ceramic—inlay, onlay, crown, bridge, or veneer made entirely of ceramic
   e. Fusing—coalescence of packed layer of particles into a single porcelain mass
   f. High-strength ceramics—ceramics that include one or more phases or strengthening mechanisms to make the composition mechanically more crack resistant than conventional porcelains
   g. Glass-ceramics—initially noncrystalline (glassy) ceramics from which some crystalline phase is precipitated for strengthening
   h. Glass-infiltrated ceramic—partially sintered ceramic particles that are infused with a glassy matrix (e.g., InCeram)

3. Classification
   a. Feldspathic porcelains—produced by traditional laboratory fabrication with porcelain particles painted into position as a water slurry (condensed) and then heated for particle coalescence (sintered)
      (1) High-fusing porcelains—for denture teeth
      (2) Medium-fusing porcelains—for jacket crowns; not commonly used
      (3) Low-fusing porcelains—veneering material for PFM restorations
   b. High-strength ceramics—produced by specialized laboratory fabrication technique
      (1) Lucite-reinforced porcelains—pressure molded
      (2) Alumina-reinforced porcelains
      (3) High-density alumina core materials
      (4) Infiltrated materials—glass or resin infiltrated
      (5) Hydroxyapatite-based materials
   c. Glass-ceramics
      (1) Mica-based glass-ceramics—used as starting blanks for CAD/CAM restorations
      (2) High-strength glass-ceramic core materials, such as lithium disilicate or lithium silicate glass-ceramic
   d. High-strength crystalline single-phase materials
      (1) Alumina
      (2) Zirconia (yttria-stabilized tetragonal zirconia)
B. Porcelain structure
1. Components
   a. Large number of oxides—principally silicon oxide (silica), aluminum oxide (alumina), and potassium oxide, created by combining clay, feldspar, and quartz raw materials
   b. Minor oxides contribute properties of opacity, translucency, and color
2. Manipulation
   a. Traditional porcelain fabrication
      (1) Porcelain powder mixed with water, padded onto substrate, compacted, and heated to produce coalescence with shrinkage
      (2) Shrinkage is approximately 30% on firing (sintering); thus porcelain layer must be made oversized and built up by several stages of application
   b. Special ceramic laboratory fabrication procedures—require specialized equipment and furnaces
   c. Milling—requires specialized equipment
C. Properties
1. Physical
   a. Excellent electrical and thermal insulation
   b. Low coefficient of thermal expansion and contraction
   c. Good color and translucency; excellent esthetics (superior to all other materials)
2. Chemical
   a. Not resistant to fluorine-containing acids and can be dissolved by contact with APF topical fluoride treatments
   b. Can be acid-etched with hydrofluoric acid or other strong acids for providing micromechanical retention for cements

3. Mechanical
  a. Harder than tooth structure and will cause opponent wear, although some glass-ceramics are comparable in hardness to enamel
  b. Can be polished with diamond pastes
  c. Poor fatigue behavior of glasses when compared with metal alloys
4. Biologic—relatively inert

Crown-and-Bridge Cements

A. General considerations (Table 13-5)
  1. Applications
    a. Luting inlays, onlays, crowns, and bridges
    b. Luting orthodontic bands and brackets
  2. Terminology—luting: attachment by gross mechanical interdigitation with crown and tooth surfaces
  3. Classification
    a. Traditional cements (typically P+L) (rarely used)—zinc oxide–eugenol (ZOE) and zinc phosphate (ZP)
    b. Polymeric cements (typically precapsulated or paste-paste)—polycarboxylate (PC), glass ionomer (GI), resin-modified glass ionomer (RMGI), resin or composite (CC), and universal cement (UC)
B. Structure
  1. Components (see Table 13-5)
    a. Traditional cements—powder (reactant; chemically basic); liquid (reactant; chemically acidic)
    b. Polymeric cements—polymer cross-linking reaction (PC, GI), polymerization reaction (RMGI, CC, UC), or both
  2. Reaction
    a. Traditional cements—acid-base reaction that forms salt; great excess of powder leaves residual powder as filler
    b. Polymeric cements—setting produced by cross-linking reactions similar to GI or composite setting reactions

3. Manipulation
  a. Traditional cements—all reactions are exothermic; reaction controlled by chilling components, chilling mixing slab, or incrementally adding powder to the liquid
  b. Polymeric cements—powder is added to liquid as quickly as possible to complete mixing in 30 seconds or mixed in triturators and used quickly; may include preplacement of bonding system as well; paste-paste systems are dispensed using auto-mix syringes
C. Properties
  1. Physical properties
    a. All luting cements are electrical and thermal insulators
    b. All luting cements have low coefficients of thermal expansion and contraction
  2. Chemical properties
    a. In acidic environments, cements tend to disintegrate
    b. PC and GI cements will adhere chemically to calcium ions on the surface of tooth structure and to oxides contained within the set cements
    c. PC and GI are most resistant to microleakage
    d. GI cements release fluoride ions (and most PC cements initially release fluoride because of small CaF_2 contents included as mixing aids)
  3. Mechanical properties—compressive strength; composite has the highest compressive strength, and ZOE has the lowest
  4. Biologic properties
    a. Eugenol-based cements produce obtundent (pain-soothing) effects
    b. PC and GI cements are most gentle to the dental pulp (when manipulated correctly)

Acrylic Appliances

A. General considerations
  1. Application—space maintenance and tooth movement for orthodontics and pediatric dentistry

TABLE 13-5 Luting Cements

Cement	Abbreviation	Powder or Filler Components	Liquid or Matrix Components
Traditional (or Conventional) Types			
Zinc oxide–eugenol (ZOE), unmodified (limited use)	ZOE	Zinc oxide	Eugenol
Zinc phosphate (ZP) (limited use)	ZP	Zinc oxide	Phosphoric acid in water
Polymeric (or Resin) Types			
Polycarboxylate	PC	Zinc oxide	Polyacrylic acid in water
Glass ionomer, conventional	GI*	Fluoro-aluminosilicate glass	Polyacrylic acid in water
Resin-modified glass ionomer	RMGI*	Fluoro-aluminosilicate glass	Copolymer acid in water; water-soluble monomers
Compomer	CM*	Fluoro-aluminosilicate glass; silicate glass	Bis-GMA–like monomers
Universal cement (esthetic resin cement, adhesive resin cement, self-adhesive resin cement, RC)	UC of RC*	Fluoro-aluminosilicate glass	Bis-GMA–like monomers

*Principal cements in use today.

2. Classification—none
B. Structure
    1. Components
        a. Powder—PMMA (polymethylmethacrylate) powder, peroxide initiator, and pigments
        b. Liquid—MMA (methylmethacrylate) monomer, hydroquinone inhibitor, cross-linking agents, and chemical accelerators (*N, N*-dimethyl-*p*-toluidine)
    2. Reaction
        a. The PMMA powder makes mixture viscous for manipulation before curing
        b. Chemical accelerators cause the decomposition of benzoyl peroxide into free radicals that initiate the polymerization of the monomer
        c. New PMMA is formed as a matrix that surrounds the PMMA powder
        d. Linear shrinkage of 5% to 7% during setting, but dimensions of appliances are not critical
    3. Manipulation
        a. The mixture of powder and liquid is painted onto the working cast to create the shape for the acrylic appliance
        b. Orthodontic wires may be part of the appliance
        c. After curing the mixture, the shape and fit are adjusted by grinding with burrs and stones, with a slow-speed handpiece
            (1) Caution—acrylic dust is irritating to epithelial tissues of nasopharynx and skin and may produce allergic dermatitis or other reactions
            (2) Grinding may heat the polymer to temperatures that depolymerize and release monomer vapor, which may be an irritant
C. Properties (see "Acrylic Denture Bases")
    1. Physical
    2. Chemical—may contain 2% to 3% unreacted monomer that can cause soft tissue irritation in approximately 4% of the population
    3. Mechanical
    4. Biologic

Acrylic Denture Bases

A. General considerations
    1. Application—used to support artificial teeth
    2. Classification
        a. PMMA/MMA dough systems
        b. PMMA/MMA injected-resin systems
        c. PMMA/MMA pour resins
        d. UDMA VLC resins
B. Structure of PMMA/MMA types
    1. Components
        a. Powder—PMMA polymer, peroxide initiator, and pigments
        b. Liquid—MMA monomer, hydroquinone inhibitor, and cross-linking agents
    2. Reaction
        a. Heat (or chemicals) used as an accelerator to decompose peroxide into free radicals

b. Free radicals initiate polymerization of MMA into PMMA
c. New PMMA is formed as a matrix around residual PMMA powder particles
d. Linear shrinkage—5% to 7% of monomer on polymerization; reduced by processing procedures
    3. Manipulation
        a. P/L mixed to form dough or fluid resin to fill mold
        b. Mold heated to start and control reaction
C. Properties
    1. Physical
        a. Thermal insulator—prevents the patient's sensations of food temperature
        b. High coefficient of thermal expansion and contraction
        c. Poor distortion resistance at higher temperatures; therefore, dentures should not be cleaned in hot water
        d. Good resistance to color change
    2. Chemical
        a. Stored in water before delivery to reach equilibrium absorption level
        b. Absorbs water and must be kept hydrated
        c. Not resistant to strong oxidizing agents
    3. Mechanical
        a. Low strength, but flexible; good fatigue resistance
        b. Poor scratch resistance; clean tissue-bearing surfaces of denture with soft brush, and do not use abrasive cleaners
    4. Biologic—occasional allergic reactions to minute residual monomer have been reported in newly processed dentures

Denture Teeth

A. General considerations
    1. Applications—complete or partial dentures
    2. Classification
        a. Porcelain teeth
        b. Acrylic resin teeth—95% of all denture teeth
        c. Abrasion-resistant teeth—composite veneered and interpenetrating network (IPN) teeth
B. Structure and properties
    1. Porcelain teeth (high-fusing porcelain)
        a. Bonded into denture base mechanically
        b. Harder than natural teeth or other restorations and are capable of abrading those surfaces
        c. Good esthetic appearance
        d. Used when clients have good ridge support and sufficient room between the arches
    2. Acrylic resin teeth—PMMA
        a. Bonded pseudo-chemically into the denture base; teeth are wetted with monomer before forming denture base
        b. Soft and easily worn by abrasive foods
        c. Good initial esthetics
        d. Used for clients with poor ridges and those who are opposed to natural teeth
    3. Abrasion-resistant teeth (composite veneered)
        a. Bonded pseudo-chemically into the denture base
        b. Much better abrasion resistance than acrylic resin teeth but poorer bonding

Denture Soft Liners

A. General considerations
1. Applications—for clients with soft tissue irritation
2. Classification
   a. Long-term liners (soft liners)—used over months for patients with severe undercuts or continually sore residual ridges
   b. Short-term liners (tissue conditioners)—used to facilitate tissue healing over several days
B. Structure
1. Soft liners—plasticized acrylic co-polymers or silicone rubber
2. Tissue conditioners—PEMA (polyethylmethacrylate) plasticized with ethanol and aromatic esters
C. Properties
1. Liners flow under low pressure, allowing adaptation to soft tissues, but are elastic during chewing forces
2. Low initial hardness, but the liner becomes harder as plasticizers are leached out during intraoral use
3. Some silicone rubber liners support the growth of yeasts

Denture Cleansers

A. General considerations
1. Applications—for removal of soft debris by light brushing and then rinsing of denture; hard deposits require professional repolishing
2. Classification
   a. Alkaline perborates—do not remove bad stains; may harm liners
   b. Alkaline hypochlorites—may cause bleaching, corrode base-metal alloys, and leave residual taste on appliance
   c. Dilute acids—may corrode base-metal alloys
   d. Abrasive powders and creams—can abrade denture surfaces
3. Techniques recommended for denture cleaning
   a. Full dentures without soft liners—immerse denture in solution of one part 5% sodium hypochlorite (Clorox) and three parts water
   b. Full or partial dentures without soft liners—immerse denture in solution of 1 tsp of sodium hypochlorite (Clorox) and 2 tsp of glassy phosphate (Calgon) in a half glass of water
   c. Lined dentures—clean any soft liner with a cotton swab and cold water; clean the denture with a soft brush
B. Properties
1. Chemical—cleansers can swell plastic surfaces or corrode metal frameworks
2. Mechanical—cleansers can scratch the surfaces of denture bases or denture teeth

Mouth Protectors (Athletic Mouthguards)

A. General considerations
1. Applications—to protect against blows to the chin, the top of the head, and the face or to prevent grinding of teeth; typically used by football, basketball, soccer, and hockey players (contact sports)
2. Terminology—mouth protectors, teeth protectors, or athletic mouthguards
3. Classification
   a. Stock protectors—least desirable because of poor fit
   b. Mouth-formed protectors ("boil-and-bite")—made by client; improved fit compared with stock type
   c. Custom-made protectors—fabrication by dentist is preferred because of durability, low levels of speech impairment, and comfort
B. Structure
1. Components
   a. Stock protectors—thermoplastic co-polymer of polyvinyl acetate–polyethylene (PVA-PE)
   b. Mouth-formed protectors—thermoplastic co-polymer
   c. Custom-made protectors—thermoplastic co-polymer or polyurethane
2. Reaction—hardening during cooling
3. Fabrication
   a. Alginate impression made of maxillary arch
   b. High-strength stone cast poured immediately
   c. Thermoplastic material is heated in hot water and vacuum-molded to cast
   d. Mouth protector trimmed to within 2 mm of labial fold, clearance provided at the buccal and labial frena, and edges smoothed by flaming
   e. Gagging, taste, irritation, and impairment of speech are minimized with properly fabricated mouth protector
4. Instructions for use—client must:
   a. Rinse before and after use with cold water
   b. Clean protector occasionally with soap and cool water
   c. Store the protector in a rigid container
   d. Protect the protector from heat and pressure during storage
   e. Evaluate the protector routinely for evidence of deterioration
C. Properties
1. Physical—thermal insulators
2. Chemical—absorbs water and stains during use
3. Mechanical—tensile strength, modulus, and hardness decrease after water absorption, but elongation, tear strength, and resilience increase
4. Biologic—nontoxic as long as no bacterial, fungal, or viral growth occurs on surfaces between uses

Veneers

A. General considerations
1. Applications—generally anterior maxillary teeth
2. Terminology
   a. Extracoronal—bonded over existing enamel, that is, no tooth preparation
   b. Intracoronal—bonded into an intraenamel cavity preparation

3. Classification by materials
   a. Direct composite veneer
   b. Indirect composite veneer (laboratory processed)
   c. Ceramic veneer (stacked or pressed ceramic)
   d. CAD/CAM ceramic veneer
B. Structure
   1. Components—composite, porcelain, or ceramic
   2. Manipulation
      a. Bonding—enamel etching and bonding
      b. Finishing and polishing must be done with care to avoid scratching the surfaces
   3. Maintenance
      a. Polishing with abrasive materials or scaling with metal instruments must be avoided
      b. The protector must be protected with petroleum jelly during topical acidulated phosphate fluoride (APF) treatments, or neutral sodium fluoride must be used
C. Properties
   1. Physical—good esthetic appearance; but some coloring may occur because of the composite resin cement used for bonding the veneer
   2. Chemical
      a. Composite veneers have good acid resistance
      b. Ceramic and CAD/CAM veneers should be protected from APF or other acids
   3. Mechanical
      a. Composite veneers are subject to scratching
      b. Ceramic and CAD/CAM veneers have good abrasion resistance
   4. Biologic—no known problems

CAD/CAM Restorations

A. General considerations
   1. Applications—inlays, onlays, veneers, crowns, bridges, implants, and implant prostheses
   2. Stages of fabrication of CAD/CAM restorations
      a. Scanning—computerized surface digitization; acquisition of surface contours and geometry, can be intraoral or scanning of impressions
      b. CAD—computer-aided (assisted) design; digital design of restoration
      c. CAM—computer-aided (assisted) machining; fabrication of restoration from block of material
   3. Classification
      a. Chairside or in-office CAD/CAM systems
      b. Laboratory CAD/CAM systems
      c. Examples of CAD/CAM systems in dentistry
         (1) CEREC (Sirona Dental Systems)
         (2) E4D Dentist (E4D Technologies)
B. Structure
   1. Materials
      a. Feldspathic porcelains (Vita Mark II, ProCAD)
      b. Machinable leucite-reinforced ceramic (IPS Empress CAD)

   c. Machinable lithium disilicate (IPS e.Max CAD) and lithium silicate (Obsidian)
   d. Machinable high-strength zirconia ceramics (BruxZir, NexxZr, Lava Plus, IPS e.Max ZirCAD)
   e. Metal alloys (limited use)
   f. Composites—CeraSmart, Lava Ultimate, Enamic
   2. Cementing
      a. Etching enamel and dentin for micromechanical retention—use of phosphoric acid or self-etching primer
      b. Bonding agent for retention to etched surface
      c. Composite as a luting cement for reacting chemically with bonding agent and with silanated surfaces of restoration
      d. Silane for wetting and chemical bonding to etched ceramic (or metal) restorations and for co-reaction with luting composite cement
      e. Hydrofluoric acid for gel etching of silica-based ceramics or sandblasting of zirconia to create spaces for micromechanical retention on surface of restoration
      f. Ceramic primer for zirconia
C. Properties
   1. Physical properties
      a. Thermal expansion coefficient well-matched to tooth structure
      b. Good resistance to plaque biofilm adsorption or retention
      c. Good esthetics (for shade matching)
   2. Chemical properties—silica-based ceramics are not resistant to hydrofluoric acid and should be protected from APF
   3. Mechanical properties
      a. Excellent wear resistance (but may abrade opposing teeth)
      b. Some wear of luting cements but self- limiting
      c. Excellent toothbrush abrasion resistance
      d. Limited fatigue resistance caused by brittleness (low-fracture toughness of some glass ceramics) and initiation and propagation of cracks
   4. Biologic properties—excellent compatibility with natural tissues

Dental Implants

See the sections on "Dental Implants" in Chapter 14 and "Advanced Instrumentation Techniques" in Chapter 17
A. General considerations
   1. Applications
      a. Single-tooth implants
      b. Abutments for bridges (freestanding, attached to natural teeth)
      c. Abutments for overdentures
   2. Terminology
      a. Endosseous—into the bone; represents more than 90% of all current types

b. Subperiosteal—below the periosteum but above the bone; second most frequently used type

c. Transosteal—through the bone

d. Endodontic—through the root canal space and into the periapical bone

e. Intramucosal—within the mucosa

3. Classification by geometric form

  a. Endosteal root forms
    (1) Screws
    (2) Cylinders
  b. Other endosteal forms
    (1) Blades
    (2) Staples
  c. Circumferential

4. Classification by materials type

  a. Metallic—titanium (majority of types; uncoated and coated), stainless steel, and chromium-cobalt
  b. Polymeric—PMMA
  c. Ceramic—hydroxyapatite, zirconia

5. Classification by attachment design

  a. Bioactive surface retention by osseo-integration—integration of bone with implant; most favored type of attachment
  b. Nonactive porous surfaces for micromechanical retention by osseo-integration
  c. Nonactive, nonporous surface for ankylosis by osseo-integration
  d. Gross mechanical retention designs (e.g., threads, screws, channels, or transverse holes)
  e. Fibro-integration by formation of fibrous tissue capsule
  f. Combinations of the above designs

B. Structure

1. Components

  a. Root (for osseo-integration)
  b. Neck (for epithelial attachment and percutaneous sealing)
  c. Intramobile elements (for shock absorption)
  d. Prosthesis (for dental form and function)

2. Manipulation

  a. Selection—based on remaining bone architecture and dimensions
  b. Sterilization—RF glow discharge leaves the biomaterial surface uncontaminated and sterile; autoclaving or chemical sterilization contraindicated for some designs
  c. Handling—must be handled with an instrument of like composition; that is, titanium instruments used to handle titanium implants to avoid metallic contamination and localized electrochemical corrosion

C. Properties

1. Physical—should have low thermal and electrical conductivity

2. Chemical

  a. Should be resistant to electrochemical corrosion
  b. Do not expose surfaces to acids (e.g., APFs)
  c. The effects of adjunctive therapies, for example, 0.12% chlorhexidine gluconate mouth rinse must be kept in mind

3. Mechanical

  a. Should be abrasion resistant and have a high modulus
  b. During scaling operations, care must be taken to avoid abrading (e.g., with metal scalers or air-abrasive systems); see the sections on "Advanced Instrumentation Techniques" and "Selective Stain Removal" in Chapter 17.

4. Biologic—depend on osseo-integration and epithelial attachment

Tissue Engineering

See the section on "Genetics" in Chapter 7.

A. General considerations

1. Applications—replacement of any orofacial tissues, particularly intraoral tissues

2. Terminology

  a. Tissue engineering—attempt to regenerate tissue for the body, either in the laboratory or in the patient, through manipulation of cellular material, biologic mediators, and natural or synthetic matrices
  b. Cells (in tissue engineering)—living cells that are either precursors of more differentiated cells or disorganized collections of cells that grow, divide, and organize into physiologically functioning tissue
  c. Signals—any physical, chemical, or biologic mediators (extracellular or intracellular) that initiate, propagate, or otherwise stimulate cellular development into fully organized tissue
  d. Scaffolds—any extracellular matrix structure (natural or synthetic, temporary or permanent, hard or soft) that provides a foundation for cells to become attached, organized, and proliferate to generate the tissue of interest

3. Classification by materials by tissue replacement therapies

  a. Autografts—from one's own body
    (1) Best chance of clinical success
    (2) Genetic match (no immunity problems)
  b. Allografts (or homografts)—from same species (usually from cadavers)
    (1) Can be antigenic (sensitize the patient)
    (2) Concerns about transmitted diseases
  c. Xenografts—from different species
    (1) Limited range of use (e.g., porcine heart valve)
    (2) Heavily treated before use
  d. Synthetics—entirely man-made
    (1) Can be metals, ceramics, polymers, or composites
    (2) Prone to long-term mechanical breakdown
    (3) Can produce a toxic response
  e. Tissue-engineered replacement—rebuilding tissues in the laboratory to be implanted, or causing the body to "rebuild the tissue" artificially in situ
    (1) Use of mixture of natural and synthetic materials
    (2) Offers the possibility of a "near-perfect" replacement
    (3) Can potentially solve transplant availability problems

B. Structure
1. Components
   a. Cells (cellular material)
      (1) Stem cells (undifferentiated)
      (2) Specific cells (e.g., osteoblasts, fibroblasts)
   b. Signals (biologic mediators)
      (1) Growth factors, such as bone morphogenic proteins (BMPs)
      (2) Genetic material
   c. Scaffolds (matrices)
      (1) Polymers—native (e.g., collagen) or synthetic (e.g., PLA/PGA)
      (2) Ceramics—native (e.g., bone chips) or synthetic (e.g., Bioglass)
      (3) Composites—combination of native and synthetic (e.g., hydroxyapatite-coated collagen fibers)
2. Manipulation

a. Design and grown human tissues outside the body for later implantation to repair or replace diseased tissues
   (1) Not necessarily patient specific
   (2) Ideal for large-volume need such as skin grafts
b. Implantation of cell-containing or cell-free devices (with appropriate signal molecules) that induce the regeneration of functional human tissues; guided tissue regeneration, for example, use of Perioglass combined with appropriate growth factors in treatment of severe periodontal disease
c. Development of external or internal devices containing human tissues designed to replace the function of diseased internal tissues
   (1) Involve use of stem cells or specific differentiated cells from the patient
   (2) Ideal for load-bearing tissues (e.g., bone, tendon)
C. Properties—physical, chemical, and mechanical properties should be similar to those of natural tissues

Website Information And Resources

Source	Website Address	Description
Clinicians Reports	http://www.cliniciansreport.org	Updates on dental materials and devices
International Association for Dental Research (IADR) Dental Materials Group	http://www.dentalresearch.org/DMG/	List of all dental materials sites and dental materials manufacturer websites
MEDLINE/PubMed	http://www.ncbi.nlm.nih.gov/sites/entrez?db=pubmed	Public access to National Library of Medicine (NLM) abstract index that includes all dental research abstracts for published articles in dental journals
The Dental Advisor	http://www.dentaladvisor.com/	Evaluation of current dental products
Dental Evaluation and Consultation Service	http://www.airforcemedicine.af.mil/decs/	List of current reviews and analyses of dental materials, instruments, and devices; evaluation of current dental products

SUGGESTED READINGS

Anusavice KJ, Phillips RW: *Phillip's science of dental materials,* ed 11, Philadelphia, 2003, Saunders.
Bayne SC, Thomson JY: *Biomaterials science [digital only],* Chapel Hill, NC, 2004, Brightstar.
Powers JM, Wataha JC: *Dental materials: properties and manipulation,* ed 10, St Louis, 2013, Elsevier-Mosby.
O'Brien WJ: *Dental materials and their selection,* ed 4, Philadelphia, 2009, Quintessence.
Sakaguchi RL, Powers JM: *Craig's restorative dental materials,* ed 13, St Louis, 2012, Elsevier-Mosby.

CHAPTER 13 REVIEW QUESTIONS

Answers and rationales to chapter review questions are available on this text's accompanying Evolve site. See inside front cover for details.

evolve

1. **Which mixing method is *not* used for dental materials?**
   a. Powder and liquid precapsulated and mixed in a triturator
   b. Powder and liquid mixed on a mixing pad
   c. Two liquids agitated together using a vibration
   d. Powder and water mixed with a spatula in a mixing bowl
   e. Two liquids mixed through a mixing nozzle
2. **What of the following is the mixing time?**
   a. Elapsed time from the beginning of mixing until the beginning of setting
   b. Elapsed time from the beginning of the working interval until the end of the setting interval
   c. The setting interval
   d. The time required by the operator to handle and place a dental material
   e. Elapsed time from the start of mixing until the end of mixing
3. **Which of the following materials does *not* set by polymerization?**
   a. Hybrid glass ionomer cement
   b. Dental stone
   c. Polyvinyl siloxane impression material
   d. Polysulfide impression material
   e. Packable dental composite

4. **Why is the linear coefficient of thermal expansion important for restorative materials?**
   a. It predicts the loss in strength of a restorative material as the temperature increases.
   b. It indicates the insulating characteristics of a restorative material.
   c. It indicates the resistance to thermal degradation of a material.
   d. It indicates the amount of expansion/contraction on polymerization.
   e. It predicts the mismatch in expansion/contraction at the interface of restorative materials.

5. **Which of the following materials involves imbibition problems?**
   a. Dental sealant
   b. Dental composite
   c. Dental cement
   d. Alginate impression material
   e. Gold restorations

6. **Which of the following is a rapid thermal conductor?**
   a. Dentin
   b. Dental amalgam
   c. Dental composite
   d. Zirconia all-ceramic inlays
   e. Dental enamel

7. **Which of the following undergoes crevice corrosion under plaque that causes pitting?**
   a. Stainless steel restorations
   b. Cast-gold restorations
   c. PFM restorations
   d. NiCr partial-denture alloys
   e. All the above

8. **Which of the following is BEST for pulpal insulation?**
   a. 1 mm of remaining dentin thickness
   b. 3 mm of composite restoration
   c. 5 mm of dental amalgam restoration
   d. Surface sealant over restoration
   e. 1 mm of calcium hydroxide liner

9. **Which of the following terms is *not* important for color matching?**
   a. Ambient lighting conditions
   b. Surface gloss
   c. Translucency
   d. Initiation
   e. Hue and chroma

10. **Which of the following is *not* associated with electrochemical corrosion events?**
    a. Crevices
    b. Stress
    c. Passivation
    d. Radiopacity
    e. Plaque

11. **Engineering stress is computed as:**
    a. Deformation divided by the volume of the object
    b. Modulus multiplied by the plastic deformation
    c. Difference between the total strain and plastic strain
    d. Deformation divided by the original length
    e. Applied load divided by original cross-sectional area

12. **Engineering strain is computed as:**
    a. Area under the stress-strain curve
    b. Load at yield divided by elastic deformation
    c. Applied load divided by the total elastic deformation
    d. Deformation divided by the original length of the object
    e. Change between the initial and final strain divided by the time

13. **What is another name for a material's stiffness?**
    a. Elastic limit
    b. Toughness
    c. Fatigue resistance
    d. Brittleness
    e. Modulus

14. **Loading of a restoration beyond the material's elastic limit causes:**
    a. Only elastic deformation
    b. Fatigue fracture
    c. Elastic and plastic deformation
    d. Stress relaxation
    e. Only plastic deformation

15. **At what point does loading produce both plastic and elastic strain at the same time?**
    a. Toughness
    b. Modulus
    c. Endurance limit
    d. Elastic limit
    e. Fracture

16. **What is the Mohs hardness value for enamel?**
    a. 2
    b. 3 to 4
    c. 5 to 6
    d. 7
    e. 9

17. **Which phase in dental amalgam restorations is MOST likely to corrode?**
    a. Ag-Sn
    b. Ag-Sn-Cu
    c. Sn-Hg
    d. Cu-Sn
    e. Ag-Hg

18. **Which phase in dental amalgam is STRONGEST?**
    a. Ag-Cu
    b. Cu-Sn
    c. Ag-Hg
    d. Ag-Sn
    e. Sn-Hg

19. **Which method for amalgam is recommended to minimize mercury vapor escape during mixing?**
    a. Friction-fit capsule
    b. Precapsulated alloy and mercury
    c. Covered mixing arm on the triturator
    d. None of the above
    e. Mortar and pestle

20. **High-copper dental amalgam alloys involve what range of copper in their composition?**
    a. 12% to 30%
    b. 6% to 12%
    c. 1% to 5%
    d. 0.5% to 1%
    e. 0.1% to 0.5%

21. **What is the major advantage of high-copper over low-copper dental amalgam restorations?**
    a. Lower coefficient of thermal expansion
    b. Greater polishability
    c. Lower corrosion tendency
    d. Lower thermal conductivity
    e. Better compressive strength

22. **What is the OSHA limit for exposure to mercury vapor in air during a 40-hour workweek?**
    a. $50 \ \mu g/m^3$
    b. $42 \ \mu g/m^3$
    c. $31 \ \mu g/m^3$
    d. $20 \ \mu g/m^3$
    e. $15 \ \mu g/m^3$

23. **What is the melting temperature of the Ag-Hg matrix phase in a set dental amalgam restoration?**
    a. 167°C
    b. 157°C
    c. 147°C
    d. 137°C
    e. 127°C

24. **What is a major problem associated with polishing a dental amalgam?**
    a. Burnishing of surface corrosion products into the amalgam
    b. Production of grayish color
    c. Localized melting of the amalgam with mercury smearing
    d. Smearing amalgam onto enamel to cause staining
    e. Creation of marginal ditching

25. **What is the estimated incidence of hypersensitivity to mercury from dental amalgam restorations in the general population?**
    a. 1 per 2000 patients
    b. 1 per 50,000 patients
    c. 1 per 3 million patients
    d. 1 per 5 million patients
    e. 1 per 100 million patients

26. **What is the principal reason for the shift away from dental amalgam use?**
    a. Environmental concerns about mercury
    b. Much improved mechanical properties of other materials
    c. Patient hypersensitivity problems to mercury released from amalgams
    d. Lower cost of procedures for alternative restorative materials
    e. Toxicity of mercury to office personnel

27. **What is the main reason for failure of a high-copper dental amalgam restoration?**
    a. Occlusal marginal ditching
    b. Creep
    c. Wear facets
    d. Interproximal caries
    e. Black or green tarnish

28. **Which restorative material is most often substituted for dental amalgam in posterior restoration applications?**
    a. Dental composite
    b. Hybrid glass ionomer
    c. Direct gold
    d. ART restorations
    e. All-ceramic

29. **Which of the following is TRUE about pit-and-fissure sealants?**
    a. Sealants should be filled to improve their mechanical properties.
    b. Tinted sealants are more useful than colorless ones.
    c. Sealant inspection is unnecessary after 2 years.
    d. Partial sealing of pits and fissures is better than no sealing at all.
    e. Uncured sealant along air-exposed surfaces will finish curing in 24 hours.

30. **Which event does *not* alter the esthetics of existing composite restorations?**
    a. Extensive tea exposure
    b. APF application
    c. Tobacco use
    d. Gum chewing
    e. Whitening techniques

31. **Which of the following is likely to be deceptive in appearance in a radiograph?**
    a. Dental composite restoration
    b. Dental sealants
    c. Temporary restorations
    d. Glass ionomer restorations
    e. Infiltrants

32. **What is the most appropriate way to manage long-term wear or discoloration of posterior dental composite restoration surfaces?**
    a. Replace the composite with a dental amalgam
    b. Repair the worn areas with resin-modified glass ionomer
    c. Resurface the old composite with new composite
    d. Replace the restoration with a new, high-strength ceramic
    e. Adjust the occlusion of the opponent tooth

33. **Which procedure does *not* require phosphoric acid etching?**
    a. Ceramic orthodontic bracket attachment
    b. Total-etch dentin bonding procedure
    c. Self-etch dentin bonding procedure
    d. Amalgam bonding procedure
    e. Dental sealant

34. **Which of the following is TRUE about the dentin smear layer?**
    a. Composed mostly of collagen and water
    b. Dissolved by acid etching during bonding procedures

c. Easily removed with air/water spray
d. Effectively seals dentin
e. 50 to 100 μm–thick debris layer

35. **What is required to produce good bond strength to dentin?**
a. Drying of dentin
b. Preapplication of chlorhexidine
c. Postcuring materials with visible light
d. Hybrid layer formation
e. Long conditioning (etching) times

36. **How do self-etching bonding systems work?**
a. Acidic monomers replace need for phosphoric acid etching.
b. New monomers chemically adhere to hydroxyapatite.
c. Phophoric acid is mixed with other components of the bonding system.
d. Chemical bonding to collagen replaces need for micromechanical bonding.
e. Wetting agent helps adaptation and replaces need for micromechanical bonding.

37. **What products most likely contain water-miscible acrylic monomers?**
a. Acidulated phosphate fluoride (APF)
b. Pit-and-fissure sealants
c. Dentin primers
d. Resin surface sealers
e. Polishing pastes

38. **Which component of the dentin bonding system is most likely to cause skin sensitization in dental personnel?**
a. HEMA
b. Ethanol
c. UDMA
d. Bis-GMA
e. Phosphoric acid

39. **What is the shorthand representation for a self-etching primer adhesive?**
a. E+PB
b. EP+B
c. EPB
d. E
e. E+P+B

40. **Which of the following restorations requires surface protection with petroleum jelly during APF applications?**
a. Amalgams
b. Dental sealants
c. Cast gold
d. Orthodontic wire
e. Porcelain ceramics

41. **Which of the following constituents may have a palliative action on the dental pulp?**
a. Calcium hydroxide
b. Bis-GMA
c. 4-META
d. Eugenol
e. HEMA

42. **What is the primary filler component composite cement?**
a. Potassium oxide
b. Silicon oxide
c. Zinc oxide
d. Calcium oxide
e. Aluminum oxide

43. **Which of the following dental cements does *not* include polymer as part of the matrix?**
a. Polycarboxylate cement
b. Glass ionomer cement
c. Resin-modified glass ionomer cement
d. Composite cement
e. Zinc oxide–eugenol (ZOE) cement

44. **What ions on tooth structure permit glass ionomer chemical adhesion?**
a. Calcium ions
b. Fluoride ions
c. Carboxylic acid ions
d. Hydrogen ions
e. Aluminum ions

45. **Which of the following materials does *not* release fluoride?**
a. Resin-modified glass ionomer
b. ART restorations
c. Provisional restorations
d. Compomer
e. Traditional glass ionomer

46. **Which of the following MOST resembles a compomer?**
a. Glass ionomer
b. Zinc phosphate cement
c. Polycarboxylate
d. Giomer
e. Composite

47. **The fluoride release from glass ionomers follows what pattern?**
a. Rapid decrease to low level after 24 hours
b. Rapid decrease over 7 to 14 days
c. Some decrease after 30 days
d. Some decrease after 6 months
e. Some decrease after 1 year

48. **What is the effectiveness of recharging glass ionomer restorations?**
a. Does not work
b. Increases fluoride release for a few days
c. Increases fluoride release for a few months
d. Increases fluoride release for 1 to 2 years
e. Permanently reestablished fluoride release from the material

49. **Which of the following applications typically involves an ART material?**
a. Class II restorations
b. Class IV restorations in permanent teeth
c. Liner under composite restorations
d. Temporary restorations
e. Class III esthetic restorations

50. **Which impression material is a hydrogel?**
a. ZOE

b. Polysulfide
c. Polyether
d. Polyvinyl siloxane
e. Alginate

51. Which of the following features does *not* apply to polyvinyl siloxane impression material?
    a. Low shrinkage on setting
    b. Dimensionally stable
    c. Accurate
    d. Contains no filler
    e. Should not be poured immediately

52. Which application typically requires the STRONGEST gypsum material?
    a. Master cast
    b. Repairing casts
    c. Removable die
    d. Denture fabrication
    e. Orthodontic model

53. What is the chemical composition of set gypsum products?
    a. Calcium sulfate dihydrate
    b. Calcium sulfate monohydrate
    c. Calcium sulfate unhydrated
    d. Calcium sulfate hemihydrate
    e. Calcium sulfate trihydrate

54. What is the chemical composition of gypsum powder that is to be mixed with water to form models?
    a. Calcium chloride
    b. Calcium sulfate hemihydrate
    c. Calcium carbonate
    d. Calcium fluoride
    e. Calcium phosphate

55. How much "water of reaction" is required for the actual setting of 100 g of calcium sulfate hemihydrate powder?
    a. 12 mL
    b. 18 mL
    c. 24 mL
    d. 32 mL
    e. 50 mL

56. What is the major difference between plaster and stone powders?
    a. Color
    b. Crystal structure
    c. Powder particle packing
    d. Sterilization techniques
    e. Hydration state

57. Why does diestone require less water for mixing than plaster?
    a. Diestone undergoes a different reaction than stone.
    b. Diestone powder particles are less porous and imbibe less water.
    c. Diestone chemical reaction generates less heat and requires less cooling.
    d. Diestone contaminants are minimized by adding less water.
    e. Diestone powder particles pack more efficiently.

58. Why should molten wax be applied slowly and in thin layers onto dies?
    a. To minimize porosity
    b. To promote wetting onto the dies
    c. To avoid distortion from thermal contraction during wax cooling
    d. To avoid sag from wax's low modulus
    e. To avoid water absorption

59. What is the role of paraffin in most dental waxes?
    a. Increase hardness
    b. Increase thermal stability
    c. Act as main low-melting component
    d. Reduce thermal expansion
    e. Increase tackiness

60. What is the main goal in the design of dental inlay waxes?
    a. Low cost
    b. Low melting temperature
    c. Complete pyrolysis on heating to CO_2 and H_2O
    d. Low coefficient of thermal expansion
    e. High hardness

61. What are the primary constituents of an investment material?
    a. Two fillers and a binder
    b. Two liquid binders
    c. Matrix, filler, and modifier
    d. Two filled pastes that are mixed
    e. Binder and accelerator

62. What is the principal advantage of phosphate-bonded investment (PBI) over gypsum-bonded investment (GBI)?
    a. Stronger
    b. Less setting expansion
    c. Faster reacting
    d. Lower cost
    e. More stability at higher temperatures

63. What is the karatage of an alloy that is 80% Au by weight?
    a. 10 karat
    b. 13 karat
    c. 16 karat
    d. 19 karat
    e. 22 karat

64. In high-gold casting alloys, which element produces a temporary protective oxide on the molten alloy surface during the casting process?
    a. Zn
    b. Ag
    c. Cu
    d. Pd
    e. Au

65. In high-gold casting alloys, which element is primarily responsible for hardness?
    a. Cu
    b. Zn
    c. Au
    d. Pd
    e. Ag

66. What element is responsible for producing the corrosion resistance of stainless steel instruments?
    a. Fe
    b. C
    c. Co
    d. Ni
    e. Cr

67. What level of chromium is required in steel alloys to produce effective passivation?
    a. 10%-14%
    b. 14%-18%
    c. 18%-28%
    d. 28%-40%
    e. >40%

68. Which one of the following terms is *not* specifically related to soldering?
    a. Brazing
    b. Joining
    c. 600 to 650 fine
    d. Precious metal content
    e. Filler metal

69. Which application does *not* use gold alloys?
    a. Cast alloy bridge
    b. Partial-denture framework
    c. Cast post and core
    d. Implant
    e. Cast alloy crown

70. Which of the following dental materials *cannot* cause nickel sensitivity?
    a. Stainless steel crowns
    b. Some PFM alloys
    c. Some partial-denture framework alloys
    d. Dental amalgam
    e. Some orthodontic wires

71. What is the approximate incidence of nickel sensitivity for men?
    a. 6%
    b. 12%
    c. 18%
    d. 24%
    e. 30%

72. What events contribute to a relatively high nickel sensitivity level in women?
    a. Contact dermatitis from nickel-based jewelry
    b. Greater contact with stainless steel
    c. Genetic differences
    d. Less protective skin and hair during contact
    e. Greater contact with metal coinage

73. What are the three principal components of dental porcelains?
    a. Alumina, zinc oxide, calcium fluoride
    b. Alumina, potassium oxide, calcium oxide
    c. Calcium oxide, magnesium oxide, chromium oxide
    d. Silica, alumina, potassium oxide
    e. Silica, calcium oxide, alumina

74. What component of dental porcelain contributes primarily to esthetics?
    a. Silica
    b. Potassium oxide
    c. Chromium oxide
    d. Titanium oxide
    e. Alumina

75. What component is involved with very-high-strength dental ceramics?
    a. Silicon carbide
    b. Potassium oxide
    c. Chromium oxide
    d. Zirconia
    e. Silica

76. Which statement is *not* true about feldspathic porcelain?
    a. Relatively low coefficient of thermal expansion
    b. Ductile
    c. Used to veneer most dental porcelains
    d. High hardness
    e. Excellent translucency

77. Which one of the following dental materials is *not* a ceramic?
    a. Silicon carbide
    b. Corundum
    c. Hydroxyapatite
    d. Zirconium
    e. Titanium dioxide

78. Which is TRUE of all traditional dental cements?
    a. Endothermic reactions
    b. Acid-base reactions
    c. Good esthetics
    d. High strength
    e. Precapsulated

79. Which of the following dental cement compositions requires staged additions of powder to the liquid during mixing on a chilled glass slab to control the reaction?
    a. Polycarboxylate cement
    b. Resin-modified glass ionomer cement
    c. Zinc phosphate cement
    d. Universal cement
    e. Compomer cement

80. What is the primary monomer involved in denture base fabrication?
    a. EMA
    b. Bis-GMA
    c. MMA
    d. UDM
    e. HEMA

81. Why are acrylic resin teeth popular for denture fabrication?
    a. Excellent wear resistance
    b. Ease of cleaning
    c. Easily bonded to denture base
    d. Lightweight
    e. Best esthetics

82. **What is the major problem for tissue conditioners over the first few days?**
    a. Discoloration
    b. Bad taste
    c. Loss of bonding
    d. Increased hardness
    e. Fungal growth

83. **Mouth protectors should be cleaned with:**
    a. Ultrasonic agitation in baking soda solutions
    b. Dilute chlorine bleach in water
    c. Denture-cleaning solutions
    d. Cool soap-and-water solutions
    e. Dilute chlorhexidine solutions

84. **Mouth protectors are typically fabricated from what material?**
    a. Thermoplastic polymer
    b. Impression material
    c. Composite
    d. Denture base resin
    e. Guttapercha

85. **Which of the following materials practically *cannot* be fabricated using CAD/CAM procedures?**
    a. Dental porcelain
    b. Gold alloys
    c. Zirconia
    d. Alumina
    e. Dental composite

86. **What process does *not* harm the protective titanium dioxide surface of dental implants?**
    a. Scaling with metal instruments
    b. Use of polishing agents
    c. Abrasive dentifrices
    d. Dental floss
    e. APF application

87. **Which one of the following dental materials fabrication processes would be classified as "additive"?**
    a. CAD/CAM machining of zirconia
    b. CAD/CAM machining of composite
    c. Inkjet printing
    d. Casting
    e. All the above

88. **What are the major requirements for tissue engineering?**
    a. Cells and bone
    b. Cells and collagen
    c. Collagen, hydroxyapatite, and signals
    d. Cells and scaffolds
    e. Cells, signals, and scaffolds

89. **Which of the following biomaterials utilizes tissue from a cadaver?**
    a. Allograft
    b. Xenograft
    c. Synthetic tissue
    d. Engineered tissue
    e. Autograft

90. **Which of the following is *not* a scaffold material for tissue engineering?**
    a. Gold mesh
    b. Polylactic acid (PLA)
    c. Bioglass
    d. Collagen
    e. Bone chips

Periodontics

Denise M. Bowen

The vast majority of periodontal needs are related to the treatment of gingivitis and early periodontitis, the prevention of periodontal disease, and the maintenance of periodontal health after therapy. The demand for these services, provided by dental hygienists, continues to grow. An understanding of periodontics is critical to the process of dental hygiene care.

BASIC FEATURES OF THE PERIODONTIUM

A. The periodontium is composed of gingiva, periodontal ligament, cementum, and alveolar bone (Fig. 14-1)
B. The function of the periodontium is to attach the teeth to the alveolar bone tissues of the mandible and the maxilla

Gingiva
Definition
A. Part of the oral masticatory mucosa that surrounds the cervical portion of the teeth and covers the alveolar process of the jaws
B. Components
1. Marginal gingiva (unattached or free gingiva)
   a. Unattached cuff-like tissue that surrounds all surfaces of the teeth
   b. Parts of marginal gingiva
      (1) Gingival margin—most coronal portion; located at or approximately 0.5 mm coronal to the cemento-enamel junction (CEJ)
      (2) Gingival groove—when present, it is located 1 to 1.5 mm apical to the gingival margin at the base of the gingival sulcus
      (3) Gingival sulcus—space formed by the tooth and the sulcular epithelium laterally and by the coronal end of the junctional epithelium (base of the sulcus) apically; a sulcular measurement of 1 to 2 mm facially and lingually and 1 to 3 mm interproximally is considered normal
      (4) Interdental gingiva—occupies the interdental space coronal to the alveolar crest (clinically, it fills the embrasure space beneath the area of tooth contact)
         (a) Interdental gingiva—consists of two interdental papillae (one facial and one lingual) that are connected by the concave interdental *col*

(b) Col is absent when teeth are not in contact
2. Attached gingiva
   a. Portion of the gingiva that is attached to the underlying periosteum of the alveolar bone and to the cementum by connective tissue fibers and the epithelial attachment
   b. Boundaries
      (1) Apically demarcated from the alveolar mucosa by the mucogingival junction
      (2) Coronally demarcated by the base of the gingival sulcus
   c. Width varies from 1.8 to 4.5 mm
      (1) Generally widest in the facial anterior maxillary areas and narrowest in the mandibular premolar facial areas
      (2) The width is not measured on the palate because it cannot be clinically distinguished from the palatal mucosa
   3. Changes in the width of attached gingiva result from changes at the coronal end

Histologic Features[1]
See the sections on "Oral Histology," "Oral Mucosa," and "Dento-Gingival Junction" in Chapter 2.
A. Epithelium
1. Sulcular (crevicular) epithelium—stratified squamous, nonkeratinized epithelium that is continuous with the oral epithelium; lines the peripheral surface of the sulcus, extending to the coronal border of the junctional epithelium
2. Junctional epithelium—stratified squamous, nonkeratinized epithelium that surrounds and attaches to the tooth on one side and attaches on the other side to the gingival connective tissue; new cells originate from the cells in the apical portion adjacent to the tooth and from the cells in contact with the connective tissue; epithelial cells are shed at the coronal end of the junctional epithelium, at the base of the gingival sulcus
   a. The junctional epithelium is more permeable the oral epithelium
   b. The junctional epithelium serves as the route for the passage of fluid and cells from the connective tissue into the sulcus and for the passage of bacteria and

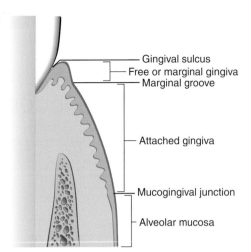

FIG 14-1 Anatomy of the periodontium.

FIG 14-2 Normal gingiva in a young adult. Note the demarcation, referred to as the mucogingival line *(arrows)*, between the attached gingival and the darker alveolar mucosa. (From Newman MG, et al: *Carranza's clinical periodontology,* ed 12, St Louis, 2015, Elsevier.)

bacterial products from the sulcus into the connective tissue

    c. The junctional epithelium is easily penetrated by the periodontal probe; penetration is increased in inflamed gingiva

    d. The length of the junctional epithelium ranges from 0.25 to 1.35 mm

  3. Epithelial attachment—basal lamina, hemidesmosomes, adhesion proteins (laminins), and anchoring fibrils that connect the junctional epithelium to the tooth surface at or slightly coronal to the CEJ

B. Connective tissue (or lamina propria)—composed of gingival fibers (connective tissue fibers), intercellular ground substance, cells, and vessels and nerves (see Chapter 2, Figs. 2-20 and 2-27)

  1. Gingival fibers—composed of collagen fibers (60% of connective tissue volume) and an elastic fiber system composed of oxytalan, elaunin, and elastin fibers; fiber bundle groups provide support for marginal gingiva, including the interdental papilla (see Chapter 2; Fig. 2-28, *B,* and the section on "Periodontal Ligament" for gingival fiber groups)

  2. Intercellular ground substance (or matrix)—similar to connective tissue in the periodontal ligament

  3. Cells

    a. Fibroblasts (predominant cells)

      (1) Produce various types of fibers found in connective tissue

      (2) Instrumental in synthesis of intercellular ground substance

        Wound healing or healing after therapy is regulated by fibroblasts (see the section on "Regeneration and Wound Healing" in Chapter 7)

    b. Other connective tissue cellular components—host defense cells

  4. Vessels and nerves (see the section on "Blood Supply, Lymph, and Innervation of the Periodontium")

Normal Clinical Features (Fig. 14-2)

A. Color—in light-skinned individuals, pale or coral pink; in dark-skinned individuals, coral pink to brown; color varies,

depending on (1) the degree of vascularity, (2) amount of melanin, (3) epithelial keratinization, and (4) thickness of epithelium

B. Texture

  1. Gingival margin—dull, smooth surface

  2. Attached—stippled, "orange peel" surface present on facial surfaces; may not always be present in health

C. Consistency

  1. Gingival margin—firm and resilient; resists displacement

  2. Attached gingiva—firmly bound to the underlying alveolar bone and cementum

D. Contour and shape

  1. Papillary contour—pointed; papilla fills proximal embrasure space to the contact point

  2. Marginal contour—most coronal edge should form a knife-like edge with a scalloped configuration mesiodistally (follows the CEJ)

  3. The contour varies with the shape and alignment of teeth and with the size and position of contacts

Periodontal Ligament

See the section on "Periodontal Ligament" and Fig. 2-27 in Chapter 2.

Functions

A. Physical—attachment of the tooth to the bone, transmission of occlusal forces to the bone, absorption of the impact of occlusal forces, and maintenance of the proper relationship of gingival tissues to teeth

B. Formative—participation in formation of cementum and bone and remodeling of the periodontal ligament by activities of connective tissue cells (cementoblasts, fibroblasts, osteoblasts)

C. Resorptive—by the activity of connective tissue cells (primarily osteoclasts)

D. Nutritive—nutrients carried through blood vessels to cementum, bone, and gingiva

E. Sensory—proprioceptive and tactile sensitivity provided by innervation to the ligament

Clinical Considerations

A. Thickness varies from 0.05 to 0.25 mm (mean, 0.2 mm), depending on the stage of eruption, the person's age, and the function of a tooth; the ligament is thickest in the apical area and is thicker in functioning than in nonfunctioning teeth and thicker in areas of tension than in areas of compression

B. Periodontal ligament cells that form collagen in ligament bundles can also remodel the ligament through secretion of new collagen (fibroblasts) and resorption of older collagen (fibroclasts), as well as lateral resorption of adjacent bone (osteoclasts) when altered forces are applied (e.g., orthodontics)

C. Accidentally exfoliated teeth can be reimplanted if handling of torn ligament is minimized before reimplantation; heal by reattachment

Cementum

See the section on "Cementum" in Chapter 2.

Clinical Considerations

A. Compensates for occlusal wear and continuous eruption by apical deposition of cementum throughout life

B. Protects the root surface from resorption during tooth movement

C. Has a reparative function, which permits reestablishment of new connective tissue attachment after certain types of periodontal therapies

D. When enamel and cementum do not meet, cervical hypersensitivity and caries are more likely

Alveolar Process

See the section on "Alveolar Bone" and Fig. 2-26 in Chapter 2.

Shape, Thickness, and Location

A. The contour of the alveolar bone follows the contour of the CEJ and the arrangement of the dentition

B. The shape of the alveolar crest is generally parallel to the CEJ of adjacent teeth; is approximately 1.5 to 2 mm apical to the CEJ

C. Cortical plates generally are thicker in the mandible than in the maxilla

D. Posterior areas—bone generally is thick, and cancellous bone separates the cortical plate from the alveolar bone proper

E. Anterior areas—bone is thin, with little or no cancellous bone separating the cortical plate from the alveolar bone proper

F. Dehiscence—situation in which the marginal alveolar bone is denuded, forming a defect extending apical to the normal level, exposing an abnormal amount of root surface

G. Fenestration—situation in which the margin of alveolar bone is intact; an isolated lack of alveolar bone on the root surface leaves it covered only by the periosteum and gingiva

Radiographic Features of the Normal Periodontium
(Fig. 14-3)

A. Alveolar crest—thin, radiopaque line continuous with the lamina dura; the shape depends on the proximity of adjacent teeth and roots and level of adjacent CEJs

FIG 14-3 Crest of interdental septum, which is normally parallel to a line drawn between the cemento-enamel junction of adjacent teeth *(arrow)*. Note the radiopaque lamina dura around the roots. (From Newman MG, et al: *Carranza's clinical periodontology*, ed 12, St Louis, 2015, Elsevier.)

B. Interdental septum—proximal alveolar bone bordered by the alveolar crest

C. Lamina dura—radiographic image of the alveolar bone proper; may or may not be present as a thin radiopaque line surrounding the bone adjacent to the periodontal ligament

D. Periodontal ligament space—thin radiolucent line surrounding each tooth between the root and adjacent alveolar bone

E. Supporting bone—radiopacity of the trabecular pattern varies, depending on the amount, pattern, and presence of cancellous and cortical bone

F. Limitations of radiographs—radiographs:
   1. Do not show the relationships between soft and hard tissues
   2. Do not show the initial signs of early bone loss
   3. Do not show bone changes on facial or lingual surfaces; these bony plates are obscured by teeth roots
   4. Do not reveal current cellular activity; only reflect past events
   5. Have their diagnostic value affected by variations in technique

Blood Supply, Lymph, and Innervation of the Periodontium[1,2]

See the section on "Blood and Lymph" and "Nerve Tissue" in Chapter 2.

A. Blood supply originates from the inferior and superior alveolar arteries

B. Lymph drains into larger lymph nodes and veins

C. The nerve supply is derived from the branches of the trigeminal nerve and thus is sensory in nature; nerve branches terminate in the periodontal ligament, on the surface of alveolar bone, and within gingival connective tissue; receives stimuli for pain (nociceptors) and for position and pressure (mechanoreceptors and proprioceptors)

DISEASES OF THE PERIODONTIUM

Classification of Periodontal Diseases[1,2]

See the section on "Periodontal Diseases" in Chapter 9.
A. Importance of disease classification
  1. Useful for dental hygiene diagnosis, prognosis, care plans, and legal documentation
  2. Classifications of periodontal diseases are changing as new information about causes, pathogenicity, and host factors continues to evolve
B. Current classifications of periodontal diseases
  1. Gingival diseases
    a. Dental plaque–induced gingival diseases—can occur on a periodontium with no attachment loss or past attachment loss that is not progressing; include dental plaque (biofilm)-associated gingivitis and gingival diseases modified by systemic factors such as hormonal disorders, blood dyscrasias, medications, and malnutrition
    b. Non–plaque-induced gingival lesions—include gingival diseases of specific bacterial, viral, fungal, or genetic origin; gingival manifestations of systemic conditions such as mucocutaneous disorders and allergic reactions; and traumatic lesions, foreign body reactions, and otherwise nonspecified gingival lesions
  2. Chronic periodontitis—localized or generalized
  3. Aggressive periodontitis—localized or generalized
  4. Periodontitis as a manifestation of systemic diseases (hematologic or genetic)
  5. Necrotizing periodontal diseases
  6. Abscesses of the periodontium
  7. Periodontitis associated with endodontic lesions
  8. Developmental or acquired deformities and conditions

Gingival Diseases[1,2]

A. Common characteristics
  1. Signs and symptoms confined to the gingiva
  2. Presence of bacterial biofilm, which initiates or exacerbates the lesion
  3. Clinical signs of inflammation
  4. No loss of attachment or stable attachment levels; possible precursor to attachment loss
B. Dental plaque–induced gingivitis
  1. Inflammation of the gingiva resulting from biofilm at the gingival margin
  2. Most common form of periodontal disease; prevalent in all age groups
  3. Change in gingival color and contour (redness, swelling, enlargement); increased sulcular temperature and gingival exudate; bleeding on provocation; reversible with biofilm removal
  4. Sensitivity or tenderness can occur, although not present in all clients
  5. Absence of attachment loss and bone loss is characteristic; after active periodontal treatment and resolution of

inflammation in periodontitis, tissue becomes healthy, but attachment loss remains; dental plaque–induced (biofilm-induced) gingivitis on a reduced periodontium can occur in these patients if gingival inflammation arises without evidence of progressive attachment loss
C. Gingival diseases associated with endocrine changes or endogenous sex hormones
  1. Periodontal tissues are modulated by androgens, estrogens, and progestin
  2. Most information exists about sex hormone–induced effects in women: menstruation, pregnancy, and puberty
  3. Gingival response requires biofilm in conjunction with steroid hormones
    a. Puberty-associated gingivitis—occurs in adolescents during puberty in both genders when the dramatic rise in hormone levels has a transient effect on gingival inflammation; signs of gingivitis exist in the presence of relatively sparse deposits
    b. Menstrual cycle–associated gingivitis—significant and observable inflammatory changes occur most frequently during ovulation, often not present
    c. Pregnancy-associated gingivitis—some of the most remarkable endocrine changes occur during pregnancy because of increased plasma hormone levels; features are similar to biofilm-induced gingivitis, but little biofilm may be present; increased prevalence and severity have been reported
    d. Pregnancy-associated pyogenic granuloma (pregnancy tumor)—pronounced response of gingiva to dental biofilm at gingival margin in the form of a sessile or pedunculated protuberant mass; most common interproximally; regresses after parturition
D. Gingival diseases associated with medications (drug-influenced gingival diseases)
  1. Drug-influenced gingival enlargement— prevalence 5% to 50%; overgrowth of the gingiva most often associated with:
    a. Anticonvulsant agents (e.g., phenytoin)
    b. Immunosuppressant agents (e.g., cyclosporine)
    c. Calcium channel blockers (e.g., nifedipine, verapamil, diltiazem, sodium valproate)
  2. Occurs most frequently in the anterior gingiva, especially in children; onset within 3 months of drug regimen
  3. Changes in gingival contour, size, and color because of enlargement; increased gingival exudate and bleeding on provocation can coexist; first occurs interproximally
  4. Found in the gingiva, with or without bone loss; not associated with attachment loss
  5. Biofilm control can limit the severity of the pronounced gingival inflammatory response
  6. Oral contraceptive–associated gingivitis—no longer considered a significant risk[3]
E. Gingival diseases associated with systemic diseases
  1. Diabetes mellitus–associated gingivitis—found in children with poorly controlled type 1 diabetes mellitus
  2. Leukemia-associated gingivitis (hematologic gingival disease)—primarily found in persons with acute leukemia

3. Both diseases manifest with pronounced inflammatory response to bacterial dental biofilm; changes in gingival color and contour; increased bleeding on provocation

4. Dental biofilm control can limit severity

F. Gingival diseases associated with malnutrition

1. Malnutrition leads to compromised host response and defense mechanisms

2. Increased susceptibility to infection may exacerbate gingival response to dental biofilm

3. Scurvy can also result from ascorbic acid (vitamin C) deficiency; the resultant gingival lesions are described as erythematous, bulbous, hemorrhagic, swollen, and spongy

G. Non–plaque-induced gingival lesions[2]

1. Infectious gingivitis—includes specific bacteria (e.g., *Neisseria gonorrhoeae*, *Treponema pallidum*), viruses (e.g., herpes simplex types 1 and 2, varicella-zoster, papillomavirus), fungi (e.g., *Candida* species), or genetic conditions (e.g., hereditary gingival fibromatosis) (see the section on "Periodontal Diseases" in Chapter 9); linear gingival erythema occurs in individuals who have acquired immunodeficiency syndrome (AIDS) or other immunocompromising diseases

a. Clinical changes—distinct band of severe erythema on marginal gingiva; can be localized or generalized; sometimes punctuated red dots are also present on attached gingiva; no ulceration or loss of attachment occurs

b. Radiographic changes—none; normal findings

c. Cause—immunosuppressed host response to biofilm microorganisms

d. Treatment—scaling and debridement with povidone-iodine irrigation for antimicrobial and topical anesthetic effect; prescription of antifungal agents if candidiasis is also present; critical importance of thorough self-care practices, including mechanical removal of dental biofilm and twice-daily 0.12% chlorhexidine rinses, 1-month reevaluation, and continued care

2. Dermatologic diseases, including lichen planus, pemphigoid, pemphigus vulgaris, erythema multiforme, psoriasis, and lupus erythematosus, also may present with gingival manifestations; the diagnosis depends on clinical findings and biopsy specimens (see the sections on "Major Aphthous Ulcers," "Skin Diseases," and "White Lesions" in Chapter 8)

3. Allergic reactions in the oral mucosa are uncommon but can be caused by dental restorations, dentifrices, mouthwashes, and food allergens; signs and symptoms do not resolve when oral hygiene is instituted

4. Foreign body reactions occur when ulceration of the gingival epithelium allows entry of a substance into the gingival connective tissue; most frequently is an amalgam tattoo

5. Mechanical trauma can be accidental, iatrogenic, or factitious; results in gingival or tooth abrasion, recession, ulceration, inflammation, or laceration

Chronic Periodontitis[1–3]

A. Slowly progressive; most common in adults; can also occur in children and adolescents

B. The disease results from the inflammatory process originating in the gingiva (gingivitis) and extending into the supporting periodontal structures; may have periods of activity and remission; has slow to moderate progression; may have periods of rapid progression

1. Can be further classified on the basis of extent and severity

a. Extent—number of sites involved

(1) Localized—30% of sites or less

(2) Generalized—more than 30% of sites

b. Severity—clinical attachment loss (CAL)

(1) Early—progression of gingival inflammation into the alveolar bone crest, with slight bone loss; with normal gingival contour, usual periodontal probing depth is 2 to 3 mm, with slight loss of connective tissue attachment and alveolar bone; average 1 to 2 mm CAL

(2) Moderate—a more advanced state of the early condition, with increased destruction of periodontal structures and noticeable loss of bone support; average probing depth of 4 to 5 mm, with normal gingival contour; average 3 to 4 mm CAL

(3) Advanced—further progression of periodontitis, with major loss of alveolar bone support greater than 30% usually accompanied by increased tooth mobility; furcation involvement in multiple-rooted teeth is likely; recession is common; average probing depth 6 mm or more, with normal gingival contour; average 5 mm or greater CAL

2. Radiographic features (see later section on "Changes in the Periodontium Associated with Disease")

3. Cause—host response to dental biofilm; the amount of destruction is consistent with the presence of local factors; subgingival calculus is frequently seen; is associated with various microbial patterns; can be associated with local predisposing factors; may be modified by systemic diseases and other risk factors

4. Treatment—nonsurgical or surgical periodontal therapy, or both, depending on extent and severity, followed by periodontal maintenance procedures

C. Chronic periodontitis can be recurrent and refractory (nonresponsive); not all cases of periodontitis have successful treatment outcomes

Aggressive Periodontitis[1–3]

A. Can occur at any age; may be localized or generalized

B. Common features

1. Occurs in persons otherwise healthy; most common in African populations

2. Rapid attachment loss and bone loss, which may or may not be self-arresting

3. Familial aggregation

4. Secondary features that are less universal include the following:

a. Bacterial biofilm inconsistent with the severity of periodontal destruction

b. Elevated proportions of *Aggregatibacter actinomycetemcomitans* and sometimes *Porphyromonas gingivalis*

c. Phagocyte abnormalities and poor antibody response

d. Progression of attachment loss and bone loss can be self-arresting

C. Localized aggressive periodontitis

1. Onset around the age of puberty is most common

2. Localized incisor and first-molar onset with interproximal attachment loss on two or more teeth (one first molar) and involving no more than two teeth other than incisors and first molars

D. Generalized aggressive periodontitis

1. Most common before age 30, but may also occur in older persons

2. Pronounced episodic nature of bone loss and attachment loss

3. Generalized interproximal attachment loss affecting at least three permanent teeth other than incisors and first molars

E. Treatment—same as for chronic periodontitis; systemic antibiotic (combination metronidazole and amoxicillin therapy) and diligent periodontal maintenance procedures

Periodontitis as a Manifestation of Systemic Diseases[1,2]

A. Systemic factors modify all forms of periodontal disease, but some systemic diseases cause periodontitis; the listing is categorized under broad headings

B. Hematologic disorders (see the section on "Blood Dyscrasias" in Chapter 8)

1. Neutrophil deficiencies cause severe destruction of periodontal tissues; leukocyte activities such as chemotaxis, phagocytosis, and killing or neutralization of ingested organisms or substances must be integrated for adequate protection

2. Quantitative leukocyte disorders

a. Neutropenia—cyclic or chronic forms involve deep periodontal pockets with extensive, generalized bone loss

b. Leukemia—most common in the acute form; symptoms include generalized gingival enlargement, swelling caused by cellular infiltrate, and uncontrolled bleeding related to associated thrombocytopenia

C. Genetic disorders[1] (see the section on "Genetics" in Chapter 7)

1. Genetic disorders usually manifest early in life and have similar signs and symptoms as those of aggressive forms of periodontitis; host genetic factors are believed to be important determinants in a person's susceptibility to periodontitis

2. Disorders associated with periodontitis include familial and cyclic neutropenia, Down syndrome, leukocytic deficiency syndrome, Papillon-Lefèvre syndrome, Chédiak-Higashi syndrome, histiocytosis syndrome, glycogen storage disease, infantile genetic agranulocytosis, Cohen syndrome, Ehlers-Danlos syndrome (types IV and VIII), and hypophosphatasia; rare conditions such as Papillon-Lefèvre syndrome, Chédiak-Higashi syndrome, and Ehlers-Danlos syndrome have the strongest evidence linking genetic mutations with periodontitis[4]

Necrotizing Periodontal Diseases[2,3]

A. Necrotizing ulcerative gingivitis (NUG)—inflammatory destructive disease of the gingiva that has a sudden onset with periods of remission and exacerbation; predisposing conditions may be preexisting (e.g., gingivitis, smoking, period of severe stress, deficient diet or sleep)

1. Clinical findings are characterized by crater-like depressions at the crest of the interdental papilla that progress into the marginal gingiva

a. Surface of the lesion(s) is covered by a gray, necrotized slough surrounded by an obvious erythematous (red) zone; interproximal necrosis

b. Bleeding may be spontaneous and will occur even when necrotic tissue is removed gently

c. Initially, moderate pain increases as the disease advances

d. Strong fetid odor and increased salivation

e. Swelling and tenderness of regional lymph nodes (especially submandibular nodes)

f. Fever and malaise may be present

2. Radiographic findings—normal, unless the disease has not been treated and has led to the destruction of supporting structures (necrotizing ulcerative periodontitis)

3. Causes—predisposing factors are present, with intermediate-sized spirochetes (*Treponema* and *Selemonas*), *Fusobacterium,* and *Prevotella intermedia* found within the tissue; the primary causative factor is uncertain; also has been associated with immunosuppression

4. Treatment

a. Debridement for dental biofilm and debris removal—initially by the clinician and then daily by the client (who may find it difficult to do because of pain); ultrasonic debridement may be beneficial

b. Reappoint in 24 to 48 hours to evaluate healing; after removal of bacterial challenge, rapid response in individuals with normal immune function; no response in the immunocompromised; complete and thorough scaling, root planing, and periodontal debridement performed at this appointment; pain is greatly reduced if healing has begun

c. The recurrent nature of NUG and the critical role of self-care practices and frequent continued-care visits must be stressed

d. Antibiotics may be prescribed for the treatment of systemic symptoms (lymphadenopathy, fever)

e. Suggest soft nutritious diet and the avoidance of spicy foods, alcohol, and tobacco

B. Necrotizing ulcerative periodontitis

1. Occurs in persons who have human immunodeficiency virus (HIV) infection or AIDS, other immunocompromising diseases, or severe malnutrition

2. Characterized by severe soft tissue necrosis and rapid destruction of periodontal attachment and bone; may lead to the exposure of alveolar bone and sequestration

3. Chief complaint may be "jaw pain" or "deep aching pain"

4. Can be localized or generalized

5. Treatment requires medical consultation and conventional periodontal therapy with povidone-iodine irrigation and

pain control; rigorous self-care practices for mechanical biofilm removal in conjunction with twice-daily 0.12% chlorhexidine mouth rinsing, judicious use of systemic antibiotics, or both; adjunctive antifungal therapy, if indicated; more frequent maintenance therapy than indicated for persons with adult periodontitis

Abscesses of the Periodontium[1]

A. Microbiology—*Streptococcus viridans* is the most common isolate; similar to microbiota found in deep periodontal pockets
B. Factors associated with abscess formation
   1. Occlusion of pocket orifices or incomplete calculus removal during treatment of a 2. periodontal pocket
   2. Furcation involvement
   3. Systemic antibiotic treatment
   4. Diabetes mellitus
C. Classification of abscesses of the periodontium
   1. Gingival abscess—a localized purulent infection involving the marginal gingiva or interdental papilla; may have bluish hue; does not involve the underlying periodontium
   2. Periodontal (or lateral) abscess—localized, purulent area of inflammation within periodontal tissue
      a. Clinical findings—the abscess may be:
         (1) In the supporting periodontal tissues lateral to the root; may result in a sinus (fistula) opening through the bone extending out to the external surface
         (2) In the soft tissue wall of a deep periodontal pocket, adjacent to a periapical lesion, or after deep scaling or periodontal debridement if incomplete
         (3) Acute or chronic
            (a) Acute—extreme pain, sensitivity, mobility, enlarged lymph nodes; the gingival area is edematous, red, and smooth with a shiny surface; exudate may be expressed from the gingival margin on pressure
            (b) Chronic—usually asymptomatic or episodes of dull pain; elevation of the tooth; desire to grind on the tooth (may have acute episodes)
      b. Radiographic findings (many variations according to the location, stage, and extent of the lesion)—typical appearance is that of a discrete radiolucent area along the lateral aspect of the root
      c. Treatment—debridement with 0.12% chlorhexidine or povidone-iodine irrigation; antibiotics if fever, swelling, or lymph node involvement is present; combined periodontic-endodontic therapy if related to periapical abscess
   3. Pericoronal abscess—inflammation of the tissue flap (operculum) surrounding the crown of a partially erupted tooth; also called *pericoronitis*; most common in third-molar areas; may be acute, subacute, or chronic
      a. Clinical findings if acute
         (1) An extremely red, swollen lesion with exudate is present
         (2) The area is painful; may radiate to the ear, throat, and floor of the mouth
         (3) A foul taste is present in the mouth
         (4) Inflammation may progress so that swelling, inability to close the jaw, fever, and malaise occur; the symptoms are less obvious when chronic
      b. Cause—accumulation of food debris and bacterial growth between the soft tissue flap and the tooth; inflammation may be compounded by trauma from the opposing tooth
      c. Treatment
         (1) Antibiotics if fever, swelling, or lymphadenopathy is present
         (2) Cleansing of the area (lavage, debridement) and creation of access for the drainage of the exudate
         (3) Frequent rinsing with warm water and return for follow-up care after 24 hours
         (4) Extraction of the involved tooth or removal (excision) of the soft tissue flap after the pain subsides and the infection is controlled

Periodontitis Associated with Endodontic Lesions[1]

Combined periodontal–endodontic lesions—either a deep periodontal pocket or an endodontic infection may be the cause or the result of the other, or both may develop independently; require combined endodontic and periodontic treatment

Developmental or Acquired Deformities and Conditions[1,3]

A. Localized tooth-related factors that modify or predispose to dental plaque–induced gingival diseases and periodontitis
   1. Tooth anatomical factors—enamel pearls, furcation, tooth position, root proximity, open contacts, root abnormalities
   2. Dental restorations and appliances—marginal discrepancies, overhangs
   3. Root fractures—periodontal lesions usually accompany vertical root fractures
   4. Cervical root resorption and cementum tears
B. Mucogingival deformities and conditions around teeth; gingival recession (or gingival atrophy)—exposure of the root surface caused by an apical shift in the position of the gingiva
   1. The severity of the recession is determined by the actual position of the gingiva
   2. The recession may be partially clinically visible and partially hidden (covered by inflamed pocket wall)
   3. The term *recession* refers only to the location of the gingiva, not to the condition of the gingiva; recession of gingiva may be inflamed or noninflamed
   4. Causes—the following factors have been implicated as possible causative factors:
      a. Gingival inflammation
      b. Faulty toothbrushing (gingival abrasion)
      c. Tooth position
      d. Location and amount of pull on margin of frenum attachment
      e. Dehiscence
      f. Advancing age

5. Clinical significance
   a. Exposed roots are susceptible to dental caries and abrasion
   b. Wearing away of cementum on the exposed surface exposes dentin, which may be sensitive to mechanical, chemical, or thermal stimuli
   c. Interproximal recession creates space for the accumulation of biofilm and debris
6. Treatment—nonsurgical or surgical
   a. Removal of causative or risk factors
   b. Daily thorough oral self-care practices and periodontal maintenance
   c. Root desensitization, if needed
   d. Gingival graft, regenerative or periodontal flap surgery may be performed
C. Mucogingival deformities or conditions on edentulous ridges—similar to dentulous areas

Epidemiology of Periodontal Diseases and Related Risks[1,3,5]

A. Basic terminology
   1. Incidence—number of new cases in an identified population during a specific period
   2. Prevalence—percentage of affected people in an identified population
   3. Extent—number or percentage of teeth or sites affected by a disease or condition
   4. Severity—degree of severity or advancement of a given disease or condition
   5. Risk factor—environmental, behavioral, or systemic characteristic or exposure that is associated strongly with a disease, without causality established; usually confirmed through longitudinal studies
   6. Risk indicator—a probable or putative risk factor that has been associated with a given condition or disease through cross-sectional studies; not confirmed in longitudinal studies
   7. Risk predictor or marker—a factor that has been associated with future development of a given disease or condition; considered potentially predictive without established causality
   8. Odds ratio—odds represent the ratio of the probability that an event will occur to the probability that the event will not occur; an odds ratio of 1.0 means that people exposed to a particular event or factor are no more likely than a normal, healthy individual to develop that disease or condition; greater than 1.0 is more likely
B. Natural history of periodontal disease
   1. Landmark studies of the natural history of periodontal disease by Löe and colleagues[6] established important features of the disease
      a. Severe disease tends to cluster in a small percentage of the population
      b. Pronounced differences in susceptibility to periodontal destruction can be independent of the environment
   2. These studies examined the course of periodontal disease during a 20-year period in two cohorts: Sri Lankan tea

workers who were generally healthy, but had never received dental care and did not know of toothbrushing, and students and academicians from Norway who had lifelong dental care and oral self-care education
3. Plaque, calculus, and gingivitis, which were common conditions in both groups, led to a slow loss of periodontal attachment with increasing age
4. Periodontal attachment loss progressed at a rate of 0.3 mm per year in Sri Lanka and 0.1 mm per year in Norway; professional care and self-care prevented or slowed the progression of disease
5. In the Sri Lankan group with no periodontal therapy, the disease patterns identified were:
   a. No progression beyond gingivitis (11%)
   b. Moderate progression of 4-mm attachment loss (81%)
   c. Rapid progression of 9-mm attachment loss (8%)
6. Periodontal diseases are most often slowly progressive; however, whereas some individuals show no progression even without care, others show rapid progression
7. Plaque, calculus, and gingival inflammation were present in both cohorts; thus, studies have identified other risk factors associated with periodontal disease
C. Current model of pathogenicity
   1. All individuals are not equally susceptible to periodontal disease
   2. Only a low percentage of sites with gingivitis will develop into periodontitis
   3. Periodontal disease is a highly complex disease, and variations in its epidemiology can be attributed to both local (environmental) factors and host susceptibility
D. Epidemiology of periodontal diseases[1,3–5]
   See also the section on "Epidemiology of Oral Diseases and Conditions" in Chapter 20.
   1. Gingivitis
      a. Prevalence—large-scale national studies in the United States have estimated that 50% of adults have gingivitis; this may be an underestimation because of study designs
         (1) Gingival bleeding in at least one site was seen in 63% of adults
         (2) Gingivitis is more prevalent, severe, and extensive in groups of participants with extensive dental deposits, low socioeconomic status, limited access to health education and dental care, less education, and low health literacy, as well as in adolescents, underserved minorities, and cognitively and developmentally challenged persons
      b. Risk factors—may be environmental or systemic
         (1) Systemic conditions that produce vascular changes, including acute leukemia, hemophilia, Sturge-Weber syndrome, and Wegener's granulomatosis
         (2) Systemic conditions that affect host response, including diabetes mellitus, Addison's disease, thrombocytopenia, combined immunodeficiency diseases, and HIV infection
         (3) Systemic conditions related to hormonal changes, such as pregnancy and puberty

(4) Environmental factors or local factors such as plaque-retentive factors (calculus, poorly fitting restorations), tooth malalignment or crowding, and smoking

c. Causative factors—cause-and-effect studied

(1) Dental biofilm is causative in gingivitis—plaque-retentive factors such as calculus, incorrect restorative margins, prostheses, and orthodontics increase risk of gingival inflammation; gingivitis is preventable in most people with frequent and effective personal and professional plaque control measures

(2) Prescription drugs can cause drug-influenced gingival enlargement, resulting, in whole or in part, from systemic drug use; these drugs can cause drug-influenced gingival enlargement, or their effects can be exacerbated by bacterial plaque

d. Possible influence of diet and nutrition

(1) No direct link has been established between nutrition and periodontal disease except in the case of scurvy and severe ascorbic acid (vitamin C) deficiency

(2) The relationship of diet and nutrition to disease susceptibility, tissue integrity, and defense mechanisms cannot be ignored

2. Chronic periodontitis[1,3,5]

a. Prevalence—varies significantly, depending on the population being treated or untreated; greatest increases in mean CAL found in untreated groups; U.S. surveys indicate as many as one in three adults over 30 years of age may have periodontitis, including only 7.3% moderate to severe forms; severity is highest in older age groups

b. Risk factors with positive association

(1) Tobacco use—strongest environmental risk factor, predicts future disease, and inhibits periodontal treatment outcomes; smokers are more likely to have periodontitis than nonsmokers; dose related: development of severe disease increases with number of cigarettes smoked per day and with years of smoking; all forms of tobacco implicated; most likely related to effects on host immune response; smoking has been found to depress the number of helper lymphocytes, impair vascularization, inhibit collagen production, increase collagenase activity, and inhibit healing after periodontal therapy; although the past effects of smoking on the periodontium are not reversed, smoking cessation is beneficial to periodontal health

(2) Diabetes mellitus—in persons with poor metabolic control and children and teenagers with type 1 diabetes; associated with more severe and rapid disease progression and with poor treatment outcomes

(3) Immunosuppression—especially when HIV converts to AIDS with CD4 counts below 200/µL and

in severely immunocompromised patients, including those with HIV infection and AIDS, immunosuppression, leukemia, hemophilia, neutropenias, uncontrolled diabetes mellitus, agranulocytosis, Wegener's granulomatosis, Addison's disease, Sjögren syndrome, Crohn disease, Sturge-Weber syndrome, Down syndrome, and others; necrotizing periodontal diseases have been associated with immunocompromised status

(4) Genetics—studies in twins have shown that genetic factors contribute significantly to the risk of chronic periodontitis

(5) Poor oral hygiene increases the risk for greater disease progression and attachment loss; poor biofilm control also is related to poor treatment outcomes

(6) Dental factors—sites previously affected by periodontitis; increased probing depth and loss of clinical attachment or multiple residual periodontal pockets after active treatment increase the risk for continued CAL

c. Risk indicators

(1) Age—rate of progression is not related to age; however, prevalence, severity, and extent are greater in older groups of people, perhaps because of the cumulative nature of the disease

(2) Gender—in developed nations, males tend to have a higher prevalence of periodontal disease than do females who have access to dental care

(3) Socioeconomic status (SES), education, and access to dental care—negative association; lower SES, education, and number of dental visits are related to more periodontal destruction

(4) Osteoporosis—most likely related to common pathways shared in the pathogenesis of periodontitis and osteoporosis

(5) Psychological stress—weakly associated; believed to be related to behavioral changes and immune system effects, especially in those who have poor coping skills

(6) Obesity—has been associated with periodontitis; both diseases also are associated with other chronic diseases, such as diabetes and heart disease

(7) Local predisposing factors can be associated with periodontal disease; tooth-related or iatrogenic factors, missing teeth, mobile teeth, mouth breathing, and areas of food impaction increase the risk of periodontal disease

3. Aggressive periodontitis

a. Prevalence—true prevalence and incidence are difficult to determine because of few longitudinal, prospective, and even careful retrospective studies, as well as variations in diagnostic criteria and protocols in larger studies; frequency of affected individuals increases between puberty and 25 years of age

b. Risk indicators

(1) Race—aggressive periodontitis seems to be more prevalent among African populations and less prevalent among Caucasians; however, it is difficult to isolate racial differences from access to care and socioeconomic factors

(2) Genetics—familial aggregation is found in siblings and offspring of those who have aggressive periodontitis; the disease is consistently present in several genetic or inherited disorders, such as leukocyte adhesion deficiency, acatalasia, Chédiak-Higashi syndrome, Ehler-Danlos syndrome, Papillion-Lefèvre syndrome, hypophosphatasia, and prepubertal periodontitis (see the section on "Genetics" in Chapter 7)

CHANGES IN THE PERIODONTIUM ASSOCIATED WITH DISEASE

See the section on "Inflammation" in Chapter 7.

A. Pathogenesis and stages of the periodontal lesion[1,3]

1. Pathogenesis—mode of origin or development of a disease; bacterial virulence factors, constituents, or metabolites that are capable of disrupting protective host mechanisms or causing disease initiation, progression, or both are required for the occurrence of periodontal disease

2. Stage I gingivitis, or initial lesion—2 to 4 days after biofilm accumulation
   a. Changes are not clinically visible; subclinical lesion
   b. Histologic changes
      (1) Brief vasoconstriction followed by "widening" of small capillaries (vasodilation), margination, emigration, and migration of polymorphonuclear neutrophils (PMNs)
      (2) Increase in leukocytes, particularly PMNs (neutrophils) and macrophages, in the connective tissue, junctional epithelium, and gingival sulcus; neutrophils are the earliest responders, or the first line of defense, in inflammation
      (3) Host systems (e.g., complement and kinin systems and arachidonic pathways)
      (4) Increase in the flow of gingival crevicular fluid into the sulcus
      (5) Inflammatory infiltrate occupies 5% to 10% of the gingival connective tissue where collagen has been lost

3. Stage II gingivitis or early lesion—begins 4 to 7 days after bacterial plaque accumulation; may persist for 21 days or longer
   a. Clinical signs of gingivitis appear (erythema, edema, and bleeding on stimulation)
   b. Histologic changes
      (1) Persistence of inflammation from initial lesion
      (2) The sulcular lining is ulcerated (allowing bleeding)
      (3) Inflammatory infiltrate in the connective tissue dominated by lymphocytes (75%); primarily T cells, with some macrophages, plasma cells, and mast cells
      (4) The junctional epithelium becomes densely infiltrated with inflammatory cells and begins to proliferate into connective tissue
      (5) Destruction of collagen fibers (especially circular and dento-gingival) in the infiltrated area; fibroblasts are altered
      (6) Migration of leukocytes, macrophages, dendritic cells, and lymphocytes into the junctional epithelium and the gingival sulcus
      (7) Gingival crevicular fluid peaks 6 to 12 days after clinical signs of gingivitis

4. Stage III gingivitis or established (chronic) lesion—the period varies; may persist for months or years without progressing to stage IV (periodontitis)
   a. Clinical changes
      (1) Erythema (redness) of the gingiva resulting from proliferation of capillaries, or a bluish hue superimposed over the reddened gingiva as a result of congested blood vessels, sluggish blood flow, or both
      (2) Bleeding may occur on probing because of thinning of the sulcular epithelium, ulceration of the sulcular epithelium, or both
      (3) Color changes begin in the gingival margin and papilla, then spread to the attached gingiva
      (4) Consistency may be soft and spongy or firm; depends on whether destructive changes or reparative changes within the gingiva are dominant
      (5) Texture may be smooth and shiny (inflammation) or stippled and nodular (reparative, fibrotic)
      (6) Increase in size of gingiva (enlargement)
      (7) Increase in depth of the gingival sulcus—may be caused by enlargement of the gingival tissue only; creates a gingival pocket or pseudopocket (Fig. 14-4)
         (a) Begins with papillary enlargement
         (b) Extends into margins, producing rounded and bulbous gingival margins
      (8) Progression of inflammation orchestrated by the progression of cytokines
         (a) May remain only within gingival tissue (gingivitis)
         (b) May extend into supporting periodontal tissue in stage IV (periodontitis)
            Note: Periodontitis must be preceded by gingivitis, but gingivitis does not always progress to periodontitis
   b. Histologic changes
      (1) Vascular proliferation and increase in number of B cells and plasma cells (produced by B lymphocytes) invade the connective tissue; blood vessels are congested, and blood flow is impaired
      (2) Widened intercellular spaces in the junctional epithelium contain lysosomes, lymphocytes, and monocytes; pathogens such as *Aggregatibacter*

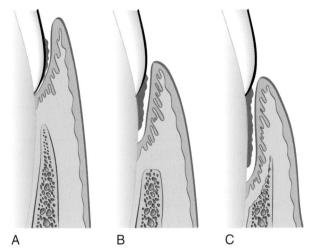

FIG 14-4 Different types of periodontal pockets. **A,** Gingival pocket. No destruction of the supporting periodontal tissues is seen. **B,** Suprabony pocket. The base of the pocket is coronal to the level of the underlying bone. Bone loss occurs horizontally. **C,** Infrabony pocket. The base of the pocket is apical to the level of the adjacent bone. Bone loss occurs vertically. (From Newman MG, et al: *Carranza's clinical periodontology,* ed 12, St Louis, 2015, Elsevier.)

actinomycetemcomitans and *Porphyromonas gingivalis* invade host tissues

   (3) Periodontal pathogens found in plaque biofilm, such as *A. actinomycetemcomitans, P. gingivalis,* and *Tannerella forsythia,* produce collagenase and elastinase, enzymes that destroy connective tissue; *A. actinomycetemcomitans, P. gingivalis,* and *Treponema denticola* also produce a trypsin enzyme that kills lymphocytes; *Prevotella intermedia, Capnocytophaga,* and *P. gingivalis* degrade antibodies

   (4) The junctional epithelium continues to protrude into the connective tissue; sulcular lining is ulcerated

   (5) Collagenase and other enzymes actively break down connective tissue, resulting in continued loss of collagen

   (6) Simultaneous proliferation of collagen fibers and epithelium (enlargement) occurs

   (7) Bone loss has not occurred

5. Stage IV—pathway of inflammation from the gingiva to supporting periodontal tissue (transition from gingivitis to periodontitis), or advanced lesion

  a. Characterized by loss of connective tissue attachment to teeth, including gingival and periodontal ligament fibers and their attachment to cementum, concurrent gingival inflammation, resorption of alveolar bone, and apical migration of the epithelial attachment along the root surface (i.e., CAL)

  b. Generally follows the course of blood vessels through soft tissues and into alveolar bone; the pattern of inflammatory pathway affects the pattern of bone destruction

  c. Initially, the inflammation penetrates and destroys gingival fibers near the gingival fiber attachment to cementum and then spreads

   (1) Interproximally—into bone and the periodontal ligament

   (2) Facially and lingually—from bone to the periodontal ligament, from the gingiva to the periosteum and periodontal ligament, and from the periosteum into bone

B. Formation of the periodontal pocket[1]

1. Persistent, chronic gingivitis may progress to periodontitis, which results in loss of connective tissue attachment, bone destruction, and periodontal pocket formation

2. Periodontal pocket—pathologic deepening of the gingival sulcus produced by the destruction of supporting tissue and apical migration of the junctional epithelium

3. Classification (see Fig. 14-4)

  a. Suprabony pocket—base of the pocket is coronal to the alveolar crest; also called *supracrestal* or *supra-alveolar pocket*

  b. Infrabony pocket—base of the pocket is apical to the alveolar crest; also called *intrabony, intra-alveolar,* or *subcrestal pocket*

4. Histopathology

  a. The gingival epithelium may show evidence of inflammatory changes

  b. Connective tissue changes

   (1) Inflammatory cells infiltrate the connective tissue and proceed through it

   (2) Degeneration of gingival connective tissue fibers; gingival cells release inflammatory mediators or chemicals that destroy bone

   (3) Tissue invasion by periodontal pathogens

  c. Changes within supporting bone as inflammatory process progresses

   (1) Cytokines and effector molecules (e.g., interleukins, prostaglandin E_2 [PGE_2], matrix metalloproteinase) have proinflammatory effects and stimulate osteoclasts that degenerate mineral content of bone; PMNs, macrophages, and mononuclear cells degenerate organic matrix of bone by producing collagenase

   (2) Bone marrow component (fatty tissue) is replaced by inflammatory cell infiltrate, fibroblastic proliferation, and deposition of collagen fibers

   (3) The cortical plate of the interdental septum (crest) is the first area to be involved

   (4) Once this central breakthrough has occurred, supporting bone is destroyed in a lateral direction; bone loss is accompanied by both resorption and formation

   (5) Periodontal pockets are constantly undergoing repair

C. Common clinical changes associated with periodontitis

1. Similar changes in the gingiva as seen in gingivitis, but usually more chronic

2. Areas of gingival recession

3. Bleeding on probing
4. Periodontal attachment loss
5. True periodontal pockets
6. Loose, extruded, or migrated teeth; diastemas may develop
7. Exudate from the gingival margin in response to pressure; suppuration (pus) is a sign of secondary infection
8. Symptoms—generally painless; client may complain of itching gums, loose teeth, food impaction, and bad taste; relief is felt with pressure applied to the gums
9. Furcation involvement

D. Radiographic changes associated with periodontitis (usually follow this sequence)
  1. Fuzziness and discontinuity off the crest of the interdental septum in the proximal area
  2. Wedge-shaped radiolucent area formed between the mesial or distal aspects of the alveolar crest and the root surface of the involved tooth; also called *triangulation*
  3. Center of the crestal portion of the interdental septum also becomes fuzzy, and faint cup-shaped areas of alveolar crest bone loss appear; bony crater
  4. Bone destruction patterns in periodontitis (Fig. 14-5 and 14-6)
    a. Horizontal bone loss is most common; bone is reduced in height but remains parallel to the CEJ of adjacent tooth surfaces
    b. Osseous defects or bone deformities
      (1) Vertical or angular defects occur in an oblique direction; most frequently, infrabony pockets accompany vertical defects
      (2) Classified by number of walls; may have one, two, or three walls
    c. Osseous craters are concavities in the crest of interdental bone, common in posterior segments
    d. Bulbous bone or bony enlargements occur as adaptations to excess function
    e. Craters result from complete loss of interdental bone without loss of radicular bone

5. Limitations of radiographs in the diagnosis of periodontitis
  a. The radiograph does not reveal minor destructive changes in bone
  b. The involvement of facial and lingual surfaces cannot be seen
  c. Angulation errors can affect radiographic image of alveolar bone
  d. The internal morphology of infrabony craters or defects cannot be seen
  e. As a general rule, bone loss is always greater than that revealed by the radiograph

E. Periodontal disease activity
  1. Refers to the stage(s) of periodontal disease characterized by loss of alveolar bone and connective tissue attachment
  2. Implies that the natural history of periodontal disease has periods of active destruction and periods of relative inactivity, although chronic inflammation persists

BACTERIAL DENTAL BIOFILM[1,3]

See the sections on "Microbiology of the Oral Cavity" and "Bacterial Plaque" in Chapter 9.

A   B

FIG 14-6 Angular defects. **A,** Circumferential vertical defect in relation to the maxillary canine and premolars. **B,** Infrabony pockets around the molars. (From Newman MG, et al: *Carranza's clinical periodontology,* ed 12, St Louis, 2015, Elsevier.)

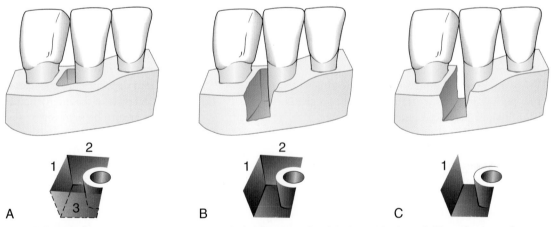

A   B   C

FIG 14-5 One-, two-, and three-wall vertical defects on the right lateral incisor. **A,** Three bony walls: *1,* distal; *2,* lingual; and *3,* facial. **B,** Two-wall defect: *1,* distal, and *2,* lingual. **C,** One-wall defect: *1,* distal only. (From Newman MG, et al: *Carranza's clinical periodontology,* ed 12, St Louis, 2015, Elsevier.)

A. Definition—complex community of bacteria that forms on any surface that is exposed to the fluids in the mouth; communication of bacteria within the biofilm allows for production of byproducts; dense, noncalcified, highly organized; firmly adherent to teeth or other hard materials within the mouth; cannot be washed off by salivary or water flow
  1. Biofilms protect bacteria housed within them (sessile), offering greater potential than freestanding (planktonic) bacteria
  2. Microorganisms produce a matrix called *glycocalyx* and extracellular proteins that encase and coat bacteria in the biofilm, providing protection from the oral environment, retentive qualities essential to being adherent to the tooth surfaces, and pathogenic byproducts (e.g., dextrans and levans, uronic acid, and others); referred to as the slime layer
  3. The matrix, or slime layer, of a biofilm provides a barrier from antimicrobial and antibiotic agents, making the biofilm resistant to chemotherapy
  4. The matrix or slime layer provides structure for the biofilm, nutritional advantages required for growth and maturation of bacteria within the biofilm, and strength against forces that attempt to detach bacteria from tooth surfaces
B. Two categories of bacterial plaque—supragingival and subgingival
C. Stages in plaque formation
  1. Acquired pellicle
  2. Bacterial plaque biofilm
    a. Complex microbial community forms, allowing for communication of bacteria within the biofilm and providing firm adherence to the tooth and other such surfaces
    b. Rate of formation varies from person to person, from tooth to tooth, and between areas on the same tooth; seen on teeth after 24 to 48 hours without oral hygiene
    c. Growth of microcolonies within the matrix and co-aggregation and adhesion of bacteria allow for increased thickness of the biofilm; shifts in the types of microorganisms occur; bacteria deep within the biofilm are more metabolically active and better protected than those on the surface that can be more easily dislodged
D. Supragingival versus subgingival plaque biofilms
  1. Supragingival plaque
    a. As plaque ages, the percentage of gram-positive organisms decreases
    b. As plaque ages, aerobic bacteria decrease and anaerobic bacteria increase
  2. Subgingival plaque
    a. Inflammatory changes in the gingival sulcus or periodontal pocket resulting from supragingival plaque modify the relationship between the gingival margin and the tooth surface, creating a protected subgingival area
    b. This environment allows subgingival bacteria to colonize and adhere to other bacteria, the tooth, or the epithelial tissue surrounding the sulcus or the pocket

c. Pathogenic anaerobic bacteria and spirochetes become well established in the subgingival plaque biofilm
d. Subgingival plaque may be attached or loosely adherent (epithelium associated)
  (1) Attached subgingival plaque (also called tooth-associated subgingival plaque)
    (a) Similar to supragingival bacterial plaque; inner layers are dominated by gram-positive rods and cocci and facultative bacteria; species of the genera *Streptococcus, Veillonella, Prevotella, Neisseria, Gemella,* and *Actinomyces*
    (b) Apical portions are dominated by gram-negative rods, with some filaments present; secondary colonizers such as *P. intermedia, Capnocytophaga* spp., *Fusobacterium nucleatum,* and *P. gingivalis* co-aggregate
  (2) Loosely adherent or unattached subgingival plaque
    (a) Extends from the gingival margin apical to the junctional epithelium, adjacent to the gingival epithelium or the pocket lumen
    (b) Primarily gram-negative rods as well as motile organisms, filaments, and spirochetes that are not highly organized; predominance of species such as *P. gingivalis, A. actinomycetemcomitans, T. denticola, P. intermedia, T. forsythia* (formerly *Bacteroides forsythus*) (pathogenic), and *Capnocytophaga ochracea* (beneficial)
e. Bacterial invasion of periodontal tissues
  (1) Bacteria have been found within diseased periodontal tissue in disease
  (2) Widened intercellular spaces in the gingival epithelium or the pocket lining may allow for the penetration of organisms from subgingival bacterial plaque
  (3) Bacterial invasion may occur, or the presence of bacteria within the tissue may be a result of displacement or manipulation rather than actual invasion
  (4) *Aggregatibacter actinomycetemcomitans* and *Porphyromonas gingivalis* are believed to be tissue-invading organisms
E. Bacterial specificity
  1. Specific plaque hypothesis—suggests that specific combinations of bacteria communicating with the biofilm cause various forms of periodontal disease; only certain microorganisms are pathogenic
  2. Research is further defining the bacterial causes and host response effects of destructive periodontal disease
F. Dental calculus—bacterial plaque that has mineralized
  1. Calculus plays a secondary role in the etiology of periodontal diseases by serving as a plaque-retentive factor; not all plaque necessarily calcifies; all calculus in humans is covered by bacterial plaque
  2. Earliest mineralization occurs along the inner surface of the plaque or in attached subgingival plaque; calcium and

phosphorus come from the saliva for the mineralization of supragingival calculus and from the gingival crevicular fluid (GCF) for the mineralization of subgingival calculus

3. Its porosity serves as a reservoir for bacteria and endotoxins that are destructive to the periodontium; impossible for the client to remove
4. Modes of attachment to teeth
   a. By acquired pellicle
   b. By direct attachment of the calculus to the tooth surface; penetrates cementum
   c. By mechanically locking into tooth surface irregularities
5. Effect on the periodontium—because bacterial plaque always covers calculus, it is primarily a bacterial irritant (not mechanical); calculus plays a significant role as a secondary, contributing factor in the pathogenesis of periodontal disease; a plaque-retentive factor

G. Pathogenic effect on periodontium (see the sections on "Acute Inflammation" and "Chronic Inflammation" in Chapter 7)
   1. Bacterial plaque biofilm contributes to periodontal breakdown by direct injury to tissue and by stimulating host-mediated responses that result in tissue injury
   2. Direct injury is caused by toxins and enzymes produced by bacteria and proinflammatory metabolic byproducts of bacterial metabolism; most significant pathologic effects during the early stages of disease
      a. Exotoxins are proteins and other metabolic byproducts such as hydrogen sulfide, uric acid, and fatty acids released by organisms that cause direct injury to tissue
      b. Endotoxins called *lipopolysaccharides* or cytotoxic agents are cellular components of gram-negative bacteria that are toxic to surrounding cells, contribute to the inflammatory process, and induce bone resorption; endotoxins are released from the cell wall on the death of gram-negative bacteria, initiating inflammation and tissue destruction
      c. Enzymes—mainly proteases, collagenase, hyaluronidase, chondroitin sulfatase, fibrinolysin, and phospholipase A—directly degrade surrounding tissue and penetrate by breaking down structural barriers
   3. Indirect toxicity results when subgingival bacteria act as antigens and a resultant local immune reaction occurs; the host response attempts to control the bacterial attack, and some destruction of tissue results by a variety of immunopathologic reactions

H. Host response—protective (see Figs. 7-1 to 7-4 in Chapter 7); host-mediated destructive processes play a role in the cause of inflammatory periodontal infections once the protective elements of the periodontium are overwhelmed
I. Host response—destructive
   1. Cytokines, including interleukins and PGE_2, participate in periodontal pathologic changes; these low-molecular-weight (LMW) proteins are produced by fibroblasts and inflammatory cells (e.g., monocytes, lymphocytes); lipopolysaccharide (LPS) stimulates cytokines

2. Collagenase and lysosomal enzymes destroy connective tissue
3. Aspartate transaminase (AST, aspartate aminotransferase)—an intracellular enzyme that indicates cell death or tissue destruction when present extracellularly
4. Elevated levels of host-derived enzymes (e.g., collagenase, AST, β-glucuronidase, elastase) in GCF can be used as markers for periodontitis
5. Tumor necrosis factor alpha (TNF-α)—an inflammatory mediator that contributes to bone resorption; shares properties with interleukins
6. Matrix metalloproteinase (MMP)—produces collagenase contributing to CAL

CLINICAL ASSESSMENT OF THE PERIODONTIUM[1,4]

A. Indices—system for documenting clinical observations to help clients become aware of their current status, to demonstrate changes in the client's health over a certain period, and to survey large populations for current status and trends in health (see Table 20-6 in Chapter 20)
B. Periodontal documentation
   1. Used to document existing periodontal status; baseline for future reference
   2. Updated periodically to determine changes in periodontal health or disease progression
   3. Necessary for care planning
   4. Serves as a guide for the clinician during treatment and evaluation
   5. Serves as a legal document; a risk management technique to reduce risks associated with failure to diagnose and treat periodontal disease
C. Periodontal assessment—complete periodontal documentation should be based on a thorough periodontal assessment, which includes the following:
   1. A description of gingival tissue—includes visual signs of inflammation
   2. Findings from examination of the periodontium with a periodontal probe (see the section on "Instrumentation for Assessment" in Chapter 17), which include the following:
      a. Presence of bleeding—widely accepted as an indicator of gingival inflammation; more sensitive than visual signs; however, inflamed sites do not always bleed, and bleeding is a poor predictor of attachment loss (only 30%), unless multiple sites are found in conjunction with deep pockets, attachment loss, or both; these combined conditions help make important risk prediction for attachment loss
      b. Probing depth (also called *sulcus* or *pocket depth*)—gives a historical record of past periodontal disease activity; useful in monitoring the success of periodontal therapy; important in determining client's ability to maintain health through plaque biofilm control; the periodontal probe remains the best diagnostic aid for detecting periodontal pockets and CAL

c. Clinical attachment level (CAL)—measures from the CEJ to the attachment; determines the amount of apical migration of the junctional epithelium or the amount of lost periodontal connective tissue attachment to the tooth; most accurate measure of severity of periodontal disease because the measurement is not influenced by the position of the gingival margin influenced by inflammation and recession, and because CEJ is a static reference point when measuring CAL
   (1) Because the gingival attachment is located slightly apical to the CEJ in a fully erupted tooth, and the gingival margin is slightly coronal to the CEJ in normal gingival contour, probing depth will be slightly greater than CAL
   (2) When gingival recession is present and the gingival margin is apical to the CEJ, the probing depth will be less than CAL; therefore, a normal sulcus depth can be present in an area of connective tissue and bone loss
   (3) If the gingival margin meets the CEJ, the probing depth and CAL are equal
d. Recession—measured from the CEJ to the gingival margin; indicates apical migration of the gingiva
e. Presence of purulent exudate (suppuration)—in response to lateral digital pressure on the gingival margin or probing; suggests advanced lesion of periodontitis and secondary infection at site
f. Adequacy of width of attached gingiva—measured from attachment to mucogingival junction; the amount varies, depending on location; adequate zone necessary to withstand stresses from mastication; if none is present, the gingival margin will move with alveolar mucosa; if inadequate, a mucogingival problem or defect exists
3. Alternatives to use of standard periodontal probe for periodontal examination[1] (see the section on "Periodontal Assessment" in Chapter 15)
   a. Periodontal screening and recording system (PSR)—provides thorough screening and recording for all clients while saving time in recording aspect of initial examination
   b. Electronic periodontal probes—increase accuracy by reducing the margin of error, standardizing pressure, or both; reduce time required for probing and recording
4. Presence and distribution of bacterial plaque and calculus (may use indices)
5. Condition of tooth proximal contacts—loose or open contacts permit food impaction
6. Degree of pathologic tooth mobility (see "Periodontal Assessment" in Chapter 15 for a specific classification system)
   a. Pathologic tooth mobility is caused by loss of periodontal support (bone loss), trauma from occlusion, inflammation extending into the periodontal ligament from the gingiva or the apex (abscesses), periodontal

surgery (temporarily), hormonal changes associated with pregnancy and sometimes menstruation or use of hormonal contraceptives, and pathologic processes of the jaws that destroy the bone or roots of teeth (e.g., osteomyelitis, tumors)
   b. Tooth mobility is usually assessed by using the blunt ends of the handles of two dental instruments (single-ended); can be measured electronically
7. Presence of furcation involvement (see "Periodontal Assessment" in Chapter 15 for a specific classification system)
8. Presence of malocclusion or malposition of teeth
9. Presence and condition of dental restorations and prosthetic appliances; missing teeth; dental implants
10. Presence of overhanging restorations (overhangs)—contributing causative factor in periodontal disease from accumulation of bacterial plaque and food impaction
11. Assessment of disease progression by longitudinal comparison of probing depths, attachment levels, and interproximal bone height (radiographic)
12. Interpretation of a satisfactory number of bitewing and periapical radiographs of diagnostic quality (see the section on "Radiographic Interpretation" in Chapter 6)
   a. Level of alveolar crest in relation to the CEJ and interdental bone
   b. Furcation areas
   c. Width of periodontal ligament space
   d. Existing dental restorations and caries
   e. Periapical disease
   f. Length, shape, and position of roots
D. Documentation of oral habits
1. Bruxing (grinding) or clenching of teeth
2. Chewing on fingernails or foreign objects
3. Smoking or drinking (alcohol) habits
4. Temporomandibular joint (TMJ) trauma (evidenced by crepitus, tenderness, or deviations)
E. Assessment of occlusion—includes:
1. Classification and anterior relationships
2. Excessive wear patterns (facets)
3. Defective prematurities—isolated occlusal contacts that cause deflection in the pathway of physiologic mandibular movement
4. Teeth, restorations, or prosthetic appliances that may interfere with the normal movements of the mandible
5. TMJ discomfort
6. Fremitus—vibration of root surfaces as the client "taps" teeth together
7. Tooth sensitivity to pressure and to hot and cold substances
F. Classification of occlusal trauma[1]
1. Primary occlusal trauma—trauma results from excessive occlusal forces when periodontal support is normal; result could be mobility, excessive wear of a tooth or teeth, sensitivity of involved teeth, or fremitus
2. Secondary occlusal trauma—the supporting periodontium is not normal (some loss of supporting structures

because of periodontitis); one or more teeth are not able to withstand even normal occlusal forces, and particularly excessive occlusal forces; could result in mobility or sensitivity

G. Additional information obtained through client interview
 1. Complete documentation of the client's past and current health status, including pharmacologic history and risk factors
 2. Complete documentation of the client's dental, fluoride, social, and cultural histories
 3. Client's daily oral hygiene routine
 4. Client's knowledge level and attitude toward oral health

H. Supplemental diagnostic tests[1]
 1. Traditional approach to periodontal diagnosis measures only the results of periodontal inflammation and destruction; the goals for developing newer diagnostic approaches include the ability to detect the presence of disease early to predict destruction before it occurs; prognostic devices or tests also are able to assess the risk of disease
 2. Validity of a diagnostic test is determined by calculating its sensitivity and specificity
  a. Sensitivity—the probability of a test being positive when a disease truly is present
  b. Specificity—the probability of a test being negative when a disease truly is not present
  c. Predictive value—refers to the probability that a disease will be present when the test is positive or not present when the test is negative; influenced by the prevalence of disease in a particular population
 3. Prognostic device or test—predicts the likelihood that a disease will occur in the future
 4. Supplemental diagnostic tests can be used for screening (to separate the diseased from healthy individuals) or to detect sites or individuals at high risk for progressive disease
 5. General categories of supplemental diagnostic tests (microbiologic monitoring)
  a. DNA (deoxyribonucleic acid) probes—paper points are inserted into specific site(s) and sent to a laboratory for analysis of presence of eight known pathogens to provide general information useful in antibiotic selection in refractory or aggressive cases
   (1) Culturing—plaque samples from specific sites are placed in a vial containing transport medium and sent to a laboratory for analysis; specific percentages of various bacterial species are identified with specific recommendations for antibiotic
   (2) Enzyme-linked immunosorbent assay (ELISA)—matches sample DNA and bacterial antigens to periodontal pathogens; used in research rather than in clinical practice
  b. Bacterial risk assessment test (BANA)—tests three anaerobes typically associated with periodontal disease risk; based on chairside incubation and testing of samples of subgingival biofilm

  c. Local measures of host response;[1] host-derived enzymes in GCF, which are produced by inflamed pocket wall and primarily composed of inflammatory cells and serum proteins as well as inflammatory mediators and tissue breakdown and bacterial byproducts (e.g., collagenase, PGE_2, AST)
  d. Genetic testing—determines genotype status through an in-office test for periodontal disease susceptibility (see the section on "Genetics" in Chapter 7)
  e. Automatic calculus detection systems
   (1) Fiberoptic probe—lights up and sounds when subgingival calculus is detected
   (2) Periodontal endoscope—a specific type of endoscopy used to explore and visualize the root surface, periodontal pocket, and furcation areas
  f. Risk assessment tool—Internet-based periodontal risk calculator that assesses a person's risk for periodontal disease on the basis of nine weighted risk factors

SYSTEMIC EFFECTS OF PERIODONTAL DISEASE[1,3]

A. Periodontal disease is a chronic inflammatory response to a given stimulus (virulent bacteria in biofilm) that has been associated with increased risk for conditions such as myocardial infarction, stroke, cardiovascular disease, peripheral vascular disease, adverse pregnancy outcomes, and pneumonia; a relationship between periodontal disease and these diseases has been documented, although a cause-and-effect connection has not been established
 1. Periodontal infection presents a chronic inflammatory burden at the systemic level
 2. Bacterial pathogens released from biofilm in the periodontal pocket enter tissues through ulcerations in the pocket epithelium and colonize other body parts; systemic exposures to these gram-negative pathogens and LPS trigger inflammatory mediator expression in the affected tissues (i.e., release of proinflammatory mediators and acute-phase proteins), contributing to systemic inflammation, atherogenesis, and other pathology
 3. Client-based clinical outcomes such as disease morbidity and mortality and surrogate markers (e.g., serum inflammatory markers such as cross-reactive protein) are used instead of traditional markers or outcomes (e.g., bleeding, pocket depth)

B. Research into the associations between periodontal diseases and the occurrence and severity of systemic diseases and conditions is ongoing.

TREATMENT[1,3,6]

Initial Care Plan

See the section on "Planning" in Chapter 15.

A. Collection of data to assess the status of the periodontium (see the previous section on "Clinical Assessment of the Periodontium")

B. Formulation of initial care plan based on data collection and assessment
1. Determination of all causative and contributing factors (risk factors and risk indicators)
2. Removal or control of etiologic and risk factors in an organized, logical sequence
   a. Plaque removal and control and removal of any plaque-retentive factors
   b. Reduction, control, or elimination of risk factors
   c. Elimination of inflammation; pocket reduction or elimination
3. Order of treatment will depend on:
   a. Severity of the client's periodontal condition and prognosis
   b. General health status of the client
   c. Client's motivation, cooperation, needs, and desires
C. Contributing factors influencing the prognosis
1. Local factors
   a. Degree of periodontal destruction (amount of attachment loss)
   b. Rate of periodontal destruction (amount of attachment loss per unit of time)
   c. Presence of contributing local factors (e.g., malocclusion, parafunctional habits, position of teeth in alveoli, malalignment, root proximity, missing teeth)
   d. Quality of restorations present
2. Risk factors—related to the client's general health (presence or absence of systemic disease), factors affecting host response, and environmental factors (stress, smoking)

Preventive Therapy or Treatment of Biofilm-Induced Gingivitis

A. Control biofilm—client co-involvement in daily self-care; remove biofilm-retentive factors
1. Address risk factors
2. Oral prophylaxis (versus nonsurgical periodontal therapy for periodontitis)
   a. The objective is to prevent the initiation of gingivitis and, failing that, to prevent the conversion of gingivitis to periodontitis; therapeutic goal of oral prophylaxis is to establish gingival health through the elimination of causative factors
   b. Performed for clients with healthy periodontium or with gingivitis; NSPT is performed for clients with loss of periodontal support
   c. Oral prophylaxis includes supragingival and subgingival debridement to remove deposits; removal or correction of biofilm-retentive factors; and coronal polishing, if necessary, for stain removal or for client satisfaction
3. The term *scaling* refers to supragingival or subgingival calculus removal without intentional removal of tooth surface
B. Nonsurgical periodontal therapy (NSPT); also called *initial therapy* or *phase I therapy*;[1,3,6] (see the section on "Concepts in Periodontal Instrumentation" in Chapter 17)
1. Objective—to treat and manage established periodontal disease and to create conditions conducive to health

2. Principles—elimination or suppression of pathogenic microorganisms through the removal and control of biofilm and its retentive factors (e.g., calculus, overhangs, food impaction, improper contacts); control of the infection and prevention of reinfection; resolution of inflammation
   a. Oral hygiene self-care, including plaque biofilm removal and control
   b. Periodontal instrumentation—scaling, root planing, periodontal debridement
   c. Adjunctive use of antiplaque and antigingivitis agents, as indicated (Table 14-1)
3. Consider and, if possible, control behavioral, systemic, and environmental host risk factors
4. Restoration or maintenance of comfort, function, and esthetics
5. Decreasing the likelihood of disease progression
C. Components of NSPT
1. Dental biofilm control—client as co-therapist: self-care, goal setting, long-term commitment; customized oral hygiene instruction, correction of biofilm-retentive factors, and supragingival and subgingival debridement; antimicrobial or antigingival agents or devices may be used as adjuncts to mechanical self-care methods; long-term success of NSPT depends on adequate biofilm control and regular periodontal maintenance visits
2. Adequate periodontal instrumentation for removal and control of biofilm and biofilm-retentive factors
   a. Rationale—periodontal instrumentation and biofilm control result in a significant reduction of gram-negative periodontal pathogens and encourage repopulation with the gram-positive microorganisms that are associated with health; a reduction in inflammatory cytokines responsible for tissue damage occurs after the bacterial composition is altered; calculus, overhanging restorations, and other biofilm-retentive factors that harbor bacterial plaque also are removed; all these components of NSPT reduce inflammation, promote tissue regeneration, and create a biologically acceptable root surface; control, alteration, or elimination of risk factors (e.g., diabetes, smoking, stress, medications) alters the host response to bacterial pathogens and has the potential to slow periodontal disease progression
   b. Supragingival and subgingival scaling, periodontal debridement, root planing, or a combination of all is performed; all these procedures are technically demanding; definitive treatment procedures are designed to remove cementum or surface dentin that is diseased, embedded with calculus, toxins, or microorganisms; treatment often requires local anesthesia; when performed thoroughly, some soft tissue removal, termed *incidental curettage,* is unavoidable; in the case of root planing, the need for extensive cementum removal to obtain a glassy, smooth surface is debatable because of a lack of clarity about its absolute necessity, the possibility of overtreatment, and resultant hypersensitivity

TABLE 14-1   Local Chemotherapy for Prevention and Control of Oral Diseases or Conditions

Agent and Delivery	Mechanism of Action	Alcohol	Directions for Use	Efficacy	Main Side Effects
Chlorhexidine 0.12% Mouthrinse	Cationic bisbiguanide ruptures bacterial cell wall; highly substantive	11.6% or 0% formulations	Rinse with 15 mL for 30 seconds 2 × daily; separate from dentifrice or fluoride by 30 minutes	45%-61% plaque and gingivitis reduction; antihalitosis	Extrinsic stain, altered taste, increase in supragingival calculus
Essential oils and phenolic compounds: Tymol 0.06% Eucalyptol 0.09% Methyl salicylate 0.06% Menthol 0.04% Mouthrinse	Antiseptic form interrupts bacterial cell wall and inhibits bacterial enzymes	21.6%-26.6% in antiseptic formulation; 0% alcohol formulation is not marketed as antigingivitis (only antihalitosis)	Rinse with 20 mL for 30 seconds 2 × daily	30%-35% reduction in plaque and gingivitis; nonalcohol formulation is antihalitosis	Burning sensation and bitter taste during use; caution with xerostomia and recovering alcoholic clients
Cetylpyridinium chloride (CPC) 0.045%-0.07% Mouthrinse	Solubilizes bacterial cell wall membrane	0%-18% (0.07% formulation has 10.8%)	Rinse with 20 mL for 30 seconds 2 × daily	Higher % CPC: small but significant reduction (14%-24%) in gingivitis; 29% reduction in plaque versus control Lower % CPC: for antihalitosis benefits	Low % CPCs have light extrinsic staining
Stannous fluoride Dentifrice (0.045%) Gel (0.04%) Mouthrinse (0.063%)	Sn (tin ion) is bacteriocidal and bacteriostatic; also desensitizing effect	0%	Apply small amount to toothbrush and brush thoroughly at least 2 × daily	18%-22% gingivitis 7%-23% plaque reductions 1100 ppm fluoride for cavity protection	Extrinsic staining light
Triclosan 0.03%/co-polymer	Inhibits bacterial metabolism; bacteristatic	0%	Apply small amount to toothbrush and brush thoroughly at least 2 × daily	59% antiplaque 32% antigingivitis 1100 ppm fluoride (0.24% sodium fluoride) for cavity protection	Small % contact dermatitis
Chlorine dioxide, zinc, or combination	Neutralizes volatile sulfur compounds (VSCs)	0% available	Available as oral spray, dentifrice, or rinse; follow manufacturer's instructions	Antihalitosis	No adverse effects known
Povidone-iodine	An iodophor effective against many bacteria, fungi, and viruses	0%	Primarily used during treatment for preprocedural rinsing or as irrigant, especially with immunocompromised status	Antimicrobial	Caution about allergy to iodine; contraindicated with allergy, thyroid dysfunction, and pregnant or lactating women
Hydrogen peroxide	Oxygenating effect is intended to affect anaerobes linked with periodontal disease	0%	Short-term use 2 × daily diluted with water		Safety concern if full-strength use — precancerous or cancerous cells; dilute 1:1 with water maximum

(1) Complete removal of calculus from root surfaces is unlikely, especially as pocket depth and inaccessibility increase; complete removal of detectible calculus remains the initial clinical end point because thorough instrumentation remains paramount to the success of therapy, whether nonsurgical or surgical

(2) The areas most susceptible to residual deposits after treatment include furcations, line angles, root concavities, and the CEJ

c. NSPT most often requires multiple appointments after assessment for treatment (e.g., four appointments 1 week apart for a quadrant therapy approach) to remove or correct all detectible deposits and plaque-retentive factors; some evidence suggests longer appointments within 24-hour and 48-hour periods for complete mouth debridement, termed *full-mouth disinfection*, are necessary to reduce cross-contamination from untreated areas to treated areas

d. Hand-activated or mechanized instruments (sonic, ultrasonic) may be effectively used for root planing and periodontal debridement; ultrasonic instruments are advocated for debridement and associated lavage

e. NSPT has been shown to be successful in treating early to moderate periodontitis, especially for initial pocket depths of 4 to 6 mm; results are less predictable in periodontal pockets more than 6 mm in depth, if tooth movement occurs, or when furcation involvement is present; NSPT is the definitive treatment for early to moderate periodontitis and an initial therapy for those expected to require surgical therapy

f. Root planing in healthy sulcus areas or shallow crevices is contraindicated; has been shown to cause a loss of attachment in crevices less than 3 mm

g. Use of lasers in periodontics appears to be equally effective to traditional instruments for scaling, root planing, and periodontal debridement

3. Initial evaluation of NSPT—occurs during and on completion of instrumentation by careful tactile exploration of tooth and root surfaces; a clear field, adequate illumination, and use of air to facilitate assessment are required

a. The term *periodontal debridement* refers to treatment of periodontal disease through mechanical removal of tooth and root surface irregularities (including biofilm, clinically detectable calculus, and all biofilm-retentive factors) depending on the health of adjacent soft tissue

b. The difference between periodontal debridement and root planing, as used in the literature, is in the desired initial end point and the extent of instrumentation; root planing is performed until root smoothness is obtained with reasonable time and effort, whereas debridement attempts to preserve tooth surface by removing only enough deposits and biofilm-retentive factors to achieve periodontal health; "periodontal debridement" is used on national certification examinations for dental hygienists

4. Ultimate evaluation of NSPT—tissue response (i.e., elimination of inflammation and bleeding)

a. Thorough reevaluation 4 to 6 weeks after scaling, root planing, or periodontal debridement to determine the need for additional therapy (e.g., surgery, physician referrals, antimicrobials, antibiotics) by means of a periodontal examination; it is critical to determine if clinical judgment regarding the extent of root planing and periodontal debridement was adequate to achieve periodontal health; if unsuccessful, retreatment is indicated; 4 to 6 weeks is considered appropriate for the resolution of inflammation and periodontal tissue healing; relevant findings of the reevaluation are documented in the patient's legal treatment record

b. Reevaluation includes:
   (1) Evaluation and reinforcement of the client's self-care
   (2) Updated periodontal assessment, including bleeding points, probing depths, and attachment levels
   (3) Reassessment of the clinical health of tissues; if areas still show signs of inflammation, the cause should be determined

c. Bacterial plaque and calculus self-care should be reviewed; perform scaling, debridement, or root planing as indicated if the condition is localized; the need for rescheduling and retreatment with active therapy should be determined if the condition is generalized
   (1) If no plaque, calculus, or inflammation is noted, the client's success is reinforced and the importance of periodontal maintenance emphasized
   (2) If the pocket depth is still moderate to severe, controlled drug delivery and surgical procedures might be warranted; the client must be referred for evaluation by a periodontist
   (3) If inflammation and bleeding are still severe, unexplained, or generalized, physical examination by a physician should be considered, including differential blood counts and complete physical examination for a possible previously undetected or undiagnosed systemic host condition

D. Use of topical antimicrobial agents as adjuncts (see the section on "Mouthrinses or Chemotherapeutics" in Chapter 16); also referred to as *local chemotherapy*; can be employed in preventive therapy, in initial or nonsurgical therapy, during the healing stage following periodontal surgery, or during continuing care for periodontal health maintenance

1. Indicated for control of supragingival biofilm and gingivitis; effectiveness in periodontitis has not been documented; used to augment oral self-care efforts that are only partially effective; also recommended for extensive restorative cases and dental implants; aids healing after periodontal surgery (see the sections on "Oral Irrigation" and "Dental Implant Maintenance" in Chapter 16)

2. Antiplaque and antigingivitis agents (see Table 14-1)

a. Chlorhexidine gluconate
   (1) Most effective antimicrobial agent for reducing plaque and gingivitis in the long term (45% to 61%); the "gold standard" for topical antimicrobial mouthrinses; 0.12% concentration in the United States and 0.2% outside the United States
   (2) High substantivity—ability to adhere to soft and hard tissues for a long duration while releasing active ingredient; a cationic bisbiguanide that ruptures bacterial cell membranes
   (3) Adverse effects—staining, reversible desquamation, poor taste or alteration of taste, increase in supragingival calculus deposits; especially with long-term use
   (4) Alcohol content 11.6%, or alcohol-free form available

(5) Twice-daily use promotes compliance; client should be instructed to use 15 mL of rinse for 30 seconds; rinse should be separate from fluoride dentifrice by 30 minutes for full effectiveness

(6) Also recommended for wound healing after surgery or as pre-rinse to reduce salivary bacterial load and aerosols during periodontal therapy and mechanized instrumentation

b. Phenolic compounds (essential oils)

(1) Antiseptic form is a safe and effective antimicrobial and antigingivitis agent (e.g., Listerine Antiseptic)

(2) Long-term studies indicate approximately 30% to 45% reduction in plaque and gingivitis

(3) Available antiseptic products have variable alcohol content (21.6% to 26.9% alcohol); thymol, menthol, eucalyptol, and methyl salicylate are active ingredients; act by bacterial cell wall disruption and inhibition of bacterial enzymes

(4) Adverse effects—burning sensation and bitter taste; some report soft tissue irritation; caution with significant xerostomia and recovering alcoholic clients; some formulations have high alcohol content; some are now alcohol free; however, they are for reduction of halitosis rather than as an antiseptic antigingivitis agent

(5) Twice-daily use promotes compliance; client should be instructed to use 15 mL of rinse for 30 seconds after brushing

(6) Also recommended as preprocedural rinse to reduce salivary bacterial load and aerosols during periodontal therapy and mechanized instrumentation

c. Triclosan

(1) Food and Drug Administration (FDA) approval as a safe and effective antimicrobial and antigingivitis agent (e.g., Colgate Total)

(2) A bisphenol that has broad-spectrum antimicrobial activity, especially when combined with zinc citrate or with a co-polymer to increase substantivity and to provide some anticalculus properties

(3) Dentifrice formulation promotes compliance; shown to reduce biofilm formation and gingivitis by 30 to 45%; can be combined with fluoride, unlike other antimicrobial agents, which often are not compatible

2. Other agents used in periodontal therapy

a. Povidone-iodine

(1) An iodophor with polyvinyl-pyrrolidone added to iodine; effective against many organisms, including bacteria, viruses, and fungi

(2) Primarily used as a preprocedural rinse or during mechanized instrumentation for antiseptic lavage or irrigation; often recommended for use during treatment of immunocompromised clients who might have multiple organisms affecting their oral

health; can be effective antimicrobial and antigingivitis agent, but only with short-term use

(3) Adverse effects—concern for iodine toxicity with prolonged use; contraindicated in those with iodine sensitivity or allergy, thyroid dysfunction and pregnant or lactating women; temporary extrinsic tooth staining

b. Stannous fluoride

(1) Antimicrobial mechanism of action appears to be related to the stannous (tin) ion rather than fluoride

(2) Long-term studies have shown significant reductions in gingivitis without concurrent significant reductions in biofilm and gingival inflammation

(3) Available in dentifrice; in gel form; or in rinses containing 0.63% concentrations; however, the dentifrice and gel forms are most effective

(4) Stannous fluoride has low to moderate substantivity, depending on concentration; twice-daily use promotes compliance

(5) Adverse effects may include unpleasant taste in the mouth and tooth staining after prolonged use (2 to 3 months) in some individuals

(6) Stannous fluoride has the American Dental Association (ADA) Seal of Acceptance for anticaries activity; the dentifrice formulation has been approved for plaque-reducing and gingivitis-reducing properties; dentifrice and gels also approved for dentinal hypersensitivity reduction

c. Quaternary ammonium compounds (cetylpyridinium chloride)

(1) The most common formulation is cetylpyridinium chloride used alone or with domiphen bromide; cationic surface active agents rupture bacterial cell walls; the compound binds to oral tissues but releases rapidly, which may limit its substantivity and therefore effectiveness in the oral cavity

(2) Six-month studies show 14% to 24% reduction in bacterial biofilm and gingivitis; the therapeutic value of the product is questionable

(3) Has benefit in reducing halitosis; often alcohol free

(4) Adverse reactions are minimal; may include possible slight staining

d. Oxygenating agents—hydrogen peroxide: anti-inflammatory properties decrease the clinical signs of inflammation, but bacterial pathogens may not be reduced; studies do not support long-term use of 100% hydrogen peroxide as oral rinse; ration with water 1:1 recommended as maximum; safety issues such as tissue injury and co-carcinogenicity have been raised with long-term use of hydrogen peroxide

e. Oxidizing agents (chlorine dioxide, zinc)—have no therapeutic value but are recommended for breath freshening and to reduce halitosis; reduce volatile sulfur compounds (VSCs) that are believed to be responsible for halitosis

3. Methods for topical delivery of antimicrobial agents

a. Mouthrinses, dentifrices, and gels deliver agents supragingivally; subgingival penetration is 0 to 1 mm—most common method

b. Oral irrigation can deliver agent subgingivally; complete plaque removal is not achieved, but periodontal pathogens found in loosely adherent plaque can be removed; recommended as an adjunct to mechanical biofilm control; often used during the maintenance of periodontal health after completion of active periodontal therapy; pulsating oral irrigators may be used as water flossers

c. Oral irrigation can be accomplished with water or antimicrobial agents; both reduce bleeding and gingivitis, but antimicrobials are more effective in removing bacterial plaque and making it less pathogenic; effect on periodontitis is not well documented

d. Depth of penetration with oral irrigation is related to type of tip used; standard jet tip is shallow; subgingival tip 6 mm or less; cannula deepest but concern for patient safety

e. Oral irrigation can have value in conjunction with daily self-care regimen for mechanical plaque biofilm removal in the treatment of gingivitis or in periodontal maintenance therapy

f. Professionally administered oral irrigation, with and without root planing and periodontal debridement, has been studied; the main benefit is from mechanical debridement; a single application of an antimicrobial irrigant has little value because of low substantivity in the periodontal pocket

E. Sustained-release, local drug delivery systems (also called *controlled drug delivery*)[1]

1. Systems are available for site-specific, sustained, local delivery of antibiotics or antimicrobials to specific subgingival sites (e.g., gels, chips, collagen film, bioabsorbable materials); the objective is to eliminate periodontal pathogens; these methods of local delivery provide the benefits of antibiotic or antimicrobial therapy with greater safety and compliance; delivery mechanisms allow the antibiotic or antimicrobial agent to be delivered for up to 14 days (varies by product) after placement; controlled delivery releases the material's active ingredient over time, maintaining a constant and sufficient release of the active ingredient

2. Controlled delivery offers the advantage of sustained release of a high concentration of the active ingredient to the site of periodontal infection without systemic involvement; can be used in conjunction with scaling, debridement, and root planing during initial periodontal therapy in pockets greater than 5 mm with bleeding on probing, at reevaluation for recalcitrant sites, or during continuing care for localized sites needing adjunctive therapy for the maintenance of periodontal health; few use these systems as a monotherapy

3. Contraindicated in the presence of allergy to the active ingredient or to any component of the delivery system and during pregnancy or lactation; not useful for treatment of generalized diseased sites

4. Studies have shown that these controlled delivery systems result in improved clinical attachment levels or probing depths of 2 mm or greater at 30% to 40% of sites treated in multiple-center, randomized clinical trials, a level considered both statistically and clinically significant

5. Examples of available sustained-release systems for subgingival application used most often in conjunction with scaling and root planing

a. Chlorhexidine chip—2.5-mg chlorhexidine gluconate in a hydrolyzed gelatin biodegradable film; self-retentive on contact with moisture, placed using cotton pliers

b. Minocycline hydrochloride microspheres (2%)—consist of antibiotic minocycline hydrochloride in a bioabsorbable polymer of poly-D, L-lactide-CO-glycolide; microspheres are dispensed subgingivally from a capsule placed in a syringe; the tip is inserted into the base of the pocket and then withdrawn after the drug has been applied

c. Doxycycline hyclate gel (10%)—solidifying liquid, biodegradable polymer that hardens after exposure to fluid in the periodontal pocket; delivered by injection from a syringe with a blunt cannula inserted into the pocket; common use is with scaling and root planing

F. Use of systemic antibiotics[1,3]—drugs that target the bacterial load

1. Sometimes used in conjunction with periodontal therapy (surgical or nonsurgical); however, no evidence that antibiotics alone arrest periodontal disease exist; may be prescribed for clients who are nonresponsive to periodontal therapy, acute periodontal infections with systemic manifestations, for prophylaxis in medically compromised clients, and in conjunction with surgical or nonsurgical therapy when systemic health or classification of periodontal disease warrants use after consideration of risks and benefits

a. Generalized recurrent or refractory periodontal disease despite appropriate treatment—often related to impaired host resistance or persistent, superinfecting microorganisms

b. Aggressive forms of periodontitis—related to neutrophil defects and tissue-invasive microorganisms (*A. actinomycetemcomitans* and *P. gingivalis*)

c. Acute, severe infections (e.g., periodontal abscess, NUG)—especially with fever, malaise, lymphadenopathy, or other systemic signs and symptoms

d. Immunocompromised status—used with extreme caution to avoid development of resistant strains

2. Not recommended for the routine treatment of gingivitis or chronic periodontitis; problems such as adverse drug reactions, drug hypersensitivity, development of antibiotic-resistant strains, interactions with other prescribed

medications taken by the client, and client nonadherence limit widespread use; the Centers for Disease Control and Prevention (CDC) recommends judicious use of antibiotics because of growing concerns about overuse and consequently the development of drug-resistant strains of bacteria, which has led to a resurgence of diseases previously well controlled by antibiotics (e.g., tuberculosis, staphylococcal infections, diphtheria); particular concerns about use in pregnant or lactating women do exist, and a higher risk of drug interactions is present with long-term use of cardiovascular disease, asthma, seizures, and diabetes medications

   a. Common side effects include nausea, vomiting, diarrhea, rashes, changes in vaginal or intestinal flora, and allergy; prolonged use can be associated with bleeding problems

   b. Specific reactions include the disulfiram (Antabuse) effect of metronidazole taken with alcohol, discoloration or deformed teeth with tetracycline use in children under 8 years of age, and increased risk of pseudomembranous colitis with clindamycin

3. Restricted use and careful selection are indicated on the basis of response to mechanical therapy, medical history analysis, possible drug interactions, and risks; indiscriminate use is prohibited; microbial analysis, antimicrobial sensitivity testing, or a combination of both before prescribing systemic antibiotics for periodontal therapy is recommended

4. Common agents include tetracylcines (doxycycline), nitroimidazoles (metronidazole), lincomycins (clindamycin), quinolones (ciprofloxacin), and macrolides (azithromycin but not erythromycin); combination therapy includes metronidazole and amoxicillin or metronidazole and ciprofloxacin; the combination is synergistic and increases the spectrum of drug activity; penicillins and cephalosporins are not considered drugs of choice

G. Use of host-modulating drugs;[1,3] host response is the target

1. While studies of nonsteroidal anti-inflammatory drugs (NSAIDs), bisphosphonates, and most recently, lipoxims and resovins have shown proof of concept, only low-dose doxycycline has been FDA approval for treatment of periodontal disease.

   a. Subantimicrobial-dose doxycycline (SDD)—used systemically in subantimicrobial doses to inhibit proteases and periodontal disease progression; downregulates the activity of MMPs that are active during periods of periodontal tissue breakdown and thus play a major role in inflammation and the destruction of collagen and bone

   b. Has not been shown to substitute for meticulous home care and periodontal maintenance

   c. Administered 20 mg twice daily (instead of the 50-mg or 100-mg dosage used as antibiotic) for 6 to 9 months or up to 12 months concurrent with periodontal therapy; a low dose eliminates most side effects, although SDD is contraindicated when known allergy to tetracyclines is present

   d. Research has shown slight but statistically significant gains in clinical attachment and reductions in probing depths

Additional Clinical Interventions

A. Gingival curettage[1,4]—a procedure to remove the ulcerated, chronically inflamed tissue lining a periodontal pocket; evidence fails to support the efficacy of this procedure

1. Studies of gingival curettage have almost always combined this technique with root planing; research indicates that gingival curettage is ineffective and that root planing alone can, in most cases, reduce inflammation, shrink tissue, and promote healing

2. In some states, gingival curettage is a legally permissible procedure that can be performed by dental hygienists

3. If new connective tissue attachment is the goal of a particular periodontal treatment plan, curettage has no justifiable application; healing occurs by means of a longer junctional epithelium and tissue shrinkage, as it does with root planing or periodontal debridement; surgical intervention is the therapy of choice when new attachment is the desired end point

B. Treatment of occlusal trauma[1]

1. Definitions

   a. Occlusal trauma—injury to the periodontal attachment apparatus resulting from occlusal forces when those forces exceed the reparative and adaptive capacity of the attachment apparatus

   b. Primary occlusal trauma—injury to the periodontium as a result of excessive occlusal forces when the periodontal attachment apparatus and the attachment level are normal

   c. Secondary occlusal trauma—injury to a compromised periodontium with loss of attachment or bone loss resulting from normal or excessive occlusal force

2. Clinical features and diagnosis

   a. When injury to the periodontal ligament occurs, collagen is destroyed, vascular elements are affected, and osteoclasts are increased on the pressure side, all of which results in a widening of the periodontal ligament space because of the lateral resorption of the bony socket wall, especially in the crestal area when the force is great enough to cause necrosis of the ligament; when a back-and-forth motion, or "jiggling," of the tooth in the socket (fremitus) occurs from occlusal trauma, changes are seen on both the tension and the pressure side, resulting in a funnel-shaped widening of the periodontal ligament and loss of bone; as such, mobility is the hallmark of occlusal trauma, and radiographic findings reveal widening of the ligament space, infrabony defects, or both; parafunctional habits such as bruxism and clenching or iatrogenic factors causing premature contacts (e.g., "high" restorations) most frequently result in occlusal trauma; tissues can regenerate on removal of the occlusal force that is causing destruction; therefore, constant evaluation and reevaluation are indicated

b. Although necrosis of the ligament and loss of bone can occur from occlusal trauma, it is important to note that attachment loss characterized by apical migration of the periodontal attachment, such as that caused by periodontitis, does not occur solely from occlusal trauma; occlusal trauma can contribute to advancing loss of attachment once attachment loss or bone loss from periodontitis has weakened tooth support

c. Positive diagnosis is made on the basis of signs and symptoms of injury (e.g., tooth mobility or migration; pain on percussion or chewing; radiographic changes such as widened periodontal ligament, crestal infrabony [angular] defects, and condensing osteitis, or root resorption; TMJ dysfunction, severe wear facets; crown or root fractures; or *fremitus* (a term used when tooth movement or vibration occurs with the teeth occluded and grinded in all functional positions); clinicians correlate clinical findings with radiographic findings; pathologic occlusion shows evidence of disease interfering with comfort, function, or esthetics that can be attributed to occlusal forces

d. Pulp vitality testing, evaluation of parafunctional habits, clinical assessment of occlusal discrepancies and bone, fremitus and mobility, radiographic assessment of the periodontal ligament and bone, and other adjunctive diagnostic procedures generally are required for differential diagnosis

3. Once diagnosed, occlusal traumatism may be treated; however, plaque-induced inflammation also must be eliminated

Surgical Interventions

A. Principles of periodontal surgery
1. Rationale
   a. Eliminate active infection
   b. Render the periodontium more cleansable by the client and maintainable by the professional
      (1) Improvement in the contours of hard and soft tissues
      (2) Pocket elimination or reduction
   c. Replace damaged or destroyed periodontium
      (1) Soft tissue replacement (gingival grafts)
      (2) Hard tissue replacement (osseous grafts)
   d. Surgery is rarely performed solely to remove inflammation or infection but, rather, in an attempt to:
      (1) Eliminate both hard and soft defects created by disease
      (2) Restore normal architecture and physiologic function
      (3) Gain regeneration or new attachment of the supporting structures
2. Case preparation (see the sections on "Implementation" and "Evaluation" in Chapter 15)
   a. Clients need to complete the initial therapy before entering the surgical phase; initial care aims to remove the causative factors, control active disease, and educate the client in the role as a co-therapist

b. Completion of initial therapy prepares tissue for surgery by reducing marginal inflammation and improving tissue tone, which allows more predictable incisions and suturing and reduces surgical bleeding

c. The prognosis is improved overall after initial preparation or therapy

d. The client's response to NSPT is assessed in relation to healing response; motivation and supplemental self-care devices may be needed for adequate healing

e. Completion of initial therapy can reduce the number of sites requiring surgery or even eliminate the need for surgery in a given sextant or quadrant

B. Types of surgical intervention
1. Resective periodontal surgery
   a. Gingivectomy—surgical procedure for pocket reduction by excision of the soft tissue pocket wall; indicated for gingival pockets composted of fibrotic enlargement or to correct gingival form; only involves the gingiva
   b. Gingivoplasty—reshaping of the gingiva to obtain a physiologic form similar to that characteristic of healthy tissue by using a rotary instrument; frequently combined with gingivectomy
   c. Periodontal flap procedures—may be used as a method of surgical curettage (e.g., modified Widman flap) or for pocket elimination by apically repositioning the soft tissue; most common form of surgery; provides access for thorough scaling and root planing when access is not possible through NSPT (deep pockets, furcation areas, or other areas of complex anatomy); can access bony deformities or craters
   d. Osseous resective surgery or osseous resection
      (1) Objectives—removal of alveolar bone to produce a more physiologic architecture or contour; ultimately, pocket reduction in one-walled infrabony or vertical defects; also for lengthening the clinical crown for root restoration; the goal is to remove a minimal amount of bone; may include ostectomy, osteoplasty, or both
   e. Root resection or hemisection—the objective is removal of the crown, root, or both to eliminate the involved furcation when osseous resection or regenerative surgery is not feasible; resection is removal of one molar root when two roots are involved to include class II or III furcations; also requires endodontics and restorative dentistry; hemisection is converting a two-rooted tooth into a single-rooted tooth by removing both one root and a portion of the crown
2. Regenerative and reconstructive surgery
   a. Bone grafts and regenerative surgery
      (1) Objective—to promote regeneration of connective tissue, periodontal ligament, cementum, and alveolar bone
      (2) Indications—two-walled and three-walled vertical defects, class II furcation defects, circumferential defects (Figs. 14-5 and 14-6)
   b. Options available

(1) Guided tissue regeneration (GTR) and guided bone regeneration (GBR)—involve using a semipermeable membrane between the epithelium and the underlying ligament and bone to prevent rapid downgrowth of the epithelium or connective tissue, which would interfere with connective tissue regrowth after surgical debridement of the defect; nonresorbable membranes most frequently used

(2) Bone grafts—involve placing bone-grafting material into a debrided defect to the level of the uninvolved crest to promote bone healing and regeneration; the graft stimulates new bone formation and thus new attachment; autografts are obtained from the same client, allografts are transferred from genetically dissimilar individuals within the same species (e.g., processed human cadaver bone that is freeze-dried or demineralized); alloplastic grafts use biologic fillers (e.g., bioactive glass ionomers, biocompatible composite polymers) or organic materials such as coral and bone; xenografts are obtained from another species

(3) Biologic and biomimicry mediators—biologic agents such as enamel matrix derivatives or synthetic biomimicry agents such as platelet-derived growth factors, platelet-rich plasma, and bone morphogenetic proteins are being studied for their potential to enhance periodontal regeneration

3. Periodontal plastic and reconstructive surgery
   a. Includes mucogingival surgery to correct defects or deficiencies in the shape, position, or amount of keratinized, attached gingiva surrounding teeth; mucogingival therapy to correct these types of defects in soft tissue and underlying bone; periodontal plastic surgery to create morphology and appearance that is acceptable to the client and the clinician, including root coverage, crown lengthening, ridge preservation, and augmentation; esthetic surgery around implants; and exposure of teeth for orthodontics
   b. Includes gingival augmentation to increase the width of the attached gingiva, establish vestibular depth, arrest progressive gingival recession, and facilitate self-care; frenectomy for the elimination of abnormal frenum often in conjunction with a soft tissue graft; alveolar ridge augmentation resulting from tooth loss; esthetic crown lengthening when anterior teeth are shorter than normal; papillary retention and reconstruction to correct deficient interproximal height of papillary gingiva; or surgical movement of impacted teeth for orthodontics

Healing Following Periodontal Therapy

See the section on "Regeneration and Wound Healing" in Chapter 7.
A. In health, periodontal tissue constantly undergoes renewal; the oral epithelium maintains thickness by the mitotic activity of epithelial cells, fibroblasts generate and regenerate connective tissue, and cementoblasts form new cementum; periodontal ligament cells and bone are continually remodeled by fibroblasts and osteoblasts
B. Basic healing processes after all forms of periodontal therapy are the same
   1. Regeneration—growth and differentiation of new cells and intercellular substances to form or re-form tissues or parts of the same type as the precursor; primary means of healing after NSPT, creating a longer junctional epithelium
   2. Repair—also referred to as *healing by scar tissue* or *fibrosis*; does not necessarily restore the original architecture or function of the tissue or part
   3. Epithelial adaptation—close adaptation of the marginal gingival epithelium without complete pocket elimination; occurs with shrinkage of the gingiva after therapy; often occurs in conjunction with the regeneration of a longer junctional epithelium
   4. New attachment—embedding of new periodontal ligament fibers into new cementum and formation of a new gingival attachment in an area previously degenerated by disease rather than repair of the periodontal attachment apparatus after an injury (reattachment)
      a. Goal of periodontal surgery—the rapid downgrowth of the epithelium must be prevented to allow the formation of connective tissue and bone; this is the basis of using a barrier in regenerative surgery
      b. Requires adequate removal of local etiologic factors through debridement; immobilization of mobile teeth and elimination of occlusal stress in a weakened periodontium are necessary

Sutures

A. Objectives
   1. Used to hold soft tissue in place until the healing process has progressed to the point at which tissue placement can be self-maintained
   2. Stabilization of the soft tissue helps:
      a. Maintain blood clotting around the wound
      b. Protect the wound area during the healing process
B. Types of suture materials
   1. Absorbable—surgical gut (from intestines of sheep); polyglactin and polyglecaprone; absorb through proteolysis by enzymes in saliva in 7 to 10 days, thus eliminating the need for removal
   2. Nonabsorbable—surgical silk most common; must be professionally removed after 7 to 10 days
C. Procedure for suture removal
   1. Grasp the knotted end of suture with cotton pliers, and gently pull it away from the tissue
   2. Insert the tip of scissors under the suture, and cut the suture material that had been in the tissue
   3. Gently pull the knotted end so that only the suture material that had previously been incorporated within the tissue will pass through the tissue during the removal process

4. Count and record the number of sutures removed, and compare this number with the suture placement record
5. Gently cleanse the wound sites, and check for bleeding; control the bleeding, as needed

Periodontal Dressings

A. The rationale for the use of periodontal dressing is to protect the tissues after surgery; have no curative properties; wound healing progresses at the same rate with or without dressings; sometimes used for client comfort or for protection of the wound area
B. Types—dressings using metallic oxide and fatty acids (noneugenol) are most common; clear, translucent light-cured dressings are preferred by some clinicians for esthetics
C. Removal of the periodontal dressing
  1. Remove the dressing within 5 to 7 days; tease the edges of the dressing away from teeth with a curette or cotton pliers; be sure that sutures are not embedded in the dressing
  2. After the pack has been removed, gently cleanse the area with warm water or dampened cotton tips; remove sutures; assess tissue healing, but do not probe sulcular areas

POSTOPERATIVE CARE

Client Instructions and Education

A. Discomfort—the client should:
  1. Expect some discomfort after the local anesthesia wears off; use the prescribed pain medication
  2. Rest and limit physical activities during the first few days to prevent excessive bleeding and promote healing
  3. Use an ice pack to prevent swelling
  4. Eliminate spicy, hot, cold, hard, or sticky foods and liquids and tobacco use to limit tissue irritants and protect the dressing
B. Home care recommendations—provide the following instructions to the client:
  1. Do not rinse the mouth on the first day because this may disturb the process of blood clotting that is necessary for wound healing
  2. After the first day, rinse gently with lukewarm water or a small amount of an antimicrobial rinse (e.g., chlorhexidine gluconate) to help control bacterial biofilm; brush and floss nonsurgical areas as usual but gently
  3. Using a soft brush and water, very gently clean the surface of the dressing
  4. Slight seepage of blood during the first few hours is normal; any unusual, persistent bleeding should be reported to the periodontist

Follow-up Care

A. Client returns approximately 7 days after surgery
B. Dressing and sutures are removed; new dressing may or may not be applied
C. Dentinal hypersensitivity may be experienced; desensitization is indicated for dentinal hypersensitivity; desensitization

methods may be prescribed (see the section on "Assessment of Dentinal Hypersensitivity" in Chapter 16)
D. Home-care instructions are provided for biofilm control
E. Long-term postoperative care requires periodic evaluation (also known as *periodontal maintenance care, continued care,* or *recare*)

Periodontal Maintenance

A. An extension of periodontal therapy; also called *periodontal maintenance*
  1. Initiated after completion of active periodontal treatment and continued at various intervals for the life of the dentition or its implant replacements
  2. Periodontal maintenance is an extension of active therapy, whether nonsurgical or surgical
B. The objectives of periodontal maintenance care is to:
  1. Minimize any recurrence and progression of periodontal disease in previously treated clients
  2. Reduce tooth loss incidence by monitoring the client's periodontal status at regular intervals
  3. Reevaluate results after active periodontal therapy (nonsurgical or surgical) over the long term
  4. Reinforce self-care instructions and encourage client's long-term protective oral health behaviors
  5. Determine the need for additional treatment in a timely manner
C. Components of periodontal maintenance care
  1. Need for the cooperation of client, dental hygienist, dentist, and periodontist
  2. Emphasis on scaling, root planing, and periodontal debridement; extrinsic stain removal; and reinstruction of client in self-care to maintain attachment levels
  3. Optimization of protective factors; minimization and elimination of risk factors
D. Periodic reevaluation and assessment
  1. Review and update of client's health, pharmacologic, and dental histories; review and control of associated risk factors
  2. Radiographic review
  3. Examination of extraoral and intraoral soft tissues
  4. Dental charting of caries, tooth mobility and fremitus, and other tooth-related problems
  5. Periodontal assessment and charting of gingival recession, probing depths, bleeding on probing; levels of plaque and calculus, furcation involvement, exudation, occlusal trauma, tooth mobility; and other signs or symptoms of periodontal disease
  6. Evaluation of client's oral self-care behavior, attitude, values, and skill
  7. Examination of dental implants and peri-implant tissues
E. Treatment—based on assessment
  1. Always encourage the client; provide oral self-care reinstruction, and reinforce client's compliance with recommended maintenance intervals
  2. Healthy periodontium—removal of supragingival deposits; no root planing indicated

3. Presence of bleeding or inflammation of the gingiva—treatment depends on the cause and pocket depths; removal of deposits and contributing factors, as necessary; possible use of an antimicrobial rinse (e.g., 0.12% chlorhexidine) or sustained-release, locally delivered antibiotic or antimicrobial agent

4. Presence of periodontal pockets—scaling, periodontal debridement, and root planing followed by reevaluation in 4 to 6 weeks to determine the need for adjunctive therapy or possible periodontal surgery

5. Determination of frequency of periodontal maintenance must be individualized
   a. The frequency increases when clients have less-than-optimal oral self-care practices
   b. Longer intervals are acceptable if clients can control bacterial plaque (dental) biofilm, unless systemic disease or advanced periodontitis exists
   c. The goal is to control the clinical signs of inflammation and to stabilize attachment levels
   d. Frequent intervals (3 months or less) are generally necessary for subgingival and supragingival plaque and calculus removal in the presence of periodontitis
   e. Generally, the shorter the interval, the greater the long-term success, particularly during the healing phase (1 year) after surgery

F. Indications for retreatment
   1. Increase in probing depth or attachment loss of 2 mm or more
   2. Bleeding on probing that does not respond to periodontal maintenance procedures
   3. Severity—to be considered in determining treatment regimens (nonsurgical or surgical); retaining questionable teeth is not recommended
   4. Generalized deterioration—systemic complication might be suspected
   5. Dental implants with bone loss or mobility

DENTAL IMPLANTS

See the sections on "Dental Implants" in Chapter 13 and "Advanced Instrumentation Techniques" in Chapter 17.

A. Definition—artificial replacements of teeth that are permanently affixed into alveolar bone by a biomedical device and usually composed of an inert metal or a metallic alloy
   1. Implants offer an alternative to removable dentures for edentulous or partially edentulous persons; single or multiple teeth can be replaced
   2. Implants provide a permanent anchor for artificial teeth by serving as an abutment for fixed or removable prostheses
      a. Implant—portion surgically placed within the bone
      b. Abutment—metallic post attached to the implant so that a restoration can be placed over it
      c. Superstructure—prosthetic replacement (e.g., crown, bridge, denture) that is affixed to the abutment or a

removable replacement tooth that the client can remove and clean
      d. Implant-assisted prosthesis—removable tissue dentures (overdentures) supported in the arch by endosseous dental implants

B. Limiting factors
   1. Systemic—age is a consideration only if the client's jaws are still growing because implants are contraindicated until full growth is attained; any condition or disease that affects an individual's ability to fight infection should be carefully considered because implant failure is often caused by infection; greater failure also occurs in poor quality and density of bone, so conditions such as osteoporosis also require careful consideration; cigarette smoking is a documented risk factor for implant failure, so tobacco cessation is essential before implant placement; factors affecting the client's ability to withstand surgery also are paramount (e.g., malnutrition, recent cardiac arrest, bleeding problems)
   2. Local—unfavorable ridge morphology or other bone quality and density changes caused by resorption; sufficient bone and soft tissue for implant positioning must be similar to that of a natural tooth within the tissue and the alveolar ridge—orthodontics and surgical augmentation or correction may be possible; severe malocclusion or parafunctional habits that would cause excessive trauma would contraindicate implants; uncontrolled periodontal disease is also a contraindication; an immobile implant generally is not attached to a natural tooth with periodontal ligament mobility

C. Implant design
   1. Systems—either two stage (submerged) or one stage (nonsubmerged)
      a. Submerged—designed to protect the implant from occlusal stress and bacterial exposure during the healing phase; the implant is placed in two steps, allowing osseo-integration for 3 to 6 months before exposing the implant to the oral cavity for abutment placement; a prosthetic device is later connected to the implant
      b. Nonsubmerged—the implant has a collar that extends through tissue and attaches the prosthesis supragingivally or slightly subgingivally at the time of placement; only one surgery is involved for client comfort and convenience
      c. Shape and size vary in either system; most common are screw-shaped, root-shaped, or cylinder-shaped implants
   2. Materials typically used for dental implants—must be biocompatible
      a. Titanium—a metallic element; pure, plasma sprayed, or titanium alloy
      b. Hydroxyapatite—plasma sprayed

D. Types of implants most frequently used
   1. Endosseous implants (inside bone)

a. The implant is placed directly into a socket, which has been prepared through a process called *trephining*; uses a series of specially prepared drills and burs

(1) Osseo-integration refers to the implant being in direct contact with bone without intervening connective tissue (i.e., no periodontal ligament or connective tissue attachment); the implant is in effect "ankylosed" within bone

(2) After initial loss of 1 to 2 mm of alveolar bone during the first year, crestal bone should be stable with no more than 0.1 to 0.2 mm per year thereafter

b. After bone and soft tissue heal, the final bridge or denture is placed

2. Transosteal implants—means "through the bone"; mandibular denture anchors are placed all the way through the mandible from under the border into the oral cavity

E. Implant-tissue interface

1. The implant-tissue interface is the basis of implant success.

2. The epithelial attachment to the implant may be similar to the attachment to a natural tooth (i.e., basal lamina and hemidesmosomes); no periodontal ligament; called *perimucosal seal*

3. Perimucosal seal, or biologic seal, is defined as the adaptation of keratinized or nonkeratinized epithelium to the abutment cylinder of an implant; critical to implant retention

4. Osseo-integration—contact established between normal and remodeled bone and the implant surface without the interposition of connective tissue

F. Criteria for successful treatment outcomes

1. Immobility of the implant

2. No peri-implant radiolucency on the radiograph

3. Width of implant

4. Width of attached gingiva

5. Medical conditions

6. Smoking

7. Absence of signs and symptoms such as pain, bleeding, infections, paresthesias, or mandibular canal involvement

8. Minimum success rate of 85% at 5 years and 80% at 10 years of observation

G. Implant management

1. Periodic evaluation of implants, surrounding tissue, and oral hygiene essential to long-term success; considerations in periodic evaluation include:

a. Extent of biofilm and dental calculus

b. Clinical appearance of peri-implant soft tissue

c. Radiographic appearance—no periodontal ligament space or bone loss; no peri-implant radiolucency

d. Absence of occlusal interference or trauma; stability of implant and prostheses—no mobility

e. Probing depths (if other signs of disease present)—gentle, careful technique

f. Absence of bleeding or exudate

g. Adequacy of maintenance interval

h. Client comfort and function

2. Goals

a. Maintenance of the health of the implant and supporting tissue

b. Prevention of loss of perimucosal seal

c. Prevention of gingivitis and, failing that, prevention of conversion of gingivitis to peri-implantitis, a periodontitis-like disease process that can affect dental implants

(1) Infectious failure—failing implants with a primarily infectious cause

(2) Traumatic failure—failing implants with a primarily traumatic cause

d. Provision of preventive and maintenance therapies with minimal damage, or surface scratching, to implants

e. Control of bacterial plaque biofilm

H. Preventive instrumentation (see the sections on "Dental Implant Maintenance" in Chapter 16 and "Instrumentation of Dental Implants" in Chapter 17)

Website Information And Resources

Source	Website Address	Description
American Academy of Periodontology	www.perio.org	Position papers, parameters of care, scientific information, and related links in periodontics as well as related information for consumers
Cochrane Collaboration	www.cochrane.org	Evidence-based health care databases; site search for "periodontal" provides excellent related systematic reviews
European Federation of Periodontology	www.efp.org	Publications, news, patient information
National Center for Dental Hygiene Research	www.usc.edu/hsc/dental/dhnet	Current topics in dental hygiene and periodontics with links to related government sites, product companies, and professional associations
University of Minnesota School of Dentistry, Division of Periodontology	www1.umn.edu/perio/tobacco/	Information on tobacco use cessation and related links

REFERENCES

1. Newman MG, Takei HH, Carranza FA: *Carranza's clinical periodontology,* ed 11, St Louis, 2012, Saunders.
2. Armitage GC: Periodontal diagnoses and classification of periodontal diseases, *Periodontology* 34:9–21, 2004.
3. Dentino A, Lee S, Mailhott J, Hefti AF: Principles of periodontology, *Periodontology* 61:16–53, 2013.
4. Darby ML, Walsh MM: *Dental hygiene theory and practice,* ed 4, St Louis, 2015, Elsevier.
5. Borrell LN, Burt BA, Taylor GW: Prevalence and trends in periodontitis in the USA: from the NHANES III to the NHANES, 1988 to 2000, *J Dent Res* 84:924–930, 2005.
6. Löe H, Anerud A, Boysen H, et al: Natural history of periodontal disease in man: the rate of periodontal destruction after 40 years of age, *J Periodontol* 49:607–620, 1978.

CHAPTER 14 REVIEW QUESTIONS

Answers and rationales to chapter review questions are available on this text's accompanying Evolve site. See inside front cover for details.

evolve

1. **Recession is noted in the mandibular anterior region, and the attached gingiva measures 0.5 mm, requiring evaluation by a dentist or periodontist. If periodontal surgery is indicated, a mucogingival surgery would be performed to correct this condition.**
   a. Both statements are TRUE.
   b. Both statements are FALSE.
   c. The first statement is TRUE; the second statement is FALSE.
   d. The first statement is FALSE; the second statement is TRUE.

2. **Smoking is a major risk factor for periodontal disease. Light, moderate, and heavy smokers are all at equal risk for more severe periodontal destruction than nonsmokers.**
   a. Both statements are TRUE.
   b. Both statements are FALSE.
   c. The first statement is TRUE; the second statement is FALSE.
   d. The first statement is FALSE; the second statement is TRUE.

3. **Which of the following devices would be MOST effective for plaque biofilm removal in the mandibular anterior region when recession has resulted in open embrasure spaces?**
   a. Dental floss
   b. Dental tape
   c. Oral irrigation
   d. Interproximal brush

4. **Systemic antibiotics are recommended in treatment of aggressive periodontitis. Locally-delivered, sustained-release antibiotics should be considered in the care plan when generalized chronic periodontitis is present.**
   a. Both statements are TRUE.
   b. Both statements are FALSE.
   c. The first statement is TRUE; the second statement is FALSE.
   d. The first statement is FALSE; the second statement is TRUE.

5. **An oxygenating mouthrinse would be beneficial for a patient with halitosis because these mouthrinses are the most effective in reducing bacterial plaque biofilm.**
   a. Both the statement and the reason are correct and related.
   b. Both the statement and the reason are correct but are NOT related.
   c. The statement is correct, but the reason is NOT correct.
   d. The statement is NOT correct, but the reason is correct.
   e. NEITHER the statement NOR the reason is correct.

6. **In addition to professional dental hygiene care and proper oral hygiene measures, which of the following procedures or agents would address a client's chief concerns about "bad breath?"**
   a. Selective stain removal
   b. Chlorine dioxide mouthrinse
   c. Tooth whitening
   d. Daily oral irrigation
   e. Daily fluoride mouthrinse

7. **Which of the following periodontal therapies would be BEST recommended for a patient who presents with probing depths of 3 to 5 mm, slight bone loss detected on the radiographs, and a history of infrequent dental hygiene care?**
   a. Regenerative periodontal surgery
   b. Gingival curettage
   c. Nonsurgical periodontal therapy
   d. Oral prophylaxis
   e. Periodontal maintenance therapy

8. **Which of the following would be the BEST indicator of treatment success at the reevaluation appointment 4 to 6 weeks after initial periodontal therapy?**
   a. Relatively free of plaque biofilm
   b. Stable periodontal probing depths
   c. Absence of gingival inflammation and bleeding
   d. No re-formed dental calculus deposits

9. **What change in alveolar bone on a dental radiograph indicates early loss of bone?**
   a. Fuzziness in the crest of the bone
   b. Faint cup-shaped areas interproximally
   c. Vertical or angular defects
   d. Furcation involvement

10. **After thorough periodontal debridement is performed, which is the first inflammatory cell to respond to avoidable resultant irritation of the gingiva?**
    a. B lymphocytes
    b. Plasma cells

c. Neutrophils

d. T lymphocytes

e. Macrophages

11. **Which of the following changes result in a false or pseudo periodontal pocket?**

a. Apical migration of the junctional epithelium

b. Apical migration of the gingival margin

c. Resorption of the alveolar bone

d. Swelling of the gingival margin without bone loss

12. **Which of the following diagnostic procedures is MOST accurate for determining severity of periodontal attachment loss?**

a. Full-mouth digital radiographic survey

b. Microbial testing of plaque biofilm

c. Detection of pathologic tooth mobility or furcations

d. Periodontal probing of all sulcular areas

e. Determining presence or absence of bleeding on probing

13. **In clients of periodontitis, what is the first area to be involved in bone resorption?**

a. Facial and lingual aspects of supporting bone

b. Cribriform plate or lamina dura

c. Cancellous portion of supporting bone

d. Cortical plate of the interdental septum

e. Bone surrounding the apical area of the tooth

14. **Which one of the following bacteria are predominant in supragingival plaque biofilm associated with gingivitis?**

a. Chromogenic bacteria

b. Gram-negative anaerobic bacteria

c. Aerobic and facultative bacteria

d. Gram-positive *Streptococcus* spp.

15. **Which of the following types of cells are responsible for resorption of cementum and bone in periodontal destruction?**

a. Cementoblasts

b. Fibroblasts

c. Osteoblasts

d. Cementoclasts

e. Osteoclasts

16. **Which of the following histologic changes in inflamed gingiva results in redness?**

a. Vasodilation within the gingival connective tissue

b. Ulceration of the sulcular lining

c. Lymphoid cell accumulation

d. Collagenase destroying the lamina propria

e. Alteration of fibroblasts in the connective tissue

17. **Tooth mobility and fremitus can be signs of occlusal trauma because trauma can result in lateral resorption of bone.**

a. Both the statement and the reason are correct and related.

b. Both the statement and the reason are correct but are NOT related.

c. The statement is correct, but the reason is NOT correct.

d. The statement is NOT correct, but the reason is correct.

e. NEITHER the statement NOR the reason is correct.

18. **Which of the following conditions can be determined by radiographic examination?** *Select all that apply.*

a. Extent and severity of bone loss

b. Height of crestal bone

c. Widening of the periodontal ligament space

d. Presence of pseudopockets

e. Presence of dental calculus on lingual surfaces

19. **Which radiographic findings will MOST LIKELY be seen in dental plaque–induced gingivitis?** *Select all that apply.*

a. A thin periodontal ligament space

b. Slight changes in the lamina dura

c. Condensing osteitis

d. Normal lamina dura and crestal bone

e. Slight fuzziness at the alveolar crest

20. **Oral examination findings for a 56-year-old woman with good general health status reports diabetes well controlled by medication and diet and taking hormonal therapy for symptoms of menopause. Clinical findings include localized 4-mm and 5-mm periodontal probing depths, with radiographic bone loss visible on teeth #3, #14, #19, #30, and #31; slight gingival inflammation in the mandibular anterior and molar regions; fair oral hygiene with generalized light deposits; and no active caries. On the basis of these findings, which of the following would be the MOST accurate preliminary diagnosis?**

a. Necrotizing ulcerative gingivitis

b. Chronic periodontitis

c. Dental plaque–induced gingivitis

d. Localized aggressive periodontitis

e. Hormone-associated gingivitis

21. **Which of the following antimicrobial and antigingivitis agent is the LEAST effective?**

a. Essential oils

b. Chlorhexidine gluconate

c. Chlorine dioxide

d. Cetylpyridinium chloride

e. Stannous fluoride

22. **Which of the following tissues consist(s) of nonkeratinized epithelium?** *Select all that apply.*

a. Crevicular epithelium

b. Attached gingiva

c. Interdental papilla

d. Junctional epithelium

e. Marginal gingiva

23. **Which of the following microbes is associated with necrotizing ulcerative gingivitis and periodontitis?**

a. *Actinomyces viscosus*

b. *Porphyromonas gingivalis*

c. *Prevotella intermedia*

d. *Treponema pallidum*

e. *Capnocytophaga ochracea*

24. **Which of the following types of drugs have been associated with fibrotic gingival overgrowth?** *Select all that apply.*

a. Oral contraceptives

b. Antidepressants

c. Calcium channel blockers

d. Antihistamines

e. Anticonvulsants

25. **Which of the following conditions can cause periodontitis as a manifestation of systemic disease?** *Select all that apply.*

a. Diabetes mellitus

b. Chédiak-Higashi syndrome

c. Papillion-Lefèvre syndrome
d. Cardiovascular disease
e. Leukemia

26. **Which of the following BEST describes the sulcular epithelium?**
a. Keratinized epithelium
b. Basal cell epithelium
c. Squamous cell epithelium
d. Simple cuboidal epithelium
e. Parakeratinized epithelium

27. **Which type of periodontal disease is characterized by gray, sloughing tissue, pain, and spontaneous bleeding with rapid connective tissue loss and exposed alveolar bone?**
a. Pericoronitis
b. Periodontal abscess
c. Necrotizing ulcerative gingivitis
d. Aggressive periodontitis
e. Necrotizing ulcerative periodontitis

28. **Which of the following indicates that periodontitis is present rather than gingivitis?** *Select all that apply.*
a. Widened periodontal ligament space on radiographs
b. Periodontal probing depth of 4 mm or greater
c. Clinical attachment loss
d. Apical migration of the alveolar bone
e. Bleeding on probing

29. **Which condition should be suspected when a radiolucent area on a radiograph occurs lateral to the root of a tooth with a 7-mm probing depth?**
a. Periodontal abscess
b. Pyogenic granuloma
c. Occlusal traumatism
d. Periapical abscess
e. Mucogingival problem

30. **Which of the following are possible causes of gingival recession?** *Select all that apply.*
a. Faulty toothbrushing
b. Bacterial plaque biofilm
c. Tissue response to medication
d. Dental caries
e. Periodontal disease

31. **All the following are risk factors associated with periodontal disease EXCEPT one. Which one is the exception?**
a. Genetics
b. Immunosuppression
c. Hormonal changes
d. Frequent fermentable carbohydrates in diet
e. Poor oral hygiene

32. **At a reevaluation appointment with a client 4 weeks after completion of nonsurgical periodontal therapy, the hygienist notes localized gingival inflammation and bleeding in the proximal surfaces of the molars. Periodontal probing depths of 5 mm remain unchanged, corresponding to the localized inflammation, but are reduced to 2 to 4 mm in most areas. Plaque control is acceptable. What is the MOST probable explanation for these findings?**
a. Residual dental calculus deposits are present.
b. Plaque removal was absent for the past 24 hours.
c. Systemic disease influencing host response is present.
d. Plaque removal was enhanced immediately before appointment.

33. **Which of the following situations would be an indication for a gingivectomy?**
a. Edematous 5-mm pseudopocket
b. Severe drug-influenced gingival enlargement
c. Infrabony pocket of 6 mm on the distal aspect of tooth #30
d. Gingival recession that extends into the alveolar mucosa
e. Periodontal abscess

34. **Which of the following is an objective of periodontal reconstructive surgery?**
a. Improve the esthetics of the client's face
b. Create gingival contour and appearance acceptable to the client
c. Remove alveolar bone to improve contour and correct defects
d. Remove enlarged tissue to assist the client in daily plaque control
e. Promote regeneration of a new attachment

35. **All the following are substances produced by the host response to bacterial plaque biofilm EXCEPT:**
a. Lipopolysaccharide (LPS)
b. Matrix metalloproteinase (MMP)
c. Cytokines
d. Interleukin-1 (IL-1)
e. Prostaglandin E_2 (PGE_2)

36. **Which of the following are necessary for new attachment after periodontal surgery?** *Select all that apply.*
a. Thorough removal of bacterial irritants
b. Immobilization of mobile teeth
c. Shrinkage of the gingival margin
d. Regeneration or generation of new tissues or parts
e. Rapid apical growth of epithelium

37. **All the following are advantages of controlled (sustained-release) drug delivery over systemic drug administration in periodontal therapy EXCEPT:**
a. Less concern about client adherence throughout indicated time frame
b. Site-specific antimicrobial action in periodontal pocket
c. High concentration delivered to the site of infection
d. Can be used when periodontal infection is generalized or severe

38. **Periodontal dressings also minimize client discomfort. These dressings make the placement of sutures unnecessary in some cases.**
a. Both statements are TRUE.
b. Both statements are FALSE.
c. The first statement is TRUE; the second statement is FALSE.
d. The first statement is FALSE; the second statement is TRUE.

39. A female patient, age 40, returns for periodontal maintenance therapy every 3 months for 1 year after nonsurgical periodontal treatment for chronic periodontitis. The inflammation has been resolved, and periodontal probing depths have decreased from 5 or 6 mm to 4 mm or less in most treated areas, with the exception of the distal surface of tooth #15, where the probing depth has increased from 4 to 6 mm. Radiographs reveal no change on tooth #15 distal. All the following explain this finding EXCEPT:
    a. Continuing clinical attachment loss
    b. Error in periodontal probing technique
    c. Calculus deposits affecting accuracy of initial reading
    d. Inaccessibility and poor visibility in pocket areas
    e. Increased inflammation of the gingival tissues

40. All the following factors could limit a recommendation for dental implants EXCEPT:
    a. Complete edentulism
    b. Tobacco habit
    c. Osteoporosis
    d. Head and neck radiation therapy

41. Which of the following materials could be used in curettes for maintaining dental implants? *Select all that apply.*
    a. Stainless steel
    b. Carbon steel
    c. Plastic resin
    d. Titanium

42. Which of the following findings would indicate a failed dental implant?
    a. Peri-implant inflammation
    b. Bleeding on provocation
    c. Alveolar bone loss
    d. Loosening of the prosthetic crown
    e. Mobility

43. Which of the following classifications of periodontal disease would be characterized by clinical attachment loss in the first molars and incisors in an adolescent patient with fair plaque control?
    a. Hormone-influenced gingivitis
    b. Localized chronic periodontitis
    c. Localized aggressive periodontitis
    d. Necrotizing ulcerative periodontitis

44. Which factors determine the severity of chronic periodontitis? *Select all that apply.*
    a. Extent of attachment loss
    b. Immune response
    c. Hormonal changes
    d. Vitamin C deficiency
    e. Frequency of periodontal maintenance therapy

45. How is clinical attachment loss measured with a periodontal probe?
    a. From the margin of the gingiva to the epithelial attachment
    b. From the cemento-enamel junction to the base of the pocket
    c. From the margin of the gingiva to the cemento-enamel junction
    d. From the cemento-enamel junction to the margin of the bone

46. In which area of the mouth would the width of the attached gingiva be expected to be the narrowest?
    a. Mandibular anterior area
    b. Mandibular premolar areas
    c. Maxillary molar areas
    d. Lingual of the maxillary teeth

47. Where is the lamina propria located in the periodontium?
    a. In the periodontal ligament
    b. In the alveolar bone
    c. At the cemento-enamel junction
    d. In the gingival mucosa

48. Which of the following changes would result in pocket reduction after periodontal debridement in an edematous pocket? *Select all that apply.*
    a. Reattachment
    b. New attachment
    c. Longer junctional epithelium
    d. Shrinkage of the gingival margin
    e. Downward growth of the junctional epithelium

49. Occlusal trauma causes clinical attachment loss and bone loss in patients with gingivitis. Occlusal trauma can contribute to attachment loss and bone loss surrounding teeth affected by periodontitis.
    a. Both statements are TRUE.
    b. Both statements are FALSE.
    c. The first statement is TRUE; the second statement is FALSE.
    d. The first statement is FALSE; the second statement is TRUE.

50. Occlusal trauma can result in all the following EXCEPT:
    a. Periodontal pockets
    b. Attrition of the tooth
    c. Temporomandibular joint discomfort
    d. Fractured teeth and restorations

51. At a reevaluation appointment following thorough periodontal debridement, what does generalized severe inflammation and bleeding in the presence of localized plaque biofilm indicate?
    a. A need for more frequent periodontal maintenance therapy
    b. Poor self-care to control plaque biofilm
    c. A possible undiagnosed systemic disease
    d. Residual calculus present

52. What does bleeding on periodontal probing indicate?
    a. Loss of crestal bone
    b. An increase in gingival vasculature
    c. Fibrosis in the connective tissue
    d. Ulceration of crevicular epithelium
    e. Apical migration of junctional epithelium

Dental Hygiene Process of Care

Laura Mueller-Joseph

The dental hygiene process of care is a systematic, problem-solving approach to the provision of quality oral health care. This process provides a framework for evidence-based decision making and sound clinical judgment while identifying and resolving client needs within dental hygiene practice.[1] The dental hygiene process is a standard of practice recognized by the American Dental Hygienists Association (ADHA) and is an educational standard of the American Dental Association (ADA) Commission on Dental Accreditation.[2,3] This chapter reviews components of the dental hygiene process of care: assessment, diagnosis, planning, implementation, evaluation, and documentation, including prognosis and legal-ethical considerations.

BASIC CONCEPTS

Dental Hygiene Paradigm[1]

A. A *paradigm* is composed of major concepts selected for study by a discipline
B. The paradigm for the discipline of dental hygiene includes four concepts[4]:
   1. Clients—recipients of dental hygiene care; include persons, families, groups, and communities from all age, cultural, gender, and economic groups
   2. Environment—external factors that affect the client's optimal oral health; includes economic, psychological, cultural, physical, legal, educational, ethical, and geographic dimensions
   3. Health and oral health—status of the overall health and the oral wellness or illness of the client
   4. Dental hygiene actions—interventions that a dental hygienist initiates to promote wellness, prevent and control oral disease, and encourage active client participation and collaboration
C. Dental hygiene practice—based on a systematic process of care that involves assessment, diagnosis, planning, implementation, and evaluation (Fig. 15-1)
D. The dental hygiene process of care provides a logical system for determining the health and disease status of a client and for selecting appropriate interventions and measuring treatment outcomes
E. The dental hygiene process of care is integrated with a client's comprehensive dental hygiene diagnosis and care plan

Human Needs Theory and Assessment[1,5–7]

See the section on "Human Behavior Principles" in Chapter 16.
A. Most widely known model in the discipline of dental hygiene—human needs conceptual model; requires assessment of each client's human needs as the framework for providing care
B. Based on the theory that human activity is dominated by behaviors aimed at need fulfillment; an internal drive exists in all humans to satisfy unmet needs; unmet needs motivate specific behaviors to eliminate the perceived deficit; the model encourages establishing an environment that is more client oriented than task oriented
C. The human needs model uses eight needs relevant to oral health that should be considered in the implementation of the dental hygiene process of care (Fig. 15-2)
D. During baseline assessment, deficits in eight human needs are identified, and a dental hygiene diagnosis is made; planning, implementation, and evaluation of dental hygiene care are carried out to address the client's unmet needs
E. Human needs assessment form—an instrument to assist in the summation and organization of gathered assessment data; used to provide a written record of unmet needs, dental hygiene diagnoses, client goals, treatment and preventive care plans, and outcome evaluation of dental hygiene care (Fig. 15-3)

Assessment

A. Definition—comprehensive and systematic collection of data used to identify a client's needs, oral health status, and general health and well-being
B. Assessment—first phase of dental hygiene process of care
C. Data collection—continuous process of collecting and documenting subjective and objective client information
D. Data are continuously updated and documented during the dental hygiene process of care
E. Data are collected by interview, questionnaire, observation, measurement, and examination
F. Data recordings are discussed with the client and other health care professionals responsible for the client's care
G. Data collection and documentation—includes comprehensive personal, health, and dental histories; pharmacologic history; identification of a client's chief concerns and human needs; clinical examination; periodontal examination and

Assessment
- Health, pharmacologic, cultural and dental history and vital signs
- Extraoral and intraoral clinical assessment
- Dentition assessment
- Periodontal and oral hygiene assessment
- Risk assessment

Diagnosis
- Synthesizing, analyzing, and interpreting client data
- Identifying unmet human need related to dental hygiene
- Formulating and validating the dental hygiene diagnosis
- Prioritizing the dental hygiene diagnosis

Evaluation
- Measure outcomes in terms of the client's goals and record an evaluative statement for each goal
- Modify plan and continue the dental hygiene process

Implementation
- Educational interventions for personal dental biofilm control, diet, preventive agents, tobacco/alcohol and other risk factors related to both oral and systemic diseases and conditions
- Professional preventive and therapeutic services for management of periodontal diseases, caries, etc.

Planning
- Establish priorities for care
- Set goals and evaluation measures related to existing dental hygiene problems
- Identify interventions appropriate for client needs
- Develop a written care plan for use during dental hygiene therapy

FIG 15-1 Dental hygiene process-of-care algorithm.

risk status; analysis of diagnostic radiographs; microbiologic or other tests for assessing periodontal status and risk levels related to dental caries[8]

HEALTH HISTORY EVALUATION

A. Health history—taken to identify and evaluate predisposing conditions and risk factors that may affect dental hygiene interventions, client management, potential for an emergency, and oral and general health outcomes;[9] such conditions and factors include, but are not limited to, allergies, chronic diseases, human immunodeficiency virus (HIV) infection, pregnancy, tobacco use, substance abuse, and medications

B. Health history form—legal document containing past and present information about a client's health[9]
   1. Provides baseline information about a client's health status and assists in medical and dental diagnoses

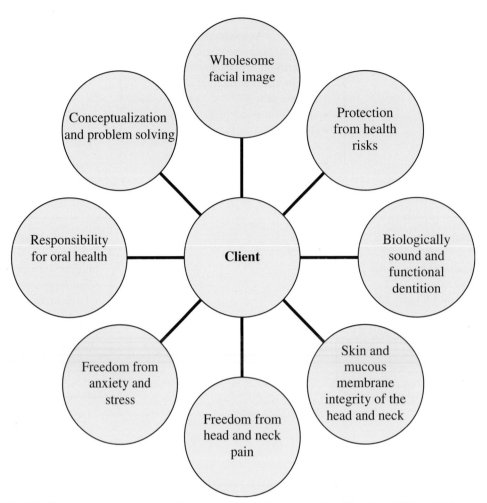

FIG 15-2 Eight human needs related to oral health and disease. (Modified from Walsh MM, Darby ML: Human needs theory and dental hygiene care. In Darby ML, Walsh MM, editors: *Dental hygiene theory and practice*, ed 4, St Louis, 2015, Saunders.)

2. Information used to assess the overall physical and emotional health of a client and allow identification of:
   a. Needed precautions to ensure a client's need for safety
   b. Potential medical emergencies
   c. Needed referrals to a physician or other health care provider
   d. Diseases, conditions, or medications that contraindicate dental or dental hygiene care
   e. Previous history of reactions to medications or drugs
   f. Infectious diseases that could endanger other individuals
   g. Physiologic state of a client, including pregnancy, puberty, menopause, and use of hormones
3. Health history questionnaire should be completed in ink, and comprehensive information should be recorded on a questionnaire form or a summary sheet; this may be a component of an electronic client record
4. The health history should be reviewed by the client and dental hygienist and updated at each dental hygiene appointment
5. The client should sign the written health history form at each appointment to confirm its accuracy; if the client is a minor, a parent or legal guardian must sign and date the

health history form; electronic signatures are used in the electronic health record
6. The dental hygienist should sign the health history form at each appointment indicating medical and pharmacologic updates were obtained and verified; electronic signatures are used in the electronic health record
7. The health history form should be thorough and concise and legible, using simple language to facilitate understanding

Health History Questions (Fig. 15-4)

A. Personal, social, and cultural histories related to health and disease
B. Dental history information should include:
   1. Main concern—why the client is seeking dental or dental hygiene care
   2. In the case of new clients, the date of the last dental or dental hygiene visit
   3. Areas of pain or discomfort identified during the health history interview, but not associated with the client's main concern

ASSESSMENT (circle signs and symptoms present)

1) WHOLESOME FACIAL IMAGE
    *expresses dissatisfaction with appearance
    –teeth –gingiva –facial profile –breath *other _____

2) FREEDOM FROM ANXIETY/STRESS
    *reports or displays:
    –anxiety about proximity of clinician, confidentiality, or
      previous dental experience
    –oral habits   –substance abuse

    *concern about:
    –infection control, fluoride therapy, fluoridation, mercury
      toxicity

3) SKIN & MUCOUS MEMBRANE INTEGRITY OF HEAD
    AND NECK
    –extra-/intra-oral lesion   –pockets ≥4 mm
    –swelling   –attachment loss ≥4 mm
    –gingival inflammation   –xerostomia
    –bleeding on probing   –other _____

4) PROTECTION FROM HEALTH RISKS
    *BP outside of normal limits   *need for prophylactic
    *potential for injury   antibiotics
                                   *risk factors
    *other _____

5) FREEDOM FROM HEAD AND NECK PAIN
    *extra-/intra-oral pain or sensitivity
    *other _____

6) BIOLOGICALLY SOUND & FUNCTIONAL DENTITION
    *reports difficulty in chewing
    *presents with:
    –defective restorations   –ill-fitting dentures, appliances
    –teeth with signs of disease –abrasion erosion
    –missing teeth   –rampant caries
    *other _____

7) RESPONSIBILITY FOR ORAL HEALTH
    *plaque & calculus present
    *inadequate parental supervision of oral health care
    *no dental exam within the last 2 years
    *other _____

8) CONCEPTUALIZATION & UNDERSTANDING
    *has questions about DH care and/or oral disease
    *other _____

DENTAL HYGIENE DIAGNOSIS (List the human need not met, then be specific about the etiology and signs & symptoms evidencing a deficit)

(Unmet Human Need)   (Etiology)   (Signs & Symptoms)
              DUE TO   EVIDENCED BY

CLIENT GOALS	INTERVENTIONS (Target etiologies)	EVALUATION (goal met, partially met, or unmet)

Appointment Schedule: _____

Continued-care recommendations:

FIG 15-3 American Dental Association (ADA) health history form. (Copyright 2011 American Dental Association. All rights reserved. Reprinted with permission.)

REQUEST FOR MEDICAL CONSULTATION

Date: _____

TO:

| | CLIENT INFORMATION |

_____

Physician's Name

RE: _____

Client's name

_____

Address

_____

Address

_____

Address

Gender:_____ Birthdate:_____

Request: It is anticipated that dental hygiene treatment will extend for (# of appointments) over (time period) (weekly/monthly) for (appointment length) hour durations. Your Client reported (or we observed) the following:

_____Cardiac arrhythmia, diagnosed _____
_____High blood pressure (readings(s)/date) _____
_____Congential heart disease (CHD)_____
_____ Anticoagulant therapy, (medication dose/name)

_____Diabetes, Type 1, glucose level _____
_____Diabetes, Type 2, glucose level_____
_____Total joint replacement (type & date replaced)
_____Other:_____

The treatment planned for _____ includes:
_____Deep scaling and root planing/debridement (hemorrhage will occur)
_____Use of local anesthesic agent
_____Use of nitrous oxide-oxygen analgesia
_____Other:_____

Our concerns for _____ include the need for:
_____Antibiotic prophylactic according to the AHA guidelines (2007)
_____Evaluation of high blood pressure prior to dental hygiene care
_____Evaluation of prothrombin time prior to dental hygiene care; INR score___
_____ Evaluation of glucose level of control. Please provide most recent diabetes laboratory test results ____ H1A$_{1c}$
_____Other:_____

_____

Dentist

_____

Registered Dental Hygienist

RECOMMENDATIONS: Please indicate the definitive diagnosis and/or level of control. Also provide applicable laboratory test results in the space provided:

_____

Physician Signature

_____

Date

Adapted with permission from Idaho State University, Department of Dental Hygiene

FIG 15-4 Request for medical consultation.

4. Nervousness or anxiety about treatment; history of an upsetting experience; the client's need for freedom from anxiety and stress should be addressed
5. Pain, swelling, or gingival bleeding
6. The client's satisfaction with his or her teeth and oral health
7. Past or current orthodontics, periodontal surgery, extractions, temporomandibular joint (TMJ) problems, occlusal equilibration, fixed and removable dentures
8. Oral habits such as clenching or grinding, biting lips or cheeks, mouth breathing, and holding foreign objects between teeth

C. Radiographic history information (see Chapter 6)
1. Purpose—the radiation exposure history of the client should be obtained to make safe decisions for radiographic prescriptions

2. Information should include:
a. Whether the client is regularly exposed to radiation in his or her work environment
b. The dates and total number of dental and medical films exposed during a 5-year period

Health History Information

See Chapters 7, 8, and 19 for more detailed discussions of health conditions.

A. Screening questions are designed to assess risk factors or undiagnosed diseases to enable a clinician to determine the need for a physician consultation or referral before dental hygiene care (Table 15-1)
B. Detailed questions are designed to identify diseases or conditions that a client previously had or currently has and to

TABLE 15-1 Health History Screening Questions

Risk Factor Category	Sample Questions	Significance of Finding
Overall health	How do you rate your general health? Has there been any change in your general health within the past year? Have you been under the care of a medical doctor during the past 2 years? What is the date of your last physical examination? Have you ever been hospitalized or had a serious illness?	Hospitalization history can provide a good record of past serious illnesses that may be significant to dental hygiene care. Knowledge of why a client was hospitalized is used to evaluate the client's ability to tolerate stress involved during treatment. Knowledge of any problems for which the client required medical intervention can increase the ability to evaluate the patient's condition before treatment
Weight fluctuation history	Have you unintentionally lost or gained more than 10 pounds in the past year? Are you on a medically recommended diet?	Unexpected weight changes may indicate heart failure, hypothyroidism, hyperthyroidism, or uncontrolled diabetes. Information may identify an underlying systemic problem, such as diabetes, hyperthyroidism, or cancer
Cardiovascular disease	When you walk up stairs or take a walk, do you ever have to stop because of pain in your chest or shortness of breath or because you are very tired? Do your ankles swell during the day? Do you require more than two pillows to sleep, or do you have an elevated bed?	Clients with cardiovascular disease are more susceptible to physical or emotional challenges during dental hygiene care. These signs may indicate possible valvular disease, arrhythmia, or congestive heart failure
Diabetes	Are you on a medically recommended diet? Do you have to urinate more than six times a day? Are you frequently thirsty? Does your mouth frequently become dry? If yes, what is the probable cause?	Determine family history or potential for diabetes; consultation with a physician may be indicated. Complications of diabetes include blindness, hypertension, kidney failure, and delayed healing
Tuberculosis or other respiratory diseases	Do you have a nonproductive persistent cough? Do you have a productive persistent cough? Do you have night sweats? Do you have difficulty breathing?	May indicate current or past history of tuberculosis. History of the disease must be defined, and medical consultation may be indicated
Hematologic disorder	Do you bruise easily? Do you have a tendency to bleed longer than normal? Have you ever had a blood transfusion?	Need to determine whether a blood disorder is present; medical consultation may be indicated. Concerns about delayed healing, prolonged bleeding, and infection
Latex allergy	Have you experienced a skin reaction (redness, rash, hives, or itching) to adhesive tape, adhesive strips, kitchen gloves, or rubber or latex products? Have you experienced swelling of the lips, tongue, or skin after dental treatment, after blowing up a balloon, or after contact with rubber or latex products? Have you experienced a runny nose, itchy eyes, scratchy throat, or difficulty breathing after contact with rubber or latex products? Do you have an allergy to bananas, kiwis, potatoes, tomatoes, avocados, chestnuts, or other foods?	Need to assess risk for reaction. May need medical consultation to determine risk of anaphylaxis. Provide a latex-reduced environment

TABLE 15-2   American Heart Association (AHA) and American Association of Orthopedic Surgeons (AAOS) Antibiotic Premedication Guidelines for Professional Oral Health Care

Dental Procedures That Require Premedication in Highest-Risk Clients*	2007 AHA Recommendations for Cardiac Conditions	2012 AAOS Recommendations for Orthopedic Conditions	Other Conditions That May Necessitate Antibiotic Premedication Based on Physician Consultation
All dental procedures that involve manipulation of gingival tissues or the periapical region of teeth, or perforation of the oral mucosa *Note:* Clients can receive antibiotic coverage within a 2-hour period if unexpected bleeding occurs,† if during treatment the client discloses additional health history information that would indicate need for premedication, or both	Highest-risk category: only people at greatest risk of bad outcomes from infective endocarditis (IE) should receive short-term preventive antibiotics before identified dental (and medical) procedures Patients at the greatest danger of adverse outcomes from IE and for whom preventive antibiotics are worth the risks include those with: — Artificial heart valves — History of having had IE — Certain specific, serious congenital heart conditions, including: — Unrepaired or incompletely repaired cyanotic congenital heart disease, including those with palliative shunts and conduits — Completely repaired congenital heart defect with prosthetic material or device, whether placed by surgery or by catheter interventions, during first 6 months after the procedure — Any repaired congenital heart defect with residual defect at the site or adjacent to the site of a prosthetic patch or prosthetic device — Cardiac transplant that develops a problem in a heart valve	Antibiotic premedication not recommended for all persons who have undergone total joint replacement Treatment decisions should be made in light of all circumstances presented by the patient Immunocompromised or immunosuppressed patients Inflammatory arthropathies (e.g., rheumatoid arthritis, systemic lupus erythematosus) Drug-induced immunosuppression Radiation-induced immunosuppression Patients with comorbidities (e.g., diabetes, obesity, human immunodeficiency virus [HIV], smoking) Previous prosthetic joint infections Malnourishment Hemophilia HIV infection Insulin-dependent (type 1) diabetes Malignancy Megaprostheses	Prophylaxis consultation recommended Renal transplants or dialysis Immunosuppressive therapy (e.g., cyclosporine) Uncontrolled diabetes Sickle cell anemia Spina bifida (ventriculoatrial shunt)

*Every attempt should be made to complete procedures and services in as few appointments as possible; follow-up appointments should be scheduled at least 9 days apart if client is premedicated.

†Clinical judgment may indicate antibiotic use in selected circumstances that may cause significant bleeding.

Modified from Committee on Rheumatic Fever, Endocarditis, and Kawasaki Disease: Prevention of infective endocarditis: Guidelines from the American Heart Association, April 19, 2007, www.americanheart.org/presenter.jhtml?identifier=3004539; and from American Academy of Orthopedic Surgeons, American Association of Orthopedic Surgeons: Prevention of orthopedic implant infection in patients undergoing dental procedures: evidence-based guidelines and evidence report, http://www.aaos.org/research/guidelines/PUDP/PUDP_guideline.pdf. Accessed July 20, 2015.

determine the need for precautionary measures, physician consultation before dental hygiene care, or need for antibiotic prophylaxis (Table 15-2)

1. When practitioner questions the client regarding his or her disease status, specific information should include:
   a. Type and onset of disease
   b. Treatment received in the past
   c. Severity of disease or extent of damage
   d. Type of current medical care
   e. Results of follow-up testing

f. Classification of the client's risk for a medical emergency using the American Society of Anesthesiologists (ASA) Physical Status Classification System (Table 15-3)

2. Questions regarding cardiovascular disease (CVD) are significant because clients with various forms of CVD are especially vulnerable to physical or emotional challenges that may be encountered during dental hygiene care; for most CVDs, the stress reduction protocol, based on the ASA system, is necessary (see the sections on "Vasoconstrictors" in Chapter 18; "Congenital Heart

TABLE 15-3   American Society of Anesthesiologists (ASA) Physical Status Classification System* and Stress Reduction Protocols

ASA Classification	Client Risk Description	Examples of Medical Conditions	Precautionary Measures for Stress Reduction
Physical status 1	Normal healthy client without systemic disease Little or no anxiety Elective dental hygiene care can be implemented	Healthy, nonsmoking, no or minimal alcohol use	Determine client's level of anxiety Schedule morning appointment Minimize waiting time Consider shorter appointments for anxious clients Optimize adequate pain control during therapy
Physical status 2	Client with mild systemic disease Healthy client with extreme anxiety Elective dental hygiene care can be implemented with minimal risk, but measures for stress reduction should be taken	Mild diseases only without substantive functional limitations; examples include current smoker, social alcohol drinker, pregnancy, obesity ($30 < BMI < 40$), well-controlled diabetes or hypertension, mild lung disease	Identify the client's medical risk potential Complete a physician consultation before starting dental hygiene care, as indicated Schedule a morning appointment time Take and record vital signs at each appointment
Physical status 3	Client with severe systemic disease that limits activity but is not incapacitating Elective dental hygiene care is not contraindicated, but risk is increased and precautionary measures for stress reduction should be taken	Substantive functional limitations; one or more moderate to severe diseases; examples include poorly controlled diabetes or hypertension, COPD, morbid obesity (BMI >40), active hepatitis, alcohol dependence or abuse, implanted pacemaker, moderate reduction of ejection fraction, ESRD patient undergoing regularly scheduled dialysis, premature infant PCA 60 weeks, history (>3 months) of MI, CVA, TIA, or CAD/stents	Optimize adequate pain control during therapy Shorter appointments, not to exceed 90 minutes Arrange appointments during the beginning of the week (Monday to Wednesday)
Physical status 4	Client with incapacitating systemic disease that is a constant threat to life Elective dental hygiene care is contraindicated until the medical condition has improved to at least ASA physical status 3	Examples include recent (within 3 months) MI, CVA, TIA, or CAD/stents; ongoing cardiac ischemia or severe valve dysfunction; severe reduction of ejection fraction; sepsis; DIC; ARD; ESRD patient not undergoing regularly scheduled dialysis	Immediate medical consultation

ARD, Acute renal disease; *BMI*, body mass index; *CAD*, coronary artery disease; *COPD*, chronic obstructive pulmonary disease; *CVA*, cerebrovascular accident; *DIC*, disseminated intravascular coagulation; *ESRD*, end-stage renal disease; *MI*, myocardial infarction; *PCA*, post-conceptual age; *TIA*, transient ischemic attack.

**Note:* Physical status 5 and 6 are used primarily in medical practice.
Modified from American Society of Anesthesiologists: ASA Physical Status Classification System, www.asahq.org/clinical/physicalstatus.htm; accessed August 20, 2015; and Malamed SF: Knowing your patients, *J Am Dent Assoc* 141:3S-7S, 2010.

Disease," "Cardiac Arrhythmias and Dysrhythmias," "Hypertensive Disease," "Ischemic Heart Disease," "Cerebrovascular Accident," and "Congestive Heart Failure" in Chapter 19; and "Vital Signs" in Chapter 21)

a. Hypertension can result in myocardial infarction (MI) and stroke (cerebrovascular accident, CVA) and contribute to arteriosclerosis, impaired kidney function, and cardiac enlargement; hypertension guidelines must be followed during professional care to reduce the risk of a medical emergency (Table 15-4)

b. When CVD is identified, it is important for the clinician to conduct a thorough interview to assess the severity and level of control of disease and to determine alterations in care (e.g., physician consultation, antibiotic prophylaxis, stress reduction protocol)

c. Clients undergoing corrective surgery for congenital heart disease and who have prosthetic material or a prosthetic device are susceptible to transient bacteremia for up to 6 months and must receive antibiotic prophylaxis; at 6 months after surgery, antibiotic prophylaxis is not usually recommended (see Table 15-2)

d. When antibiotic prophylaxis is necessary, 9 to 10 days should be scheduled between appointments to allow oral bacteria to return to the original state; clients currently following an antibiotic regimen must use an alternative regimen of antibiotic therapy; if antibiotic medication is inadvertently missed, administer within 2 hours after the procedure

3. Questions regarding diseases of the immune system and blood disorders assess a client's potential risk for infection in dental hygiene care and his or her ability to handle stress through the appointment; primary concerns include prolonged bleeding, delayed healing, and secondary infections; physician consultation may be required for more chronic or involved conditions

TABLE 15-4 Classification of Adult Blood Pressure (BP) and Precautionary Measures

Category	Systolic (mm Hg)		Diastolic (mm Hg)	Dental Management Considerations
Normal	<120	and	<80	Routine dental management
				Recheck at continued-care (recare) visit
Prehypertension	120-139	or	80-89	Routine dental management
				Advise client of status and recommend lifestyle management
				Recheck at recare visit
Stage I hypertension	140-159	or	90-99	Monitor BP at consecutive appointments
				If all exceed these guidelines, seek medical consultation
				Stress reduction protocol
				Recheck at recare visit
Stage II hypertension	≥160-170	or	≥100-110	Recheck BP in 5 minutes
				If BP still elevated within this range, seek and receive medical consultation before dental hygiene therapy
				Noninvasive care only
				Definitive emergency care only if BP is less than 180/110 mm Hg
				Stress reduction protocol
				Continue to monitor BP at consecutive appointments
				Recheck at each visit
Hypertensive crisis	>180	or	>110	Recheck BP in 5 minutes
				If BP still elevated, immediate medical consultation is indicated
				No dental or dental hygiene care, elective or emergent, until BP is decreased
				Noninvasive emergency care with drugs: analgesics or antibiotics are indicated
				Refer to hospital for immediate invasive dental care

Modified from Little JW, Miller C, Rhodus NL, Falace D: *Dental management of the medically compromised patient*, St Louis, 2008, Mosby; and US Department of Health and Human Services, National Institutes of Health, National Heart, Lung, and Blood Institute, National High Blood Pressure Education Program: JNC 7 Express, Seventh Report of the Joint National Commission on Prevention, Detection, Evaluation, and Treatment of High Blood Pressure, Bethesda, Md, NIH Pub No 03-5233, 2004, http://www.nhlbi.nih.gov/guidelines/hypertension/jnc7full.htm; accessed August 20, 2015.

a. For clients with diabetes, concerns exist about a hypoglycemic incident, susceptibility to oral infections (abscesses, periodontal diseases), impaired wound healing, and impaired glycemic control because of the presence of periodontal disease; consultation with a physician is indicated in most cases, and referral is based on health history, dialogue, and oral conditions

b. Oral assessment should be initiated to determine the presence of infections and the extent of periodontal disease before consultation with a client's physician; glycated hemoglobin values (A_{1c}) and blood glucose levels are requested from the physician; the client should be asked to bring his or her glucometer, or a glucometer should be available in the oral care facility (Box 15-1)

c. In clients with well-controlled diabetes, no alteration of the care plan is indicated unless complications of diabetes such as hypertension, congestive heart failure (CHF), MI, angina, or renal failure are present

d. Clients with controlled diabetes should eat before appointments; appointments should be scheduled no later than midmorning, and a sugar source must be available in the oral care facility in case of an episode of hypoglycemia or hyperinsulinism

4. Metabolic syndrome (MetS) is closely associated with insulin resistance, in which the body cannot use insulin efficiently; patients with MetS are at increased risk of coronary heart disease, stroke, peripheral vascular disease, and type 2 diabetes

a. MetS is identified by the presence of three or more components: obesity measured by waist circumference (men >40 inches and women >35 inches), fasting blood triglycerides (>150 mg/dL), blood high-density lipoprotein (HDL) cholesterol (men <40 mg/dL and women <50 mg/dL), blood pressure (>130/ 85 mm Hg), and fasting glucose (>100 mg/dL)

b. Physician referral, medical consultation, or both may be required for clients who do not have regular medical care, to determine the presence of associated conditions or the level of control of existing conditions

5. Questions regarding respiratory disease or chronic obstructive pulmonary disease (COPD) assess the level of compromised respiratory function; clinicians should use precautionary measures to avoid further depression of respiration (see the section on "Chronic Obstructive Pulmonary Disease" in Chapter 19)

6. Musculoskeletal system disorders may be associated with chronic use of salicylates or nonsteroidal antiinflammatory drugs (NSAIDs), which can alter blood clotting and corticosteroid therapy and increase the risk of acute adrenal insufficiency

BOX 15-1   Glycemic Management for Adults (Nonpregnant) with Diabetes

Blood Glucose Level (mg/dL)

<70	Tendency toward hypoglycemia; give 15 g* of carbohydrate, and wait 15 minutes; monitor again to assess whether the treatment should continue; notify client's physician
70-130 (Preprandial)	Acceptable
<180 (Peak postprandial)†	
180-239	Risk for infection
>240	Unacceptable for treatment; refer to a physician, and reschedule or postpone treatment until the client reports control and acceptability of treatment
Glycosylated hemoglobin	Level periodically determined to assess plasma glucose control during the preceding 1 to 3 months
Hemoglobin A_{1c} (HbA_{1c})	Normal range <6.5%

*15 g = 3 glucose tablets, a tube of glucose gel, or 4 ounces of fruit juice.
†Postprandial glucose measurements should be made 1 to 2 hours after the beginning of the meal.
Modified from American Diabetes Association: Standards of medical care in diabetes 2015, *Clin Diabetes* 33(2):97-111, 2015.

7. Neurologic and psychological disorders must to be identified and the degree of control determined; medications used to control seizures can cause drug-influenced gingival enlargement, and psychiatric drugs have the potential to interact adversely with the vasoconstrictors in local anesthetic agents

8. Other disorders, such as glaucoma, sexually transmitted infections (STIs), herpes, chemical dependency, and tobacco use, have significant implications for treatment; in clients with glaucoma, anticholinergics are contraindicated because these agents increase intraocular pressure; chemical dependency and tobacco use are risk factors for infectious diseases, malignancies, CVD, pulmonary diseases, and periodontal diseases; dental hygiene care for clients with active herpes or STIs should be postponed until the disease is no longer active

9. The physiologic state of women identifies their status related to pregnancy and endocrine changes

10. The identification of the risk of latex allergy is essential to reduce the chances of an allergic reaction; types of reactions include irritant contact dermatitis, allergic contact dermatitis (delayed hypersensitivity), and latex allergy
    a. Irritant contact dermatitis—the most common reaction; causes dry, itchy areas of irritation on the skin
    b. Allergic contact dermatitis (type IV hypersensitivity reaction)—results from exposure to chemicals added to latex during harvesting of rubber, processing, or manufacturing
    c. Latex allergy, or immediate allergic urticaria (type I hypersensitivity reaction)—results from certain proteins in latex rubber; symptoms range from skin redness, rash, hives, or itching to runny nose, itchy eyes, asthma, and anaphylaxis
    d. Clients at risk for latex reaction should be treated in a latex-reduced environment; physician consultation is indicated for clients with risk of an anaphylactic reaction

11. Listing of current medications—used to determine medications taken by the client and possible interactions with other medications; these medications may be the only clue to the client's existing condition (*Physicians' Desk Reference* or *Mosby's Dental Drug Reference* can help with the identification of adverse reactions, precautions, contraindications, and dental considerations)

12. Identification of medication allergies informs health care professionals of the client's previous adverse reactions to medications

13. Vital signs (see the section on "Vital Signs" in Chapter 21)
    a. Vital signs are values given to measurements of blood pressure (BP), respiration, pulse, and temperature; serve as a baseline in a medical emergency
    b. Abnormal or elevated BP values should be brought to the client's immediate attention; on the basis of the BP values, monitoring of BP at every appointment or a physician consultation may be required before initiation of dental hygiene care (see Table 15-4)
    c. BP, respirations, and pulse are measured and recorded before the administration of local anesthetic agents or nitrous oxide–oxygen (N_2O-O_2) analgesia

14. Conditions being treated with medications—may influence or contraindicate certain procedures; for example, anticoagulant therapy may require a lower dose; antihypertensive drugs may alter the choice of local anesthetic; antipsychotic medications may alter the choice of N_2O-O_2 analgesia (see the sections on "Anticoagulants" in Chapter 11; "Toxicity," "Vasoconstrictors," and "Conscious Sedation with Nitrous Oxide–Oxygen" in Chapter 18; and Chapter 21)

15. Physician consultations—may be necessary, depending on the information obtained from health history or physical examination; written documentation from the physician is necessary (see Fig. 15-1)
    a. Written informed consent is obtained from the client before submitting the request for physician consultation
    b. Medical consultation can be faxed or mailed to the physician's office

C. Health history information is gathered through interviews, written questionnaires, or a combination of both
   1. The interview method allows the dental hygienist to develop client rapport and ensures that the client understands the questions
   2. The self-administered written questionnaire is the most common format used to gather information pertaining to the client's health status

3. Use of both the interview and the written questionnaire is the best approach to collect accurate and comprehensive health information

EXTRAORAL AND INTRAORAL ASSESSMENT

A. Purpose—to assess and recognize deviations from normal conditions significant to a client's health
B. Establishment of an assessment sequence that is followed systematically—skills used in performing extraoral and intraoral examination include direct observation, palpation, auscultation, and olfaction
   1. Direct observation—visual inspection techniques used to examine a client's movement, body symmetry, color, texture, contour, consistency, and form of skin and mucous membrane
   2. Palpation—sense of touch used to examine for tenderness, texture, masses, and variations in structure and temperature within the head and neck region
      a. Digital palpation—use of single (index) finger to move or press against the tissue of the floor of the mouth or hard palate
      b. Bidigital palpation—use of one or more fingers and thumb to move or compress the tissue of lips, tongue, cheeks, and vestibule
      c. Bimanual palpation—simultaneous use of the index finger of one hand and the fingers and thumb of the other hand to move or compress the tissue of the floor of the mouth
      d. Manual palpation—use of all the fingers of one hand to move and compress tissue to assess cervical lymph nodes
      e. Bilateral palpation—use of both hands simultaneously to move or press the tissue on the contralateral sides of the head to assess the submandibular nodes, TMJ, inferior border of mandible, and temporalis and masseter muscles
      f. Circular compression—use of fingers that move in a rotating, circular motion while slight pressure is applied
   3. Auscultation—listening to and detecting sounds made by the body, such as clicking (crepitation) of the TMJ; speech disorders; and vocal hoarseness
   4. Olfaction—use of the olfactory sense to detect variations in breath odors, such as alcohol breath, fruity ketosis (diabetic acidosis), and halitosis associated with dental caries, periodontitis, and necrotizing ulcerative gingivitis

Extraoral Examination Procedure

See also Chapter 4.
A. Head, neck, and face—the overall appearance of client should be assessed via visual inspection
B. The symmetry of skin, eyes, nose, and ears should be observed; areas of unusual discoloration should be inspected
   1. Skin (see the section on "Skin Diseases" in Chapter 8)
      a. Normal texture is continuous, firm, and pigmented in relation to normal variations associated with race and ethnicity
      b. Abnormal textures or pigmentations should be recorded (e.g., scarring, swelling, moles, freckles, pallor, redness, severe acne, tumors, jaundice)
      c. Abnormal lesions should be measured and documented in writing, with details about color, size, shape, and surface texture
   2. Face
      a. Face and head should be symmetrical and have normal function
      b. Asymmetry or lack of function may be associated with injury, Bell's palsy, tumor, abnormal growth and development, difficulty swallowing, Parkinson's disease, Tourette syndrome, and abuse
      c. Facial expression can indicate the client's general frame of mind (e.g., anxious, happy, sad, angry)
   3. Eyes (see the section on "Visual Impairment" in Chapter 19)
      a. Clarity of the sclera should be noted; a yellowing color may indicate the presence of jaundice
      b. Excessively dry or irritated eyes may be a result of medication side effects
   4. Nose
      a. Breathing should be assessed; flared nostrils or ragged breath could indicate difficulty breathing
      b. An enlarged, bulbous, and red nose may be associated with an overgrowth of sebaceous and sweat glands from alcohol abuse (rhinophyma)
   5. Ears (see the section on "Hearing Impairment" in Chapter 19)
C. The symmetry of bones, muscles, lymph nodes, and salivary glands should be observed
   1. The inferior border of the mandible should be assessed for asymmetry by using bimanual palpation from the midline to the posterior angle
   2. The TMJ and the muscles of mastication should be inspected
      a. The TMJ should be assessed for deviation, pain, crepitus, grinding, and reduced range in opening or closing; evaluated through client interview and bilateral palpation with index fingers anterior to outer meatus; client is asked to open and close the mouth slowly several times; any deviation or symptomatology is recorded
      b. Masseter and temporalis muscles are assessed for overdevelopment, pain, swelling, and unusual hardness by using bilateral circular compression; client is asked to clench the teeth together while the muscles are palpated
   3. The mentalis muscle is assessed for overdevelopment and smoothness of contraction during the swallowing movement; evaluated by digital palpation; tissue is moved over the mandible, and client is asked to swallow
   4. The larynx is assessed for unrestricted movement by bimanual palpation; the larynx is gently moved from side to side to check movement
   5. Lymph node chains are assessed (Fig. 15-5)
      a. Occipital lymph nodes are assessed for pain, swelling, enlargement, unusual hardness, or fixed position by using bilateral palpation

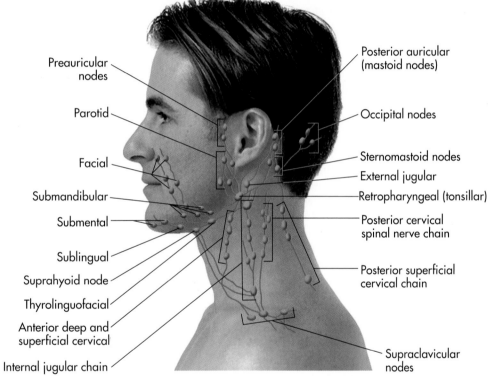

FIG 15-5 A, Location of the thyroid gland and major muscle groups. **B,** Lymph nodes of the head and neck region. (Modified from Ball JW, et al: *Seidel's guide to physical examination,* ed 8, St Louis, 2015, Elsevier.)

b. Auricular and parotid lymph nodes are examined for pain, swelling, enlargement, unusual hardness, or fixed position by using bilateral palpation

c. Superficial cervical lymph nodes are assessed for pain, enlargement, unusual hardness, and fixed position by placing client's head to one side with the chin slightly lowered and by palpating with fingers along the sternocleidomastoid muscle

d. Deep cervical lymph nodes are examined for pain, enlargement, unusual hardness, and fixed position by placing client's head upright and by palpating deep tissues along the sternocleidomastoid muscles with the thumb and fingers

6. Submental and submandibular glands are examined for asymmetry, noncontinuous borders, pain, tenderness, swelling, enlargement, unusual hardness, or difficulty in swallowing by bilateral digital palpation

7. The thyroid gland is assessed for asymmetry and enlargement by a combination of bidigital palpation and circular compression; client is asked to sit upright and to swallow (see Fig. 4-8 in Chapter 4)

8. Parotid glands are examined for pain, swelling, enlargement, and hardness by using bilateral circular compression; salivary flow can be observed at the opening of Stensen's duct when the gland is compressed

Intraoral Examination Procedure

A. Screen the client to detect lesions that may be pathologic, particularly lesions that may be cancerous

B. Prevent the development of advanced, irreversible, or untreatable oral disease through early recognition of initial lesions

C. Oral piercing is a popular form of body art
1. Inspect the tongue, lips, cheeks, frenum, and uvula for piercings
2. Barbells and rings are the most common types of jewelry
3. Complications from piercing include excessive hemorrhage; transmission of communicable diseases; nerve damage; infection; bacteremia; Ludwig's angina; cracked, fractured, or abraded teeth; recession; dehiscence; and aspiration or ingestion of jewelry[10]
4. Jewelry should be removed during the radiography procedure

D. The oral mucosa, lips, floor of the mouth, tongue, salivary ducts, hard and soft palates, and oropharynx should be examined and evaluated (see Table 5-1 and Figs. 5-1 to 5-8 in Chapter 5)
1. The lips are examined by visual inspection and palpation for:
   a. Changes in size—may be caused by swelling or allergic reaction
   b. Chapping—may be caused by mouth breathing or nutritional deficiency
   c. Blistering—may be associated with herpetic lesions
   d. Cracking—may be associated with angular cheilosis, candidiasis, or vitamin B deficiency (see the section on "Vitamins" and Table 12-4 in Chapter 12)
   e. Scar tissue or irritations—may be associated with habitual lip biting or trauma; bruising at commissures may indicate binding or gagging associated with physical abuse
   f. Abnormal texture, lack of moistness or firmness—may be associated with dehydration and excessive sun exposure
   g. Limitations of opening; muscle elasticity, and muscle tone—may be associated with stroke or TMJ dysfunction
2. Labial and alveolar mucosa and the gingiva are examined by using bilateral and bidigital palpation
   a. Signs of tissue trauma from biting, toothbrush abrasion, burns, or physical abuse; lacerated or torn frenum (tissue tags) may indicate binding, gagging, or forced feeding
   b. Ulcerated lesions such as herpetic lesions or aphthous ulcers
   c. Tight or low frenum attachments, which can cause gingival defects such as recession and loss of attached gingiva
   d. "Spit tobacco" lesion (leukoplakia), hyperkeratinized tissue; white, sometimes corrugated in appearance; client should be taught self-assessment techniques
   e. Amalgam tattoo, blue-and-black coloration, size variations—can be found on any area of soft tissue (see section on "Conditions of Oral Soft Tissues" in Chapter 8)
   f. Fordyce granules—ectopic sebaceous glands

3. The buccal mucosa is assessed by using bidigital palpation; the mouth mirror is used to reflect light and to inspect the buccal mucosa
   a. The buccal mucosa is examined for color and texture
   b. The parotid papilla and duct (Stensen's duct) are evaluated; the duct is palpated to assess salivary function
   c. Atypical findings include traumatic lesions related to cheek biting, linea alba adjacent to occlusal plane, ectopic sebaceous glands (Fordyce granules)

4. Hard and soft palates and alveolar ridges are examined by visual inspection; the mouth mirror is used to reflect light; digital palpation is used on the hard palate and alveolar ridges; palpation is not recommended for soft palate to avoid triggering the gag reflex
   a. The hard palate, including the incisive papilla, rugae, and palatine fovea, is examined and assessed for:
      (1) Shape of the palate—low, high, narrow vault; alterations in shape may require alteration in oral radiographic techniques
      (2) Petechiae, torus palatinus, trauma (food burns, denture irritation), stomatitis (nicotine, ulcerative, necrotizing, and denture), fistulas from draining abscesses, denture-related candidiasis (see Chapter 8)
   b. The soft palate is assessed for inflammation, petechiae, trauma, stomatitis, and bifid uvula
   c. Alveolar ridges are assessed for impacted third molars, scarring from third-molar extractions, opercula, and exostosis

5. Oropharynx is assessed by visual inspection with a mouth mirror
   a. Client is asked to say "ah" to relax and lower the posterior portion of the tongue
   b. Anterior and posterior pillars are assessed for inflammation, petechiae, trauma, stomatitis, and enlarged tonsillar tissues

6. Floor of the mouth is examined by visual inspection and bimanual palpation
   a. Function of the submandibular gland is tested by wiping each Wharton's duct with gauze and compressing it with a gloved finger to observe salivary flow
   b. Entire floor of the mouth is palpated; the finger of one hand and the finger and thumb of the other hand are placed under client's chin to palpate
   c. Enlargement or masses, Wharton's duct, sublingual caruncle, and lingual frenum are assessed
   d. Varicosities, tight frenum attachment (ankyloglossia), and blocked salivary duct are inspected
   e. Exostosis along lingual surface of mandible and mandibular tori—significant if interfering with prosthetic appliances

7. The tongue is examined by visual inspection and digital palpation
   a. The dorsal surface is inspected; the entire tongue is palpated, and the lateral borders of the tongue are examined by using gauze to gently hold the tongue

b. The ventral surface is examined by having client touch the palate with the tongue
c. The tongue is assessed for:
   (1) Coating on the dorsal surface and the condition of papillae; the extent is assessed
   (2) Size; macroglossia associated with Down syndrome or cretinism (see the section on "Down Syndrome" in Chapter 19)
   (3) Lingual frenum; tight frenum restricting movement (ankyloglossia)
   (4) Fissured tongue; deep grooves and crevices along the lateral borders and the dorsal surface; the lateral borders are common sites of oral cancer
   (5) Geographic tongue—benign condition in which a sporadic migration of dorsal papilla occurs; tenderness is assessed
   (6) Nutritional deficiencies; burning or glossy tongue (see the section on "Abnormalities Affecting the Tongue" in Chapter 8)
   (7) Black hairy tongue related to proliferation of filiform papillae; caused by irritants such as smoking, alcohol, and rinsing with hydrogen peroxide (see the section on "Abnormalities Affecting the Tongue" in Chapter 8)
   (8) Hairy leukoplakia caused by extensions of keratin on the lateral borders of the tongue; associated with HIV infection
   (9) Atypical lesions, including aphthous ulcerations, trauma-associated fibroma, hemangiomas, and white plaque

ASSESSMENT OF DENTITION

A. Purpose—to assess and document the position and condition of teeth, restorations, and dental caries, noting normal and abnormal findings on a detailed dentition chart
   1. Used for care planning, communication with client, legal documentation, forensic use, and financial audits
   2. Components include study models, occlusion assessment, dentition charting, pulp vitality testing, and strain assessment
B. Study models—impressions for study models taken to obtain visual reproduction of teeth, gingiva, and adjacent intraoral structures and to assist with dentition and periodontal charting
C. Occlusion assessment—presence of malocclusion or tooth position determined; signs of parafunctional habits resulting in occlusal traumatism noted (see the sections on "Intra-arch and Interarch Relationships" in Chapter 5 and "Clinical Assessment of the Periodontium" in Chapter 14)
D. Dentition charting—graphic representation of a client's teeth at assessment (see Table 15-5)
   1. Includes developmental anomalies and defects, condition of teeth, dental caries activity, restorative history, and other problems; a combination of radiographs and direct visual inspection is used to assist with accurate recording of tooth assessment (Box 15-2)

2. Office guides and professional organizations' dentition charting symbols may be adopted for use; the ADA's National Board Dental Examination (NBDE) provides a dental charting symbol key in each client case used
3. Universal Numbering System—most widely used notation system; permanent teeth numbered from 1 to 32 and primary teeth lettered from A to T; 1 to 16 or A to J are located on the maxillary arch, moving right to left; 17 to 32 or K to T are located on the mandibular arch, moving left to right (from client's perspective)
4. Developmental anomalies that affect enamel and dentin, developmental defects that affect tooth shape, number of teeth, and tooth size are noted (see the section on "Abnormalities of Teeth" in Chapter 8)
5. Tooth positions, eruption patterns, and missing teeth are recorded (see the sections on "Eruption" and "Intra-arch and Interarch Relationships" in Chapter 5)
6. Tooth damage that results in loss of integrity of tooth surface is recorded; common forms of damage include attrition, abrasion, erosion, fracture, and dental caries (see the section on "Abnormalities of Teeth" in Chapter 8)
7. Dental caries is an infectious, transmittable, and multifactorial disease of bacterial origin; carious lesions are classified by the type and location of the lesion by using visual inspection with magnification, laser fluorescence, light fluorescence, digital imaging, fiberoptic transillumination, gentle probing, and radiographic examination with standard bitewing or digitized view[11]
   a. Classification for carious lesions includes rate, direction, and type of disease progression; used to determine level of priority for restorative therapy
      (1) Rampant caries—a rapidly progressive decay process that affects the smooth surfaces of numerous teeth and requires urgent intervention; frequently found with early-childhood caries (formerly called *nursing bottle syndrome*)
      (2) Chronic caries—slow progressive decay process
      (3) Arrested caries—carious lesion that has been reversed because of the remineralization process
      (4) Backward caries—lateral spread of decay at the dentino-enamel junction through an undermining process; the surface lesion appears small, but destruction is extensive underneath[12]
      (5) Recurrent or secondary caries— new decay located around existing restorations
   b. Carious lesions described by specific location on tooth surface (see the section on "Dental Caries" in Chapter 9)
      (1) Pit-and-fissure caries—develop in the pits and grooves of the occlusal surfaces of premolars and molars, lingual pits of maxillary incisors, buccal grooves of mandibular molars, and lingual grooves of maxillary molars; pit-and-fissure sealants are an effective preventive strategy to protect tooth surfaces (see the sections on

TABLE 15-5	**Periodontal Assessment Symbols**	
Term	**Procedure**	**Symbol**
Gingiva Blunted papilla	Indicate by placing a straight horizontal line in the affected interproximal space	
Cratered papilla	Indicate by drawing the shape of the crater in the affected interproximal space from the buccal or lingual space	
Inadequate amount of attached gingiva	Indicate when less than 1 mm of attached gingiva is present; calculate by measuring from the margin of free gingiva to the mucogingival junction, and subtract from the pocket depth measurement	NAG | IAG NAG = no attached gingiva IAG = inadequate attached gingiva
Recession	Measure the amount of recession in millimeters from the margin of the free gingiva to the cemento-enamel junction; draw the gingival margin	
Loss of attachment	Measure the amount of recession in millimeters from the margin of the free gingiva to the cemento-enamel junction; add to the depth of the pocket	PD 222 212 / LOA 4 3
Frenum pull	Indicate any abnormal muscle pull on the gingiva, attachment of the free gingiva, or tight frenums by placing a symbol in the area where it occurs	
Exudate Probing depth	Indicate by placing an X above the affected tooth Measure from the margin of the free gingiva to the junctional epithelium; record all readings and all areas of hemorrhage	X

DATE 1/6/02 PD 645 434 423 / PD / LOA / AG

TABLE 15-5   Periodontal Assessment Symbols—cont'd

Term	Procedure	Symbol
Pathology		
Furcation involvement (class I, II, III, or IV)	Use Roman numerals on the affected area to depict the extent of the furcation from the buccal or lingual bifurcation or trifurcation, or use a triangle in the furcation area showing class I (partial triangle), class II (complete triangle unfilled), or class III (triangle completely filled in)	
Mobility (class 1, 2, or 3 or I, II, or III)	Record on the basis of degree of tooth movement	
Periodontal pathology	Outline the affected area, approximating the size and location of the radiolucency observed on the radiograph	
Other Factors		
Marginal ridge discrepancy	Place an N in the area of the occlusal contact when adjacent marginal ridges are not equal in height	
Food impaction	Indicate by placing a zigzag arrow in the interproximal space	
Deficient contacts	Indicate a loose contact by drawing a single vertical line in the interproximal space Indicate an open contact by drawing two vertical lines in the interproximal space	

BOX 15-2   Systematic Approach for Dentition Charting Sequence

Complete a general appraisal of teeth, and note developmental anomalies and defects affecting tooth shape, number of teeth, tooth size, and presence of partial or complete dentures (e.g., generalized moderate fluorosis, amelogenesis imperfecta, peg laterals, number of teeth present, mandibular partial denture)

Chart all missing or erupted supernumerary teeth before recording specific tooth-by-tooth information

Using radiographs, chart all unerupted or impacted teeth

Chart teeth indicated for extraction

Chart existing restorations (amalgam, tooth-colored, and temporary restorations; inlays, onlays, and gold foils; crowns, veneers, and bridges)

Chart signs of tooth damage (dental caries, risk areas, attrition)

Chart areas of plaque-retentive factors and defective restorations needing replacement (overhangs, deficient margins, unpolished amalgam restorations, fractured restorations, improper anatomical contour, occlusal surfaces indicated for pit-and-fissure sealants)

When treatment has been completed on teeth indicated for restorative or supportive care, update the chart using a different color to quickly identify teeth that were restored after original baseline charting

Update the dentition charting at each recare visit, and record any areas of change

---

"Pit-and-Fissure Sealants" in Chapter 13 and "Dental Sealants" in Chapter 16)

(2) Smooth surface caries—found on the facial, lingual, mesial, and distal surfaces of teeth

(3) Root caries—found on exposed root surfaces

c. G.V. Black's classification of dental caries and restorations provides a precise description of the types and location of caries and restorations

(1) Class I—pits and fissures on the occlusal, buccal, and lingual surfaces of posterior teeth and the lingual surfaces of anterior teeth

(2) Class II—proximal surface of posterior teeth, usually involving the occlusal surfaces

(3) Class III—proximal surfaces of incisors and canines, not including the incisal edge

(4) Class IV—proximal surfaces of incisors and canines, including the incisal edge

(5) Class V—gingival third of facial or lingual surfaces of any tooth

(6) Class VI—cusp tips of posterior teeth and the incisal edge of anterior teeth

8. Charting of existing restorations, treatment procedures (endodontics, apicoectomy), and tooth replacement methods (implants, crown, bridge) completed by using accepted dental symbols

a. Restorations should be charted with G.V. Black's classification system and should reflect the actual restoration

b. The restoration morphology, margin quality and location, and biocompatibility of restorative material with soft tissue are evaluated[13]

(1) The restoration and the surrounding tooth structure are assessed for new or recurrent dental caries

(2) The marginal and structural integrity assessed for open margins or signs of restorative material fatigue or fractures; the appropriate margin is smooth to tactile evaluation and does not show any overhang

(3) The interproximal and occlusal contours and the proximal contact are assessed; the appropriateness of faciolingual and occlusocervical dimensions are determined; indication for amalgam polishing or recontouring to improve restoration is assessed

(4) Surface finish is assessed to determine whether it meets the functional and esthetic requirements of the client; indication for amalgam polishing or finishing is assessed

c. Faulty restorations are usually in need of replacement because of the presence of recurrent dental caries, fractures, or factors that encourage microbial plaque biofilm retention and may contribute to the development of secondary caries, periodontal disease, and dentinal hypersensitivity

d. Overhangs on class II restorations should be assessed for removal (margination procedures) to correct defective margins and to provide a smooth surface that will not harbor bacterial plaque biofilm[13,14]

(1) Type I overhang—less than one third of the interproximal space; treated with margination procedure and repolishing of restoration; may be detected radiographically

(2) Type II overhang—one third to one half of the interproximal embrasure space; treated with margination procedure if the predicted final result is good (prognosis for the tooth, complexity, and cost of replacement are considered); usually radiographically and clinically detectable

(3) Type III overhang—more than half of the interproximal embrasure space; treated with replacement of restoration; clinically and radiographically detectable

9. Implant identification (see the sections on "Dental Implants" in Chapters 13 and 14)—to assess for peri-implantitis and the stability of the implant

10. Prosthetic appliances—assessed for stability and functionality

E. Pulpal vitality testing—when applicable (see the section on "Pulpal Vitality and Testing Devices" in Chapter 16)

F. Stain assessment (see the section on "Selective Stain Removal" in Chapter 17)—to determine the extent and type of stain present

1. Stains are primarily factors related to esthetics; result from deposits of chromogenic bacteria, foods, and chemicals

2. Heavy tobacco stains encourage bacterial plaque biofilm retention

PERIODONTAL ASSESSMENT

See the section on "Clinical Assessment of the Periodontium" in Chapter 14.

A. Recognition of oral health, gingivitis, or periodontitis must occur through systematic and comprehensive periodontal examination to determine whether oral prophylaxis, non-surgical periodontal therapy (NSPT), periodontal maintenance (PM), or other periodontal therapy is indicated and to what extent[15] (Table 15-5)

B. During general periodontal examination, anatomical features such as position, size, and shape of gingiva and interdental papillae and position of frena must be recorded
1. The presence, location, and severity of gingival inflammation are assessed—soft tissue description (color, texture, consistency, marginal and papillary shape)
2. Mucogingival relationships are evaluated to identify the deficiencies of keratinized tissue, abnormal frenum insertions, and other tissue abnormalities, such as clinically significant gingival recession (e.g., recession, loss of attachment/clinical attachment level, attached gingiva)

C. Periodontal probing is done to assess the probing depth and to provide information on the health of subgingival areas, including the presence of bleeding on probing (see the section on "Clinical Assessment Using Periodontal Probes" in Chapter 17)
1. Probing depths are measured on six tooth sites (distofacial, facial, mesiofacial, distolingual, lingual, mesiolingual) and recorded on the periodontal chart
2. Clinical pocket depth measurements and loss of attachment readings are used to determine the presence of pseudopockets (false or gingival pockets) or periodontal pockets

D. Periodontal soft tissues, including peri-implant tissues, should be examined

E. The presence of purulent exudates and gingival crevicular fluid (GCF) should be determined; increased GCF and purulent exudate indicate inflammatory changes within the pocket wall; these are considered risk factors for disease progression and require further assessment to determine cause and to plan interventions

F. The presence and amount of bleeding on probing is noted to assist in the determination of disease severity

G. The presence and distribution of bacterial plaque biofilm and calculus—location, extent, and tenacity of deposits are identified to assist with appropriate care planning and instrument selection (see the section on "Clinical Assessment with Dental Explorers" in Chapter 17)

H. Degree of mobility of teeth and dental implants
1. Mobility—risk factor for periodontal disease progression; should be measured when moderate to advanced disease is present
2. Measured by bidigital evaluation when teeth are not occluded and by direct observation (fremitus) when teeth are occluded; classified by degree of movement
   a. Class 1 or I—slight mobility, greater than normal
   b. Class 2 or II—moderate mobility, greater than 1 mm
   c. Class 3 or III—severe mobility, tooth can move in all directions and can be depressed into the socket
3. Contributing factors—trauma from occlusion, inflammation in periodontal ligament, periodontal surgery, physiochemical changes (pregnancy or hormonal changes) in periodontal tissues, and pathologic conditions (tumors)[16]

I. The presence, location, and degree of clinical furcation involvement are determined
1. Occurs when loss of attachment extends into bifurcation or trifurcation of multi-rooted teeth; classified by degree of involvement
   a. Class I—exposure of furcation; but bone remains between roots
   b. Class II—loss of some bone between roots; but not complete communication from one surface to another
   c. Class III—through-and-through involvement with complete loss of bone between roots; opening covered by gingiva
   d. Class IV—through-and-through involvement with complete loss of bone between roots; entrance clearly visible
2. Furcation involvement—risk factor in predicting periodontal breakdown; compromises the prognosis of a tooth; detection and thorough periodontal debridement essential at the earliest point

J. Bacterial culturing, genetic testing, deoxyribonucleic acid (DNA) or ribonucleic acid (RNA) probes, antibody and enzyme markers should be used, when indicated (see the section on "Clinical Assessment of the Periodontium" in Chapter 14)
1. Microbial assessments are not recommended routinely because tests fail to identify specific diseases or predict disease progression; however, microbiologic monitoring may be used in clients who continue to experience disease progression despite regular NSPT, surgical intervention, and effective oral self-care; those at high risk for disease progression or medically compromised clients with aggressive periodontitis may benefit from microbiologic monitoring
2. Commercially available genetic tests assess susceptibility to chronic periodontitis and assist in risk assessment
3. Salivary diagnostic advances allow for identification of periodontal bacteria and genetic testing; although use in clinical practice is limited, this diagnostic assessment tool is expanding[17]

RADIOGRAPHIC EVALUATION

See the sections on "Radiology Techniques: Intraoral and Extraoral" and "Radiographic Interpretation" in Chapter 6.

A. A satisfactory number of diagnostic-quality periapical and bitewing radiographs are exposed and interpreted during the assessment phase of therapy

B. Depending on the diagnostic needs of the client, current radiographs are used for the proper evaluation and interpretation of the status of the dentition, periodontium, and dental implants

C. Any radiographic abnormalities are noted in the client's chart, and appropriate follow-up or referral is done

D. Digital subtraction radiology is used to detect and measure small changes in living bone (progressive bone loss or bone fill) that would otherwise go unnoticed with traditional technology

ORAL HYGIENE ASSESSMENT

A. Oral hygiene assessment—review of current home care practices, adherence levels, oral health and hygiene knowledge, skill levels, and psychosocial factors that might influence behaviors and oral habits; assists in the development of effective self-care educational sessions during the implementation phase of care (see Chapter 16)

B. Indices—tools to measure and score periodontal assessment factors such as plaque biofilm, calculus, and bleeding for the benefit of both the clinician and the client (see the section on "Clinical Assessment of the Periodontium" in Chapter 14 and Table 20-11 in Chapter 20)

C. Oral self-care methods—used by a client to remove or reduce bacterial biofilm both supragingivally and subgingivally (1 to 3 mm); oral hygiene measures, oral home care, plaque biofilm control, and mechanical plaque biofilm removal are synonymous with oral self-care methods (see the sections on "Dental Plaque Biofilm Detection," "Mechanical Plaque Biofilm Control on Facial, Lingual, and Occlusal Tooth Surfaces," "Interdental Plaque Biofilm Control," and "Care of Fixed and Removable Prostheses" in Chapter 16)
   1. Determination of the use, frequency, and methods of plaque biofilm removal devices, dentifrices, mouthrinses, and fluorides
   2. Determination of the frequency of tobacco use, oral habits, and sugar intake
   3. Assessment of a client's skill level for oral self-care
      a. Skill deficiency—present if the client does not have the knowledge and the psychomotor ability to perform mechanical plaque biofilm removal
      b. Management deficiency—present if the client possesses the ability but does not perform plaque biofilm removal effectively on a daily basis
   4. Assessment of a client's motivation and readiness for behavior change

D. Evaluation of dietary risk factors for dental caries; recommendations offered to reduce total sugar clearance time per day (see the section on "Nutritional Assessment and Counseling" in Chapter 12)

RISK FACTOR ASSESSMENTS

A. Risk factors—factors that significantly increase the risk for the onset or progression of a specific disease; include systemic disease, oropharyngeal cancer, caries, and periodontal disease risk factors

B. Systemic disease—risk factor for periodontal disease, and in some cases, periodontal disease is considered a contributing factor for systemic conditions; CVD, diabetes mellitus, respiratory disease, osteoporosis, and preterm low birth weight (see Chapter 14); when these conditions are present, consider the following American Academy of Periodontology recommendations[18,19]
   1. Diagnose the periodontal condition, and inform the client of his or her risk for systemic disease
   2. Consultation with client's physician may be indicated to advise the physician about the client's periodontal status and the proposed care plan
   3. Determine the level of control or the status of disease, such as gestational period, medications used, and glycemic control
   4. Provide self-care education regarding the relationship of periodontal infection to systemic health and of systemic health to periodontal disease
   5. Provide adequate NSPT, and encourage the client to commit to periodontal maintenance care

C. Oral and pharyngeal cancer risk—determined by evaluating risk factors such as socioeconomic status, tobacco use, race, alcohol use, sun exposure, gender, and age to formulate appropriate care plan and intervention to reduce risk: use the ADHA's tobacco cessation initiative Ask, Advise, Refer based on U.S Department of Health and Human Services Clinical Practice Guidelines[20]

D. Caries risk—determined by assessing protective and causative factors (e.g., frequency of sugar intake, high cariogenic bacteria count, biofilm removal ability, salivary dysfunction, biofilm-retentive factors, recare and fluoride history) to formulate appropriate care plan to reduce the client's risk (Table 15-6)
   1. Sugar intake assessment includes determining the form and frequency of exposure and offering appropriate recommendations to reduce exposure
   2. Plaque-retentive factors (restoration overhangs, defective and poorly fitting crown margins, dental caries, exposed root surfaces, excess cement, xerostomia) should be identified and eliminated or minimized
   3. Use of topical fluoride or chemotherapeutic agents (e.g., antimicrobial mouthrinses and dentifrices, products with xylitol) should be assessed and prescribed if not already being used by the client
   4. Recare regularity is evaluated and adjusted on the basis of the level of caries risk

E. Periodontal risk—assessed by determining dental and host-environmental risk factors and risk indicators (e.g., history of previous aggressive disease, increased pocket probing depth, loss of clinical attachment, infrequent dental visits, stress, poor oral hygiene, specific bacterial pathogens, tobacco use, diabetes mellitus with poor glycemic control, inherited risk) and by determining signs and symptoms of disease to assist with the formulation of accurate diagnosis and plan of care (see the section on "Changes in the Periodontium Associated with Disease" in Chapter 14)

TABLE 15-6   Classification of Caries Risk

Risk Level	Children (0 to 5 years)	Children (6 years and older) and Adults
Low	*No evidence of:* – Carious or incipient lesions, restorations, or tooth loss caused by caries in past 2 years – Caries activity in the mother or other siblings in the past 2 years – Dental or orthodontic appliances – Plaque biofilm present – Inadequate salivary flow – Special care health needs – Not eligible for government programs *Evidence of:* – Optimal fluoride exposure – Regular recare intervals – Eating sugary or starchy foods or drinks with meals or infrequent exposure	*No evidence of:* – Carious or incipient lesions, restorations, or tooth loss caused by caries in past 3 years – Caries activity in the mother or other siblings in the past 2 years – Interproximal restorations or restorations with plaque-retentive factors or open contacts – Dental or orthodontic appliances – Exposed root surfaces – Plaque biofilm present – Special care health needs – Chemotherapy or radiation therapy – Smokeless tobacco use – Eating disorders – Drug/alcohol abuse *Evidence of:* – Adequate salivary flow – Optimal fluoride exposure – Regular recare intervals – Eating sugary or starchy foods or drinks with meals or infrequent exposure – Low count of cariogenic bacteria – Well-coalesced pits and fissures
Moderate	*No evidence of:* – Fluoride exposure – Regular recare or dental home *Evidence of:* – Caries activity in the mother or other siblings in the past 7 to 23 months – Frequent or prolonged exposure to sugary or starchy foods or drinks between meals – Dental or orthodontic appliances – Visible plaque biofilm	*No evidence of:* – Fluoride exposure – Regular recare or dental home *Evidence of:* – One or two new carious or incipient lesions, restorations, or tooth loss caused by caries in the past 3 years – Caries activity in the mother or other siblings in the past 7 to 23 months – Interproximal restorations or restorations with plaque-retentive factors or open contacts – Dental or orthodontic appliances – Exposed root surfaces – Visible plaque biofilm – Special care health needs – Smokeless tobacco use – Eating disorders – Drug or alcohol abuse – Deep pits and fissures or developmental defects
High	*No evidence of:* – Fluoride exposure – Regular recare or dental home *Evidence of:* – Caries activity in the mother or other siblings in the past 6 months – Carious or incipient lesions – Restorations or tooth loss caused by caries in the past 2 years – Bottle or sippy cup at bedtime with juice or sugar (cariogenic agent) – Eligibility for government program – Special care health needs – Inadequate saliva flow related to hyposalivary medications, cancer treatment, or genetic factors	*No evidence of:* – Fluoride exposure – Regular recare or dental home *Evidence of:* – Three or more carious or incipient lesions, restorations, or tooth loss caused by caries in the past 3 years – Caries activity in the mother or other siblings in the past 6 months – High levels of cariogenic bacteria *Streptococcus mutans* (105 CFU/mL) and lactobacilli (103 CFU/mL) – Frequent or prolonged exposure to sugary or starchy foods or drinks between meals – Special care health needs – Chemotherapy or radiation therapy – Inadequate saliva flow related to hyposalivary medications, cancer treatment, or genetic factors

CFU/mL, Colony-forming units per milliliter.

Modofied from American Academy of Pediatric Dentistry: Guideline on caries-risk management for infants, children, and adolescents, *Pediatr Dent* 35(5):E157-E164, 2013; and American Dental Association, Councils on Dental Practice and Scientific Affairs: Caries risk assessment form. http://gsa.ada. org/search?as_sitesearch=www.ada.org/sections/professionalResources/docs&q=caries+risk&searchButton.x=0&searchButton.y=0& site=ADAorg_Collection&client=ADAFrontEnd&proxystylesheet=ADAFrontEnd&output=xml_no_dtd&ie=UTF-8&ip=24.117.153.112&access=p& sort=date%3AD%3AL%3Ad1&entqr=3&oe=UTF-8&ud=1. Accessed August 20, 2015.

DIAGNOSIS

A. Definition—clinical diagnosis by licensed dental hygienist that identifies actual or potential unmet human needs (deficits) related to oral health or disease that a dental hygienist is educated and licensed to treat or refer for care;[7] the second phase in the dental hygiene process of care (see Fig. 15-1)

B. Dental diagnosis identifies a specific oral disease, whereas dental hygiene diagnosis identifies human needs deficits related to dental hygiene care

C. Interpretation of collected data during assessment phase of care is necessary to identify significant findings, recognize deviations from normal, describe abnormalities, and analyze significance of the abnormalities
   1. Analysis of assessment data used to identify deviations from normal values and to identify patterns or relationships within data
   2. Synthesis combines elements from data to develop explanations for symptoms
      a. Inductive reasoning finds possible patterns in observations to predict new information
      b. Deductive reasoning begins with generalizations and proceeds to discover specific facts

D. Identification of unmet human needs related to oral health or systemic problems provides a unique focus for the provision of dental hygiene care

E. Validation allows for the recognition of errors and discrepancies, the need for additional information from the client or from other health care professionals, or the reinterpretation of documented evidence

F. Diagnostic statements are formulated after data analysis and validation; become framework for planning, implementation, and evaluation phases of care; Fig. 15-6 shows three major components of written diagnostic statements:
   1. Condition or problem, or potential problem, as identified by unmet human needs (diagnosis) related to dental hygiene care; used to formulate client goals
   2. Identification of contributing or causative factors related to unmet human needs; used to determine appropriate dental hygiene interventions
   3. Signs and symptoms (evidence) of unmet human needs that support existence of problem; used to evaluate outcomes of dental hygiene care

PROGNOSIS

A. Definition—prediction of duration, course, and termination of disease and response to treatment; usually determined after diagnosis and before care is planned

B. Overall prognosis considers both oral and systemic health and the significance of factors present (e.g., type of periodontal disease, age, socioeconomic status, systemic conditions, malocclusion, periodontal status, complicated prosthesis, tobacco use, cooperation of client)

C. Prognosis for individual teeth made after overall prognosis is determined and relates to mobility, periodontal pockets, adequacy of attached gingiva, mucogingival involvement, furcation involvement, tooth morphology, status of teeth serving as abutments, bone level surrounding tooth, and extensive caries

D. Level of prognosis established through collaboration of the dental hygienist and the dentist after comprehensive assessment[21]
   1. Excellent prognosis—no bone loss, excellent gingival conditions, and adequate client commitment to care
   2. Good prognosis—adequate remaining bone support, adequate possibilities to control causative and risk factors, and adequate client commitment to care
   3. Fair prognosis—less-than-adequate remaining bone support, some tooth mobility, grade I furcation involvement, adequate maintenance possible, and acceptable client commitment to care
   4. Poor prognosis—moderate to advanced bone loss, tooth mobility, grade I and II furcation involvement, difficult areas to maintain, and doubtful client commitment to care

FIG 15-6 Dental hygiene diagnosis. (Modified from Darby ML, Walsh MM: Application of the human needs conceptual model to dental hygiene practice, *J Dent Hyg* 74(3):233, 2000.)

5. Questionable prognosis—advanced bone loss, grade II and III furcation involvement, tooth mobility, and inaccessible areas

6. Hopeless prognosis—advanced bone loss, areas not maintainable, and extraction or extractions indicated

EVIDENCE-BASED DECISION MAKING[22,23]

A. Health care professionals must be able to assess the value of the information available in scientific literature and to use current best evidence when providing dental hygiene care

B. Evidence-based decision making integrates clinical expertise, client values, and best evidence into the decision-making process to achieve successful therapeutic outcomes

C. Evidence-based decision making begins during the process of care when a client presents with a specific clinical question or when a question arises during dental hygiene care; the four elements of an evidence-based question (PICO) are:
   1. Patient, or problem
   2. Intervention, cause, or prognosis
   3. Comparison, or control
   4. Outcome, or outcomes

D. The hygienist develops a well-defined clinical question (PICO) related to the diagnosis, therapy, prognosis, cause, or harm to answer the client-related question (Table 15-7)

E. A computerized literature search is conducted to answer the PICO question—randomized controlled clinical trials (RCTs), systematic reviews, or meta-analysis studies provide the best evidence for answering the question

F. Evidence obtained from literature search is critically evaluated to determine validity and clinical applicability—studies are reviewed to identify the results and determine whether they are valid and whether they apply to the client

TABLE 15-7   Asking the Clinical Question: PICO Mnemonic

Element (PICO)	Descriptive Question(s) to Ask	Example
Patient, or problem	How would I describe a group of clients similar to mine? What are the most important characteristics for this client?	A client with generalized marginal biofilm and inflammation
Intervention, cause, or prognosis	Which main intervention or prognostic factor am I considering for this client?	A powered toothbrush
Comparison, or control	What is the main alternative to compare with the intervention?	Compared with a manual toothbrush
Outcome, or outcomes	What can I hope to accomplish, measure, or improve?	Decrease marginal biofilm and inflammation

Modified from Forest JL, Miller SA: Translating evidence-based decision making into practice: EBDM concepts and finding the evidence, *J Evid Based Dent Pract* 9:(2):59-72, 2009.

G. Evidence gathered from literature appraisal is applied to clinical practice by discussing the findings with client and offering recommendations for treatment

H. The process and the clinician's performance are evaluated

PLANNING

A. Definition—identification and prioritization of current and potential dental and dental hygiene care needs, establishment of client goals, and determination of interventions and outcomes to meet these needs

B. Clients are more likely to express their wants, needs, and desires and to commit to a care plan if they are actively involved in the development of goals, priorities, interventions, and appointment planning

C. Assessment data and diagnosis should be used to develop a logical plan of therapy to eliminate disease, slow disease progression, and maintain and promote health[15]

D. Four components to consider when completing written care plan:
   1. Establish priorities for care that require a collaborative approach among the client, the dental hygienist, and the dentist; address the following:
      a. Needs of the client based on conditions that pose the greatest threat to comfort, life, health, and safety
      b. Main concerns or preferences of the client (chief complaint)
      c. Motivational level of the client
   2. Set client-oriented goals and evaluation measures that reflect the expected and desired outcomes of dental hygiene care
      a. For each dental hygiene diagnosis, at least one goal and intervention should be established; some diagnoses may require multiple interventions
      b. Goals should focus on the cognitive, affective, or psychomotor domain and contain a subject, verb, measurement criteria, and specific time element:
         (1) Cognitive goals focus on increasing knowledge level
         (2) Affective goals focus on changes in beliefs, attitudes, and values
         (3) Psychomotor goals focus on skill development when skill deficiencies are present
      c. Expected outcomes and evaluation measures are used to determine whether goals are being met during care or after completion of therapy; when indicated, modify the diagnosis or care plan if goals are not being met; two forms of evaluation should be considered when planning care:
         (1) Evaluation that occurs throughout the implementation phase of care
         (2) Evaluation or reevaluation that occurs after the completion of initial therapy
   3. Identify interventions as part of care planning that specifically address the dental hygiene diagnosis (Table 15-8)
      a. Traditional phases of dental care planning include[24]:
         (1) Preliminary phase—focuses on treating periodontal or dental emergency needs

TABLE 15-8　Components of Dental Hygiene Care

Component	Elements
General assessment	Medical and dental history
	Chief concern
	Clinical examination
	Radiographic analysis
	Microbiologic, genetic, and biochemical diagnostic tests
	Extraoral and intraoral examinations
Periodontal and restorative assessment	Risk assessment
	Plaque or biofilm, calculus
	Dental restorations
	Caries assessment
	Dental implants
	Probing depth (bleeding and suppuration)
	Clinical attachment level and gingival recession
	Furcation status
	Prosthetic appliances
	Occlusion (mobility, occlusal discrepancy, fremitus)
	Proximal contact relationships
	Periodontal-systemic interrelationships
Self-care education	Risk factors
	Disease theory education
	Skill enhancement
	Behavior interventions (nutrition counseling, tobacco cessation, medical referral)
Instrumentation and supportive therapy	Pain and anxiety control methods
	Plaque biofilm and calculus removal
	Restoration overhang removal
	Desensitization for dentinal hypersensitivity
	Fluoride therapy
	Sealant application
	Local or systemic chemotherapeutic agents
	Implant maintenance
	Mouthguard fabrication
Selection of polishing procedures	Selective stain removal (polishing)
	Restoration enhancement (finishing, polishing)
Referrals	Medical consultation
	Restorative therapy
	Periodontal surgery
	Orthodontics
	Endodontics
	Oral surgery
	Oral pathology diagnosis

Modified from American Academy of Periodontology: Statement on comprehensive periodontal therapy, 2010, http://www.perio.org/resources-products/posppr3-4.html, accessed August 20, 2015.

(2) Phase I therapy—focuses on controlling the risk factors responsible for disease; includes self-care education, diet control, removal or correction of biofilm-retentive factors, antimicrobial therapy, and dental caries management

(3) Phase II therapy—focuses on surgical care; includes periodontal surgery, placement of implants, and endodontic therapy

(4) Phase III therapy—focuses on prosthetic treatment and final management of dental caries, along with periodontal examination to reevaluate response to restorative procedures

(5) Phase IV therapy—focuses on long-term periodontal maintenance therapy; includes assessment, self-care education, deposit removal, and evaluation of continued-care (recare) interval

b. Common system of periodontal disease classification; includes overall disease extent (localized and generalized), severity (case type), and activity (chronic, aggressive, or necrotizing) (see the section on "Diseases of the Periodontium" in Chapter 14)

c. Interventions for common forms of periodontal disease include:

(1) Therapy for gingivitis (case type I)—includes oral self-care education, supragingival and subgingival debridement, antimicrobial agents, and correction of plaque biofilm–retentive factors completed during a 1-hour appointment; may include reevaluation at another appointment if extensive bleeding occurs on probing or pseudopockets are present

(2) Therapy for mild periodontitis (case type II)—includes elimination, modification, or control of systemic diseases and other risk factors; oral self-care education; and supragingival and subgingival debridement, including scaling and root planing with a quadrant approach, during four 60- to 90-minute appointments, and reevaluation

(3) Therapy for moderate periodontitis (case type III)—includes elimination, alteration, or control of systemic diseases and other risk factors; oral self-care education; and supragingival and subgingival debridement, including scaling and root planing with a sextant or quadrant approach, during four to six 60- to 90-minute appointments, and reevaluation for surgery

(4) Therapy for advanced periodontitis (case type IV)—includes elimination, modification, or control of systemic diseases and risk factors; oral self-care education; debridement, including scaling and root planing; subgingival microbial sampling; and extraction of teeth that have a poor prognosis with a sextant approach during six 60- to 90-minute appointments, and reevaluation for surgery

(5) Therapy for refractory periodontitis—includes self-care education, debridement, scaling and root planing, control of risk factors, systemic antibiotics, locally delivered antibiotics, microbial diagnostic testing, and antimicrobial therapy, with a sextant or quadrant approach, based on number of sites involved; reevaluation for surgery; and periodontal maintenance therapy

4. Written care plan provides permanent documentation and becomes a contract between the dental hygienist and a client; elements of care plan include:

a. Procedure—course of action or procedures to be rendered; associated risks and benefits
b. Alternative treatment options
c. Appointment sequence—order in which therapy will be given
d. Approximate time for each procedure and total time for each appointment
e. Expected outcomes and limitations of care

CASE PRESENTATION

A. Definition—presentation of assessment data to include dental and dental hygiene diagnosis and proposed care plan
B. Purpose—to satisfy legal and ethical responsibilities for care, reach agreement for therapy, and obtain informed consent
C. A collaborative approach between client and clinician should be encouraged
D. Case presentation should be accurate, direct, and concise; should describe:
   1. Existing oral conditions and related causative and contributing factors presented in terms that are understandable to the client
   2. Treatment procedures and how therapy may differ from previous appointments (e.g., number of appointments, length, purpose of each appointment, services to be incorporated, description of services)
   3. Desired outcomes of treatment and provisional prognosis
   4. Risks and benefits of all treatment options involved
   5. Consequences of rejecting treatment or not proceeding with all components of care
   6. Alternative approaches to care, if any exist (e.g., mechanized vs. hand-activated instrumentation; NSPT vs. surgery when advanced disease is present)
   7. Client's responsibility as a co-therapist (e.g., commitment to self-care and continued-care recommendations)
   8. Client's right to decline care by providing an opportunity to initially consent for care and to withdraw from treatment at any time
   9. Time and cost involved in professional care

INFORMED CONSENT

A. Definition—process by which a client agrees to a proposed treatment after a complete case presentation (see Chapter 22)
B. Includes use of a written informed consent form, signed by the client or guardian, the clinician, and a witness, stating that all treatment descriptions, risk, benefits, outcomes of treatment, alternative treatments, and an opportunity for questions and answers were provided; should be completed before implementation of care plan
C. An *informed refusal form* is completed when a client declines some or all of the care plan; includes:
   1. Proposed dental and dental hygiene care planned
   2. Risks involved without treatment
   3. List of procedures being refused

   4. Date the informed refusal form was signed
   5. Signature of the client, the dental hygienist or the dentist, and a witness

IMPLEMENTATION

See the section on "Preventive Therapy or Treatment of Biofilm-Induced Gingivitis" in Chapter 14.
A. Definition—delivery of preventive and therapeutic procedures identified in an individualized care plan to meet a client's human needs (see Table 15-8)
   1. Activities—reduction or elimination of risk factors for disease, health promotion, self-care education, mechanical and mechanized instrumentation, pharmacotherapeutic interventions, pain control strategies, selective polishing; supporting interventions include overhang removal, desensitization, dietary assessment and counseling, dental caries management, and occlusal therapy
   2. Modifications to the initial care plan are made as new assessment criteria become available during the implementation of care (i.e., improved self-care, increase in healing response time)
B. Self-care education—teaching disease control, health maintenance, and health promotion strategies to target the client's diagnosed problems; should occur at each appointment before instrumentation procedures; strategies are those implemented by the client at home (see Chapter 16)
C. Pain and anxiety control should be used when indicated to prevent or manage apprehension and pain and promote the client's cooperation and compliance; includes local anesthetic agents, N_2O-O_2 analgesia, topical anesthetic agents, and psychosomatic methods (see Chapter 18)
D. Instrument selection—based on intraoral conditions discovered in the assessment phase of care: periodontal pocket depth, furcation involvement, root concavities, deposit size, configuration, mode of attachment, and location (see Chapter 17)
   1. Hand-activated instrumentation—use of sharp curets and files, with fundamental instrumentation principles during scaling and debridement
   2. Mechanized instrumentation—ultrasonic and sonic scaling equipment and techniques for scaling and debridement
E. Polishing procedures—use of abrasive agents, prophy angle, low-speed handpiece, toothbrush, or air abrasion unit to remove bacterial plaque biofilm and stain and to produce a smooth, lustrous tooth surface
   1. Selective polishing—esthetic procedure accomplished with a rubber cup and paste or air-polishing unit (air abrasion) to remove extrinsic stain remaining after periodontal instrumentation (see the section on "Selective Stain Removal" in Chapter 17)
   2. Therapeutic polishing—prophylaxis pastes may include supplemental ingredients for added benefits, including fluoride, xylitol, and calcium phosphate compounds[25]
   3. Polishing and finishing restorations prevent recurrent caries and deterioration of restorations, maintain periodontal health, and prevent occlusal problems

F. Maintenance therapy (formerly known as *supportive therapy*)—a term used for interventions directed at sustaining oral health and controlling disease progression (e.g., debridement for control of periodontal diseases and maintenance of periodontal health, fluoride therapy, sealant application, occlusal appliance fabrication, oral irrigation, desensitization, local or systemic antibiotics, implant maintenance) (see the section on "Periodontal Maintenance" in Chapter 14 and "Oral Irrigation," "Fluorides," "Mouthrinses or Chemotherapeutics," "Dental Sealants," "Care of Fixed and Removable Prostheses," "Dental Implant Maintenance," "Tobacco Use Interventions," and "Assessment of Dentinal Hypersensitivity" in Chapter 16.

G. *Ergonomics* focuses on the prevention of exposure to injury within the work environment; involves clinician and client positioning, tasks and procedures performed, equipment design and use, and impact of these actions on musculoskeletal health
   1. Cumulative trauma disorders (also known as *repetitive strain disorders*)—musculoskeletal and nerve impairments caused by repetitive work activities, especially when performed aggressively, in awkward positions, or both
   2. Prevention of ergonomic hazards—involves daily application of ergonomic principles while providing dental hygiene care (e.g., posture, grasp, properly fitted gloves, instrument and equipment design, exercise for hand and body, positioning of equipment and materials in the environment)

CLIENT MANAGEMENT WITH EFFECTIVE COMMUNICATION

A. Communication—giving or exchanging information, signals, or messages through facial expression, behavior, talking, gestures, and writing; effective communication is essential in creating an environment conducive to modifying a client's psychomotor skills, level of knowledge, values, attitudes, and lifestyle

B. Intrapersonal communication—processing a message within oneself; often affected by one's personal life experiences, culture, beliefs, and values

C. Interpersonal communication—messages between two or more people; focuses on the interaction and interpretation of a conversation with nonverbal behaviors and spoken words; effective interpersonal communication may reduce the incidence of miscommunication and client management problems and increase the client's commitment to care
   1. Nonverbal behaviors—nonspoken messages, including body orientation, posture, facial expressions, gestures, touch, distance, voice tone, and hesitation in speech
   2. Verbal behaviors—spoken messages, including language, active listening, paraphrasing, and reflective responding
      a. The language used in communication should be carefully selected based on the client's characteristics and presented in a straightforward and nonthreatening manner

      b. Active listening requires maintaining eye contact and concentration and focusing on what the client is communicating
      c. Paraphrasing is restatement or summary of what the client said; provides the opportunity to correct any misunderstandings
      d. Reflective responding addresses the actual feelings of the client; response is presented in manner that restates, rewords, or reflects what the client said

D. Enhancement of client–dental hygienist relationship through confidence and trust requires:
   1. Acceptance—accepting the client without judgment
   2. Comfort—ability to deal with embarrassing or emotionally painful topics related to an individual's health
   3. Concreteness—communicating in a clear and precise manner with terms understandable to a client
   4. Empathy—listening and understanding the emotions and feelings of an individual
   5. Genuineness—communicating in an open and honest manner
   6. Respect—ability to convey honor and esteem for an individual
   7. Responsiveness—ability to reply to messages at the very moment they are sent
   8. Self-disclosure—sharing personal experiences with a client
   9. Warmth—displaying personal feelings and empathy

EVALUATION

See the sections on "Treatment" and "Periodontal Maintenance" in Chapter 14.

A. Definition—measurement of extent to which client has achieved specified goals in care plan and determination of success of interventions; ensures that high-quality care has been provided

B. The quality of dental hygiene care is assessed by certain criteria and standards
   1. Criteria—qualities or characteristics by which the knowledge, skill, or oral health status of a client is measured through descriptions of acceptable levels of performance of client or dental hygienist (e.g., probing attachment levels are reduced by 1 to 2 mm and no sites with bleeding on probing)
   2. Standards—acceptable and expected levels of performance by the dental hygienist or other health care professionals, established through national consensus[2]

C. Measurement of outcomes of dental hygiene interventions involves collecting evaluation data to determine whether the client's goals established during the planning phase of care have been met, partially met, or not met

D. *Supervised neglect* occurs when the client needs further professional care to achieve higher levels of oral wellness or to prevent or control oral disease process, but has been discharged from care under the false assumption that a healthy state was achieved

E. Two forms of evaluation:
   1. Evaluation—occurs continually throughout implementation phase of care; provides the mechanism for modifying the care plan as new assessment criteria become available during treatment (e.g., improved client self-care, increase in healing response time)
   2. Reevaluation—occurs 4 to 6 weeks after therapy is completed to evaluate response to initial care and to recommend additional therapy as needed (e.g., decrease in probing depths, elimination of bleeding points)
F. Elements of reevaluation appointment include components of the dental hygiene process of care: assessment, diagnosis, planning, and implementation
   1. Assessment
      a. Reassessment of initial assessment data and periodontal status to evaluate improvement, such as effective self-care methods, reduction of 1 to 2 mm in probing measurements, no bleeding on probing, and healthy-appearing gingival tissue
      b. Determination of the presence of residual deposits, newly accumulated deposits, or unresponsive areas indicated by bleeding on probing or gingival inflammation
      c. Reevaluation of the client's self-care practices
   2. Diagnosis—reevaluation of dental or dental hygiene diagnosis, if indicated, based on assessment data
   3. Planning—care plan developed on the basis of assessment findings; includes, when indicated, modification to self-care practices, localized debridement, chemotherapy, appropriate referrals, and establishment of continued-care schedule or periodontal maintenance therapy
   4. Implementation—provision of self-care education; removal of residual deposits and plaque biofilm–retentive factors; debridement of nonresponsive areas; provision of indicated therapy, and reassessment of continued-care schedule
G. The continued-care (recare) schedule is determined on the basis of individual client needs, degree of risk for oral disease, and disease progression; client is informed of the rationale for and the importance of continued care[24]
   1. Continued-care schedules with intervals of 1 to 3 months are recommended to clients who display poor results after therapy, have significant risk factors, have advanced or aggressive disease, have poor self-care, have furcation involvement, or have complicated prostheses
   2. Intervals of 3 months are recommended to clients who complete routine NSPT with uneventful healing and demonstrate moderate to high risk for oral diseases and disease progression
   3. Intervals of 3 to 4 months are recommended to clients who have maintained generally good results for 1 year or longer after therapy but display significant risk factors (e.g., inconsistent or poor oral hygiene, heavy calculus formation, systemic disease or condition, tobacco use, localized pockets, occlusal problems, complicated prostheses, ongoing orthodontic therapy, dental caries activity, localized teeth with less than 50% of alveolar bone support)

   4. Intervals of 6 months to 1 year are recommended to clients who maintain excellent results for 1 year or longer and have been able to eliminate or control risk factors for oral disease (e.g., good oral hygiene, minimal calculus, no occlusal problems, no complicated prosthesis, no remaining pockets, no teeth with less than 50% of alveolar bone remaining, low risk for dental caries)
H. Documenting the outcomes of dental hygiene care aids in preventing possible legal charges related to inadequate documentation and client feeling inadequately informed about his or her oral health status; should include:
   1. Status and prognosis for the case, sites at risk for disease progression, and sites with disease progression
   2. Sites with plaque biofilm and calculus, bleeding, and areas of inflammation
   3. Need for restorative and periodontal treatment and for referral to a specialist
   4. Discussion that took place with the client regarding his or her health or disease status
   5. Past commitment of the client and recommendations suggested by the clinician
   6. Time interval required for the next appointment (continued-care interval)
   7. Acceptance or rejection of any further needed therapy

DOCUMENTATION

A. Definition—the process of accurately recording all aspects of the process of care, including assessment data, diagnosis, care plan, treatment rendered, client education, and evaluation findings, for the purpose of establishing the client's health record
B. Accurate documentation of all assessment findings is the legal responsibility of all clinicians (see Table 15-8)
C. Assessment findings should be clearly recorded and dated using ink on appropriate data collection forms: health history forms, extraoral and intraoral examination forms, dentition and periodontal charting forms, and radiographic interpretation forms
   1. Documentation and monitoring of abnormal lesions must be followed; if after 1 week to 10 days the lesion or abnormality remains, procedures should be implemented to diagnose the condition (e.g., excisional or incisional biopsy, brush biopsy) (see the section on "Diagnostic Tools for Oral Cancer Detection" in Chapter 16)
   2. Active disease or any deviations from normal should be documented and monitored
D. Additional information that was assessed (e.g., risk factors) and discussed with the client, but not charted, should be recorded on a record-of-services form
E. Diagnostic report documentation includes clearly written statements that connect assessment findings with possible causes that can be prevented, reduced, or resolved by dental hygiene interventions
F. Care-planning documentation, as previously mentioned, should outline all interventions needed to address client needs, including the estimated number of appointments

G. Implementation documentation is the recording of all treatments and educational interventions administered to the client, with the appropriate date of service; must include the signature of the provider of care

H. Documentation of evaluation includes the resulting outcomes of the interventions provided as well as any updated information found during the reassessment process; next steps are communicated to the client and detailed in the client's permanent record

ETHICAL, LEGAL, AND SAFETY ISSUES

Provision of comprehensive, quality care by licensed dental hygienists includes legal, ethical, and safety issues that require consideration.

A. Ethical issues that place hygienist at risk are:
1. Failure to refer to a medical professional or other dental specialist when indicated
2. Failure to maintain client confidentiality
3. Failure to perform a thorough case presentation so that a client can make an informed decision about the dental hygiene care
4. Failure to perform comprehensive assessment to detect oral diseases and abnormalities and degree of client risk for disease or disease progression

B. Legal issues that place hygienist at risk are:
1. Failure to comply with the Health Insurance Portability and Accountability Act (HIPAA); the clinician must verify that clients have read the HIPAA policy and obtain a written Acknowledgment of Receipt of the Notice from the client
2. Failure to assess, diagnose, treat, or refer for disease; even when under the supervision of a dentist, a licensed dental hygienist is accountable and responsible for client care
3. Failure to obtain written informed consent before initiating care
4. Failure to provide necessary care on the basis of assessment findings; constitutes "supervised neglect"
5. Failure to provide evidence-based care
6. Failure to document assessment, care plan, informed consent, services rendered, and client response to care

C. Safety issues that place the dental hygienist and the client at risk are:
1. Failure to protect a client from harm during care
2. Failure to assess accurately the client's health and pharmacologic history and to make necessary physician referrals
3. Failure to allow time during appointment for the provision of adequate care
4. Failure to evaluate therapy after completion of care or to recommend an appropriate continued-care interval
5. Failure to follow established protocol that protects the clinician and the client during therapy (e.g., standard precautions; see Chapter 10)
6. Failure to use instrumentation in effective and responsible manner (e.g., not using sharp instruments, not selecting appropriate instruments based on conditions present, and causing tissue trauma)
7. Failure to follow the manufacturer's instructions in the use of equipment, devices, and dental materials

Website Information and Resources

Source	Website Address	Description
Medline and PubMed	www.ncbi.nlm.nih.gov/pubmed/	Used for evidence-based decision making
Medline Plus	www.nlm.nih.gov/medlineplus/	Patient information on health topics and medication; medical encyclopedia
National Center for Dental Hygiene Research	www.usc.edu/hsc/dental/dhnet/	Focus for many dental hygiene research-related topics and links
Healthfinder	www.healthfinder.gov	Patient information on health topics, special population topics, health care, directory
Dimensions of Dental Hygiene	www.dimensionsofdentalhygiene.com/	Online journal with dental and dental hygiene–related topics
National Institutes of Health	www.nih.gov	Health topics, funding, news, events
American Academy of Periodontology	www.perio.org	Association website; parameters of practice and position papers related to the treatment of periodontal diseases
National Institute of Dental and Craniofacial Research	www.nidcr.nih.gov	Oral health information, educational resources and research
National Guideline Clearinghouse	www.guideline.gov	Evidence-based clinical practice guidelines
Centers for Disease Control and Prevention	www.cdc.gov	Health and safety topics, publications, data and statistics
Occupational Safety and Health Administration	www.osha.gov	Information on the health and safety of employees
RxList	www.rxlist.com/script/main/hp.asp	Information related to prescription medications
Merck Manual	www.merck.com	Information related to medical conditions
MyMedicineList	www.safemedication.com	Database containing important medication information
Aetna InteliHealth (Harvard Medical School-Intelihealth Partnership)	www.intelihealth.com	Consumer information related to health and medicine
U.S. Department of Health and Human Services	www.hhs.gov/ocr/privacy/	Health information privacy

REFERENCES

1. Darby ML, Walsh MM, editors: *Dental hygiene theory and practice,* ed 4, St Louis, 2015, Saunders.
2. American Dental Hygienists Association: *Standards for clinical dental hygiene practice,* Chicago, 2008, ADHA.
3. Commission on Dental Accreditation: *Accreditation standards for dental hygiene education programs,* Chicago, 2013, American Dental Association.
4. American Dental Hygienists Association: *Policy manual: ADHA framework for theory development—1,* Chicago, 2005, ADHA.
5. Darby ML, Walsh MM: A proposed human needs conceptual model for dental hygiene. Part I, *J Dent Hyg* 67(6):326–334, 1993.
6. Darby ML, Walsh MM: Application of the human needs conceptual model of dental hygiene to the role of the clinician. Part II, *J Dent Hyg* 67(6):335–346, 1993.
7. Darby ML, Walsh MM: Application of the human needs conceptual model to dental hygiene practice, *J Dent Hyg* 74 (3):230–237, 2000.
8. American Academy of Periodontology: Statement on comprehensive periodontal therapy, 2010: http://www.perio.org/resoures-products/posppr3-4. Accessed July 24, 2015.
9. Pickett AF: Personal, dental and health histories. In Darby ML, Walsh MM, editors: *Dental hygiene theory and practice,* ed 4, St Louis, 2015, Saunders.
10. Pires IL, Cota LO, Oliveira AC, Costa JE: Association between periodontal conditions and use of tongue piercing, *J Clin Periodontol* 37(8):712–718, 2010.
11. Fontana M, Young DA, Wolff MS, et al: Defining dental caries for 2010 and beyond, *Dent Clin North Am* 54(3):423–440, 2010.
12. Pimlott JF, Leakey JD: Assessment of the dentition. In Darby ML, Walsh MM, editors: *Dental hygiene theory and practice,* ed 4, St Louis, 2015, Saunders.
13. Hinrichs JE: The role of dental calculus and other predisposing factors. In Newman MG, Takei HH, Klokkevold PR, Carranza FA, editors: *Clinical periodontology,* ed 12, St Louis, 2015, Saunders.
14. Chan DCN, Chung AKH: Management of idiopathic subgingival amalgam hypertrophy: the common amalgam overhang, *Operat Dent* 34(6):753–758, 2009.
15. American Academy of Periodontology: Guidelines for periodontal therapy, *J Periodontol* 72:1624–1628, 2001.
16. American Academy of Periodontology: Parameter on occlusal traumatism in patients with chronic periodontitis, *J Periodontol* 71:873–875, 2000.
17. Giannobile WV: Salivary diagnostics for periodontal diseases, *J Am Dent Assoc* 143(10 Suppl):6–11, 2012.
18. Lockhart P, Bolger A, Papapanou P, et al: Periodontal disease and atherosclerotic vascular disease: does the evidence support an independent association? AHA Scientific Statement, *Circulation* 125:2520, 2012.
19. American Academy of Periodontology: Parameter on systemic conditions affected by periodontal diseases, *J Periodontol* 71:880–883, 2000.
20. Fiore MC, Bailey WC, Cohen SJ, et al: Treating tobacco use and dependence: clinical practice guideline, Rockville, Md, 2000, US Department of Health and Human Services, Public Health Service.
21. Novak KF, Goodman SF, Takei HH: Determination of prognosis. In Newman MG, Takei HH, Klokkevold PR, Carranza FA, editors: *Clinical periodontology,* ed 12, St Louis, 2015, Saunders.
22. Forrest JL: Introduction to the basics of evidence-based dentistry: concepts and skills, *J Evid Based Dent Pract* 9(3):108–112, 2009.
23. Forrest JL, Miller SA: Translating evidence-based decision making into practice: EBDM concepts and finding the evidence, *J Evid Based Dent Pract* 9(2):59–72, 2009.
24. Merin RL: Supportive periodontal treatment. In Newman MG, Takei HH, Klokkevold PR, Carranza FA, editors: *Clinical periodontology,* ed 12, St Louis, 2015, Saunders.
25. Pence S: Polishing particulars, *Dimens Dent Hyg* 11(6):24–28, 2013.

SUGGESTED READINGS

American Academy of Periodontology: Guidelines for the management of patients with periodontal diseases, *J Periodontol* 77 (9):1607–1611, 2006.

Beemsterboer PL: *Ethics and law in dental hygiene,* ed 3, Philadelphia, 2010, Saunders.

Featherstone J, Roth JR: Curing the silent epidemic: caries management in the 21st century and beyond, *J Calif Dent Assoc* 35(10):681–685, 2007.

Featherstone J, Young DA, Domejean-Orliaguet S: Caries risk assessment in practice for age 6 though adult, *J Calif Dent Assoc* 35 (10):703–713, 2007.

Forrest JL: Introduction to the basics of evidence-based dentistry: concepts and skills, *J Evid Based Dent Pract* 9(3):108–112, 2009.

Forrest JL, Miller SA: Translating evidence-based decision making into practice: EBDM concepts and finding the evidence, *J Evid Based Dent Pract* 9(2):59–72, 2009.

Friedewald VE, Kornman KS, Beck JD, et al: The *American Journal of Cardiology* and *Journal of Periodontology* Editors' Consensus: Periodontitis and atherosclerotic cardiovascular disease, *J Periodontol* 80:1021–1032, 2009.

Little JW, Miller C, Rhodus NL, Falace D: *Dental management of the medically compromised patient,* ed 7, St Louis, 2008, Mosby.

Malamed SF: *Medical emergencies in the dental office,* ed 6, St Louis, 2007, Mosby.

Mealey BL, Oates TW: Diabetes mellitus and periodontal diseases, *J Periodontol* 77:1289–1303, 2006.

Miller SA, Forrest JL: Translating evidence-based decision making into practice: appraising and applying the evidence, *J Evid Based Dent Pract* 9(4):164–182, 2009.

Ramos-Gomez F, Crall J, Gansky S, et al: Caries risk assessment appropriate for the age 1 visit (infants and toddlers), *J Calif Dent Assoc* 35(10):687–702, 2007.

Wartenberg D, Thompson WD: Privacy versus public health: the impact of current confidentiality rules, *Am J Public Health* 100 (3):407–412, 2010.

Wun E, Dym H: How to implement a HIPAA compliance plan into a practice, *Dent Clin North Am* 52(3):669–682, 2008.

CHAPTER 15 REVIEW QUESTIONS

Answers and rationales to chapter review questions are available on this text's accompanying Evolve site. See inside front cover for details.

evolve

CASE A

A 44-year-old man presents as a new client for dental hygiene care. His medical history reveals type 2 diabetes, high blood pressure (BP) controlled with medication, and a hip replacement. He reports no blood glucose monitoring and controls diabetes with diet and exercise. He had a physical examination last year but is not sure of the examination results. He assumes "everything is fine." You record his BP reading at 150/102 mm Hg.

Use Case A to answer questions 1 to 4.

1. **Which of the following should be considered before implementing dental hygiene care for this client?**
   a. Dental hygiene care can be implemented immediately without any considerations.
   b. Dental hygiene care can be started immediately as long as the client consents to treatment.
   c. Consult with client's physician to establish a definitive diagnosis of diabetes and level of control for diabetes and hypertension before initiating dental hygiene care.
   d. Appointments should be longer than normal to reduce the number of appointments needed and to reduce stress.

2. **What is this client's ASA physical status (PS) classification?**
   a. PS1
   b. PS2
   c. PS3
   d. PS4

3. **What is the BEST course of action for the dental hygienist related to the BP reading?**
   a. Recheck BP in 5 minutes; if it is still elevated within that range, dismiss the client and seek immediate consultation with physician
   b. Recheck BP at each appointment; if it is still within range for three consecutive appointments, refer to physician
   c. Recheck BP in 5 minutes; if it is still elevated within that range, continue with noninvasive care only and consult with physician before dental hygiene therapy
   d. Recheck BP in 5 minutes, and continue with dental hygiene care

4. **Which human need should be considered during the dental hygiene process of care?**
   a. Freedom from head and neck pain
   b. Protection from health risks
   c. Skin and mucous membrane integrity of head and neck
   d. Wholesome facial image

CASE B

A 25-year-old female presents for dental hygiene care. Her records indicated that 10 months have lapsed since receiving dental hygiene care, and she scheduled the appointment because her teeth are sensitive when she eats candy and her "gums" hurt when she brushes her teeth. She reports an arrhythmia but is not sure of the type or cause and irregularly takes the prescribed medication for its treatment. Her vital signs are within normal limits. During the dental and periodontal assessment, you record generalized marginal gingival inflammation, generalized moderate interproximal subgingival calculus deposits, generalized bleeding on probing, with 2-mm to 4-mm probing depths. Existing restorations include teeth #14-MO, #4-MOD, #13-MO, #18-MO, and #19-B. Radiographs reveal no evidence of bone loss, proximal carious lesions on #29 D, #30 M, and #19 M and restoration overhangs on #14 M and #4 D. She brushes once a day and does not use an interproximal cleaning aid.

Use Case B to answer questions 5 to 11.

5. **Which of the following conditions represents the MOST accurate periodontal disease classification?**
   a. Case type I—gingivitis
   b. Case type II—mild periodontitis
   c. Case type III—moderate periodontitis
   d. Case type IV—advanced periodontitis

6. **All the following human need categories relate to the client's current conditions EXCEPT one. Which one is the *exception*?**
   a. Protection from health risks
   b. Freedom from anxiety and stress
   c. Skin and mucous membrane integrity of head and neck
   d. Biologically sound and functional dentition

7. **All the following are related to the overhanging restorations EXCEPT:**
   a. Increase bacterial plaque biofilm retention
   b. Restorations should be replaced
   c. Restorations are risk factors for periodontal disease
   d. Restorations are treated using margination procedures

8. **Based on the oral assessment findings, what is the classification of caries risk for this client?**
   a. Low risk
   b. Moderate risk
   c. High risk
   d. Insufficient data to determine

9. **The restoration on tooth #14 would be BEST classified as a:**
   a. Class I restoration

b. Class II restoration
c. Class III restoration
d. Class IV restoration

10. **Based on the periodontal assessment, what is the BEST reevaluation interval for this client?**
   a. 1 to 2 weeks
   b. 4 to 6 weeks
   c. 3 to 4 months
   d. 6 months to 1 year

11. **What is the overall prognosis for this client after phase I therapy?**
   a. Excellent
   b. Good
   c. Fair
   d. Poor

CASE C

A heavy tea drinker just purchased over-the-counter whitening strips to see if her discolored teeth could be whitened. She wants to know if using whitening strips is better than using the professional custom tray bleaching system at home. You want to provide an evidence-based answer, based on a search of the research literature.

Use Case C to answer questions 12 and 13.

12. **Which of the following would be an example of a well-developed question to help narrow your research literature search?**
   a. For clients with discolored teeth, are whitening strips the best method to increase whitening?
   b. Are whitening strips the best method to increase whitening?
   c. Are whitening strips more effective than custom tray bleaching systems?
   d. For clients with tooth discoloration from tea stain, are whitening strips more effective in increasing teeth whitening compared with professional at-home custom tray bleaching?

13. **Which type of study will provide the BEST evidence to answer the client's question?**
   a. Case-control studies
   b. Randomized controlled clinical trials
   c. In vitro research
   d. Case reports

14. **A dental hygienist records a client's blood pressure as 152/85 mm Hg. What blood pressure category is represented?**
   a. Prehypertension
   b. Stage I hypertension
   c. Stage II hypertension
   d. Stage III hypertension

15. **What phase of dental care focuses on periodontal surgery?**
   a. Preliminary phase
   b. Phase I
   c. Phase II
   d. Phase III

16. **The written care plan includes all the following components EXCEPT:**
   a. Appointment sequence for therapy to be provided
   b. Approximate time for each appointment
   c. Cost of each presented procedure
   d. Expected outcomes and limitations of care

17. **When localized bleeding on probing is noted during a 4- to 6-week reevaluation appointment, all following procedures are required EXCEPT:**
   a. Determining presence of residual or new deposits
   b. Establishment of continued-care (recare) interval
   c. Evaluation of self-care practices
   d. Referral to physician

18. **Which is a CORRECT statement regarding the assessment phase of care?**
   a. It includes the comprehensive collection, analysis, and permanent documentation of client data.
   b. It involves the collection of only subjective information.
   c. Assessment data should be updated only during continued-care (recare) appointments.
   d. Data should *not* be discussed with the client or appropriate health care providers.

19. **When reviewing a health history, the client has indicated that he has allergies to kiwis, avocados, and bananas. For what condition is this client at risk?**
   a. Acute adrenal insufficiency
   b. Asthma
   c. Diabetes
   d. Latex allergy

20. **The American Academy of Periodontology (AAP) classification for advanced periodontitis is:**
   a. Case type I
   b. Case type II
   c. Case type III
   d. Case type IV

21. **All the following factors are considered when providing dental hygiene care for diabetic clients EXCEPT:**
   a. Cardiovascular conditions
   b. Continued-care (recare) interval
   c. Susceptibility to oral infection
   d. Rapid healing

22. **Individuals with stable angina pectoris, COPD, and/or mild congestive heart failure are in which ASA physical status (PS) classification category?**

    a. PS1
    b. PS2
    c. PS3
    d. PS4

23. **What phase of the dental hygiene process of care immediately follows diagnosis?**
    a. Assessment
    b. Evaluation
    c. Implementation
    d. Planning

24. **All the following are components of assessment EXCEPT:**
    a. Health history
    b. Intraoral photographs
    c. Periodontal probing
    d. Self-care education

25. **After a comprehensive assessment, findings show chronic periodontitis with moderate bone loss, generalized pocket depths of 4 to 6 mm with bleeding, light subgingival biofilm and calculus on the maxillary arch, and moderate to heavy subgingival biofilm and tenacious calculus on the mandibular arch. Based on these findings, what would be a realistic approach to nonsurgical periodontal therapy (NSPT) for this client?**
    a. A 60-minute appointment consisting of oral self-care education and supragingival and subgingival debridement
    b. Two 60-minute appointments consisting of oral self-care education, debridement, and scaling and root planing
    c. Five 60- to 90-minute appointments consisting of oral self-care education, debridement, scaling and root planing, and reevaluation
    d. Six 60- to 90-minute appointments consisting of oral self-care education, debridement, scaling and root planing, and reevaluation

26. **When client-oriented goals are developed during the planning phase of care, to what do affective goals relate?**
    a. Increasing client's knowledge level about bacterial biofilm
    b. Influencing changes in beliefs and attitudes
    c. Providing information related to bacterial biofilm
    d. Modifying a toothbrushing method

27. **When reviewing a health history, the client has indicated that she urinates more than six times a day, she is frequently thirsty, and her mouth is always dry. What condition manifests these characteristics?**
    a. Asthma
    b. Diabetes mellitus
    c. Hypertension
    d. Thyroid disease

28. **Which of the following conditions is indicated by yellow sclera of the eye?**
    a. Difficulty breathing
    b. Drug abuse
    c. Jaundice
    d. Medical emergency status

29. **What is the G.V. Black classification of dental caries and restoration located on the gingival buccal third of tooth #18?**
    a. Class II
    b. Class III
    c. Class IV
    d. Class V

30. **A client presents with a type III overhang on an amalgam restoration. Which of the following statements related to this overhang is CORRECT?**
    a. Covers less than one third of interproximal space
    b. Restoration indicated for replacement
    c. Indicated for a margination procedure
    d. Clinically not detectable

31. **All the following represent standard client assessment information that is necessary for planning comprehensive dental hygiene care EXCEPT:**
    a. Extraoral assessment
    b. Current self-care practices
    c. Dentition evaluation
    d. Fluoride varnish application

32. **A 53-year-old client presents for a periodontal maintenance appointment. When developing a dental hygiene care plan, which of the following should be addressed first?**
    a. Chlorhexidine stain on teeth
    b. Localized light plaque
    c. Pain on tooth #28
    d. Smoking habit

33. **Which of the following is the BEST method for examining the mentalis muscle?**
    a. Circular compression
    b. Digital palpation
    c. Indirect vision
    d. Auscultation

34. **Which of the following is LEAST significant when determining the continued-care (recare) interval for periodontal maintenance therapy?**
    a. Presence of light plaque biofilm
    b. Elimination of pocket depths
    c. Bleeding on probing
    d. Cost of care

35. **Assessment findings reveal that an 11-year-old client has deep pits and fissures, generalized areas of heavy plaque, marginal gingival inflammation, and incipient carious lesions on teeth #3 and #14, #19, and #30. Given these findings, what would be the degree of caries risk?**
    a. Low
    b. Moderate
    c. High
    d. No risk

36. **A client cannot correctly demonstrate the use of the threader with floss. The discrepancy in performance is MOST likely the result of which of the following?**
    a. Management deficiency
    b. Motivation
    c. Readiness to learn
    d. Skills deficiency

37. **To engage in effective verbal behaviors, which one of the following skills is necessary?**
    a. Appropriate voice tone
    b. Gestures
    c. Paraphrasing
    d. Posture

38. **All the following are included in the case presentation EXCEPT:**
    a. Desired outcomes of treatment
    b. Alternative approaches to care
    c. Risks of all proposed therapeutic options
    d. Treatment outcome guarantee

39. **Which of the following BEST identifies the procedure that is immediately followed after a client declines a component of the dental hygiene care plan?**
    a. Alternative approaches to care are suggested.
    b. Outcomes of therapy are explained.
    c. Informed refusal form is completed.
    d. Client's right to decline care is clarified.

40. **What would be a reasonable prognosis for a client with chronic periodontitis and moderate bone loss with localized areas of grade II furcation involvement, improvable oral self-care methods, and irregular continued-care (recare) intervals?**
    a. Excellent
    b. Good
    c. Fair
    d. Poor

41. **Failure to refer a client to a medical professional when indicated constitutes which one of the following?**
    a. Ethical issue
    b. Legal issue
    c. Safety issue
    d. Breach of contract

42. **When implementing a tobacco cessation program into practice, the second step is:**
    a. Ask
    b. Advise
    c. Assist
    d. Arrange

43. **When providing dental hygiene care, all the following relate to safe practice issues EXCEPT:**
    a. Failure to obtain written informed consent
    b. Failure to provide comprehensive care
    c. Failure to follow infection control protocol
    d. Failure to use proper instrumentation during the provision of dental hygiene care

44. **What is a grade III furcation involvement?**
    a. Exposure of furcation with bone remaining between roots
    b. Complete loss of bone between roots
    c. Loss of some bone between roots
    d. Severe bone loss and furcation clearly visible

45. **To determine a care plan that is BEST for a client, which of the following actions should be addressed FIRST?**
    a. Periodontal debridement for the entire mouth
    b. Consultation and treatment for areas of pain
    c. Tobacco cessation counseling
    d. Consultation for periodontal surgery

46. **When reviewing the health history, the client indicates that he has a persistent cough that is nonproductive, difficulty breathing, and night sweats. What condition is manifested by these characteristics?**
    a. Acute adrenal insufficiency
    b. Asthma
    c. Tuberculosis
    d. Common cold

47. **Which of the following conditions is often related to a nutritional deficiency?**
    a. Black hairy tongue
    b. Burning tongue
    c. Geographic tongue
    d. Macroglossia

48. **The term *prognosis* refers specifically to which of the following?**
    a. Diagnosis
    b. Care planning
    c. Evaluation
    d. Prediction

49. **What recare interval is recommended for a client who has maintained good results for the first year following routine nonsurgical periodontal therapy, but displays localized pockets?**
    a. 1 to 2 months
    b. 3 to 4 months
    c. 4 to 6 months
    d. 6 months

50. **The submental glands are BEST examined using which type of palpation?**
    a. Bilateral digital
    b. Circular compression
    c. Digital palpation
    d. Auscultation

51. **Which of the following conditions requires prophylactic antibiotic premedication for dental hygiene care?**
    a. Rheumatic heart disease
    b. Functional heart murmur
    c. Prosthetic heart valve
    d. Mitral valve prolapse with regurgitation

Strategies for Oral Health Promotion and Disease Prevention and Control

*M. Anjum Shah**

The promotion of oral health and the prevention of oral diseases are fundamental to dental hygiene practice and distinguish the profession from other health disciplines. As a provider of preventive and therapeutic services, a dental hygienist must use evidence-based strategies and interventions that support prevention-oriented health care. The success of a preventive oral health program depends on a client's self-care behaviors. Therefore, a dental hygienist must be knowledgeable about behavior change theories and be able to employ behavior change models designed to motivate client adherence to appropriate self-care regimens. This chapter focuses on the dental hygienist's role in health promotion at the individual level.

PREVENTIVE CARE PLANNING

Basic Concepts

A. Initiation and progression of oral diseases depend on the interaction of host, agent, and environmental factors; thus, prevention and control of these diseases require attention to all primary and modifying factors in each category.

B. Dental caries and inflammatory periodontal diseases are complex disease states that involve colonization by specific pathogenic bacteria in dental plaque biofilm; none will occur in the absence of pathogenic bacteria in biofilm; thus the control of plaque biofilm is essential in any oral disease prevention program

C. The discipline of dental hygiene is based on disease prevention, halting disease progression, and maintenance of oral health

D. Effective preventive programs assess disease risk and identify active disease; clients at high risk for dental caries, periodontal disease, and oral lesions require multiple preventive strategies applied frequently and aggressively (see the sections on "Epidemiology of Periodontal Diseases and Related Risks" in Chapter 14 and "Risk Factor Assessments" and Table 15-6 in Chapter 15)

E. The prevention of oral disease requires the participation of clients who understand oral disease processes and personal level of risk; skills in implementing oral self-care, health literacy, and the motivation to practice preventive behaviors to

decrease the level of risk also are key to preventing oral disease

F. Many strategies can facilitate changes in the health behaviors of clients; a grasp of the basic concepts underlying educational, motivational, and behavioral theory is necessary to understand the variables influencing a person's oral health beliefs, attitudes, values, and behaviors

G. Assisting clients in adopting effective oral care practices follows the dental hygiene process-of-care model

BEHAVIOR CHANGE THEORY[1]

Human Behavior Principles

A. Values
1. Values form the basis for behaviors
2. Clients come to the dental hygienist with existing values
3. Conflicts between clients' existing values and those values that support and enable preventive oral health care practices must be recognized and resolved
4. Clients who have value systems that support preventive health behaviors will adopt new behaviors that fit readily into their existing value system

B. Motivation
1. Definition—a desire to fulfill an unmet human need (deficit); an inner force that causes a person to act; motivation may be internally or externally generated
   a. Internally generated motivation focuses on one's own perceived needs; generally longer lasting
   b. Externally generated motivation is based on offers of reward or punishment; generally of shorter duration

Maslow's Hierarchy of Needs[2]

A. Theory about human nature that is used to explain the motivational process; Maslow suggested that inner forces (needs) drive a person to action; he classified needs in a pyramid according to their importance to the client, his or her ability to motivate self, and the importance placed on the needs being satisfied; only when a client's lower needs are met will a client become concerned about higher-level needs; once the needs have been met, they no longer function as motivators (Fig. 16-1)

B. Hierarchy of needs
1. Physiologic—survival needs are the most powerful and must be met before any others; include the components

---

*M. Anjum Shah and the publisher acknowledge the past contributions of Catherine Mary Dean and Jacquelyn L. Fried to this chapter.

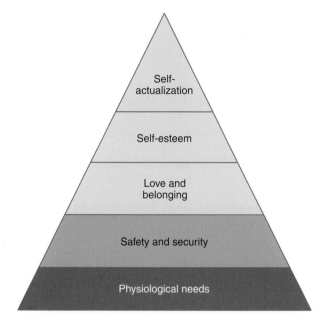

FIG 16-1 Maslow's hierarchy of needs. (From Darby ML, Walsh MM: *Dental hygiene theory and practice,* ed 4, Philadelphia, 2014, Saunders. Modified from Potter PA, Perry AG: *Fundamentals of nursing,* ed 8, St Louis, 2012, Mosby.)

necessary for body homeostasis, such as food, water, oxygen, sleep, temperature regulation, and sex
2. Security and safety—these needs are required for protection against physical or psychological damage and are more cognitive than physiologic in nature; include shelter, a job for economic self-sufficiency, and a well-organized and stable environment
3. Social—once the physiologic and security needs have been met, then the needs for love and social belonging become prime motivators; include belonging to a group and having the chance to give and receive friendship and love
4. Esteem or ego—of the two categories of needs that exist at this level, one involves feelings of worth, such as competence, achievement, mastery, and independence; the other involves gaining the esteem of others and triggers learning and the desire to acquire status, power, and higher-level skills
5. Self-actualization or self-realization—these needs drive the client to reach the very top of his or her field; based on positive actions toward development, growth, and self-enhancement
C. Application—assessment of a client's level of needs may aid in the identification of motivational factors that can be targeted for enhancing behavior change

Health Belief Model[3]

A. Based on the concept that one's beliefs direct behavior; the model is used to explain and predict health behaviors and acceptance of health recommendations; the emphasis is on the perceived world of a client, which may differ from objective reality

B. Components
1. Susceptibility—clients must believe that they are susceptible to a particular disease or condition
2. Severity—clients must believe that if they contract the particular disease or condition, the consequences will be serious
3. Asymptomatic nature of disease—clients must believe that a disease can be present without their being fully aware of it
4. Benefit of behavior change—clients must believe that effective means of preventing or controlling the potential or current problem exist, and that action on their part will produce positive results
C. Cues to action—once these beliefs have been accepted, the client will act on them, when necessary; the stronger the beliefs, the greater the potential that appropriate action will occur

Trans-Theoretical Model[3,4]

A. Conceptualizes behavior change through a series of steps; progression through the steps depends on the balance of the advantages and disadvantages of the decision
B. Provides a framework to determine and select appropriate interventions to assist clients in improving their health behaviors
C. Stages of change include:
1. Precontemplation—the client has no intention of making a change within the next 6 months
2. Contemplation—the client intends to make a change within the next 6 months
3. Preparation—the client intends to make a change within the next 30 days and has taken some behavioral steps in this direction
4. Action—the client has practiced changed behaviors for less than 6 months
5. Maintenance—the client has practiced changed behaviors for more than 6 months

Motivation Theories[3]

A. Locus of control
1. Internal locus of control—clients believe that they have control over their own outcomes and that their behavior will make a difference; they are most likely to adopt preventive health behaviors
2. External locus of control—clients believe that the outcomes are out of their control and that whatever they do will not affect the outcomes; they are less likely to change behaviors and rely more on the dental professional to take care of their problems
B. Attribution theory
1. Involves explanations given for performance; influences client's feelings about self
2. The success or failure at performing a behavior is influenced by the client's thoughts[1]
3. Self-efficacy—the client's level of self-confidence affects his or her belief in the success of performing a behavior

Motivational Interviewing: Evidenced-Based Approach[5–8]

A. Motivational interviewing (MI)—form of collaborative conversation for strengthening a person's motivation and commitment to change
1. Client-centered counseling style for addressing the common problem of ambivalence about change
2. Designed to strengthen an individual's motivation for and movement toward a specific goal by eliciting and exploring the person's own reasons for change within an atmosphere of acceptance and empathy
3. Shown to have positive effects on health behavior change related to smoking, exercise and weight reduction, diabetes management, medication adherence, condom use, and oral health
B. Using the guiding principles of MI, the dental hygienist asks open-ended questions designed to elicit a client's desire, ability, reasons, and need for change ("change talk");
1. Collaborative exploration accomplished through four key principles of MI:
   a. Resisting the righting reflex (refraining from trying to fix the problem)
   b. Understanding the client's motivation
   c. Listening to the client
   d. Empowering the client
2. Identifying the client's stages of change is also an important component in the use of MI
3. Use of these principles enables the client to express his or her view of the pros and cons associated with a particular behavior and to determine what action, if any, to take
4. Ultimately, the decision to change resides within the client, not the clinician; in this sense, the dental hygienist allows the client to have complete autonomy in the decision-making process

Concepts of Effective Teaching

See Table 19-14 for dental management considerations for clients who have special needs.
A. Effective teaching involves the facilitation of learning to help make positive changes in a person's behaviors
B. To maximize learning, these four principles apply to the design of an educational plan:
1. Small step size—present only what person can assimilate in one session; provide conceptual or factual information when the "need to know" is evident
2. Active participation—provide time and opportunity for the person to ask questions; offer suggestions and monitor the practicing of new skills to enhance learning and retention
3. Immediate feedback—provide the learner with early and frequent information regarding progress; make suggestions for improvement, and use positive reinforcement to support and encourage learning
4. Self-pacing—recognize that each person will progress at a different pace; recognize the learner's needs, and establish an instructional pace tailored to each client

C. Visual aids enhance verbal instructions
1. Use of visual aids available in print or on the Internet can enhance client comprehension of oral hygiene instructions
2. Demonstration of dental plaque biofilm control techniques on models before intraoral demonstration may be helpful
3. Written instructions and illustrated pamphlets reinforce in-office instructions
4. Use of an intraoral camera that projects images on a monitor enables clients to see the conditions in their mouth

Factors Influencing Client Adherence to Preventive Regimen

A. Client-clinician relationship
1. The quality of communication and the relationship between the client and the hygienist is critical to achieving client adherence
2. Clients must be encouraged to share the responsibility for their oral health
3. Authoritarian or autocratic verbal and nonverbal messages from the dental hygienist will be less effective than messages that allow for genuine client involvement and assumption of responsibility
4. The dental hygienist must recognize that established behaviors are difficult to change because they generally satisfy needs; new behaviors are adopted slowly
B. Health literacy[9]
1. The ability to comprehend health, medical, dental, and overall health information
2. Clients who exhibit greater understanding of information provided in the health care setting are more likely to be compliant in home care instructions
3. Low dental health literacy is considered a barrier to good oral health outcomes
4. Clinicians need to explain health related information in an easily understandable vocabulary
5. Screening instruments are available to evaluate a client's health literacy
C. Client's support systems
1. Client's lifestyle and significant others influence the client's willingness and ability to carry out self-care regimens
2. Support systems are important, especially with children and clients with disabilities, who must depend on caregivers to carry out home care practices
D. Complexity of therapy
1. Clients must agree that time and effort required to practice preventive behaviors are reasonable
2. Changes in basic lifestyle are more difficult to achieve than modest modifications to existing behaviors
3. Product cost and availability affect adherence to oral self-care regimens

Prevention Principles for Children

A. Proactive counseling of parents about anticipated developmental changes in their children

---

BOX 16-1   Tips for Dental Hygienists Working with Children

When a child visits your practice, your priority is to create a positive dental experience. The child is more important than his or her teeth. Incorporating the ideas from this fact sheet as you interact with children will help them to become both comfortable and compliant.

Make the reception area a friendly, colorful place. Include toys, games, and videos. Books about visiting a dental office and a doll dressed as an oral health care provider will help children discuss any fears they may have.

Each staff member should greet the child by name in a friendly and welcoming manner. Bend down or squat so that you are at the level of the child's head, and listen to what the child has to say.

The treatment room should be decorated in a way that is visually accessible and appealing to children. Show the child the instruments you will be using, and explain how they are used. Make everything that looks unfamiliar look friendly. For example, you might draw friendly faces on masks used for demonstration, and some practitioners like to call the suction "Mr. Thirsty." Demonstrate the buttons on the chair and how it moves up and down, but do not put the chair back if doing so makes the child nervous.

Allow the parent into the treatment area if the child desires, especially for the first visit. Both you and the room will look less frightening with a familiar face present.

Explain exactly what you are going to do during the appointment. Use age-appropriate terms to explain why it is so important that teeth be kept healthy.

Turn the appointment into a game. For example, count eyes, ears, and fingers before moving on to counting teeth. Always give the child a choice of flavors. Write down preferences so that you will have all the child's favorites ready for the next visit. If the light shines in the child's eyes, produce a pair of sunglasses and say how cool he or she looks.

Use a new toothbrush presented during the brushing lesson. Apply fluoride varnish. Let the child know that you are in control, with a fast solution to every problem.

Praise the good, but don't criticize the bad. A child may take "these teeth don't look so good" very personally and feel he or she has done something wrong. Concentrate on teaching the proper way to take care of teeth.

Don't use tricks or lie; keep your promises. If you say, "Just let me do one more thing," do it and let the child go. If a child will not cooperate, try again another day.

When the visit is over, let the child pick a treat from a "treasure box." Praise good behavior, and let the child give the parent the "good news" about the child's teeth.

Snap a picture of the child's sparkling smile and create a gallery of photos in the office. Seeing his or her own picture is something a child can look forward to at the next appointment.

Modified from American Dental Hygienists' Association: Tips for dental hygienists working with kids [members-only section, requires registration and password].

B. Information provided to parents or caregivers in appropriate-sized "bites" on the basis of the developmental milestone anticipated in their children

C. Guidance is based on the rationale that people are ready to apply information that is most relevant to them and their children

D. Box 16-1 provides suggestions for obtaining compliance from pediatric clients

DENTAL PLAQUE BIOFILM DETECTION

General Considerations

A. Because dental plaque biofilm is relatively invisible and tooth surfaces are not easily accessed, teaching clients dental disease-control skills can be challenging

B. Agents that make biofilm visible supragingivally can enhance the teaching-learning process by:
   1. Demonstrating a relationship between the presence of plaque biofilm and the clinical signs of disease
   2. Guiding the development of skills that are applied before biofilm removal
   3. Allowing evaluation of the effectiveness of skills that are applied after biofilm removal
   4. Promoting self-evaluation of skills that are applied by the client at home

C. The presence of subgingival plaque biofilm cannot be demonstrated by using disclosing agents

D. The plan for disease control education should include establishing the associations among the presence of plaque, clinical signs of disease such as bleeding, the presence of risk factors, and possible links to systemic disease

E. Subgingival biofilm detection by the client is best managed when the client has an understanding of the gingival sulcus (or pocket) and of the clinical changes that occur with ineffective plaque biofilm removal

Disclosing Agents

A. Erythrosin (FD&C Red No. 3 or No. 28)
   1. A red dye available in tablet or solution form; most widely used agent
   2. Can be dissolved into a solution or chewed to dissolve in mouth
   3. Tends to stain soft tissues, making postapplication evaluation of gingiva difficult

B. Fluorescein dye (FD&C Yellow No. 8)
   1. Plaque biofilm stained with sodium fluorescein; visible only with use of an ultraviolet light source
   2. More expensive to use but has the advantage of not interfering with gingival assessment or leaving a visible stain on oral tissues

C. Two-tone dyes (FD&C Red No. 3 and Green No. 3)
   1. Combination solution; has the advantage of differentiating mature plaque biofilm (stains blue) from new plaque biofilm (stains red)
   2. Discloses plaque biofilm but not gingival tissues

D. Precautions
   1. Avoid staining restorative materials that may be susceptible to permanent discoloration
   2. Dispense the solution into a disposable cup; do not contaminate the solution by introducing applicators into the storage container bottle

3. To avoid staining the lips, apply a light coat of nonpetroleum or water-based lubricant (e.g., K-Y jelly)
4. Avoid using the agent before application of a dental sealant
5. Avoid any risk of staining clothing, that is, provide appropriate protective drapes to the client, and use small amounts of the solution

Plaque and Gingival Indices

Recording a plaque score at consecutive appointments enables the client to see progress (see Table 20-11 for information on indices and computing indices).

MECHANICAL PLAQUE BIOFILM CONTROL ON FACIAL, LINGUAL, AND OCCLUSAL TOOTH SURFACES

Basic Concepts

A. Microbial population of dental plaque biofilm contributes to the initiation of dental caries and periodontal diseases
B. Mechanical disruption of organized plaque biofilm colonies, both supragingivally and subgingivally, is effective and widely used to prevent and control dental diseases
C. Toothbrushing—most widely used and effective means of controlling plaque biofilm
D. Toothbrushes are available in many shapes, sizes, and textures
E. The selection of the type of toothbrush should be based on the client's needs, oral characteristics, and preferences
F. Special attention to subgingival plaque biofilm control in areas greater than 3 mm is essential; toothbrushes are generally ineffective in depths greater than 3 mm and in furcations; additional tools must be selected
G. Toothbrushes should be replaced after 2 to 3 months of use and when filaments become bent or splayed
H. Clients who are immunosuppressed, debilitated, or diagnosed with a known infection and those about to undergo surgery should disinfect their toothbrushes or use disposable ones

Manual Toothbrushes

A. Description
   1. Parts include the handle, head, and shank; the head, or the working end, holds clusters of bristles (tufts) in a pattern
   2. Design variables
      a. Handle can be in the same plane with the head or offset at an angle
      b. The length varies, with adult brushes being longer than those recommended for children
      c. Tuft placement can be in two to four rows, with 5 to 12 tufts per row; bristles may be of varying lengths
      d. The brushing planes can be even, flat, or uneven
      e. Many brushes have contoured or thick handles, angled shanks, and flexible heads

   3. Bristle characteristics
      a. Nylon bristles, or filaments, are manufactured for uniformity in texture, shape, and size; nonabsorbent nylon bristles are easily cleaned, dry quickly, and are durable
      b. Relative stiffness—the diameter and length of filaments determine whether the brush will be ranked hard, medium, soft, or extra-soft; variations exist among products from different manufacturers
B. Desirable characteristics of toothbrushes
   1. Conform to individual requirements in size, shape, and texture
   2. Easily and efficiently manipulated
   3. Readily cleaned and aerated
   4. Impervious to moisture
   5. Durable and inexpensive
   6. Flexible and soft
   7. Contain rounded-end filaments
C. Factors in toothbrush selection and recommendations
   1. Oral health status
   2. Recommended method of brushing
   3. Periodontal status
   4. Client's age, dexterity, and ability to use the brush in an effective, nontraumatic manner
   5. Client's preference and motivation
   6. Unique, special needs of the client (e.g., arthritis, Parkinson's disease; see Chapter 19)
D. Soft brush head design is important for effective plaque removal and minimal likelihood of trauma to soft and hard tissues[4]
E. Both angled and standard toothbrush designs have little impact on plaque removal capacity; both designs prevent gingival recession as long as soft-bristled toothbrush is used

Manual Toothbrushing Methods[1]

Although the Bass (sulcular) method is widely recognized as being the most effective and most often recommended, it is helpful to know all the major toothbrushing methods. The method selected should disrupt both supragingival and subgingival plaque biofilm to the extent possible. Although a horizontal scrub technique is often used, it is not recommended because of potential trauma to hard and soft tissues.

In all the following methods, the handle is placed parallel to the occlusal plane for posterior (facial and lingual) and anterior facial surfaces and parallel to the long axis of the tooth (using the toe of the brush) for anterior lingual surfaces. Occlusal surfaces are cleaned with a scrubbing motion.

A. Bass or sulcular brushing method
   1. Technique—direct the bristles into the sulcus at a 45-degree angle to the long axis of the tooth; vibrate the bristles in a short, back-and-forth motion
   2. Indications—plaque biofilm disruption at and under the gingival margin; good gingival stimulation; widely recognized as an effective control technique
B. Stillman's method
   1. Technique—position the bristles on the attached gingiva, and direct them apically at a 45-degree angle to the long

axis of the tooth; use firm, gentle vibration, holding the bristles stationary
   2. Indication—gingival stimulation
C. Roll method
   1. Technique—place the sides of the bristles on the attached gingiva and direct them apically; turn the wrist to roll or sweep the bristles over the gingiva and the tooth
   2. Indications—facial and lingual tooth surfaces; often combined with the Bass, Charters', or Stillman's method
D. Charters' method
   1. Technique—position the bristle tips toward the occlusal surfaces at a 45-degree angle to the long axis of the tooth; move the bristles in a short, back-and-forth motion
   2. Indications—cleaning orthodontic appliances, fixed appliances; after periodontal surgery when sulcular brushing must be avoided to allow wound healing
E. Fones (circular) method
   1. Technique—with upper and lower teeth together, place the bristles perpendicular to the buccal tooth surfaces; use a wide circular motion to cover the gingiva and tooth surfaces of both arches; on the lingual surfaces, use smaller circles to brush each arch separately
   2. Indications—when technique must be easy to learn and execute; can be mastered by children
F. Combination methods
   1. Modified-Bass method—combination of Bass and roll methods
   2. Modified-Stillman's method—combination of Stillman's and roll methods

Power Toothbrushes

A. General description
   1. Brush heads contain bundles of bristles arranged on a variety of brush head shapes; toothbrushes with different brush head shapes are available on the market
   2. The bristles can have flat, bilevel, or multi-level trims; designed for occlusal and smooth surfaces or interdental proximal surface cleaning
   3. The handles are larger than those of manual brushes
   4. Power toothbrushes move in directions and at speeds unattainable by manual toothbrushes
   5. Power toothbrushes have timers to ensure adequate brushing duration and a pressure sensor to monitor the force applied on the toothbrushes
B. Power source—electric rechargeable handle-base; replaceable, rechargeable, and nonreplaceable batteries
C. Motion—distinctly different stroke movement from the motion of manual toothbrushes; motions occur in one of the following directions:
   1. Side-to-side, arcuate, or back-and-forth
   2. Oscillating or rotating
   3. Rotating or counter-rotating
   4. High-frequency pulsating, combined with an oscillating or rotating movement
   5. Sonic vibratory motion from low-frequency acoustic energy

D. Indications for use—recommended for all clients because of the effectiveness of power toothbrushes in removing plaque biofilm and reducing gingivitis; especially valuable to those who:
   1. Lack the manual dexterity, discipline, or motivation to master an effective manual toothbrushing technique, especially children and adolescents who are physically and mentally challenged (recommended to the caregivers who may be doing the toothbrushing for these children and adolescents)
   2. Have orthodontic appliances or implants
   3. Are prone to dental stain
   4. Are aggressive brushers, or exhibit abrasion, erosion, abfraction, or gingival recession
   5. Have periodontal disease or are undergoing periodontal maintenance therapy
E. Power toothbrushes, especially those with oscillating-rotating brushes reduce gingival bleeding and inflammation[10]
F. Power toothbrushes reduce plaque biofilm and gingivitis better than the manual toothbrush can, with or without floss[10]

Single-Tufted Brushes

A. Design—flat or tapered
B. Suggested use—to remove plaque biofilm from surfaces not accessible with larger brushes, including areas of crowded or malpositioned teeth, distal surfaces of terminal molars, around pontics, in furcations, and on lingual surfaces of molars; also used on type II or III embrasure (depending on design) and fixed dental prosthesis[1]
C. Technique—tufts are positioned at or just under the gingival margin, and a sulcular brushing stroke is used; placement of the tapered angled side against teeth allows for the insertion of the bristles several millimeters subgingivally

Factors in Toothbrushing Effectiveness

A. Sequence
   1. A methodical, systematic approach enhances effectiveness
   2. Suggested sequence—begin systematic, overlapping strokes at the facial aspect of the maxillary right or left terminal tooth; continue around the arch to the terminal tooth on the opposite side; switch to the lingual aspect, and begin working back toward the starting side; use the same pattern for the mandible, and then brush the occlusal surfaces
B. Duration
   1. Monitor the brushing time in an area by counting strokes or seconds after each time the brush is moved
   2. The total manual brushing time of 2 minutes is often recommended; the average brushing time is 1 minute or less
C. Frequency
   1. Thorough removal of plaque biofilm every day is the goal of client self-care and for maintenance of oral health
   2. Toothbrushing should be performed twice daily; however, the frequency should be increased when gingival

or periodontal conditions warrant it or when caries risk is high

3. Thoroughness in daily brushing is more important than frequency
4. Emphasis should be placed on effective oral cleaning, not just toothbrushing

D. Skill level
1. Careful attention should be given to evaluating skill development in all components of toothbrush manipulation, including grasp, placement, activation, wrist movement, and amount of pressure applied
2. Control of toothbrush placement and motion is essential for effectiveness

Improper Toothbrushing

A. Need to assess
1. Improper toothbrushing—may result from lack of education in proper technique, incorrect application following instruction, or long-established habits
2. The dental hygienist should evaluate the client's toothbrushing technique and monitor the conditions of hard and soft tissues at each continued-care visit
3. Faulty placement, overly vigorous motion or pressure, and use of a brush with frayed, splayed, or broken bristles can lead to unwanted consequences

B. Acute consequences—soft tissue injuries such as denuded attached gingiva, lesions that appear "punched out" and red, and clusters of small ulcerations at the gingival margin

C. Chronic consequences
1. Soft tissue—loss of gingival tissue or change in contour; malpositioned or prominent teeth and an inadequate band of attached gingiva are predisposing factors
2. Hard tissue—loss of tooth structure and creation of a wedge-shaped defect at the cervical third of tooth (noncarious cervical lesion)

Toothbrush Maintenance

A. Toothbrushes should be rinsed clean after each use and then allowed to air-dry in the upright position

B. Toothbrushes should be replaced when the bristles splay or lose resiliency; generally, should not be used longer than 2 to 3 months

C. Some toothbrushes have color-indicator bristles to alert the user about replacement time

D. After an acute illness and an oral infection, toothbrushes should be replaced or disinfected with 0.12% chlorhexidine gluconate; power toothbrushes with a built-in sanitizer unit help control toothbrush contamination[1]

INTERDENTAL PLAQUE BIOFILM CONTROL

Basic Concepts

A. Toothbrushes—effective in removing plaque biofilm from facial, lingual, and occlusal surfaces of teeth; relatively ineffective on proximal surfaces

B. Interdental cleaning devices—designed for access to interproximal surfaces; essential for effective control of plaque biofilm

C. Interdental col area—protected area that harbors microorganisms that can initiate disease

D. Anatomy of the interdental area—significant factor in both disease initiation and disease control

Factors to Consider When Selecting Interdental Cleaning Methods

A. The level of oral health or disease, teeth positioning, and condition of the gingiva and attachment should be considered when recommending interdental aids (Fig. 16-2); three types of embrasures[1]:
1. Type I embrasures are occupied by interdental papillae
2. Type II embrasures have slight to moderate recession of interdental papillae
3. Type III embrasures have extensive recession or complete loss of interdental papillae

B. Client manual dexterity, adherence, skill development, and personal preferences must be considered

Flosses

A. Dental floss—most frequently recommended device for interdental cleaning of type I embrasures[1] (Fig. 16-3)

B. Flossing may precede or follow brushing in a home care regimen

C. As gingival recession increases, as in type II and type III embrasures, the effectiveness of flossing decreases; other interdental plaque-control aids should be selected

D. Agents to enhance color, taste, and therapeutic value have been incorporated into the dental floss; evidence to confirm the effectiveness of the addition of fluoride and whitening agents is limited

E. Floss type

FIG 16-2 Interproximal embrasure types and corresponding interdental cleansers. **A,** Type I—no gingival recession: dental floss. **B,** Type II—moderate papillary recession: interdental brush. **C,** Type III—complete loss of papillae: uni-tufted brush. (From Darby ML, Walsh MM: *Dental hygiene theory and practice,* ed 4, St Louis, 2014, Saunders. Modified from Newman MG, et al: *Carranza's clinical periodontology,* ed 12, St Louis, 2015, Elsevier.)

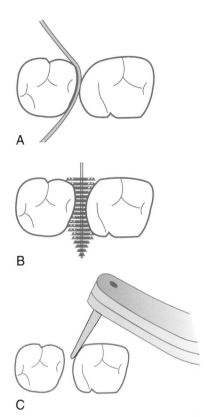

FIG 16-3 Use of interdental plaque biofilm control devices. **A,** Dental floss. **B,** Interdental brush. **C,** Toothpick in holder. (From Darby ML, Walsh MM: *Dental hygiene theory and practice,* ed 4, St Louis, 2015, Saunders.)

1. Unwaxed—unbound filaments are spread on the tooth and have more friction for cleaning; filaments hold plaque and debris for easier removal; the floss slips through contacts more easily
2. Waxed—resists tearing and shredding on faulty restorations or when moved through very tight contacts
3. Polytetrafluoroethylene (PTFE) floss—slides through contacts easily; does not fray

Flossing Technique

A. Floss length—varies with holding technique; 10 to 15 inches when forming a loop; 12 to 24 inches when wrapping around fingers
B. Holding technique
   1. Ends may be tied together to form a loop, wrapped around middle fingers, or tucked into the palm of the hand
   2. With equal tension in both hands, grasp with both thumbs or with the thumb and the forefinger for use on the maxilla or with both forefingers for use on the mandible; leave 1-inch to 2-inch length between fingers
C. Insertion
   1. Approach the embrasure space obliquely, and ease the floss past the contact with a back-and-forth motion
D. Adaptation and stroke
   1. Position fingers such that the floss wraps securely against the proximal surface and forms a C shape against the tooth

2. Slide beneath the gingival margin, and move in an apico-coronal direction several times

Improper Flossing

A. Acute consequences—snapping through contacts, failure to curve the floss against the proximal surfaces, and application of excessive pressure can result in floss cuts of interdental papillae
B. Chronic consequences
   1. Soft tissue—excessive pressure applied submarginally can be destructive to soft tissue
   2. Hard tissue—repeated heavy sawing movements in a facio-lingual direction can abrade proximal tooth structure

Flossing Aids

A. Types of aids
   1. Floss holders
      a. General description—the floss is threaded through and held on a double-pronged plastic device, forming a span between the prongs
      b. Technique—the prepared holder is positioned for insertion, then adapted and activated in much the same manner as the handheld floss; special care should be taken not to snap the floss through the contacts
      c. Indications for use—client's lack of dexterity to floss properly and client preference
   2. Floss threaders
      a. General description—firm, flexible, blunt-ended devices for moving the floss through closed contacts or under pontics or orthodontic wires; a variety of designs are available
      b. Technique—position the floss in the threader with even lengths on each side; pass the threader through the embrasure from the buccal aspect to the lingual aspect, leaving sufficient length on the buccal aspect; remove the threader and use the floss in the normal manner; slide through the space to remove it

Interdental Brushes

A. General description
   1. Soft nylon filaments are twisted onto a stainless steel wire to form a tapered or a nontapered small brush; the wire may be plastic coated for use around dental implants and for client comfort
   2. Interdental brushes must be used with a special handle; some have small handles, and some have contra-angled handles
   3. Interdental brushes provide excellent access to root concavities, furcation areas, and proximal surfaces where papillae do not fill the interdental spaces, as in type II and type III embrasures (see Fig. 16-3)
   4. Interdental brushes come in a variety of sizes, with thin wires and a tapered brush to remove interproximal plaque biofilm from all types of embrasures
B. Technique
   1. Choose a brush of appropriate size, insert interproximally, and use an in-and-out motion from the buccal aspect to the lingual aspect, and vice versa

2. Brushes may be used in furcation areas in a similar manner
3. Access into the interproximal pockets may be achieved with careful vertical placement and movement

C. Precautions
1. Avoid forcing through tight, tissue-filled areas to prevent trauma
2. Do not aim the wire into tissue
3. Discard the tip when the filaments lose their original shape
4. Do not use a brush with a stainless steel wire on an implant; the brush must have a plastic-coated wire to prevent damage to the implant

Toothpicks[1]

A. Suggested use—for proximal surfaces and concavities and in exposed furcation areas
B. Technique—round toothpicks can be used alone or inserted into special holders; moisten the tip with saliva, and adapt it to the surface to be cleaned; subgingivally, use a 45-degree angle to the tooth; move the toothpick in and out several times for cleaning the interproximal surfaces, and follow the tooth contour on the facial or lingual surfaces
C. Precautions—rigid pointed tips can cause injury if forced into tight tissue areas; over time, papillae will abrade if toothpicks are used improperly

Interdental Wedges[1]

A. Suggested use—for cleaning the proximal surfaces or just under the gingival margin; triangular in cross section; should be used interproximally only when adequate space for insertion is available (e.g., type II and III embrasures)
B. Technique—moisten the tip, position the flat base of the triangle at the gingival border, insert with the tip angled slightly toward the occlusal surface, and move the wedge in and out, with moderate pressure against the surface
C. Precautions—discard tips as soon as splaying occurs; repeated insertion with the tip perpendicular to the long axis of the tooth may cause blunting of interdental papillae

Interdental Tip

A. Suggested uses—for proximal surfaces, in exposed furcations, and under gingival margins; conical or pyramidal, flexible rubber or plastic tip; may be used to maintain interproximal gingival contours or to recontour papillae following periodontal surgery; rubber tips are also used for massaging the gingiva to improve blood circulation, increase keratinization, and provide epithelial thickening[1]
B. Technique
1. Dental plaque biofilm removal—trace the gingival margin with the tip aimed into the sulcus; move the tip in and out in a buccolingual direction along the proximal tooth surface apical to contact areas
2. Contouring gingiva—place the tip, without forcing it, into the interdental contour, being careful to follow the gingival form; press the side of the tip against the gingiva, and use a firm rotary motion to apply intermittent pressure

C. Precaution—avoid flattening interdental papillae; use of interdental tips made from rubber should be avoided in clients with latex sensitivity

Power Interdental Cleaning Devices

A. Power flossing devices are available to make interdental cleaning easier; include flossers, interdental brushes, and dental water jets
B. Technique—usually the unit comes with an attachment (similar to a floss holder, interdental brush, or single-tufted or end-tufted brush); the brush is activated by turning it on after attaching the brush handle; requires only one hand to operate; the tip is aimed into the interproximal space
C. Suggested use—alternative to the handheld floss; client preference

Dental Water Jet[1]

A. General description—motor-driven pulsating device with a reservoir and specially designed tips to deliver the irrigant to the gingival pocket; depending on the size of the tip selected, this device has the ability to reach deep periodontal pockets; dental water jets produce a steady stream of fluid
B. Technique—the reservoir is filled with water or an antimicrobial agent; after inserting the appropriate tip into the handle, the pressure gauge is adjusted to the client's comfort setting; starting with posterior teeth, the tip is placed at a 90-degree angle to the long axis of the tooth, following each tooth along the gingival margin
C. Indications for use—clients with fixed orthodontics, dental implants, crowns, and bridges; those with gingivitis; and persons in periodontal maintenance program; research suggests that the use of oral irrigation does not reduce plaque biofilm; however, it does improve gingival health compared with regular oral hygiene[11]
D. Precaution—each manufacturer's product differs; follow each model's instructions for use

DENTIFRICES

Basic Concepts

A. Definition—toothpaste used with a toothbrush
B. Purposes
1. Cosmetic—tooth surfaces are cleaned and polished; breath is freshened
2. Cosmetic and therapeutic—certain nontherapeutic substances augment the efficiency of brushing in the removal of plaque biofilm, debris, and stain
3. Therapeutic—vehicle for transporting biologically active ingredients such as fluoride, which inhibits tooth demineralization and promotes remineralization, to the tooth and its environment
C. Basic ingredients[1]
1. Detergents—lower surface tension to loosen debris and stain; provide foaming characteristic; sodium lauryl sulfate, a common foaming agent, has been implicated in causing aphthous ulcers in susceptible clients

2. Cleaning and polishing agents—abrasives that help remove stain, plaque biofilm, and debris from tooth surfaces and give a luster to the tooth surface; should provide maximal cleaning benefit with minimal abrasion; examples include calcium carbonate, silica, calcium pyrophosphate, aluminum oxide, insoluble calcium metaphosphate, magnesium carbonate, and bicarbonate

3. Humectants—retain moisture to ensure a chemically and physically stable product; for example, glycerin, mannitol, sorbitol, synthetic cellulose, vegetable oils, and propylene glycol

4. Binding agents—prevent separation by increasing the consistency of a mixture of liquid and solid ingredients; for example, mineral colloids, natural gums, and seaweed colloids

5. Flavoring and sweetening agents—provide a pleasant and refreshing flavor and aftertaste, and cover unpleasant flavors; for example, peppermint, cinnamon, wintergreen, and noncariogenic artificial sweeteners such as glycerin, sorbitol, menthol, and xylitol

6. Coloring agents—contribute to the product's attractiveness and desirability; vegetable dyes and titanium dioxide

7. Preservatives—prevent bacterial growth and prolong shelf life of the product; for example, alcohol, benzoates, and dichlorinated phenols

Therapeutic and Active Ingredients

A. Definition—biologically active ingredients that produce a beneficial effect on hard or soft tissue; dentifrices claiming therapeutic effects are eligible for acceptance by the American Dental Association (ADA) Council on Scientific Affairs; all products with the ADA Seal of Acceptance are listed at www.ada.org

B. Remineralizing agents
   1. Fluoride—substantial data exist to show that approved fluoride dentifrices reduce the incidence of dental caries; fluorides currently used in dentifrices are sodium fluoride (NaF), stannous fluoride (SnF_2), SnF_2–sodium hexametaphosphate, and sodium monofluorophosphate $(Na_2\text{-}PO_3F)$[1]
   2. Amorphous calcium phosphate (ACP)—calcium and phosphate were traditionally added to dentifrices as abrasives and lubricants and now for caries control
   3. Xylitol—a sugar substitute, which has anticaries and antiplaque properties; *Streptococcus mutans* cannot metabolize xylitol, which allows a less acidic environment for tooth demineralization[1]

C. Antimicrobial agents—triclosan is the primary agent used in the United States; its antigingivitis and antiplaque efficacy has been demonstrated

D. Desensitizing agents— desensitization agents work in one of two ways; they either block dentinal tubules (high concentration of fluoride, calcium phosphates, and oxalate salts) or block nerve repolarization (potassium salts, including potassium nitrate and potassium citrate); potassium nitrate is the primary agent used in desensitizing dentifrices[1]

E. Anticalculus agents—function by interfering with the calcium phosphate bond in the calculus matrix; effective only against the formation of supragingival calculus on enamel surfaces
   1. Pyrophosphate system—pyrophosphate has a negative charge, attracts positively charged calcium ions, and interferes with calculus formation
   2. Zinc system—zinc has a positive charge, attracts negatively charged phosphate ions, and interferes with calculus formation

F. Whitening agents—several dentifrices are marketed for their ability to remove or bleach stains; several whitening dentifrices have low abrasive levels; may be effective for the maintenance of cosmetic restorations; whitening agents include papain (Citroxain), silica, hydrogen peroxide, and carbamide peroxide

Guidelines for Dentifrice Selection

A. Products selected should carry the ADA Seal of Acceptance or the Canadian Dental Association (CDA) Seal of Recognition; this ensures that adequate evidence of safety and efficacy has been demonstrated in controlled clinical trials, that advertising claims comply with ADA and CDA standards for accuracy and truthfulness, and that the therapeutic ingredient will be bioavailable when the dentifrice is used

B. All ADA-accepted and CDA-recognized dentifrices have safe levels of abrasiveness

C. Dentifrices containing fluoride are granted acceptance on the basis of their caries-reducing properties

D. Desensitizing dentifrices that carry ADA and CDA seals have gained acceptance for their proven efficacy in the control of dentinal hypersensitivity

Guidelines for Dentifrice Use

A. Daily use of fluoride dentifrice should be recommended to all clients, regardless of caries risk, because these products promote tooth remineralization

B. Young children (under age 6) should be supervised when using a fluoride dentifrice—use of a small, pea-sized amount of a toothpaste because children under 6 will most likely swallow the dentifrice

CONTROLLING ORAL MALODOR[12]

A. Identifying malodor
   1. Oral malodor (bad breath, or halitosis)— common problem that originates approximately 90% of the time from the mouth and from the oropharynx region (tongue coating, gingivitis, periodontitis, pharyngitis, and tonsillitis); systemic causes account for 10% of oral malodor
   2. Malodors are produced by microorganisms on the tongue and teeth; proteolytic activity results in foul-smelling compounds or volatile sulfur compounds (VSCs)
   3. Oral dryness (xerostomia) exacerbates malodor; smoking, medications, alcohol, and caffeine increase oral dehydration
   4. Bad breath caused by high levels of VSCs is often associated with periodontal infections and overnight denture wearing

5. Malodor can be measured by sensory or organoleptic (smell) instruments such as gas chromatography (GC) that monitor VCSs (hydrogen sulfide, methyl mercaptan, methyl sulfide)

B. Controlling malodor
   1. Improve oral hygiene by including tongue cleaning in the process
   2. Abstain from tobacco and alcohol use
   3. Avoid caffeine
   4. Stimulate salivary flow by chewing sugarless gum with xylitol
   5. Use ADA-accepted or CDA-recognized antimicrobial mouthrinses
   6. Use saline nasal sprays and humidifiers to control dryness of throat and nasal passages
   7. Use sugar-free (with xylitol) breath sprays, breath fresheners, or drops

ORAL IRRIGATION

Basic Concepts

Oral irrigation can be a valuable adjunct to maintaining oral cleanliness and health. Oral irrigating devices force a steady or pulsating stream of water over gingival tissue and teeth, with the goals of removing unattached debris and reducing the concentration of microorganisms and cellular end products that may be present; irrigators also are used to deliver antimicrobial agents supragingivally and subgingivally.

Home Irrigation

A. Home uses
   1. Before toothbrushing and flossing to remove debris or retained food particles, or after toothbrushing to deliver antimicrobial agents
   2. Debridement of recessed areas of fixed prosthetic or orthodontic appliances; around dental implants
   3. Flushing of periodontal pockets with a controlled, low-intensity, pulsating stream of water

B. Types of irrigators
   1. Hand syringes—blunt tip, side-port cannula; requires high level of dexterity and motivation; not recommended for most clients
   2. Power-driven device—unit with a water reservoir; plugs into an electrical outlet to create a pulsating jet of water; water pressure is regulated by an adjustable dial or sliding switch
   3. Water pressure–driven device—attaches directly to a faucet to deliver a constant stream of water; pressure is controlled by regulating water flow from the faucet
   4. Tips—standard jet tip or flexible subgingival tip; tips with a side-port design or an end-port design show similar effectiveness

C. Use with antimicrobial agents[1,13]
   1. Some studies have documented greater benefits with the addition of antimicrobial agents
   2. Since standard irrigation tips are unable to access periodontal pockets completely, no significant benefits in treating periodontitis is found; demonstrated benefits are limited to parameters such as plaque and bleeding indices, gingivitis, and reduction of bleeding on probing
   3. The use of water alone is as effective as the use of chemotherapeutic agents

D. Precautions—contraindications to use
   1. Clients should be trained in the proper use of irrigating devices and be monitored for adverse effects
   2. Transient bacteremias may occur following oral irrigation, particularly when untreated disease is present; persons at highest risk for infective endocarditis can use irrigation as part of their oral self-care
   3. Use of low pressure prevents gingival tissue trauma and allows better access to the base of the pocket

E. Antimicrobial agents
   1. Stannous fluoride—1.64% SnF_2; dispense equal parts of 3.28% SnF_2 concentrated gel and distilled water; use a fresh mixture for each client
   2. Chlorhexidine digluconate—0.12% in the United States and 2% in Europe; may be diluted to 0.06% concentration; may become less effective in the presence of sodium laurel sulfate, fluoride, blood, and protein
   3. Essential oils mouthrinse; may be diluted with equal parts water for use in a power irrigator, but most studies use it at full strength

CARE OF FIXED AND REMOVABLE PROSTHESES

Dental prostheses are replacements for one or more teeth or other oral structures, ranging from a single tooth to a complete denture. Clients wearing fixed or removable dental prostheses have unique needs that require specific procedures for maintaining the prosthesis as well as retained natural teeth; relevant terminology follows[1]:

A. Appliance—in dentistry, a general term referring to a device used to provide a functional or therapeutic effect
B. Abutment—tooth, root, or dental implant used for the support and retention of a fixed or removable dental prosthesis
C. Clasp—retains and stabilizes the denture by attaching it to the abutment teeth
D. Denture—artificial substitute for missing natural teeth and adjacent tissues
E. Pontic—artificial tooth on a fixed, partial denture or isolated tooth on a removable, partial denture that replaces lost natural tooth, restores its function, and usually occupies space previously occupied by a natural crown
F. Fixed prosthesis—dental prosthesis firmly attached to natural teeth, roots, or dental implants usually by a cementing agent; cannot be removed by client
G. Obturator—maxillofacial prosthesis that includes an intraoral structure that replaces all or part of the palate or the maxilla; it may also have a palatal lift that aids in speech or swallowing
H. Overdentures—dentures with retained natural teeth or dental implants
I. Removable prosthesis—dental prosthesis that can readily be placed in the mouth and removed by the wearer

J. Orthodontic bracket—a small metal attachment fixed to a band that serves as a means of fastening the archwire to the band

K. Orthodontic band—a thin metal ring that secures orthodontic attachments to a tooth

L. Orthodontic wire—a slender, pliable rod or thread of metal used as a source of force to direct teeth to move in desired directions

M. Implant, or dental implant—a device surgically inserted into the jawbone to be used as a prosthodontic abutment; may be used to support complete dentures

N. Grills ("grillz," fronts)—a decorative, jewel-encrusted encasement for teeth in hip-hop culture; usually made of precious metals (e.g., gold, platinum)

Fixed-Prosthesis Maintenance

A. Fixed prostheses such as fixed bridges and orthodontic bands and wires increase the potential for plaque biofilm and debris retention and make access to the proximal surfaces more difficult

B. Home care armamentarium
1. Floss threaders—allow the floss to move beneath pontics and between pontics and abutments
2. Interdental brushes—access interdental spaces apical to closed contacts
3. Special brushes and toothpicks
   a. Orthodontic bilevel toothbrushes—three rows wide, with shorter middle row; moves into and around orthodontic appliances; adapts to areas between the orthodontic appliance and the gingival margin
   b. Two-row brushes—for cleaning of sulci; adapt to narrow areas between brackets and gingivae
   c. Toothpick holders—for cleaning type II embrasures, furcations, and margins of appliances, brackets, and sulci
   d. Single-tuft or end-tuft brushes—for use in type III embrasure areas, furcations, margins of appliances and brackets, and single-teeth abutments
   e. Oral irrigators—flushing action removes loose debris and food material

Removable-Prosthesis Maintenance

A. Clients with removable appliances, including orthodontic appliances, must be taught about the importance of conscientious home care

B. Debris, stain, plaque biofilm, and calculus will collect on removable appliances, if the appliances are not cleaned regularly

C. Inadequate cleaning may contribute to the development of soft tissue lesions underlying the appliance or of carious lesions on abutting tooth surfaces; chronic *Candida albicans* infection also may result

D. Removable prostheses can be maintained by:
1. Brushing with dentifrice after each meal and before retiring to bed at night
   a. Special denture brushes have two different arrangements of filaments to access both the inner curved surface and the outer and occlusal surfaces

   b. Special clasp brushes have a narrow, tapered cylindrical design that can adapt to the inner clasp surface, a prime site for plaque biofilm formation and retention
2. Immersion in a solvent that chemically loosens or removes stains and deposits is recommended; the appliance should be brushed after soaking it to remove residual debris and chemicals
3. Antifungal denture solutions help prevent candidiasis

E. Removable appliances should be taken out at night and stored in a covered container with one of the solvents or denture solutions listed above

F. Cleansing procedures
1. Hold the appliance securely to avoid dropping and breaking it
2. When brushing, hold the appliance over a sink partly filled with water or lined with a cushioning material
3. Avoid overzealous brushing and use of strong abrasives; the plastic resin material can be scratched or abraded to the extent of compromising denture fit
4. If any denture adhesive material is used, it should be removed from the appliance and the underlying mucosa several times a day
5. Brush the underlying mucosa at least once daily with a soft toothbrush
6. Solutions used for cleansing or soaking a denture should be renewed for each use

G. All removable appliances and prostheses, including fluoride carriers, night guards, mouthguards, and bleaching trays should be cleaned on a regular basis and appropriately stored after use[1]

Dental Implant Maintenance

See the sections on "Dental Implants" in Chapters 13 and 14 and "Instrumentation of Dental Implants" in Chapter 17.

A. Osteo-integrated implants and superstructures require special home maintenance, products, and techniques; clients must learn the techniques for plaque biofilm control that prevent damage to the implant material and superstructure

B. The home care armamentarium may include:
1. Soft-bristled, multi-tufted nylon toothbrushes
2. Interdental brushes with nylon coating over metal wire cores; coating prevents scratching of the implant material (usually titanium)
3. Flat and tapered end-tuft brushes
4. Dental floss
5. Implant flossing aids—braided nylon filaments with a hook leader for insertion is recommended; flat cotton floss; or floss containing a soft filament brush component
6. Rubber tip stimulator; wood sticks
7. Disclosing tablets or liquid; may be most useful during initial education on plaque biofilm control
8. Antimicrobial mouthrinse; chlorhexidine used twice daily is the rinse of choice after treatment; other antimicrobial mouthrinses may be used for long-term treatment
9. Small amount of ADA-approved or CDA-recognized gel or fine-abrasive, fluoridated toothpaste; abrasive

toothpastes must be avoided; anticalculus formulas are acceptable

10. Oral irrigators may be used on the lowest setting, with the tip directed perpendicular to the long axis of the tooth or implant; water, chlorhexidine 0.12%, phenol-based, or plant alkaloid mouthrinses may be used

C. Skill development in plaque biofilm control
   1. Clients must be shown how to control plaque biofilm on all areas of the implant and the superstructure
   2. Sufficient supervised practice will ensure adequate skill development
   3. Plaque biofilm control must be monitored at each continued-care appointment and techniques modified, as indicated
   4. Research indicates that tobacco use increases implant failure[14]

CARIES MANAGEMENT

Caries Management by Risk Assessment[15]

Caries management by risk assessment (CAMBRA) is an evidence-based approach to the prevention or treatment of dental caries in the earliest stages. The dental hygienist identifies a client's level of risk by determining the balance between pathologic and protective risk factors. Once the clinician identifies a client's caries risk (low, moderate, high or extreme), a therapeutic and/or preventive plan is implemented. (See Table 15-6 in Chapter 15.)

A. Caries disease indicators—uses acronym WREC to describe:
   1. White spots lesions
   2. Restorations placed within the past 3 years as a result of caries
   3. Enamel proximal lesions
   4. Cavitation of carious lesions penetrating into dentin
B. Pathologic factors
   1. Medium or high level of streptococci and lactobacilli counts
   2. Presence of heavy biofilm on teeth
   3. Frequent snacking between meals
   4. Deep pits and fissures
   5. Recreational drug use
   6. Inadequate salivary flow caused by medication, radiation, or systemic diseases
   7. Exposed roots
   8. Orthodontic appliance
C. Protective factors—biologic or therapeutic factors related to the client's practice of oral hygiene that can counterbalance the challenge presented by caries risk factors
   1. Drinks fluoridated water on a regular basis
   2. Uses a fluoride toothpaste once or more daily
   3. Uses fluoride-containing mouthrinse daily
   4. Has had fluoride varnish applied in the past 6 months
   5. Has received an in-office topical fluoride treatment in the past 6 months
   6. Has used prescription chlorhexidine daily for 1 week in each of the past 6 months
   7. Has used xylitol gum or lozenges four to five times daily in the past 6 months
   8. Has used calcium and phosphate supplement during the past 6 months
   9. Has adequate salivary flow

Fluorides[16,17]

See the sections on "Topical Fluorides and Fluoride Varnishes" in Chapter 13 and "Preventing and Controlling Oral Diseases and Conditions" in Chapter 20.

General Considerations

A. Most effective agent for the prevention and control of dental caries, especially on smooth surfaces
B. A multi-therapeutic approach is most effective; three categories of administration:
   1. Systemic—community water supplies, institutional water supplies, and dietary supplementation
   2. Professional application—gels and varnishes
   3. Self-applied—dentifrices, rinses, and gels
C. Safe when used in recommended amounts and concentrations; dental hygienists must be alert to the potential for acute and chronic adverse effects
   1. Large quantities of fluoride products should not be stored in the home
   2. Institutions that have fluoride programs must handle and store fluoride products safely
   3. Parents and caregivers must be educated about supervising home use of products containing fluoride by young children to prevent acute toxic reactions or long-term effects (e.g., dental fluorosis)
   4. Products intended for topical application should not be swallowed
   5. If excessive amounts have been ingested, vomiting should be induced immediately with ipecac or manually; calcium solution or milk should be administered to slow the absorption rate; emergency medical care should be obtained (see the section on "Drug-Related Emergencies and Poisoning" in Chapter 21)
   6. Fluoride therapy is based on the client's risk assessment

Ingested Fluorides

A. Drinking optimally fluoridated water (0.7 ppm) during tooth formation and then later as a topical fluoride from drinking the water provides a significant decrease in the overall percentage of dental caries in both children and adults
B. Maximum benefits are obtained when fluoride is provided from the onset of tooth development until tooth eruption is complete and then used continuously for drinking
C. Fluoride works primarily and most effectively via topical (surface) mechanisms (whether delivered in the drinking water, foods, beverages, or products) to inhibit demineralization, enhance remineralization, and inhibit plaque bacteria
D. The dental hygienist has a key role in educating parents, caregivers, and children about the value of fluoride and its topical benefits

Fluoride Agents for Professional Application

A. Neutral sodium fluoride (NaF)
   1. Characteristics—first fluoride used for topical application; available in 2% concentration foam or gel and 5% concentration varnish
   2. Application
      a. Applications of 2% NaF at 6-month intervals as a substitute for acidulated phosphate fluoride when porcelain or certain types of composite restorations are present have not been substantiated in the literature; 4-minute application
      b. Fluoride varnish—contains a 5% NaF concentration, approved by the U.S. Food and Drug Administration (FDA) for use as a desensitizing agent and cavity liner; the varnish is used as a topical fluoride treatment; painted on teeth; the varnish is retained on the tooth surface for 3 to 4 hours
   3. Advantages—safe for use in dentition with porcelain crowns and composite restorations; varnish is easily applied on the teeth of young children; research highly supports the efficacy of fluoride varnish for caries prevention compared with other professional fluoride methods[16]
B. Acidulated phosphate fluoride (APF)
   1. Characteristics—available as foam, gels, and thixotropic gels; 1.23% NaF with 1 molar (M) orthophosphoric acid concentration
   2. Application intervals—every 6 months, or more frequently when caries risk is high; 4-minute application
   3. Advantages—high level of client acceptance; nonirritating to soft tissues; does not discolor tooth structure; highest documented efficacy; most common in-office treatment; 1-minute application not supported by the research literature
   4. Disadvantages and precautions—low pH of 3.5 for enhanced fluoride uptake may cause etching of dental sealants and porcelain and some composite restorations; sealants, porcelains, and composites should be protected with a water-based lubricant, or use NaF as an alternative

Indications for Professional Application

A. Topical fluoride therapy is an accepted part of the prevention-oriented care plan
B. Assessment of client's risk for dental caries will determine a client's fluoride therapy plan
C. Therapy regimen may include both professionally applied and self-applied agents
D. Inclusion of topical fluoride in client's care plan should be based on the following criteria[16]:
   1. For children and adults at moderate, high, or highest risk for dental caries—fluoride varnish or fluoride gel is the treatment of choice at continued-care intervals
   2. Less than optimally fluoridated drinking water
   3. Fair or poor oral hygiene
   4. Decalcification, white spots, or incipient lesions are present; secondary or recurrent caries; active caries
   5. Following root instrumentation, dentin can be exposed and dentinal tubules opened; hypersensitive root surfaces that often result can be controlled by fluoride application
   6. Fluoride application reduces incidence of root caries and dentinal hypersensitivity associated with exposed root surfaces resulting from gingival recession
   7. Irregular professional dental visits
   8. Inappropriate dietary practices (e.g., frequent sugar intake)
   9. When xerostomia is present as a result of irradiation to the head and neck, certain medications, or salivary gland dysfunction, resulting in changes in quality and quantity of saliva; caries destruction occurs rapidly and is generalized when salivary production is minimal; multiple fluoride treatments are used to control high risk for dental caries associated with xerostomia
   10. Clients wearing orthodontic, prosthodontic, or any other oral appliances

Application Principles—General Guidelines for Client Preparation

A. Explain the indication(s), the steps involved, and the time required for the procedure, the need to control salivary flow and to avoid ingestion, and postapplication instructions
B. Position the client to facilitate salivary control and reduce potential for gagging
C. Calculus, extrinsic stains, materia alba, and heavy plaque biofilm should be removed before the application of fluoride

Application Methods

Tray Systems

A. Designed for use with fluoride gels; trays cover all teeth in an arch, come in a variety of materials, shapes, and sizes; tray systems are not appropriate for solutions because they cannot be adequately retained within tray boundaries
B. Tray examples—most frequently used
   1. Disposable polystyrene (Styrofoam)—used for professional fluoride application; ADA and CDA do *not* recommend the use of fluoride foam because of lack of sufficient scientific evidence for its efficacy in caries prevention; ADA and CDA recommend only 4-minute fluoride gel application[16]
   2. Custom-fitted polyvinyl—used by the client for self-application of fluoride gel; provides excellent coverage; must be remade as the dentition matures; relatively expensive
C. Application procedure
   1. Assemble the armamentarium—trays, fluoride, a saliva ejection device, gauze squares, and a timer or clock
   2. Protect the dental sealants and the porcelain or composite restorations with a water-based lubricant for APF application, or, preferably, use neutral NaF
   3. Thoroughly dry each arch; this prevents dilution of the material and controls for a potential salivary barrier
   4. Insert the tray(s); one or two trays can be inserted at once; tray type, client variables, and clinician preference will influence the method selected
   5. Insert the saliva ejection device, which reduces the potential for ingestion, nausea, and vomiting

6. Adapt the tray(s); the dental hygienist or the client can gently press on the trays to close any small anterior gaps

7. Have the client apply gentle biting pressure to force the gel interproximally

8. Remove the tray(s); if only one tray was inserted initially, insert the second tray at this point; do not allow the client to rinse between insertions

9. Clear any excess agent from the mouth; instruct the client to expectorate and swab the tongue, teeth, and soft tissues with gauze squares

10. Provide post-treatment instructions; clients are instructed not to eat, rinse, or drink for at least 30 minutes; this increases the total contact time of fluoride exposure

Self-Applied Fluorides

A. Frequent, low doses of fluoride exposure to tooth surfaces are important for enamel remineralization and prevention of demineralization

B. Rinses—available by prescription, except as noted
1. Daily use—low potency, high frequency
   a. 0.044% APF rinse supplement
   b. 0.05% NaF (available over the counter [OTC])
   c. 0.1% SnF_2 rinse (0.63% plus water)
2. Weekly use—high potency, low frequency
   a. 0.2% NaF
   b. Most common concentration used for school-based fluoride rinse programs
3. Many commercially prepared fluoride rinses contain alcohol and should *not* be recommended for persons with a history of alcoholism or xerostomia; use alcohol-free rinses with children and clients who need to avoid exposure to alcohol
4. Fluoride rinses are not recommended for children under 6 years old; swallowing small doses of fluoride over a period may lead to dental fluorosis

C. Gels—available OTC and by prescription
1. 0.4% SnF_2 (brush-on or tray application)
2. 1.1% NaF (brush-on or tray application, also available in paste)
3. 0.05% APF (tray application)

D. Some studies indicate that SnF_2 may have antiplaque, antihypersensitivity, and anticaries effects

Amorphous Calcium Phosphate[18,19]

A. Amorphous calcium phosphate (ACP) contains the same minerals as the hydroxyapatite crystals of tooth enamel

B. Casein phosphopeptide–amorphous calcium phosphate (CPP-ACP), a milk protein peptide, is usually added to stabilize and localize the calcium and phosphate ions on the tooth surface, promoting remineralization of enamel

C. Products that contain ACP should *not* be substituted for fluoride therapy; ACP should be used in conjunction with fluoride to enhance fluoride uptake

D. Several professionally applied and OTC self-applied products, including dentifrices, tooth-whitening agents, prophylaxis paste, and fluoride varnish, contain ACP

Xylitol for Dental Caries Prevention[20,21]

A. Xylitol is a noncariogenic artificial sweetener; *Streptococcus mutans* cannot metabolize xylitol, which causes a decrease in *S. mutans* infections

B. Xylitol inhibits the attachment and transmission of *S. mutans,* reduces plaque biofilm formation, and stimulates salivary secretion

C. Research does not support the effectiveness of xylitol in preventing dental caries

D. Xylitol-containing salivary stimulants can be beneficial for people with xerostomia and diabetes

E. Several products contain xylitol (e.g., chewing gum, lozenges, mints); when used for therapeutic purposes, products must contain 1.55 g of xylitol and must be used at least four or five times daily

MOUTHRINSES OR CHEMOTHERAPEUTICS[22,23]

A. May have cosmetic and therapeutic value

B. Effectiveness of many mouthrinses is limited to dislodging gross debris, temporarily reducing microorganisms, and providing a feeling of freshness

C. One category of commercial mouthrinses is approved by the ADA Council on Scientific Affairs: phenol-related essential oils compounds gained acceptance for control of both plaque biofilm and gingivitis and carry the ADA Seal of Acceptance
1. Chlorhexidine gluconate (Peridex, PerioGard, Pro Dentx, PerioRx)
   a. Available by prescription only
   b. 0.12% concentration in an aqueous solution containing 11.6% alcohol, pH 5.5; also made without alcohol for persons who cannot use alcohol (ask the pharmacist)
   c. Clinical effects are comparable with 0.2% mouthrinse used for many years outside the United States; extensive clinical research has documented its efficacy
   d. Review of numerous studies has established chlorhexidine's safety, stability, and substantivity, which make it effective in preventing and controlling plaque biofilm and reducing and inhibiting gingivitis
   e. May cause brownish yellow stain and supragingival calculus
   f. Unpleasant taste may hinder client acceptance
   g. Recommended for short-term use only; one 2-ounce, 30-second rinse, twice daily for 6 months
   h. Available in alcohol-free formulation
2. Phenol-related essential oils (Listerine and many equivalent generic store brands)
   a. Available without a prescription
   b. Contains thymol, menthol, eucalyptol, and methylsalicylate in a hydroalcohol solution, 21.6% to 26.9% alcohol, pH 5.0
   c. Low substantivity
   d. Listerine's efficacy in inhibiting bacterial plaque biofilm and gingivitis has been documented

e. Various flavors available to enhance client acceptance and adherence to manufacturer's recommendation for a 30-second rinse twice daily

f. Essential oils mouthrinses, using basically the same formula as Listerine, are marketed under many store brand names and are also accepted by the ADA Council on Scientific Affairs as having antiplaque and antigingivitis effects

g. Can be used as preprocedural mouthrinses before aerosol-producing procedures; or as a preprocedural subgingival irrigant

h. Anticalculus formulation of Listerine containing zinc chloride; inhibits supragingival calculus accumulation; has the ADA Seal of Acceptance

i. Available in alcohol-free formulation

D. Mouthrinses are recommended as adjuncts to, not replacements for, mechanical plaque biofilm control

E. Effective on supragingival biofilm only, unless delivered subgingivally with irrigators

F. Approved mouthrinses should be considered for clients with the following conditions:
1. Inability to achieve acceptable mechanical plaque biofilm control
2. Fixed splinting, prostheses, dental implants, and overdentures
3. Orthodontic appliances
4. Postperiodontal or other oral surgery
5. Clients at high risk for dental caries
6. Medication-induced gingival enlargement
7. Immunosuppression
8. Preprocedural application to minimize bacteremia and disease transmission

G. Commercially prepared mouthrinses may contain alcohol or may be alcohol free; other ingredients are water, flavoring, coloring, sweetening agents, and a variety of active ingredients such as:
1. Antimicrobials to reduce or inhibit biofilm activity (cetylpyridinium chloride, chlorhexidine, sanguinarine, phenolic compounds, triclosan)
2. Oxygenating agents to debride and release oxygen (hydrogen peroxide)
3. Astringents to shrink tissue (citric acid, zinc chloride)
4. Anodynes to alleviate pain
5. Buffering agents to reduce acidity, dissolve mucinous films, and relieve soft tissue pain
6. Deodorizing (sodium bicarbonate) and oxidizing (chlorine dioxide) agents to neutralize odors and eliminate volatile sulfur compounds
7. Fluorides to decrease dental caries risk (see the previous section on "Self-Applied Fluorides")
8. Whitening agent such as hydrogen peroxide to reduce intrinsic stains

H. Inexpensive mouthrinses may be prepared by the client (not recommended for clients on a low-salt or sodium-free diet) and used following thorough periodontal debridement
1. Isotonic (normal) saline solution: 1/2 teaspoon salt in 8 ounces of water
2. Hypertonic saline solution: 1/2 tsp salt in 4 oz water
3. Sodium bicarbonate solution: 1/2 tsp sodium bicarbonate (baking soda) in 8 oz warm water

I. Mouthrinse use should be monitored by both the client and the dental hygienist; any adverse effects indicate that use should be evaluated and possibly discontinued

J. The dental hygienist should teach clients how to be wise consumers of mouthrinses, helping clients to recognize the benefits, limitations, and appropriate therapeutic regimens for mouthrinses

DENTAL SEALANTS

General Considerations

See the section on "Pit-and-Fissure Sealants" in Chapter 13.

A. Although systemic and topical fluorides provide increased resistance to carious destruction, the pit-and-fissure surfaces do not benefit from fluoride use to the same degree as do smooth surfaces

B. Sealants are a thin resin or glass ionomer coating placed in the pits and fissures of teeth to act as a physical barrier to oral bacteria
1. Preventive sealant—placed in caries-free pits and fissures
2. Therapeutic sealant—placed in pits and fissures with incipient carious lesions to halt caries process

C. Pits and fissures allow for the accumulation and stagnation of fermentable substrates and serve as accumulation sites for acidogenic microorganisms capable of demineralizing tooth tissue

D. The effectiveness of dental sealants in the prevention of pit-and-fissure caries has been clearly demonstrated in research settings

E. Protection from caries approaches 100% when pits and fissures remain completely sealed; numerous clinical trials have documented the efficacy of sealants

F. Comprehensive prevention programs incorporate the complementary use of sealants and fluorides

G. Sealants classified by method of polymerization
1. Auto-polymerizing—chemically cured or self-curing
2. Photo-polymerizing—cured by visible light

H. Sealants classified by filler content
1. Filled sealant—composite resin sealant containing particles of glass and quartz
2. Unfilled sealants—composite resin sealant without particles; less resistant to long-term wear
3. Glass ionomer—salivary control not a critical factor; ideal for teeth when moisture control is an issue
4. Fluoride releasing—promotes remineralization
5. Calcium phosphate—promotes remineralization

I. Sealants classified by color—available in clear, tinted, and opaque color; the color aids in detection and in monitoring retention

Indications for Application

A. Factors to consider
1. Dental caries activity, risk, and pattern
2. Depth of pits and fissures

3. Dietary patterns
4. Current and past fluoride exposure
5. Eruption status
6. Frequency of preventive services

B. Procedure for sealant placement[1]
   1. Clients or guardians should be informed about sealants as a primary preventive measure
   2. Clients who can benefit from sealant application:
      a. Children with newly erupted teeth with pits and fissures
      b. Persons whose lifestyle, behavior patterns, physical or emotional development, or lack of fluoride exposure put them at high risk for dental caries
      c. Children and adults whose teeth have deep pits and fissures
      d. People with xerostomia or persons with orthodontic appliances
      e. Other persons who desire sealants as a preventive measure to protect pits and fissures

C. Teeth with questionable or incipient carious lesions should be sealed; incipient lesions are arrested after sealant placement[24]

Contraindications to Sealant Application

A. Presence of frank carious lesion on occlusal surface
B. Presence of carious lesion on proximal surface that necessitates preparation of occlusal surface
C. Previously restored tooth, except as noted in item C above
D. Life expectancy of the primary tooth predicted to be short

Application Guidelines[1]

A. Mechanical cleansing of enamel
   1. Debride the pit-and-fissure surface of plaque biofilm and surface debris
   2. Cleansing agents include:
      a. Toothbrush
      b. Air polishing, rubber cup polishing
      c. Dental explorer
B. Isolating
   1. Salivary contamination of etched enamel surfaces is a major reason for resin sealant failure
   2. Isolation—using a rubber dam or cotton rolls and bibulous (absorbent) pads is essential for consistent success
C. Drying
   1. Dry isolated tooth thoroughly in preparation for the application of conditioner or etchant
   2. Avoid water contamination if using air/water syringe
D. Conditioning or etching
   1. Acid conditioning etches enamel surface before the application of resin or glass ionomer (sealant) material; etching removes a layer of enamel and increases the total surface area by rendering the deeper enamel regions porous; the sealant's resin material fills the enamel micropores, producing a mechanical "lock" when polymerized
   2. Acid conditioning agents (30% to 50% phosphoric acid)—available in solution or gel form
      a. Apply the solution by gently dabbing the enamel surface with a saturated cotton pellet or brush; avoid

rubbing the surface because it causes a breakdown of lattice-like micropores
      b. Gels are applied with a special applicator, brush, cotton tip, or cotton pellet
      c. Whether using gel or solution, cover all susceptible surfaces and cuspal inclines with the etchant
      d. Contact between the etching agent and soft tissues should be avoided
      e. Etch the tooth surface for 10 to 20 seconds; check the manufacturer's instructions for etching time

E. Rinsing the conditioned tooth
   1. Thoroughly rinse the etched enamel surfaces by using a water syringe and a high-speed evacuation system; do not allow the client to swish; rinsing time may need to be increased to ensure complete removal
   2. Salivary contamination at this point results in substantial reduction in resin sealant bond strength
      a. Do not allow client to close the mouth, rinse, or touch the conditioned surface with the tongue
      b. When using cotton rolls or bibulous (absorbent) pads, change them as needed, being careful to avoid salivary contamination

F. Drying the conditioned tooth
   1. Prepare the tooth for resin sealant application by drying it thoroughly with compressed air for at least 10 seconds; a completely dry tooth surface is essential for effective application of the resin sealant; it is not as critical when using glass ionomer sealants
   2. Examine the conditioned surface; properly etched surfaces will appear dull and chalky; re-etch the tooth surface when these changes are not seen or salivary contamination occurs

G. Applying the sealant material—all susceptible pits and fissures, including the buccal pits of mandibular molars and the lingual grooves of maxillary molars, should be sealed, when possible
   1. Visible light–cured sealants—the resin sealant is applied to the etched surface; the tip of the light source is placed 2 mm from the sealant (see the manufacturer's instructions)
      a. Light must be delivered for polymerization to occur and for the prevention of sealant failure
      b. Once polymerization is complete, the sealant should be wiped with a wet cotton roll or pellet to remove any air-inhibited layer of nonpolymerized resin; failure to remove this layer will result in an unpleasant taste
      c. The sealant material is delivered in a variety of ways; unit dose dispensers contain enough sealant for one quadrant; this method reduces the risk of cross-contamination, when used properly
   2. Chemical or self-curing sealants—the catalyst and the sealant are mixed and then placed immediately onto the prepared tooth surface with a brush or a custom dispenser; working time from mixing to setting is 1 to 3 minutes; it is important not to disturb the layer of applied sealant during polymerization

3. The sealant material should be allowed to flow into all areas to minimize entrapment of air bubbles
4. Applying excess sealant to the occlusal surface should be avoided because this could alter the client's occlusion

H. Evaluating the results
   1. Examine the sealant to determine the adequacy of bond strength and the absence of voids, underextensions, over-extensions, or undercuring
   2. The sealed surface should feel completely smooth
   3. Floss teeth to ensure that the sealant has not flowed into interproximal spaces
   4. For the filled-type sealant material, occlusion should be checked with articulating paper; frank high spots should be reduced with a finishing bur or fine stone; in the case of unfilled-type sealant materials, high spots self-adjust after a few days
   5. Evaluate sealant retention at each appointment; replace the material, as needed
   6. Most sealant failures result from "operator error," for example, oil, debris, or moisture contamination, or from not following manufacturer's instructions

I. Document on client's chart the type of sealant used and the teeth sealed

TOBACCO USE INTERVENTIONS

General Considerations[25,26]

A. The two types of tobacco are smoked tobacco and unsmoked tobacco
   1. Examples of smoked tobacco include *bidis,* cigars, pipes, cigarettes, water pipe *(hookah),* and clove cigarettes
   2. Unsmoked tobacco is also known as *spit tobacco, snuff,* or *smokeless tobacco*

B. Tobacco cessation is considered to have occurred when an individual permanently discontinues the use of tobacco

C. Smoking is a primary risk factor for:
   1. Lung cancer
   2. Chronic obstructive lung disease
   3. Heart disease
   4. Head and neck, oropharyngeal, and other cancers
   5. Periodontal disease

D. Oral effects of tobacco use: oral and pharyngeal cancer, failure of periodontal therapy, failure of dental implants, dental caries, tobacco abrasion, extrinsic stain, halitosis, attrition, delayed wound healing, nicotine stomatitis, oral leukoplakia, and tooth loss

E. From a host response perspective, smoking has been found to interfere with the normal function of helper lymphocytes critical to antibody production, impair revascularization in both soft and hard tissues, inhibit collagen production, and increase collagenase activity

F. Spit tobacco use is associated with oral, laryngeal, and pharyngeal cancers
   1. Oral mucosal lesions and gingival recession are mostly observed in individuals using spit tobacco
   2. Oral mucosal lesions often disappear after spit tobacco use is discontinued

G. Dental hygienists must assume the responsibility for helping clients abstain from tobacco use and to encourage and appreciate nonusers

H. Nicotine itself is not a carcinogen, but it is physiologically addictive; clients trying to quit may experience withdrawal symptoms (e.g., insomnia, irritability, weight gain); embedded social and psychological factors also contribute to the challenge

I. Dental hygienists should take an active role in the community and in legislative efforts to reduce all tobacco use

Tobacco Cessation Interventions[25-28]

A. Oral care and all other health care facilities should be tobacco free

B. Oral health care professionals should strive to quit all tobacco-related habits and serve as positive role models

C. Tobacco use by all clients should be addressed, assessed, and documented in clients' permanent records

D. The Agency for Healthcare Research and Quality's Clinical Practice Guideline on Treating Tobacco Use and Dependence recommends five components for successful client-provider interaction[28]:
   1. Ask—at every visit of every client, identify and document tobacco use status
   2. Advise—a clear, strong, personalized message to refrain from all tobacco use should be communicated to each client who uses tobacco
   3. Assess—determine if the client is willing to make an attempt to quit
   4. Assist—if client is willing to make an attempt to quit, counseling and pharmacotherapeutic agents should be used; FDA-approved pharmacotherapeutic agents include:
      a. Nicotine reduction therapy—nicotine transdermal patch, gum, lozenge, nasal spray, and oral inhaler
      b. Nonnicotine agents for managing nicotine addiction—sustained-release bupropion hydrochloride (Zyban) tablets and varenicline (Chantix)
   5. Arrange—a follow-up contact should be scheduled within the first week following the quit date

E. The American Dental Hygienists' Association Smoking Cessation Initiative (SCI) recommends three steps:
   1. Ask—ask every client about his or her tobacco use at every visit; ask if the client is a current, former, or never tobacco user
   2. Advise—advise every tobacco user to quit; advise those who have tried and not succeeded to try again; employ the teachable moment by linking clinical findings with advice
   3. Refer—refer the client to QUITLINES, websites, and local cessation programs; find programs and assistance at www.smokefree.gov, www.askadviserefer.org, or call 1-800-QUIT NOW (1-800-784-8669); these websites and telephone numbers provide resources to use at the chairside

F. Teenagers, preteens, and children should be considered potential users of smoked and spit tobacco products; interventions include:

1. Questioning them about tobacco use (e.g., cigarettes, cigars, pipes, water pipes [hookahs], chewing tobacco, snuff)
2. Educating them about the health risks of tobacco use[27]
3. Educating them about the negative effects of tobacco on their physical appearance and athletic prowess
4. Encouraging them to resist peer pressure and media messages to start using tobacco

G. Tobacco-use assessment should be part of history taking; assessment should include:
  1. Form of tobacco used
  2. Amount used
  3. Duration of habit
  4. Previous quit attempts
  5. Reasons for quitting or abstaining from tobacco use

H. Client readiness for cessation—clients should be asked if they are ready to quit; the trans-theoretical model can be used to assess stages of readiness to quit; clients should set their own quit date[27] (see Table 20-16 in Chapter 20)

I. Typically, smokers try to stop multiple times before they succeed

PERIODONTAL DISEASE RISK ASSESSMENT[29]

A. Periodontal risk assessment
  1. Involves the identification of clients and populations at risk of developing periodontal disease
  2. Purpose of risk assessment
    a. Reduce the need for complex periodontal therapy
    b. Improve client outcome
    c. Reduce risk of chronic systemic diseases
  3. Identification of risk factors and taking steps that can reduce the risk will help prevent periodontal disease; identification of risk factors does not imply cause and effect

B. Common risk factors for periodontal disease
  1. Tobacco use
    a. Heat from smoking enhances attachment loss and increases calculus formation, which in turn creates favorable environment for plaque biofilm retention
    b. Nicotine negatively affects collagen synthesis, protein secretion, and bone formation, leading to impaired bone healing
    c. Use of tobacco products increases production of cytokines because of lower oxygen levels, which cause breakdown periodontal tissues
    d. Tobacco history is assessed during health and social histories
  2. Systemic diseases
    a. Have been associated with oral diseases (e.g., periodontal disease, dental caries, salivary gland dysfunction and xerostomia, burning mouth syndrome) and increased susceptibility to oral infections
    b. Evidence shows a high chronic systemic inflammatory response in clients with metabolic syndrome
  3. Genetic factors
    a. Interleukin-1 (IL-1) polymorphism studies have indicated that IL-1 genotype–positive clients have greater

chance of periodontal disease than IL-1 genotype–negative clients
    b. Oral disease and tooth loss in the family are assessed during the health history
  4. Poor oral hygiene—lack of plaque biofilm removal encourages an environment conducive to the survival of periodontal disease pathogens
  5. Metabolic syndrome[29,30]
    a. Group of disorders that increase the risk of heart disease, stroke, and diabetes, including high blood pressure, elevated plasma glucose, excess body fat around the waist and abdominal area, and high cholesterol level
    b. Studies show link between periodontal disease and metabolic syndrome

ORAL CANCER RISK ASSESSMENT

Many oral cancers, unfortunately, are not detected until they have invaded deep tissues and require radical surgery, extensive chemotherapy, irradiation, or all three interventions. Early detection and early treatment are the best ways to manage oral cancer; self-examination can supplement a thorough in-office head and neck, extraoral, and intraoral examination. Clients can potentially benefit from self-examination skills. It is especially important to educate high-risk persons.

A. Clients need to be taught mutable and nonmutable risk factors for oral cancer
  1. Mutable risk factor—can be changed or eliminated (e.g., smoking, sun exposure, or drinking behavior)
  2. Nonmutable risk factor—cannot be changed or eliminated (e.g., genetic makeup, gender)

B. Strategies for reducing risk factors should be part of the dental hygiene care plan

High-Risk Factors[31,32]

A. Tobacco use
  1. Clients who smoke are estimated to be at greater risk than nonsmokers
  2. Clients who use snuff and spit tobacco are prone to squamous cell carcinomas at or near the site where the tobacco is held

B. Alcohol use—the combination of smoking and alcohol use is responsible for the majority of head and neck cancers[1]

C. Virus—certain viruses, such as human immunodeficiency virus (HIV) and human papillomavirus (HPV), are linked to the development of cancers of the nasopharynx, cervix, and lymphatic system

D. Sun exposure—clients who work outdoors, especially those with a fair complexion, are at higher risk for basal cell tumors of the skin (predominating around the face and lips)

Examination Technique
Materials Needed

A. Large mirror and adequate light source are essential for self-examination procedures

B. A flashlight, mouth-sized mirror, and gauze or tissue squares help to access and visualize intraoral structures

Systematic Approach

A. Face and neck
1. Symmetry—one-sided irregularities should be further investigated; right and left sides should have the same outline and shape; lesions that fail to heal within 2 weeks should be suspect
2. Skin—have the client remove eyeglasses; check for sores, bumps, and discoloration
3. Neck—palpate lymph chains for lumps or tender areas
B. Visually examine and palpate lips and gums
1. Have the client remove full or partial dentures
2. Retract the lips; look for sores or color changes
C. Cheek
1. Retract the right side and then the left side to visualize the inner surface; look for red, white, brown, or speckled patches
2. Palpate for lumps or tenderness
3. Run a finger over the inside surface to check for rough or raised places
D. Roof of mouth
1. Tilt the head back and use a flashlight for better visualization
2. Look for sores or color changes; feel for lumps or areas of tenderness
E. Tongue
1. Have the client extend the tongue, and look at the dorsum
2. Grasp the tongue with a gauze square; pull and roll the tongue to the right side and then to the left side
3. Look for sores, color changes, and irregularities
4. Feel for lumps, areas of tenderness, or roughened surfaces
F. Floor of mouth
1. Have the client place the tip of the tongue against the roof of the mouth
2. Look for any asymmetry, sores, or color changes
3. Place the fingers of one hand under the client's jaw, and use the index finger of the other hand to compress structures
4. Check for lumps, tenderness, or irregularities
G. Provide the client with an assessment of his or her mutable and nonmutable risk factors; help the client to reduce the risks for oral cancer
H. Provide the criteria for determining significant deviations from normal
1. Sores that fail to heal within 2 weeks
2. Appearance of white, red, or dark-colored patches
3. Presence of swellings, lumps, bumps, or growths
I. Define the oral health professional's role in interpreting findings; the client should report unusual findings, but should not self-diagnose
J. Establish the concept that self-examination is not meant to be a substitute for periodic regular professional evaluation

DIAGNOSTIC TOOLS FOR ORAL CANCER DETECTION

General Considerations

A. The combination of visual examination and palpation is the main approach to detecting epithelial changes in the oral mucosa
B. Routine examination for the detection of oral cancer should be completed for each client (see the section on "Extraoral and Intraoral Assessment" in Chapter 15)
C. Routine oral cancer screenings can reduce oral cancer incidence and mortality rate[30]
D. The diagnosis of a suspicious lesion is established by traditional biopsy

Brush Biopsy

Definition

A. Transepithelial oral biopsy—samples the superficial, intermediate, and basal epithelial layers to detect oral cancer at its earliest stages (Fig. 16-4); indicated for small, innocuous-appearing lesions
B. The dental hygienist's role is to identify red, white, or mixed lesions as well as ulcerated, thickened, traumatized, or irritated oral epithelium to be evaluated using brush biopsy
C. Dental hygienists should consult their state regulatory board or state statutes to determine whether they are legally permitted to perform brush biopsies
D. Accurate detection of precancerous or cancerous areas requires scalpel biopsy

Advantages

A. Easy, chairside test to evaluate epithelial changes and lesions that may have received only a clinical follow-up before this test became available
B. Rapid results, generally within 3 days to detect dysplasia or carcinoma
C. Minimally invasive

FIG 16-4 Brush biopsy technique being used in evaluation of a suspect intraoral lesion. (Photo courtesy of Oral CDx, Suffern, New York.)

D. Each specimen is evaluated by both computer-assisted analysis and a pathologist

Disadvantages

A. Costs for both obtaining and analyzing the specimen are incurred by the client
B. As with any biopsy method, false-negative results are possible
C. Brush biopsies with negative results require careful follow-up

Procedure

A. Armamentarium (see www.oralcdx.com)
   1. Sterile brush instrument for biopsy
   2. Microscope specimen slide
   3. Fixative
   4. Laboratory forms
B. Obtaining and preparing the sample
   1. Using the client's saliva, moisten the biopsy brush
   2. Firmly press the biopsy brush against the lesion
   3. While pressing, rotate the brush over the surface of the lesion until pink tissue or pinpoint areas of bleeding occur; number of rotations will vary, depending on the thickness of the lesion
   4. Use of topical anesthesia is contraindicated because it may distort the sample
   5. To prepare the glass slide, transfer as much of the cellular sample as possible by rotating and dragging brush lengthwise on the slide
   6. Apply the fixative to cover the slide thoroughly; allow drying for 15 minutes
   7. Package the sample and send it to the laboratory for evaluation

Laboratory Findings for Brush Biopsy

A. Classification categories
   1. Unsatisfactory—specimen is not adequate for diagnosis
   2. Class I: Normal—only normal cells are present
   3. Class II: Atypical—some cellular changes may be present; no suggestion of malignancy is present
   4. Class III: Intermediate—changes may suggest malignancy, but findings are not clear; biopsy is recommended
   5. Class IV: Suggestive of cancer—cells with malignant characteristics are present; biopsy is mandatory
   6. Class V: Positive for cancer—cells are obviously malignant; scalpel biopsy is mandatory
B. Follow-up needs
   1. Unsatisfactory—the client should be scheduled for another smear or brush biopsy
   2. Class I or II findings—the client should be monitored for healing of lesion or reevaluated if the lesion fails to resolve; as with all biopsy methods, false-negative reports are possible; a healed lesion is the best reassurance for reports in categories I and II
   3. Class III, IV, or V findings—the client should be referred for scalpel biopsy

ViziLite

A. Definition—an FDA-approved technology that screens for oral abnormalities potentially indicative of oral cancer
   1. This tool helps oral health care professionals identify lesions before they appear on oral tissue surfaces
   2. ViziLite illumination cannot distinguish keratotic, inflammatory, malignant, or possibly malignant lesions; clinical judgment, and scalpel biopsy are essential for proper patient care[33]
B. Procedure
   1. The client rinses with a solution
   2. The oral health care professional activates a patented light stick intraorally
   3. The light stick illuminates any suboral lesions during the oral cancer screening examination (www.vizilite.com)
C. Studies have shown inconsistent results with the use of ViziLite

VELscope

A. Definition—an FDA-approved handheld device that uses oral fluorescence technology to identify precancerous and cancerous lesions in the oral cavity[33]
   1. The fluorescence technology shows healthy tissue as green and potentially cancerous lesions as dark magenta, brown, or black
   2. Changes in tissue can be detected while the change is still subepithelial and otherwise not visualized during conventional oral examination
   3. Surgical margins can be determined, which will help guide complete removal of oral cancers in the operatory
B. This device should be used as an adjunct to clinical screening; clinical judgment and scalpel biopsy are essential for the diagnosis of oral cancer lesions
C. There is higher risk of false-positive results; VELscope does not provide a definitive diagnosis

Other Devices and Oral Examination

A. Other oral cancer detection devices are available, such as Identafi; however, these devices are unable to provide definitive diagnosis
B. Routine oral cancer visual and tactile examination is still the "gold standard" for identification of oral cancer lesions[33]

ASSESSMENT OF DENTINAL HYPERSENSITIVITY

A. Definition—abnormal condition that occurs when vital dentin is exposed to the environment of the oral cavity; the result is painful stimuli that can reach the pulp and cause pain
   1. Thermal, evaporative, tactile, osmotic, or chemical stimuli can cause fluid movement within the dentinal tubule, exciting the nerve and signaling the pulp to respond
   2. Gingival recession and loss of enamel should be minimized to avoid dentinal hypersensitivity
   3. Treatment of dentinal hypersensitivity is a valuable client service; symptoms cause considerable discomfort to the

client and may interfere with both control of plaque biofilm and professional treatment

B. Characteristics
1. Rapid onset
2. Sharp pain
3. Short duration
4. Response to stimuli

ETIOLOGY

A. Primary causes of hypersensitivity are exposed dentin and open dentinal tubules
B. Dentin exposure occurs:
1. In 10% of all teeth; during development, enamel and cementum do not join
2. When enamel or cementum is lost through abrasion, erosion, abfraction, dental caries, or overinstrumentation
3. When soft tissue is lost because of gingival recession, periodontal surgery, or an aggressive toothbrushing technique
4. When diet exposes the dentin to foods and beverages with a low pH; soft drinks, sport drinks, coffee, and fruit juices/drinks; citrus fruits; yogurt; and some alcoholic beverages; plaque biofilm acids
C. Loss of hard and soft tissues is believed to be accelerated from the combined use of mechanical brushing and a dentifrice applied immediately after exposure to acidic food or drink

Pain Mechanism

A. Hydrodynamic theory—the most widely accepted
B. Explains the following:
1. Dentinal tubules are exposed
2. Pain-producing stimuli are present
3. Pain-producing stimuli initiate the flow of lymphatic fluid within dental tubules
4. Odontoblasts and their processes act as receptors and transmitters of sensory stimuli
5. The movement of tubular fluids causes nerve endings at the pulpal wall to be stimulated and produce pain

Pain Stimuli

A. Thermal or evaporative stimuli—foods and liquids at extreme temperatures, cold air, and too-rapid drying of a tooth surface; cause a concurrent rapid drop in tooth temperature; are more problematic than hot-air changes
B. Mechanical stimuli—instrumentation, home care devices, eating utensils, and friction from removable prosthetic or orthodontic devices
C. Chemical stimuli—foods high in acid or sugars; some topical medications; plaque acids

Desensitizing Agents

A. Modes of action—desensitizers:
1. Seal dentinal tubules by surface precipitation of ions, subsurface incorporation of ions, or stimulation of secondary dentin

2. Decrease the excitability of sensory nerves, thereby making the nerve less sensitive to stimuli
B. Optimal characteristics—professionally applied desensitizing agents should act rapidly and should be nontoxic, easy to apply, and have consistent outcomes and long-term effects

Types of Desensitizing Treatments

A. No single desensitizing agent or form of treatment is effective for all persons
B. Numerous agents have varying degrees of success, including:
1. Solutions, gels, or pastes of fluoride in varying compounds and percentages, stannous fluoride, calcium hydroxide, strontium chloride, potassium nitrate, sodium citrate, formaldehyde, glutaraldehyde, arginine and insoluble calcium, casein phosphopeptide–amorphous calcium phosphate complex, or potassium or ferric oxalate
2. Adhesive, varnish, or bonding materials
3. Polymerizing agents[1]
   a. Glass ionomer cements (GICs)—used in cervical abrasion and abfraction; the sensitive area is etched with 50% citric acid, rinsed with water, and dried before application of GIC
   b. Adhesive resin primers—reduces dentin permeability by occluding open tubules; the material is rubbed on the sensitive area for approximately 30 seconds and air-dried
4. Iontophoretic devices—technique sensitive
   a. Iontophoresis is the application of an electrical current to impregnate tissues with ions from dissolved salts
   b. Fluoride iontophoresis is thought to result in the increased uptake and penetration of fluoride ions into dentin
5. Laser therapy—one-time treatment that reduces or eliminates dentin sensitivity by sealing dentinal tubules; sensitive dentin treated with laser is found to be harder than untreated dentin
6. Restorations—restoration may be placed on the surface where dentin is exposed to help reduce sensitivity

Desensitization Methods

A. Self-care regimens
1. Effective plaque biofilm control strategies are important in gaining and maintaining control of hypersensitivity; modifications to minimize aggressive brushing are critical
2. Specially formulated toothpastes containing 5% potassium nitrate to desensitize the nerve are often combined with fluoride, which promotes remineralization
3. Daily use of a fluoride gel or rinse is advisable when the problem is generalized or recurrent
B. Professionally delivered regimens should support and enable self-care regimens
1. General guidelines
   a. Remove all deposits; involved surfaces must be free of barriers to the agent
   b. Local anesthesia is appropriate when instrumentation procedure or application of the agent is too painful

c. Isolate the sensitive tooth and control saliva

d. Dry the affected tooth with cotton pellets or gauze; avoid using an air syringe

e. Apply the agent according to the manufacturer's instructions for method and time required

   (1) Pastes are usually burnished in with a wooden point, whereas solutions, gels, or varnishes are painted or bathed on

   (2) Some clients may experience an acute pain reaction to the agent; immediately remove the agent, wait a few minutes, and then attempt reapplication

f. Remove any excess agent to avoid ingestion by the client

g. Test for change in pain reaction; this will not be possible with anesthetized areas

h. Plan for future reapplication if desensitization has not occurred

2. Precaution—some agents have very high concentrations of fluoride; to prevent nausea, use proper application and techniques to control salivary flow

PULPAL VITALITY AND TESTING DEVICES

Basic Concepts

A. Teeth may become nonvital from bacterial invasion of the pulp associated with caries or periodontal disease or from injuries such as mechanical or thermal trauma

B. Any tooth suspected of being nonvital should be tested for pulpal vitality

C. The preferred method of testing provides a *qualitative* assessment

D. Tests should correlate with or mimic the client's chief complaint

E. Palpation, percussion, and radiographic findings (e.g., widened periodontal ligament) are other sources of data for pulpal assessment

Laser Doppler Flowmetry[34]

A. Noninvasive, painless, semi-quantitative method; measures pulpal blood flow through assessment of the vascular supply by the passage of light through a tooth; monitors blood flow in response to pressure changes and administration of local anesthesia

B. Useful in young children whose responses are usually unreliable

C. Studies have shown that blood circulation is the most accurate determinant in assessing pulp vitality[34]

D. Laser Doppler flowmetry is more reliable at identifying vital and nonvital teeth earlier than other pulp vitality tests

Traditional Electrical Testing Devices

A. The electrical pulp tester (also known as a *vitalometer*) and the digital pulp tester use gradations of electrical current to excite a response in pulpal tissue and thus assess response to stimulus

1. Pulp testers have either a portable battery or a plug-in electrical power source

2. All testers have rheostats, with a scale (e.g., 1 to 10 or 1 to 50) that indicates the relative amount of current being applied; digital pulp testers provide a digital reading

3. Electrical pulp testers can be used safely on clients with implanted cardiac devices

B. Procedure

1. Armamentarium

   a. Testing device

   b. Cotton rolls

   c. Toothpaste or other conducting medium

2. Client preparation

   a. Explain the procedure to the client; use the minimal stimulation necessary to evoke a response

   b. Instruct the client to raise a hand when the slightest warmth or tingling sensation is felt

3. Obtaining a reading

   a. Isolate and dry the teeth to be tested; this prevents the conduction of current into the soft tissue

   b. Apply a small amount of toothpaste, or an alternative conductor, to the tester tip

   c. Place the tip on sound tooth structure, within the middle third of the crown for a single-rooted tooth and within the middle third of each cusp for a multi-rooted tooth; a clip resting on the client's lip and attached to the handpiece is necessary to create a closed electrical circuit and to activate the tester

   d. Avoid any contact with restorations and soft tissue

   e. Slowly advance the rheostat from zero to increasingly higher numbers until a sensation is felt by the client; the rheostat should not be moved above that point for that tooth

4. Documentation

   a. Two readings should be taken for each tooth tested and the readings averaged

   b. For all teeth tested, record the lowest average reading, the type of testing device and conductor used, and any client actions or reactions that may have affected the results

C. Variables affecting results

1. Pulpal conditions may vary from early inflammation to complete necrosis; client responses vary with each condition; the pulp of the tooth that is tested is considered to be degenerating when, compared with a control, much more current is required to gain a response

2. Metallic restorations conduct electrical charges more rapidly than tooth structure and can produce false readings

3. Teeth with splints, bridges, or proximal restorations may produce false-positive reactions because the circuit can be transferred from adjacent vital teeth

4. Multi-rooted teeth may have some combination of vital and nonvital canals and may give false-positive results

5. Pain reactions are influenced by the client's attitude, age, gender, anxiety, emotions, fatigue, culture, and medications

Thermal Testing

A. Employs a hot or cold stimulus to test for pulpal response

B. The cold test is used most often

C. The heat test is useful when an unidentified tooth is heat sensitive

ETHICAL, LEGAL, AND SAFETY ISSUES

A. Dental hygienists must have knowledge of evidence-based preventive products and strategies to provide optimal care
B. A combination of frequent review of the literature; focus on information from controlled clinical trials and systematic review articles; the practitioner's knowledge, clinical experience, and judgment; and client preferences leads to appropriate evidence-based decision making and best practices
C. Thorough, accurate, and confidential chart documentation is essential; adherence to the regulations of the Health Insurance Portability and Accountability Act (HIPAA) is mandatory

D. The client's progress with regard to self-care should be documented in the client record and should include the client's response, knowledge, adherence, involvement, skills, and measurable oral changes
E. The dental hygienist should discuss all the procedures with clients on an appropriate level for comprehension, obtain informed consent, and encourage client participation in the dental hygiene care plan
F. Dental hygiene interventions are offered within the scope of dental hygiene practice and within the legal jurisdiction of the employment setting
G. Clients have the right to accept or reject the dental care plan and still retain the respect of the dental hygienist
H. Clients have the right to receive individualized, cutting-edge, evidence-based recommendations and care

Website Information and Resources

Source	Website Address	Description
National Center for Dental Hygiene Research	http://www.usc.edu/hsc/dental/dhnet/	Dental hygienists' resources and links
American Academy of Periodontology	http://www.perio.org	Periodontics resources and position papers
Campaign for Tobacco Free Kids	http://www.tobaccofreekids.org/index.php	Information and initiatives to keep kids tobacco free
ADHA Ask. Advise. Refer. Campaign	http://www.askadviserefer.org	Information about smoking cessation
American Lung Association—Freedom from Smoking	http://www.lungusa.org/	Information about lung diseases and tobacco cessation

REFERENCES

1. Darby ML, Walsh MM: *Dental hygiene theory and practice,* ed 4, Philadelphia, 2014, Saunders.
2. Maslow AH: A theory of human motivation, *Psychol Rev* 50 (4):370–396, July 1943. http://dx.doi.org/10.1037/h0054346.
3. Karen G, Barbara KR, Viswanath K: *Health behavior and health education: theory, research, and practice,* ed 4, San Francisco, 2008, Jossey-Bass.
4. Hollister MC, Anema MG: Health behavior models and oral health: a review, *J Dent Hygiene* 78(3):6, Summer 2004.
5. Bray KK, Catley D, Voelker MA, Liston R, Williams KB: Motivational interviewing in dental hygiene education: curriculum modification and evaluation, *J Dent Educ* 77(12):1662–1669, 2013.
6. Johansson AC, Johannsen G, Uhlin L, Johannsen A: Dental hygienist students' learning about motivational interviewing, *Dentistry J* 2(2):65–77, 2014.
7. Miller WR, Rollnick S: *Motivational interviewing: helping people change,* ed 3, New York, 2013, Guilford Press.
8. Rollnick S, Miller WR, Butler C: *Motivational interviewing for health care professionals,* New York, 2007, Guilford Press.
9. Lee JY, Divaris K, Baker D, Rozier RG, Vann WF: The relationship of oral health literacy with oral health status and dental neglect, *Am J Public Health* 102(5):923–929, 2012.
10. Grender J, Williams K, Walters P, Klukowska M, Reick H: Plaque removal efficacy of oscillating-rotating power toothbrushes: review of six comparative clinical trials, *Am J Dent* 26(2):68–74, 2013.
11. Husseini A, Slot DE, van der Weijden GA: The efficacy of oral irrigation in addition to a toothbrush on plaque and the clinical parameters of periodontal inflammation: a systematic review, *Int J Dent Hyg* 6(4):304–314, 2008.

12. Nachnani S: Oral malodor: causes, assessment, and treatment, *Comp Cont Educ Dent* 32(1):22–32, 2011.
13. Kato K, Tamura K, Nakagaki H: Quantitative evaluation of the oral biofilm-removing capacity of a dental water jet using an electron-probe microanalyzer, *Arch Oral Biol* 57(1):30–35, 2012.
14. Kasat V, Ladda R: Smoking and dental implants, *J Int Soc Prev Community Dentistry* 2(2):38–41, 2013.
15. Hurlbutt M: CAMBRA: best practices in dental caries management. *RDH* October 2011:9-108. http://www.rdhmag.com/etc/medialib/new-lib/rdh/site-images/volume-31/issue-10/1110RDH095-109.pdf. (Accessed 23.03.15.)
16. Weyant RJ, Tracy SL, Anselmo TT, et al: Topical fluoride for caries prevention: executive summary of the updated clinical recommendations and supporting systematic review, American Dental Association Council on Scientific Affairs Expert Panel on Topical Fluoride Caries Preventive Agents, *J Am Dent Assoc* 144 (11):1279–1291, 2013.
17. Ten Cate JM: Contemporary perspective on the use of fluoride products in caries prevention, *Br Dent J* 214(4):161–167, 2013.
18. Cochrane NJ, Reynolds EC: Calcium phosphopeptides: mechanisms of action and evidence for clinical efficacy, *Adv Dent Res* 24(2):41–47, 2012.
19. Azarpazhooh A, Limeback H: Clinical efficacy of casein derivatives: a systematic review of the literature, JADA Continuing Education, *J Am Dent Assoc* 139(7):915–924, 2008.
20. Fontana M, Gonzalez-Cabezas C: Xylitol lozenges were not effective in overall dental caries prevention in adults, *J Evid Based Dent Pract* 13(3):97–99, 2013.
21. Bader JD, Vollmer WM, Shugars DA, et al: Results from the Xylitol for Adult Caries Trial (X-ACT), JADA Continuing Education, *J Am Dent Assoc* 144(1):21–30, 2013.

22. Swango PA: Regular use of antimicrobial mouthrinses can effectively augment the benefits of oral prophylaxis and oral hygiene instructions at 6-month recall intervals in reducing the occurrence of dental plaque and gingivitis, *J Evid Based Dent Pract* 12(2):87–89, 2012.

23. Gunsolley JC: Clinical efficacy of antimicrobial mouthrinses, *J Dent* 38(1):S6–S10, 2010.

24. De Assunção IV, da Costa Gde F, Borges BC: Systematic review of noninvasive treatments to arrest dentin non-cavitated caries lesions, *World J Clin Cases* 2(5):137–141, 2014.

25. Centers for Disease Control and Prevention: Tobacco industry and products, August 21, 2014. http://www.cdc.gov/tobacco/basic_information/tobacco_industry/. (Accessed 20.10.14.)

26. Mishra S, Mishra MB: Tobacco: its historical, cultural, oral, and periodontal health association, *J Int Soc Prev Community Dentistry* 3(1):12–18, 2013.

27. Wisconsin Dental Association: Treating tobacco use and dependence: a toolkit for dental office. http://www.ctri.wisc.edu/HC.Providers/dentists/toolkit.pdf. (Accessed 24.06.14.)

28. Fiore MC, Anderson JE, Jorenby DE, Scott WJ: *Treating tobacco use and dependence: 2008 update, 2008: Clinical practice guidelines,* Rockville, Md, 2008, US Department of Health and Human Services http://www.ahrq.gov/professionals/clinicians-providers/guidelines-recommendations/tobacco/clinicians/update/treating_tobacco_use08.pdf (Accessed 22.10.14.).

29. Genco RJ, Borgnakke WS: Risk factors for periodontal disease, *Periodontology* 62:59–94, 2000. June 2013.

30. Halpern A, Mancini MC, Magalhães ME, et al: Metabolic syndrome, dyslipidemia, hypertension and type 2 diabetes in youth: from diagnosis to treatment, *Diabetol Metab Syndr* 2:55, August 2010.

31. Foulkes M: Oral cancer: risk factors, treatment and nursing care, *Nurs Standard* 28(8):49–57, 2013 (Royal College of Nursing [Great Britain] 1987).

32. González-Ramírez I, Irigoyen-Camacho M, Ramírez-Amador V, et al: Association between age and high-risk human papilloma virus in Mexican oral cancer patients, *Oral Dis* 19(8):796–804, 2013.

33. Messadi DV: Diagnostic aids for detection of oral precancerous conditions, *Int J Oral Sci* 5(2):59–65, June 2013.

34. Vaghela D, Sinha A: Pulse oximetry and laser Doppler flowmetry for diagnosis of pulpal vitality, *J Interdisciplinary Dentistry* 1 (1):14–21, 2011.

SUGGESTED READINGS

Harris NO, Garcia-Godoy F: *Primary preventive dentistry,* ed 8, Upper Saddle River, NJ, 2013, Pearson Prentice Hall.

Kenneth M: A new treatment alternative for sensitive teeth: a desensitizing oral rinse, *J Dentistry* 41(1):S1–S11, 2013.

Pockey JR, Song E, Sutfin EL, et al: The need for tobacco cessation in a free clinic population, *Addict Behav* 37(12):1299–1302, 2012.

Schmidt BL: Current topics in oral cancer research and oral cancer screening, *J Dent Hygiene* 86:7–8, February 2012.

Wilkins EM: *Clinical practice of the dental hygienist,* ed 11, Philadelphia, 2013, Lippincott Williams & Wilkins.

Yasuhiro N, Katsura S, Yuuji K, et al: Examination of denture-cleaning methods based on the quantity of microorganisms adhering to a denture, *Gerodontology* 29(2):e259–e266, 2012.

CHAPTER 16 REVIEW QUESTIONS

Answers and rationales to chapter review questions are available on this text's accompanying Evolve site. See inside front cover for details.

evolve

1. **Which behavior change theory stresses the importance of patient autonomy in decision-making?**
   a. Human Needs Model
   b. Trans-theoretical Model
   c. Health Belief Model
   d. Motivational Interviewing

2. **Which of the following theory states that the client's basic needs must be met before they can be motivated to achieve higher-level needs, such as purchase of a power toothbrush?**
   a. Health Belief
   b. Maslow's hierarchy of needs
   c. Motivation theory
   d. Trans-theoretical model

3. **Ms. Murphy, 30 years old, presents to clinic with a chief complaint of bleeding gums when brushing. On probing, the dental hygienist notices generalized calculus with 5-mm to 6-mm pocket depths. The dental hygienist plans to perform four-quadrant scaling and root planing. Performing scaling and root planing falls under which of the following steps of the dental hygiene process of care?**
   a. Assessment
   b. Planning
   c. Implementation
   d. Documentation

4. **Which of the following products would you recommend for plaque removal under a pontic to a client with severe rheumatoid arthritis?**
   a. End-tuft brush
   b. Super-floss
   c. Proxy brush
   d. Waxed floss

5. **All the following are risk factors for oral cancer EXCEPT one. Which one is the *exception*?**
   a. HPV
   b. Tobacco use
   c. Alcohol use
   d. Periodontitis

6. **All the following interventions are aimed at the prevention of oral cancer EXCEPT:**
   a. Oral cancer screening at each visit
   b. Tobacco cessation counseling
   c. Biofilm removal education

d. Nutritional counseling

7. **A client with periodontal disease can benefit from using all the following products EXCEPT:**
   a. Antimicrobial mouthrinse
   b. Power toothbrush
   c. Dentifrices with potassium nitrate
   d. Interdental brush

8. **For proper oral care, a toothbrush should be regularly disinfected and replaced every 3 months of use. Toothbrushes should be changed after a cold, the flu, a mouth infection, or a sore throat.**
   a. Both statements are TRUE.
   b. Both statements are FALSE.
   c. The first statement is TRUE; the second statement is FALSE.
   d. The first statement is FALSE; the second statement is TRUE.

9. **Which of the following ingredients in oral products helps in the remineralization of a tooth surface?**
   a. Amorphous calcium phosphate
   b. Casein phosphopeptide–amorphous calcium phosphate
   c. Fluoride
   d. All the above

10. **All the following are TRUE statements about 5% fluoride varnish EXCEPT:**
    a. Approved for caries control
    b. Can be applied to teeth in both children and adults
    c. Recommended for clients with high caries risk
    d. Available over the counter for caries prevention

11. **All the following mouthrinses can be recommended to clients with periodontal disease EXCEPT:**
    a. 0.12% chlorhexidine gluconate
    b. 0.05% sodium fluoride
    c. Essential oils
    d. Cetylpyridinium chloride

12. **One of the main causes of oral malodor is plaque biofilm accumulation on the dorsal surface of the tongue. Clients struggling to control oral malodor should seek professional oral health care combined with daily interdental cleaning, tongue brushing, and use of antimicrobial mouthrinse.**
    a. Both statements are TRUE.
    b. Both statements are FALSE.
    c. The first statement is TRUE; the second statement is FALSE.

d. The first statement is FALSE; the second statement is TRUE.

13. **Which of the following is NOT a risk factor for root caries?**
    a. Dental recession
    b. Xerostomia
    c. Plaque biofilm
    d. Diastema

14. **Triclosan as an added ingredient to dentifrices falls under which of the following categories?**
    a. Therapeutics
    b. Humectants
    c. Preservatives
    d. Binding agents

15. **All the following are risk factors for dental implants failure EXCEPT:**
    a. Tobacco use
    b. Heavy plaque biofilm
    c. Periodontal disease
    d. Dental calculus

16. **An individual can be in the "high-risk" or "low-risk" category for development of dental caries. All the following factors are low-risk factors in the development of dental caries for adults EXCEPT:**
    a. Normal salivary flow
    b. Use of fluoride mouthrinse
    c. Sealants in pits and fissures
    d. Poor manual dexterity

17. **Which of the following clients would be an ideal candidate for dental sealants?**
    a. Client with periodontal disease
    b. Client who uses fluoride
    c. Client with incipient carious lesions
    d. Client with habitual bruxism

18. **Stimuli causes fluid movement within the dentinal tubule, exciting the nerve and signaling the pulp to respond as dentin hypersensitivity. Pain stimuli can only be thermal, such as hot or cold foods and liquids.**
    a. Both statements are TRUE.
    b. Both statements are FALSE.
    c. The first statement is TRUE; the second statement is FALSE.
    d. The first statement is FALSE; the second statement is TRUE.

CASE A

Ms. McDonald, age 59, is a regular patient at the dental office. She has been recently diagnosed with breast cancer and is scheduled to have double mastectomy in 1 month. She takes valsartan (Diovan HCT) for hypertension and naproxen for rheumatoid arthritis. She experiences dry mouth and reports brushing twice daily with a soft toothbrush. She states she knows she should floss more often, but only flosses occasionally. Ms. McDonald has moderate levels of interproximal plaque biofilm. She is missing teeth #1, #3, #14, #16, #17, and #32. She has occlusal amalgam restorations on teeth #2, #29 and #3.

Use Case A to answer questions 19 to 23.

19. **According to the Trans-theoretical model, what stage of change is Ms. McDonald in with regard to flossing?**
    a. Precontemplation
    b. Contemplation

c. Preparation
d. Action

20. **How would you categorize Ms. McDonald's caries risk assessment after radiation therapy?**
    a. Low caries risk

b. Moderate caries

c. High caries risk

d. Severe caries risk

21. **What American Society of Anesthesiologists (ASA) Physical Status Classification is applicable to Ms. McDonald?**
    a. ASA I
    b. ASA II
    c. ASA III
    d. ASA IV

22. **What interdental device would the dental hygienist recommend to Ms. McDonald?**
    a. Dental floss
    b. Floss threader
    c. Interdental brush
    d. Toothbrush

23. **Which of the following over-the-counter products can the dental hygienist recommend to Ms. McDonald for remineralization of her teeth?**
    a. Fluoride mouthrinse
    b. Essential oil mouthrinse
    c. 5% fluoride varnish

d. Dentifrices with triclosan

24. **A client with high caries risk would manifest all the following EXCEPT:**
    a. Moderate plaque biofilm
    b. Xerostomia
    c. Generalized restorations
    d. Fluorosis

25. **In addition to proper toothbrushing technique, daily use of all the following may help a client with calculus prevention EXCEPT:**
    a. Dental floss
    b. Dentifrice with triclosan
    c. Fluoride mouthrinse
    d. Antimicrobial mouthrinse

26. **Clients with all the following conditions can benefit from daily use of oral irrigation EXCEPT those with:**
    a. Osteoarthritis
    b. Hypertension
    c. Parkinson's disease
    d. Periodontal disease

CASE B

Ms. Thompson, age 35, is a new patient who presents to clinic today. Her health history reveals she is taking metformin for type 2 diabetes and the anticonvulsant phenytoin for prevention of seizers. She smokes one-half pack of cigarettes daily. Intraoral assessment reveals a coated tongue; a white, asymptomatic, 3-mm lesion on the left lateral border of the tongue; generalized brown extrinsic stains covering most of the lingual surfaces; moderate gingival hyperplasia; and light calculus around the cervical third of premolars. Periodontal assessment reveals generalized 6-mm probing depths with no recession. When asked about the lesion on her tongue, Ms. Thompson states, "It has been there for at least a month."

Use Case B to answer questions 27 to 37.

27. **Which of the following is contributing to Ms. Thompson's gingival hyperplasia?**
    a. Phenytoin
    b. Plaque biofilm
    c. Smoking
    d. Both a and b

28. **Which of the following may be signs of periodontal disease?**
    a. Bleeding on probing
    b. Gram-negative anaerobic bacteria
    c. Probing depths
    d. All the above

29. **Which of the following clinical examination methods should the dental hygienist use when examining Ms Thompson's tongue?**
    a. Probing and transillumination
    b. Observation and palpation
    c. Radiographs and exploration
    d. Transillumination and palpation

30. **What is MOST likely contributing to Ms. Thompson's white spot lesion on the tongue?**
    a. Phenytoin
    b. Smoking
    c. Plaque biofilm
    d. Diabetes

31. **State statutes do not permit the dental hygienist to perform biopsies. How best can the dental hygienist deal with Ms. Thompson's tongue lesion?**
    a. Refer to oral pathologist for definite diagnosis
    b. Leave the lesion alone, since it is asymptomatic
    c. Use ViziLite for immediate diagnosis
    d. Perform scalpel biopsy

32. **Which of the following dentifrices can Ms. Thompson use for whitening her teeth?**
    a. Dentifrice containing triclosan
    b. Dentifrice with sodium fluoride
    c. Dentifrice with potassium nitrate
    d. Dentifrice with hydrogen peroxide

33. **Ms. Thompson can benefit from all the following measures to control her gingival hyperplasia EXCEPT:**
    a. Floss threader
    b. Dentifrice with triclosan
    c. Antimicrobial mouthrinse
    d. Daily oral irrigation

34. **When discussing maintenance of Ms. Thompson's white smile, the dental hygienist should include all the following EXCEPT:**
    a. Smoking cessation
    b. Tooth-whitening methods
    c. White spot lesion on the tongue
    d. Desensitizing treatments

35. **How best can the dental hygienist document 6 mm probing depths using the American Academy of Periodontology (AAP) classification system?**
    a. AAP Case Type I
    b. AAP Case Type II
    c. AAP Case Type III
    d. AAP Case Type IV

36. **Dental stains are classified as exogenous/endogenous and extrinsic/intrinsic. Tobacco stains on Ms. Thompson's teeth are considered to be endogenous and intrinsic.**
    a. Both statements are TRUE.
    b. Both statements are FALSE.
    c. The first statement is TRUE; the second statement is FALSE.
    d. The first statement is FALSE; the second statement is TRUE.

37. **Which of the following educational pamphlets will the dental hygienist recommend to Ms. Thompson for prevention of oral cancer?**
    a. Risk of tobacco use
    b. Oral self-examination
    c. Management of nicotine addiction
    d. All the above

38. **Which of the following antimicrobial and antigingivitis agents is known for its high substantivity?**
    a. Essential oils
    b. Chlorhexidine gluconate
    c. Cetylpyridinium chloride
    d. Stannous fluoride

39. **When evaluating gingival characteristics, how would the clinician describe an enlarged gingival margin with the formation of a life saver–like gingival prominence?**
    a. Coral pink
    b. Festooned
    c. Stippled
    d. Firm

40. **Both mutable and nonmutable risk factors for oral cancer can be changed. Examples of mutable risk factor include smoking, sun exposure, and high alcohol intake.**
    a. Both statements are TRUE.
    b. Both statements are FALSE.
    c. The first statement is TRUE; the second statement is FALSE.
    d. The first statement is FALSE; the second statement is TRUE.

41. **Which of the following mouthrinses is available only as a prescription?**
    a. 0.12% Chlorhexidine gluconate
    b. 0.05% Sodium fluoride
    c. Essential oils
    d. Cetylpyridinium chloride

42. **In which of the following toothbrushing methods are the toothbrush bristles placed on the attached gingiva and directed apically at 45-degree angle to the long axis of the tooth?**
    a. Bass method
    b. Charters' method
    c. Stillman's method
    d. Fones method

43. **All the following are desirable characteristics of toothbrushes EXCEPT:**
    a. Durable
    b. Impervious to moisture
    c. Flexible and soft
    d. All the above

44. **Clients with removable appliances should be educated on the proper cleaning and storage of the oral appliance. Inadequate cleaning of oral appliances can contribute to which of the following oral conditions?**
    a. *Candida albicans* infection
    b. Amelogenesis imperfecta
    c. Dental fluorosis
    d. Fordyce granules

45. **Which of the following is NOT a removable oral appliance?**
    a. Obturator
    b. Partial denture
    c. Dental implant
    d. Mouthguard

46. **Which of the following is a GOOD characteristic of professional desensitizing agents?**
    a. Fast acting
    b. Easy application
    c. Nontoxic
    d. All the above

47. **What is the number-one reason for the failure of resin-based pit-and-fissure dental sealants?**
    a. Incomplete dry tooth surface
    b. Conditioning or etching
    c. Glass ionomer cements
    d. Photo-polymerization

48. **All the following are therapeutic ingredients in dentifrices EXCEPT:**
    a. Amorphous calcium phosphate
    b. Triclosan
    c. Sodium fluoride
    d. Sodium laurel sulfate

49. **All the following dentifrice ingredients would help control calculus formation EXCEPT:**
    a. Zinc citrate
    b. Pyrophosphate
    c. Triclosan
    d. Potassium citrate

50. **All the following types of dentifrices will be beneficial for a client with generalized demineralization EXCEPT:**
    a. Stannous fluoride
    b. Carbamide peroxide
    c. Amorphous calcium phosphate
    d. Sodium fluoride

51. **Which one of the following statements is FALSE when recommending the use of oral irrigation systems?**
    a. Improves gingival bleeding
    b. Reduces pocket depths
    c. Replaces dental floss
    d. Removes loose biofilm

Periodontal Instrumentation for Assessment and Care

Jill S. Gehrig, Rebecca A. Sroda

This chapter focuses on the use of periodontal instruments for assessment and nonsurgical periodontal instrumentation. The primary objective of nonsurgical periodontal instrumentation is to restore periodontal tissue to health by removing plaque biofilm, its byproducts, and biofilm-retentive factors from tooth surfaces and from within the tooth pocket space. Successful professional care depends on reducing biofilm to a level that is acceptable to the tissue; therefore, instructing and supervising the client's daily self-care precedes, continues with, and follows instrumentation by the dental hygiene practitioner.

INSTRUMENT DESIGN

Parts of an Instrument

A. Handle—the part of a periodontal instrument that the clinician holds; various shapes, weights, sizes, and surface serrations (smooth, ribbed, or knurled) exist
  1. Types
    a. Single-ended—one working end
    b. Double-ended—two working ends; working ends may be unpaired (dissimilar working ends) or paired (mirror-image working ends)
  2. Handle design characteristics
    a. Small-diameter ($\frac{3}{17}$-inch) handles, with smooth or flat texture, decrease the user's control and increase muscle fatigue
    b. Large-diameter ($\frac{3}{8}$-inch) handles that are lightweight and have bumpy texturing maximize the user's control and reduce muscle fatigue
B. Shank—connects the working end with the handle; usually bent in one or more places to facilitate placement of the working end against the tooth surface
  1. Functional shank—the part of the shank that allows the working end to be adapted to the tooth surface; begins below the working end and extends to the last bend in the shank nearest the handle
    a. Instruments with short functional shanks are used on teeth crowns
    b. Instruments with long functional shanks are used on both the crown and the root (Fig. 17-1)
  2. Lower (terminal) shank—the bent portion of the functional shank nearest to the working end (Fig. 17-1)

3. Extended lower shank—3 mm longer than a standard lower shank; provides additional leverage, acting as a fulcrum, and is ideal for working in deep periodontal pockets
4. Simple shank—bent in one plane (front to back); used primarily on anterior teeth; also called a *straight shank*
5. Complex shank—bent in two planes (front to back and side to side) to facilitate instrumentation of posterior teeth; this design is necessary to reach around the crown and onto the root surface; also called an *angled shank* or *curved shank*
C. Working end—the part of the dental instrument that contacts the tooth (explorer, curet) or soft tissue (probe) to perform the work of the instrument; begins where the instrument shank ends; an instrument may have one or two working ends
  1. Parts of the working end—identified as the face, back, lateral surfaces, toe, and tip; on a hand-activated periodontal instrument, a cutting edge is formed by the union of a lateral surface and the face of the working end
  2. Application of the working end—the tooth surfaces or areas of the mouth on which an instrument can be used
    a. Anterior use—one single-ended instrument (e.g., anterior sickle scaler, such as a Jacquette 33) can be used to perform procedures on the facial, lingual, mesial, and distal surfaces of anterior teeth
    b. Posterior use—one double-ended instrument (e.g., posterior sickle scaler, such as a Jacquette 34/35) can be used to perform procedures on the facial, lingual, mesial, and distal surfaces of posterior teeth
    c. Universal use—one double-ended instrument (e.g., universal curet, such as a Columbia 13/14) can be used to perform procedures on both anterior and posterior teeth
    d. Area-specific use—an instrument that can be applied only to specific surfaces and areas of the mouth; a set of area-specific instruments (e.g., area-specific curets, such as the Gracey series) is needed for procedures on the entire dentition
  3. Function of the working end
    a. Assessment of teeth, soft tissue, or both
    b. Instrumentation of tooth surfaces (the removal or disruption of calculus deposits and plaque biofilm)

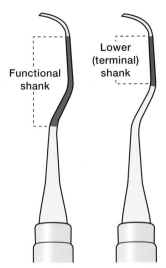

FIG 17-1 Functional shank and lower (terminal) shank. (From Nield-Gehrig JS: *Fundamentals of periodontal instrumentation and advanced root instrumentation,* ed 6, Philadelphia, 2013, Lippincott Williams & Wilkins.)

Design Characteristics

A. Instrument balance—a balanced instrument has working ends that are aligned with the long axis of the handle
   1. During a work stroke—for example, in calculus removal; balance ensures that finger pressure applied against the handle is transferred to the working end, which results in pressure against the tooth
   2. An instrument that is not balanced is more difficult to use and increases stress on the muscles of the user's hand and arm
B. Instrument identification—the unique design name and number that identify each periodontal instrument
   1. Design name—identifies the school or individual responsible for the original design or development of an instrument or group of instruments (e.g., ODU 11/12 periodontal explorer, in which the ODU stands for Old Dominion University; and the TU-17, in which TU stands for Tufts University School of Dental Medicine)
   2. Design number—the number designation of the working end that, when combined with the design name, provides the exact identification of the working end (e.g., Gracey 11, in which Gracey is the design name, and 11 is the design number)
   3. Identification of the working ends of a double-ended instrument—a double-ended instrument will have two design numbers, one number for each working end of the instrument
      a. If the design name and number are stamped along the length of the handle, each working end is identified by the number closest to it
      b. If the design name and number are stamped across the handle, the first number identifies the working end at the top of the handle, and the second number identifies the working end at the bottom

TABLE 17-1 Use of Hand-Activated Instruments

Classification	Purpose
Calibrated probe	Measurement of pocket depths, clinical attachment level, width of attached gingiva, gingival recession, and intraoral lesions; evaluation of gingival tissue for consistency and presence of bleeding or exudate
Furcation probe	Detection of furcation involvement in multi-rooted teeth
Explorer	Detection of calculus deposits, tooth surface irregularities, defective margins on restorations
Sickle scaler	Removal of medium-sized to large-sized calculus deposits from enamel surfaces; provides good access to the proximal surfaces on anterior crowns and the enamel surfaces apical to the contact areas of posterior teeth; should NOT be used on cementum
Periodontal file	Used to crush large calculus deposits and prepare burnished calculus before removal with another instrument; should NOT be used directly on cemental surfaces
Universal curet	Instrumentation of crown and root surfaces; removal of light to medium-sized supragingival and subgingival calculus deposits; some designs have long functional shanks that allow access to the cervical and middle thirds of root surfaces
Area-specific curet	Instrumentation of crown and root surfaces; removal of light supragingival and subgingival calculus deposits; some designs have extended shanks that allow access to the middle and apical thirds of root surfaces

From Nield-Gehrig JS: *Fundamentals of periodontal instrumentation and advanced root instrumentation,* ed 6, Philadelphia, 2013, Lippincott Williams & Wilkins.

HAND-ACTIVATED INSTRUMENTS

Classifications

A. Hand-activated nonsurgical periodontal instruments are classified as periodontal probes, explorers, sickle scalers, periodontal files, universal curets (or curettes), and area-specific curets (Table 17-1); hoes and chisels are rarely used because their functions have been largely replaced by ultrasonic and sonic devices
B. Periodontal instruments are divided into classifications based on the specific design characteristics of the working end
   1. Design of the cutting edges, back, lateral surfaces, and shank
   2. Cross section of the working end
   3. Relationship of the face to the lower shank
C. In selecting an instrument for a specific task, one of the most important considerations is the classification of the working end

Dental Mirror

A. Characteristics
   1. The working end has a reflecting (mirrored) surface
   2. Types
      a. Front surface—the reflecting surface is on the front surface of the glass; produces a clear mirror image with no distortion

b. Concave—the reflecting surface is on the front surface of the mirror lens; produces a magnified but slightly distorted image

c. Plane—the reflecting surface is on the back surface of the mirror lens; this type of surface is less easily scratched than a front surface mirror and produces a double or "ghost" image

B. Uses

1. Indirect vision—the mirror's reflecting surface provides a view of the tooth surface or intraoral structure that cannot be seen directly

2. Retraction—using the mirror to hold the client's cheek or tongue to view tooth surfaces or other structures that are otherwise hidden by the cheeks or tongue

3. Indirect illumination—reflecting light from the mirrored surface into a dark area of the mouth

4. Transillumination—reflecting light from the mirrored surface through anterior teeth

Probe

A. Characteristics

1. Assessment instrument that is used to evaluate the health of periodontal tissue

2. Two types: calibrated and furcation probes

B. Types

1. Calibrated probe (e.g., Williams, PSR screening probe) has a slender, rod-shaped, blunt working end marked in millimeter increments; can be used as a miniature ruler for making intraoral measurements, such as for measuring sulcus and pocket depths, clinical attachment levels, width of attached gingiva, or the size of oral lesions; also used to assess for the presence of bleeding or purulent exudate (pus)

2. Furcation probe (e.g., Nabers 1 N) is a curved, blunt-tipped instrument used to detect and assess bone loss in the furcation areas of bifurcated and trifurcated teeth

C. Calibrations—millimeter marks at intervals that are specific for each probe design

1. Calibrated probes

a. Probe designs may differ in millimeter markings (Table 17-2); only certain millimeter increments may be indicated on the probe (e.g., 1—2—3—5—7—8—9—10 mm), or each millimeter may be indicated (e.g., 1—2—3—4—5—6—7—8—9—10—11—12—13—14—15 mm)

b. Color-coded probes are marked in bands (often black), with each band being several millimeters in width (e.g., 3 to 5 mm and 8 to 10 mm)

2. Furcation probes

a. Most furcation probes do not have millimeter markings

b. Some furcation probes are marked in bands (usually black), with each band being several millimeters in width (e.g., 3 to 6 mm and 6 to 9 mm); these probes usually are used in research investigations to facilitate investigators' calibration

TABLE 17-2 Examples of Probe Markings

Type	Marking Pattern	Increments (mm)
UNC15	All mm marked	1 to 15
Glickman 26G	No mark at 6 mm	1–2–3–5–7–8–9–10
Goldman Fox	No mark at 6 mm	1–2–3–5–7–8–9–10
Merritt	No mark at 6 mm	1–2–3–5–7–8–9–10
Williams	No mark at 6 mm	1–2–3–5–7–8–9–10
Maryland Moffitt	No mark at 6 mm; ball-end	1–2–3–5–7–8–9–10
Michigan "O"	Marks at 3, 6, and 8 mm	3–6–8
PSR Screening	Colored band from 3.5–5.5; marks at 8.5 and 11.5 mm; ball end	3.5–5.5–8.5–11.5
CP-18	Colored bands from 3–5 and 8–10	3–5–8–10
CP-11	Colored bands from 3–6 and 8–11	3–6–8–11
CP-12	Colored bands from 3–6 and 9–12	3–6–9–12
Hu-Friedy Novatech	Right-angled probe; available in a wide variety of designs	Available in various increments

From Nield-Gehrig JS: *Fundamentals of periodontal instrumentation and advanced root instrumentation,* ed 6, Philadelphia, 2013, Lippincott Williams & Wilkins.

Explorer

A. Characteristics

1. Assessment instrument with a fine, flexible wire-like working end

2. Provides the best tactile information to the clinician's fingers; used to locate calculus deposits, tooth surface irregularities, and defective margins on restorations

B. Design (Fig. 17-2)

1. The working end is 1 to 2 mm in length and is referred to as the tip; the side of the tip, rather than the actual point, is used for detecting calculus

2. Circular in cross section, the explorer may have paired or unpaired working ends

FIG 17-2 Design characteristics of a dental explorer. (From Nield-Gehrig JS: *Fundamentals of periodontal instrumentation and advanced root instrumentation,* ed 6, Philadelphia, 2013, Lippincott Williams & Wilkins.)

C. Types—available in a variety of design types; not all design types are well suited to subgingival use; therefore, the clinician must be knowledgeable about the recommended use of each design type
  1. Shepherd hook (e.g., #23 and #54 explorers)—an unpaired explorer with a short, highly curved shank and a sharp point; used for supragingival examinations to detect irregular margins of restorations; not recommended for calculus detection because subgingival use could result in tissue trauma
  2. Straight explorer (e.g., 6, 6A, 6 L, 6XL)—an unpaired explorer with a short lower shank and a sharp point; used for examinations to detect irregular margins of restorations; not recommended for subgingival calculus detection
  3. Curved explorer (e.g., 3, 3A)—an unpaired explorer with a curved shank and a sharp point; limited for use in examining normal sulci or shallow pockets; may be used for calculus detection; however, care must be taken not to injure the junctional epithelium when the working end is used subgingivally
  4. Orban-type explorer (e.g., TU-17, Orban 20)—an unpaired explorer with a straight lower shank that can be used in deep pockets with only slight tissue displacement (stretching of the tissue wall away from the tooth); the explorer tip is bent at a 90-degree angle to the terminal shank, which allows the back of the tip (instead of the point) to be directed toward the junctional epithelium; useful for detecting subgingival calculus on anterior teeth or on the facial and lingual surfaces of posterior teeth; however, the straight lower shank makes it difficult to adapt to the line angles and proximal surfaces of posterior teeth
  5. Pigtail or cowhorn explorer (e.g., 3MI, 3CH, 2A)—a paired universal explorer with a short, broadly curved lower shank and a sharp point; the curved lower shank causes considerable tissue displacement; useful for detecting calculus in normal sulci or shallow pockets extending no deeper than the cervical third of the root
  6. The 11/12-type explorer (e.g., ODU 11/12, 11/12 AF)—a paired universal explorer with an extended lower shank and a tip that is bent at a 90-degree angle to the terminal shank; the tip design allows the back of the tip to be applied to the pocket base without lacerating the junctional epithelium; this effective explorer design adapts well to all surfaces throughout the mouth and is equally useful when exploring a shallow sulcus or a deep periodontal pocket

Sickle Scaler

A. Characteristics
  1. Calculus removal instrument; limited for use on enamel surfaces
  2. Anterior and posterior designs
B. Design (Fig. 17-3)
  1. Cutting edges—two cutting edges that meet in a point
  2. Back—sharp, pointed back; some types of scalers are made with flattened backs

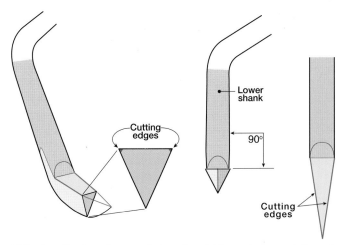

FIG 17-3 Design characteristics of a sickle scaler, consisting of two-level cutting edges that meet in a point and an instrument face that is at a 90-degree angle to the lower shank. (From Nield-Gehrig JS: *Fundamentals of periodontal instrumentation and advanced root instrumentation,* ed 6, Philadelphia, 2013, Lippincott Williams & Wilkins.)

  3. Cross section—triangular; lateral surfaces meet the instrument face at an internal angle between 70 and 80 degrees
  4. Face—perpendicular to the lower shank so that the cutting edges are level with each other; level cutting edges require that the lower shank be tilted slightly toward the tooth surface to establish correct angulation
  5. The anterior sickle scaler has an unpaired working end and a simple shank; primarily used on anterior teeth (e.g., Jacquette 33)
  6. The posterior sickle scaler has paired working ends, with complex shanks; primarily used on posterior teeth but may be used on anterior teeth (e.g., Jacquette 34/35)
C. Uses
  1. Removal of medium-sized to large calculus deposits from enamel tooth surfaces
  2. Provides good access to the proximal surfaces on anterior crowns and to the enamel surfaces apical to the contact areas of posterior teeth
D. Limitations
  1. The pointed tip and the straight cutting edges do not adapt well to rounded root surfaces and concavities
  2. The pointed back is not suited to subgingival use (may injure the junctional epithelium)

Periodontal File

A. Characteristics
  1. Calculus removal instrument used to prepare calculus deposits before removal with another instrument
  2. Anterior and posterior designs
B. Design
  1. Cutting edges—multiple cutting edges at a 90- to 105-degree angle to the lower shank

2. Working end—thin in width with a large circumference at the base; the base may be round, oval, or rectangular in shape
3. Area-specific application—each working end is designed for use on a single surface (four working ends are needed for procedures on all tooth surfaces); files with simple shanks work best on anterior teeth; those with complex shanks work best on posterior teeth

C. Uses
1. Preparation of burnished calculus deposit (a deposit with a smooth outer surface) before definitive removal of the deposit with a curet; a file is used to scratch the surface of a burnished deposit so that it can be removed with another instrument
2. Crushing of a large calculus deposit; once a deposit has been crushed with a file, it is easier to remove with a curet
3. Smoothing overextended or rough amalgam restoration in sites where the file can be effectively adapted

D. Limitations
1. Limited to use on enamel surfaces or to applications on the outer surface of a calculus deposit; gouging could result if a file is used on root surfaces
2. The working ends have straight cutting edges on a flat base; do not adapt well to curved tooth surfaces

Universal Curet

A. Characteristics
1. One of the most frequently used and versatile of all the instruments for calculus removal
2. Used both supragingivally and subgingivally; two curets usually are paired on a double-ended instrument (the paired working ends are mirror images of each other)

B. Design (Fig. 17-4)
1. Cutting edges—two cutting edges that converge in a rounded toe
2. Back—the rounded back is ideal for subgingival use

3. Cross section—semi-circular; lateral surfaces meet the instrument face at an internal angle between 70 and 80 degrees
4. Face—perpendicular to the lower shank so that the cutting edges are level with each other; the level cutting edges require that the lower shank be tilted slightly toward the tooth surface to establish correct angulation
5. Universal use—one double-ended instrument can be applied to all tooth surfaces in the anterior and posterior regions of the mouth

C. Uses
1. Calculus removal from crown and root surfaces
2. Removal of small to medium-sized calculus deposits

D. Limitations
1. The toe is wider than a pointed tip and therefore may be more difficult to adapt for use beneath the contact areas of anterior teeth
2. The level cutting edges require that the lower shank be tilted slightly toward the tooth for correct angulation

Area-Specific Curet

A. Characteristics
1. Calculus removal instrument with one cutting edge (only one cutting edge per working end is used for procedures); a set of curets is needed to perform procedures throughout the mouth
2. The curet is used supragingivally and subgingivally; especially well suited for instrumentation of roots within periodontal pockets
3. Designs include area-specific curets with flexible and rigid shanks

B. Design (Fig. 17-5)
1. Cutting edge—one working cutting edge per working end; only the lower, longer cutting edge is used

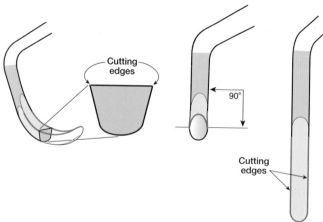

FIG 17-4 Design characteristics of a universal curet, consisting of two-level cutting edges and an instrument face that is at a 90-degree angle to the lower shank. (From Nield-Gehrig JS: *Fundamentals of periodontal instrumentation and advanced root instrumentation,* ed 6, Philadelphia, 2013, Lippincott Williams & Wilkins.)

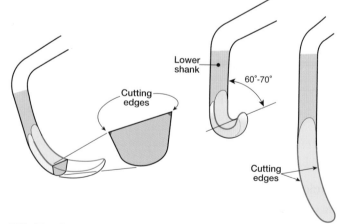

FIG 17-5 Design characteristics of an area-specific curet, consisting of one cutting edge, an instrument face at a 70-degree angle to the lower shank, and one cutting edge positioned lower than the other, nonworking cutting edge. (From Nield-Gehrig JS: *Fundamentals of periodontal instrumentation and advanced root instrumentation,* ed 6, Philadelphia, 2013, Lippincott Williams & Wilkins.)

2. Back—rounded back; ideal for subgingival use
3. Cross section—semi-circular; the lateral surfaces meet the instrument face at an internal angle between 70 and 80 degrees
4. Face—tilted at a 60- to 70-degree angle in relation to the lower shank, making one cutting edge (the working cutting edge) lower than the other; this tilted relationship makes the working cutting edge "self-angulated"; that is, when the lower shank is parallel to the tooth surface, the cutting edge is at the correct angulation
5. Area-specific use—each working end is limited to use only on certain teeth and on certain surfaces

C. Uses
  1. Instrumentation of crown and root surfaces
  2. Removal of small deposits of calculus and biofilm

D. Limitations
  1. The toe is wider than a pointed tip and is therefore more difficult to adapt to the proximal surfaces of anterior crowns
  2. A single working cutting edge per working end means exchanging instruments more frequently

Advanced Root Instrumentation

A. Characteristics
  1. The treatment of clients with periodontitis requires specialized instruments with longer shank lengths and miniature working ends for instrumentation of root concavities and furcation areas
  2. Designs include area-specific curets with miniature working ends, extended shanks, flexible and rigid shanks, and diamond-coated working ends

B. Examples of advanced periodontal instruments—a variety of periodontal instruments have been developed to increase treatment effectiveness on root surfaces within deep periodontal pockets
  1. The 11/12-type periodontal explorer—an 11/12 AF (After Five) explorer has an extended shank and is ideal for use in deep periodontal pockets
  2. Advanced curet designs—several curets are ideal for instrumentation within deep periodontal pockets
     a. Vision Curvette curet series—have a working end that is shortened to half the length of a standard Gracey curet, a curved working end, and an extended lower shank
     b. Modified Gracey curets
        (1) Several varieties of modified Gracey curets—include modified Gracey curets with extended shanks, miniature Gracey curets, and micro Gracey curets
        (2) Design features for modified Gracey curets—include extended lower shank length, thinner working ends, and working ends that are shorter in length than in a standard Gracey curet
     c. Quétin (kee'-tan) furcation curets—specialized instruments that are used to debride furcation areas and root concavities; each miniature working end has a single, straight cutting edge with rounded corners; the working ends are available in either 0.9-mm or 1.3-mm size

d. O'Hehir debridement curets—area-specific curets that are designed to remove light residual calculus deposits and bacterial contaminants from root surfaces
   (1) The working end of an O'Hehir curet is a tiny circular disc; the entire working end is a cutting edge; the working end curves into the tooth for easy adaptation in furcation areas and developmental grooves
   (2) These curets have extended lower shanks
e. Instruments with diamond-coated working ends
   (1) The working ends of these instruments do not have cutting edges; instead, they are coated with a very fine diamond grit; for example, a version of the Nabers furcation probes is diamond coated
   (2) Diamond-coated instruments can be used to remove light, residual calculus deposits
   (3) Because of the abrasive nature of their working ends, these instruments should be used with light, even pressure against the root surface to avoid gouging or grooving

PRINCIPLES OF INSTRUMENTATION

Position of the Clinician

A. Neutral, seated position (Fig. 17-6)

FIG 17-6 Neutral seated position for the clinician. (From Nield-Gehrig JS: *Fundamentals of periodontal instrumentation and advanced root instrumentation*, ed 6, Philadelphia, 2013, Lippincott Williams & Wilkins.)

1. Head—tilt of 0 to 15 degrees
2. Shoulders—in a horizontal line
3. Back—straight or leaning forward slightly from the waist or hips
4. Thighs—hips slightly higher than the knees
5. Upper arms—parallel to the long axis of the torso
6. Elbows—at waist level; held slightly away from body
7. Forearms—parallel to the floor; raised or lowered, if necessary, by pivoting at the elbow joint rather than by raising the elbows
8. Feet—seat height should be positioned low enough so that the heels of the feet can rest on the floor

B. Relationship to the client and the dental unit
 1. The client's chair should be positioned such that the tip of the client's nose is at a level slightly lower than clinician's elbows; clinician should not have to raise the elbows above his or her waist level to reach the client's mouth; lower arms should be in a horizontal position or raised slightly so that the angle formed between the lower and upper arm is slightly less than 90 degrees
 2. All instruments and equipment should be positioned within easy reach of the clinician

Stabilization During Instrumentation

A. Modified pen grasp—the recommended grasp for holding a periodontal instrument that allows precise control of the working end; precise placement of the fingers in the modified pen grasp is important to be successful in instrumentation technique
 1. Finger placement and function (Fig. 17-7)
  a. Index finger and thumb—finger pads hold the instrument handle
  b. Middle finger—the side of the finger pad rests on the instrument's shank; the clinician's fingers should be able to feel the vibrations in the instrument's shank as the working end encounters roughness on the tooth surface
  c. Ring finger—fingertip rests on a stable surface, usually the occlusal or incisal tooth surface, which stabilizes the hand for control and strength
 2. Technique
  a. A light grasp is needed for increased tactile sensitivity during assessment procedures (e.g., subgingival use of explorer or probe)
  b. A firm grasp is used with hand-activated instruments during calculus removal
 3. Glove fit—proper fit of sterile gloves is important in avoiding muscle strain during instrumentation
  a. Select right-hand and left-hand fitted gloves rather than ambidextrous gloves
  b. Select gloves that come in a range of numbered sizes (e.g., 5½, 6, 6½) rather than those marked in size ranges of small, medium, and large

B. Fulcrum and finger rest
 1. Definitions
  a. Fulcrum—the point of support on which the clinician rests the hand; used to stabilize the clinician's hand

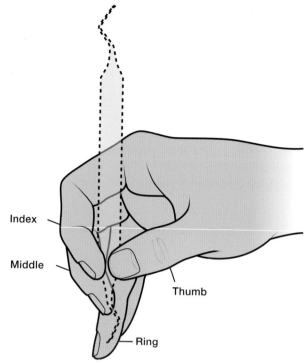

FIG 17-7 Finger placement in the modified pen grasp. The index finger and the thumb hold the instrument handle. The middle finger rests on the instrument shank. The ring finger acts as a support for the hand and instrument. (From Nield-Gehrig JS: *Fundamentals of periodontal instrumentation and advanced root instrumentation,* ed 6, Philadelphia, 2013, Lippincott Williams & Wilkins.)

during instrumentation; the pad of the ring finger serves as the fulcrum finger during instrumentation to control stroke pressure and length
  b. Finger rest—the place where the fulcrum finger rests during instrumentation
 2. Types of fulcrums
  a. Basic intraoral fulcrum
   (1) The finger rest is placed on a tooth, close to the tooth being worked on; should not be positioned in the line of the instrument's stroke to prevent instrument stick
   (2) The intraoral fulcrum is considered the most desirable because it provides the greatest stability and strength for calculus removal
  b. Basic extraoral fulcrum—placed outside the client's mouth, usually on the chin or cheek
  c. Advanced fulcrums—variations of the basic fulcrum that may be required for access to posterior teeth or root surfaces within periodontal pockets; advanced fulcrums require greater skill and stroke control than the basic intraoral fulcrum
 3. Advanced fulcrum techniques
  a. Piggybacked—intraoral fulcrum in which the middle finger is stacked on top of the ring finger
  b. Cross-arch—intraoral fulcrum in which the finger rests on the side of the mouth opposite the treatment

area (treatment area is mandibular right quadrant, finger rest on mandibular left quadrant)

   c. Opposite arch—intraoral fulcrum in which the finger rests on the arch opposite to the treatment area (treatment area on mandibular arch, finger rest on maxillary arch)

   d. Finger-on-finger—intraoral fulcrum in which the finger of the nondominant hand serves as the resting point for the ring finger of the dominant hand

   e. Stabilized—intraoral or extraoral fulcrum in which a finger of the nondominant hand is used to concentrate lateral pressure against the tooth surface and to help control the instrument stroke

Adaptation

A. Definition—positioning the first 1 or 2 mm of the lateral surface of the instrument's working end in contact with the tooth surface

B. Characteristics

   1. Explorer—the first few millimeters of the tip (not the point) are adapted to the tooth surface for calculus detection

   2. Probe—the side of the probe tip is maintained against the tooth surface, with the length of the probe almost parallel to the tooth surface being probed

   3. Sickles and curets—the leading one third of the cutting edge is positioned to conform to the tooth surface

Angulation

A. Definition—the relationship between the instrument face and the tooth surface to which the working end is applied

B. Principles

   1. For insertion beneath the gingival margin—the face-to-tooth surface angulation is between 0 and 40 degrees

   2. For calculus removal—the face-to-tooth surface angulation is between 45 and 90 degrees; a 60-degree angulation works well for biofilm removal, whereas a 70- to 80-degree angulation is ideal for calculus removal (Fig. 17-8)

Activation

A. Definition—moving an instrument to produce a stroke; it is the action of an instrument in the performance of the task for which it was designed

B. Types

   1. Hand-forearm activation

      a. Made by rotating the hand and forearm as a unit to provide the power for the instrumentation stroke; similar to the action of turning a doorknob

      b. Uses the power of the hand and arm to move the instrument; recommended for calculus removal with hand-activated instruments

   2. Digital (finger) activation

      a. Created by flexing the thumb, index, and middle fingers to move the instrument

      b. Used whenever physical strength is not required during a task, such as when using ultrasonic or sonic instruments, probes, and explorers

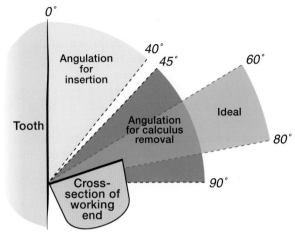

FIG 17-8 Angulation for calculus removal should be between 45 and 90 degrees. An angulation between 60 and 80 degrees is ideal for calculus removal. (From Nield-Gehrig JS: *Fundamentals of periodontal instrumentation and advanced root instrumentation*, ed 6, Philadelphia, 2013, Lippincott Williams & Wilkins.)

C. Stabilization and lateral pressure

   1. Definitions

      a. Stabilization—preparing for an instrument's stroke by locking the joints of the ring finger and pressing the fingertip against the tooth surface to provide control for the stroke

      b. Lateral pressure—applying pressure equally with the index finger and the thumb inward against the instrument's handle to engage the working end apical to a calculus deposit before and throughout a calculus removal or assessment stroke

   2. Stroke pressure

      a. Pressure during stroke activation—stroke pressure is applied in a coronal direction; the pressure ranges from light to firm, depending on the amount of pressure needed for the particular task (e.g., assessment, calculus removal)

      b. Pressure between strokes—finger muscles should be relaxed as the working end is repositioned, using light stroke pressure

D. Maintaining adaptation during stroke production

   1. Hand pivot—turning the hand and arm slightly while resting on the fulcrum to maintain adaptation; used when moving around line angles and onto proximal surfaces

   2. Handle roll—rolling the instrument handle slightly between the thumb and the index finger to maintain adaptation as the instrumentation strokes advance around the tooth surface; either the thumb or the index finger is used to roll the instrument

E. Neutral wrist position—correct wrist position is important to avoid muscle discomfort and injury during the procedure; the wrist should be aligned with the long axis of the forearm; bending the wrist up, down, or to the side should be avoided

Instrumentation Strokes

A. Types of strokes
1. Assessment strokes—used to evaluate a subgingival root surface or the health of periodontal tissue
   a. Used with probes, explorers, curets
   b. Angulation—50 to 70 degrees
   c. Lateral pressure—in contact with the tooth surface; light pressure
   d. Character—fluid strokes of moderate length
   e. Number—many strokes used to cover the entire root surface
2. Work strokes for calculus removal
   a. Used with hand-activated sickle scalers, curets, and files
   b. Angulation—70 to 80 degrees
   c. Lateral pressure—moderate to firm
   d. Character—powerful strokes; short in length
   e. Number—the number of strokes should be limited to the areas where needed
3. Work strokes for removal of residual calculus deposits and biofilm removal
   a. Used with hand-activated curets
   b. Angulation—60 to 70 degrees
   c. Lateral pressure—light to moderate
   d. Character—lighter strokes of moderate length
   e. Number—many strokes used to cover the entire root surface
B. Stroke direction
1. Vertical—parallel to the long axis of the tooth; used on facial, lingual, and proximal surfaces of anterior teeth and on the mesial and distal surfaces of posterior teeth
2. Oblique—diagonal to the long axis of the tooth; used most often on facial and lingual surfaces
3. Horizontal—perpendicular to the long axis of the tooth; used at the line angles of posterior teeth, furcation crotch areas, and within pockets that are too narrow to allow vertical or oblique strokes
4. Multi-directional—a combination of vertical, oblique, and horizontal strokes, one by one, used in succession on of a subgingival tooth surface
C. Stroke characteristics
1. Length—short, powerful stroke for calculus removal; longer, lighter stroke for removal of residual calculus deposits and biofilm
2. Overlap—strokes should overlap to ensure complete coverage; long ridges of calculus are treated in sections, in overlapping scaling zones
3. Pattern
   a. Large calculus deposits should be removed in sections with a series of short, firm strokes
      (1) A calculus deposit should not be removed in layers because removing the outermost layer will leave the deposit with a smooth surface (burnished surface)
      (2) A burnished calculus deposit may be indistinguishable (when explored) from the tooth surface
   b. For subgingival instrumentation, it is helpful to imagine that the root surface is divided into a series of narrow, diagonal instrumentation zones
      (1) Each instrumentation zone is only as wide as the toe-third of the cutting edge
      (2) Deposits are removed in each zone, from the junctional epithelium to the gingival margin, before progressing to the next zone

STEPS FOR CALCULUS REMOVAL WITH HAND-ACTIVATED INSTRUMENTS

A. Position the dental mirror, and establish a finger rest
B. Grasp the instrument in a modified pen grasp
C. Establish a finger rest
1. Locate the finger rest near the site of instrumentation in the dental arch; precise control of the instrument's stroke becomes more difficult as the finger rest is moved farther away from the site of the procedure
2. Select the correct working end of the instrument
D. Adjust the hand-wrist-forearm as a unit
1. Position the thumb and the index finger across from each other on the instrument handle, near the junction of the handle and shank
2. Lightly rest one side of the middle finger pad on the instrument shank
3. Place the other side of the middle finger pad against the ring finger to allow the hand to function as a unit during the production of the stroke
4. Balance the tip of the ring finger on an occlusal or an incisal surface to support the weight of the hand and instrument
5. Position the wrist in a neutral position so that it is aligned with the long axis of the forearm (Fig. 17-9)
E. Adapt the cutting edge
1. If working subgingivally, close the face of the working end toward the tooth, and slide the working end to the junctional epithelium; use a light grasp while positioning the working end
2. Adapt the toe-third of the cutting edge to the tooth surface just apical to the deposit
3. Establish the instrument face-to-tooth surface angulation of 70 and 80 degrees
4. Fine-tune the grasp and the wrist position

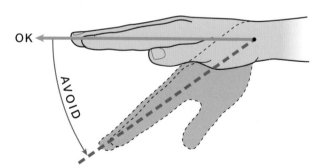

FIG 17-9 Neutral wrist position. The wrist should be aligned with the long axis of the forearm. (From Nield-Gehrig JS: *Fundamentals of periodontal instrumentation and advanced root instrumentation*, ed 6, Philadelphia, 2013, Lippincott Williams & Wilkins.)

F. Stabilize the grasp, and apply lateral pressure
   1. Press down with the ring finger against the finger rest
   2. Apply pressure against the instrument handle with the index finger and the thumb
G. Activate a pulling stroke away from the junctional epithelium
   1. Use hand-forearm activation for strength and control
   2. Activate instrumentation strokes in a coronal direction to prevent particles of calculus from being pushed into soft tissue
   3. Use vertical and oblique strokes in most areas; supplement these strokes with horizontal strokes, as needed
   4. Use short, powerful strokes for calculus removal and longer, lighter strokes for removal of residual calculus deposits and biofilm
   5. Use overlapping strokes to ensure complete coverage of the entire root surface
H. Pause briefly at the end of a stroke
   1. Relax the grasp, the finger rest, and the lateral pressure
   2. Use a relaxed grasp to reposition the working end of the instrument for the next stroke
I. Check the instrumentation area frequently with an explorer

INSTRUMENTATION FOR ASSESSMENT

Basic Concepts

A. Thorough assessment involves examining all aspects of the periodontium and teeth
B. Client preparation, based on information from the personal, comprehensive health and dental histories, is essential for safe instrumentation
C. Successful treatment depends on well-developed assessment skills, before instrumentation for dental hygiene care planning and during and after instrumentation for evaluating treatment outcomes

Assessments with Periodontal Probes

A. Purposes of the periodontal examination
   1. Aid in planning dental hygiene care by determining gingival characteristics, probing depth, level of attachment, and presence of bone loss
   2. Determine the extent of inflammation in conjunction with the probing depth and attachment level; bleeding resulting from probing is an early clinical sign of inflammation (Fig. 17-10)
   3. Evaluation of treatment outcomes according to:
      a. Tissue response to the client's self-care and nonsurgical periodontal therapy
      b. Evidence of health determined by the probe
         (1) No bleeding on gentle probing
         (2) Clinical attachment levels remain the same or decrease in depth
B. Factors that may affect probing accuracy
   1. Probe design
      a. Calibration—the probe must be clearly and accurately marked and easy to read; the clinician must be knowledgeable about the calibration pattern
      b. Thickness—a thinner probe causes less distention of the sulcus or the pocket wall; use a probe no larger than 0.5 mm in diameter

FIG 17-10 Assessment for the presence of bleeding. Bleeding on probing is an early clinical sign of inflammation. (From Nield-Gehrig JS: *Fundamentals of periodontal instrumentation and advanced root instrumentation,* ed 6, Philadelphia, 2013, Lippincott Williams & Wilkins.)

   2. Influence of tissue health and related factors
      a. Tissue resistance—with light pressure, the probe is inserted until it meets the physical resistance of the base of the sulcus or the periodontal pocket
         (1) Normal tissue—the junctional epithelium offers more resistance; probing is stopped by the coronal portion of the junctional epithelium
         (2) Gingivitis and early periodontitis—the junctional epithelium offers less resistance; the probe tip passes farther into the junctional epithelium
         (3) Advanced periodontitis—the junctional epithelium offers little or no resistance; the probe tip may penetrate the junctional epithelium to reach the attached connective tissue fibers
      b. Dental calculus—large calculus deposits can hinder the placement of the probe
   3. Concepts of probing technique
      a. Adaptation—place the side of the probe tip against the tooth surface, with the length of the probe positioned as parallel as possible to the tooth surface; to assess the col region, tilt the probe so that the tip reaches under the contact area
      b. Stroke technique—strokes must be close to each other as the probe is "walked" along the entire circumference of the junctional epithelium
      c. Pressure—a light pressure of 10 to 20 g should be sufficient

Probing Technique

A. Parallelism—the probe is positioned as parallel as possible to the tooth surface being probed
B. Adaptation—the side of the probe tip is maintained in contact with the tooth at all times
C. Activation—digital (finger) activation may be used with the probe because only light pressure is used when probing

D. Walking strokes—a series of bobbing strokes made within the sulcus or the pocket while keeping the probe tip against the tooth
1. The junctional epithelium is continuous around a tooth, and the probing depth may vary considerably on different surfaces; for complete evaluation, the entire circumference of the sulcus or the pocket base should be assessed with a series of probing strokes
2. The probe is gently inserted under the gingival margin, holding the side of the tip against the tooth with a light lateral pressure; the probe tip is moved gently in an apical direction along the tooth surface until it encounters the resistance of the junctional epithelium
3. The tip is moved up and down in short bobbing strokes of 1 to 2 mm while progressing forward in small, 1-mm to 2-mm steps around the circumference of the tooth; with each downward stroke, the probe tip returns to gently touch the junctional epithelium
4. The base of the sulcus or pocket will feel soft and resilient; if the resistance on the probe feels hard, the probe tip has encountered a large calculus deposit before reaching the junctional epithelium
5. The probe should not be removed from the sulcus or the pocket after each instrumentation stroke; repeated insertion and removal is unnecessary and can cause trauma to the free gingival margin
E. Proximal surface probing—the probe is walked across the proximal surface until it touches the contact area; the probe is slanted slightly so that the tip reaches under the contact area; with the probe in this position, it is gently pressed downward to touch the junctional epithelium to take a reading
F. Sequence of steps for probing by quadrants
1. Insert the probe at the distal line angle of the posterior-most tooth in the quadrant; walk the probe in a distal direction, adapting the probe around the line angle and across the distal surface, slightly past the midline of the distal surface (because this is the distal-most tooth in the quadrant, no contact area is present to contend with)
2. Reinsert the probe at the distal line angle, and proceed in a mesial direction, across the distal surface, around the line angle, and across the mesial surface, slanting under the mesial contact area, as needed
3. Remove the probe from the sulcus or the pocket, and reinsert at the distal line angle of the next tooth in the quadrant; assess each tooth in the quadrant in a similar manner, ending with the mesial surface of the central incisor
4. After probing the facial aspect of the quadrant, assess the lingual aspect of the same quadrant
G. Calculus—when a large calculus deposit is encountered, the probe should be moved outward from the tooth and around the deposit and guided back to the tooth, proceeding in an apical direction
H. Recording probing depths—for the purpose of documentation, each tooth is divided into six areas (three on the facial aspect and three on the lingual aspect)
1. The six areas are:
a. Distofacial line angle to the midline of the distal surface

b. Facial surface
c. Mesiofacial line angle to the midline of the mesial surface
d. Distolingual line angle to the midline of the distal surface
e. Lingual surface
f. Mesiolingual line angle to the midline of the mesial surface
2. Only one reading per area is recorded—if the probing depths vary within an area, the deepest reading obtained in that area is recorded (e.g., when readings for an area range from 3 to 6 mm, only the 6-mm reading is entered on the chart for that area)
3. Depths are recorded in millimeters and rounded up (e.g., a reading of 4.5 mm is recorded as a 5-mm reading)

Clinical Assessment Using Periodontal Probes

A. Bleeding on probing
1. Rationale
a. Bleeding on probing is a significant clinical indicator of inflammation and is an earlier clinical sign of disease than marginal redness
b. Bleeding on probing correlates with an increase in motile bacterial organisms, especially spirochetes, in the pocket
c. Bleeding may indicate an area nonresponsive to nonsurgical periodontal treatment
d. No bleeding on probing is a criterion for healthy tissue
2. Technique
a. Insert the probe a few millimeters into the pocket (tip should not be in contact with the junctional epithelium)
b. Make horizontal sweeping strokes along the pocket wall, using light pressure with the side of the probe
c. Spongy tissue of a pocket wall will usually bleed near the gingival margin; firm chronic pocket linings usually do not bleed until sweeping strokes are made in the deep part of the pocket (bleeding may not be evident for a few seconds)
d. Bleeding on probing usually is recorded on the periodontal chart; often indicated by a red dot on the chart
B. Measurement of recession of the gingival margin
1. Definition and rationale
a. Gingival recession is the movement of the gingival margin from its normal position, slightly coronal to the cemento-enamel junction (CEJ), leading to exposure of a portion of the root surface to the oral cavity
b. Gingival recession indicates the apical migration of the junctional epithelium
2. Procedure
a. Position a calibrated probe parallel to the tooth surface with the toe of the probe touching the gingival margin
b. Measure the extent of recession in millimeters from the CEJ to the gingival margin with a calibrated periodontal probe
C. Measuring probing depths
1. Definition—the distance in millimeters from the gingival margin to the base of the sulcus or the pocket, as measured with a calibrated probe

2. Rationale
   a. Used in mathematically calculating clinical attachment levels
   b. Useful in prescribing client self-care regimens and in educating clients
3. Limitations—in the presence of gingival recession, probing depth measurements are not an accurate indication of loss of attachment or level of bone support to the tooth
4. Technique
   a. With the probe in a vertical position and in contact with the attached tissue, record the distance from the gingival margin to the base of the sulcus or the pocket
   b. When the gingival margin contacts the probe between the millimeter marks, use the higher number for the final reading
D. Measuring clinical attachment levels (CALs)
   1. Definition—the position of the attached tissue at the base of the sulcus or the pocket, as measured from a fixed point, usually the CEJ
   2. Rationale
      a. Probing depths are not reliable indicators of the position of the junctional epithelium because the measurement is made from the gingival margin; the position of the gingival margin changes with recession and edema
      b. Measurements are taken from a fixed point on the tooth; the CEJ usually is used because it provides a more reliable indication of the level of the attached tissue
      c. When evaluating treatment outcomes, measurements taken from a fixed point provide a better way of monitoring whether the level of the attached tissue has remained the same, decreased, or increased in depth
   3. General concepts
      a. Two measurements are made and then used to calculate the clinical attachment; the measurements include:
         (1) The probing depth
         (2) The distance from the CEJ to the gingival margin
      b. Three possible relationships exist between the CEJ and the gingival margin; the clinician must understand how to calculate the CAL for each of these relationships
         (1) Visible gingival recession (gingival margin is apical to the CEJ) (Fig. 17-11)
         (2) Gingival margin is coronal to the CEJ
         (3) Gingival margin is approximately level with the CEJ
   4. Calculation technique in areas of visible gingival recession
      a. Measure and record the probing depth (distance from the gingival margin to the base of the pocket)
      b. Measure and record the amount of gingival recession (distance from the CEJ to the gingival margin)
      c. Calculate the CAL by adding the probing depth and the measurement of gingival recession

5. Calculation technique in areas where gingival margin is coronal to the CEJ
   a. Measure and record the probing depth
   b. Apply the probe, and determine the location of the CEJ by tactile sensitivity; measure the distance from the gingival margin to the CEJ
   c. Calculate the CAL by subtracting the distance from the gingival margin to the CEJ from the probing depth
6. Calculation technique in areas where the gingival margin is level with the CEJ—when the gingival margin is within 0.5 mm apical or coronal to the CEJ, the probing depth and the CAL are the same measurement
E. Mucogingival examination
   1. Rationale—to determine the width of the attached gingiva
   2. Procedure for determining the amount of attached gingiva
      a. On the external (outer) surface of the gingiva, measure the distance in millimeters from the gingival margin to the mucogingival junction; this is the total width of the gingiva (free and attached gingiva)
      b. Measure the probing depth

Gingival Margin Below CEJ

FIG 17-11 Comparison of the probing depth and the clinical attachment level (CAL) when the gingival margin is apical to the cemento-enamel junction *(CEJ)*. The CAL provides an accurate estimation of the level of the attached tissues. (From Nield-Gehrig JS: *Foundations of periodontics for the dental hygienist,* ed 3, Philadelphia, 2010, Lippincott Williams & Wilkins.)

c. Calculate the width of the attached gingiva by subtracting the probing depth from the total width of the gingiva

3. Significance of finding
   a. If the probing depth is equal to or greater than the width of the total gingiva, no attached gingiva (NAG) exists
   b. If the probe tip passes the mucogingival junction, mucogingival involvement exists in this area

F. Furcation involvement
   1. Definition—furcation involvement occurs when periodontal infection invades the area between and around the roots of a bifurcated or trifurcated tooth, and the bone level is apical to the furcation crotch area
   2. Classification—furcation involvement is classified according to the extent of bone loss
      a. Class I—early, or incipient, involvement; the anatomy of the root surfaces can be felt by moving the probe from side to side, passing over the root into the concavity of the furcation area, and up the opposite side to the adjacent root
      b. Class II—moderate involvement; bone has been destroyed to an extent that allows the probe to partially enter the furcation, which extends approximately one-third the width of the tooth between the roots
      c. Class III—severe, or advanced, involvement; in mandibular molars, the probe can pass between the roots, through the entire furcation; in maxillary molars, the probe can pass between the mesiobuccal and distobuccal roots to touch the palatal root
      d. Class IV—same as class III; also, the furca is visible clinically because of the presence of tissue recession
   3. Access to furcation area
      a. Bifurcated roots (two roots)
         (1) Mandibular molars—to examine between the mesial and distal roots, probe midfacial and mid-lingual aspects (Fig. 17-12)

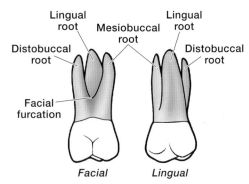

FIG 17-13 Furcation morphology on a maxillary molar (mesiobuccal, distobuccal, and palatal roots). The furcation can be examined from the facial, mesial, and distal aspects. (From Nield-Gehrig JS: *Fundamentals of periodontal instrumentation and advanced root instrumentation,* ed 6, Philadelphia, 2013, Lippincott Williams & Wilkins.)

         (2) Maxillary first premolars—to examine between the buccal and palatal roots, probe from the mesial and distal aspects, apical to the contact area
      b. Trifurcated roots (three roots)—maxillary molars; to examine around the palatal root and the two facial roots, probe from the midfacial, mesial, and distal aspects (Fig. 17-13)

G. Evaluation of oral deviations—a calibrated periodontal probe is used to determine the size of an oral lesion or deviation; when documenting measurements, anatomical terminology such as anteroposterior or superoinferior, is used, rather than terms such as length or width

Clinical Assessment with Dental Explorers

A. Purposes and uses
   1. Dental explorers detect, by tactile response, the texture and character of tooth surfaces before, during, and after treatment, to assess the progress and thoroughness of instrumentation
   2. Dental explorers examine tooth surfaces for:
      a. Dental calculus
      b. Cemental changes that may have resulted from pocket formation
      c. Anomalies
      d. Anatomical features such as grooves, curvatures, and furcation areas
   3. Dental explorers define the extent of instrumentation for treatment procedures of the tooth surface, including:
      a. Removal of calculus deposits and biofilm
      b. Removal of overhanging restorations
      c. Sealant placement

B. Dental calculus (see the sections on "Bacterial Plaque" in Chapter 9 and "Bacterial Dental Biofilm" in Chapter 14)
   1. Definition
      a. Calcified or mineralized plaque biofilm is a hard, tenacious mass that forms on tooth surfaces and on dental prostheses

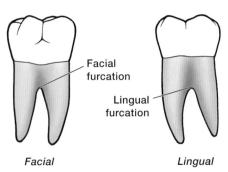

FIG 17-12 Furcation morphology on a mandibular molar (mesial and distal roots). The furcation can be examined from the facial and lingual aspects. (From Nield-Gehrig JS: *Fundamentals of periodontal instrumentation and advanced root instrumentation,* ed 6, Philadelphia, 2013, Lippincott Williams & Wilkins.)

b. The surface of calculus is rough and is covered by a layer of plaque biofilm

2. Types, distribution, and shape
   a. Supragingival (supramarginal) calculus
      (1) Located coronal to (above) the gingival margin
      (2) Distribution—localized, usually not generalized throughout the mouth
      (3) Most common locations include the lingual surfaces of mandibular anterior teeth, facial surfaces of maxillary molars, teeth out of occlusion, or overlapping teeth
   b. Subgingival (submarginal) calculus
      (1) Located apical to (beneath) the gingival margin
      (2) Distribution—may be localized or generalized; heaviest on proximal surfaces
      (3) Extends along the root surface almost to the base of the pocket; the newest, less calcified calculus is at the most apical area, near the soft tissue attachment
      (4) Shape—flattened to conform to pressure from the gingival pocket wall; forms may include combinations of the following:
         (a) Nodular deposits (spicules)
         (b) Ledge-like or ring-like formations
         (c) Thin, smooth veneers
         (d) Finger-like and fern-like formations

3. Modes of attachment—calculus is more easily removed from some tooth surfaces than from others; the difficulty in removal usually is related to the manner in which the calculus is attached to the tooth; on any one tooth, more than one mode of attachment can occur
   a. Attachment to acquired pellicle (thin acellular layer on tooth surface)—most common mode of calculus attachment to enamel; calculus may be removed readily because no interlocking of calculus to the tooth exists
   b. Attachment by "locking" into minute irregularities in the tooth surface
   c. Attachment of the calcified calculus matrix to the tooth surface by interlocking of inorganic crystals of the tooth with the mineralizing plaque biofilm

C. Calculus detection
   1. Supragingival assessment—unnecessary supragingival exploration should be avoided; adequate light combined with the use of a dental mirror and compressed air will reveal most supragingival deposits
   2. Subgingival assessment and adaptation
      a. Instrument grasp and lateral pressure—a relaxed grasp and light lateral pressure are used to enhance tactile sensitivity; pressure with the middle finger against the instrument shank should be avoided, because this reduces tactile sensitivity
      b. Activation—a combination of hand-forearm and digital activation
      c. Strokes—many, overlapping, fluid strokes are used to thoroughly cover the entire root surface

D. Carious lesions
   1. Historically, the use of tactile examination of a tooth surface, with firm application of a sharp tip of an explorer into a suspected site of caries, was a common method of carious lesion detection, but this approach is no longer recommended
   2. Research has shown this technique to be unreliable for carious lesion detection and to be potentially harmful
   3. Firm application of a sharp explorer tip into a carious pit or fissure on a tooth surface may actually cause additional damage to the tooth surface and interfere with subsequent attempts at remineralization of the caries lesion (see Chapter 16)

CONCEPTS IN PERIODONTAL INSTRUMENTATION

Instrumentation Terminology

A. Instrumenting—using a periodontal instrument for a task
B. Biofilm management—the disruption or removal of subgingival plaque biofilm and its byproducts from cemental surfaces and the pocket spaces
C. Tactile sensitivity—the ability to feel vibrations transferred from the instrument's working end, shank, and handle to the clinician's fingers
D. Assessment—examination of a tooth and periodontium to determine anatomy and detect biofilm-retentive factors, and oral disease status
E. Nonsurgical periodontal instrumentation—removal of hard and soft deposits from the tooth crown, root surfaces, and pocket space to the extent needed to reestablish periodontal health and restore a balance between the bacterial flora and the host's immune responses
F. Overhang removal—recontouring procedures that correct defective margins of restorations to provide a smooth surface that will deter bacterial accumulation
G. Supragingival—located coronal to (above) the gingival margin
H. Subgingival—located apical to (beneath) the gingival margin
I. Biofilm-retentive factors—conditions that foster the establishment and growth of biofilm, such as calculus deposits and overhanging restorations

Rationale for Nonsurgical Periodontal Instrumentation

A. Arrests the progress of disease
B. Induces positive changes in the subgingival bacterial flora (count and content)
C. Creates an environment that permits the gingival tissue to heal, thereby eliminating inflammation
   1. Converts the pocket from an area experiencing increased loss of attachment to one in which the CAL remains the same or decreases
   2. Eliminates bleeding
   3. Improves integrity of tissue attachment
D. Increases the effectiveness of client self-care

E. Permits reevaluation of periodontal health status; surgery may then be unnecessary, lessened in extent, or confined to specific areas

F. Prevents recurrence of disease through frequent periodontal maintenance therapy

Rationale for Removal of Overhangs

A. Eliminates irregular surfaces where biofilm can collect

B. Induces positive changes in the microflora of the pocket when the overhang extends subgingivally

C. Encourages resolution of inflammation

D. Facilitates interdental biofilm removal and control by the client

End Point of Instrumentation

A. The goal of instrumentation is to render the root surface and pocket space acceptable to tissue so that healing occurs

B. Tissue healing occurs slowly, and it is not possible to assess tissue response for at least 1 month after completion of instrumentation
   1. The client's appointment for reevaluation should be scheduled 4 to 6 weeks after completion of instrumentation
   2. During reevaluation, a periodontal assessment should be completed that includes probing depths, CALs, and bleeding on probing
   3. Nonresponsive sites are those that show continued loss of attachment and may exhibit clinical signs of inflammation or bleeding, or both, on probing; nonresponsive sites may require:
      a. Removal of new or residual calculus deposits; or other biofilm-retentive factors
      b. Thorough subgingival biofilm removal, preferably with an ultrasonic instrument or glycine-powder air polishing with a specially designed subgingival nozzle tip
   4. Consideration should be given to other risk factors that might be contributing to the disease process (host response, systemic, and local factors)

Steps for the Preparation for Instrumentation

A. Protect client safety
   1. Review the client's personal and health histories for indications of special needs; prepare for a possible emergency
   2. Assess vital signs
   3. Observe the client for signs of stress

B. Use standard precautions (see Chapter 10)
   1. Postpone treatment for a client with a communicable disease or an open oral lesion
   2. Provide the means for lowering the bacterial count of the client's oral surfaces
      a. Provide the client with a preprocedural antimicrobial mouthrinse or antimicrobial irrigation to lower the count of oral microorganisms
      b. Discuss oral self-care with client (e.g., plaque control) before any instrumentation

SHARPENING OF HAND-ACTIVATED INSTRUMENTS

A. Sharp cutting edges are vital to achieve efficient periodontal instrumentation with minimal tissue trauma

B. Sharp cutting edges help provide more efficient treatment because of easier calculus removal, fewer strokes, improved stroke control, increased client comfort, and reduced clinician fatigue

C. To sharpen instruments correctly, the clinician must understand the design of the working end
   1. A sharp cutting edge is a line without width; a dull cutting edge is a rounded surface
   2. The internal angle formed between the face and lateral surface of a sickle scaler or curet is between 70 and 80 degrees
   3. Most sickle scalers have pointed tips and backs; curets have rounded toes and backs
   4. Sickle scalers and universal curets have two working cutting edges per working end; area-specific curets have one working cutting edge per working end

D. Instruments should be sharpened at the first sign of dullness—the cutting edge of the instrument dulls at various rates because of:
   1. Number of working strokes used
   2. Amount of lateral pressure used
   3. Hardness and tenacity of the deposit
   4. Composition of the metal of the instrument

E. Equipment
   1. A stable, well-lighted work surface
   2. Heat-sterilized rectangular sharpening stone or sharpening tool and plastic sharpening test stick (Table 17-3)
   3. Water or oil to lubricate the stone (depending on the type of stone)
   4. Protective eyewear, facemask, and household gloves (when sharpening contaminated instruments)

ULTRASONIC AND SONIC INSTRUMENTATION

A. Description
   1. Powered ultrasonic and sonic devices use rapid vibrations of a fluid-cooled instrument tip to fracture and dislodge supragingival and subgingival calculus deposits from the teeth and to cleanse the environment within the periodontal pocket
   2. Ultrasonic devices (magnetostrictive and piezoelectric)
      a. High-frequency electrical energy is converted into mechanical energy in the form of ultrasonic vibrations; instrument tip vibrations range from 25,000 to 50,000 cycles per second (cps, hertz [Hz])
      b. Heat that is produced must be dissipated by a constant flow of water through the handpiece; antimicrobial solutions may be used instead of water in certain units
      c. Ultrasonic instruments provide efficient removal of all types of calculus deposits (old, new, supragingival and subgingival, light and heavy deposits)

TABLE 17-3 Sharpening Stones and Tools

Type	Abrasiveness	Description	Purpose	Lubricant	Sterilization*
Ceramic	Fine	Synthetic stone	Routine sharpening of metal and some plastic implant instruments	Water	All methods
Arkansas	Fine	Natural stone	Routine sharpening of metal instruments	Mineral oil	All methods†
India	Medium	Synthetic stone	Sharpening of metal instruments that are dull	Water or oil	All methods
Composition	Coarse	Synthetic stone	Sharpening of metal instruments that are extremely dull or that need reshaping	Water	All methods
Nievert Whittler	—	Tungsten carbide steel	Routine sharpening of metal instruments	Water	All methods
Reciprocating honing device	—	—	Sharpening of metal instruments	—	—

*Includes autoclave, dry heat, or chemical sterilization.
†Natural stones become brittle over time with heat exposure.
Modified with permission from Nield-Gehrig JS: *Fundamentals of periodontal instrumentation and advanced root instrumentation*, ed 6, Philadelphia, 2013, Lippincott Williams & Wilkins.

3. Sonic instruments
   a. Air pressure also is used to create rapid mechanical vibrations; sonic instrument tip vibrations range from 3000 to 8000 cycles per second (Hertz)
   b. No heat is generated; although water cooling is not necessary, a water coolant is indicated to obtain the benefits of water lavage
   c. Because of the lower frequency of vibration, sonic instruments are less efficient in removing calculus deposits and have a limited ability to remove tenacious deposits; they function well for the removal of newly formed and light deposits
B. Definitions
   1. Fluid lavage—the fluid stream within the periodontal pocket, produced by the constant flow of fluid through the handpiece, near the instrument's tip; when the fluid strikes the vibrating instrument tip, it creates a spray composed of millions of tiny bubbles
   2. Cavitation—the energy release that occurs when the tiny bubbles in the fluid spray collapse, producing shock waves that may alter or destroy bacteria by tearing the bacterial cell walls
   3. Stroke—the maximum distance the powered instrument tip moves during one cycle of vibration
C. Instrument tip design
   1. Working ends of ultrasonic/sonic instruments have no cutting edges to cut or tear tissue; less tissue trauma can result in faster healing rates for sites treated with ultrasonic or sonic instruments
   2. The entire length of the working end is active; therefore, adaptation is not limited to a single region on the working end
   3. Tip selection
      a. Ultrasonic tip selection varies, depending on the manufacturer; the availability of a full range of tip designs is an important criterion when purchasing a mechanized device
      b. Tips may range in size from large, broad tips (standard size), to medium-sized tips to slim-diameter slender tips

c. Standard tips (ultrasonic and sonic designs)
   (1) Broad, large tips are used to remove heavy, supra-gingival deposits
   (2) Medium-sized tips are used to remove medium and light deposits; some may be used subgingivally if the tissue permits easy insertion of the tip
d. Slim-diameter ultrasonic tips
   (1) Similar in diameter to periodontal probes, and significantly smaller in size than the working end of a curet
   (2) Approximately 40% thinner than a standard-sized ultrasonic tip
   (3) Available in straight, right-paired, and left-paired styles
   (4) Used for biofilm and light calculus removal; provide excellent access to deep pockets and furcation areas
4. Energy dispersion—ultrasonic instrument tips are active on all surfaces; by adapting the appropriate tip surface, the clinician can control energy dispersion and client sensitivity during the procedure
   a. Point—generates the most energy; should not be used directly against the tooth surface
   b. Face (concave surface)—second most powerful surface (generates less energy than the point); usually not recommended for use against the tooth surface
   c. Back (convex surface)—generates less energy than the face; follow the manufacturer's recommendations regarding direct use on the tooth surface
   d. Lateral surfaces (sides)—generate the least amount of energy; may be used directly against the tooth surface; adaptation of a lateral surface is recommended for calculus removal and deplaquing
5. Fluid delivery—ultrasonic instruments require a constant stream of fluid running through the handpiece, which disperses in a fine spray at or near the instrument tip to prevent overheating of the vibrating instrument tip
   a. Fluid delivery to the tip
      (1) The external flow tube is adjacent to the instrument's shank

FIG 17-14 Active tip area of a mechanized instrument. The active tip area ranges in length from 2 to 3 mm and is the portion of the instrument tip that is capable of doing the work. (From Nield-Gehrig JS: *Fundamentals of periodontal instrumentation and advanced root instrumentation*, ed 6, Philadelphia, 2013, Lippincott Williams & Wilkins.)

      (2) In the internal fluid flow system, the fluid flows directly through the instrument tip

    b. Water is the most common fluid used; some ultrasonic units have an independent fluid reservoir that can deliver distilled water or other fluid solutions (e.g., sterile saline, stannous fluoride, chemotherapeutic agents) to the instrument tip

  6. Tip frequency—the number of times per second that the tip moves back and forth during one cycle

    a. Active tip area—the portion of the tip that is capable of doing work; ranges from 2 to 4 mm in length (Fig. 17-14)

    b. Manual ultrasonic units allow the clinician to adjust the tip frequency by turning an adjustment knob on the unit; automatic ultrasonic units control the tip frequency automatically; sonic instruments have a preset frequency that cannot be controlled by the clinician

D. Several factors influence the force produced by the powered instrument tip

  1. Exposure time—sufficient time must be allowed for the tip to do its work (e.g., ultrasonic instruments are effective, but even they do not instantaneously remove calculus); powered instrument tips work by creating microfractures in a calculus deposit; the tip should be moved back and forth repeatedly over the deposit to allow time for the microfractures to develop

  2. Angle of adaptation—an angle of between 0 and 15 degrees is recommended for direct adaptation to tooth surfaces

  3. Sharp or dull tip—only dull tips are recommended; sharpened tips emit high energy levels that could damage the tooth

  4. Lateral pressure—tips function most effectively with light lateral pressure against the tooth or calculus deposit; moderate or firm lateral pressure decreases or even stops the vibrations of the tip

E. Uses of modern ultrasonic instruments

  1. Removal of attached and unattached plaque biofilm from root surface and pocket space

  2. Removal of supragingival and subgingival calculus

  3. Removal of toxins from root surfaces

  4. Smoothing down overextended or rough amalgam restorations, removing extrinsic stains for esthetic considerations, and removing orthodontic cement (using standard tips)

F. Contraindications

  1. Client with a communicable disease that can be disseminated by aerosols

  2. Immunocompromised client with high susceptibility to an infection who could be exposed to microorganisms in contaminated water or aerosols or by other means (e.g., debilitated clients, those with uncontrolled diabetes, immunosuppressed clients)

  3. Client with respiratory disease or difficulty breathing (e.g., history of emphysema, cystic fibrosis, asthma); the client is at increased risk of respiratory infection if septic material or oral microorganisms are aspirated

  4. Client who has difficulty swallowing or is prone to gagging (e.g., multiple sclerosis, amyotrophic lateral sclerosis, muscular dystrophy, paralysis)

  5. Client with a cardiac pacemaker; the dental clinician should check with the client's cardiologist if the device is shielded or unshielded

  6. Client with primary or newly erupted teeth—danger of heat being conducted to large pulp chambers

  7. Direct contact between the instrument tip and porcelain jacket crowns, composite resin restorations that could be damaged by the vibration or the tip, and demineralized enamel surfaces (conservation of demineralized enamel surfaces is indicated) should be avoided

  8. Direct contact with titanium implant surface should be avoided, unless the instrument tip is covered with a specially designed plastic sleeve

G. Precautions

  1. The handpiece and the working end of ultrasonic instruments must be cooled with constant flow of water to dissipate heat

  2. Aerosols produced may be contaminated with pathogens; use of barriers, surface disinfectants, protective clothing, and laminar airflow systems is recommended

  3. The client may experience sensitivity

  4. Shifts in hearing sensitivity have been reported; the effect of ultrasonic and sonic equipment on the hearing of clinicians who frequently use these instruments has not been studied well

H. Preparation

  1. Employ universal precautions, and ensure that protective attire is worn by the clinician, the assistant, and the client

  2. Have the client use a preprocedural antimicrobial mouthrinse, or irrigate the treatment area to reduce the number of airborne microorganisms in aerosols created by water spray

  3. Monitor the condition of the equipment

  4. Replace the instrument tip as soon as it shows signs of wear or damage

    a. Tip wear—1 mm of wear results in approximately 25% loss of efficiency; tips should be discarded at 2 mm of wear; some manufacturers offer wear guides that make it easy to determine tip wear; precision-thin tips must be replaced more frequently than standard tips

    b. Metal stacks of magnetostrictive insert—replace if the stacks are bent or separated, or if the insert does not slide easily into the ultrasonic handpiece

5. Instrument tips and handpieces should be sterilized according to manufacturer's instructions; use surface disinfectant and barriers on an ultrasonic unit

I. Technique

1. Biofilm control in water tubing—flush the water tubing of stagnant water for 2 minutes at the start of the day, and for 30 seconds between clients; use units with an independent fluid reservoir or waterline point-of-use filter, or both

2. Tip selection—select the appropriate instrument tip for the task at hand
   a. Broad, standard tips for removal of heavy and medium-sized supragingival calculus
   b. Medium-sized standard tips for moderate and light supragingival use; also may be used subgingivally if the tissue permits easy insertion of the tip
   c. Slim-diameter tips for removal of light deposits and deplaquing

3. Power setting—use standard instrument tips at medium-power or low-power setting, and slim-diameter tips at low-power setting; high-power setting is no more effective than medium power and is not recommended

4. Grasp—use light, relaxed grasp, even during calculus removal

5. Finger rest—use an intraoral or extraoral rest; advanced fulcrum techniques may be helpful for gaining access to posterior pockets

6. Lateral pressure—use light stroke pressure for effective calculus removal

7. Activation—use digital activation as recommended

8. Fluid adjustment and containment
   a. Adjust the water spray around the instrument tip to create a light mist or halo effect, with no excess dripping of water; insufficient water flow over an ultrasonic tip can result in trauma to the pulp; a warm handpiece is a sign of inadequate fluid flow through the handpiece
   b. Use high-volume suction or a saliva ejector for fluid control; position the suction tip at the corner of the mouth where the fluid will pool; deactivate the instrument tip occasionally to prevent large amounts of fluid accumulation
   c. Use the client's lips and cheeks as barriers to deflect fluid back into the client's mouth

9. Tip adaptation
   a. Adaptation to the tooth surface—position the tip with the point directed toward the junctional epithelium and the length of the tip at a 0- to 15-degree angle to the tooth surface; never apply the point of the tip directly to the tooth surface
   b. Adaptation to a calculus deposit—place the tip directly against the uppermost or outermost edge of the calculus deposit; the lateral surface of a tip may also be adapted to a calculus deposit

10. Instrumentation strokes
    a. Motion—use a tapping motion against large-sized calculus deposits and a sweeping, eraser-like motion against small deposits and for biofilm removal from root surfaces
    b. Pressure—use light pressure; firm pressure decreases effectiveness
    c. Direction—use overlapping vertical, oblique, and horizontal strokes; subgingival strokes should cover the entire root surface for calculus removal and deplaquing

11. Calculus removal
    a. Sequence—work in a coronal-to-apical direction, beginning at the gingival margin and working toward the junctional epithelium (this is the reverse of the sequence for calculus removal with a curet)
    b. Technique for removing stubborn deposits
       (1) Use an adequate number of strokes—move the tip repeatedly over the deposit or tap against the deposit; keep the tip in constant motion
       (2) Select the proper tip for the type of calculus; for example, do not use slim-diameter tips for medium-sized or large deposits
       (3) Approach the deposit from different aspects (e.g., approach an interproximal deposit from both the facial and the lingual aspect)
       (4) Do not apply firm stroke pressure; use of light pressure is most effective
       (5) Increase the frequency on a manually calibrated unit
       (6) Increase the power setting from low to medium

ADVANCED INSTRUMENTATION TECHNIQUES

Instrumentation of Dental Implants

A. Definition—dental implant: a nonbiologic device surgically inserted into or onto the jawbone to replace a missing tooth or to provide support for an implant superstructure (e.g., a fixed bridge or denture)

B. General guidelines
1. Special instruments are recommended for assessment and instrumentation of implants; plastic instruments are used most often because the plastic material is softer than the implant material
2. Metal instruments (e.g., stainless steel, carbon steel, and metal ultrasonic instruments) may leave scratches on the surface of the implant
   a. Scratches or surface roughness on an implant may promote accumulation of biofilm
   b. Surface coating of an implant may be disturbed, thereby reducing the biocompatibility of the implant with the surrounding tissues
3. Some plastic instruments may be sterilized by autoclaving; follow the manufacturer's instructions for sterilization and reuse

C. Design of the working end of plastic instruments
1. Wrench-shaped, crescent-shaped, and hoe-shaped working ends—useful for instrumentation of an implant's superstructure

2. Working ends that are similar in design to conventional metal probes, sickle scalers, and curets—useful for the assessment and instrumentation of the implant abutment

D. Use of plastic, calibrated probe for assessing peri-implant tissues (soft tissues that surround the dental implant)
   1. Peri-implant probing depths are related to the thickness of the mucosa around the implant; deeper probing depths are found in conjunction with a thicker mucosa
   2. Probing depths and CALs are important parameters for the longitudinal monitoring of peri-implant tissue stability
   3. Considerations
      a. Probing may be invasive because the probe may penetrate the weakly adherent biologic seal and could introduce bacteria into peri-implant tissue
      b. Accurate probing depths may be difficult to obtain because of the constricted "cervical" area of some implants
      c. Radiographs are more accurate than probing depths for detecting the absence or presence of bone loss around implants

E. Instrumentation for calculus removal
   1. Calculus is removed easily from implants because no interlocking or penetration of the deposit exists within the implant surface
   2. Light lateral pressure with a plastic scaler or curet is recommended; care must be taken not to scratch the surface of the implant
   3. Instrumentation should be restricted to supragingival deposit removal

SELECTIVE STAIN REMOVAL

A. Definitions
   1. Intrinsic—stains that occur within the tooth substance; the process of removal is performed by a dentist using bleaching techniques or prosthetic coverage with a crown
   2. Extrinsic—stains that occur on the external surface of the tooth; removed by client self-care and professional procedures such as scaling and rubber cup and brush scaling, rubber cup/brush, and conventional air polishing

B. Significance of dental stains
   1. No detrimental effects have been shown to result from the presence of dental stains; research shows that stains do not directly contribute to periodontal disease, dental caries, or any oral disease; however, stains may contribute to biofilm retention
   2. Removal of unsightly dental stains on anterior teeth may benefit the client's appearance and self-esteem

C. Rationale for selective stain removal
   1. Polishing is viewed as a cosmetic procedure with limited application; stain removal provides no therapeutic benefit to the client and has numerous detrimental effects on teeth and soft tissue
   2. Decision to include stain removal in a client's care plan can best be made after client self-care education and after complete periodontal instrumentation because much of the stain may be removed along with calculus deposits

D. Contraindications to polishing
   1. Dental contraindications
      a. Tooth surfaces that have no extrinsic stains or have stains that are not visible when client smiles or engages in conversation
      b. Areas of dentinal hypersensitivity—application of fluoride is one treatment for tooth sensitivity; protective fluoride must be left undisturbed (see the section on "Assessment of Dentinal Hypersensitivity" in Chapter 16)
      c. Restored tooth surfaces—gold and other restorative materials may be scratched by the abrasive agent
      d. Titanium implants—polishing could scratch the titanium abutment
      e. Areas of demineralization—conservation of demineralized enamel surfaces is indicated
      f. Gingiva that is enlarged, soft, spongy, or bleeds easily—polishing is not recommended because paste can enter the tissue, and the action of the rotating cup can further traumatize the tissue
   2. Systemic contraindications
      a. Client with a communicable disease that could be spread by aerosols
      b. Client with a high susceptibility to infection who could inhale contaminated aerosols (e.g., client with respiratory or pulmonary disease, debilitated client)
      c. Client who has a history of renal insufficiency, Addison's disease, Cushing syndrome, or metabolic alkalosis; is taking mineralocorticosteroids, antidiuretics, or potassium supplements; air polisher use should be avoided
      d. Client who has a history of hypertension or a sodium-restricted diet; air polishing using a sodium-containing powder is contraindicated; air polishing can be used with one of the newer, sodium-free polishing powder products, such as those composed of aluminum trihydroxide or calcium carbonate

E. Adverse effects of polishing
   1. Aerosol production and spatter from power-driven polisher
      a. Contaminated aerosols present a hazard to the clinician, other dental personnel, and other clients in the oral health care environment; polishing splatter is composed of polishing paste, microorganisms, and saliva
      b. Components of commercial prophylaxis pastes may include various chemicals that can cause a severe inflammatory response in the eye
   2. Iatrogenic damage to tooth surfaces
      a. Enamel surfaces—stain removal with an abrasive agent removes the surface layer of tooth structure where the fluoride content is greatest and most protective; polishing the teeth for 3 minutes with pumice removes 3 to 4 micrometers (μm) of enamel; over time, the loss of enamel can be significant
      b. Cemental surfaces—exposed surface near the CEJ has a thin cementum or dentin surface that can be abraded or removed with an abrasive agent

c. Heat production—care must be taken to use a wet polishing agent with minimal pressure and low speed to prevent overheating of a tooth, particularly the pulp tissues of small children; primary teeth have large pulp chambers, which make them particularly vulnerable to heat generated by power-driven handpieces

3. Tissue trauma—during polishing, abrasive paste is forced into the gingival sulcus and even into the tissue itself; some individuals experience a negative tissue response to abrasive particles or chemicals in the paste, which can delay tissue healing

F. Power-driven polisher (rubber cup polishing)
   1. Description
      a. Handpiece—connects to the dental unit's low-speed handpiece line
      b. Prophylaxis angle—attaches to the handpiece; holds polishing cups and bristle brushes
      c. Attachments
         (1) Polishing cups—used for stain removal from tooth surfaces and for polishing restorations
         (2) Bristle brushes—used for stain removal from occlusal surfaces; not for use near the gingival margin or on cementum or dentin, where the brush could denude the epithelium or remove cementum
   2. Technique considerations
      a. Application of polishing agent—apply agent only to individual teeth requiring stain removal for esthetic purposes
      b. Use the lowest possible handpiece speed
      c. Apply the cup to the tooth with a light, intermittent pressure
         (1) The edges of the cup should just barely flare from the tooth surface
         (2) Use of continuous motion—avoid holding the cup on a single spot for too long to prevent buildup of frictional heat

G. Conventional supragingival air polishing
   1. Definition—an air-powered device using air and water pressure to deliver a controlled slurry of powder to the tooth surface
   2. Technique
      a. Wear protective attire
         (1) Client—provide a plastic apron, hair cover, eye protection, and lip lubrication
         (2) Clinician and assistant—wear a paper or cloth long-sleeved garment, facemask, hair cover, eye protection, and gloves
      b. Administer a preprocedural mouthrinse to lessen contaminated aerosols; have the client rinse with an antibacterial mouthrinse
      c. Direct the powder spray away from the gingival tissue, never direct the spray into the sulcus or pocket space; establish the recommended angulation of the tip to the tooth surface
         (1) Facial and lingual surfaces—position the nozzle tip at a 60- to 80-degree angle to the tooth

         (2) Occlusal surfaces—position the nozzle at a 90-degree angle to the surface of the tooth
      d. Direct the spray in constant motion for only 3 to 5 seconds at any area on the enamel surface

H. Postoperative procedures for mechanical and air polishing
   1. Remove particles of abrasive at the contact areas with dental floss
   2. Loosen and remove particles in sulci or pockets by irrigation and aspiration with central suction

ETHICAL, LEGAL, AND SAFETY ISSUES

A. Provision of quality care by licensed dental hygienists includes ethical, legal, and safety issues

B. A comprehensive review of the client's medical health and pharmacologic histories is essential to assess the degree of client risk for dental procedures and to make necessary physician or specialty referrals

C. Adherence to the Health Insurance Portability and Accountability Act (HIPAA) is necessary; thorough, accurate, and confidential chart documentation is essential

D. A comprehensive client assessment is essential to detect oral diseases and abnormalities and determine the degree of client risk for caries, periodontal disease, or disease progression

E. Failure to provide necessary care based on assessment findings constitutes supervised neglect; the licensed dental hygienist is accountable and responsible for client care

F. A thorough case presentation is essential so that the client can make an informed decision about recommended dental hygiene care; written informed consent should be obtained before beginning care; discussion of all procedures with clients, using everyday language the client can understand, and encouragement of client participation are essential

G. The dental hygienist has an obligation to provide evidence-based care

H. The dental hygienist has an obligation to protect the client from harm during care

I. The dental hygienist has an obligation to follow established protocol that protects the clinician and the client during treatment

J. It is essential to allow sufficient time during appointments for provision of adequate care

K. Nonsurgical periodontal instrumentation should be performed in an effective and responsible manner; use of sharp instruments and selection of appropriate instruments for the task are essential

L. It is important to evaluate the success of nonsurgical periodontal instrumentation at appropriate continued-care intervals

M. The dental hygienist has a legal obligation to document thoroughly and accurately the assessment, care plan, informed consent, services provided, and the client's response to care

Website Information and Resources

Source	Website Address	Description
American Academy of Periodontology	http://www.perio.org	Parameters of care, position papers, scientific information, related links
Cochrane Collaboration	http://www.cochrane.org	Evidence-based health care database
National Center for Dental Hygiene Research	https://dent-web10.usc.edu/dhnet	Current topics in dental hygiene; links
Hu-Friedy	http://www.hu-friedy.com	Online catalogue of periodontal instruments; ultrasonic and air-polishing devices; white papers, material safety data sheets (MSDS), instrument care, articles
Premier Dental	http://www.premusa.com	Online catalogue of periodontal instruments; fluoride; continuing education seminar information
Deldent Ltd. Air Polishers	http://www.deldent.com	Information about the products marketed by Deldent
Dentsply Ultrasonic Units	http://www.dentsply.com	News articles, career and legal information, and information about Dentsply products
KaVo America	http://www.kavousa.com	Information about KaVo dental products
Parkell Ultrasonic Scalers	http://www.parkell.com	Information about Parkell dental products

SUGGESTED READINGS

Darby ML, Walsh MM: Instruments and instrumentation theory. In Darby ML, Walsh MM, editors: *Dental hygiene theory and practice*, ed 3, Philadelphia, 2010, Saunders.

Nield-Gehrig JS: *Fundamentals of periodontal instrumentation and advanced root instrumentation*, ed 7, Philadelphia, 2013, Lippincott Williams & Wilkins.

▌ CHAPTER 17 REVIEW QUESTIONS

Answers and rationales to the review questions are available on this text's accompanying Evolve site. See inside front cover for details.

evolve

▌ CASE A

Synopsis of Patient History
Age: 57
Sex: M
Height: 6'3"
Weight: 220 lb

Vital Signs
Blood pressure: 150/95
Pulse: 76 bpm
Respiration: 15 rpm

1. Under the care of a physician: x YES   ____ NO
2. Hospitalized within the last 5 years: x YES   ____ NO
3. Has or had the following condition:
   Hypertension
   On a physician-directed sodium-restricted diet
4. Current medications:
   Lisinopril 20 mg/day
5. Smokes or uses tobacco products: x YES   ____ NO
   Cigarettes and cigars for 35 years

Medical History
History of hypertension diagnosed 5 years ago

Dental History
Missing with no replacement: #1, #2, #13, #16, #17, #31, #32
Several large amalgams and tooth-colored anterior restorations
Recurrent caries apical to class V amalgam on F #19
Pocket depth range 3-6 mm with class II furcation involvement on F #3 and #18

6-mm pocket depth on M #14, which has drifted mesially
6-mm pocket depth on D #15
Significant recession on F #19, D and F #14
Heavy tobacco stain
Fibrotic gingival tissues with generalized slight bleeding on probing

Social History
Real estate agent
Deacon at his church

Chief Complaint
Wants teeth to look whiter and wants to replace the "gap" on the upper left

Current Oral Hygiene Status
Generalized subgingival calculus deposits in anterior and posterior sextants
Heavy generalized plaque biofilm on gingival thirds of teeth
Radiographs confirm bone loss and furcation involvement in posterior sextants

Use Case A to answer questions 1 to 10.

1. **The best way to remove tobacco stain is to use:**
   a. The toe of a universal curet
   b. An air polisher with coarse, abrasive sodium bicarbonate slurry
   c. A Nabers diamond-coated file (similar to Nabers furcation probe with diamond coating)
   d. A standard ultrasonic tip

2. **Which of the following instruments would be the BEST choice to initiate removal of the moderate calculus deposits?**
   a. Standard ultrasonic tip
   b. Ultrasonic slim-diameter tip with a straight working end
   c. Set of rigid Gracey curets 1/2, 11/12, and 13/14
   d. Quétin furcation curet

3. **Tooth #3 has class II furcation involvement on the facial aspect. Which of the following instruments would be the BEST choice for light calculus removal and deplaquing of the furcation area?**
   a. Slim-diameter ultrasonic tip with a curved working end
   b. Periodontal file
   c. Standard Gracey curet 1/2
   d. Universal curet with an extended lower shank

4. **You are working on the mesial of tooth #14, which has drifted mesially, and having difficulty keeping the instrument's lower shank parallel to the long axis of the tooth. You are using an After Five (AF) Gracey 11/12 with a miniature working end with a standard intraoral finger rest. Which of the following would MOST LIKELY improve access on this mesial surface?**
   a. Switch to an advanced fulcrum
   b. Use a straight, slim-diameter ultrasonic tip
   c. Use a universal curet with an extended shank
   d. Use a rigid Gracey curet instead

5. **Which instrument would be BEST to detect furcation involvement on multi-rooted teeth?**
   a. Furcation probe, such as a Nabers probe
   b. Periodontal file
   c. Miniature Gracey curet
   d. Calibrated periodontal probe

6. **All the following statements are TRUE about ultrasonic instrumentation EXCEPT:**
   a. The side of the tip should maintain contact with the tooth at all times.
   b. Cavitation creates tiny bubbles that collapse and kill bacteria.
   c. You should never use digital motion.
   d. There are no cutting edges on the ultrasonic tip.

7. **To determine the deepest pocket depth on the distal surface of the *facial* aspect of tooth #15, the clinician should:**
   a. Place the probe tip at the distofacial line angle, slide it down to the base of the pocket, take a reading, and record this as the probing depth for the facial aspect distal surface
   b. Insert the probe to the base of the pocket, use a series of walking strokes from the distofacial line angle to the midline of the distal surface, and record the deepest reading as the probing depth for the facial aspect of the distal surface
   c. Use the probe to measure the point where the col would be if tooth #16 were still present and record this depth
   d. Slant the probe so that the tip crosses the midline of the distal surface, insert the probe, and take and record this reading for the facial aspect of the distal surface

8. **On a tooth with class III furcation involvement, which of the following instruments would you use from the facial aspect to instrument the distal half of the mesial root?**
   a. Universal curet
   b. ODU 11/12 explorer
   c. Miniature Gracey 11/12 curet
   d. Miniature Gracey 13/14 curet

9. **Tooth #19 has significant recession of the gingival margin. If there were light tobacco stain on the root surface, what would be the BEST way to remove it?**
   a. Use a straight, slim-diameter ultrasonic tip with light overlapping strokes
   b. Do not remove the stain, because it is not visible when the patient smiles, and stain does not contribute to periodontal disease or dental caries
   c. Use a rigid Gracey 11/12 curet with light pressure
   d. Use a motor-driven polisher with fine pumice

10. **A periodontal probe can be used to assess all the following EXCEPT:**
    a. Width of attached gingiva
    b. Clinical attachment level
    c. Degree of recession
    d. Extent of carious lesions

CASE B

Synopsis of Patient History
Age: 27
Sex: F
Height: 5'4"
Weight: 120 lb

Vital Signs
Blood pressure: 118/74
Pulse: 70 bpm
Respiration: 16 rpm

1. Under the care of a physician:	x YES	___ NO
2. Hospitalized within the last 5 years:	x YES	___ NO
	(childbirth)	
3. Has or had the following condition: Asthma		
4. Current medications: Prenatal vitamins		
5. Smokes or uses tobacco products:	x YES	___ NO
6. Is pregnant:	x YES	___ NO
	(5 months)	

(Continued)

Medical History

Pregnant with second child

Asthma controlled with albuterol inhaler; last attack about a year ago and has not used it since becoming pregnant

Dental History

All third molars have been surgically extracted

Tooth-colored filling on occlusal #31 and lingual of #7

Gingival tissues red and slightly enlarged on maxillary and mandibular anterior teeth

Social History

Academic advisor at nearby university

Chief Complaint

Wants teeth cleaned

Current Oral Hygiene Status

Light calculus on proximal and lingual surfaces of #22 to #17 and facial surfaces of #3 and #14

Generalized moderate plaque biofilm

Use Case B to answer questions 11 to 19.

11. **Access to the light subgingival calculus deposits on the proximal surfaces of the anterior teeth is difficult because of papillary enlargement of the gingival tissues. Which of the following is the BEST approach for thorough subgingival calculus removal from the proximal surfaces?**
    a. Use a universal curet
    b. Try to remove the deposit with an explorer since the working end is so tiny
    c. Apply a topical anesthetic, then use a calculus removal stroke subgingivally with an anterior sickle
    d. Use an ultrasonic slim-diameter tip and approach the deposit from both facial and lingual aspects

12. **Clinical examination shows that the gingival tissues are red and slightly enlarged on maxillary and mandibular anterior teeth. Which of the following should the hygienist consider as an etiologic factor(s) in the tissue inflammation and enlargement?**
    a. Moderate plaque biofilm is present.
    b. The patient is pregnant.
    c. The patient is asthmatic.
    d. Both a and b

13. **Which of the following instruments would be the MOST effective in removing a small subgingival calculus deposit on the lingual aspect of tooth #24?**
    a. Gracey 1/2 curet with a miniature working end and an extended lower shank
    b. Anterior sickle scaler
    c. Periodontal file designed for use on the lingual aspect
    d. Standard Gracey 1/2 curet

14. **Calculus assessment reveals light calculus deposits on the mandibular anterior teeth and maxillary first molars and generalized plaque biofilm. Of the following instruments, which would you be most likely NOT to use in treating this client?**
    a. Universal curet
    b. Anterior sickle scaler
    c. ODU 11/12 explorer
    d. Standard Gracey curet

15. **While removing the light calculus on the lingual surfaces of lower anterior teeth, you would be using your mirror for all the following purposes EXCEPT:**
    a. Retraction

    b. Direct vision
    c. Indirect illumination
    d. Indirect vision

16. **Which of the following is TRUE regarding use of a universal curet for this client's treatment?**
    a. It can be used in the anterior and posterior sextants for removal of supragingival and subgingival calculus deposits.
    b. It is the most efficient instrument for removing small calculus deposits just below the contact areas of the mandibular anterior teeth.
    c. The pointed tip is effective in removing calculus interproximally.
    d. If used in areas of gingival inflammation, the curet will cause undue discomfort for the patient.

17. **When removing calculus deposits on the facial aspect of a maxillary posterior sextant, where would you place your fulcrum for best stability?**
    a. On the facial surface of a tooth near the tooth being instrumented
    b. On the opposite arch (mandibular arch)
    c. On the occlusal surface of a tooth near the one being instrumented
    d. On the occlusofacial or occlusolingual line angle of a tooth near the tooth being instrumented

18. **What is the correct sequence in steps for executing a calculus removal stroke?**
    a. Adjust instrument grasp, establish a finger rest, position the mirror, adapt the cutting edge to the tooth
    b. Position the mirror, establish a finger rest, adjust instrument grasp, adapt the cutting edge to the tooth
    c. Establish a finger rest, adjust instrument grasp, position mirror, adapt cutting edge to the tooth
    d. Position the mirror, establish a finger rest, adapt the cutting edge to the tooth, adjust instrument grasp

19. **The facial surface of tooth #3 is coated with a thin layer of supragingival calculus. All the following instruments will remove this calculus deposit efficiently EXCEPT a:**
    a. Posterior sickle scaler
    b. Gracey curet
    c. Universal curet
    d. Standard ultrasonic tip

CASE C

Synopsis of Patient History
Age: 87
Sex: M
Height: 5'9"
Weight: 188 lb

Vital Signs
Blood pressure: 122/86
Pulse: 59 bpm
Respiration: 14 rpm

1. Under the care of a physician: x YES   ____NO
2. Hospitalized within the last 5 years: x YES   ____NO
                      (placement of cardiac stent)
3. Has or had the following conditions:
    Hyperlipidemia
    Hypertension
4. Current medications:
    Crestor 20 mg/day, used to treat high cholesterol
    Metroprolor 50 mg/day, used to treat angina
    (chest pain) and hypertension
5. Smokes or uses tobacco products: ____YES   x NO

Medical History
Sees a physician every 3 months for monitoring of cardiac condition and cholesterol levels
Is compliant in taking medication and monitors fat intake
Client reports that it is typical for his blood pressure to "run a little high"

Dental History
Missing all third molars and #14 and #18
Two Maryland bridges on 6/7 and 10/11 replace congenitally missing laterals
Gold onlay on #3 and gold inlays on #13 and #20
Large class II amalgams on #30 and #19 with overhangs on both M and D of both teeth
Gingival tissues are inflamed and bleed easily on probing; moderate bleeding interproximally in all posteriors
Tissue in mandibular anterior and premolar teeth is thin and tears easily

Social History
Retired pilot for United Airlines
Had a second career for 10 years as a salesman for sheet metal

Chief Complaint
Has noticed bleeding when brushing and was told by his friend at the retirement community he should have his teeth cleaned
Reports mouth has become very dry

Current Oral Hygiene Status
Moderate generalized interproximal calculus
Moderate plaque biofilm at gingival third
Probing depths range 4-7 mm with deepest readings in mandibular left and maxillary right
Clinical attachment levels confirm generalized bone loss

Use Case C to answer questions 20 to 29.

20. **While checking for subgingival calculus deposits on the mandibular anterior teeth with an ODU 11/12 explorer, the clinician finds it difficult to insert the explorer without unduly distending the tissue. Which** of the following techniques might cause less tissue distention?
    a. Switch to an Orban-type explorer
    b. Aim the point of the ODU 11/12 explorer toward the base of the sulcus so that less of the working end is inserted in the sulcus
    c. Switch to a pigtail explorer
    d. Use a calibrated periodontal probe to locate calculus deposits

21. **One of the client's chief complaints is that his medication makes his mouth dry. All the following are useful suggestions for the client to minimize effects of xerostomia EXCEPT:**
    a. Increase intake of caffeine beverages to stimulate saliva production
    b. Use toothpastes and mouthrinses specially designed for individuals with xerostomia
    c. Chew sugarless gum to increase the flow of saliva
    d. Replace lost saliva with saliva substitutes

22. **You are using hand instruments to remove the calculus deposits from the client's teeth. After 30 minutes, your hand muscles are noticeably fatigued. Potentially, all the following can cause hand fatigue EXCEPT:**
    a. Glove fit is too big
    b. Instrument handles are of small diameter
    c. Instrument is not balanced
    d. Using finger motion instead of wrist motion activation

23. **A large piece of burnished calculus is present on the distal aspect of tooth #2. Which instrument would be MOST effective in preparing the burnished deposit for eventual removal with another periodontal instrument?**
    a. Beavertail ultrasonic tip
    b. Rigid Gracey 13/14
    c. Periodontal file
    d. Miniature Gracey 13/14 curet with an extended shank

24. **The client has defective margins (overhangs) on the amalgam restorations on two posterior teeth, reducing his ability to keep the area clean with floss and resulting in chronic inflammation. What can you do to help mitigate the circumstance?**
    a. Use a standard Gracey to pop off the extra amalgam
    b. Use a sturdy posterior sickle apical to the overhang to try and remove it
    c. Use an ultrasonic tip designed to smooth defective margins on restorations
    d. Use a Quétin curet to smooth the extra amalgam

25. **The client is missing teeth #14 and #16. What might be challenging when trying to remove subgingival calculus deposits from the mesial surface of tooth #15?**
    a. Keeping the instrument's functional shank parallel to the long axis of the tooth
    b. Finding a secure intraoral fulcrum
    c. Establishing 0-degree insertion with an area-specific curet
    d. Probing the col

26. **The client has two bridges to replace congenitally missing maxillary lateral incisors. All the following statements are TRUE regarding patient treatment EXCEPT:**
    a. There is no reason to probe around teeth #7 and #10
    b. Since calculus does not form on pontics, there is no need to check the pontics for calculus deposits
    c. Avoid using the motor-driven polisher so as not to scratch the restoration
    d. Instrumentation of the abutment teeth is necessary to remove all calculus deposits

27. **Tooth #15 has supererupted, causing an exposed root surface. Which of the following instruments is the BEST choice for removal of light calculus deposits from the facial surface of the root?**
    a. Universal curet
    b. Posterior sickle scaler
    c. Gracey 11/12 curet
    d. Periodontal file

28. **After working for 15 minutes on the distal of tooth #3, the calculus deposit remains. You decide to take a minute to assess your instrumentation technique. Ensuring all the following steps will help you effectively remove the deposit EXCEPT:**
    a. The instrument working end angulation is 70 to 80 degrees.
    b. Only the toe-third of the working end is adapted to the tooth.
    c. The instrument's lower shank is parallel to the long axis of the tooth.
    d. Your middle finger is on top of the handle to allow for greater pressure against the tooth.

29. **The client has dark-coral, friable tissue in the mandibular anterior area. After instrumentation of the lower mandibular anterior teeth, there is evidence of tissue trauma. All the following practices may cause tissue trauma EXCEPT:**
    a. Using a standard versus miniature area specific curet
    b. Using a cowhorn explorer instead of an Orban-type explorer
    c. Repeatedly removing the working end from the sulcus or pocket space and reinserting it again beneath the gingival margin after each stroke
    d. Adapting the anterior third of the working end

Use Case D to answer questions 30 to 33.

30. **In addition to controlling local oral factors—biofilm and calculus deposits—the dental team should consider the all the following to assist Michael in improving his oral health EXCEPT:**
    a. Consultation with Michael's primary care or endocrinologist
    b. Explain the connection between poor glycemic control and poor oral health
    c. Recommend a gingivectomy to control the marginal gingivitis
    d. Brainstorm with Michael about alternative methods of biofilm control that he would be more likely to use on a daily basis, such as a water flosser instead of dental floss

31. **The client's mandibular anterior teeth are crowded and in linguoversion, making it challenging to remove calculus deposits from the lingual surfaces. Which of the following patient-positioning suggestions is BEST to ensure an ergonomic instrumentation technique?**
    a. Ask the client to lower his chin (chin-down position)
    b. Lower the back of the chair until it is parallel to the floor
    c. Ask the client to keep his chin in an upward position (chin-up position)
    d. Put the chair in an upright position so the clinician can work from a standing position

32. **Before calculus removal, an explorer is used to determine the type, amount, and location of calculus deposits. Which of the following explorers is NOT recommended for calculus detection?**
    a. ODU 11/12
    b. Shepherd's hook
    c. Orban type
    d. Pigtail or cowhorn

33. **During instrumentation for calculus removal using hand instruments, your hand becomes fatigued. Self-assessment indicates you have been using finger motion. Digital activation is acceptable for all the following situations EXCEPT:**
    a. Using an ultrasonic for debridement
    b. Using a calibrated probe to measure pocket depth
    c. Looking for calculus using an ODU 11/12 explorer
    d. Using a universal curet for calculus removal

CASE D

Michael is a precocious, 15-year-old high school senior with type 1 diabetes mellitus who struggles to keep his blood glucose levels stable. His doctor has advised him to lose 30 pounds, but his weight has plateaued at 250 pounds for his 5-foot, 8-inch frame. He presents for his appointment with generalized marginal gingivitis, moderate bleeding on probing, light calculus, and heavy plaque biofilm. Dental examination revealed four new class V carious lesions on the facial of mandibular molars. He admits to drinking four cans of soda (Mountain Dew) a day.

CASE E

Stacy accepts a new position as dental hygienist for a large dental conglomerate, replacing an employee who held the position for the previous 12 years. On her first day, Stacy notices that almost all the instruments in her cassettes are dull and that a few have broken tips. The instrument handles are narrower in diameter than the large-diameter handles she previously used. In addition, the selection of instruments in each cassette is limited to one anterior sickle, a standard Gracey 11/12, and a standard Gracey 13/24.

Use Case E to answer questions 34 and 35.

34. Using a dull instrument inhibits efficient patient treatment. All the following statements are TRUE about the importance of using a sharp versus a dull instrument EXCEPT:
a. Calculus is more easily removed.
b. Heavier lateral pressure is applied.
c. Fewer strokes are necessary.
d. Stroke control is much improved.

35. At the end of the workday, Stacy notices muscle fatigue in her dominant hand. All the following may cause muscle fatigue EXCEPT:
a. Narrow-diameter handles cause the clinician to use more grip pressure, thus causing muscle fatigue.
b. A limited selection of instruments forces the clinician to use an instrument that is not appropriate for the task at hand, such as using a Gracey 11/12 to remove a heavy calculus deposit.
c. Dull instruments are not effective in removing calculus deposits.
d. Relaxing the fingers in the grasp after each calculus removal stroke is inefficient and stresses the hand muscles.

CASE F

Candy is a healthy 4-year old preschooler who presents at your office for her 6-month recare appointment. Her mother assists with daily toothbrushing and states that the family uses Colgate toothpaste and ACT mouthwash. On examination, you do not identify any new carious lesions. There are no visible calculus deposits, but there is light plaque along the gingival margins. The lingual surfaces of the teeth have light stain from the fruit juice that Candy drinks daily.

Use Case F to answer questions 36 to 38.

36. All the following instruments can be used during treatment of a pediatric patient EXCEPT:
a. Anterior sickle
b. Pigtail explorer
c. Universal curet
d. Ultrasonic instrumentation

37. Which of the following approaches to biofilm removal is likely to be of MOST benefit to the patient's ongoing oral health?
a. Guiding the child as she removes the biofilm herself during the appointment
b. Using a universal curet to remove the biofilm
c. Using a rubber cup and prophy paste to remove the biofilm
d. Using a toothpick holder (Perio-Aide) to remove the biofilm

38. All the following are TRUE about power-driven polishing (rubber cup polishing) EXCEPT:
a. Using a dry polishing agent with high speed can heat up the large pulp chambers in primary teeth.
b. Only teeth requiring stain removal for esthetic purposes should be polished with polishing agent.
c. Bacteremia can be induced during rubber cup polishing.
d. All teeth in the dentition should be polished with a rubber cup polisher until all surfaces are shining.

CASE G

Shirley, age 92, suffers from dementia. Her husband, also 92, drove her to the appointment and sits in a corner of the treatment room to assist in explaining the procedures to his wife. Shirley does not seem aware of her surroundings, and although she has been your patient for the past 3 years, she does not know who you are or what you are doing. She presents with generalized posterior recession of the gingival margin and bone loss and moderate subgingival calculus.

Use Case G to answer questions 39 to 41.

39. You decide to use ultrasonic instrumentation for calculus removal. Which of the following statements is TRUE about the correct technique with ultrasonic instrumentation?
a. Keep the tip stationary and on top of a calculus deposit until you feel or see it release.
b. Use moderate to firm pressure against a calculus deposit for more effective removal.
c. Move the tip repeatedly over a calculus deposit, using light stroke pressure, for efficient calculus removal.
d. Always set the power level to the highest setting for use with all ultrasonic tips, because the high power setting is much more effective than a medium power setting.

40. The client's medical history presents a few challenges, so a thorough assessment must be conducted. At what stage of treatment should you assess the client for signs of anxiety?
a. After instrumentation of a few teeth
b. After reviewing the medical history and before beginning instrumentation
c. While explaining what to expect during ultrasonic instrumentation
d. Before taking radiographs

41. All the following are ethical and legal concerns when treating this client EXCEPT:
a. Obligation to protect the client from harm or injury during care
b. Following standard of care protocol for her treatment
c. Assessing for physician or specialty referrals
d. Having the patient's daughter present at all times during treatment

42. Which of the following instruments would be BEST to remove moderate to heavy calculus on the distal of tooth #29?
a. Rigid Gracey 13/14 curet
b. Posterior sickle
c. Quétin curet
d. Universal curet

43. Removing the medium-sized subgingival calculus deposits from the mandibular anterior teeth would be BEST accomplished using:
a. Straight ultrasonic tip
b. Anterior sickle
c. Standard Gracey 1/2
d. Universal curet

44. Tooth #32 has drifted into the open space with a tilt, making it challenging to assess the mesial surface accurately. When detecting calculus with an ODU 11/12 explorer, it is important to take all the following steps to ensure accuracy EXCEPT:

a. Maintain the explorer's lower shank parallel to mesial tooth surface
b. Use a fulcrum for stability
c. Instead of using the working-end normally used on a mesial surface, switch to the opposite working-end for easier access
d. Use overlapping strokes to assess carefully the entire mesial surface with the explorer

45. The calculus deposit on the distal of tooth #18 has been burnished. Which of the following hand instruments would be your FIRST choice when beginning calculus removal?
a. Periodontal file
b. Standard Gracey 13/14
c. Posterior sickle
d. Universal curet

46. Which of the following instruments is BEST for calculus removal from a dental implant?
a. Plastic curet
b. Plastic periodontal probe
c. Standard Gracey curet
d. Miniature Gracey curet

47. The patient's periodontal diagnosis is chronic generalized periodontitis. Teeth #28 and #29 have heavy calculus deposits. Which of the following is NOT recommended for removing these calculus deposits?
    a. Begin calculus removal using a powered tip of a sonic device
    b. Begin with a standard ultrasonic tip, approach the deposits from both the facial and the lingual aspect of the sextant
    c. Assess the amount, type, and location of the calculus deposits with a periodontal explorer, such as an ODU 11/12
    d. Once the heavy and medium-sized deposits have been removed, use a slim-diameter ultrasonic tip to complete calculus removal

48. Which instrument would be most efficient in removing supragingival interproximal calculus deposits from the anterior teeth that exhibit crowding?
    a. Universal curet
    b. Anterior sickle scaler
    c. Gracey miniature 1/2 curet
    d. Beavertail ultrasonic tip

49. The client has multiple teeth restored with porcelain-fused-to-metal crowns, many of which have defective margins. Which of the instruments would you use FIRST to begin removal of the moderate calculus deposits?
    a. Thin ultrasonic tip
    b. Gracey miniature 11/12 and 13/14 curets
    c. Posterior sickle scaler
    d. A universal curet

50. **The distal of tooth #18 has a large piece of calculus. When probing, what is the BEST way to obtain accurate probing depth?**
   a. Insert the probe until it is obstructed by the calculus deposit; record this measurement as the probing depth
   b. To obtain an initial reading, move the probe over and around the deposit and insert the probe to the base of the sulcus or pocket; record this as an initial depth
   c. Once the calculus deposit has been removed, use the probe to obtain an accurate probing depth
   d. Answers b and c would obtain the most accurate reading

Management of Pain and Anxiety

Gwen L. Hlava, Todd N. Junge

Subject Matter Consultants: Margaret J. Fehrenbach, Demetra Daskalos Logothetis

As clinicians, dental hygienists must be able to manage the client's pain and anxiety. This requires mastery of head and neck anatomy, physiology, pharmacology, medical emergencies, and clinical technique. Local anesthetic administration is within the legal scope of dental hygiene practice in most jurisdictions in the United States. This chapter reviews four methods to relieve and manage pain and anxiety: (1) local anesthesia with standard syringe, (2) topical anesthesia, (3) computer-controlled local anesthesia delivery device, and (4) nitrous oxide–oxygen conscious sedation.

CHARACTERISTICS AND PHYSIOLOGY OF PAIN

A. Definitions
   1. Pain—sensation of discomfort resulting from the stimulation of specialized nerve endings called *nociceptors* (free nerve endings)
   2. Pain perception—process whereby the sensation of pain is transmitted from the periphery to the central nervous system
   3. Pain reaction—result of pain perception; what a person will do about the perceived pain
   4. Pain-reaction threshold—amount of pain one must experience before exhibiting a reaction
B. Pain reactions and pain-reaction thresholds vary from individual to individual and within the same individual from day to day
C. Pain perception
   1. Functional unit—neuron, or nerve cell
   2. Types of nerve cells
      a. Unipolar
      b. Bipolar—transmits dental pain perception
      c. Multi-polar
   3. Sensory neuron characteristics (Fig. 18-1)
      a. Cell body
      b. Nucleus
      c. Axons (fibers, processors)
      d. Free nerve endings (nociceptors)

Gwen L. Hlava, Todd N. Junge, and the publisher acknowledge the past contributions of Danielle Leigh Ryan to this chapter.

   4. Fiber diameter—varies; determines speed of impulse conduction and type of pain perceived
      a. A fibers—3 to 20 micrometers (μm, microns)
         (1) Myelinated
         (2) Rapid conduction (rate of 100 meters per second [m/s])
      b. C fibers—0.5 to 1 μm
         (1) Nonmyelinated
         (2) Slow conduction (rate of 0.5 to 2 m/s)
   5. Nerve trunk versus ganglia—a nerve trunk is an extremely large bundle of nerve fibers or axons; a ganglion is the site where cell bodies are bundled
D. Resting nerve cell membrane
   1. Membrane potential—the difference in the electrical charges across the nerve membrane
   2. Membrane potential maintained by:
      a. The sodium-potassium pump
      b. The permeability of the cell membrane
   3. Ions essential to nerve conduction
      a. Potassium (K^+) ions (predominately intracellular)
      b. Sodium (Na^+) ions (predominently extracellular)
   4. Sodium-potassium pump; resting state polarized (unstimulated)

$$\text{Outside cell } Na^+$$
$$\frac{+ + + + + + + + + + + +}{- - - - - - - - - - - -}\text{cell membrane}$$
$$\text{Inside cell } K^+$$

   5. Permeability of the cell membrane—impermeable to sodium (at rest)
E. Minimal threshold stimulus
   1. Stimulus—an environmental change that can be chemical, thermal, mechanical, or electrical in nature
   2. Minimal threshold stimulus—the magnitude of the stimulus required to initiate a nerve impulse
   3. "All-or-none" law—either the nerve fires as strongly as possible or it does not fire at all
F. Excitation
   1. When a minimal threshold stimulus excites the nerve:
      a. The permeability of the cell membrane changes
         (1) Influx—Na^+ enters the cell
         (2) Efflux—K^+ diffuses to the outside of the cell

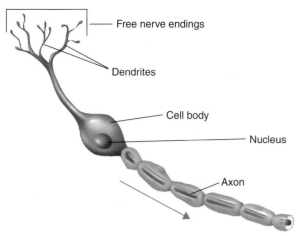

FIG 18-1 Sensory neuron showing the direction of impulse travel *(red arrow)*. (From Patton KT, Thibodeau GA: *Anatomy and physiology*, ed 8, St Louis, 2013, Mosby.)

b. Reversed polarity

Outside cell K$^+$

$-\ -\ -\ -\ -\ -\ -\ -\ -\ -\ -$ cell membrane
$+\ +\ +\ +\ +\ +\ +\ +\ +\ +\ +$
Inside cell Na$^+$

2. Depolarization—the time interval that exists while ionic concentrations are reversing
3. Reversed polarity—the result of a reversal in ionic charges
4. Repolarization—occurs after reversed polarity; the membrane becomes hyperpermeable to K$^+$ and impermeable to Na$^+$; polarity is reestablished
5. Action potential—rapid sequence of changes in the membrane potential (negative to positive, and positive back to negative); the stages are:
   a. Depolarization—resulting in reversed polarity
   b. Repolarization
6. Absolute refractory period—the period during depolarization and reversed polarity when the cell membrane cannot be reexcited
7. Relative refractory period—during repolarization, the nerve cell membrane can be reexcited, but it requires a greater stimulus than the stimulus required for excitation from the resting state
G. Pain intensity determined by:
   1. Number of fibers stimulated—depends on:
      a. Anatomy of the area
      b. Dimensions of the area being stimulated
   2. Frequency of excitation—depends on duration of the stimulus
H. Pain reaction—determined by a person's pain-reaction threshold
   1. High pain-reaction threshold produces hyporeactive behavior

2. Low pain-reaction threshold produces hyperreactive behavior
3. Factors affecting the pain-reaction threshold
   a. Emotional state—most consistently reported, variable; greater anxiety and negativity results in lower pain-reaction threshold
   b. Fatigue—greater fatigue results in lower pain-reaction threshold
   c. Age—younger people experience a lower pain-reaction threshold
   d. Gender—variable

LOCAL ANESTHESIA ARMAMENTARIUM

A. Definition—all items essential for the administration of a local anesthetic agent
B. Armamentarium categories
   1. Needle
      a. Components (Fig. 18-2)
      b. Composition—stainless steel
      c. Gauge (ga)—the diameter of the lumen is indicated by a number
         (1) The larger the gauge number, the smaller the lumen diameter
         (2) The 25-, 27-, and 30-ga needles are the most common in dentistry
      d. Length—measured from hub to the point of bevel
         (1) Short = 1 inch
         (2) Long = 1⅝ inches

FIG 18-2 Components of a hypodermic needle. *A*, Shaft or shank, the working end of the needle. *B*, Bevel, or angulation, of the tip. *C*, Lumen, the hollow interior of the shaft. *D*, The hub holds the shaft and is threaded onto the adapter of the syringe. *E*, The syringe end enters the anesthetic cartridge. *F*, The protective shield sleeve (colored end) covers the needle shaft. *G*, The protective shield guard (clear or white) covers the syringe end of the needle. *H*, The security seal holds the protective shield sleeve and guard together until the hub is assembled and attached to the syringe.

Aluminum cap

Drug identifying
color-coded band

Plunger
indented from
rim of glass

Neck   Cylinder

Rubber
diaphragm

Inscription

Silicone rubber
plunger/stopper

FIG 18-3 Components of the glass cartridge for the dental local anesthetic. (Modified from Malamed SF: *Handbook of local anesthesia*, ed 6, St Louis, 2013, Mosby.)

e. Method of sterilization—disposable needles come pre-sterilized, with a security seal
2. Anesthetic cartridge
   a. Components (Fig. 18-3)
      (1) Metal cap end is directed toward the needle when the cartridge is loaded into the syringe
      (2) Round rubber diaphragm—the syringe end of the needle penetrates this diaphragm and enters the cartridge
      (3) Cylinder—glass tube containing the anesthetic solution
      (4) Inscription—legally required information on the cartridge, which includes:
         (a) Volume—1.8 mL
         (b) Anesthetic agent—generic and brand names
         (c) Percentage of drug
         (d) Vasoconstrictor
         (e) Concentration ratio of vasoconstrictor
         (f) Manufacturer
         (g) Lot number
         (h) Expiration date
      (5) Rubber stopper—seals the opposite end of cartridge; it is the movable component of the cartridge
   b. Ingredients in the anesthetic solution
      (1) Anesthetic drug
      (2) Vasoconstrictor
      (3) Preservative (sodium bisulfite)
      (4) Sodium chloride—makes the solution isotonic
      (5) Distilled water—inert ingredient
   c. Method of storage—away from direct sunlight and ultraviolet light, and maintained at room temperature (68 °F to 77 °F; 20 °C to 25 °C) or slightly cooler
3. Anesthetic syringe (Fig. 18-4)
   a. Components
      (1) Adapter—the hub of the needle is threaded onto this part of the syringe
      (2) Barrel—holds the anesthetic cartridge
      (3) Harpoon—the fishhook-shaped tip is forced into the rubber stopper

Needle
adaptor

Piston rod with
harpoon

Spool finger grip

Syringe
barrel

Thumb ring

A

Needle
adaptor

Window

B

FIG 18-4 A, Assembled breech-loading, metallic, cartridge-type syringe. **B,** Disassembled local anesthetic syringe. (Modified from Malamed SF: *Handbook of local anesthesia*, ed 6, St Louis, 2013, Mosby.)

      (4) Piston rod—connects the harpoon to the thumb ring; can be advanced to expel the solution or retracted to aspirate
      (5) Large window—faces the operator during injection; rubber stopper speed, positive aspirations, and volume are observable
      (6) Small window—aids in removing the used cartridge
      (7) Spool finger grip—place of rest for the index and middle fingers
      (8) Thumb ring—enables the operator to aspirate or express fluid from the cartridge
   b. Method of syringe sterilization—the bioburden is removed; the syringe is dried, packaged, and sterilized
   c. Auxiliary materials—hemostat or cotton pliers; used if the needle breaks
C. Record keeping and documentation in client dental record
   1. Documentation requirements vary by state law
   2. Documentation includes:
      a. Time of administration
      b. Type and percentage of drug administered
      c. Type and ratio of vasoconstrictor
      d. Amount of drug administered in milligrams
      e. Name of injection(s) administered and the region of the mouth in which the injection(s) is administered
      f. Reactions to drug (if any)
      g. The American Dental Association (ADA) Code D9215 for health insurance reimbursement

LOCAL ANESTHETIC AGENTS (TABLE 18-1)

Chemical Structure

A. Chemical components
   1. Aromatic lipophilic group—for diffusion into the lipid nerve membrane
   2. Intermediate chain—determines if the agent is an ester or an amide; also determines the potential for any allergic reaction
   3. Hydrophilic group—required for diffusion into water-soluble tissues
B. Allergies related to chemical structure
   1. A considerable amount of documentation on allergic reactions to esters is available; because of their potential for causing allergic reactions, esters are no longer used
   2. Cross-reactivity occurs with esters; thus, if a client is allergic to one ester, an allergic reaction will occur with all other ester derivatives
   3. No substantiated cases, to date, of allergic reactions to amides
   4. Cross-reactive allergic reactions do not occur among amides
   5. In cases where the agent cannot be identified, the client should be referred to an allergist for testing

Mechanism of Action

A. Physiologic effect—local anesthetics prevent cell membrane permeability to sodium
B. Properties of local anesthetics
   1. Salt
      a. Water soluble (hydrophillic)
      b. Acidic
      c. Charged, cation RNH+ (ionized)
      d. Active form at site of action
      e. Form present in dental cartridge (pH 3.3-6.0)
   2. Free Base
      a. Fat soluble (lipophillic)
      b. Unstable
      c. Alkaline
      d. Uncharged, anion RN, nonionized
      e. Penetrates nerve tissue
      f. Form present in tissue (pH 7.4)
C. Dissociation—the ability of a drug to separate or part
   1. Solution in cartridge is predominately acidic pH 3.3-6
   2. Once injected into basic tissue pH 7.4 dissociation (loss of H+ molecule) of cation RNH+ (acid) to anion RN (base) occurs to penetrate the nerve
   3. Once in axoplasm molecules regain a H+ ion and revert back to active RNH+ (ionized) form to block nerve conduction
D. Effects of inflammation—decreased anesthetic effect in areas of inflammation; caused by three factors:
   1. Decreased pH of tissues—causes dissociation to occur more slowly or not at all
   2. Edema—dilutes concentration of local anesthetic
   3. Increased vascularity—facilitates rapid removal of drug from area

E. Nerve fiber susceptibility
   1. Smaller, nonmyelinated fibers (C fibers) are the first to be blocked; however, sensation is regained last in these fibers
   2. Large, myelinated fibers (A fibers) are the last to be blocked; however, sensation is regained first in these fibers

Potency

A. Definition—lowest concentration of drug needed to consistently produce adequate anesthesia
   1. Potency is related directly to lipid solubility
   2. If a local anesthetic drug is highly potent, lower concentrations are effective in achieving adequate anesthesia
   3. Greater potency also equals greater chance of systemic toxicity (see Table 18-1)

Toxicity

A. Definition—the amount of drug capable of causing adverse systemic reactions in normal persons; adverse reactions occur when the rate of drug absorbed is greater than the rate of *biotransformation,* the body's ability to metabolize the drug
B. True toxic reactions occur immediately—the most profound effects of toxic reaction are on the central nervous system (CNS) and the cardiovascular system
   1. CNS effects
      a. CNS stimulation phase—the person becomes extremely talkative, restless, and anxious
      b. CNS depression phase—convulsions may occur, in extreme cases, unconsciousness may result
   2. Cardiovascular effects
      a. During the stimulation phase—the person's blood pressure and pulse rise rapidly
      b. During the depression phase—the person's blood pressure and pulse drop significantly
   3. Respiratory failure is the primary cause of death
   4. Vital functions must be supported until the drug is eliminated by biotransformation

Biotransformation (Metabolism)

A. Definition—process whereby the drug is broken down, changed, or combined with other substances to render it physiologically inactive
B. Biotransformation (according to chemical group)
   1. Esters—metabolized in plasma through the process of hydrolysis; inactivated by plasma cholinesterase (an enzyme)
   2. Amides—metabolized in the liver; history of cirrhosis, alcoholism, liver disease or liver transplantation, and jaundice may affect the rate of biotransformation
      a. Lidocaine, mepivacaine, and bupivacaine are metabolized in the liver
      b. Prilocaine is metabolized in the liver and lungs
      c. Articaine is metabolized 95% in the plasma and 5% in the liver

TABLE 18-1 Comparison of Frequently Used Local Anesthetic Agents in Dentistry

Generic Name	Brand Name	Color Code	Concentration	Chemical Classification	Vasoconstrictor	Concentration of Vasoconstrictor	Onset of Action	APPROXIMATE DURATION — Without Vasoconstrictor	APPROXIMATE DURATION — With Vasoconstrictor	Toxicity*	Method of Metabolism	Milligram/Cartridge	MAXIMUM SAFE DOSAGE FOR NORMAL ADULT CLIENT — Milligram	MAXIMUM SAFE DOSAGE FOR NORMAL ADULT CLIENT — Cartridge
Lidocaine	Xylocaine	Green	2%	Amide	Epinephrine	1:50,000	2-3 min		Pulpal = 60 min / Soft tissue = 3-5 hr	100%	Liver	36	500 mg	13.8
		Red	2%	Amide	Epinephrine	1:100,000	2-3 min		Pulpal = 60 min / Soft tissue = 3-5 hr	100%	Liver	36	500 mg	13.8
Mepivacaine	Carbocaine	Brown	2%	Amide	Neo-Cobefrin	1:20,000	1½-2 min		Pulpal = 60 min / Soft tissue = 3-5 hr	75%	Liver	36	400 mg	11.1
		Tan	3%	Amide			2-4 min	Pulpal = 20-40 min / Soft tissue = 2-3 hr		75%	Liver	54	400 mg	7.4
Prilocaine	Citanest Forte	Yellow	4%	Amide	Epinephrine	1:200,000	2-4 min		Pulpal = 60-90 min / Soft tissue = 3-8 hr	60%	Liver and lung	72	600 mg	8.3
	Citanest	Black	4%	Amide			2-4 min	Pulpal = 40-60 min / Soft tissue = 2-4 hr		60%	Liver and lung	72	600 mg	8.3
Articaine	Septocaine	Gold	4%	Amide	Epinephrine	1:100,000	2-2½ min		Pulpal = 60-75 min / Soft tissue = 3-6 hr	100%	Plasma and liver	72	None listed	***
		Silver	4%	Amide	Epinephrine	1:200,000	2-2½ min		Pulpal = 45-60 min / Soft tissue = 2-5 hr	100%	Plasma and Liver	72	None listed	***
Bupivacaine	Marcaine	Blue	0.5%	Amide	Epinephrine	1:200,000	6-10 min		Pulpal = 90-180 min / Soft tissue = 4-9 hr	>400%	Liver	9	90 mg	10

*Reference value = Lidocaine@100%

Topical Anesthetic

A. Purpose—reduces the discomfort associated with the initial penetration of the needle through the mucosa
B. Controversy exists with regard to widespread use
   1. Dosage control—impossible to standardize because of variability in factors such as operator, client, and area of operation
   2. The concentration of the topical anesthetic used exceeds that which is administered by injection (e.g., 5%, 10%, 20% topical anesthetic vs. 2%, 3%, or 4% local anesthetic)
   3. Except for 5% lidocaine (Xylocaine), all other topical anesthetics are esters
   4. Lidocaine and prilocaine periodontal gel (Oraqix) is an amide; used in adults who require limited pain control during root debridement in periodontal pockets
   5. Cetacaine—a combination of benzocaine, butamben, and tetracaine hydrochloride—is an ester topical indicated in adults who require preinjection, deep scaling, and suture removal anesthesia (available in spray, liquid, or gel form)
C. Esters have a greater incidence of allergic reactions and cross-reactivity than amides
D. Topical agents have indications and contraindications; can interact with other medications; clinicians must always assess for potential allergies, side effects, and adverse effects and take appropriate precautions

Calculation of Maximum Recommended Dose for Local Anesthetics

A. Maximum recommended dose (MRD)—maximum amount of drug administered that does not produce a toxic reaction and is based upon mg per pound or mg per kilogram
B. Maximum recommended doses of local anesthetic agents per appointment for healthy patients
   1. Lidocaine: 3.2 mg/lb, 7.0 mg/kg, 500 mg max
   2. Mepivacaine: 3.0 mg/lb, 6.6 mg/kg, 400 mg max
   3. Prilocaine: 4.0 mg/lb, 8.8 mg/kg, 600 mg max
   4. Articaine: 3.2 mg/lb, 7.0 mg/kg, no max listed
   5. Bupivacaine: 0.9 mg/lb, 2.0 mg/kg, (based on Canadian recommendations, no US weight based recommendations), 90 mg max
C. Steps to calculating maximum recommended dose and maximum cartridges

Step 1: Obtain necessary patient information
Step 2: Calculate number of mg of anesthetic in one cartridge
   Take the percentage of solution and multiply by 10.
   Take the answer and multiply by 1.8 (mL in one cartridge) = mg of anesthetic per cartridge.
   (2% lidocaine: $20 \times 1.8 = 36$ mg/cartridge)
Step 3: Convert pounds to kilograms if using this unit of measurement $lb \div 2.2 = kg$.
   Multiply kilograms by mg/kg or pounds by mg/lb
   $120 \div 2.2 = 54.5$ kg $\times 7$ (mg/kg) $= 381.5$ mg (MRD)
   or
   120 lb $\div 3.2$ (mg/lb) $= 384$ mg (MRD)
   This number may be different for each anesthetic and provides the maximum recommended dose (MRD) in mg for the patient, based on his/her weight.
Step 4: Divide the MRD (Step 3) by the number of mg of the selected anesthetic per cartridge (Step 2) = maximum number of cartridges.
   384 mg $\div 36 = 10.6$ cartridges
D. Calculating milligrams of anesthetic administered
   1. Multiply number of cartridges administered by the number of mg of anesthetic in each cartridge.
   Administered 2.5 cartridges of 4% articaine: 2.5×72 (mg of articaine in one cartridge) $= 180$ mg administered

Vasoconstrictors (Table 18-2)

A. Vasoconstrictors are combined with local anesthetics to counteract the vasodilating properties of local anesthetics.
B. Description—all vasoconstrictors can be referred to as *adrenergic drugs* or *sympathomimetic amines*
   1. Adrenergic drug—capable of producing the same effects as those of adrenalin
   2. Sympathomimetic amine—mimics the sympathetic nervous system and contains an amine group within its chemical structure, which is characteristic of vasoconstrictors
   3. All vasoconstrictors can be produced synthetically; two naturally occurring vasoconstrictors, epinephrine and norepinephrine, are produced in the adrenal medulla and the sympathetic postganglionic nerve fibers
   4. There are two vasoconstrictors that are added to local anesthetic drugs available in the US, epinephrine and levonordefrin.

TABLE 18-2 Vasoconstrictors Available in the United States

Generic Name	Brand Name	Concentration Used In Dentistry	Pressor Potency	Milligram/ Milliliter (mg/mL)	Milligram/ Cartridge (mg/cart)	Maximum Recommended Dose (MRD) (Healthy Adult)		MRD (Cardiac Dose)		Approx % of α/β Activity
Epinephrine	Adrenalin	1:50,000	1	0.02	0.036	0.2 mg	5.5 cart	0.04 mg	1.1 cart	50/50
		1:100,000		0.01	0.018	0.2 mg	11.1 cart	0.04 mg	2.2 cart	
		1:200,000		0.005	0.009	0.2 mg	22.2 cart	0.04 mg	4.4 cart	
Levonordefrin	Neo-Cobefrin	1:20,000	⅙	0.05	0.09	1.0 mg	11.1 cart	0.2 mg	2.2 cart	75/25

C. Benefits of Vasoconstrictor:
1. Reduce systemic absorption of the local anesthetic agent
2. Decrease risk of systemic toxicity
3. Reduce blood flow through the area (hemostasis)
4. Increase duration of action of the anesthetic
5. Increase in the effectiveness of the local anesthetic by decrease in diffusion
6. Lower dose of the local anesthetic agents required

D. Mode of action—stimulate α-adrenergic receptors located in the walls of arterioles
1. α-Adrenergic receptors—responsible for arterial constriction
2. β-Adrenergic receptors—responsible for dilation
3. Each type of vasoconstrictor possesses varying degrees of response of both α- and β-adrenergic activity (see Table 18-2); although epinephrine exhibits the most β-adrenergic activity, to achieve the same amount of vasoconstriction as epinephrine, the concentration of all other vasoconstrictors must be increased

E. Termination of action—Once absorbed, the action of epinephrine is terminated primarily by the reuptake action of adrenergic nerves, any epinephrine that escapes the reuptake action is inactivated by enzymes catechol-O-methyltransferase (COMT), and monoamine oxidase (MAO) in the blood.

F. Pressor potency—the ability of a drug to produce vasoconstriction
1. Epinephrine—the most potent vasoconstrictor; pressor potency value = 1
2. Levonordefrin—another type of adrenergic vasoconstrictor; pressor potency value = $\frac{1}{6}$
3. Concentrations of all vasoconstrictors must be increased to obtain the same vasoconstrictive potency as that of epinephrine

G. Vasoconstrictors in solution—unstable; preservative (e.g., sodium bisulfite) is added to prevent oxidation

H. Toxicity—toxicity resulting from vasoconstrictor overdose is caused by constriction of blood vessels, which raises blood pressure and cardiac rate from β-adrenergic receptor stimulation
1. Symptoms
   a. Increased blood pressure
   b. Increased heart rate (tachycardia >150 beats/min)
   c. Talkativeness
   d. Restlessness
   e. Palpitations or irregular heartbeat
   f. Headache
2. Prevention of cardiac emergencies—strict adherence to MRD in the case of persons with cardiac disease (see Chapter 21)

I. Maximum recommended dose for vasoconstrictor drugs
1. Based on recommendations from the American Heart Association and the New York Heart Association.

a. Based on "healthy" or "compromised" individuals, and not weight dependent
b. See Table 18-2 for "healthy" and "cardiac" doses

J. Steps to calculating vasoconstrictor drug doses (using 1:100,000 epinephrine as the example)
Step 1: Obtain necessary patient information
Step 2: Calculate mg of vasoconstrictor in one cartridge of anesthetic
Example 1:100,000
1 g = 1000 mg/100,000 mL of solution = 0.01 mg vasoconstrictor/1 mL of solution
To obtain amount in 1 cartridge multiply 0.01 × 1.8 mL (mL in one cartridge) = 0.018 mg in one cartridge
Step 3: Convert MRD of vasoconstrictor to cartridges
Divide MRD by number of mg of vasoconstrictor per cartridge of anesthetic (Step 2)
Healthy MRD = 0.2 mg ÷ 0.018 = 11.1 cart
Cardiac MRD = 0.04 mg ÷ 0.018 = 2.2 cart

K. Limiting drug (see Table 18-1)
1. When determining the safety of administering a specific quantity of a particular anesthetic solution, you must calculate both the MRD of the anesthetic drug and the MRD of the vasoconstrictor
2. In any local anesthetic solution containing a vasoconstrictor, either the anesthetic drug or the vasoconstrictor drug will reach its MRD first; when you have determined which of the drugs limits the total amount of solution to be administered, you have determined the limiting drug
3. Example: 150 pound healthy patient for 2% lidocaine 1:100,000
For the local anesthetic (lidocaine)
2% = 20 mg/mL × 1.8 mL = 36 mg (in one cartridge of lidocaine) 150 × 3.2 mg/lb = 480 mg MRD
480 mg ÷ 36 mg = 13.3 cartridges of lidocaine maximum
For the vasoconstrictor (epinephrine) calculation
1:100,000 = 1 mg/100 mL = 0.01 mg/1 mL × 1.8 mL = 0.018 mg (in one cartridge of 1:100,000 epinephrine dilution)
0.2 mg (MRD of vasoconstrictor for healthy patient) ÷ 0.018 mg = 11.1 cartridges maximum
Because 11.1 is lower than 13.3, epinephrine is the limiting drug in this example.

LOCAL ANESTHESIA INJECTIONS
Basic Injection Procedure
A. Steps to providing a successful injection
1. Preanesthetic patient assessment and consultation
2. Select anesthetic and dosage based upon preanesthetic patient assessment
3. Confirm care plan

4. Obtain informed consent
5. Select injection(s) based upon the areas needing to be anesthetized, presence of infection, and the need for hemostatis
6. Prepare and check equipment
7. Position patient in a supine position
8. Apply topical anesthetic
9. Dry tissue and visualize or palpate the penetration site to determine any needle access problems
10. Establish a fulcrum
11. Make tissue taut
12. Keep syringe out of patient's sight
13. Gently insert needle and slowly move toward target
14. Aspirate, if negative, slowly deposit anesthetic at a rate of 1 mL of solution per minute
15. Observe the patient
16. Document the procedure

Injection Types

A. Supraperiosteal injection or *local infiltration*—anesthetizes small area, usually one or two teeth and associated structures by injection near apices
   1. Can be administered on any tooth of either dental arch
   2. Increased clinical effectiveness in maxillary arch more than mandibular arch and mandibular anterior teeth than mandibular posterior teeth
   3. Target area—superior (or inferior) to apex (apices) near terminal nerve endings
   4. Injection site—needle should be inserted parallel to long axis of tooth usually the height (or depth) of mucobuccal fold or lingual tissue with bevel orientation of needle toward alveolar process
B. Nerve block (see next sections for Maxillary Nerve Blocks and Mandibular Nerve Blocks, see Tables 18-3 and 18-4)—usually affects larger area of anesthesia than supraperiosteal injection and thus additional teeth
   1. Increased level of clinical effectiveness when compared to supraperiosteal injection and can be administered at a distance away from localized inflammation or infection
   2. Fewer injections and lesser amounts of agent can be used for anesthesia within a quadrant
   3. Target area—Near larger nerve trunks

TRIGEMINAL NERVE: MAXILLARY NERVE, SECOND DIVISION (V_2)

See the section on "The Nervous System" in Chapter 4.

Maxillary Nerve Innervation

A. V_2 branches within pterygopalatine fossa
   1. Zygomatic nerve—fibers for lacrimal gland via lacrimal nerve
      a. Zygomaticofacial nerve
      b. Zygomaticotemporal nerve
   2. Pterygopalatine nerves
      a. Orbital branches

   b. Nasal branches—including nasopalatine (NP) nerve (relevant branch for local anesthesia)—both right and left nerves via incisive foramen (with incisive papilla)
   c. Palatine branches—communication between nerves at junctions of distribution
      (1) Greater palatine (GP) nerve (relevant branch for local anesthesia)—via GP foramen
      (2) Lesser palatine nerve—via LP foramen; possible gag reflex by default when soft palate anesthetized with GP nerve
   d. Pharyngeal branch
3. Posterior superior alveolar (PSA) nerve (relevant branch for local anesthesia)—via superior dental plexus; join with IO nerve or maxillary nerve
   a. External branch—innervation of maxillary molars
   b. Internal branch—via PSA foramina
4. Infraorbital (IO) nerve (relevant branch for local anesthesia)—largest contributor via IO foramen; joins PSA nerve or maxillary nerve directly
   a. Anterior superior alveolar (ASA) nerve—via superior dental plexus; possibly involved in crossover-innervation; joins with IO nerve in IO canal
   b. Middle superior alveolar (MSA) nerve—via superior dental plexus in only 28% of cases; joins with IO nerve in IO canal
   c. Lateral nasal nerve
   d. Superior labial nerve
   e. Inferior palpebral nerve

Maxillary Nerve Blocks (See Table 18-3 and Fig. 18-5)

TRIGEMINAL NERVE: MANDIBULAR NERVE, THIRD DIVISION (V_3)

See the section on "The Nervous System" in Chapter 4.

Mandibular Nerve Innervation

A. V_3 branches from undivided main nerve trunk within infratemporal fossa
   1. Meningeal branches (sensory)
   2. Medial pterygoid nerve (motor)
B. V_3 branches from divided nerve trunk
   1. Anterior trunk
      a. Lateral pterygoid nerve (motor)
      b. Masseter nerve (motor)
      c. Anterior deep temporal nerve (motor)
      d. Posterior deep temporal nerve (motor)
      e. (Long) buccal nerve (sensory)—relevant branch for local anesthesia—does not serve buccinator muscle
   2. Posterior trunk
      a. Auriculotemporal nerve (sensory) (relevant brand for local anesthesia)—can get anesthetized with IA nerve
      b. Lingual nerve (sensory) (relevant branch for local anesthesia)—can get damaged with oral surgery and local anesthesia

TABLE 18-3 Maxillary Nerve Blocks

Injection	Structures Anesthetized	Target Area	Injection Site	Needle Length	Amount Deposited
ASA	Maxillary anterior teeth Labial periodontium and gingiva of anterior teeth, labial mucosa, and upper lip	ASA nerve superior to apex of maxillary canine approximately 5-6 mm of short needle	Height of mucobuccal fold of maxillary canine and just medial to and parallel to canine eminence	27-gauge short needle	0.9 to 1.2 mL or one-half to two-thirds of cartridge Wait 3-5 min
MSA	Maxillary premolars and mesiobuccal root of maxillary first molar in 28% of the population Buccal periodontium and gingiva of maxillary premolars and mesiobuccal root of first molar, buccal mucosa and upper lip	MSA nerve superior to apex of maxillary second premolar approximately 5 mm of short needle	Height of maxillary mucobuccal fold of maxillary second premolar	27-gauge short needle	0.9 to 1.2 mL or one-half to two-thirds of cartridge Wait 3-5 min
IO	Maxillary anterior teeth and premolars as well as the mesiobuccal root of maxillary first molar in approximately 28% of cases Facial periodontium and gingiva of anesthetized teeth; upper lip to midline; medial part of cheek; side of nose; lower eyelid	Infraorbital nerve at IO foramen at approximately 10 mm inferior to midpoint of IO rim with zygomaticomaxillary suture Approximately 16 mm or one-half depth of long needle	Height of maxillary mucobuccal fold of maxillary first premolar	27-gauge long or 27-gauge short for children (or small adults)	0.9 to 1.2 mL or one-half to two-thirds of cartridge Wait 3-5 min
PSA	Maxillary molars in approximately 72% of cases; however, the mesiobuccal root of maxillary first molar is not anesthetized in approximately 28% of cases due to possible presence of MSA nerve Buccal periodontium and gingiva of anesthetized teeth as well as buccal mucosa and upper lip	PSA nerve at PSA foramina on infratemporal surface of maxilla and posterosuperior on maxillary tuberosity Approximately three-fourths the depth of short needle	Height of maxillary mucobuccal fold of maxillary second molar, distal to zygomatic process of maxilla by inserting needle upward at a 45° angle to maxillary occlusal plane, inward at a 45° angle to maxillary occlusal plane, and backward at 45° angle	25- or 27-gauge short needle	0.9 to 1.8 mL or one-half to full cartridge Wait 3-5 min
GP	Posterior hard palate and palatal periodontium and gingiva of ipsilateral maxillary posterior teeth Palatal mucosa to midline	GP nerve at GP foramen at junction of the alveolar process of maxilla and hard palate Approximately 4 to 6 mm depth of short needle or until contact with palatine bone	Palatal tissue 1 to 2 mm slightly anterior to greater palatine foramen using pressure anesthesia	27-gauge extra-short or short with standard syringe or 30-gauge extra-short or short with computer-controlled local anesthetic delivery device	0.45 to 0.6 mL or one-fourth to one-third of cartridge until blanching of tissue Wait 2-3 min
NP	Anterior hard palate and palatal periodontium and gingiva of maxillary anterior teeth Palatal mucosa in anterior hard palate	Nasopalatine nerves at incisive foramen on anterior hard palate approximately 4 to 5 mm depth of short needle or until gentle contact	Palatal tissue lateral to incisive papilla and palatal to maxillary central incisors using pressure anesthesia on opposite side of overlying incisive papilla	27-gauge extra-short or short with standard syringe or 30-gauge extra-short or short with computer-controlled local anesthetic delivery device	0.45 mL or one-fourth of cartridge Wait 2-3 min

ASA, Anterior superior alveolar; *MSA,* middle superior alveolar; *IO,* infraorbital; *PSA,* posterior superior alveolar; *GP,* greater palantine; *NP,* nasopalantine.
Data from Logothetis DD: *Local anesthesia for the dental hygienist,* ed 2, St Louis, 2017, Mosby.

c. Inferior alveolar nerve (mixed) (relevant branch for local anesthesia)—travels in mandibular canal; via mandibular foramen; can be bifid with two mandibular foramina
   (1) Mylohyoid nerve (motor but may provide accessory sensory innervation for mandibular first molar)
   (2) Mental nerve (sensory) (relevant branch for local anesthesia)—via mental foramen
   (3) Incisive nerve (sensory) (relevant branch for local anesthesia)—travels in mandibular incisive canal; via mental foramen; possibly involved in crossover-innervation

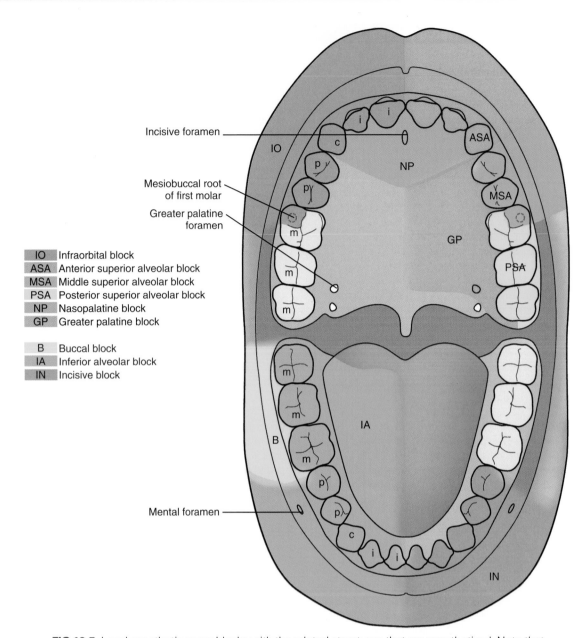

Incisive foramen

Mesiobuccal root of first molar

Greater palatine foramen

IO	Infraorbital block
ASA	Anterior superior alveolar block
MSA	Middle superior alveolar block
PSA	Posterior superior alveolar block
NP	Nasopalatine block
GP	Greater palatine block
B	Buccal block
IA	Inferior alveolar block
IN	Incisive block

Mental foramen

FIG 18-5 Local anesthetic nerve blocks with the related structures that are anesthetized. Note that the anterior middle superior alveolar, the mental, and the Gow-Gates or Vazirani-Akinosi mandibular blocks are not included (see also Table 18-3 and Table 18-4). (From Fehrenbach MJ, Herring SW: *Illustrated anatomy of the head and neck*, ed 5, St Louis, 2017, Elsevier.)

Mandibular Nerve Blocks (Table 18-4)

COMPUTER-CONTROLLED LOCAL ANESTHESIA DELIVERY DEVICE (CCLADD)

CCLADD System Components

A. Three main components (Table 18-5):
   1. Drive unit
   2. Disposable plastic handpiece and tubing
   3. Foot control that activates the unit and controls the two slow/fast flow rates
      a. Slow flow rate:
         (1) Delivers 1 drop every 2 seconds
      (2) 1.8 mL of anesthetic is delivered in 2 minutes
      b. Rapid flow rate:
         (1) Delivers a steady stream (30-gauge) or rapid drip (27-gauge)
         (2) Takes 1 minute to deliver the contents of cartridge

Basic CCLADD Procedure

A. Decreases main causes of pain associated with dental injections that include:
   1. Initial tissue puncture
   2. Depositing volume of fluid too rapidly into a confined space

TABLE 18-4   Mandibular Nerve Blocks

Injection	Structures Anesthetized	Target Area	Injection Site	Needle	Amount Deposited
IA	Mandibular teeth to midline Facial periodontium and gingiva of the mandibular anterior teeth and premolars to midline Lingual periodontium and gingiva to midline Lower lip Anterior two-thirds of tongue Floor of the mouth to midline	IA nerve at mandibular foramen on medial surface of mandibular ramus overhung by lingula; lingual nerve by diffusion; at two-thirds to three-fourths distance from coronoid notch to posterior border of mandibular ramus (where pterygomandibular raphe (fold) turns superior towards soft palate) Approximately 20 to 25 mm or two-thirds to three-fourths of a long needle until bone is gently contacted	Center of pterygomandibular space (triangle) at 6-10 mm superior to occlusal plane of mandibular molars	25-gauge long needle	Approximately 1.8 to 3.6 mL (one to one and a half to two cartridges); save portion for administration of the buccal block, if needed Wait 3-5 min
B	Buccal periodontium and gingiva of mandibular molars Skin of cheek	(Long) buccal nerve as it passes over anterior border of mandibular ramus in the area of retromolar pad (triangle) Approximately 2 to 4 mm of needle length until bone is gently contacted	Buccal mucosa distal and buccal to most distal mandibular molar	25-gauge long (same needle as IA block administered immediately following in most cases) or 27-gauge short (if administered alone in fewer cases)	Approximately 0.3 mL or one-eighth cartridge Wait 1 min
M	Facial periodontium and gingiva of mandibular anterior teeth and premolars to midline Lower lip Skin of chin to midline	Mental nerve at mental foramen at depth of mandibular mucobuccal fold inferior to the apices of the mandibular premolars or location determined by radiographs and/or palpation Approximately 5 - 6 mm of short needle	At mental foramen at depth of mandibular mucobuccal fold inferior to apices of the mandibular premolars or location determined by radiographs and/or palpation	27-gauge short needle	Approximately 0.6 mL or one-third of cartridge Wait 2-3 min
I	Mandibular anterior teeth and premolars to midline Facial periodontium and gingiva of anesthetized mandibular teeth to midline Lower lip Skin of chin to midline	Same as Mental Nerve Block Following injection must massage solution into the mental foramen for 2 minutes	Same as Mental Nerve Block	27-gauge short needle	Approximately 0.6 mL or one-third of cartridge Wait 2-3 min
G-G	Mandibular teeth to midline Lingual periodontium and gingiva of anesthetized mandibular teeth Facial periodontium and gingiva of anesthetized mandibular anterior teeth and premolars to midline and possibly buccal periodontium and gingiva of anesthetized mandibular molars Lower lip, anterior two-thirds of tongue and floor of the mouth to midline Skin over zygomatic bone and posterior part of buccal and temporal regions	IA nerve, lingual nerve, (long) buccal nerve (75% of cases), mental nerve, incisive nerve, mylohyoid nerve, auriculotemporal nerve at anteromedial border of neck of mandibular condyle	Buccal mucosa on medial surface of mandibular ramus, just distal to height of mesiolingual cusp of maxillary second molar using pathway that parallels imaginary extraoral line connecting intertragic notch and ipsilateral corner of the mouth while keeping mouth wide open as well as after for 1 to 2 minutes	25-gauge long	Approximately 1.8 mL or full cartridge Wait 3-5 minutes

(Continued)

TABLE 18-4 Mandibular Nerve Blocks—cont'd

Injection	Structures Anesthetized	Target Area	Injection Site	Needle	Amount Deposited
V-A	Mandibular teeth to midline Lingual periodontium and gingiva of anesthetized mandibular teeth Facial periodontium and gingiva of anesthetized mandibular anterior teeth and premolars to midline and possibly buccal periodontium and gingiva of anesthetized mandibular molars Lower lip, anterior two-thirds of tongue, and floor of the mouth to midline	IA nerve, lingual nerve, (long) buccal nerve (75% of cases), mental nerve, incisive nerve, mylohyoid nerve at center of pterygomandibular space and at approximately equidistant between the mandibular foramen and neck of mandibular condyle as well as being adjacent to maxillary tuberosity	Medially past coronoid process and then into buccal mucosa on medial surface of mandibular ramus at same height as mucogingival junction of maxillary third or second molar directly across way and with bevel oriented away from the bone of mandibular ramus so it faces toward the midline	25-gauge long	Approximately 1.8 mL or full cartridge Wait 5 minutes

IA, inferior alveolar nerve block; *B*, buccal nerve block; *M*, mental nerve block; *I*, incisive block; *G-G*, Gow-Gates mandibular block; *V-A*, Vazirani-Akinosi mandibular block.

Data from Logothetis DD: *Local anesthesia for the dental hygienist*, ed 2, St Louis, 2017, Mosby.

TABLE 18-5 Comparison of Standard Syringe to Computer-Controlled Local Anesthesia Delivery Device (CCLADD)

	Standard	CCLADD
Grasp and needle control	Palm grasp Relies on large muscles of wrist, forearm, and shoulder Weighs 80 grams Held 9 inches from insertion site	Pen grasp Control is transferred to small muscles of fingers and thumb Weighs few grams Held within 2 inches of insertion site
Fluid delivery	Thumb is used to start and stop flow of agent	Uses a foot control to deliver flow of agent
Fluid metering	Pressure and volume cannot be separated; thus is operator dependent	Maintains constant pressure and controlled volume
Aspiration	Relies on operator control	Automatic (on demand) by releasing foot control
Needles	Threaded hub in most cases; luer-lok in fewer cases 25-gauge, long and short 27-gauge, long and short	Luer-Lok hub Smaller gauge and length preferred 30-gauge 30-gauge, short 27-gauge, long
Path of insertion	Linear insertion (straight push through tissues, possibly causing needle deflection)	Bi-rotational insertion (180°) between the thumb and index finger to overcome needle deflection

B. Advantages of CCLADD (Table 18-5)
  1. Eliminates initial pain from needle penetration by establishing anesthetic pathway
  2. Eliminates pressure pain by constant pressure and controlled volume

C. Anesthetic pathway—anesthetic drip precedes the path of the needle and can be used for any injection
D. Prepuncture technique used for palatal injections to increase comfort
  1. Place bevel of needle against the tissue
  2. Use cotton-tipped applicator on the top to seal bevel to tissue surface
  3. Initiate a rate of anesthetic for 2 to 3 seconds to force anesthetic through surface epithelium before actual tissue penetration of palatal tissue
E. Complications—postinjection pain, swelling, necrosis when administered too rapidly and with too much agent

Computer-Controlled Local Anesthesia Delivery Device (CCLADD) Injections

(Note: GP nerve block and NP nerve block can also use this device effectively as well as other nerve blocks)
A. Anterior middle superior alveolar (AMSA) nerve block—palatal approach
  1. Teeth anesthetized—maxillary anterior teeth and premolars within one maxillary quadrant; covering area served by ASA, MSA, GP, NP blocks
  2. Other structures anesthetized—facial periodontium and gingiva of anesthetized teeth to midline; hard palate and palatal periodontium and gingiva of the ipsilateral maxillary posterior teeth and maxillary anterior teeth bilaterally; no regional soft tissue anesthesia of upper lip and face but will need to administer PSA nerve block to complete maxillary quadrant
  3. Not as effective anesthesia for nonsurgical periodontal therapy due to multi-tooth and pulpal anesthesia delivered from a single injection increased deposition time, variable anesthesia, reduced hemostatic control but with

no numbness of lips and of muscles of facial expression so used in cosmetic dentistry

4. Target area—pores in maxilla of hard palate allowing diffusion of agent
5. Injection site—area on palate superior to apices of maxillary premolars and midway between palatal gingival margin and median palatal raphe (suture)
6. Amount—approximately 1.4 to 1.8 mL until blanching of tissue
7. Flow rate—slow flow rate
8. Needle—30-gauge extra-short or short

B. Palatal–anterior superior alveolar (P-ASA) nerve block
1. Teeth anesthetized—maxillary central incisors, lateral incisors, and canines (lesser degree) in maxillary anterior sextant; covering area served by bilateral ASA and NP blocks
2. Associated labial as well as palatal periodontium and gingiva bilaterally
3. Not as effective anesthesia for nonsurgical periodontal therapy due to multi-tooth and pulpal anesthesia delivered from single injection with increased deposition time, variable anesthesia, reduced hemostatic control but with no numbness of lips and facial muscles of facial expression so used in cosmetic dentistry
4. Target area—anterior part of superior dental plexus and NP nerve
5. Injection site
   a. Contralateral to incisive papilla
   b. Needle should be reoriented to gain access to incisive canal (and advance needle to bony wall and aspirate)
6. Amount—1.4 to 1.8 mL
7. Aspiration—required
8. Duration—60 to 90 minutes
9. Flow rate—slow flow rate
10. Needle—30-gauge extra-short or short

C. Periodontal ligament (PDL) injection
1. Teeth anesthetized—single tooth
2. Other structures anesthetized—associated periodontium and gingiva of selected tooth
3. Pulpal anesthesia for single tooth or supplemental injection to block or supraperiosteal injection or local infiltration
4. Target area—nearby terminal nerve endings at apex (or apices) so agent can also flow into marrow spaces of alveolar bone proper
5. Injection site—maxillary and mandibular teeth
   a. Long axis of tooth either mesial or distal with single-rooted tooth; mesial or distal to each root for multi-rooted tooth
   b. Into depth of gingival sulcus and then into alveolar bone proper
6. Aspiration—not necessary
7. Duration—1 hour
8. Flow rate—slow flow rate
9. Needle
   a. 27-gauge extra-short or short for premolars and molars
   b. 30-gauge extra-short or short for incisors

D. Intraseptal injection
1. Structures anesthetized—interdental periodontium and gingiva of two adjacent teeth
2. Target area—terminal nerve endings within marrow of interdental bone of alveolar process associated with adjacent periodontium and gingiva of two or more teeth
3. Injection site—inject few drops and then use pressure to push needle into interdental bone center of interdental papilla adjacent to selected teeth
4. Aspiration—required
5. Duration—variable
6. Flow rate—slow flow rate
7. Needle—27-gauge short

LOCAL ANESTHESIA COMPLICATIONS

See Table 18-6

CONSCIOUS SEDATION WITH NITROUS OXIDE–OXYGEN

A. Synonymous terms
1. Conscious sedation
   a. The client is always awake and able to respond to verbal commands
   b. Protective reflexes are intact, including the ability to maintain an open airway, breathe automatically, and cough, to avoid aspiration
2. Inhalation sedation—nitrous oxide and oxygen gases are inhaled through the nose
3. Nitrous oxide psychosedation—acts on the CNS in such a way that pain impulses are not relayed to the cerebral cortex, or the interpretation of pain impulses is altered
4. Relative analgesia
   a. Refers to the state of sedation produced
   b. Alters the mood and increases the pain reaction threshold but does not totally block pain sensations

B. Chemistry
1. Nitrous oxide (N_2O) properties
   a. Stored as a liquid at 650 to 900 pounds per square inch (psi) in a blue cylinder and delivered as a gas
   b. The contents of the N_2O cylinder cannot be determined by the pressure gauge until it is almost empty
   c. Colorless
   d. Tasteless
   e. Sweet smelling
   f. Nonexplosive
   g. Supports combustion
2. Oxygen (O_2)
   a. Stored as a gas in a green cylinder and delivered as a gas
   b. Contents of the O_2 cylinder can be determined by reading the pressure gauge (full = 2100 psi)

TABLE 18-6 Local Complications Associated with the Administration of Local Anesthetics

Complication	Causes	Prevention	Management
Needle breakage	Sudden, unexpected movement; Poor technique	Patient communication Long, large-gauge needle Do not bend needle Advance needle slowly Never force needle No sudden direction changes Never insert to hub	Remain calm Keep hands in patient's mouth to prevent closure Remove needle fragment if visible Refer to oral surgeon Document incident
Pain during injection	Careless technique Dull needle Barbed needle Hitting bone Rapid deposit	Proper technique Sharp needles Topical anesthetic Sterile anesthetics Inject slowly Room temperature solutions	Good communication Reassure patient that pain is only temporary
Burning during injection	Contamination of local anesthetics Heated anesthetic Expired solution Rapid deposit	Never store in disinfecting solution Store at room temperature Check expiration date Do not use cartridge warmers Inject slowly Consider buffering the local anesthetic	Reassure patient that burning will last only a few seconds
Hematoma	Inadvertent puncturing of a blood vessel Overinsertion of needle during posterior superior alveolar (PSA) block Improper technique Multiple needle penetrations	Short 25-gauge needle for PSA Know dental anatomy Modify injection technique for patient size Minimize the number of needle insertions Maintain good technique	Swelling; apply direct pressure Apply ice to the region; warm packs the next day Discuss possibility of soreness and limited movement to patient Instruct patient that swelling and discoloration will disappear after 7–14 days Dismiss patient when bleeding has stopped
Transient facial paralysis	Inadvertent deposition of local anesthetic in parotid salivary gland during inferior alveolar (IA) block or Vazirani-Akinosi (V-A) block Parotid salivary gland is located on the posterior border of the mandibular ramus and fifth cranial or facial nerve travels through gland Temporary loss of function of muscles of facial expression due to anesthesia of facial nerve	Use proper technique for IA or V-A block Contact bone on the medial surface of the mandibular ramus before depositing agent for the IA or V-A block Redirect barrel of syringe more posteriorly if bone is not contacted	Reassure patient that paralysis is temporary and will last only a few hours Ask patient to remove contact lenses if applicable Close eyelid manually Document
Paresthesia	Irritation to nerve following injection of contaminated agent (less nerve fascia) Edema places pressure on nerve Trauma, electrical shock, or even hemorrhage around nerve sheath Higher concentrations of local anesthetic agent may increase risk for paresthesia Controversy on role of articaine	Store dental cartridges properly Avoid placing cartridges in disinfectant solution Use proper technique: do not move needle around in deep tissue, change needle directions when needle is almost completely withdrawn from tissue Use conservative approach by not using articaine for IA block Use alternative blocks to IA block	Reassure patient Arrange examination with dentist Consultation with oral surgeon Record incident Inform insurance carrier of incident
Trismus	Trauma to muscles in infratemporal space Multiple needle insertions Using contaminated needles Depositing contaminated agent Depositing large amounts of agent in restricted areas Hemorrhage Low-grade infection	Store anesthetic properly Use sharp, sterile, needles Use appropriate injection technique Use minimal amount of agent Deposit agent slowly	Arrange for exam with dentist Heat therapy Jaw exercises Infection; antibiotic treatment Severe pain; refer to oral surgeon Record incident

TABLE 18-6 Local Complications Associated with the Administration of Local Anesthetics—cont'd

Complication	Causes	Prevention	Management
Infection	Contamination of the anesthetic needle before injection Improper handling of local anesthetic Administration of contaminated agent Improper tissue preparation Administering local anesthetics through areas of dental infection (needle tract)	Sterile needle Sheath needle before and immediately after injection Be aware of the location of the uncovered needle at all times Use appropriate infection protocols Store anesthetic properly Wipe off diaphragm Topical antiseptic Do not administer local anesthetics through areas of dental infection	Treat initially as trismus; if patient does not respond in 3 days, systemic antibiotic therapy may be prescribed by their dentist or physician
Edema	Trauma during injection Administration of contaminated agent Hemorrhage Infection Allergic response; may produce airway obstruction	Appropriate infection control Appropriate technique Adequate preanesthetic assessment	Usually resolves within several days without any required treatment Edema caused by infection may require systemic antibiotics
Soft tissue injuries	Lips, tongue, cheeks traumatized by patient while numb Typically seen in children and in special needs patients	Select anesthetic with appropriate duration for treatment Warn patient not to eat, drink hot fluids, or test anesthesia by biting Instruct parent or guardian of danger Place cotton rolls between teeth and soft tissue Warning stickers can be used to remind patient and guardian of dangers associated with being numb Consider administering phentolamine mesylate	Analgesics for pain Antibiotics should be prescribed for infections Recommend warm saline rinses to decrease swelling and discomfort Petrolatum can be used to coat the lips to minimize discomfort
Tissue sloughing	Prolonged use of topical anesthetics Sterile abscess may develop after prolonged ischemia, usually on palate caused by vasoconstrictor	Use topical agent for only 2 to 3 minutes and in a small area Avoid high concentrations of vasoconstrictors	Usually requires no treatment
Postanesthetic intraoral lesions	Trauma to area of injection	Use appropriate administration techniques	Topical anesthetic agents or pastes for discomfort

From: Logothetis DD, *Local anesthesia for the dental hygienist*, ed 2, St Louis, 2017, Mosby.

3. Blood-gas solubility coefficient
   a. The blood-gas solubility coefficient of N_2O is 0.47, which means that 100 mL of blood dissolves 47 mL of N_2O
   b. This blood-gas solubility coefficient accounts for the rapid onset and recovery from the effects of the analgesic
   c. N_2O is 15 times more soluble in the blood than nitrogen; N_2O displaces nitrogen in blood
   d. N_2O does not compete with O_2 and carbon dioxide (CO_2) in combining with the hemoglobin molecule

C. Pharmacology
   1. N_2O has no effect on heart rate, blood pressure, and the liver or the kidneys, as long as an adequate amount of O_2 is delivered simultaneously
   2. N_2O affects all sensations (e.g., hearing, touch, pain, warmth)
   3. N_2O reduces the gag reflex but does not eliminate it

D. Physiology
   1. N_2O works by depressing the CNS

2. The exact mechanism of action is unknown; however, the effect either alters the relay of nerve impulses to the cerebral cortex or causes them to be interpreted differently
3. The client experiences reduced anxiety and increased tolerance to pain
4. Pain perception is not blocked
5. N_2O does not combine with any body tissues; it is the only anesthetic that is not metabolized
6. The N_2O molecule enters the bloodstream through the lungs, where it displaces nitrogen and is eventually exhaled, unchanged, through the lungs
7. Toxic reaction associated with too much N_2O is hypoxia (lack of O_2 to the tissues), characterized by headache and nausea

E. Stages of anesthesia
   1. Stage I: Analgesia stage—client feels pain but is not bothered by it; this stage has three planes; the first two planes are appropriate for dental hygiene care

2. Stage II: Delirium or excitement stage—hyperresponsiveness to stimuli; exaggerated inhalations and loss of consciousness
3. Stage III: Surgical anesthesia—used in oral and maxillofacial surgery; this stage has four planes
4. Stage IV: Respiratory paralysis—the patient is no longer breathing independently
F. Indications for use
1. Mild apprehension
2. Refusal of local and general anesthesia
3. Allergy to local anesthesia
4. Hypersensitive gag reflex
5. Intolerance for long appointments
6. Cardiac conditions
7. Hypertension
8. Asthma
9. Cerebral palsy
10. Intellectual and developmental disabilities
G. Relative contraindications to use
1. Pregnancy
2. Communication difficulties
3. Nasal obstruction
4. Emphysema
5. Multiple sclerosis
6. Emotional instability
7. Epilepsy
8. Negative response to past experience
H. Advantages and disadvantages of use
1. Advantages
a. History of cardiovascular disease—O_2 enrichment coupled with stress reduction
b. Simple, relatively safe procedure to perform
c. Minimal equipment
d. No restraining straps or pharyngeal airways
e. The client is awake and responsive
f. Rapid onset of and recovery from the effects of the anesthetic
g. No need for the client to be accompanied by someone to the appointment
h. No preoperative tests or food intake restrictions required
i. No need for the patient to spend time in a recovery room
2. Disadvantages
a. Oversedation causes vertigo, nausea, or vomiting
b. Difficult behavioral problems cannot always be managed
c. Instrumentation in the maxillary anterior region difficult because of the presence of the mask over the nose of the client
I. Signs and symptoms of N_2O-O_2 sedation
1. Objective signs—directly observed by the clinician in the client
a. Being awake
b. Lessened pain reaction
c. Drowsy, relaxed appearance
d. Normal eye reaction and pupil size
e. Normal respiration

f. Normal blood pressure and pulse
g. Minimal movement of limbs
h. Flushing of skin
i. Perspiration
j. Lacrimation
k. Little or no gagging or coughing
l. Speech infrequent and slow
2. Subjective symptoms—reported by the client
a. Mental and physical relaxation
b. Indifference to surroundings and passage of time
c. Lessened pain awareness
d. Floating sensation
e. Drowsiness
f. Warmth
g. Tingling or numbness
h. Sounds seeming distant
J. Equipment
1. Cylinders—blue indicates N_2O; green indicates O_2
2. Gas machine
a. Yokes
b. Flowmeter
c. Pressure gauge
d. Reservoir bag
e. Gas hose
3. Mask
a. Only masks with two-hose scavenging systems reduce the N_2O exhaled into the air and breathed in by the operator
b. Scavenging systems reduce environmental N_2O contamination from 900 to 30 parts per million (ppm)
c. Maximum allowable contamination in health care environments is 50 ppm
K. Safety measures
1. Color-coded tanks—blue (N_2O) versus green (O_2)
2. Pin Index System—ensures that the N_2O cylinder does not fit into the yoke that holds the O_2 cylinder, and vice versa
3. Diameter Index System—the diameter of the hole at the top of the cylinder (O_2 or N_2O) fits only with corresponding cylinder head
4. Audible alarm system—emitted when O_2 runs out
5. Automatic turnoff—occurs when O_2 is depleted
6. Oxygen maintained at 2 to 3 L at all times in most units
7. Oxygen flush—fills the reservoir bag with 100% O_2
L. Record keeping and documentation in the client's dental record
1. Documentation will vary according to the laws of the state or the legal jurisdiction
2. Documentation includes:
a. Tidal volume (TV) in liters (L)
b. Amount of N_2O in liters or percentage
c. Amount of O_2 in liters or percentage
d. Duration of sedation
e. Oxygenation period (5 minutes O_2/15 minutes N_2O delivered)
f. Client's response
g. ADA Code D9230 for health insurance reimbursement

Website Information and Resources

Source	Website Address	Description
Essential Skeleton 4	https://itunes.apple.com/us/app/essential-skeleton-4/id623811668?mt=8	Study bony landmarks, nerves, and muscles pertaining to the administration of local anesthesia
Dental—Head and Neck Anatomy	https://play.google.com/store/apps/details?id=com.jass.refapp8	Same as above

SUGGESTED READINGS

American Dental Association (ADA): *Glossary of dental clinical and administrative terms* CDT 2011–2012, Chicago, IL.

Fehrenbach MJ, Herring SW: *Illustrated anatomy of the head and neck*, ed 5, St. Philadelphia, 2017, Saunders/Elsevier.

Logothetis DD: *Local anesthesia for the dental hygienist*, ed 2, St Louis, 2017, Elsevier.

Malamed SF: *Handbook of local anesthesia*, ed 6, St Louis, 2013, Mosby.

Walsh MM: Nitrous oxide-oxygen analgesia. In Darby ML, Walsh MM, editors: *Dental hygiene theory and practice*, ed 4, Philadelphia, 2015, Saunders.

Walsh MM, Darby ML: Local anesthesia. In Darby ML, Walsh MM, editors: *Dental hygiene theory and practice*, ed 4, Philadelphia, 2015, Saunders.

CHAPTER 18 REVIEW QUESTIONS

Answers and rationales to review questions are available on this text's accompanying Evolve site. See inside front cover for details.

evolve

1. **The potency of an anesthetic agent is primarily a result of its:**
   a. Water solubility
   b. Protein solubility
   c. Lipid solubility
   d. Carbohydrate solubility

2. **The nerve that travels the mental foramen is a branch of the:**
   a. Inferior alveolar nerve
   b. Middle superior alveolar nerve
   c. Lingual nerve
   d. Posterior superior alveolar nerve

3. **Sodium bisulfite is added to a cartridge of anesthetic to increase the stability of the:**
   a. Distilled water
   b. Vasoconstrictor
   c. Hydrochloride salt
   d. Plasma cholinesterase

4. **Which of the following explains why the administration of a local anesthetic into an area of inflammation has a decreased effect?**
   a. Inflamed tissue has a high pH.
   b. The local anesthetic remains in the salt form (ionized).
   c. Vascularity is decreased in the area of the inflammation.
   d. The local anesthetic is converted to the free base (unionized).

5. **All the following statements are TRUE about lidocaine EXCEPT:**
   a. It is an amide-linked compound.
   b. It is used in 2% concentrations.
   c. It forms a salt with a strong acid that is water soluble.
   d. Its lipophilic portion is ester-linked to the amino group.

6. **Which of the following gauge numbers indicates the needle with the smallest lumen?**
   a. 30

   b. 27
   c. 5
   d. 23

7. **The maxillary division of the trigeminal nerve is:**
   a. Sensory only
   b. Motor only
   c. Sensory and motor simultaneously
   d. Mostly sensory and minimally motor

8. **The type and size of a nerve plays an important part in the development of adequate anesthesia. All the following are TRUE about nerves and anesthesia EXCEPT:**
   a. Myelinated nerves require a greater concentration to be blocked.
   b. Myelinated nerves require less time to be blocked.
   c. Smaller nerve fibers are the last to regain sensation.
   d. Smaller nerve fibers are blocked before the larger ones.

9. **Anesthetics decrease or limit the sensation of pain by:**
   a. Decreasing the firing threshold
   b. Preventing depolarization
   c. Repolarizing the nerve membrane
   d. Causing hyperpolarization

10. **Saltatory conduction refers to:**
    a. Rapid transmission of nerve impulses along a myelinated nerve fiber
    b. Diffusion of sodium into the nerve cell during impulse conduction
    c. Conduction of an impulse along a nonmyelinated nerve fiber at the nodes of Ranvier
    d. None of the above

11. **The sensory receptors responsible for the initiation of pain perception are:**
    a. Meissner's corpuscles
    b. Ruffine's end organs
    c. Free nerve endings
    d. Pacini's corpuscles

12. **When does depolarization of a nerve fiber occur?**
    a. During the resting state of the fiber
    b. Because of the sodium pump
    c. During the relative refractory period
    d. Between the polarization stage and reverse polarity

13. **An environmental change capable of initiating a nerve impulse is termed:**
    a. Minimal threshold stimulus
    b. Initiation stimulus
    c. Firing mechanism
    d. The "all or none" law

14. **The anesthetic solutions injected into the tissues are:**
    a. Acidic salts
    b. Strong acids
    c. Weak bases
    d. Alkaloids

15. **The lipophilic portion of an anesthetic molecule allows the anesthetic solution to:**
    a. Diffuse through the nerve tissue
    b. Diffuse through osseous tissue
    c. Diffuse through the interstitial tissues
    d. Be absorbed by the blood supply

16. **Which acid is most often combined with a local anesthetic drug?**
    a. Sodium bisulfite
    b. Sodium chloride
    c. Acetic acid
    d. Hydrochloric acid

17. **The patient's medical history indicates past liver damage. Why is the amount of amide-based anesthetic solution a relative contraindication?**
    a. Amides increase the risk of an allergic reaction.
    b. Amides undergo biotransformation in the liver.
    c. Without action by the liver, amides will be reabsorbed.
    d. Amides are absorbed much slower at the injection site.

18. **All the following ingredients are contained within an anesthetic solution EXCEPT:**
    a. Sodium chloride
    b. Sodium bisulfate
    c. Water
    d. Vasoconstrictor

19. **Local anesthetic drugs are bases; the local anesthetic solution injected into the tissues are weak bases.**
    a. Both statements are TRUE.
    b. Both statements are FALSE.
    c. The first statement is TRUE; the second statement is FALSE.
    d. The first statement if FALSE; the second statement is TRUE.

20. **The lipophilic portion of an anesthetic molecule allows the anesthetic solution to diffuse through the interstitial tissues; the hydrophilic portion allows the solution to diffuse through the nerve membrane.**
    a. Both statements are TRUE.
    b. Both statements are FALSE.
    c. The first statement is TRUE; the second statement is FALSE.

    d. The first statement is FALSE; the second statement is TRUE.

21. **Vasoconstrictors are added to local anesthetic agents to increase duration and:**
    a. Reduce toxicity by increasing the efficiency of the heart
    b. Reduce toxicity by slowing absorption
    c. Extend the overall shelf life
    d. Help speed up the detoxification process

22. **Where are vasoconstrictors metabolized?**
    a. Liver
    b. Plasma
    c. Bloodstream
    d. Kidneys

23. **For what purpose is epinephrine added to either prilocaine or lidocaine local anesthetic agent?**
    a. Prolongation of anesthesia
    b. Reduction of hemorrhage in field of operation
    c. Constriction of blood vessels in area of injection
    d. Prevention of toxic effects from too-rapid absorption
    e. All the above

24. **Which of the following vasoconstrictor agents is used with mepivacaine (Carbocaine) 3%?**
    a. Neo-Cobefrin
    b. Epinephrine
    c. Levophed
    d. Benzocaine
    e. None of the above

25. **After starting the root-plaing procedure, you encounter considerable bleeding from the client's sulcular tissues. After consulting with the dentist, it is decided to administer a local anesthetic for hemostasis. Which component of the local anesthetic will help to achieve hemostasis?**
    a. Anesthetic salt
    b. Vasoconstrictor
    c. Sodium bisulfite
    d. Distilled water

26. **What is the pressure in a FULL tank of oxygen (O_2)?**
    a. 700-800 psi
    b. 900-1100 psi
    c. 1400-1600 psi
    d. 1800-2100 psi

27. **What is the pressure in a FULL tank of nitrous oxide (N_2O)?**
    a. 650-900 psi
    b. 900-1100 psi
    c. 1400-1600 psi
    d. 1800-2100 psi

28. **What is the pressure of a HALF-FULL tank of O_2?**
    a. 700-800 psi
    b. 900-1100 psi
    c. 1400-1600 psi
    d. 1800-2100 psi

29. **What is the pressure in a HALF-FULL tank of N_2O?**
    a. 650-900 psi
    b. 900-1100 psi
    c. 1400-1600 psi
    d. 1800-2100 psi

30. **Which of the following is TRUE concerning N₂O?**
    a. A full tank would read approximately 2100 psi.
    b. It exists as a gas in the tank and is delivered as a gas.
    c. It can be administered and monitored by dental hygienists in all states.
    d. It may induce nerve damage if used chronically.

31. **The use of a scavenging system with N₂O sedation equipment is desirable because it:**
    a. Removes the odor of nitrous from the room
    b. Assists the patient's respiration
    c. Removes any potentially toxic waste gas from the environment
    d. Allows the patient to inhale room air through the nosepiece

32. **Which of the following patients would NOT be a good candidate for the use of N₂O?**
    a. "Gagger"
    b. Pediatric patient
    c. Patient with heart disease or a heart attack
    d. Patient with chronic obstructive pulmonary disease

33. **In monitoring the use of N₂O, the patient should be in which stage of general anesthesia?**
    a. Stage I
    b. Stage II
    c. Stage III
    d. Stage IV

34. **The ideal concentration range of N₂O is:**
    a. 10% to 25%
    b. 30% to 50%
    c. 50% to 60%
    d. 60% to 70%

35. **The dental hygienist administered 2.4 cartridges of 3% mepivacaine. How many milligrams were administered?**
    a. 129.6 mg
    b. 135.7 mg
    c. 138.4 mg
    d. 125.2 mg

36. **How many cartridges of lidocaine 2% 1:100,000 epinephrine anesthetic agent can be safely administered to a 120-lb patient taking tricyclic antidepressants?**
    a. 1.1 cartridges
    b. 2.2 cartridges
    c. 3.3 cartridges
    d. 4.4 cartridges

37. **How many cartridges of prilocaine 4% anesthetic agent can a healthy 130-lb patient receive?**
    a. 6.8 cartridges
    b. 7.2 cartridges
    c. 7.8 cartridges
    d. 8.3 cartridges

38. **What is the target area for the inferior alveolar nerve block?**
    a. Mandibular foramen
    b. Lateral surface of mandibular ramus
    c. Anteromedial border of neck of mandibular condyle
    d. Retromolar pad or triangle

39. **What is the injection site for the posterior superior alveolar nerve block?**
    a. Retromolar pad or triangle
    b. Maxillary tuberosity
    c. Pterygopalatine fossa
    d. Superior to maxillary canines

40. **How can you determine a positive aspiration with the computer-controlled local anesthetic delivery device?**
    a. Blood will be noticed in the glass cartridge.
    b. Blood will be noticed in the plastic tubing only.
    c. Blood will be noticed at the needle hub.
    d. The unit will beep rapidly if aspiration is positive.

CASE A

Synopsis of patient history
Age:40
Sex: F
Height: 5'6"
Weight: 160 lb

Vital Signs
Blood pressure: 125/82 mm Hg
Pulse: 75 bpm
Respiration: 16 rpm
1. Under the care of a physician: x YES ___NO
2. Hospitalized within the last 5 years: x YES ___ NO
   Reason: _____
3. Has or had the following conditions:

   _____

   _____

4. Current medications:
   Occasional aspirin
   Daily OTC multi-vitamin
5. Smokes or uses tobacco products: x YES ___ NO
6. Is pregnant: ___ YES x NO

Medical History
Client has a history of smoking ½ pack of cigarettes for the past 20 years.

Dental History
Client's oral hygiene is fair.
AAP classification = III

Social History
Client is a single divorced mother who works two jobs and has three young children.

Chief Complaint
Client recently acquired dental insurance and wants teeth cleaned and an examination.

Current Oral Hygiene Status
1. Client brushes 1-2 times a day
2. Never flosses
3. Interproximal bleeding generalized

Supplemental Oral Examination Findings
1. Previously extracted teeth #1, #16, #17, and #32
2. Mandibular anterior teeth have crowding
3. Attrition on anterior teeth with moderate supragingival calculus
4. Moderate to slight interproximal subgingival deposits throughout

Use Case A to answer questions 41 to 50.

41. **Which nerve is involved when anesthetizing the palatal gingiva of the maxillary lateral incisor?**
    a. Middle superior alveolar nerve
    b. Nasopalatine nerve
    c. Infraorbital nerve
    d. Anterior superior alveolar nerve
    e. Inferior alveolar nerve

42. **After administering a posterior superior alveolar nerve block, the maxillary first molar remains sensitive, but the maxillary second and third molars are anesthetized. Which of the following would be the BEST explanation?**
    a. Anesthetic agent was deposited too high
    b. Not enough anesthetic agent was deposited
    c. Mesiobuccal root is normally not anesthetized by posterior superior alveolar nerve block
    d. Anesthetic agent was deposited too low

43. **Which nerve is involved when anesthetizing the facial gingiva of the maxillary canine?**
    a. Middle superior alveolar nerve
    b. Nasopalatine nerve
    c. Infraorbital nerve
    d. Anterior superior alveolar nerve
    e. Inferior alveolar nerve

44. **When lingual nerve is anesthetized, which of the following tissue will NOT be affected?**
    a. Anterior two-thirds of the tongue
    b. Floor of the mouth
    c. Lingual gingiva
    d. Palatal periodontium
    e. Lower lip

45. **The soft tissue of alveolar process of the mandible is innervated by:**
    a. Buccal and lingual nerves only
    b. Buccal and mental nerves only
    c. Buccal, lingual, and mental nerves
    d. Buccal and inferior alveolar nerves only

46. **Which injection anesthetizes the palatal gingiva and palatal mucosa of tooth #14?**
    a. Middle superior alveolar nerve block
    b. Posterior superior alveolar nerve block
    c. Anterior middle superior alveolar nerve block (palatal approach)
    d. Greater palatine nerve block

47. **Which nerve is involved when anesthetizing the mandibular first premolar?**
    a. Middle superior alveolar nerve
    b. Nasopalatine nerve
    c. Infraorbital nerve
    d. Anterior superior alveolar nerve
    e. Inferior alveolar nerve

48. **To prepare the maxillary right premolars for nonsurgical periodontal therapy, which of the following nerves need to be anesthetized?**
    a. Right buccal nerve only
    b. Right MSA and greater palatine nerves
    c. Right ASA only
    d. Right PSA only

49. **When anesthetizing the mental nerve, which of the following tissues will be affected?**
    a. Facial gingiva of mandibular molars and mandibular second premolar
    b. Floor of the mouth as well as lower lip
    c. Lingual gingiva of mandibular teeth
    d. Facial gingiva of mandibular anterior teeth and mandibular first premolar
    e. Skin of upper cheek as well as lower chin

50. **Following the administration of local anesthesia to anesthetize teeth numbers 1 - 3 you notice a faint bluish discoloration on her cheek. You check introrally and find the same discoloration near the injection site along with swelling. What is the most probable cause of this mark?**
    a. The anesthetic cartridge was contaminated with alcohol
    b. The needle created a tear in the blood vessel
    c. The hygienist used a needle of too fine a gauge
    d. The hygienist injected too rapidly

Dental Hygiene Care for Clients with Special Care Needs

Susan Lynn Tolle

Every person has unique abilities and needs. Two of every five clients treated in the oral health care environment may require a modified care plan because of special care needs. These special care needs may be transient, such as pregnancy or a broken foot, or may be lifelong, such as end-stage renal disease or intellectual and developmental disabilities. With ongoing health care reforms and improved access to care for underserved populations, dental hygienists will be serving increased numbers of persons with special care needs in a variety of settings. The National Institute of Dental and Craniofacial Research describes persons requiring special care as those with genetic or systemic disorders that affect oral, dental, or craniofacial health; whose medical treatments cause oral problems; or whose intellectual or physical disabilities complicate oral hygiene or dental treatment.

GENERAL CONSIDERATIONS

Life Span Approach to Care

A. Principles of growth, development, and maturation
1. Growth includes physical and functional maturation
2. Growth is generally a continuous and orderly process but can be modified by numerous factors (e.g., nutritional deficiencies)
3. Different parts of the body grow and mature at different rates
4. Critical periods exist in growth and development
5. Hormonal changes can alter:
   a. Physical stature and function
   b. Mental state and mood
   c. Oral status
   d. Immunity and host response
6. During growth and maturation, a person's perception of self and of self in relation to others changes
7. Health status generally progresses from acute illness to chronic illness
8. Transition from one life stage to another is gradual and not necessarily based on chronologic age
9. Biologic age is not synonymous with chronologic age
10. Signs of aging can appear at any age
B. The U.S. health care system (see the section on "Provision of Oral Health Care" in Chapter 20)
1. The current system is categorical, with many gaps in services

2. A continuum of services through people's life stages must ensure:
   a. Universal access
   b. Continuity of care
   c. A comprehensive philosophy of care
   d. A system of planned change
3. Health care providers should consider:
   a. Heterogeneity of persons bearing the same label
   b. Individualized approach to care
4. Oral health needs and approaches to care can differ throughout a person's life cycle (Table 19-1)

Incidence and Prevalence of Individuals with Special Needs

A. National statistics on incidence and prevalence figures are difficult to compile because of:
1. Unreliable reporting systems
2. Variable and changing definitions of conditions
3. Differences between acute conditions versus chronic conditions
4. Overlap in data when dealing with multiple conditions
B. More than 60 million persons (1 in 5 persons) are considered "disabled" as defined by the Americans with Disabilities Act; of these, approximately 1 million are children younger than 6 years
C. In the United States, 38.3 million persons are considered to have a severe disability
D. Table 19-2 identifies the most common chronic conditions in the older adult population
E. The most common disabilities in the United States are caused by cardiovascular disease, stroke (CVA), obesity, arthritis, cancer, and diabetes
F. The prevalence of disability increases with age
1. Of persons in the United States age 5 to 15, 6% are disabled
2. Of persons in the United States age 16 to 64, 12% are disabled
3. Of persons in the United States age 65 and older, 41% are disabled
G. Of individuals with developmental disabilities, 80% live in community-based residences or at home with families

TABLE 19-1 Life-Span Approach to Oral Health Care

Life Stage	General Care Concerns	Usual Oral Concerns
Early childhood	Teaching parents and caregivers oral care skills	Oral infections
	Preventing early occurrence of caries or trauma (protecting developing teeth)	Dental caries
	Controlling risk factors	Dental development
	Preventing vertical and horizontal disease transmission	
Childhood	Developing positive dental attitudes and behaviors	Dental caries
	Teaching self-care skills	Dental development
	Controlling risk factors	Gingivitis
	Preventing vertical and horizontal disease transmission	
Adolescence	Motivating toward self-responsibility for seeking and receiving care	Dental caries
	Controlling risk factors for disease	Periodontal diseases
	Preventing oral injuries	Dental development
	Tobacco use cessation	
Young adult	Decreasing barriers and integrating oral health care into daily schedule	Periodontal diseases
	Tobacco use cessation	
Midlife	Maintaining status and preventing deterioration	
	Controlling risk factors	
	Tobacco use cessation	
Older adult	Motivating to continue preventive care and accept new theories and interventions	Periodontal diseases
	Decreasing barriers to care	Dental caries
	Controlling risk factors	Oral cancer
	Tobacco use cessation	
Elderly adult	Maintaining status and function and preventing infections and tooth loss	Periodontal diseases
	Controlling risk factors	Dental caries
	Tobacco use cessation	Oral cancer
		Fractures, tooth loss
		Oral infections

TABLE 19-2 Leading Chronic Conditions in the Older-Adult Population

Noninstitutionalized Older Adults	Nursing Home Residents
Arthritis	Arthritis
Hypertension	Heart disease
Hearing impairments	Mental illness
Heart disease	Paralysis

The Dental Hygienist and Individuals with Special Needs

A. Recognize physical, mental, medical, social, and oral needs
B. Communicate with clients and caregivers in a positive, appropriate, nondiscriminatory manner
C. Communicate with other professionals and team members to facilitate planning, implementation, and coordination of care
D. Plan, implement, and evaluate community-based and office-based programs
E. Adapt dental hygiene care plans, interventions, and evaluations to meet clients' special needs, considering:
   1. Barriers to care
   2. Resources
   3. Personal skills and abilities
   4. Cultural values and beliefs
F. Identify and eliminate potential barriers to care
G. Assess one's own attitudes, values, and commitment to provision of oral health services to these clients
H. Evaluate local, state, regional, and national trends for their potential impact on the provision of oral health care
I. Advocate oral health promotion and disease-prevention programs, full use of dental hygienists, and development of sound research so that evidenced-based care is provided in oral health care programs

General Definitions

These definitions tend to change frequently and often overlap.
A. Labeling—the process of classifying persons for educational, medical, or financial reasons
B. Barrier-free environment—facilities that are physically accessible to everyone
C. Normalization—making available patterns and conditions of everyday life that are as close as possible to the norms and patterns of mainstream society
D. Mainstreaming—integration of persons with special needs into community-based programs and services
E. Access to oral health care—opportunity for each individual to enter into the oral health care system and use needed services

Goals of Normalization for Persons with Special Care Needs

A. Ensure the same legal and civil rights as others
B. Guarantee appropriate education for continued learning

C. Increase or maintain social skills and problem-solving abilities
D. Increase employment options and decrease employer discrimination
E. Ensure comprehensive network of community resources

Potential Barriers to Oral Health Care

A. Accessibility
  1. Financial
    a. One fourth of the older adult population has an inadequate income level; percentages are higher for women, ethnic minorities, and single heads of household
    b. Between 65% and 85% of disabled persons live near the poverty level
    c. Medicaid coverage for oral health care is extremely variable across states and often does not cover older-adult care
    d. Medical and pharmaceutical expenses for many persons with disabilities consume a major portion of their income
    e. Many individuals with special needs who have limited incomes cannot afford standard private practice fees for dental care, have no health insurance, or are underinsured
  2. Transportation and geography
    a. More than 50% of the disabled and older adult population live in urban settings; the remainder live in small rural communities or on farms
    b. Public transportation is often unreliable, confusing, unaffordable, or nonexistent
    c. Clients with special care needs often rely on others for transportation to dental appointments, which increases their dependence and makes scheduling and compliance difficult
    d. Homebound, hospitalized, or institutionalized clients frequently cannot be transported for care in the community
  3. Physical facilities
    a. Minimum standards for accessibility must be met by dentists according to the Americans with Disabilities Act of 1993
    b. External barriers include parking lots and spaces, walkways, curbs, stairs, narrow doors and entryways, heavy or pressurized doors, and small-print signs
    c. Internal barriers include narrow passageways or doors, cluttered rooms or hallways, loose rugs or heavy shag carpets, abrupt changes in floor textures, and bathrooms without grab-bars or other modifications
B. Psychosocial concerns
  1. More than 50% of persons in the United States express positive attitudes toward older adults and persons with disabilities, and yet most really perceive these populations as "different" and "inferior"
  2. Society perceives disabilities, differences, and disease states before recognizing similarities
  3. Feelings of guilt, anxiety, apathy, inadequacy, embarrassment, depression, anger, and resentment about special needs interfere with attempts to seek care
  4. Fear of or inability to comprehend dental procedures, antisocial or atypical behavior, or dependency on oral health care providers interferes with provision of care
  5. Basic daily needs and activities are often overwhelming and can lower the priorities for oral health care
  6. Perception of self-image and worth can affect care planning
C. Provider philosophy and provision of care
  1. The Americans with Disabilities Act requires that public and private dental offices serve persons with disabilities, that treatment is provided on the same basis as for nondisabled persons, and that dentists make reasonable modifications to facilitate access
  2. Despite the Americans with Disabilities Act, surveys indicate some dentists are unwilling to treat persons who are physically or mentally challenged
  3. Reasons given for not treating individuals with special needs include:
    a. Inadequate facilities and equipment
    b. Inadequate training (knowledge and competencies)
    c. Not wanting to expose "normal" clients to "special" clients
    d. Inability to collect adequate fees
    e. Additional effort and time required
    f. Personal discomfort about perceived "differences" of special clients
    g. Treatment of medically complex persons increases insurance premiums
D. Communication and cultural concerns
  1. Sensory impairments (hearing, visual) limit the client's ability to transmit and receive communications when scheduling or undergoing oral care or participating in oral health care education
  2. The use of technical terminology or inappropriate language level may interfere with understanding
  3. Differences in communication styles (eye contact, physical proximity and contact, formal vs. informal speech, cultural variations, use of nonverbal cues and verbal language) can impair effective communication
  4. Use of condescending voice tones or language levels closes off communication lines
  5. Foreign language barrier may deter a client from seeking care or reduce effectiveness of care
  6. Inadequate numbers of health care providers possess cross-cultural competence
E. Medical concerns
  1. Situations compromising the provider or client
    a. Inadequate infection control procedures
    b. Inadequate or inaccurate health histories
    c. Inadequate precautions for potential emergencies
    d. Inadequate knowledge of systemic conditions and their treatments

F. Mobility and stability concerns
1. Impaired ambulation or use of assistive devices may hinder access to care
2. Uncontrolled or sudden movements may interfere with home care or dental hygiene interventions
3. Uncontrolled or aggressive behavior may endanger the care providers and the client
4. Spatial disorientation may interfere with client relaxation in the dental chair or with oral care procedures

SPECIFIC CONDITIONS

See Chapters 8 and 9.

Developmental and Cognitive Challenges

A. Definition
1. Subaverage intellectual functioning originating during the developmental period and associated with impairment in adaptive behavior (formerly known as "mental retardation")
2. Not the same as mental illness
3. Label represents a highly heterogeneous group of persons
4. Most common developmental disability
B. Incidence—2% to 3% of the U.S. population (57.7 million total), depending on criteria
C. Levels of intellectual disabilities—intelligence quotient (IQ)
1. Mild—approximate IQ 50 to 70 (89%)
2. Moderate—approximate IQ 40 to 55 (6%)
3. Severe—approximate IQ 25 to 40 (3.5%)
4. Profound—IQ below 20 (1.5%)
D. Etiology—acquired (12%), inherited (13%), unknown (75%)
1. Viral infections and toxemias (rubella, meningitis, lead poisoning)
2. Trauma and physical or chemical agents (child abuse; fetal alcohol syndrome)
3. Disorders of metabolism or nutrition (phenylketonuria, PKU)
4. Gross brain disease (atrophy or neoplasms)
5. Genetics
6. Gestational disorders (Rh incompatibility, anoxia, prematurity)
7. Environmental (lack of stimulation)
E. Signs, symptoms, and clinical manifestations
1. Variable, depending on etiology and individual circumstances
2. Unusual difficulty in learning and applying what is learned to issues of daily living
3. Skull or other craniofacial anomalies may exist
   a. Microcephaly—small cranium that restricts brain growth
   b. Hydrocephaly—expansion of the cranium from excessive accumulation of cerebrospinal fluid
   c. Malformation or asymmetry of growth
4. General developmental delays
5. Other possible manifestations include motor incoordination, mental deficiencies, visual or hearing disorders, specific learning disabilities, maladaptive behaviors,

emotional disturbances, medical disabilities, and self-injurious behaviors
F. Oral manifestations
1. Most oral health problems are not inherent to the disability but are related to extrinsic factors (e.g., neglect by caregivers or lack of coordination leading to poor oral disease control)
2. Decayed-missing-filled surfaces (DMFS) scores comparable with those of the general population, but the "decayed" component may be higher because of lack of professional treatment (Fig. 19-1)
3. Higher prevalence of periodontal conditions, probably related to poor oral hygiene and lack of regular care
4. Higher incidence of malocclusion and deviations in tooth eruption is associated with craniofacial syndromes and growth abnormalities (Figs. 19-2 and 19-3)
5. Some cases of enamel dysplasia more frequently seen in those with severe mental deficiency resulting from prenatal or perinatal defect or insult
6. Thick flaccid lips, microglossia, bruxism, tooth anomalies such as microdontia and abnormal eruption patterns

FIG 19-1 High incidence of dental caries is common and most likely related to neglect. (From National Oral Health Information Clearinghouse, National Institute of Dental and Craniofacial Research: *Oral conditions in children with special needs: a guide for health care providers,* March 2011.)

FIG 19-2 Delayed tooth eruption is a common oral condition in children with developmental disabilities. (From National Oral Health Information Clearinghouse, National Institute of Dental and Craniofacial Research: *Oral conditions in children with special needs: a guide for health care providers,* March 2011.)

FIG 19-3 Malocclusion is a common oral finding in children with developmental disabilities. (From National Oral Health Information Clearinghouse, National Institute of Dental and Craniofacial Research: *Oral conditions in children with special needs: a guide for health care providers,* March 2011.)

FIG 19-4 Tooth anomalies showing variations in eruption patterns and size and shape of the teeth. (From National Oral Health Information Clearinghouse, National Institute of Dental and Craniofacial Research: *Oral conditions in children with special needs: a guide for health care providers,* March 2011.)

Fetal Alcohol Spectrum Disorders (FASD)

A. Definition
1. An umbrella term describing a pattern of malformations caused by maternal alcohol consumption during pregnancy
2. Characterized by prenatal and postnatal growth deficiency, dysmorphic facial features, and central nervous system (CNS) dysfunction
3. FASD include fetal alcohol syndrome (FAS), alcohol-related neurodevelopmental disorders (ARND), and partial fetal alcohol syndrome (PFAS)

B. Incidence and prevalence
1. Incidence of FASD is 0.3 to 1.5 per 1000 live births
2. Leading known preventable cause of mental impairments and birth defects in the United States

C. Etiology
1. Severity of fetal alcohol effects is dose dependent
2. No safe amount of alcohol known during pregnancy
3. Effects related to differences in blood alcohol content and differences in tissue susceptibility
4. Alcohol affects the cell membrane and cell migration, thus altering the organization of embryonic tissue
5. The fetal brain is most susceptible during the third trimester
6. Metabolic disturbances can impair fetal cell division and growth

D. Signs, symptoms, and clinical manifestations can range from mild to severe
1. Premature or postnatal (or both) growth retardation—results in short stature, slight build, small head, low body weight
2. Craniofacial dysmorphia—short eye openings, short upturned nose, smooth philtrum, flat midface, thin upper lip
3. Nonspecific abnormalities in any organ system, depending on the time of alcohol insult
4. Wide IQ range, many within the developmental/cognitive-challenged range

5. Limited ability to read and write, but with minimal comprehension; also language problems
6. Poor social judgment and socialization skills
7. Hyperactivity and short attention span
8. Problems with heart, kidneys, and bones
9. Skeletal and ear disorders

E. Oral manifestations
1. The majority of children with developmental and cognitive challenges have oral problems related to tooth eruption, malformations, or malpositioning of teeth (usually class II or III malocclusion) (Fig. 19-4)
2. Some may have V-shaped or cleft palate
3. Moderate to severe gingivitis is seen

Down Syndrome

A. Definition and etiology
1. Mental or intellectual disorder
2. Associated with an anomaly of chromosome 21 (trisomy 21) in all or some body cells

B. Incidence—most common chromosomal abnormality (1 in 691 live births; but varies with maternal age); approximately 400,000 individuals in the United States affected

C. Signs, symptoms, and clinical manifestations
1. Mild to profound developmental and cognitive challenges
2. Poor muscular development, with hyperflexibility and hypotonia during childhood
3. Short stature, with delay in skeletal maturation
4. Short neck; extremities with broad stubby fingers
5. High incidence of congenital heart defects (30% to 50%); language, vision (60%), and hearing problems (75%); risk of leukemia (less than 1%), thyroid problems, and immunologic defects
6. Abnormal craniofacial features
   a. Small brachycephalic skull
   b. Round flat facies
   c. Small nasomaxillary complex
   d. Ocular hypotelorism (eyes closer together than normal)

FIG 19-5 Common facial characteristics shown in a person with Down syndrome. (From Regezi JA, Sciubba JA, Jordan CK: *Oral pathology: clinical pathologic correlations,* ed 7, St Louis, 2017, Elsevier.)

FIG 19-6 Discoloration and enamel dysplasia associated with developmental defects. (From Regezi JA, Sciubba JA, Jordan CK: *Oral pathology: clinical pathologic correlations,* ed 7, St Louis, 2017, Elsevier.)

FIG 19-7 High-arched palate with decreased width and length. (From Regezi JA, Sciubba JA, Jordan CK: *Oral pathology: clinical pathologic correlations,* ed 7, St Louis, 2017, Elsevier.)

     e. Epicanthal folds

     f. Strabismus (convergent eyes)

     g. Simian crease (single transverse palmar crease)

     h. More susceptible to infection because of poor immune response

D. Oral manifestations (Fig. 19-5)

  1. Relative mandibular prognathism as a result of a small nasomaxillary complex

  2. Dry skin and thick, dry, fissured lips

  3. Open-mouth posture, with a protrusive, fissured tongue

  4. Hyperplasia of the adenoids and tonsils

  5. Altered salivary gland mechanism (decreased flow)

  6. Increased susceptibility to severe periodontal disease of early onset, especially in anterior areas; may be related to host immune defects (e.g., periodontitis as manifestation of systemic disease)

  7. Delayed eruption of teeth and abnormal tooth development

  8. Higher incidence of congenitally missing teeth

  9. Small tooth crowns with short crown/root ratio

  10. Enamel dysplasia (Fig. 19-6)

  11. Malocclusion—anterior open bite or cross-bite, posterior cross-bite, malocclusion common

  12. Attrition

  13. High palatal vault (Fig. 19-7)

E. Risk of associated conditions—increased risk for congenital heart defects, leukemia, respiratory conditions, and Alzheimer's disease

Autism Spectrum Disorders (ASD)

A. Definition

  1. A group of developmental disorders that affect the functioning of the brain, resulting in specific behavioral and communicative difficulties; speech, language and communication, social interaction, sensory impairments, play, and repetition of behaviors are key areas affected

  2. Wide range of symptoms and behaviors with considerable individual variation

B. Incidence and prevalence

  1. Incidence not completely known; prevalence rate of autism is increasing 10% to 17% annually

  2. Unclear if the increase is real or reflects better diagnostic practices

  3. Occurs in as many as 1 in 68 children

  4. Five times more common in boys (1 in 42 vs. 1 in 189 girls)

  5. Appears during the first 3 years of life

C. Etiology—different theories
1. Psychogenic theories
2. Genetic theories
3. Biochemical deficit theories
4. Neurophysiologic theories
D. Signs, symptoms, and clinical manifestations
1. Great variability in expression; no standard type
2. Extreme aloneness; failure to develop eye contact, to cuddle as infants normally do, to develop social relationships, or to perceive others' feelings
3. Language disturbances—repetitious speech, pronoun reversals, lack of ability to use gestures; failure to develop functional speech in 50%
4. Comprehension problems, especially with verbal directions
5. Obsessive about maintaining routines and sameness of the environment (resistance to change)
6. Abnormal response to stimuli; may not respond to pain; or may have constant movement and repetitious activity
7. Sensitivities to sight, hearing, touch, smell, and taste
8. May be aggressive or self-abusive
E. Oral manifestations
1. None directly associated with the syndrome; difficult behaviors, feeding problems, and poor cooperation are challenges to dental care
2. Oral care may be neglected because of issues with communication, physical limitations, sensory stimulation, and socialization

Attention Deficit Hyperactivity Disorder (ADHD)

A. Definition
1. Developmental and behavioral disorder affecting specific areas of learning or impulse control that can cause problems in acquiring new skills
2. Relates primarily to vision, hearing, language, attention, and touch
B. Incidence and prevalence
1. Much controversy over diagnosis and treatment
2. One of most common neurobehavioral disorders of childhood and occurs in 11% of school-age children 4 to 7 years old
3. More than 6.4 million persons have been diagnosed with ADHD
4. More common in boys at 13.2% than girls at 5.6%
5. Affects up to 60% of adults who had ADHD in childhood
C. Etiology—unknown, but may be related to:
1. Neurologic deficits or neurochemical imbalances
2. Emotional factors
3. Environmental toxins
4. Genetic factors
D. Categories—areas of CNS function affected
1. Input—receiving, recognizing, and decoding messages (e.g., auditory-perceptual or visual-perceptual problems)
2. Organization—information storage, integration with other information, and prompt retrieval (e.g., short-term memory problem)
3. Output—management of movement or utterances (e.g., hyperactivity, apraxia)

E. Signs, symptoms, and clinical manifestations
1. Hyperactivity and inattentiveness
2. Irritability, impulsiveness, and need for immediate satisfaction
3. Problems with concentration and memory
4. Immaturity, clumsiness
5. Lack of sense of direction, position, or time
6. Problems in reading, writing, or math
F. Oral manifestations—none directly associated

Emotional Disturbance and Mental Illness

A. Definition
1. Any disease or condition affecting the brain that impairs thinking, feeling, behavior, or all of these functions
2. Leading cause of disability in the United States
3. Many suffer from more than one mental disability at any given time
B. Incidence and prevalence
1. Approximately 57.7 million persons in the United States over age 18 affected (26.2% of population)
2. At some point in life, 10% of all adults will need or benefit from some form of mental health intervention
3. Major depression, bipolar disorder, schizophrenia, and obsessive-compulsive disorder are among top 10 leading causes of disability
C. Etiology—depends on the type of disturbance
1. Heredity (genetics)
2. Environmental stressors (e.g., death, divorce, financial problems, dysfunctional family life)
3. Biology (dysfunctional neurotransmitters and neurologic chemical imbalances)
4. Psychological trauma
D. Classification—three common classes:
1. Psychoneuroses—anxiety, depressive, obsessive, or conversion reactions
2. Personality disorders—situational or adjustment reactions
3. Psychoses—schizophrenia
E. Signs, symptoms, and clinical manifestations—depend on the type of disorder
1. Inner tensions create anxiety, frustration, fears, and impulsive behavior
2. Examples of behavior
   a. Translation of fears or anxieties into physical symptoms
   b. Regression to earlier forms of behavior
   c. Displays of hostility or aggression
   d. Withdrawal into fantasy (e.g., daydreaming)
   e. Fear of failure and criticism
   f. Development of substitute fears, phobias, or compulsions
F. Oral manifestations
1. None directly associated
2. May see intraoral trauma resulting from unusual habits or aggressive behavior
3. May have xerostomia as a side effect of medications
4. With compulsive behavior, may have immaculate oral hygiene

Disorders of Eating

See signs and symptoms of disordered eating in the section on "Energy Balances and Weight Control" in Chapter 12.

A. Definitions
  1. Anorexia nervosa
     a. Psychophysiologic condition characterized by suppression and denial of sensation of hunger
     b. Person may be socially isolated and relatively asexual
     c. Consumption of only 300 to 600 calories per day is common
     d. Often come from middle-class to upper-class families with high parental or societal expectations
     e. Perfectionists, competitive, and overachievers
     f. Deny their emaciated appearance
     g. Diagnosis based on person's refusal to maintain normal body weight for height and age; intense fear of becoming fat despite being underweight; denial of the seriousness of the starvation and a distorted body image
  2. Anorexia bulimia
     a. Syndrome involving episodic binge eating and purging
     b. Purging involves self-induced vomiting and use of laxatives, diuretics, or enemas
     c. Often occurs after failed attempts to lose weight through dieting
     d. May be of normal weight
     e. Usually outgoing and sexually active
     f. Calories consumed during bingeing range from 3500 to 20,000
     g. Vomiting episodes may last from 5 to 30 minutes
     h. Diagnosis of bulimia if there are at least two bulimic episodes per week for 3 months

B. Incidence and prevalence
  1. About 90% are female; 1.1% to 4.5% of the U.S. population have eating disorder in their lifetime; rate is increasing yearly
  2. Occurs in 1 in 200 white adolescent females
  3. Occurs in 3% to 20% of college students
  4. Most common age group is 12 to 35 years; also occurs in older adults
  5. From 27% to 42% of persons with anorexia indulge in bulimia
  6. Mortality rate of 9%

C. Etiology—multiple interactive causes
  1. Depressive illnesses
  2. Fear of obesity
  3. Endocrine changes at puberty
  4. Feelings of low self-esteem and poor body image

D. Signs and symptoms
  1. Anorexia nervosa
     a. Intense fear of becoming obese; refusal to maintain normal weight
     b. Disturbance of body image
     c. Weight loss of at least 25% of original body weight, not caused by physical illness
     d. Downy growth of body hair (lanugo)
     e. Periods of overactivity
     f. Dry, flaky skin
     g. Lowered blood pressure, body temperature, and pulse
     h. Episodes of bulimia
     i. Complications include cardiac arrhythmia from reduced heart muscle mass and electrolyte imbalance from dehydration
  2. Anorexia bulimia
     a. Awareness that eating pattern is abnormal
     b. Depression and self-deprecating thoughts
     c. Repeated attempts to lose weight
     d. Recurrent bingeing (rapid intake of food in a short period), usually high-calorie, easily ingested food
     e. Inconspicuous eating
     f. Termination of episodes by purging with self-induced vomiting, laxatives, diuretics, and enemas
     g. Weight fluctuation more than 10 pounds
     h. Dehydration
     i. Electrolyte imbalance

E. Oral manifestations
  1. Esophageal lacerations and chronic sore throat from repeated vomiting
  2. Parotid gland swelling and xerostomia
  3. Burning sensation in the tongue
  4. Perimyolysis (dental erosion), dentinal hypersensitivity, and margination of amalgams from acid erosion of vomiting; lingual surfaces of maxillary incisors most often affected
  5. Rampant caries from high consumption of sucrose, xerostomia, and dehydration
  6. Irritated soft tissues from vomiting, dehydration, and vitamin deficiencies
  7. Dentinal hypersensitivity and vitamin deficiencies

Alzheimer's disease

A. Definition
  1. Progressive irreversible brain disorder characterized by intellectual and cognitive disturbance, behavioral changes, and eventually a state of complete dependence
  2. Three types:
     a. Early onset—diagnosis before age 65
     b. Late onset—occurs after age 65
     c. Familial—entirely inherited; onset often in the 40s

B. Incidence and prevalence
  1. Estimated 5.2 million cases in the United States
  2. About 1 in 9 older Americans has Alzheimer's disease
  3. Estimated 130% increase expected by 2050

C. Signs, symptoms, and clinical manifestations—different parts of the brain affected in varying degrees but reflect neuronal degeneration
  1. Early
     a. Memory loss and inability to concentrate
     b. Anxiety, irritability, withdrawal, petulance
     c. Abnormal sleep patterns
     d. Motor abnormalities, including exaggerated reflexes and gait disturbances
  2. Later
     a. Apathy, depression

b. Disorientation, lack of judgment and understanding
c. Incontinence
D. Risk factors
1. Age—greatest risk factor
2. Family history
3. Mild cognitive impairment
E. Oral manifestations
1. None specific to the condition
2. Disease states usually are a result of neglect, the aging process, or any accompanying chronic illnesses

Seizure Disorders

See the section on "Seizures and Convulsive Disorders" in Chapter 21.
A. Definitions
1. Not a disease; the term *seizure disorders* is used to describe symptoms of recurrent or chronic brain dysfunction
2. Characterized by discrete, recurring behavioral manifestations that include disturbances of balance, sensation, behavior, perception, or consciousness
3. Should not be confused with one-time seizures that result from drug overdoses, brain tumors, or other problems
4. Seizure—an episode of cerebral dysfunction produced by abnormal excessive neuronal discharge; not necessarily a recurring condition
5. Convulsion—a broad range of behavioral manifestations, including seizure activity
6. Aura—a specific sensation preceding a seizure, lasting from one to several seconds and manifested as:
   a. Numbness, tingling
   b. Unusual smell perception
   c. Peculiar sound perception
   d. Feeling of nausea or fear
7. Status epilepticus
   a. Continuous convulsion lasting longer than 5 minutes
   b. May lead to death from heart failure, kidney failure, or both
   c. Constitutes a medical emergency
B. Incidence and prevalence
1. Affect almost 3 million people in the United States
2. About 200,000 new cases of seizure and epilepsy are diagnosed in the United States each year
3. Prevalence is highest among children, with occurrence of 5.2 to 7.3 per 1000 school-age children
4. About 10% of Americans will have at least one seizure in their lifetime
C. Etiology
1. Prenatal
   a. Maternal infections
   b. Fetal growth abnormalities or prematurity
   c. Chromosomal disorders
   d. Toxicity or damage from drugs or radiation
   e. Genetic influences
2. Perinatal
   a. Delivery problems
   b. Anoxia

3. Postnatal
   a. Degenerative brain disease
   b. Injury
   c. Tumors
   d. Prolonged high fever
   e. Parasitic infections
   f. Toxic agents (including alcohol and drugs)
4. Unknown
D. Types—can be classified by the origin of the seizure, the cause, or the type of seizure activity
E. Signs, symptoms, and clinical manifestations
1. Generalized tonic-clonic (grand mal)
   a. May experience an aura
   b. Loss of consciousness
   c. Tonic movements (voluntary muscles experience continuous contractions)
   d. Clonic movements (intermittent muscular contraction and relaxation)
   e. Interruption of respiration and dilation of pupils
   f. Loss of bladder or bowel control
   g. Seizure activity usually lasts 1 to 3 minutes
   h. Lethargy and disorientation follow the return of consciousness
   i. May occur any time during the day or only during sleep
2. Generalized absence (petit mal)
   a. Transient loss of consciousness
   b. May have minor motor movements of the eyes, head, or extremities
   c. Lasts 5 to 30 seconds
   d. Person may not be aware of having had a seizure
3. Complex partial (psychomotor)
   a. May be preceded by an aura
   b. Transient clouding of the consciousness
   c. Behavioral alterations
   d. Purposeless, repetitive, and stereotypical movements or actions
   e. Changes in affect or perception
   f. May become antisocial
   g. Person usually does not remember the incident
4. Atonic
   a. Type of seizure that consist of a brief lapse in muscle tone
   b. Caused by temporary alterations in brain function
   c. Seizures are brief, usually less than 15 seconds
   d. Originate in childhood and may persist into adulthood
F. Oral manifestations
1. Orofacial trauma—lips, tongue, buccal mucosa, teeth, facial bones, or jawbone
2. Drug-induced gingival enlargement from phenytoin (Fig. 19-8)
   a. More marked in anterior regions and facial surfaces
   b. Does not occur in edentulous areas
   c. Correlated with poor oral hygiene
   d. Characteristically pale, pink, and fibrous
   e. Aesthetic concerns caused by gingival enlargement
   f. Severe gingival enlargement may displace teeth, create malocclusion, and compromise esthetics

FIG 19-8 Drug-induced gingival enlargement associated with medication taken to control seizures. (From Regezi JA, Sciubba JA, Jordan CK: *Oral pathology: clinical pathologic correlations,* ed 7, St Louis, 2017, Elsevier.)

    g. Superimposed inflammation occurs from food retention or mouth breathing

    h. Can sometimes be alleviated through meticulous oral hygiene, surgery, or pressure appliances

Visual Impairment

A. Definitions
1. Visual impairment—when visual acuity in the best eye is no better than 20/200 after correction, or if central or peripheral vision impairment is present
2. Legally blind—visual acuity of less than 20/200 with correction

B. Incidence and prevalence
1. Approximately 0.6 in 1000 persons in the United States is legally or totally blind
2. Visual impairments occur in 12.2 in 1000 persons under age 18
3. About 5 million persons in the United States over age 65 have severe visual impairment
4. Leading cause of vision loss in those 25 to 74 years old is diabetic retinopathy

C. Etiology—congenital, perinatal, postnatal, aging
1. Trauma
2. Disease (infections, inflammation, toxicity)
3. Structural or developmental defects
    a. Nearsighted
    b. Farsighted
    c. Astigmatism
4. Retrolental fibroplasia—high concentration of oxygen in the incubators of premature infants causes hemorrhage of retinal blood vessels, scarring, and retinal detachment
5. Macular degeneration (loss of central vision)
6. Retinitis pigmentosa—night blindness and loss of peripheral vision
7. Diabetic retinopathy—retinal hemorrhages
8. Glaucoma—failure of liquid in the eye to drain, resulting in increased pressure, pain, and destruction of the optic nerve
9. Cataracts—clouding and opacity of the lens blocking light perception (mainly associated with aging or congenital problems)

D. Signs, symptoms, and clinical manifestations
1. Wears glasses or contact lenses
2. Awkward ambulation or bumping into objects
3. Eye pain
4. Constant tearing
5. Unusual squinting or blinking
6. Use of a guide dog or cane
7. Deliberate, slow actions
8. Attention to details and orderliness
9. Cloudy or fuzzy vision
10. Problems with glare
11. Double vision (diplopia)

E. Oral manifestations
1. No particular dental problems
2. Gingivitis, if the person cannot see the gingiva to monitor gingival health
3. Trauma to the orofacial area if the person experiences frequent accidents or falls

Hearing Impairment

A. Definitions
1. Hearing impairment—defective but functional hearing
2. Deaf—unable to understand speech, even with the use of an aid
3. Frequency—length of the sound wave (vibrations per second, or cycles per second [cps, hertz]; human range is 16,000 to 30,000 cps/Hz)
4. Intensity—measured in decibels (dB); human range is 1 to 100 dB

B. Incidence and prevalence
1. Approximately 31.5 million deaf and hearing-impaired persons in the United States (10% of population); 66% of those affected are age 65 or older; 1 in 6 persons age 41 to 59 have a hearing impairment
2. Two to three cases of congenital hearing loss in 1000 live births
3. Hearing loss is associated with a number of other disabling conditions
    a. Cleft palate (90%)
    b. Cerebral palsy (20%)
    c. Down syndrome (70%)
4. Environmental causes are increasing

C. Classifications—usually by severity of loss, as measured in decibel loss (Table 19-3)

D. Types of hearing loss (Table 19-4)
1. Conductive hearing loss
    a. Injury or disease interferes with organs that conduct sound waves through the outer or middle ear
    b. Usually consistent over the entire range of sound
    c. The person benefits most from the use of a hearing aid (sound conducted by bone)
    d. Speech is soft and low; the person hears own voice louder than that of others
    e. Usually caused by obstruction of the ear canal by cerumen or a foreign object, perforated eardrum, otitis media, otosclerosis, or congenital malformations of the ear

TABLE 19-3 Hearing Loss and Probable Outcomes

Classification	Loss (dB)	Hearing Status without Amplification (Hearing Aid)
Normal range	0-15	All speech sounds
Slight loss	15-25	Hears vowel sounds clearly; may miss unvoiced consonant sounds
Mild loss	25-40	Hears only louder-voiced speech sounds
Moderate loss	40-65	Misses most speech at normal conversational level
Severe loss	65-95	Misses all speech at normal conversational level
Profound loss	>95+	Hears no speech or sounds

TABLE 19-4 Description of Hearing Problems

Condition	Characteristics
Acoustic neuroma	Benign tumor of the auditory nerve; causes gradual hearing loss, tinnitus, and dizziness
Mastoiditis	Inflammation of the air cells of the mastoid
Ménière's disease	Condition of the inner ear characterized by hearing loss, tinnitus, and vertigo
Otitis media	Inflammation of the middle ear caused by infection
Otosclerosis	Disease characterized by formation of spongy bone in bone surrounding the inner ear; results in gradual loss of hearing
Presbycusis	Progressive hearing loss that occurs with age
Tinnitus	Sensation of sound in the head (e.g., roaring, hissing, buzzing)
Transient	Temporary hearing shifts associated with noise exposure

2. Sensorineural hearing loss
   a. Malfunction of organs that perceive sound (sensory hair cells of inner ear, auditory nerve, auditory center in brain)
   b. Most common causes—aging process (presbycusis), hereditary disease, noise damage, childhood viral infections, skull fractures, intracranial tumors, oxytoxic drugs, and Rh incompatibility
   c. Involves loss of sensitivity and acuity in one or more frequencies (usually higher frequencies and consonants)
   d. If the individual wears a hearing aid, sound is conducted by air
   e. Speech is loud; the person cannot hear own voice
E. Etiology
   1. Prenatal or congenital
      a. Genetic defects
      b. Infections (rubella accounts for 20% of congenital types), influenza, and syphilis
      c. Rh incompatibility
      d. Certain drugs, including thalidomide, streptomycin, aspirin, erythromycin, kanamycin, neomycin, indomethacin, furosemide (Lasix)
      e. Unknown causes (10% to 20% of cases)
      f. Environmental noise (more than 30% of cases)
   2. Acquired
      a. Infections (e.g., mumps, measles, poliomyelitis, chronic serous otitis media)
      b. Hereditary conditions
      c. Trauma
      d. Chronic use of certain drugs (e.g., aspirin, streptomycin)
      e. Noise exposure
      f. Pathology (e.g., brain tumor, stroke)
F. Signs, symptoms, and clinical manifestations
   1. May lip-read or focus attention on other facial or nonverbal expressions (speech reading); but can generally only understand 26% to 40% of what is said
   2. Speech may be characterized by aberrant modulations, pronunciations, or grammatical structures
   3. May use sign language—American Sign Language (ASL) or finger spelling (American or manual alphabet)
   4. May turn the head to one side if the loss is unilateral
   5. May frequently ask others to repeat phrases, or may provide an unrelated response to a question or comment
   6. May not acknowledge having hearing loss
G. Oral manifestations
   1. Not generally seen with hearing impairments unless associated with a syndrome (e.g., rubella syndrome)
   2. Prematurity or rubella may result in enamel dysplasia
   3. Bruxism may be evident

Cleft Lip or Palate

A. Definition—disturbances in embryologic formation resulting in incomplete closure of the lip, the palatal area, or both
B. Incidence and prevalence
   1. About 2650 babies are born with a cleft palate and 4440 with a cleft lip with or without a cleft palate
   2. Occurs in 1 in 1000 Caucasian live births in the United States; twice as common in Asian Americans; half as common in African Americans
   3. One of the most common congenital malformations of the face and mouth
   4. Cleft lip more common in males; cleft palate more common in females
   5. One in 2000 babies born with cleft palate, but without cleft lip
C. Classifications of cleft involvement
   1. Tip of the uvula
   2. Bifid uvula
   3. Soft palate
   4. Soft and hard palates
   5. Unilateral lip and palate (Fig. 19-9)
   6. Bilateral lip and palate
D. Etiology
   1. Genetic in most cases
   2. Other risk factors include maternal nutritional deficiencies, alcohol use, infectious diseases, and smoking during pregnancy
   3. Cleft lip occurs during gestational weeks 4 to 7
   4. Cleft palate occurs during gestational weeks 8 to 12
   5. Folic acid supplementation for the mother during pregnancy may reduce risk

FIG 19-9 Cleft lip. (From Regezi JA, Sciubba JA, Jordan CK: *Oral pathology: clinical pathologic correlations,* ed 7, St Louis, 2017, Elsevier.)

E. Signs, symptoms, and associated problems
1. Orofacial deformities
2. Ear disease with resultant hearing loss
3. Speech difficulties are a major disability caused by:
    a. Palatal insufficiency
    b. Missing or malpositioned teeth
    c. Hearing loss
4. Feeding problems
5. Predisposition to upper respiratory tract infections
F. Oral manifestations
1. High incidence of missing or maldeveloped teeth in the line of the cleft, usually affects lateral incisors
2. High incidence of malocclusion resulting from structural defects
3. Oral-motor dysfunction
4. Scar tissue from surgery

Cerebral Palsy

A. Definition—static, nonprogressive neuromuscular condition comprising a series of syndromes that result from damage to the brain
B. Incidence
1. Approximately 764,000 persons in the United States have some degree of cerebral palsy
2. About 10,000 babies born each year will develop cerebral palsy; 40% to 50% of children born with cerebral palsy are premature, low birth weight, or both
C. Etiology
1. Prenatal—genetic or congenitally acquired (e.g., anoxia, infections, alcohol or drug abuse, Rh incompatibility, metabolic disturbances, lack of folic acid)
2. Natal—anoxia, hemorrhage
3. Postnatal—head injury, infections, neoplasms, anoxia
D. Classification
1. Motor disorders
    a. Spasticity (50% to 75%)—slight stimulus causes exaggerated muscle contraction; stiff and jerky movements
    b. Athetosis (15% to 25%)—muscles contract involuntarily; difficulty bringing the body to the upright position
    c. Ataxia (10%)—muscles respond to a stimulus but cannot complete a contraction; low muscle tone and poor coordination

FIG 19-10 Person with spastic-type cerebral palsy, in which limbs are in a severely flexed posture. (From Porter SR et al: *Medicine and surgery for dentistry,* Philadelphia, 1999, Churchill Livingstone.)

    d. Hypotonia (less than 10%)—unable to respond to a volitional stimulus
    e. Rigidity (less than 10%)—increased initial muscle resistance; gives way with minimal force
    f. Mixed (5% to 20%)—two or more types appearing in the same person
2. Limbs involved
    a. Monoplegic—one limb
    b. Hemiplegic—both limbs on the same side of the body
    c. Paraplegic—lower limbs
    d. Diplegic—like parts on either side of the body (e.g., both lower limbs, both upper limbs)
    e. Quadriplegic—all four limbs
    f. Triplegic—three limbs
E. Signs, symptoms, and clinical manifestations (Fig. 19-10)
1. Characterized by paralysis, weakness, muscle spasms, incoordination, or other aberrations of motor function, especially involving voluntary muscles
2. Joint immobility and contractures increase with age
3. Retained primitive reflexes (e.g., asymmetrical or symmetrical tonic neck reflex)
4. Other associated conditions
    a. Speech and language disorders (60%)
    b. Hearing disorders (20%)
    c. Visual defects (40%)
    d. Developmental and cognitive challenges (40%)
    e. Seizures (40%)
5. Wide range of limitations, from mild to totally dependent

FIG 19-11 Example of extreme bruxism in a child with a developmental disability. (From National Oral Health Information Clearinghouse, National Institute of Dental and Craniofacial Research: *Oral conditions in children with special needs: a guide for health care providers*, March 2011.)

FIG 19-13 Person with Bell's palsy, in whom the left side of the face is paralyzed. (From Trend P, Swash M, Kennard C: *Neurology: color guide*, Edinburgh, 1998, Churchill Livingstone.)

FIG 19-12 Example of oral trauma. (From National Oral Health Information Clearinghouse, National Institute of Dental and Craniofacial Research: *Oral conditions in children with special needs: a guide for health care providers*, March 2011.)

D. Signs, symptoms, and clinical manifestations (Fig. 19-13)
   1. Abrupt paralysis without preceding pain
   2. Occurs unilaterally
   3. Corner of the mouth droops, causing drooling
   4. Eyelids will not close; lower eyelid droops; predisposes the eyes to infections
   5. Speech and chewing are difficult
   6. Spontaneous remission may occur in 2 to 8 weeks, or permanent paralysis
E. Oral manifestations—ora--motor difficulties can cause food retention and the potential for increased caries or gingivitis

F. Oral manifestations—marked variation among individuals
   1. Higher incidence of bruxism (Fig. 19-11), dental caries, enamel dysplasia, malocclusion, and periodontal diseases
   2. Drug-induced gingival enlargement if phenytoin is used
   3. Oral-motor dysfunction (e.g., impaired swallowing), mouth breathing
   4. Temporomandibular joint (TMJ) disorders
   5. Increased gag reflex
   6. Drooling
   7. Trauma resulting from incoordination and frequent falls (Fig. 19-12)
   8. Attrition and possible TMJ disturbances from mouth sticks
   9. Increased dental caries as a result of surgery to control saliva and drooling

Bell's Palsy

A. Definition—paralysis of facial muscles that are innervated by cranial nerve VII (facial nerve)
B. Incidence and prevalence
   1. About 40,000 persons in the United States are affected annually
   2. After age 50; more common in males
C. Etiology
   1. Unknown
   2. Associated with bacterial and viral infections (herpes simplex), trauma from oral extractions, or surgery on the parotid gland

Myasthenia Gravis

A. Definition—autoimmune neuromuscular disease characterized by variable weakness or fatigue of striated, voluntary muscles
B. Incidence and prevalence
   1. Most often affects women younger than 40
   2. If late onset after 60, men affected more often
   3. Affects approximately 2 in 100,000 persons
C. Etiology—autoimmune mechanism causing a defect in nerve impulse transmission at the neuromuscular junction
D. Signs, symptoms, and clinical manifestations
   1. First symptoms usually affect muscles of the eyes (blurred or double vision, drooping of one or both eyelids, weakness of muscles affecting the eyeball, facial expression, mastication, and swallowing)
   2. Breathing and speech are disturbed (weak, muffled voice)
   3. Fatigue and weakness of muscles vary widely but tend to be worse at the end of the day
   4. Myasthenic crisis—weakness affects muscles that control breathing; usually transient but life threatening
     a. Precipitated by:
       (1) Emotional excitement, stress
       (2) Surgical procedures
       (3) Fatigue or loss of sleep
       (4) Infections

b. Symptoms
   (1) Unable to clear secretions from the throat
   (2) Impaired breathing; assisted ventilation may be needed
   (3) Double vision
E. Medications that may cause muscle weakness and must therefore be avoided:
  1. β-Adrenergic blockers
  2. ᴅ-Penicillamine
  3. Interferon-α
  4. Calcium channel blockers
F. Oral manifestations
  1. Oral-motor dysfunction
  2. Retention of food increases susceptibility to dental caries and periodontal problems
  3. Weakness of masticatory muscles causes the mouth to continuously hang open
  4. Chewing and swallowing difficulties
  5. Furrowed and flaccid appearance of the tongue

Parkinson's Disease

A. Definition—progressive disorder of the CNS causing loss of postural reflexes, slowness of spontaneous movement, tremors, and muscle rigidity
B. Incidence and prevalence
  1. Develops between ages 40 and 60
  2. At age 60 or older, 1 in 100 persons affected
  3. Higher incidence in men than in women (2:1)
  4. Approximately 1.5 million persons in the United States affected; 7 to 10 million worldwide
C. Etiology
  1. Cause unknown
  2. Imbalance of dopamine and acetylcholine
D. Signs, symptoms, and clinical manifestations
  1. Mild, diffuse muscular pain
  2. Tremors of the extremities, occurring mainly at rest
  3. Shuffling, slow gait, with arms held to the side
  4. Slurred, indistinct speech
  5. Staring, mask-like facial expression
  6. Excessive salivation or dryness of mouth (side effects of medications)
  7. Intellect not usually affected

8. Tremors in the lips, tongue, or neck; difficulty swallowing; can lead to aspiration
9. Feelings of stiffness and rigidity (particularly of the large joints)
10. Sensitivity to heat
E. Oral manifestations
  1. Impaired oral-motor functions and home care skills may increase the incidence of dental caries, periodontal disease, and perioral skin irritation
  2. Side effects of medications (e.g., xerostomia) may increase the incidence of dental caries and periodontal disease and negatively affect dental prosthesis retention
  3. Rigidity and tremors can induce orofacial pain, TMJ discomfort, and trauma to soft and hard tissues

Arthritis

A. Definition
  1. Term used to describe more than 100 disorders that cause pain in the joints and connective tissue
  2. Joint inflammation
  3. The term *polyarthritis* refers to the involvement of many joints
B. Major types (Table 19-5)
  1. Osteoarthritis (affects 21 million U.S. adults)
  2. Rheumatoid (adult type) (affects three million adults)
  3. Rheumatoid (juvenile type)
  4. Others include gout, fibromyalgia, ankylosing spondylitis, lupus
C. Incidence and prevalence: common in all age groups
  1. More than one in five U.S. adults is affected
  2. Affects more than 22% of the U.S. population
  3. Affects 55% of the population age 65 or older
  4. More common in women than men
D. Etiology (see Table 19-5)—cause unknown
E. Signs, symptoms, and clinical manifestations—these affect various sites in different ways; most are chronic (see Table 19-5)
F. Oral manifestations
  1. Bruxism and occlusal imbalances
  2. TMJ pain and limited ability to open the mouth
  3. Masking of inflammation by prolonged steroid therapy
  4. Delayed healing and excess bleeding with long-term aspirin therapy

TABLE 19-5	**Characteristics of Arthritis**		
	Osteoarthritis	**Rheumatoid (Adult Type)**	**Rheumatoid (Juvenile Type)**
Etiology	Unknown or from trauma, infection, or joint abnormality	Cause unknown; theories include autoimmunity, hereditary or psychosomatic factors, and infection	Same as adult type
Sites affected	Weight-bearing joints (hips, knees, vertebrae)	First affects fingers, hands, and knees; TMJ later	Involves many joints, especially fingers, knees, wrists, vertebrae, and TMJ
Signs and symptoms	Pain, aggravated by temperature changes; joint stiffness after inactivity; develops gradually; swelling rare; does not usually limit range of motion	Fatigue, loss of appetite, low-grade fever, migratory joint pain and swelling, stiffness after periods of inactivity, paresthesias, subcutaneous nodules, joint deformities, TMJ involvement, muscle atrophy near joints	Joint enlargement, stiffness, and pain; onset is acute with fever, rash, spleen and lymph node enlargement, tachycardia, and limited oral opening

TMJ, Temporomandibular joint.

5. Mucosal ulcerations or secondary oral infections (especially of the gingiva) if gold salts are administered
6. Monitor need for antibiotic premedication

Fibromyalgia Syndrome (FMS)

A. Definition—neurosensory disorder characterized by widespread musculoskeletal pain
  1. Pain accompanied by persistent fatigue, sleep disturbances, and memory and mood issues
  2. Most common cause of chronic pain in the United States
B. Incidence and prevalence
  1. FMS can affect any person regardless of age, gender, or ethnicity; however 75% to 90% of those diagnosed are women
  2. Prevalence of fibromyalgia is higher at middle age (30 to 50 years) or over age 50
  3. Worldwide incidence of FMS is 6.88 per 1000 males and 11.28 per 1000 females
C. Etiology
  1. This complex syndrome is linked to a multifactorial etiology
  2. Suspected causes of FMS include abnormalities in pain pathways, neuroendocrine system, and autonomic nervous system, as well as genetic and environmental factors such as physical trauma and psychosocial factors such as abuse
D. Signs, symptoms, and clinical manifestations
  1. Widespread pain—exacerbated by physical or emotional stress, nonrestorative sleep, strenuous activity, and changes in weather
  2. Sleep disturbances, including nonrestorative sleep, insomnia, and poor-quality sleep
  3. Fatigue, cognitive deficiency, tenderness on mild palpation
  4. Can result in severe disability and loss of function, making daily tasks, including oral self-care, difficult or unmanageable
E. Oral manifestations
  1. Severe pain when opening; limited opening
  2. TMJ disorder
  3. Burning tongue
  4. Difficulty discerning pain from oral disease from FMS pain
  5. Taste distortion
  6. Xerostomia

Scleroderma

A. Definition
  1. Group of chronic connective tissue disorders
  2. Autoimmune rheumatic condition with excessive collagen deposition and vascular hyperreactivity and dysfunction
B. Incidence and prevalence
  1. Mainly affects women, 4:1 over men, with onset between ages 30 and 50
  2. Approximately 20 per 1 million individuals affected
C. Etiology—unknown, but presents with vascular dysfunction that manifests as injury to the endothelial cells; immunologic activation of T cells, cytokines, inflammation; and fibrosis
D. Signs and symptoms
  1. Localized scleroderma affects only the skin—areas of the skin become thickened, hard, and discolored, with hair loss over affected areas
  2. Diffuse scleroderma also harms structures beyond the skin, such as blood vessels, internal organs, and digestive tract
    a. Skin eventually binds with underlying structures, and painful ulcerations occur at the joints
    b. Esophageal dysmotility, renal disease, cardiac dysfunction, and pulmonary disease manifest
    c. Caused from chronic hardening and sclerosis of the connective tissue within these organ systems, with life-threatening consequences
E. Oral manifestations
  1. Limited mouth opening
  2. Fibrosis at the hard and soft palate
  3. Widening of the periodontal ligament space
  4. Mandibular resorption
  5. Trigeminal neuropathy
  6. Increased risk for periodontal disease and caries disease

Multiple Sclerosis

A. Definition—chronic degenerative disease of the CNS
  1. Myelin is destroyed through the formation of sclerotic tissue called *plaque*
  2. Nerve impulses to the brain are disrupted or not transmitted
  3. Scattered plaque accumulation causes inflammation and widespread and varied symptoms with periods of exacerbation and remission
B. Incidence and prevalence
  1. Approximately 500,000 persons affected in the United States; more than 2.5 million worldwide
  2. Varies geographically; more common in northern regions
  3. Two to three times more common in women than men
  4. Onset occurs at any age, but usually between 20 and 50
C. Etiology
  1. Unknown, although genetic markers have been found
  2. Possibly an autoimmune reaction or associated with viral infections
D. Signs and symptoms
  1. Result from the location of lesions (Table 19-6)
  2. Precipitating factors
    a. Infections
    b. Stress and emotional trauma
    c. Injury
    d. Heavy exercise and fatigue
    e. Pregnancy
    f. Heat
  3. Periods of remission in some; chronic progression in others
  4. Death is usually the result of an infection

E. Oral manifestations
   1. Most are the result of poor oral hygiene or the side effects of drugs
      a. Ulcerations
      b. Xerostomia
      c. Drug-induced gingival enlargement (phenytoin administered for pain)
   2. Facial pain and TMJ dysfunction and pain

TABLE 19-6 Symptoms Associated with Lesions in the Central Nervous System

Location of Lesions	Possible Symptoms
Spinal cord	Numbness
	Loss of sensitivity in appendages
	Sensitivity to heat
	Unsteady gait; muscle stiffness
	Loss of strength in the legs
	Impaired eye-hand coordination resulting in difficulty in fine motor movements
Brainstem	Blurred vision, double vision, or both
	Difficulty in swallowing or chewing
	Diminished gag reflex
	Slurred speech
Cerebrum (lesions in the cerebrum usually occur in the later stages of the disease process)	Disruptions in thinking
	Euphoria
	Depression
	Disruptions in behavior

From Lange BM, Enwistle BM, Lipson LF: *Dental management of the handicapped: Approaches for dental auxiliaries*, Philadelphia, 1983, Lea & Febiger.

Muscular Dystrophies

A. Definition—group of progressive chronic diseases of the skeletal (striated) muscles characterized by the degeneration of muscle cells with replacement by fat or fibrous tissue
B. Incidence and prevalence
   1. Affects approximately 220,000 persons in the United States
   2. Two thirds of cases are children; 400 to 600 males are born with this disease each year in the United States
C. Etiology—inherited; defective gene leading to a protein abnormality
D. Types (Table 19-7)
E. Signs, symptoms, and clinical manifestations—vary by site and type (see Table 19-7)
F. Oral manifestations
   1. Weakness in masticatory muscles leads to decreased maxillary biting force
   2. Higher incidence of mouth breathing, open bite, and overexpansion of the maxilla
   3. In facio-scapulo-humeral type, the lips appear thick because of involvement of the orbicularis oris muscle
   4. Increase in dental disease if oral hygiene has been neglected

Spinal Cord Injuries

A. Definition
   1. Fracture, dislocation, hyperextension, compression, or severance of components of the spinal column
   2. Occurs most often in the cervical and lumbar curves
   3. Cord damage can occur above or below the level of bone injury

TABLE 19-7 Types and Characteristics of Muscular Dystrophies

	Duchenne's	Limb Girdle	Facio-Scapulo-Humeral	Myotonic
Onset	Mainly affects boys; occurs before age 10 years	Occurs later (average age 20); affects both males and females	Males and females equally affected; usually occurs around puberty	Both genders affected; appears in early adulthood
Severity	Most severe and destructive form	Slower progression in most cases	Least destructive and progresses at slower rate; least common type	Weakening spreads steadily; shortened life span
Etiology	Sex-linked recessive trait with high mutation rate	Autosomal recessive trait	Autosomal dominant trait	Autosomal dominant trait
Sites affected	Pelvis, abdomen, hip, and spine affected first; spreads to trunk, extremities, and myocardium (cranial nerves not affected); osteoporosis also noted	Initial weakness in pelvic girdle, then in shoulder	Facial muscles affected first; weakness is asymmetrical; progresses to shoulder girdle and upper arm	Weakness of lower legs and arms and facial muscles
Limitations	Becomes confined to wheelchair and bed within a few years of diagnosis; may develop scoliosis, obesity, and cardiopulmonary problems; death usually occurs during adolescence	May be severely disabled by midlife, with decreased life span	May remain in a state of indefinite remission, with some people living symptom-free, normal life span	Walking difficult; may be severely disabled; cataracts may develop
Signs and symptoms	Clumsiness, frequent falls resulting from precarious balance, toe-walking, weakness of hips, lordosis, cramping of legs and abdomen, Gowers' sign, enlargement of calves, decreased stamina	Begins as pain after exercise; then total muscle involvement	Mask-like, wrinkle-free, expressionless facial features; difficulty in closing eyes; muscles above elbow atrophy, below elbow are normal ("Popeye effect"); difficulty in raising arms	Stiffness, drooping eyelids and jaw, frequent tripping and falling

B. Incidence and prevalence
  1. Affects approximately 450,000 persons in the United States
  2. Annually, 15 to 40 new cases per 1 million population
  3. About 82% of cases are males age 16 to 30
C. Etiology—acquired injury from accidents
  1. Automobile or motorcycle crashes cause 50% of injuries
  2. Occupational accidents cause 25% of injuries
  3. Sporting accidents cause 18% of injuries
  4. Falls, gunshot wounds, or other trauma cause 7% of injuries
D. Signs, symptoms, and clinical manifestations
  1. Depend on severity and level of injury
  2. Prognosis
    a. First-aid measures performed at the site of the accident
    b. Type and level of injury to the spinal cord
    c. Survival is increasing with advances in emergency care and rehabilitation
    d. Restoration of function still very limited
  3. *Paraplegia* refers to an injury below the cervical level that results in paralysis of the lower portion of the body
  4. *Quadriplegia* refers to an injury occurring in the cervical region that results in paralysis of all four limbs and the trunk
  5. Most frequent cause of death is kidney stones or infection
  6. Functional limitations and specific manifestations depend on the level of the lesion (Tables 19-8 and 19-9)

Spina Bifida

A. Definition
  1. Neural tube defect of the spinal column
  2. Vertebrae fail to close completely around the spinal cord
B. Incidence and prevalence
  1. Affects 166,000 persons in the United States in some form
  2. Each year, about 1500 babies are born with spina bifida
  3. A major cause of paraplegia in children
C. Etiology—specific cause unknown; but multiple factors, including genetic and environmental factors, are suspected; folic acid supplements taken during pregnancy can prevent this
D. Types (Fig. 19-14)
  1. Spina bifida occulta
    a. Small defect in a vertebra not involving the spinal cord
    b. Often undetected
  2. Meningocele—bony defect that allows meninges and cerebrospinal fluid (CSF) to form a sac that protrudes from the vertebral column
  3. Meningomyelocele (also myelomeningocele)—severe defect in which the spinal cord also protrudes into the sac
E. Signs, symptoms, and clinical manifestations
  1. Potential exposure of the nervous system to the external environment results in an increased chance for further damage from trauma or infection
  2. Loss of motor function in the lower half of the body
    a. Differential involvement of muscle groups causes muscle imbalance, leading to spinal and limb deformities

Area Affected	Clinical Manifestations
Muscles (limb and trunk)	Innervation and perception of pain and touch disturbed; leads to muscle atrophy
	Concerns for safety around varying temperatures
	Formation of decubitus ulcers (pressure sores) caused by breakdown of tissue from immobilization, bruises, or braces
	Decreased or absent self-care skills
	Spasticity and tremors
	Adaptive equipment required, especially for:
	—Wrist stability
	—Pencil grasp
	—Arm movements
Respiration	Intercostal muscles may be paralyzed, resulting in need for diaphragmatic breathing or tracheostomy and total or partial dependence on a respirator
Bowel and bladder	Limited innervation, resulting in incontinence and encopresis or retention
	Can lead to infections, particularly of kidneys
	Autonomic hyperreflexia can occur (medical emergency)
	Caused by sudden constriction of blood vessels
	Symptoms—rapid increase in blood pressure (e.g., 280/80 mm Hg), low pulse, pounding headache, skin blotching and sweating above site of injury, cold goose bumps below site of injury
Bones and joints	Contractures from spasticity and immobilization
	Heterotopic ossifications (bony accumulations) may develop around joints
Metabolism	Regulation of body temperature impaired
Social and emotional status	Problems associated with coping with a debilitating acquired injury
	May experience stages of shock, denial, anger, depression, mobilization, and coping

TABLE 19-8 Clinical Manifestations of Spinal Cord Injuries

    b. Loss of sensation to pain, touch, and temperature creates safety hazards and pressure sores
    c. Loss of bladder and bowel control
    d. Ambulation may be affected, creating a need for orthopedic devices or a wheelchair
  3. Deformity of the brain
    a. Most have normal intelligence but experience learning disabilities, especially visual-perceptual problems
    b. Some develop seizure disorders
    c. In about 80–90% of spina bifida cases, there is a cyst with parts of the spinal cord and spinal wall present. This is called a myelomeningocele. This type of spina bifida can happen in a relatively high or low position on one's back. It often causes problems with bladder and bowel functioning, and sometimes paralysis or limb weaknesses.
      (1) CSF accumulates in the ventricles of the brain
      (2) Pressure expands the brain and skull
  4. Latex allergy is common in this population
F. Oral manifestations
  1. None directly associated

TABLE 19-9 **Functional Significance of Cervical, Thoracic, and Lumbar Lesion Levels**	
Lesion Level	**Functional Expectations for Complete Lesions**
Cervical Lesions	
C1-C3	Respirator dependent; totally dependent
C4	Incapable of voluntary function in arms, trunk, or legs; poor respiratory reserve; totally dependent
C5	Can stabilize and rotate neck; has function of rhomboids and deltoids, allowing some shoulder movement, elbow flexion; biceps and brachioradialis partially innervated
C6	Can move shoulders well; strong elbow flexion; wrist muscles allow weak closure of hand; can use large-handled, lightweight objects; can sit up in bed with help and roll over; still needs attendant; can drive van with hand controls
C7	Can lift own body weight; can use hands, which are weak and lack dexterity; can eat independently, with some assistance; confined to wheelchair; can live independently and manage self-care in wheelchair-accessible environment without attendant
Thoracic Lesions	
T1	Independent in bed, self-care (short of lifting weights); lacks trunk stability, respiratory reserve, and trunk fixation of arm prime movers
T6	Capable of heavy lifting (because of thoracic musculature); increased respiratory reserve; independent transfers, self-application of braces
T12	Can ambulate with crutches and braces, but still uses wheelchair as primary means of mobility
Lumbar Lesions	
L4	Complete independence in all phases of self-care and ambulation—usually aided by crutches or canes

From Schubert MM, Snow M, Stiefel DJ: *Dental management of patients with CNS and neurologic impairment: spinal cord injury.* DECOD series, Seattle, 1989, University of Washington.

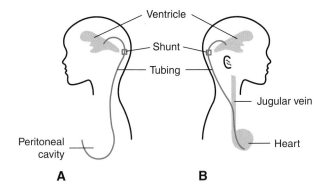

FIG 19-15 Types of shunts.

2. Evaluate for premedication if person has a ventriculoatrial shunt (Fig. 19-15)

Cystic Fibrosis

A. Definition—inherited disorder of the exocrine glands
B. Incidence and prevalence
   1. Occurs in 1 in 3000 live births in the United States
   2. Between 2% and 5% of the population are carriers
   3. Affects approximately 30,000 persons in the United States; 10 million or more are carriers of the gene for cystic fibrosis
   4. Most common cause of chronic lung disease in Caucasian children
   5. Mean survival about 37.4 years
C. Etiology—autosomal recessive disorder; defect in gene on chromosome 7 that results in phenylalanine deletion and problem with chloride ion transport
D. Signs, symptoms, and clinical manifestations—include increased viscosity of mucus (obstructs the pancreatic ducts, leading to cyst formation, impaired metabolism, and progressive deterioration)

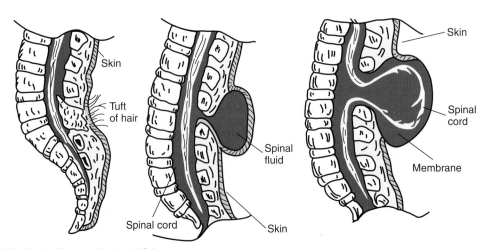

FIG 19-14 Types of spina bifida.

1. Accumulation of mucus in the lungs interferes with oxygen exchange
   a. Interferes especially with exhalation, causing a barrel-chested appearance
   b. Air sacs collapse and infections occur, often leading to suppurative bronchitis, pneumonia, and obstructive emphysema
   c. Clubbing of fingers and toes
   d. Chronic cough
2. Sweat glands affected, leading to high levels of sodium in the sweat ("salty sweat")
3. Salivary glands also affected
4. Other findings and complications include a small gallbladder, cirrhosis of the liver, and sterility in men
5. Delayed linear growth and bone development
6. Insufficient pancreatic function can lead to diabetes
7. Death usually occurs in early adulthood
E. Oral manifestations
   1. Lower dental caries rate and plaque accumulation with increased calculus deposits; probably a result of alterations in saliva and long-term use of antibiotics
   2. Enlargement of the salivary glands
   3. Intrinsic staining of the teeth, if tetracycline is administered during the formative years
   4. Mouth breathing, if sinuses are occluded

Chronic Obstructive Pulmonary Disease (COPD)

A. Definitions
   1. General term for pulmonary disorders characterized by obstruction of airflow during respiration
   2. Consists of two or more disease processes that may coexist
   3. Bronchitis—obstruction caused by narrowing or loss of airways
   4. Emphysema—loss of elasticity and collapse of overinflated air sacs; loss of gas exchange surface area; causes obstruction during expiration
B. Incidence, prevalence, and etiology
   1. Chronic bronchitis affects 10% to 25% of U.S. adults
   2. More common in males and in persons age 60 or older
   3. Most important risk factor is smoking, accounting for 80% to 90% of persons with COPD
   4. Can be a hereditary defect in pulmonary tissue; may be caused by severe respiratory illnesses during childhood
C. Signs, symptoms, and clinical manifestations
   1. Dyspnea and wheezing on exertion or at rest; orthopnea
   2. Chronic cough, mucus, respiratory infections, and cyanosis in bronchitis
   3. Use of accessory muscles of respiration
   4. Chest pain
   5. Advanced complications are heart failure and pulmonary failure
D. Oral manifestations—no associated oral manifestations unless a side effect of the medications

Bronchial Asthma

See the section on "Asthma" in Chapter 21.
A. Definition
   1. Chronic clinical state of hyperreactivity of the tracheobronchial tree characterized by recurrent paroxysms of dyspnea and wheezing
   2. Results from bronchospasm, bronchial wall edema, inflammation, and hypersecretion by mucous glands
   3. Status asthmaticus—persistent exacerbation of asthma despite drug therapy (life threatening); causes excessive strain on the circulatory and respiratory systems
B. Incidence and prevalence
   1. Affects approximately 25.9 million persons in the United States
   2. Initial symptoms usually occur in the first 5 years of life
   3. Approximately 50% of affected children become asymptomatic before adulthood
   4. From 75% to 85% also have allergies
C. Etiology—unknown, but precipitating factors and their effects are known
   1. Extrinsic factors—smoking, dust, mold, pollen, smoke, animal dander, household sprays, wool, certain foods, air pollutants, sulfiting agents
   2. Other factors—respiratory tract infections, aspirin and other anti-inflammatory drugs, overexertion
D. Signs, symptoms, and clinical manifestations
   1. Wheezing, dyspnea, coughing, chest pain, sneezing, sputum production, fatigue, anxiety
   2. Expiratory phase of breathing is slower and more pronounced
   3. Facial (sinus) pain, conjunctivitis, otitis media
   4. More severe symptoms—syncope, respiratory failure, cyanosis, hyperexpansion of the chest
E. Oral manifestations
   1. β-Adrenergic agonists may impair salivary secretions, increasing caries risk
   2. Mouth breathing
   3. *Candida* infections from inhalant use

Congenital Heart Disease

A. Definition
   1. Anomalies of heart structure
   2. Usually develops during the first 9 weeks in utero
B. Incidence and prevalence
   1. Occurs in 8 to 10 of 1000 births in the United States
   2. Affects approximately 500,000 adults
C. Etiology
   1. Generally unknown
   2. Genetic (e.g., Down syndrome)
   3. Environmental (maternal)
      a. Fetal hypoxia, endocarditis, or immunologic abnormalities
      b. Rubella infection (German measles) or other viruses
      c. Nutritional deficiencies (especially vitamin deficiencies)

d. Drugs (e.g., lithium, alcohol, cocaine)

e. Radiation

f. Metabolic disorders (PKU or diabetes)

D. Types of malformations

1. Cause initial left-to-right shunting of blood (e.g., atrial septal defect, ventricular septal defect, patent ductus arteriosus)

2. Initial right-to-left shunting (e.g., tetralogy of Fallot)—causes significant cyanosis

3. Malformations that obstruct blood flow (e.g., pulmonary stenosis)

E. Signs, symptoms, and clinical manifestations

1. Dyspnea, fatigue, weakness (most common symptoms)

2. Cyanosis, dizziness, syncope, or ruddy color, leading to congestive heart failure

3. Clubbing of fingers or toes

4. Heart murmurs

5. Delayed growth and development

6. Complications—brain abscess, bacterial endocarditis, congestive heart failure, acute pulmonary edema, bleeding problems

F. Oral manifestations

1. Bluish mucosa, if cyanotic; ruddy color, if person has polycythemia

2. Developmental defects of teeth sometimes seen

3. Slight hemorrhage secondary to trauma, if bleeding problems are present

4. May have decreased ability to fight oral infections

Cardiac Arrhythmias and Dysrhythmias

A. Definition

1. Irregular heartbeat manifested as abnormal pulse rates or rhythms

2. Produces alterations in the normal sequence of contractions, leading to inadequate blood flow, and produces aberrant electrical depolarization

3. Adversely affects the ventricular rate

B. Types

1. Bradycardias—slowed heart rate (less than 60 beats/min)

2. Tachycardias—increased heart rate (more than 100 beats/min)

3. Isolated ectopic beats—premature impulses resulting in premature atrial beats

4. Preexcitation syndrome

5. Cardiac arrest

C. Signs, symptoms, and clinical manifestations (may also be asymptomatic)

1. Abnormal pulse

2. Palpitations

3. Breathlessness, pallor, fatigue

4. Syncope or dizziness

5. Cyanosis

6. Pain

7. Cardiac failure

8. Cardioversion through defibrillation

D. Oral manifestations—may have side effects from medications, such as xerostomia, taste changes, or cyanotic oral tissues

Hypertensive Disease

See the section on "Vital Signs" in Chapter 21.

A. Definitions

1. Hypertension—abnormal elevation of arterial blood pressure when constricted blood vessels increase resistance to blood flow, causing an increase in pressure against blood vessel walls

2. Hypertensive heart disease—sustained elevation of the blood pressure, creating an increased workload for the heart, resulting in left ventricular hypertrophy and in late-stage kidney disease

3. Four hypertension categories (see Table 15-5 in Chapter 15; see the section on "Cardiac Emergencies" in Chapter 21)

a. Normal—less than 120/80 mm Hg

b. Prehypertension—120/80 to 139/89 mm Hg

c. Stage 1—140/90 to 159/99 mm Hg

d. Stage 2—160/100 mm Hg or higher in either number

e. Hypertensive crisis—higher than 180/110 mm Hg in either number

B. Incidence and prevalence

1. Incidence is increasing, with hypertension affecting approximately 1 in 3 (or 74.5 million) persons in the United States; more remain undiagnosed

2. Prevalence increases with age and is greater in men before age 55 and in women after age 55

C. Etiology

1. Most cases are of unknown cause (essential hypertension)

2. From 5% to 10% are secondary to other conditions, such as renal disease and endocrine disorders

3. Risk factors include prehypertension, race (African American), age, stress, smoking, overweight and obesity, oral contraceptives, and excess salt and fat in the diet

4. Chronic hypertension causes cardiac enlargement and eventual congestive heart failure

D. Signs, symptoms, and clinical manifestations

1. Early—occipital headache, dizziness, tingling of the extremities, vision changes, tinnitus, dyspnea

2. Advanced—cardiac enlargement, ischemic heart disease, congestive heart failure, renal failure, stroke

E. Oral manifestations

1. Generally no direct oral manifestations

2. Facial palsy from some drugs

3. Oral lesions, taste changes or xerostomia from drugs

4. Many side effects and precautions associated with drugs; some calcium channel blockers cause drug-induced gingival enlargement

Ischemic Heart Disease (Coronary Heart Disease)

A. Definition—coronary atherosclerotic heart disease that is symptomatic

B. Incidence and prevalence

1. Affects 17.6 million persons in the United States

2. Leading cause of death after age 40

3. Incidence and severity increase with age; more than 50% who die suddenly have no previous evidence of disease

C. Etiology
1. Risk factors are the same as for hypertensive disease
2. Periodontitis may be a significant risk factor related to elevated levels of cross-reactive protein and growth acceleration of lipids in blood vessels because of increased inflammatory mediators associated with periodontal gram-negative bacteria
3. Accumulation of atherosclerotic plaque inside blood vessels impairs blood flow and thus the oxygen supply to the heart
D. Signs, symptoms, and clinical manifestations
1. Angina pectoris—transient and reversible oxygen deficiency; classified as stable or unstable
   a. Pain—crushing or paroxysmal, usually less than 10 minutes; often mistaken for indigestion
   b. Sweating, anxiety, pallor, difficulty breathing
   c. Relieved by administration of nitroglycerin or rest
2. Myocardial infarction (MI)—an infarct or ischemic necrosis caused by a sudden reduction or arrest of blood flow
   a. Pain in the sternum, radiating to the left arm; lasts longer than angina
   b. Not relieved by nitroglycerin
   c. Same symptoms as angina, with nausea and vomiting, palpitations, and lowered blood pressure
   d. Often leads to sudden death from ventricular fibrillation
   e. Symptoms vary between males and females
E. Oral manifestations
1. None directly associated
2. Oral lesions or xerostomia may result as a drug side effect
3. Pain may be radiated to the mandible, palate, or tongue
4. Drug-induced gingival enlargement may result as a side effect of some calcium channel blockers

Congestive Heart Failure (CHF)

A. Definition
1. Represents a symptom complex that involves the failure of one or both ventricles (usually the left ventricle)
2. Imbalance between the demand placed on the heart and its ability to respond
3. Results in an inadequate supply of blood and oxygen throughout the body and in congestion of blood within the vascular system
B. Incidence and prevalence
1. Most common cause of death in the United States
2. Prevalence is 5.1 million persons; incidence is 400,000 cases each year; incidence of 5% occurs in persons under age 40
C. Etiology
1. Underlying causes
   a. Heart valve damage; ventricular failure; overload of blood in the ventricles
   b. Obstructive lung disease
   c. Damage to the walls of the heart muscle
2. Precipitating causes that place an additional demand on the heart
   a. Hypertensive crises

   b. Pulmonary embolism
   c. Arrhythmia
D. Signs, symptoms, and clinical manifestations
1. Dyspnea, irregular breathing pattern, coughing, weakness; the person cannot breathe unless sitting up
2. Swollen ankles late in the day, pitting edema, ascites
3. Cyanosis, anxiety, fear
4. Paleness, sweating, cold skin
5. Decreased urine output
6. Frothy pink or white sputum
7. Weak pulse
8. Confusion from decreased cardiac output, thus decreased oxygen to the brain
E. Oral manifestations—infections, gingival bleeding, and petechiae if displaying polycythemia

Cerebrovascular Accident (CVA, Stroke)

A. Definition—sudden loss of brain function resulting from interference with the blood supply to a portion of the brain
B. Incidence and prevalence
1. Affects 4.6 million persons in the United States, 75% in persons age 66 or older
2. Third leading cause of death in the United States; leading cause of serious disability
3. African Americans are at greater risk than Caucasians
4. Men are at greater risk than women
5. Likelihood of having a stroke increases with age
C. Etiology
1. Intracranial hemorrhage
2. Blockage of vessels by thrombi or emboli (most common cause)
3. Vascular insufficiency
4. Predisposing conditions and risk factors
   a. Cerebral arteriosclerosis
   b. Dehydration
   c. Trauma
   d. Hypertension
   e. Diabetes
   f. Cigarette smoking
   g. Periodontitis
D. Signs, symptoms, and clinical manifestations—depend on the area of the brain involved and the extent of damage (Table 19-10)
1. Immediate
   a. Syncope, headache, chills, convulsions, nausea, and vomiting
   b. Changes in level of consciousness
   c. Transient paresthesias
   d. Mood swing
2. Residual or chronic
   a. Paralysis—hemiparesis or localized paralysis
   b. Speech problems and aphasia (reduced capacity for interpretation and formulation of language)
   c. Alterations in reflexes, especially the oral-motor reflexes
   d. Functional disorders of the bladder or bowel
   e. Visual impairments
   f. Seizures

TABLE 19-10 Functional Limitations in Stroke (CVA) Victims

Right Hemiplegia (L-CVA*)	Left Hemiplegia (R-CVA)
Language problems	Spatial-perceptual task difficulties—
Decreased auditory memory (cannot remember a long series of instructions)	inability to judge distance, size, position, rate of movement, form, and relation of parts to a whole
Vocabulary problems	Often thought to be unimpaired
Slow, cautious, disorganized	because able to speak and
Anxious	understand
	Visual field cuts; angles, etc. cannot be perceived
	Cannot use mirrors
	Cannot sequence tasks, such as toothbrushing
	Decreased visual memory (loses place when reading)
	Cannot monitor self (keeps talking even though answered questions already)
	May neglect left side
	Tendency to be impulsive and unaware of deficits; spatial-perceptual difficulties are easy to miss

CVA, Cerebrovascular accident.
From Schubert MM, Snow M, Stiefel DJ: *Dental management of patients with CNS and neurologic impairment: spinal cord injury*. DECOD series, Seattle, 1989, University of Washington.

E. Oral manifestations
  1. Oral-motor dysfunction
  2. Increased incidence of dental caries or periodontal disease caused by oral-motor problems and poor oral hygiene
  3. Anticoagulant therapy to prevent clot formation creates bleeding issues and physician consults required

Sickle Cell Disease

A. Definitions
  1. Defect of hemoglobin that causes red blood cells to become sickle shaped
  2. Sickle cell trait—individual shows no symptoms unless experiencing abnormally low concentration of oxygen
  3. Sickle cell disease—progressively deteriorating and complex disease with multiple symptoms
B. Incidence and prevalence
  1. Found in African Americans and other nonwhite persons; occurs in both genders
  2. Two million persons in the United States are carriers of the sickle cell trait
  3. Approximately 80,000 persons in the United States have full-blown sickle cell anemia
  4. About 1 in 1400 Hispanic American children born with sickle cell anemia
  5. Babies do not show symptoms until age 6 months

C. Etiology
  1. Mutation in the globin gene of hemoglobin
  2. Sickle cell trait—the person has half normal hemoglobin and half sickled hemoglobin
  3. Sickle cell anemia—the person receives a sickle hemoglobin gene from both parents; sickle cell anemia is autosomal recessive
D. Signs, symptoms, and clinical manifestations
  1. Young children
    a. Can develop enlarged spleen, septicemia, and meningitis
    b. Swelling of the feet and hands, anemia, pallor, tiredness, fever, pneumonia
    c. Severe pain crises affecting the extremities
    d. Stroke occurs in 10% of those affected
  2. Children and adolescents
    a. Can develop gallstones, enlarged hearts, and lung infarctions
    b. Bones degenerate as a result of repeated sickling
    c. Delayed growth and late puberty
    d. Increased chance for stroke, impaired kidney and liver function with jaundice, and arthritis
    e. Continued pain crises
  3. Adulthood
    a. Hemorrhage in the eye, detached retina
    b. Pain crises—variable in each person
    c. Lung and kidney damage, gallstones
    d. Leg ulcers and bone changes
    e. Infection is a major cause of death and also precipitates crises
E. Oral manifestations
  1. Sore, painful, red tongue
  2. Loss of taste sensation
  3. Osteoporosis
  4. Decreased radiodensity (ground-glass appearance) with coarse trabecular bone pattern and large marrow spaces
  5. Mucosal pallor
  6. Delayed eruption of teeth
  7. Hypoplastic enamel—pain in the mandible
  8. Bone loss can be significant in children

Cancer

A. Definition—cells that multiply at an abnormally rapid rate, invading and destroying healthy tissue
  1. Metastasis—spread of cancer to distant sites
  2. Invasion—spread of cancer to local sites
B. Incidence and prevalence
  1. Estimated 1,248,900 new cases of oral cancer per year; less than 50% alive after 5 years
  2. About 201 in 100,000 persons will die of cancer each year in the United States
  3. Approximately 75% of all head and neck cancers begin in the oral cavity
  4. The tongue is the most common intraoral location (30%) (Fig. 19-16)

FIG 19-16 Squamous cell carcinoma on the lateral border of the tongue. (From Regezi JA, Sciubba JA, Jordan CK: *Oral pathology: clinical pathologic correlations,* ed 7, St Louis, 2017, Elsevier.)

FIG 19-17 A and **B,** Radiation-associated cervical caries. (From Regezi JA, Sciubba JA, Jordan CK: *Oral pathology: clinical pathologic correlations,* ed 7, St Louis, 2017, Elsevier.)

C. Etiology of oral cancer
   1. Tobacco
   2. Alcohol
   3. Human papillomavirus (HPV)
   4. Ultraviolet light
   5. Genetics
D. Warning signs of oral cancer
   1. Unexplained swelling, lump, or growth with or without pain
   2. White scaly patches or red areas
   3. Any sore that does not heal in 2 weeks
   4. Unexplained numbness or tingling
   5. Difficulty opening mouth or swallowing
   6. Prolonged hoarseness
E. Oral manifestations—side effects of treatment and depend on type of cancer and treatment
   1. Oral ulcerations and mucositis
   2. Candidiasis
   3. Anemia
   4. Xerostomia
   5. Radiation caries (Fig. 19-17)
   6. Loss of taste
   7. Osteoradionecrosis (Fig. 19-18)
   8. Tooth sensitivity
   9. Muscular dysfunction and trismus
   10. Spontaneous gingival bleeding
   11. Cosmetic disfigurement

Leukemia

A. Definition
   1. Progressive malignant neoplasms characterized by an overproduction of abnormal leukocytes
   2. Abnormal leukocytes displace hematopoietic tissue in the bone marrow, leading to decreased production of platelets, erythrocytes, and normal leukocytes
B. Classification—chronicity
   1. Acute form (A)—large numbers of immature nonspecific leukocytes are produced; accounts for 25% more cases than the chronic form

FIG 19-18 Osteoradionecrosis of the lingual mandible. (From Regezi JA, Sciubba JA, Jordan CK: *Oral pathology: clinical pathologic correlations,* ed 7, St Louis, 2017, Elsevier.)

   2. Chronic form (C)—leukocytes are well differentiated and able to mature; but immunologic capacity is decreased
C. Incidence and prevalence
   1. Estimated 44,790 new cases each year in the United States
   2. About 33% of cancers in children are leukemia
   3. Seventh leading cause of cancer death in adults; leading cause of cancer death in children
   4. Five-year survival rate is approximately 46%
D. Etiology
   1. Specific cause unknown
   2. Predisposing factors—genetic factors, ionizing radiation, chemical agents, exposure to human T cell lymphotrophic virus type I

FIG 19-19 Gingival conditions associated with monocytic leukemia. (From Regezi JA, Sciubba JA, Jordan CK: *Oral pathology: clinical pathologic correlations,* ed 7, St Louis, 2017, Elsevier.)

E. Signs, symptoms, and clinical manifestations
1. Acute form appears suddenly and severely; chronic form is insidious
2. Fatigue, weakness, pallor, weight loss
3. Ecchymosed skin and nosebleeds
4. Fever
5. Headache, nausea, and vomiting
F. Oral manifestations (Fig. 19-19)
1. Initial
a. Leukemic infiltrate of the pulp and gingiva
(1) Causes pain in teeth
(2) Enlarged, bluish red, spongy, blunted papilla
(3) Ulceration and necrosis
b. Mucositis, mucosal atrophy, and mucosal pallor
c. Areas of spontaneous hemorrhage (intermittent oozing) and petechiae
d. Loss of lamina dura, resorption of alveolar bone, cancellous bone destruction
2. Secondary
a. Mucosal infections (e.g., *Candida, Pseudomonas*) and periapical infections
b. Necrotizing ulcerative gingivitis
c. Viral infections
d. Osteomyelitis
3. Tertiary (treatment effects)
a. Painful oral ulcerations
b. Stomatitis
c. Xerostomia and dental caries
d. Jaw pain with Bell's palsy
e. Secondary infections

Congenital Disorders of Coagulation: Hemophilias

See the section on "Hemophilia" in Chapter 8.
A. Definition—congenital disorder of the blood-clotting mechanism
B. Incidence and prevalence
1. More than 18,000 persons in the United States have hemophilia; 400 births yearly
2. Hemophilia A accounts for 80% to 85%; hemophilia B for 10% to 15%

3. About 90% of patients are under age 25
4. Vast majority of those affected are men
C. Classification
1. Type
a. Hemophilia A (factor VIII deficiency)—1.9 in 10 persons with hemophilia have type A
b. Hemophilia B (factor IX deficiency)—Christmas disease
c. Von Willebrand's disease (lack of plasma)—von Willebrand's factor is required for primary hemostasis
2. Severity—level of clotting factor (normal level is 50% to 100%)
a. Severe—have less than 1% of clotting factor; may bleed spontaneously or from minor trauma
b. Moderate—have 5% to 25% of clotting factor; hemorrhage only with trauma
c. Mild—have 25% to 50% of clotting factor; bleed only after severe injury or surgery
D. Etiology
1. Hemophilia A and B
a. Sex-linked recessive mode of inheritance (female carrier and manifested in males)
b. High mutation rate
2. Von Willebrand's disease—transmission by dominant autosomal gene; occurs with equal frequency in both genders
E. Signs, symptoms, and clinical manifestations
1. Bleeding and bruising from minor cuts or pressure
a. Ecchymoses and hematomas
b. Oozing
c. Intramuscular bleeding causes pain
2. Hemarthroses—bleeding into the soft tissues of joints, leading to pain, swelling, and permanent joint contractures
3. Renal function is impaired; exposure to hepatitis during transfusions
4. Intracranial hemorrhages can cause seizures or other neurologic disorders
F. Oral manifestations
1. Ecchymoses, hematomas, and gingival oozing can be problems
2. Oral trauma is more evident and can be serious

Diabetes Mellitus

See the section on "Diabetes Mellitus" in Chapter 21.
A. Definition—hereditary disease of metabolism with:
1. Inadequate production and action of insulin from the pancreas
2. Disorders in carbohydrate, protein, and fat metabolism
3. Body cells unable to use glucose, leading to hyperglycemia
4. Alternating extremes of hypoglycemia and hyperglycemia found in the person with "brittle" (very poorly controlled) diabetes
B. Incidence and prevalence
1. Diabetes mellitus affects 23.6 million persons in the United States, with approximately 8 million undiagnosed

TABLE 19-11   Comparison of Type 1 and Type 2 Diabetes Mellitus

Characteristic	Type 1	Type 2
Age of onset	Young, usually before or during puberty, but may appear later	Adult, usually after 30 years, but may occur at younger age
Body weight	Normal or thin	Obesity is most important risk factor
Ethnicity	More common in Caucasians	More common in African Americans, Asian Americans, Hispanic Americans, and Native Americans
Hereditary	Yes, but less frequent occurrence in families than type 2	Much more frequent occurrence in families
Lifestyle	Restrictions very difficult for young persons	More frequent in sedentary individuals with high-fat diets
Onset of symptoms	Rapid, abrupt symptoms of hyperglycemia	Slow, insidious progression over years
Symptoms	Weight loss; weakness; polyuria; polydipsia; polyphagia; blurred vision; mimic flu; frequent/recurrent infections; slow healing; tingling/numb extremities; fatigue; eye/kidney/cardiovascular problems	Any type 1 symptom; kidney/cardiovascular problems
Severity	Severe, life-threatening	Early mild but progressively serious
Complications	Acute hypoglycemic or hyperglycemic emergencies and chronic long-term complications common	Acute complications rare; chronic long-term complications common
Stability	Unstable, difficult and much effort to control	More stable, easier to manage
Exogenous insulin required	All	Some
Chronic manifestations	Uncommon before 20 years; prevalent and severe by 30 years	Develop slowly at later ages
Ketoacidosis	Common	Rare
Prevention	None (because of multiple factors)	Prevent or delay with lifestyle changes

Modified from Wilkins EM: *Clinical practice of the dental hygienist*, ed 10, Philadelphia, 2009, Lippincott Williams & Wilkins.

2. Third leading cause of death in the United States
3. Much higher in Hispanic Americans and Native Americans
4. Approximately 800,000 new cases diagnosed yearly
C. Major types (Table 19-11)
   1. Type 1—insulin dependent
   2. Type 2—non–insulin dependent (92% of cases)
   3. Prediabetes—impaired glucose tolerance; higher than normal levels but not yet diagnostic for diabetes; at risk for atherosclerotic disease
   4. Gestational diabetes—occurs in 2% of pregnant women during the second or third trimester; the condition returns to normal after delivery in most cases, but 30% to 40% may develop type 2 diabetes later in life
D. Etiology
   1. Genetic disorder
   2. Destruction of the insulin-producing cells of the pancreas resulting from inflammation, viruses, cancer, or surgery
   3. Secondary to endocrine disorders (e.g., hyperthyroidism)
   4. Iatrogenic disease after administration of steroids
   5. Obesity
E. Signs, symptoms, and clinical manifestations (Table 19-12)
   1. Cardinal symptoms are those associated with hyperglycemia
   2. An overdose of insulin or inadequate glucose intake to balance the insulin intake can result in insulin shock (hypoglycemia)
   3. Chronic complications include:
      a. Atherosclerosis and other cardiovascular problems
      b. Renal failure
      c. Motor, sensory, and autonomic neuropathies
      d. Glaucoma and cataracts leading to blindness

TABLE 19-12   Clinical Manifestations of Diabetes Mellitus

Hyperglycemia	Hypoglycemia
Polydipsia	Early stage
Polyphagia	—Diminished cerebral function
Polyuria	—Changes in mood
Loss of weight	—Decreased spontaneity
Fatigue	—Hunger
Headache	—Nausea
Blurred vision	More severe stage
Nausea and vomiting	—Sweating
Tachycardia	—Tachycardia
Florid appearance	—Piloerection
Hot and dry skin	—Increased anxiety
Kussmaul respiration	—Bizarre behavior patterns
Mental stupor	—Belligerence
Loss of consciousness	—Poor judgment
	—Uncooperativeness
	Later severe stage
	—Unconsciousness
	—Seizure activity
	—Hypotension
	—Hypothermia

Modified from Malamed SF: *Medical emergencies in the dental office*, ed 6, St Louis, 2013, Mosby.

   e. Associated with increased incidence of large babies, stillbirths, miscarriages, neonatal deaths, and congenital defects
F. Treatment—no known cure
   1. Management of acute symptoms
   2. Exercise and diet plan (food exchange system)

FIG 19-20 Gingival tissues exhibiting spontaneous bleeding, inflammation, and edema in an adult client with diabetes. (From Newman MG, et al: *Carranza's clinical periodontology,* ed 12, St Louis, 2015, Elsevier.)

TABLE 19-13   Clinical Features of Thyroid Disease

HYPOTHYROIDISM		
Cretinism	**Myxedema**	**Hyperthyroidism**
Dwarfism and obesity	Obesity	Weight loss
Coarse hair	Hair loss	Fine, friable hair
Eyes set apart	Puffy eyelids	Puffy eyelids
Muscle weakness	Muscle weakness	Exophthalmos
Dry, cold skin	Dry, cold skin	Tremors
Decreased sweating	Decreased sweating	Warm, moist skin
Cold intolerance	Cold intolerance	Increased sweating
Lethargy	Lethargy	Heat intolerance
Bradycardia	Bradycardia	Hyperactivity
Delayed tooth eruption		Tachycardia
Small jaws and malocclusion		Accelerated tooth eruption
		Large jaws
		Osteoporosis of alveolar bone
		Rapidly developing dental caries and periodontal disease

G. Oral manifestations
1. Seen more often in persons with uncontrolled diabetes
2. Delayed wound healing and inability to manage oral infections (e.g., *Candida*), periodontal abscesses
3. Decreased salivary flow may lead to increased caries; may have parotid gland enlargement
4. Predisposition to aggressive periodontal disease in both types of diabetes, even in children and adolescents; magenta hue with edematous glassy tissue, enlarged papilla, mobility, alveolar bone loss (Fig. 19-20)
5. Periodontitis can make blood glucose levels more difficult to control
6. Poor blood glucose control greatly increases risk for periodontal breakdown, bone loss, and loss of attachment
7. Children with diabetes may have accelerated tooth eruption and enamel hypoplasia

Thyroid Disease

A. Definitions
1. Hyperthyroidism (thyrotoxicosis)—excess of thyroid hormones in the bloodstream
2. Graves disease—type of hyperthyroidism; toxic goiter
3. Hypothyroidism—inadequate thyroid hormones in the bloodstream
   a. Cretinism—childhood onset (congenital)
   b. Myxedema—adult onset (acquired)
B. Incidence and prevalence
1. Thyroid disease affects 28 million persons in the United States, with up to one half undiagnosed
2. Hyperthyroidism—disease is seven times more common in women; especially manifested during puberty, pregnancy, or menopause
3. Hypothyroidism
   a. Rare
   b. Myxedema is five times more common in females; most common between ages 30 and 60
   c. Permanent congenital hypothyroidism occurs in 1 in 3500 to 4500 births

C. Etiology
1. Hyperthyroidism (Graves disease)
   a. Cause is unknown
   b. Autoimmune cause or familial tendency is postulated
2. Hypothyroidism
   a. Disease of the thyroid gland
   b. Myxedema may follow thyroid gland or pituitary gland failure resulting from irradiation, surgery, or excessive antithyroid drug therapy
D. Signs, symptoms, and clinical manifestations—results of underproduction or overproduction of thyroid hormone (Table 19-13)
E. Oral manifestations—primarily delayed or accelerated dental development or deterioration of alveolar bone (Fig. 19-21 and Table 19-13)

Chemical Dependency

See the section on "Substance Abuse" in Chapter 11.
A. Definitions
1. State of psychological or physical dependence (or both) after administration of a drug on a periodic or continuous basis
2. Drug use—when the effects of a drug can be realized with minimal hazard
3. Drug misuse—when the drug or amount taken makes it more dangerous than necessary to produce the desired effect
4. Drug abuse—continual misuse of a drug, loss of control over its use, or disruption of family, social, or job responsibilities
5. Tolerance—use of larger doses of a drug to experience the same effects over time

FIG 19-21 A, Radiograph of mandibular radiolucencies associated with hyperparathyroidism. **B,** Radiograph of loss of lamina dura associated with hyperparathyroidism. (From Regezi JA, Sciubba JA, Jordan CK: *Oral pathology: clinical pathologic correlations,* ed 7, St Louis, 2017, Elsevier.)

6. Recovery—overcoming physical and psychological dependence; commitment to drug-free life
B. Incidence and prevalence
   1. Several drugs or drug categories cause the most concern: cocaine, heroin and other opiates, marijuana, stimulants, barbiturates and other depressants, hallucinogens (psychedelics), tranquilizers, volatile solvents, and other inhalants
   2. Alcohol is a major problem (see next section); 70% of persons in the United States drink at least on a social basis

3. Nitrous oxide and prescription drug abuse is of most concern to dental professionals
4. Routes of administration—oral ingestion, inhalation, injection, snorting, buccal, suppositories
5. In the United States, 41.7% of those over age 12 have used illegal drugs at least once

C. Etiology
   1. Stressful social, psychological, or economic environment
   2. Peer pressure
   3. Gateway drugs—alcohol, tobacco, marijuana

D. Signs and symptoms—vary with the agent involved and route of administration
   1. Affect autonomic, central, and peripheral nervous systems
   2. Drug interactions have additive, inhibitory, and synergistic effects
   3. Duration of effects ranges from 1 hour to many days
   4. Withdrawal symptoms reported for all drug categories except hallucinogens
   5. Possible effects of some drug categories
      a. Narcotics—euphoria, drowsiness, respiratory depression, constricted pupils, nausea
      b. Depressants—slurred speech, disorientation, intoxicated behavior
      c. Stimulants—alertness, excitation, euphoria, increased pulse rate and blood pressure, insomnia, loss of appetite
      d. Hallucinogens—illusions and hallucinations, poor perception of time and distance
      e. Marijuana—euphoria, relaxed inhibitions, increased appetite, disoriented behavior

E. Oral manifestations
   1. Oral trauma—if the person engages in aggressive behavior or fights or has accidents
   2. Xerostomia—if dehydrated
   3. Mucosal lesions and leukoplakia from irritants smoked or used orally
   4. Increased caries typically seen at the cervical area; periodontal disease prevalent if oral hygiene is neglected or the person consumes high-carbohydrate diet
   5. Advanced cervical caries associated with heavy methamphetamine use
   6. Tooth abrasion
   7. Increased risk for oral and esophageal cancers
   8. Reduced tolerance to pain
   9. Bruxism

Chronic Alcohol Abuse and Dependence

A. Definition and etiology
   1. Chronic impairment in physical, mental, or social functioning caused by frequent ingestion (more than two drinks per day) of alcohol
   2. Can become dependent on alcohol ingestion and develop a tolerance to increasing amounts
   3. Genetically transmitted susceptibility to alcoholism
   4. Often induced by a psychiatric disorder or stress

B. Incidence and prevalence
   1. Estimated 5.1 million persons in United States suffer from alcohol abuse

2. About 1 in 13 U.S. adults abuses alcohol or is an alcoholic (7.42% of persons age 18 and older)
3. Alcohol problems are higher among young adults age 18 to 29
4. Normal activities are maintained by 90%
5. Approximately 80% are heavy smokers

C. Signs, symptoms, and clinical manifestations
   1. Alcoholic breath
   2. Unexplained tremors
   3. Nausea and vomiting, gastrointestinal problems, ulcers
   4. Cutaneous lesions (redness, acne, spider angiomas)
   5. Edema of the eyelids and other parts of the body
   6. Nutritional deficiencies (vitamin B, protein, calcium)

D. Long-term complications
   1. Hypertension and other types of heart disease
   2. Increased risk for various types of cancers
   3. Hepatitis, cirrhosis, and hypoglycemia
   4. Interference with secretion of pancreatic enzymes
   5. Bleeding tendencies
   6. Altered enzyme functioning and malabsorptive syndromes of the small intestine
   7. Irritation of the gastric mucosa leading to bleeding, inflammation, and ulceration
   8. Fetal alcohol syndrome (pregnant women)

E. Oral manifestations—increased incidence of:
   1. Caries caused by nausea and vomiting, neglected oral hygiene, and xerostomia
   2. Periodontal disease caused by an impaired immune system and the effects on white blood cells
   3. Glossitis and angular cheilitis from nutritional deficiencies
   4. Leukoplakia and oropharyngeal cancer (use of alcohol and tobacco products increases risk of oropharyngeal cancer)
   5. Swelling of the parotid glands leads to decreased salivation and increased caries incidence
   6. Trauma during inebriated states (accidents or fights)
   7. Attrition secondary to bruxism

End-Stage Renal Disease

A. Definition
   1. Progressive bilateral deterioration of renal function, resulting in uremia and eventual death
   2. Uremia is the toxic condition produced by retention of urinary constituents in the blood

B. Incidence and prevalence
   1. Chronic kidney disease affects approximately 20 million persons in the United States, or 1 in 9 adults; over 5-year period, the number of patients with kidney failure averaged about 90,000 annually
   2. More than 485,000 persons in the United States are being treated for end-stage renal disease; of these, more than 341,000 are patients receiving dialysis and 140,000 have undergone kidney transplantation
   3. More common in Caucasians (61%), followed by African Americans (31.7%), Hispanic (14%), Asians (4.5%), Native Americans (1.3%), and other (1.5%)

C. Etiology
1. Infectious diseases (e.g., nephritis, viral and fungal infections)
2. Hypersensitivity states (e.g., glomerulonephritis)
3. Developmental defects of the kidneys
4. Circulatory disturbances (e.g., hypertension, hemorrhages)
5. Metabolic diseases (e.g., diabetes)
6. About 10% of new cases may result from analgesic misuse

D. Signs, symptoms, and clinical manifestations
1. Mental slowness or depression
2. Swelling and edema
3. Muscular hyperactivity
4. Hyperpigmentation of the skin (brownish yellow)
5. Anorexia, vomiting, and diarrhea
6. Anemia
7. Possible functional defect in factor VIII protein, leading to hemorrhagic episodes
8. Hypertension, congestive heart failure
   a. Blood runs from the artery to the dialysis machine, is filtered, and then is returned to the vein
   b. Heparin is added to prevent blood clotting
   c. Patient is at risk for acquiring hepatitis B, hepatitis C, and hepatitis D viruses from commercial blood products
9. Kidney transplantation—problems with graft rejection and infection; use steroids, antibiotics, and immunosuppressives such as cyclosporine

E. Oral manifestations
1. Painful oral ulcerations and stomatitis from drugs
2. Candidiasis or herpetic lesions from immunosuppression
3. Increased calculus deposits
4. Anemic mucosa
5. Oral petechiae and hemorrhage
6. Ground-glass appearance of alveolar bone caused by leaching of calcium (uremic bone disease)
7. Bad taste and halitosis from urea in saliva
8. Enamel hypoplasia
9. Immunosuppressed patient who has received a transplant may have increased risk for cancer
10. Drug-influenced gingival enlargement from cyclosporine (an immunosuppressant) or nifedipine (a calcium-channel blocker)
11. Delayed eruption in primary teeth
12. Monitor for premedication needs with physician
13. Schedule appointment 24 hours after dialysis

Older Adults

A. Definition
1. Age 55 and older
2. Older/elderly adults age 68 and older

B. Incidence and prevalence
1. Approximately 13% of the U.S. population age 66 or older; fastest-growing segment of population
2. It is estimated that 20% of U.S. population will be age 65 or older by 2030
3. About 47% of older adults live in nursing home
   a. 1% of persons age 65 to 74
   b. 20% of persons age 85 or older

C. Systemic manifestations
1. Disease response—increased severity, longer course, and slower healing
2. Decreased metabolism
3. Reduced elasticity of tissues, diminished reparative ability
4. Thin, dry, wrinkled skin; delayed healing
5. Special senses
   a. 13% of persons age 70 to 74 and 31% of persons age 85 or older have a visual impairment
   b. 26% of persons age 70 to 74 and 49% of persons age 85 or older have a hearing impairment
6. Musculoskeletal changes
   a. Osteopenia and osteoporosis
   b. Osteoarthritis
   c. Loss of muscle function and tone
7. Increase in cardiovascular diseases
   a. High blood pressure
   b. Coronary heart disease
   c. Valvular disease

D. Common chronic conditions
1. Arthritis
2. Hypertension
3. Cardiovascular disease
4. Diabetes

E. Oral manifestations
1. Soft tissues
   a. Dry, purse-string lips with opening difficulties; angular cheilitis (Fig.19-22)
   b. Capillary fragility, hyperkeratosis of oral mucosa
   c. Fissures, sublingual varicosities, reduced taste from loss of taste buds of tongue
   d. Increased incidence of oral cancer

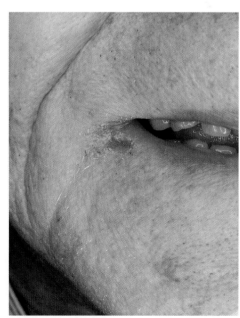

FIG 19-22 Angular cheilitis is a common oral finding in older adults because of nutritional deficiencies. (From Ibsen OAC, Phelan JA: *Oral pathology for the dental hygienist,* ed 6, St Louis, 2014, Elsevier.)

2. Hard tissues
   a. Abrasion, attrition, dark color of teeth
   b. Root caries
   c. Decreased tooth sensitivity
   d. Decreased pulp chamber size

OVERALL DENTAL MANAGEMENT CONSIDERATIONS FOR SPECIAL CARE CLIENTS

A. Personal and professional prerequisites (Table 19-14)
   1. Interview the client in a sensitive manner to gather accurate data; initiate dental hygiene process
   2. Analyze and summarize data in oral or written formats
   3. Use problem-solving skills to develop alternative strategies to manage problems
   4. Evaluate client and professional goals and progress for appropriateness and effectiveness
   5. Remain current of new conditions, new protocols for medical management, and advances in dental and dental hygiene care
   6. Apply new knowledge or techniques from other areas to dental management of special clients
   7. Apply research principles and techniques to acquire clinical data that serve as the basis for care planning and decision making
B. Office management issues
   1. Stress a team concept, with cooperation among members and coordination of information and activities; dental hygiene procedures may require the help of a dental assistant
   2. Identify and anticipate client needs and problems before initiation of care; use of a previsit questionnaire is helpful (Fig. 19-23)
   3. Obtain informed consent for treatment from the client or an appropriate representative
   4. Explain office policies, procedures, and philosophy to the client or guardian before or at the first appointment
   5. Determine financial limitations that may affect care planning or payment procedures
      a. Assess additional resources available from other sources (e.g., community organizations)
      b. Attempt to provide flexible payment alternatives
   6. If the client is unable to receive care in the office because of physical limitations or geographic distance, determine if care can be provided in the home or community setting with portable equipment
   7. If office facilities do not comply with accessibility guidelines, discuss ways to:
      a. Make them physically accessible
      b. Accommodate client needs, or refer the client to a provider who can provide access
   8. Ensure that office layout and environment are not safety hazards or health hazards for some clients
   9. Keep scheduling somewhat flexible to allow for transportation or other problems; block appointments are helpful when dealing with groups
   10. Be prepared to implement wheelchair transfers

C. Medical issues
   1. Obtain a health history from the client or caregiver, with supplemental information from other professionals or agency records
   2. Update the health history at each visit
   3. Because many standard health history forms are inadequate for the multiple conditions and problems of some clients, ask supplemental questions
   4. Obtain specifics regarding medical treatment regimens or other therapies that may affect scheduling or treatment
   5. Obtain names, addresses, and phone numbers for all the client's physicians who might provide helpful data (e.g., generalist, cardiologist, orthopedist, endocrinologist) with permission to release information
   6. Be particularly alert to the client's physical status during initial assessment
   7. Monitor vital signs, as indicated
   8. Record all medication information; update at each visit
   9. Note any indications or contraindications to treatment or premedication
   10. Maintain records of all medical advice, prescriptions, or drugs given
   11. If clients refuse to disclose medical information or do not follow recommended standard procedures for their own protection (e.g., antibiotic premedication), have them sign a statement to that effect for the records
D. Treatment adaptations
   1. Demonstrate understanding and acceptance of conditions or problems to the client and to caregivers or family
   2. Determine which special needs require provider adaptations versus client adaptations
   3. Demonstrate empathy, not sympathy
   4. Discuss before implementation:
      a. Behavioral expectations
      b. Overview of the entire care plan
      c. Procedures that will be performed at the appointment
      d. Approximate time required
      e. Communication techniques to be used during the appointment
   5. Introduce clients to the oral health care setting gradually by using desensitization, modeling, "show-tell-do," or other methods
   6. Ensure client comfort in the dental chair through frequent assurance, positioning, and supportive measures as needed (e.g., pillows)
   7. Explain carefully any need for client body restraint or stabilization for behavioral or stability purposes to ensure the clinician's safety and the client's safety while in the chair; Velcro® straps similar to safety belts are helpful for stability (Fig. 19-24); ensure the following:
      a. Obtain informed consent to use these aids
      b. Ensure least restrictive restraint is used
      c. Clearly document restraint used
      d. Check state regulations to ensure proper compliance

TABLE 19-14   Dental Management Considerations for Clients with Special Needs

Condition	Medical Issues	Barriers to Care	Other Associated Health Issues	Treatment Considerations*	Prevention/Education/Health Promotion Issues
Developmental and cognitive challenges (formerly called "mental retardation")	Syndrome Associated medical conditions and other disabilities Treatment regimens	Limited financial resources Degree of reliance on others Limited mental ability	Oral-motor dysfunction General incoordination Cariogenic foods and reinforcers Self-abuse Resistant behavior	Short, midmorning appointments Gagging: radiographs, instrument placement, positioning Consult caregiver for behavioral management approaches Mental impairment: communication, cooperation, stability in chair, limited attention span, minimize distractions Limited finances: alternative treatment plans	"Tell-show-do" approach Simple language Frequent repetition and positive reinforcement Frequent continued-care intervals, minimize distractions Alternatives for snacks and food reinforcers Chlorhexidine mouthrinses or spray, sealants ADA-approved or CDA-recognized antimicrobial mouthrinse daily
Fetal alcohol spectrum disorders (FASD), fetal alcohol syndrome (FAS)	Which organs affected? Heart? Brain Growth deficiency	Family may be dysfunctional Behavioral problems May have mental disabilities	Attention deficit disorders Dental malformations	Behavior and attention: short, structured appointments Family problems: ensure that follow-up care is understood Compliment cooperative behavior	Ensure adequate supervision for oral hygiene care Use same methods as for children with learning disabilities or developmental and cognitive challenges ADA-approved or CDA-recognized antimicrobial mouthrinse daily based on level of cooperation
Down syndrome	Possible congenital heart defect (prophylactic antibiotic premedication) Hearing and vision problems Decreased resistance to infection; frequent respiratory infections	Same as for developmental and cognitive challenges	Same as for intellectual and developmental disabilities	Same as for developmental and cognitive challenges plus small oral area: oral access for procedures Hearing and vision disorders: communication Avoid use of powered instruments with respiratory problems	Same as for developmental and cognitive challenges plus stress oral hygiene and periodontal maintenance care
Autism spectrum disorders (ASD)	No major problems unless self-abusive	Behavior Degree of reliance on others Communication, minimal Language skills	Disordered eating or fetishes Resistant behavior	Dependence on "routines"; procedure sequencing, desensitization appointment Lack of useful language: communication Learning disabilities and sensitivity to stimuli: communication, limit distractions Avoid light in eyes	Combine verbal and nonverbal communication techniques and positive reinforcers Teach toothbrushing as a "motion" rather than a function Avoid metaphors and complex language structures
Learning disabilities, attention deficit hyperactivity disorder (ADHD)	Medications and potential side effects	Depends on type of disability	Depends on disability Oral-motor dysfunction General incoordination Hyperactive behavior	Depends on disability Disorientation/hyperactivity; stability in chair; short appointments; physical contact can be alarming Minimize distractions	Focus on strengths Use combination of teaching approaches Maintain attention through eye contact and physical contact; involve caregiver Consistency important

(Continued)

TABLE 19-14 Dental Management Considerations for Clients with Special Needs—cont'd

Condition	Medical Issues	Barriers to Care	Other Associated Health Issues	Treatment Considerations*	Prevention/Education/Health Promotion Issues
Emotional disturbance or mental illness	Medications and potential side effects; Psychological causes of reported symptoms or diseases, fears	Limited financial resources in some cases; Emotional concerns and fears; Disturbed thought processes	Depends on nature of disturbance; Inadequate diet or strange food practices; Phobias about oral care; Self-abuse; Side effects of medications	Anxiety, fear, aggression: stability in chair, cooperation, communication, safety for patient and clinician	Reality orientation techniques; Possible dietary counseling; Involve caregivers; Positive reinforcement and repetition; For xerostomia, recommend a dry-mouth management protocol that includes saliva substitutes, ice chips and drinking water, daily use of xylitol-containing products, fluoride therapy, and calcium phosphate therapy; ADA-approved or CDA-recognized antimicrobial mouthrinse daily
Disordered eating	Symptoms; Amount of weight loss; Presence and frequency of bulimia; Medical and psychological interventions; Eating patterns	Psychological status; Denial of symptoms; Length of treatment; Compliance with appointments	Eating patterns; Frequent vomiting; Xerostomia; Depression; Life-threatening risk factors: conflict, life crises, major life changes, need for control and approval	Plan for referral and coordinated care with physicians, nutritionist, and psychologist; Carious or eroded teeth: restorations, margination of restorations; Anxiety: psychosedation; Pit-and-fissure sealants if appropriate; Study models to monitor progression of tooth structure loss	Rinsing with sodium bicarbonate after vomiting rather than using toothbrush; Neutral-pH sodium fluoride rinses or stannous fluoride gels used daily; Frequent continued-care intervals; For xerostomia, recommend a dry-mouth management protocol that includes saliva substitutes, ice chips and drinking water, daily use of xylitol-containing products, fluoride therapy, and calcium phosphate therapy; ADA-approved or CDA-recognized antimicrobial mouthrinse daily
Alzheimer's disease	Multiple medical problems; Medications; Reduced bowel and bladder control; Fatigue from abnormal sleep patterns; Wheelchair	Behavior: uncooperative; Finances may be limited by disability and medical problems; Dependence on others	Oral-motor dysfunction; Depression or disorientation leading to oral neglect; General motor dysfunction; Potential for injury	Dental consult as soon as possible after diagnosis; Fluctuating moods and disorientation: short appointments, communication, cooperation, safety; Motor problems: oral access, radiographs, stability in chair; Memory loss: data collection; Never leave unattended; May need sedation; Do not force client to have treatment	Involve caregivers; Involve client when most lucid and positive; Simple instructions and frequent repetition; Positive reinforcement; Frequent continued-care intervals; Prevent oral injury; Aggressive preventive program; Powered oral hygiene aids
Seizure disorders	Medications and side effects; Drug induces leukopenia and thrombocytopenia; Seizure information; Type of disorder; Frequency and how well controlled; General management; History of status epilepticus	Disturbance in self-image; Transportation if cannot drive; Embarrassment	Side effects of medications; Potential for orofacial trauma during seizures	Seizure activity: precipitating factors, treatment planning, appointment scheduling, stability in chair, communication; stop procedures if seizure occurs; Avoid NSAIDs and aspirin; Replace missing teeth with fixed not removable appliances; Drug-influenced gingival enlargement from phenytoin; Prolonged bleeding time from valproic acid; Assess if medications are taken as prescribed	Optimal oral hygiene and frequent continued-care intervals to control gingival enlargement from phenytoin; First-aid instructions for oral trauma; Positive reinforcement and self-image building; Chlorhexidine mouthrinses or spray; For xerostomia, recommend a dry-mouth management protocol that includes saliva substitutes, ice chips and drinking water, daily use of xylitol-containing products, fluoride therapy, and calcium phosphate therapy

Condition				
Visual impairment	Degree of impairment / Sensitivity to light / Treated versus untreated conditions / Degree of dependence on others / Attitudes and stereotypes about disability and toward guide dogs / Physical obstacles to or in office	Difficulty monitoring oral status	Determine level of assistance needed / Sight impairment: appointment scheduling, explanation of procedures, communication, positioning of light, mobility in clinic, data collection; Guide dog: role and placement in office / Use other senses to connect with client	Large print with written instructions / Demonstrate procedures on finger / "Tell-show-do" approach / Precede actions with clear verbal descriptions / Have client explore own mouth prior to oral hygiene instructions / Involve caregiver when necessary / Use audio aids or physical models for teaching / ADA-recognized or CDA-recognized antimicrobial mouthrinse daily
Hearing impairment	Degree of impairment / Use interpreter or other assistive devices / Functioning of hearing aid / Degree of dependence on others / Communication: sign language, lip reading, inaccurate pronunciation	No specific factors	Hearing impairment appointment scheduling, explanation of procedures, clinician position, use of normal tone of voice for lip reader, communication, data collection, noise interference, use of hearing aid during appointment / Many pretend to hear out of embarrassment / Remove mask when talking or use clear face shield because may be lip reader	Determine appropriate communication techniques / Provide paper and pencil, if desired / Involve interpreter if needed / Watch facial expressions / Demonstrate when possible / Make cards with frequently used phrases / Use physical models for teaching / ADA-approved or CDA-recognized antimicrobial mouthrinse daily
Cleft lip or palate	Hearing impairment / Upper respiratory tract infections / Prosthetic appliances / Medications / Diet / Fear of health care providers / Self-image problems	Missing or malaligned teeth / Oral-motor dysfunction / Feeding disorders	Cleft: clear communication, instrument positioning or fulcruming, suctioning and prevention of aspiration / Fear: dental procedures, cooperation	Instruct in cleaning any prosthetic aids / Involve caregiver, when necessary / Dietary counseling, if needed
Cerebral palsy	Associated disorders / Medications / Other therapies / Respiration impaired? / Presence of primitive reflexes / Degree of impairment / Communication / Transportation if in wheelchair or cannot drive / May have limited financial resources / Degree of dependence on others for care / Mobility issues if in wheelchair / Provider attitudes toward condition / Self-image problems	Oral-motor dysfunction / General motor dysfunction / Special diets	Primitive reflexes: client or clinician position, instrument positioning or fulcruming, stability, oral access, suctioning and amount of water used / Treatment based on what client can tolerate / Avoid use of powered instruments / Radiographs (few at a time) / Wheelchair transfers; calm treatment environment: relaxation needed to avoid muscle spasms / Do not force arms and legs in unnatural positions / May need sedation or muscle relaxants for extensive treatment / Minimize distractions / Softly cradle client's head during treatment	Modified or powered toothbrush / Involve caregivers as appropriate / Be patient with slowness of responses and progress / Use combination of communication methods with consistency and repetition / Assess need for adaptive aids for home care / Frequent continued care / Fluoride therapy, sealants, and antimicrobials if needed / Simple, concrete instructions / Involuntary movements and safety issues, may need restraints (consent necessary) / ADA-approved or CDA-recognized antimicrobial mouthrinse daily
Bell's palsy	Therapies, especially prednisone / Duration of condition / Possible surgery to achieve facial symmetry / Language skills / Self-image problems	Oral-motor dysfunction / anesthesia used or opposite side affected precautions needed	Lack of eye closure: protection of eyes (goggles) / Oral-motor dysfunction: protection of airway / Corticosteroid therapy	Caution regarding effects of anesthesia / Frequent rinsing or toothbrushing for food retention of affected side / Antimicrobial mouthrinse daily

(Continued)

TABLE 19-14 Dental Management Considerations for Clients with Special Needs—cont'd

Condition	Medical Issues	Barriers to Care	Other Associated Health Issues	Treatment Considerations*	Prevention/Education/Health Promotion Issues
Myasthenia gravis	Medications; History of radiation therapy or surgery; History of myasthenic crises	Communication; Client may hold chin to help during speaking	Oral-motor dysfunction; Choking risk myasthenia crisis from stress	Weakness increases during day: schedule short appointments in morning; Drug interaction; Amide types of local anesthetics used; Oral-motor dysfunction, paralysis, and impaired breathing: protection of airway, use of rubber dam, suctioning, chair position, mouth props; Difficulty retaining dentures; Be prepared for emergency; Avoid use of powered instruments	Frequent continued-care intervals to prevent infection; Frequent rinsing or toothbrushing for food retention; Fluoride therapy, if needed; Modified toothbrush or powered oral hygiene aids; ADA-approved or CDA-recognized antimicrobial mouthrinse daily
Parkinson's disease	Medications and side effects; Rigidity of larger muscles; Tremors; Sensitivity to heat	Mobility to and in office; Communication	Oral-motor dysfunction; Side effects of drugs; Xerostomia; Possible inadequate diet; Hypersalivation	Tremors: stability, instrumentation, radiographs; Sensitivity to heat: temperature of operatory; Muscular pain and joint rigidity: chair position, appointment length; Slurred speech: communication	Frequent continued care; Frequent rinsing and toothbrushing; Adaptive equipment or assistance if needed; Fluoride therapy; Counseling about side effects of medications; Antimicrobial mouthrinse daily
Arthritis	Medications; Degree of impairment; Joints affected: pain; Joint replacement (premedication may be needed); Potential for adrenal suppression with long-term corticosteroid use	Mobility to and in office; Limited finances, if disabled; Weakness or fatigue decreases motivation to seek care	General motor impairment; Drug-related complications such as prolonged bleeding and bone marrow suppression	Steroid therapy; Joint pain: chair position, appointment length; Limited oral opening: positioning, instrumentation, radiographs, TMJ assessment; Joint replacement: antibiotic premedication; Long-term aspirin therapy: prolonged bleeding	Adaptive equipment or assistance is needed; Counseling about side effects of medications; Prevent sources of oral infection
Fibromyalgia syndrome (FMS)	Biophysical issues, fatigue, sleep, depression, stress, cognitive impairments, comorbidities of migraines, Sjögren syndrome, cystitis, chronic fatigue	Muscle pain; Discomfort in supine position; Decreased platelet formation from large doses of NSAIDs	Side effects of medications; Comorbidities: depression, chronic facial muscle pain, migraines, irritable bowel syndrome, fatigue	May not be able to endure long appointments; Pain or fatigue in orofacial region limits opening: TMJ pain; Chair position: discomfort with supine position; Last-minute cancellations due to pain; Four-handed dentistry to promote efficacy in time; Stress-free appointment; Cervical pillows	Dietary counseling; Frequent continued care; Modified oral care devices; Written self-care instructions; Xerostomia management
Scleroderma	Extensive and often rapidly progressive skin indurations as well as involvement of multiple internal organ systems; Overall range of motion becomes highly compromised	Mobility	May need premedication because of immunosuppressive therapies	Prone to oral disease; Early treatment intervention are important complications when implementing dental hygiene care; As disease worsens, more problems opening mouth; Swallowing problems; avoid powered instruments; Four-handed dentistry	Xerostomia management; Oral self-care modifications; Frequent continued care; Oral stretching exercises; Avoid powered instruments with swallowing issues

Condition				
Multiple sclerosis	Medications and side effects Degree of facial pain Degree of impairment Sensitivity to heat Mobility to and in office, especially if in wheelchair Depression or moodiness Limited finances if disabled	Special diets Side effects of drugs Fine motor coordination problems Oral-motor dysfunction Infection Fatigue, stress, and pain	Weakness and numbness: wheelchair transfer, stability, appointment length Oral-motor dysfunction: protection of airway Mood changes: communication, acceptance of treatment, cooperation Sensitivity to heat: room temperature Periods of exacerbation or remission: appointment scheduling	Oral care: adaptive equipment or assistance may be needed More frequent rinsing and brushing Assistance in dietary counseling Fluoride therapy Antimicrobial mouthrinse daily More frequent continued-care intervals to prevent infections Refer for TMD assessment Importance of healthy periodontium: infection can cause exacerbation of multiple sclerosis
Muscular dystrophies	Medications Other therapies Type and degree of involvement Prognosis Obesity, scoliosis, or cardiopulmonary involvement? Depends on type Mobility to and in office, especially if in wheelchair Limited financial resources Weakness and possible decreased life span	Balance issues Oral-motor dysfunction General motor weakness and incoordination Dietary inadequacies Mouth breathing	Facial muscle weakness can interfere with appointment length and self-care Depends on type and degree of involvement Muscle weakness: stability in chair, wheelchair transfers, radiographs, instrumentation, appointment length Oral-motor dysfunction: protection of airway, communication Incoordination: restorative treatment planning and possible emergency care Limited life span: treatment planning, motivation	Frequent continued care More frequent brushing and rinsing Fluoride therapy ADA-approved or CDA-recognized antimicrobial mouthrinse daily Adapted equipment or physical assistance for oral care Powered oral hygiene aids
Spinal injuries	Depends on level of injury Medications Respiratory involvement Decubitus ulcers Incontinence and encopresis Contractures Heterotopic ossifications Body temperature regulation Potential for autonomic hyperreflexia Type of adaptive equipment Mobility to and in office, especially if in wheelchair or on respirator Limited financial resources Psychosocial concerns or depression Poor self-image	Depends on level of injury Oral-motor dysfunction Limited or total dependence on others Special diets	Psychological state: communication, cooperation Spasticity, tremors: stability Paralysis: mobility, wheelchair transfers, stability in chair, length of appointment, graphs Impaired respiration and oral-motor dysfunction: chair position, use of rubber dam, protection of airway, instrumentation Mouth stick appliance	Powered or adaptive equipment or physical assistance needed Fluoride therapy ADA-approved or CDA-recognized antimicrobial mouthrinse daily Emphasize self-care to degree possible
Spina bifida	Depends on type Similar to spinal injuries Shunt for hydrocephalus (consult physician for antibiotic premedication) Seizure disorders Depends on type and degree of impairment Similar to spinal injuries	Similar to spinal injuries, except oral-motor dysfunction not apparent	Similar to spinal injuries, although psychological state not as poor Latex sensitivity	Learning disabilities influence dental health education methods Powered oral hygiene aids
Acquired immunodeficiency syndrome (AIDS; see	Systems involved Degree of impairment Consult with physician Kaposi's sarcoma Treatment regimens Finding dentist who will treat Fear of rejection and discrimination	Oral infections Debilitated state	Oral infections (e.g., candidiasis); transmission potential Kaposi's sarcoma: treatment planning Psychological state: communication, motivation Gingivitis should be treated to prevent necrotizing ulcerative periodontitis	Palliative care for oral infections and oral ulceration Increased attention to oral hygiene ADA-approved or CDA-recognized antimicrobial mouthrinse daily

(Continued)

TABLE 19-14   Dental Management Considerations for Clients with Special Needs—cont'd

Condition	Medical Issues	Barriers to Care	Other Associated Health Issues	Treatment Considerations*	Prevention/Education/Health Promotion Issues
Chapters 8 and 9)	Predisposition to multiple opportunistic infections Immunosuppressive medications	Stigma associated with disease Decreased motivation or depression Limited finances if unemployed, underinsured, or uninsured		Povidone-iodine: use with initial debridement with necrotizing ulcerative periodontitis Antibiotic may be needed	Frequent recare
Cystic fibrosis	Degree of impairment and prognosis Dietary changes Treatment regimens Chronic pulmonary disease Abnormal viscous secretions causing damage to major organs, such as lungs, pancreas, and liver	Small stature may cause embarrassment Prognosis may decrease motivation Finances may be limited Short life span	Decreased resistance to infections Pulmonary complications compounded by problems of malabsorption and malnutrition Recurrent attacks of pneumonia, bronchiectasis	Mucus accumulations and impaired breathing: chair position, appointment scheduling and length, coughing, protection of airway, use of rubber dam Avoid use of air polisher and ultrasonic scaler Cooperation and scheduling issues Susceptibility to infections: appointment scheduling Tetracycline staining: esthetics, treatment planning	For xerostomia, recommend a dry-mouth management protocol that includes saliva substitutes, ice chips and drinking water, daily use of xylitol-containing products, fluoride therapy, and calcium phosphate therapy Frequent oral care because of mouth breathing Low-fat diet Recommend tartar-control products ADA-approved or CDA-recognized antimicrobial mouthrinse daily
Chronic obstructive pulmonary disease (COPD)	Single or coexisting conditions Degree of impairment Medications or need for oxygen	Portable oxygen Fear of procedures that impair breathing	Side effects of medications	Impaired respiration: upright position, suctioning and coughing, no nitrous oxide–oxygen sedation in severe cases rubber dam, orthopnea Medications: avoid those that depress respiration, N_2O-O_2 may be used, drug interactions Avoid use of air polisher and ultrasonic scaler	Same as for bronchial asthma
Bronchial asthma	Type and severity of asthma Frequency and severity of attacks Precipitating factors Treatment regimens History of hospitalizations or status asthmaticus Instruct patient to bring inhalers if used Screen for sensitivity to NSAIDs	Fear of medical and dental environments Allergens in office	No specific risk factors Maxillofacial growth altered with childhood asthma	Anxiety: possible premedication or relaxation techniques Type of asthma, history of attacks Medications and precipitating factors: contraindications to prescribing or using certain drugs such as aspirin or β-blockers Avoid use of air polisher and ultrasonic scaler Medical emergency preparedness, eliminate allergens Have bronchodilator present Use of local anesthetic without epinephrine or levonordefrin in some cases; N_2O-O_2 contraindicated Avoid aspirin-containing medications and NSAIDs	Stress-free environment For xerostomia, recommend a dry-mouth management protocol that includes saliva substitutes, ice chips and drinking water, daily use of xylitol-containing products, fluoride therapy, and calcium phosphate therapy ADA-approved or CDA-recognized antimicrobial mouthrinse daily

Condition					
Congenital heart disease	Type and if repaired Extent of limitations Medications Prognosis Need for antibiotic premedication Physician consult	Financial constraints from medical bills Frequent illness Possibly debilitated state Overprotective attitude of parents	Decreased resistance to infections	Bleeding potential in some cases: treatment planning, need for laboratory tests, possible referral to specialist Prophylactic antibiotic premedication, stress management protocols, chair position	Emphasize danger of intraoral infections in terms of aggravating heart condition Frequent continued-care intervals Prevention of infective endocarditis ADA-approved or CDA-recognized antimicrobial mouthrinse daily
Rheumatic fever and heart disease	Residual effects of rheumatic fever	No specific barriers	Rheumatic fever Pharyngeal infection with group A streptococci	Consult with cardiologist Antimicrobial rinse before treatment	Stress oral hygiene to prevent oral infections and self-induced bacteremias Antimicrobial mouthrinse daily No specific preventive regimens
Cardiac arrhythmias and dysrhythmias	Symptoms Medications and side effects Presence of pacemaker and type	Excessive bleeding if taking blood thinner Avoidance of certain electromagnetic equipment with older pacemakers	No specific risk factors Development of dysrhythmias or arrhythmias from cocaine-epinephrine interactions in cocaine abusers	Only treat for preventive measures if stable Pacemaker: if not shielded, may need to avoid electromagnetic equipment: check with physician Limit epinephrine to less than 2 carpules of 1:100,000 Patient taking digoxin: no epinephrine Blood thinner: INR 3.5 or less Set upright: minimize x-ray films Arrhythmia: stress management protocol, drug precautions, bleeding potential from medications	For xerostomia, recommend a dry-mouth management protocol that includes saliva substitutes, ice chips and drinking water, daily use of xylitol-containing products, fluoride therapy, and calcium phosphate therapy
Hypertensive disease	Vital sign monitoring Physician consult or referral Medications and side effects and other treatment regimens Cause: primary or secondary Predisposing or general risk factors Severity, symptoms Possibility of orthostatic hypotension	Anxiety about oral health care	Side effects of medications Potential for stroke, myocardial infarction, and renal failure Potential for adverse drug interactions between vasoconstrictors and antihypertensive drugs Limit use of vasoconstrictor in anesthetics	Hypertension: stress management protocols, chair position, treatment planning, monitoring vital signs, short appointment Overly stressed: terminate appointment Medications: drug interactions Limit epinephrine to less than 2 anesthetic carpules of 1:1000,000 Bleeding potential, pain control, xerostomia, gingival enlargement BP 180/110 mm Hg: delay treatment and refer to physician	Counseling regarding reducing general risk factors Palliative care for oral infections from medications For xerostomia, recommend a dry-mouth management protocol that includes saliva substitutes, ice chips and drinking water, daily use of xylitol-containing products, fluoride therapy, and calcium phosphate therapy Create stress-free environment Prevent postural hypertension
Ischemic heart disease (coronary atherosclerotic heart disease)	Physician consult Angina or myocardial infarction episodes Hospitalizations Medications and side effects Surgery	Possible debilitated state Medical and other expenses Anxiety about dental treatment	Side effect of medications Susceptibility to infections if debilitated Limit use of vasoconstrictor in anesthetics	Heart condition: same considerations as for hypertensive disease and preparation for medical emergency, contraindications to treatment if unstable or recent attack (within 3 to 6 months) Medications: same as for hypertensive disease; pain control Aspirin use: bleeding concerns, INR less than 3.6	Palliative care for side effects of medications Counseling on decreasing general risk factors Special oral hygiene instructions if hospitalized or bedridden Frequent maintenance visits Create stress-free environment Educate about increased risk for myocardial infarction in clients with periodontitis Antimicrobial mouthrinse daily

(Continued)

TABLE 19-14 Dental Management Considerations for Clients with Special Needs—cont'd

Condition	Medical Issues	Barriers to Care	Other Associated Health Issues	Treatment Considerations*	Prevention/Education/Health Promotion Issues
Congestive heart failure	Same as for severe ischemic or hypertensive heart disease	Mobility Debilitated Labored breathing	Pulmonary congestion and edema Limit use of vasoconstrictor in anesthetics	Avoid use of air polisher and ultrasonic scaler Prone to nausea and vomiting during oral health care Keep client upright in chair	Frequent continued-care intervals Create stress-free environment ADA-approved or CDA-recognized antimicrobial mouthrinse daily
Cerebrovascular accident (CVA, stroke)	Type of involvement, degree of limitation Medications and side effects Other therapies	Communication Accessibility if need adaptive equipment or wheelchair Degree of dependence on others	Oral-motor dysfunction Side effects of medications Impaired general motor coordination Dietary inadequacies Transient ischemic attacks Previous stroke, hypertension, cardiac abnormalities, atherosclerosis, diabetes mellitus, elevated blood lipid levels	Dental treatment could precipitate CVA Memory and speech impairment: communication, data collection Oral-motor dysfunction or paralysis: radiographs, instrumentation, jaw stability, treatment planning Impaired emotional control: cooperation, communication Evaluate calcifications in carotid artery with panoramic radiographs Short, morning appointments General paralysis: mobility, possible wheelchair transfers, stability in chair Minimize use of epinephrine Avoid elective dental care for 6 months Potential bleeding problems	Use combination of teaching approaches Reinforce and repeat instructions Frequent continued care Fluoride therapy, if needed ADA-approved or CDA-recognized antimicrobial mouthrinse daily Adaptive aids or supervision for oral care Avoid sensory overload Reorient client to situation; rinsing difficult or impossible Use one-step instructions Educate about increased CVA risk in clients with periodontitis
Sickle cell disease	Precipitating factors for crises Symptoms and severity Associated conditions Transfusions? Lab tests needed Physician consult regarding need for antibiotic premedication	Periods of pain Debilitated condition at times Fear of dental environment Limited financial resources because of medical bills	Susceptibility to infections Low stress tolerance	Sickle cell crises: emergency care only Susceptibility to infections: periodontal maintenance, physician consult for prophylactic antibiotic premedication Reduce patient stress Consultation with physician Avoid medications that depress respiration Limit epinephrine	Dietary counseling Frequent maintenance care because of associated alveolar bone problems and need to control oral infection Involvement of others in client's care Create a stress-free oral health care environment Emphasis on optimal oral health care behaviors because periodontitis can cause a crisis Antimicrobial mouthrinse daily
Cancers	Parts of body affected, treatment regimens, medications and side effects, potential for bleeding and anemia Physician consult regarding need for antibiotic premedication	Frequent hospitalization or medical appointments Debilitated states Financial burdens Reliance on others Depression	Side effects of medications Oral infections and ulcerations Metastasis to oral cavity Weakness for self-care	Radiation therapy: care before and after Prevention and palliative care for oral infections and ulcerations Short appointments and frequent active follow-up Potential bleeding problem Prompt treatment of dental-related infections Evaluate need for antibiotic premedication	Radiation therapy: care before and after With cues, if bleeding is a problem Fluoride therapy Antimicrobial mouthrinse daily Oral hygiene aids Help with oral care, if needed Monitor removable appliances Frequent maintenance care For xerostomia, recommend a dry-mouth management protocol that includes saliva substitutes, ice chips and drinking water, daily use of xylitol-containing products, fluoride therapy, calcium phosphate therapy, and antifungals, as needed

Condition				
Leukemias	Type Treatment regimens, frequency Presence of anemia Monitor bleeding time Thrombocytopenia and infection Immunosuppression from therapy	Stages of acute disease versus remissions Fear of dental environment	Side effects of chemotherapy or radiation therapy Candidiasis Susceptibility to infections Oral hemorrhage	Bleeding potential: platelet count status needed—avoid treatment if less than 50,000/mm^3 Appointment scheduling, physician consult, surgical procedures Susceptibility to infections: periodontal maintenance, antibiotic premedication Ideally, provide invasive care before chemotherapy or radiation therapy Acute versus remission stages: treatment planning, appointment scheduling Chemotherapy or radiation therapy: treatment planning Consultation with oncologist	Palliative care for oral lesions Frequent continued-care intervals Fluoride therapy program Involvement of others in care program For xerostomia, recommend a dry-mouth management protocol that includes saliva substitutes, ice chips and drinking water, daily use of xylitol-containing products, fluoride therapy, and calcium phosphate therapy Eliminate potential sources of oral infection Meticulous oral hygiene ADA-approved or CDA-recognized antimicrobial mouthrinse daily
Congenital disorders of coagulation: hemophilias	Type and severity Frequency and location of bleeds Treatment regimens Joint replacements Hepatitis AIDS? Seizures Inhibitor status Laboratory tests needed	Finding dentist who will treat Resources for emergency care	Potential for oral bleeds Potential to acquire hepatitis, cirrhosis, or AIDS-associated disease with frequent clotting-factor replacement therapy	Bleeding potential: preappointment laboratory tests, surgery, physician consult, clotting-factor replacement therapy, instrumentation, radiographs, use of rubber dam, suctioning, use of aminocaproic acid (Amicar) or tranexamic acid (Cyklokapron) Joint replacements: prophylactic antibiotic premedication Hepatitis carrier: disease transmission procedures Avoid use of aspirin	Use extra-soft–bristled brush ADA-approved or CDA-recognized antimicrobial mouthrinse daily Counseling regarding first aid for oral trauma Frequent continued-care intervals Educate about role of oral infection and increased bleeding
Diabetes mellitus	Type and severity Medication regimens Poor wound healing Dietary regimen Complications Hypertension and other heart conditions Frequency of episodes of hypoglycemia or hyperglycemia	Finding dentist who will treat if have chronic complications	Susceptibility to infections (e.g., oral candidiasis) Decreased salivary flow Recalcitrant periodontal disease Slow healing Complications associated with disturbances in vision and kidney function	Insulin-sugar balance: potential for medical emergency, appointment scheduling, stress management protocol Susceptibility to infection: periodontal maintenance, possible antibiotic premedication Monitor hemoglobin A$_{1c}$ status Avoid elective treatment, if uncontrolled HbA$_{1c}$ greater than 9 15 g of oral carbohydrate available for hypoglycemia reaction	3- to 6-month continued-care intervals Dietary analysis For xerostomia, recommend a dry-mouth management protocol that includes saliva substitutes, ice chips and drinking water, daily use of xylitol-containing products, fluoride therapy, and calcium phosphate therapy Need for excellent bacterial biofilm control Antimicrobial mouthrinse daily Minimize stress Control of oral infections Prevention of insulin shock or diabetic coma Role of periodontitis in blood glucose control

(Continued)

TABLE 19-14   Dental Management Considerations for Clients with Special Needs—cont'd

Condition	Medical Issues	Barriers to Care	Other Associated Health Issues	Treatment Considerations*	Prevention/Education/Health Promotion Issues
Thyroid disease	Type and cause Symptoms and severity Medications Cardiac arrhythmias/dysrhythmias	No specific barriers Swelling of tongue in hypothyroidism may cause difficulty in speech communication	Abnormal dental development Thyroid crisis is life threatening Osteoporosis	Sensitivity to drugs: treatment planning, postoperative instruction, preparation for medical emergency Developmental and cognitive challenges in some (see previous entry) Abnormal dental development: treatment planning Heat or cold intolerance: room temperature, length of appointment "Thyroid storm" or thyroid crisis precipitated by surgery, infection, trauma, or uncontrolled thyroid disease Exaggerated response to central nervous system depressants	Prevention of infection ADA-approved or CDA-recognized antimicrobial mouthrinse daily Prevention of thyroid crisis Create a stress-free environment
Chemical dependency	Obtaining adequate history Types of drugs used Symptoms Treatment interventions Potential for drug interactions or overdose Emotional stability during appointment At risk for AIDS, hepatitis	Emotional state Denial of drug problem Demanding requests for use of nitrous oxide or pain medications Disoriented behavior	Neglect personal hygiene Potential for oral trauma Potential link (not documented) to oral cancer Potential drug interaction if local anesthetic with epinephrine is injected into blood vessel	Coordinated care: professional team and family if in treatment program Use of drugs for procedure: restrict Strict guidelines for keeping appointments necessary Avoid local anesthesia with epinephrine for 6 hours after cocaine or methamphetamine use Complete as much treatment as possible per visit Drug use can alter anesthesia effectiveness Avoid prescribing controlled medications	Encourage to seek medical care Frequent brushing and flossing Teach oral self-examinations Avoid mouthrinses containing alcohol Topical fluoride program
Chronic alcohol abuse and dependence	Client's perception of severity of problem Nutritional deficiencies Chronic complications Degree of liver impairment At risk for tuberculosis	Potential for no-show appointments or intoxication at appointment	Susceptibility to infection Nutritional deficiencies Nausea and vomiting Potential for oral trauma	Liver impairment and bleeding potential: preappointment laboratory testing, drug metabolism, instrumentation, treatment planning Inebriated states: emergency care, appointment scheduling, treatment planning, data collection Use only alcohol-free medicaments Recommend alcohol-free mouthrinses	Nutritional counseling Frequent continued-care intervals Fluoride therapy and alcohol-free antimicrobials Frequent soft tissue evaluation for oral cancer Counseling regarding oral trauma For xerostomia, recommend a dry-mouth management protocol that includes saliva substitutes, ice chips and drinking water, daily use of xylitol-containing products, fluoride therapy, and calcium phosphate therapy Instill responsibility for oral care Counsel to avoid alcohol prior to premedication

Condition					
End-stage renal disease	Symptoms and severity Hypertension Dialysis? Transplantation? Special diets Need for antibiotic premedication Excretion of drugs Electrolyte and fluid imbalance	Finding dentist who will treat Debilitated condition at times Limited finances Fear of oral health care environment	Susceptibility to oral infection Dietary inadequacies Viral hepatitis Drug-influenced gingival enlargement from cyclosporine	Physician consult Hypertension and kidney failure: vital signs, drug interactions; avoid use of drugs metabolized by the kidney Bleeding tendency: preappointment blood tests, consult with patient's physician Schedule dental treatment the day after dialysis Atrioventricular fistula: consult physician for antibiotic premedication; take blood pressure in arm without fistula Dialysis: scheduling Transplants: elective care postponed for 6 months posttransplant Prophylactic antibiotic premedication: amoxicillin and metronidazole	3- to 6-month continued-care interval because of increased calculus Prevent infection Palliative care for oral lesions Daily home fluoride therapy Tartar control dentifrices Chlorhexidine mouthrinses
Pregnancy	Trimester Side effects Nutritional status Rise in progesterone levels Significant changes in the immune response	Frequent sickness Physical comfort Nausea and sensitivity to various odors	Possible dietary inadequacies Vulnerability of fetus during first trimester Increased incidence of gingivitis	Fetal sensitivity: avoidance of drugs and elective dental procedures and elective x-ray films; use paralleling techniques for necessary exposures with lead apron on patients front and back Chair position: orthostatic hypotension (turn on left side to alleviate pressure) Safest period to provide routine care is second trimester Short appointments Caution with nitrous oxide; 30 minutes at 50% oxygen	Prenatal counseling Optimal oral hygiene to decrease gingival inflammatory changes Education on relationship among oral biofilm, hormone level, and periodontal disease Education on increased risk for preterm and low-birth-weight delivery in clients who are pregnant and have periodontitis Education on relationship between caries process and gastric acids from vomiting Education on vertical and horizontal disease transmission, care of infant's oral cavity, and causes of early childhood caries (may need to initiate xylitol protocol) Daily home fluoride therapy and sodium bicarbonate mouthrinses (before toothbrushing if episodes of vomiting) Healthy diet Antimicrobial mouthrinse daily
Older adult	Medications and potential side effects Chronic diseases Joint replacements Sensory impairments Reduced disease resistance	Transportation problems Finances may be limited Person may be depressed	Side effects of medications Physical side effects of chronic diseases Anatomical changes of gingiva	Identify side effects of medications Sensory impairments Short appointments in midmorning Increased risk for root caries Assess need for sodium fluoride therapy (home and in office) Assess need for antibiotic premedication	Instruct person about oral cancer self-examination and risk factors Instruct in oral hygiene and modifications of oral hygiene devices For xerostomia, recommend a dry-mouth management protocol that includes saliva substitutes, ice chips and drinking water, daily use of xylitol-containing products, fluoride therapy, and calcium phosphate therapy Make suggestions gradually Antimicrobial mouthrinse daily

*Standard precautions for infection control are used at each appointment.

ADA, American Dental Association; CDA, Canadian Dental Association; NSAIDs, nonsteroidal anti-inflammatory drugs; TMJ, temporomandibular joint; TMD, temporomandibular disorder; INR, international normalized ratio.

Name_____ Telephone_____

Address_____ Age _____

Name and address of contact person (if different)   Telephone _____

_____

_____

_____

Physician _____ Specialty _____ Telephone _____

Physician _____ Specialty _____ Telephone _____

Medical problems or disabling conditions _____

_____

Potential barriers:

Transportation _____

Finances _____

Communication _____

Psychosocial _____

Cultural _____

Medical _____

Mobility/stability _____

Other _____

Scheduling limitations _____

Other data _____

FIG 19-23 Previsit questionnaire for gathering preliminary data about individuals with special needs.

8. Pharmacologic restraints such as oral, intramuscular, intravenous, or inhalation sedation may be needed; general anesthesia is sometimes necessary when a client is not easily stimulated or has partial or complete loss of protective reflexes

9. Be aware that adaptations for specific procedures require problem solving and experimentation among the provider, client, and caregiver, if appropriate; Fig. 19-25 displays a variety of mouth props

10. Discuss the mechanisms for wheelchair transfers with each client; preferences and techniques vary

11. Protect the client's airway through use of a rubber dam, adequate suctioning, and other means; this is of paramount importance because of the frequency of impaired oral reflexes

12. Some pediatric clients' behavior may improve if they bring comfort items such as a stuffed animal or a blanket; asking the caregiver to sit nearby or hold the child's hand may be helpful as well

13. For the most part, keep appointments short and positive

14. Fluoride therapies (varnishes) and antimicrobial rinses are important preventive measures

15. Stress the importance of good oral health being part of good general health

E. Preventive measures

1. Identify risk factors for oral disease to plan preventive programs that:
   a. Maximize positive health behaviors
   b. Eliminate risk factors
   c. Eliminate existing disease

FIG 19-24 The Rainbow® Stabilizing System. **A,** Adult on large hinged board. **B,** Child with elbow and knee stabilizers that prohibit movement of joints. **C,** Head stabilizer. **D,** Safety belts for securing the client safely in the dental chair. (Used with permission from Specialized Care, Hampton, NH.)

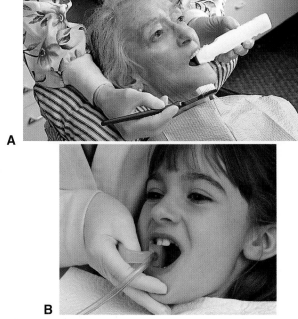

FIG 19-25 A, Clinician shown using the OpenWide® Disposable Mouth Prop on an adult. **B,** Clinician shown using the OpenWide® Re-Usable Mouth Prop that allows for a saliva ejector to be kept in place with the bite block. (Used with permission from Specialized Care, Hampton, NH.)

2. Common risk factors
   a. Inappropriate nursing and feeding habits
   b. Transfer of oral pathogens from mother or caregiver to infant (vertical transmission); usually from sharing food and eating utensils; can also occur among siblings or playmates (horizontal transmission)
   c. Nutritionally inadequate diet
   d. Frequent intake of cariogenic foods
   e. Suboptimal fluoride supplementation
   f. Oral-motor dysfunction (e.g., hyperactive gag reflex or impaired tongue control)
   g. General motor dysfunction interfering with oral hygiene care
   h. Crisis orientation to care
   i. Preoccupation with one's disability; depression
   j. Previous negative experience with health care
   k. Limited income and education
   l. Different cultural values and beliefs
3. Develop individualized programs to reduce or eliminate the risk factors and increase the protective factors
4. Consider the client's limitations when recommending home care procedures
   a. Problems with fluoride or antimicrobial rinses or disclosing tablets if the client has oral-motor problems

b. Problems performing the sequence of toothbrushing strokes if the client has memory or general motor impairment; Fig. 19-26 displays a modified toothbrush for easier accessibility

c. Problems picking up and using a toothbrush and toothpaste if the client has paralysis or control problems

d. Power toothbrushing and flossing devices can work well, but some patients may respond poorly since they can be frightened by the noise

5. Provide anticipatory guidance to parents on milestones and preventive measures at each developmental stage

6. Schedule frequent maintenance care appointments

7. Coordinate preventive efforts in the home, school, day care, workplace, or oral health care settings

8. Encourage the establishment of a dental home

FIG 19-26 The Surround® Toothbrush has a unique head that surrounds the tooth to clean all surfaces at the same time; ideal aid for caregiver brushing another person's teeth. (Used with permission from Specialized Care, Hampton, NH.)

Website Information and Resources

Source	Website Address	Description
American Academy of Pediatric Dentistry	http://www.aapd.org	Information, education, policies, and guidelines on working with all children, including those with special care needs
National Maternal and Child Oral Health Resource Center	http://www.mchoralhealth.org/default.html	Information on working with children with disabilities
National Institute of Dental and Craniofacial Research	http://www.nidcr.nih.gov	Information, education, and strategies on providing care to patients with special care needs
National Institute of Neurological Disorders and Stroke	http://www.ninds.nih.gov	Health information and resources for patients and professionals related to a wide variety of neurologic disorders
National Institute on Disability and Rehabilitation Research	http://www.ed.gov/programs/nidrr	Support related to rehabilitation of individuals with disabilities
University of Washington; School of Dentistry; Patients with Special Needs	http://dental.washington.edu/oral-medicine/special-needs/patients-with-special-needs/	Health and dental information for caregivers and professionals related to patients with special care needs

SUGGESTED READINGS

American Dental Education Association: *Oral health for independent older adults.* http://www.adea.org/publications/Documents/CurriculumResourceGuide.pdf. Accessed Oct 20, 2014.

Cawson RA, Odell EW: *Oral pathology: clinical pathologic correlations,* ed 6, Philadelphia, 2012, Elsevier.

Darby M, Walsh M: *Dental hygiene theory and practice,* ed 4, Philadelphia, 2015, Elsevier.

Faulks D, Freedman L, Thompson S, et al: The value of education in special care dentistry as a means of reducing inequalities in oral health, *Eur J Dent Educ* 16(4):195–201, 2012.

Fikleman M, Stark P, Tao W, Morgoa J: Relationship between duration of treatment in oral health in adults with intellectual and developmental disabilities, *Spec Care Dent* 34(4):171–175, 2014.

Little JW, Falace DA: *Dental management of the medically compromised patient,* ed 8, St Louis, 2013, Elsevier.

Mayo Clinic Website: *Diseases and conditions.* www.mayoclinic.com/invoke.cfm. Accessed Oct 24, 2014.

National Oral Health Information Clearinghouse: *Practical oral care for people with developmental disabilities, Making a difference series,* NIH Pub No 04-5193.

Simmer-Beck M: Providing care to individuals with special healthcare needs, *Dimens Dent Hygiene* 8(5):64–67, 2010.

CHAPTER 19 REVIEW QUESTIONS

Answers and rationales to review questions are available on this text's accompanying Evolve site. See inside front cover for details.

evolve

1. **The seizure type characterized by continuous intermittent contractions and relaxation of voluntary muscles and loss of consciousness is termed:**

a. Complex partial

b. Generalized absence

   c. Generalized tonic-clonic

   d. Atonic

2. **All the following are common clinical manifestations found with Down syndrome EXCEPT one. Which one is the *exception*?**

   a. Long neck with thin, long fingers

   b. Tranverse palmar hand crease

   c. Eyes closer together than normal

   d. Microcephaly of the head

3. **Which of the following is the leading cause of preventable mental impairments in the United States?**

   a. Nutritional deficiencies

   b. Alcohol consumption

   c. Exposure to toxic waste

   d. Sensorineural malfunctioning

4. **Which trimester of pregnancy is considered the safest for routine dental care?**

   a. First

   b. Second

   c. Third

   d. None

5. **Which of the following is the progressive hearing loss that occurs with age?**

   a. Otitis media

   b. Presbycusis

   c. Mastoiditis

   d. Acoustic neurinoma

6. **Which of the following is a nonprogressive neuromuscular condition caused by damage to the immature brain and affecting the ability to control posture and movement?**

   a. Parkinson's disease

   b. Scleroderma

   c. Trigeminal neuralgia

   d. Cerebral palsy

7. **All the following are common oral findings associated with bulimia EXCEPT:**

   a. Esophageal lacerations

   b. Submandibular gland swelling

   c. Enamel erosion

   d. Burning tongue

8. **Drug-influenced gingival enlargement is often associated with which of the following antiseizure medications?**

   a. Carbamazepine (Tegretol)

   b. Valproic acid (Depakote)

   c. Topiramate (Topamax)

   d. Phenytoin (Dilantin)

9. **Which of the following is a chronic degenerative disease of the central nervous system that destroys myelin?**

   a. Myasthenia gravis

   b. Spina bifida

   c. Fibromyalgia

   d. Multiple sclerosis

10. **Which of the common manifestations of Down syndrome is an indication for antibiotic premedication prior to dental hygiene care?**

   a. Hearing impairment

   b. Shunt

   c. Congenital heart defect

   d. Thyroid problem

11. **Which of the following is an internal barrier to physical facilities for the person with a disabling condition?**

   a. Armless chairs with wheels

   b. Bathroom with grab bars by the commode

   c. 36-inch-wide doorways

   d. Nonslip floors

12. **Which of the following is a common oral manifestation in the client with Down syndrome?**

   a. Early eruption patterns

   b. Large tooth crowns with long crown/root ratio

   c. Enamel dysplasia

   d. Low palatal vault

13. **In which of the following conditions is retention of food common, causing increased susceptibility to oral disease?**

   a. Fibromyalgia

   b. Myasthenia gravis

   c. Spina bifida

   d. Bronchial asthma

14. **Body stability maintenance during dental hygiene care is of great concerns for patients with:**

   a. Scleroderma

   b. Sjögren syndrome

   c. Addison's disease

   d. Cerebral palsy

15. **In which of the following conditions would oral paralysis be found?**

   a. Cystic fibrosis

   b. Bell's palsy

   c. Pemphigus vulgaris

   d. Multiple sclerosis

16. **Latex allergy is common in patient with:**

   a. Spina bifida

   b. Parkinson's disease

   c. Congenital heart disease

   d. Hyperthyroidism

17. **Powered scaling devices would be *contraindicated* for use in patients with all the following conditions EXCEPT:**

   a. Myasthenia gravis

   b. Cystic fibrosis

   c. Emphysema

   d. Pernicious anemia

18. **A dental hygienist should expect physical mobility limitations in patients with all these disabling conditions EXCEPT:**

   a. Parkinson's disease

   b. Muscular dystrophy

   c. Epilepsy

   d. Cerebral palsy

19. **A stroke survivor should postpose elective dental hygiene treatment for:**

   a. 2 months

   b. 3 months

c. 4 months

d. 6 months

20. **When being escorted, an adult blind patient holds the arm of the dental hygienist just below the wrist. The blind patient then walks beside and slightly behind the hygienist.**
    a. Both statements are TRUE.
    b. Both statements are FALSE.
    c. The first statement is TRUE; the second statement is FALSE.
    d. The first statement is FALSE; the second statement is TRUE.

21. **Which of the following is an appropriate action for the dental hygienist when a blind patient brings a guide dog to the appointment?**
    a. Pet the dog to make "friends"
    b. Have "dog treats" ready to ensure the dog will behave
    c. Ask the patient to leave the dog in the waiting room
    d. Ignore dog, since it is working

22. **Which is the most common chronic illness found in the elderly population?**
    a. Renal dysfunction
    b. Arthritis
    c. Visual disturbances
    d. Diabetes

23. **Which is the most serious complication of radiation therapy to the head and neck area?**
    a. Xerostomia
    b. Radiation caries
    c. Osteoradionecrosis
    d. Increased severity of periodontal disease

24. **Which of the following conditions represents a medical emergency for someone with a: spinal injury?**
    a. Incontinence
    b. Tremors
    c. Deficit in acetylcholine
    d. Autonomic dysreflexia

25. **In which of the following conditions would mouth opening be a potential problem for oral hygiene implementation?**
    a. Cystic fibrosis
    b. Multiple sclerosis
    c. Scleroderma
    d. Myelomeningocele

26. **Antibiotic premedication would be indicated before dental hygiene treatment for the client with which of the following conditions?**
    a. Artificial heart valve
    b. Generalized tonic-clonic seizure
    c. Chronic obstructive pulmonary disease
    d. Angioplasty and stent placement

27. **Use of local anesthetic with epinephrine is contraindicated in patients with coronary heart disease, since the epinephrine in limited amounts can precipitate a myocardial infarction.**
    a. Both parts of the statement are TRUE.

b. Both parts of the statement are FALSE.

c. The first part of the statement is TRUE, but the second part is FALSE.

d. The first part of the statement is FALSE, but the second part is TRUE.

28. **Which of the following functional limitations is common in patients who have experienced a right CVA (cerebrovascular accident)?**
    a. Disorganization
    b. Inability to use mirrors
    c. Inability to see angles
    d. Inability to judge distance

29. **Patients with all the following conditions should see a dentist immediately after diagnosis to help manage their oral disease and condition EXCEPT those with:**
    a. Alzheimer's disease
    b. Diabetes
    c. Sickle cell disease
    d. Oral cancer

30. **Which of the following drugs is *contraindicated* to control dental pain in a patient who is pregnant?**
    a. Acetaminophen
    b. Naproxen
    c. Codeine
    d. Morphine

31. **A renal transplant patient should have routine dental care postponed for 6 months after the transplant, since the organ transplant is still being monitored for signs of rejection.**
    a. Both parts of the statement are TRUE.
    b. Both parts of the statement are FALSE.
    c. The first part of the statement is TRUE, but the second part is FALSE.
    d. The first part of the statement is FALSE, but the second part is TRUE.

32. **All the following conditions may complicate the patient's ability to perform oral self-care EXCEPT:**
    a. Scleroderma
    b. Parkinson's disease
    c. Arthritis
    d. Hypothyroidism

33. **A ground-glass appearance of the alveolar bone would be seen on radiographs in the patient with which condition?**
    a. End-stage renal disease
    b. Ischemic heart disease
    c. Myasthenia gravis
    d. Lichen planus

34. **An alcoholic patient may have delayed healing after scaling and root debridement because of:**
    a. Chronic swelling of glands
    b. Deceased endocrine hormones
    c. Decreased white blood cell count
    d. Increased platelet count

    Use Case A and Figs. 19-27 through 19-32 to answer questions 35 to 45.

SYNOPSIS OF PATIENT HISTORY	Age	25	VITAL SIGNS	
	Sex	female	Blood Pressure	130/80
	Height	5 feet 3 inches	Pulse Rate	60 bpm
	Weight	165 pounds	Respiration Rate	16 rpm

CHIEF COMPLAINT:
My teeth hurt and my gums bleed

MEDICAL HISTORY:
Under care of a physician:

Yes ☒   No ☐

Condition(s): epilepsy
_____
_____

Has or had the following conditions:

Mild mental impairment

Seasonal allergies
_____
_____

Current Medications: 200 mg Tegretol (carbomaze)
10 mg Allegra (fexofenadine HCL)
_____

1. Smokes or uses tobacco products:

   Yes ☐   No ☒

DENTAL HISTORY:
Patients' dental visit have been limited; mainly emergency care with extractions. Patient has no memory of having their teeth cleaned or ever receiving self care instructions

SOCIAL HISTORY:
Patient lives in a group home with 5 other adults with mental impairments. She works in a sheltered workshop sorting small tools and screws.

CURRENT ORAL HYGIENE STATUS:
Heavy biofilm; generalized bleeding on probing; moderate calculus

SUPPLEMENTAL ORAL EXAMINATION FINDINGS:
1 and 16; partially erupted

Clinically visible caries need to draw in caries on mesial 6 and mesial, facial and distal of 7,8,9,10,11 and mesial of 12

Clinically missing tooth draw in missing teeth

Furcation

"Through and through" furcation

Adult clinical examination

Probe 2/1	1	2	3	4	5	6	7	8	9	10	11	12	13	14	15	16
	434	434	423	✕	324	233	323	323	323	323	424	233	✕	434	524	535

Facial

R

Palatal

Probe 1/2	424	425	✕	424	323	232	323	233	323	323	✕	435	425	535

Probe 2/1	525	✕	525	424	423	324	423	323	222	232	323	423	324	525	✕	434

Lingual

R

Facial

Probe 1/2	434	✕	525	424	324	323	323	323	232	234	323	545	✕	525

| 32 | 31 | 30 | 29 | 28 | 27 | 26 | 25 | 24 | 23 | 22 | 21 | 20 | 19 | 18 | 17 |

FIG 19-27 Case A: anterior teeth.

FIG 19-29 Lingual teeth.

35. **In which blood pressure category would this patient's reading today be placed?**
    a. Normal
    b. Prehypertension
    c. Stage 1
    d. Stage 2

36. **The apices of the roots are not present on the maxillary right molar view? What is the most likely cause of this error?**
    a. Incorrect placement of film-holding device
    b. Too much horizontal angulation
    c. Too little vertical angulation
    d. Too little horizontal angulation

FIG 19-30 Right lateral teeth.

FIG 19-28 Full mouth radiographs.

FIG 19-31 Maxillary lingual teeth.

FIG 19-32 Left lateral teeth.

37. All the following teeth have radiographic signs of subgingival calculus EXCEPT:
a. #2
b. #12
c. #28
d. #30

38. Which of the following medications is the patient taking to help manage the symptoms of fibromyalgia?
a. Symbicort
b. Lyrica
c. Glucophage
d. Zocar

39. The patient's chief complaint of having jaw-opening problems is most likely related to which of her medical conditions?
a. Diabetes type 2
b. Hyperlipidemia
c. Fibromyalgia syndrome
d. Asthma

40. Which of the following medical emergencies is most likely to occur with this patient?
a. Seizure
b. Hyperglycemia
c. Angina
d. Anaphylaxis

41. Which American Society of Anesthesiologists (ASA) Physical Status (PS) Classification would be most appropriately assigned to this patient?
a. PS1
b. PS2
c. PS3
d. PS4

42. All the following treatment modifications may be warranted for this patient EXCEPT:
a. More upright chair position
b. Cervical neck pillow
c. Back and leg supports
d. Longer appointments

43. The patent reports an HbA$_{1c}$ value of 7%. This means that the level of diabetes control is rated as:
a. Well controlled
b. Moderately controlled
c. Uncontrolled
d. Life threatening

44. What is the clinical attachment loss on the facial of tooth #24?
a. 4 mm
b. 5 mm
c. 6 mm
d. 8 mm

45. Which of the following oral hygiene aids would be BEST recommended for cleaning the area between teeth #8 and #9?
a. Floss
b. Balsa wooden wedge
c. Interproximal brush
d. End tuft brush

Use Case B and Figs. 19-33 through 19-38 to answer questions 46 to 52.

SYNOPSIS OF PATIENT HISTORY		VITAL SIGNS	
Age	54	Blood Pressure	140/98
Sex	female	Pulse Rate	80 bpm
Height	5 feet 3 inches	Respiration Rate	20 rpm
Weight	175 pounds		

MEDICAL HISTORY:

Under care of a physician:

Yes ☒   No ☐

Condition(s): *Diabetes type 2; patient reports HbA1c of 7 %*

Hyperlipidemia

Fibromyalgia Syndrome

Asthma

Has or had the following conditions: *Diabetes type 2*

Hyperlipidemia

Fibromyalgia Syndrome

Asthma

Slipped disc

Current Medications: *budesonide and formoterol inhalation (Symbicort) 160/4.5 mcg*

pregabalin (Lyrica) 150 mg

metformin (Glucophage) 500 mg 2 x day

simvastin (Zocar) 10 mg

1. Smokes or uses tobacco products:

   Yes ☒   No ☐

DENTAL HISTORY:

The patient went to a dentist 2 months ago for two tooth extractions. She states she has not had a dental cleaning in at least 8 years.

SOCIAL HISTORY:

The patient works part time at a local day care center

CHIEF COMPLAINT:

My gums are bleeding and I have bad breath; I am having problems opening my jaw

CURRENT ORAL HYGIENE STATUS:

Generalized bleeding; heavy subgingival calculus

SUPPLEMENTAL ORAL EXAMINATION FINDINGS:

Mandibular facial anterior areas of 24 and 22 exhibits 4 mm of facial recession

Adult clinical examination

	1	2	3	4	5	6	7	8	9	10	11	12	13	14	15	16
Probe 2/1			436	535	545	344	434	323	434	343	443	345	524	655	645	

Facial

Palatal

| Probe 1/2 | | | 545 | 654 | 645 | 454 | 434 | 434 | 434 | 434 | 444 | 554 | 645 | 565 | 545 | |

| Probe 2/1 | | | 747 | 747 | 545 | 535 | 434 | 424 | 444 | 444 | 324 | 434 | 545 | 745 | 646 | |

Lingual

Facial

| Probe 1/2 | | | 545 | 324 | 545 | 545 | 434 | 434 | 444 | 444 | 456 | 535 | 426 | 635 | 635 | |
| | 32 | 31 | 30 | 29 | 28 | 27 | 26 | 25 | 24 | 23 | 22 | 21 | 20 | 19 | 18 | 17 |

 Clinically visible caries

 Clinically missing tooth

 Furcation

 "Through and through" furcation

FIG 19-33 Case B: full-mouth series.

FIG 19-34 Maxillary anterior teeth.

FIG 19-35 Left lateral teeth.

FIG 19-36 Mandibular lingual teeth.

FIG 19-37 Right lateral teeth.

FIG 19-38 Maxillary lingual teeth.

46. **What G.V. Black classification of caries is found on the mesial of tooth #8?**
    a. Class I
    b. Class II
    c. Class III
    d. Class IV

47. **On the radiographs, the arrow is pointing to what radiopaque structure on the maxillary left molar image?**
    a. Internal oblique ridge
    b. Floor of the maxillary sinus
    c. Coronoid process
    d. Nutrient canal

48. **As you are working on the patient, she displays a blank, staring look and is nonresponsive for about 30 seconds, but quickly returns to normal. What type of seizure is she experiencing?**
    a. Generalized tonic-clonic
    b. Myoclonic
    c. Generalized absence
    d. Simple motor partial

49. **The radiopaque area in the mandibular anterior image apical to teeth #23 and #24 is:**
    a. Sclerotic bone
    b. Tori
    c. Genial tubercles
    d. Nutrient foramen

50. **What is the technique error associated with the left premolar periapical radiograph?**
    a. Beam-indicating device alignment
    b. Incorrect placement of film-holding device
    c. Incorrect horizontal angulation
    d. Incorrect vertical angulation

51. **All following are acceptable approaches for teaching this patient oral self-care EXCEPT:**
    a. "Show-tell-do" approach
    b. Explanation of bone loss using radiographs
    c. Demonstration of proper use of disclosing tablets
    d. Use of powered toothbrushing techniques

52. **Which of the following oral rinses would the patient MOST benefit from?**
    a. Chlorhexidine
    b. Phenolic-related essential oils
    c. Cetylpyridinium chloride
    d. Chlorine dioxide

Community Oral Health Planning and Practice

Christine French Beatty, Connie E. Beatty, and Charlene B. Dickinson

Assessment, diagnosis, planning, implementation, and evaluation—the dental hygiene process of care—are used in community oral health practice, program development, and outcomes assessment. Community health extends the role of the dental hygienist from a traditional health care setting to the community as a whole. In a sense, the community can be viewed as the client and the oral care environment as the neighborhood health center, extended care facility, hospital, school, agency, or country. One of the characteristics of community health is the use of a team approach. Concerns for the oral health of the population has renewed an interest in expanding the roles and responsibilities of dental hygienists in order to increase access to oral health care for underinsured and underserved patients. Expanding roles in community-based care settings require that the dental hygienist possess the knowledge and skills for developing public health programs, research and epidemiologic methods, prevention and control of oral diseases, provision and financing of oral health care, and the adaptation of care and programs to diverse populations.

BASIC CONCEPTS

A. Health—community health practice requires a broad view of health that includes the following:
   1. Complete physical, mental, and social well-being; not just the absence of disease or infirmity
   2. Anatomical, physiologic, and psychological integrity
   3. Ability to perform personally valued family, work, and community roles to achieve individual and society goals
   4. Ability to deal with physical, biologic, psychological, and social stress
   5. Freedom from the risk of disease and untimely death
   6. Extent to which an individual or a group is able to realize aspirations and satisfy needs and to change or cope with the environment
   7. Emphasis on social and personal resources as well as physical capabilities
B. Oral health—status of the oral cavity, encompassing all features, normal and abnormal, of the oral, dental, and craniofacial complex
C. Wellness—high-level wellness is described as a dynamic process in which the individual is actively engaged in moving toward fulfillment of his or her human needs and potential; it reflects the following:
   1. A change in the perceptions of health and wellness from the medical model of health care that is treatment oriented
   2. A prevention preference that examines the relationships among the host, agent, environment, and preventive strategies
   3. A health promotion orientation aimed at creating an environment that enables individuals to increase control over and improve current and future health status
D. Determinants of health—consist of social and economic factors, the physical environment, and the person's individual characteristics and behaviors
   1. Many determinants are nonmodifiable
   2. Risk factors are modifiable determinants that can be changed through education, preventive therapies, public health policies, and modifications in the structure of health care delivery
E. Public health—the combination of sciences, skills, and beliefs directed at maintaining and improving the health of all persons by preventing disease, improving the quality of life, and promoting physical and mental health through collective or social actions in the community; characteristics include a collaborative approach, preventing rather than curing disease, dealing with population health rather than individual health, social responsibility for oral health, use of epidemiology and a multifactorial approach to controlling and preventing disease, and application of biostatistics
   1. Aggregate health of a group, community, state, nation, or group of nations
   2. Public health seen as people's health
   3. Concerned with four broad areas:
      a. Lifestyle, behavior, and culture
      b. Environment
      c. Human biology
      d. Organization of health programs and systems
F. Dental public health—science and art of preventing and controlling oral diseases and promoting oral health through organized community efforts; the form of dental practice that serves the community as a client rather than the individual; concerned with the oral health education of the public, applied dental research, and administration of group

oral health care programs, as well as the prevention and control of oral diseases on a community basis; the application of public health and all its characteristics to oral health

G. Community—any group with common traits, shared features, or communal experiences; not strictly defined by traditional geographic boundaries; as broad as a region or a state or as focused as a specific institution or agency, such as a nursing home community, including administrators, staff, residents, and caregivers

H. Community health—generally synonymous with *public health*; full range of health services, environmental and personal, including major activities such as health education of the public and the social context of life as it affects the community; efforts that are organized to promote and restore the health and quality of life of the people; uses a population-based approach for identifying and addressing community-based problems

I. Community oral health—services directed toward developing, reinforcing, and enhancing the oral health status of people, either as individuals or as groups and communities for the purpose of enhancing the oral health of the population; Table 20-1 presents a comparison of private health care practice to community health care practice

J. Access—an individual's or group's ability to obtain appropriate health care services

K. Prevention—primary focus of community oral health is prevention; the wellness model focuses educational and behavioral efforts and programs toward prevention of disease and maintenance of an optimum state of well-being; three levels of prevention:
  1. Primary—prevention of disease before it occurs; for example, placement of dental sealants
  2. Secondary—early disease control, including early identification and prompt treatment before the individual is aware of a problem; for example, restoration of caries identified through a routine dental examination
  3. Tertiary—provision of services that prevent further disability; for example, restoration of a fractured tooth caused by severe caries

L. Comparison of private health care practice to community health care practice—steps are presented in Table 20-1; the focus of public health is on the population rather than on any individual patient, yet similarities exist in the process of care

M. Criteria for identifying a public health problem
  1. A condition, practice, or situation is widespread and an actual or potential cause of morbidity (disease) or mortality (death)
  2. The public, nongovernmental agency, government, or public health personnel perceive the condition is a public health problem and direct efforts at a solution
  3. Public health solution—a solution to a public health problem that is directed to the community at large; preventive strategies possess as many characteristics of an ideal public health solution as possible (Box 20-1)

N. Core functions of public health—nationally identified; form the foundation of all community health activities
  1. Assessment—regular and systematic collection, assembling, and analysis of data related to the health of the population and making the data available for use by various agencies; for example, oral disease data collected through the National Oral Health Surveillance System
  2. Policy development—development of comprehensive public health policies based on scientific evidence; for example, adoption of *Healthy People 2020* objectives and Centers for Disease Control and Prevention (CDC) recommendations for water fluoridation
  3. Assurance—provision of services necessary to achieve agreed-on health goals related to improving the health of the public; for example, provision of services and programs that are publicly funded

TABLE 20-1 Comparison of Private Dental Practice and Community Oral Health Practice*

Private Dental Practice	Community Oral Health Practice
Assessment of client's dental, health, pharmacologic, and sociocultural history and oral health status	Survey of community oral health status; situation analysis including assessment of population demographics, culture, mobility, economic resources, and infrastructure (community profile)
Diagnosis of client's oral health needs	Analysis of survey data to determine the oral health needs of the population
Treatment plan based on diagnosis, professional judgment, client's needs, and priorities	Program plan based on data analysis, community priorities, and resources available
Treatment plan initiated; primary dentist may coordinate treatment with other providers (e.g., dental hygienists, specialists)	Program operation implemented by varied, sometimes interdisciplinary, personnel
Payment methods determined	Financing throughout process; funds may be from a combination of government (local, state, and federal), philanthropic and/or community agencies
Evaluation during treatment, at specific intervals, on completion of treatment, or at all these times	Ongoing and varied evaluation and appraisal conducted in terms of effectiveness, efficiency, appropriateness, and adequacy

*Education occurs at all levels to facilitate anticipated outcomes.

BOX 20-1 Characteristics of an Ideal Public Health Solution

1. Safe; not hazardous to life or function
2. Effective in reducing or preventing a targeted disease, condition, or practice
3. Easily and efficiently implemented
4. Potency maintained for a substantial time period
5. Attainable regardless of socioeconomic status (SES), education, or income
6. Effective immediately on application
7. Affordable, cost-effective, and within the means of a community

O. Governmental levels of public health—each level provides various services, meets different needs of the population, and supports the functions of other levels; for example, the federal departments support state agencies, and local programs are often funded by grants or contracts from the state or federal levels

1. Local—responsible for direct administration of educational resources, preventive care, and patient care programs
2. State—consultation to the local level and other agencies; channels federal and state funds such as Medicaid and Children's Health Insurance Program (CHIP); coordinates programs throughout the state; conducts programs in rural areas that do not have local public health agencies
3. Federal—numerous national public health government agencies are involved in public health issues of national significance; Box 20-2 describes significant agencies and organizations that act as a resource for community programming

---

BOX 20-2 Federal Governmental Agencies of Interest in Community Oral Health

Public Health Service (PHS)—the primary operating division of the U.S. Department of Health and Human Services (DHHS), responsible for the protection and advancement of the American population's physical and mental well-being. Various agencies and programs (e.g., CDC, NIH, IHS, FDA) accomplish the goals of coordinating and implementing national health policy on the state and local levels; conducting medical and biomedical research; addressing issues related to access, quality, and cost of health care; and enforcing laws to ensure the safety of drugs and medical devices and to protect the public against impure foods and cosmetics. Goals are carried out by the Commissioned Core of health officers led by the Surgeon General, who also staff federal clinics (e.g., in federal prisons, Indian Health Service programs, and some armed services) and respond to national crises.

National Institutes of Health (NIH)—conducts epidemiologic research, provides science transfer, and publishes and distributes educational materials. Several institutes are relevant to oral health, such as National Institute of Dental and Craniofacial Research (NIDCR), National Cancer Institute (NCI), and National Institute on Aging (NIA) (e.g., tobacco cessation); and provides surveillance data (e.g., water fluoridation).

Indian Health Service (IHS)—provides direct patient care and community health programming for Native American populations.

Centers for Disease Control and Prevention (CDC)—provides expertise, information, tools, and community collaboration to assist agencies with community programming; formulates recommendations for evidence-based practice (e.g., infection control and use of fluoride varnish); develops educational programs for local implementation.

Department of Defense (DoD) and *Veterans Administration* (VA)—provide direct care for specific armed services populations.

Centers for Medicare and Medicaid Services (CMS)—manages the federal Medicare and Medicaid programs to assist citizens with health care.

Administration for Children and Families (ACF)—involved in programs that promote the economic and social well-being of families, children, individuals, and communities; manages the Head Start program.

Data from Beatty CF: *Community oral health practice for the dental hygienist*, ed 4, St Louis, 2017, Elsevier Saunders.

---

4. International—the World Health Organization (WHO) is the best-known and largest international health agency; primarily serves developing countries but also monitors health conditions and establishes programs to coordinate health care throughout the world; the Pan-American Health Organization (PAHO) is the regional office of WHO for the Americas

P. Key national documents relevant to community oral health programming—classic documents continue to provide a basis to prioritize programs and target specific population groups; newer documents update the vision and strategies for implementation with a broader focus within the medical community; the documents complement each other as they categorize population oral health needs, priorities, and strategies and stress the importance of improving access to oral health care and reducing oral health disparities in the population; based on the three core public health functions of assessment, policy development, and assurance

1. *Oral Health in America: a Report of the Surgeon General*, 2000—the key points are:
   a. Oral health is more than just healthy teeth
   b. Oral health is integral to general health for all Americans
   c. General health factors (e.g., tobacco use, poor diet, obesity, diabetes) affect oral and craniofacial health
   d. Oral health can be achieved by all Americans
   e. Disparities exist in the oral health of Americans
2. *A National Call to Action to Promote Oral Health*—developed by a broad collaboration of private and public health agencies and organizations led by the Surgeon General's office; includes five principles and implementation strategies designed to result in programs that will more effectively contribute to the goal of optimum oral public health:
   a. Change perceptions about oral health
   b. Build the science and accelerate the transfer of the science
   c. Increase collaborations (partnerships, coalitions)
   d. Increase workforce diversity, capacity, and flexibility
   e. Overcome barriers by replicating effective programs
3. *Healthy People (HP) 2020*—a comprehensive list of approximately 1200 disease prevention and health promotion objectives in 42 health topic areas
   a. Developed by a federal interagency workgroup led by the U.S. Department of Health and Human Services (DHHS) with input from various health organizations
   b. Includes developmental objectives that as yet have no baseline data source; objectives are revised each decade based on outcomes from previous decade
   c. Current objectives establish the health agenda for the United States and provide priorities for community programming for the current decade
   d. Oral health is one of the topic areas; there are 17 Oral Health objectives (Table 20-2); objectives that relate to oral health are also contained in other *HP* topic areas, such as cancer, diabetes, older adults, and tobacco use

TABLE 20-2   *Healthy People (HP) 2020* Objectives and Targets, with Outcomes in Last Decade

HP 2020 Oral Health (OH) Objective	Baseline Data for *HP 2020* Goal	Target for *HP 2020* Goal[1]	Baseline versus Final % Change, 2000 to 2010	% Targeted Change Achieved, 2000 to 2010
Oral Health of Children and Adolescents				
OH-1 Reduce proportion of children and adolescents with dental caries experience				
OH-1.1 Young children ages 3 to 5 years, primary teeth	33.3%	30.0%	33.3% increase	☹[2]
OH-1.2 Children ages 6 to 9 years, primary and permanent teeth	54.0%	49.0%	1.9% increase	☹[2]
OH-1.3 Adolescents ages 13 to 15, permanent teeth	53.7%	48.3%	8.2% decrease	50% ☺[2]
OH-2 Reduce proportion of children and adolescents with untreated dental caries				
OH-2.1 Young children ages 3 to 5 years, primary teeth	23.8%	21.4%	18.8% increase	☹[2]
OH-2.2 Children ages 6 to 9 years, primary and permanent teeth	28.8%	25.9%	3.6% increase	☹[2]
OH-2.3 Adolescents ages 13 to 15, permanent teeth	17.0%	15.3%	10.0% decrease	40% ☺[2]
Oral Health of Adults				
OH-3 Reduce proportion of adults with untreated dental caries				
OH-3.1 Ages 35 to 44, untreated dental caries	27.8%	25.0%	3.7% increase	☹[2]
OH-3.2 Ages 65 to 74, untreated coronal caries	17.1%	15.4%	DNA[3]	DNA[3]
OH-3.3 Ages 75 and older, untreated root surface caries	37.9%	34.1%	DNA[3]	DNA[3]
OH-4 Reduce proportion of adults with an extracted tooth from caries or periodontal disease				
OH-4.1 Ages 45 to 64 years, no permanent tooth loss	76.4%	68.8%	26.7% improved[4]	80% ☺[2]
OH-4.2 Ages 65 to 74 years, complete tooth loss	24.0%	21.6%	17.2% improved	71.4% ☺[2]
OH-5 Reduce proportion of adults with destructive periodontal disease				
OH-5 Ages 45 to 74 years, moderate or severe periodontitis	12.8%	11.5%	27.3% decrease	75.0% ☺[2]
OH-6 Increase proportion of oral and pharyngeal cancers detected at earliest stage				
OH-6 Increase early detection	32.5%	35.8%	8.3% decrease	☹[2]
Access to Preventive Services				
OH-7 Increase proportion of children, adolescents, and adults who used the oral health care system in past year				
OH-7 Increase in use of oral health care system	44.5%	49.0%	2.3% decrease	☹[2]
OH-8 Increase proportion of low-income children and adolescents who received any preventive dental service during past year				
OH-8 Increase in receipt of preventive dental services	30.2%	33.2%	24% increase	14.6% ☺[2]
OH-9 Increase proportion of school-based centers with an oral health component				
OH-9.1 That includes provision of dental sealants	24.1%	26.5%	100% increase	400% *[2]
OH-9.2 That includes provision of dental care	10.1%	11.1%	11.1% increase	50% ☺[2]
OH-9.3 That includes provision of topical fluoride	29.2%	32.1%	DNA[3]	DNA[3]
OH-10 Increase the proportion of local health departments and Federally Qualified Health Centers (FQHCs) that have an oral health program				
OH-10.1 Increase FQHCs with an oral health care program	75.0%	83.0%	44% increase	100% *[2]
OH-10.2 Increase local health departments with oral health prevention or care programs	25.8%	28.4%	DNA[3]	DNA[3]
OH-11 Increase proportion of patients who receive oral health services at FQHCs each year				
OH-11 Increase in patients served at FQHCs	17.5%	33.3%	DNA[3]	DNA[3]
Oral Health Interventions				
OH-12 Increase proportion of children and adolescents who have received dental sealants				
OH-12.1 Ages 3 to 5 years, one or more sealed primary molars	1.4%	1.5%	DNA[3]	DNA[3]
OH-12.2 Aged 6 to 9 years, one or more sealed permanent first molars	25.5%	28.1%	39.1% increase	33.3% ☺[2]
OH 12.3 Ages 13 to 15 years, one or more sealed permanent second molars	19.9%	21.9%	40.0% increase	17.1% ☺[2]
OH-13 Increase proportion of population served by community water systems with optimally fluoridated water				
OH-13 Increase in proportion	72.4%	79.6%	16.1% increase	76.9% ☺[2]
OH-14 (Developmental) Increase proportion of adults who receive preventive interventions in dental offices[4]				
OH-14.1 (Developmental) Provision of information by dentist or dental hygienist focused on reducing tobacco use or smoking cessation	N/A[5]	N/A[5]	DNA[3]	DNA[3]
OH-14.2 (Developmental) Oral and pharyngeal cancer screening by dentist or dental hygienist	N/A[5]	N/A[5]	38.5% increase[6]	71.4% ☺[2]
OH-14.3 (Developmental) Testing or referral for glycemic control by dentist or dental hygienist	N/A[5]	N/A[5]	DNA[3]	DNA[3]

TABLE 20-2 *Healthy People (HP) 2020* **Objectives and Targets, with Outcomes in Last Decade—cont'd**

HP 2020 Oral Health (OH) Objective	Baseline Data for *HP 2020* Goal	Target for *HP 2020* Goal	Baseline versus Final % Change, 2000 to 2010	% Targeted Change Achieved, 2000 to 2010
Monitoring, Surveillance Systems				
OH-15 (Developmental) Increase the number of states and the District of Columbia that have a system for recording and referring infants and children with cleft lips and cleft palates to craniofacial anomaly rehabilitative teams				
OH-15.1 (Developmental) Increase number of systems for recording of cleft lips and cleft palates	N/A[5]	N/A[5]	106.3% increase[6]	48.6% ☺[2]
OH-15.2 (Developmental) Increase number of systems for referral for cleft lips and cleft palates to rehabilitative teams	N/A[5]	N/A[5]	DNA[3]	DNA[3]
OH-16 Increase number of states and the District of Columbia that have an oral and craniofacial health surveillance system				
OH-16 Increase in number of states	32	51	Could not be calculated	84.3% ☺[2]
Public Health Infrastructure				
OH-17 Increase health agencies that have a dental public health program directed by a dental professional with public health training				
OH-17 Proportion of state and local agencies serving 250,000 or more persons	23.4%	25.7%	38.5% increase	750% *[2]
OH 17.2 Increase number of Indian Health Service Areas and tribal health programs that serve 30,000 or more persons	11	12	11.1% increase	Met at baseline *[2]

Data from Department of Health and Human Services: Healthy people 2020, http://www.healthypeople.gov/2020/topicsobjectives2020/default.aspx; and National Center for Health Statistics: Healthy people 2010 final review: overview and selected findings, PHS Pub No 2012-1038, Hyattsville, Md, 2012, http://www.cdc.gov/nchs/data/hpdata2010/hp2010_final_review.pdf.

[1]Target setting method was 10% improvement for most *HP 2020* goals (OH-11 and OH-16 were exceptions).
[2]☹ = Moved away from target; ☺ = Moved toward target; * = Met or exceeded target.
[3]DNA = Data not available. These are new goals for 2020.
[4]This goal for 2010 was for ages 35 to 44 years rather than the current age range of 45 to 64 years in the 2020 goal.
[5]N/A = Not applicable: baseline data and targets are not set for developmental goals.
[6]*HP 2010* goal existed for this subgoal without other subgoals of the 2020 goal.

4. *Advancing Oral Health in America*—developed by the Institute of Medicine (IOM); established the following new recommendations, called a New Oral Health Initiative, to build and enhance the current systems that are in place:
   a. Establish high-level accountability
   b. Emphasize disease prevention and oral health promotion
   c. Improve oral health literacy and cultural competence
   d. Reduce oral health disparities
   e. Explore new models for payment and delivery of care
   f. Enhance the role of nondental health care professionals
   g. Expand oral health research and improve data collection
   h. Promote collaboration among private and public stakeholders
   i. Measure progress toward short-term and long-term goals and objectives
   j. Advance the goals and objectives of *HP 2020*
5. *Improving Access to Oral Health Care for Vulnerable and Underserved Populations*—report of IOM focused on integrating oral health into overall health care, including emphasis on changes needed in laws and regulations such as scope of practice laws, improving dental education in relation to treating diverse populations in various settings, reducing financial and administrative barriers, and expanding capacity

Q. Roles of the dental hygienist reflect various activities in public health; all should be based on sound scientific information (evidence-based practice):
   1. Clinician—provides direct client care
   2. Educator—uses valid educational theories to present scientific information to individuals and groups to prevent disease and promote oral health
   3. Advocate—promotes change and advances the health of the public through legislation and public policy
   4. Researcher—determines which procedure, products, and programs most effectively promote oral health and prevent disease, and communicates those findings
   5. Administrator/manager—administers and manages programs aimed at promoting oral health

EPIDEMIOLOGY

A. Definitions
   1. Epidemiology—study of health-related conditions and diseases in human populations and how these states are influenced by the environment and ways of living, including the nature, cause, control, and determinants of health and disease as well as related factors; concerned with factors and conditions that determine the occurrence and distribution of health, disease, defects, disability, and deaths among individuals and groups; characterized by the use of statistical and research

Epidemiology is derived from three Greek root words:
- *epi*: upon or among—"upon the body; among the people"
- *demos*: people or district—"demographics"
- *logos*: study, word or discourse—"the study of"
1. A branch of medical science that deals with the incidence, distribution, and control of disease in a population
2. The sum of the factors controlling the presence or absence of a disease or pathogen
3. The study of the distribution and determinants of disease frequency

Data from http://www.merriam-webster.com/dictionary/epidemiology; and What is epidemiology? http://www.helsinki.fi/science/bgs/epidemiology.pdf.

BOX 20-4   **Uses of Epidemiology**

1. To study
   - Describe normal biologic processes
   - Establish a history of disease in a population
   - Measure the distribution of diseases in populations; detect patterns of disease among groups
   - Analyze trends in chronic disease and social epidemiology
   - Identify nondisease entities such as accidents, suicide, or injury
   - Recognize syndromes and precursors
2. To assess
   - Collect data to describe and measure disease or health conditions within a community
   - Identify current public health policies, activities, and health services that relate to disease in the community
3. To identify:
   - Identify risk factors, risk indicators, risk markers, and other determinants of disease such as health literacy
   - Estimate risk of diseases among population groups
   - Detect cause-and-effect relationships of diseases and various factors to help in the diagnostic processes of disease identification, as well as planning of preventive strategies
4. To control
   - Limit causes of diseases, conditions, injury, disability, or death for prevention and/or elimination
   - Contain diseases within the population
5. To plan
   - Develop appropriate health services and public health programs
   - Design mechanisms to evaluate effectiveness of services and programs
6. To evaluate
   - Calculate how well public health policies, intervention and preventive strategies, and programs control disease and improve the health status of the population
   - Appraise the appropriateness and utility of health services
7. To research
   - Test hypotheses for the effectiveness of measures to prevent and control disease
   - Determine the success of disease prevention and control measures in populations

methods to focus on comparisons between groups or defined populations (Box 20-3)
2. Applied epidemiology—the application or practice of epidemiology to address public health issues
B. Uses of epidemiology (Box 20-4)
C. Characteristics of epidemiology
   1. Groups rather than individuals are studied
   2. A multifactorial approach is used to study disease (multiple causation); modifiable risk factors are controlled to control the disease or condition
   3. Determinants—risk factors or events that are capable of bringing about a change in health; the various factors that make up the multifactorial approach to a disease or health condition
   4. Epidemiologic triad (epidemiologic triangle)—the traditional model of infection or disease causation used to study the occurrence and distribution of disease; includes a susceptible host, an external agent (etiologic agent), and an environment that brings the host and agent together so that disease occurs, as well as the time dimension required for disease to occur; the ongoing interaction among these factors affects disease or health status (Fig. 20-1)
   5. Burden of disease—cumulative effect of a broad range of harmful disease consequences on a community; includes the full scope of the health, social, and economic effects of disease
   6. Preventive intervention—a strategy to eliminate risk factors and reduce the occurrence of disease
D. General epidemiology concepts—ideas that must be grasped to comprehend epidemiology (Table 20-3)
E. Concepts related to measurement of disease and its distribution
   1. General measurement concepts (Table 20-4)
   2. Surveillance/monitoring
      a. Surveillance—ongoing, constant, systematic observation; use of repeated surveys to analyze and evaluate health data to monitor changes in populations related to disease, conditions, injuries, disabilities, or death trends, for the purpose of program planning; essential feature of epidemiology
      b. National Oral Health Surveillance System (NOHSS)—a collaborative effort between the CDC Division of Oral Health and the Association of State and Territorial

Dental Directors (ASTDD) to track oral health indicators on a state and national level using a variety of clinical and nonclinical methods (e.g., NHANES)
   c. Oral health indicators are routinely assessed, based on the *Healthy People* objectives (see Table 20-2); 26 of the hundreds of *HP 2020* objectives are deemed the leading health indicators, considered to be the most critical to the health of the population; two of the 26 leading *HP 2020* health indicators relate to oral health:
      (1) Increase dental utilization (Oral Health topic objective)
      (2) Reduce adult and adolescent cigarette smoking (Tobacco Use topic objective)
   d. National Health and Nutrition Examination Survey (NHANES)—routinely conducted national health surveys carried out by the National Center for Health Statistics of the CDC to monitor the health and nutritional status of U.S. adults and children of all ages; conducted through interviewing and direct physical and dental examinations

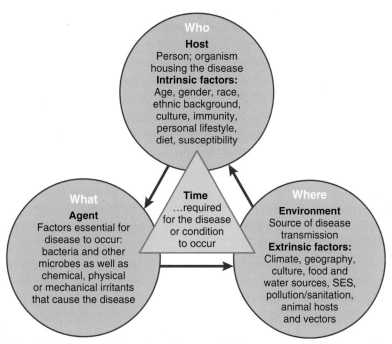

FIG 20-1 Epidemiologic triangle. (Data from Centers for Disease Control and Prevention: Lesson 1, Understanding the epidemiologic triangle through infectious disease. http://www.cdc.gov/bam/teachers/documents/epi_1_triangle.pdf.)

TABLE 20-3	**General Epidemiologic Concepts**
Term	**Definition**
Acute disease	Beginning abruptly with marked intensity, and then subsiding after a relatively short period; often treatable
Chronic disease	Developing slowly and persisting for a long period, often for the remainder of the lifetime of the individual
Cluster	Aggregate of cases of a disease or other health-related conditions, particularly cancer or birth defect, closely grouped in time or space
Endemic	Continuing problem involving normal disease prevalence; the expected number of cases native to a population or geographic area
Epidemic	A disease of significantly greater prevalence than normal (more than the expected frequency); rapid spread of a disease through a population
Pandemic	An epidemic that crosses international borders to affect a large proportion of the geographic population of a continent, people, or the world
Population at risk	Includes persons in the same community or population group who can acquire a disease or condition
Mortality	Death from a disease or condition
Morbidity	Presence or extent of disease, injury, or disability in a defined population
Status	Current state of a disease or health related condition in the population
Trend	Long-term changes or movements in disease patterns and health-related conditions in the population determined by examining surveillance data
Eradication	The elimination of the infectious disease agent through surveillance and containment
Socioeconomic status (SES)	Includes education, income, occupation, attitudes, and values and how SES relates to health-associated characteristics in the population

TABLE 20-4	**Measurement Concepts in Epidemiology**
Term	**Definition**
Basic screening	Rapid assessment accomplished in a short time by visual detection and providing information about gross dental and oral lesions; accomplished with a tongue blade, dental mirror, and appropriate lighting
Epidemiologic examination	Detailed visual tactile assessment; accomplished with dental instruments and a light source, provides more detailed information than basic screening; differs from a clinical examination in that is does not involve a clinical diagnosis that results in a treatment plan
Count	The actual number of cases of a disease or condition occurring in a population; simplest measure of a disease or condition; for example, the number of children with a toothache
Rate	Expression of disease in a population using a standardized denominator and including a time dimension; allows for valid comparisons; for example, the percentage of people diagnosed with cancer during a specific year, or the percentage of children with caries in 2014
Incidence	Rate of new cases of a disease (number of new cases/population at risk) during or over a specific period; measures how fast a disease is spreading; for example, the number of children with new carious lesions out of the entire school population during the school year

(Continued)

TABLE 20-4	Measurement Concepts in Epidemiology—cont'd
Term	**Definition**
Prevalence	Rate of the total number of all existing cases of a disease or health condition in a population measured at a given time, in relation to the number of individuals in the population; expressed as a proportion; can be expressed as a percentage; does not include a time period as incidence does; for example, the percentage of children with untreated caries at the time of a survey
Occurrence	General term of frequency of disease; does not distinguish between incidence and prevalence
Ratio	Expression of the magnitude of one occurrence of disease exposure in relation to another with a fraction, obtained by dividing one quantity by the other; often compares two rates; for example, if 4% of male and 2% of female infants were born with cleft palate, the ratio of cleft palate in male versus female infants would be 2:1
Prospective	Observations of disease or disease related factors made forward in time (into the future)
Longitudinal	Observations of disease progression made over a long period (length of time depends on condition being studied)
Retrospective	Disease related data collected in the past; ex post facto, causal comparative, or case control
Validity	The accuracy of a measure; produced by measuring what is supposed to be measured
Sensitivity	The ability of a test to accurately identify the presence of a disease or condition when disease is, in fact, present
Specificity	The ability of a test to accurately identify the absence of a disease or condition
Predictive value	The ability of a diagnostic test to accurately measure both the presence and the absence of disease
Reversal; negative reversal	A change of diagnosis in an illogical direction over a period, in contrast to a positive reversal, which is a change of the measurement made in error in a logical direction
Reliability	Consistency or reproducibility of a measurement over time
Inter-examiner (rater) reliability	Agreement among two or more examiners as they apply an index or instrument to measure a disease or condition
Intra-examiner (rater) reliability	Consistency of a single examiner in applying an index or instrument over time to measure a disease or condition
Calibration	Standardization of examiners to increase reliability as they apply epidemiologic measurements

(1) Began in the 1960s and has evolved to the current periodic program that focuses on a variety of health and nutrition measurements used to determine the health status of the population and assess progress on *Healthy People* objectives

(2) Survey examines a nationally representative sample of about 5000 persons each year, located in counties across the United States; oral health is one of the areas of diseases and health indictors monitored by NHANES

EPIDEMIOLOGY AND RESEARCH

A. Evidence-based practice (EBP)
1. Involves the conscientious, explicit, and judicious use of current evidence to inform decisions during the care of individual clients in relation to their oral and medical conditions
2. Evidence alone is not sufficient to make decisions; the clinical expertise of the professional and client preferences and values are combined with the best available external clinical evidence from a body of rigorous research findings to make EBP decisions (Fig. 20-2)
3. Evidence is ranked according to the design of the research study (Fig. 20-3)
4. EBP relates to the practice of a dental hygienist in all roles and settings, not just clinical; has implications for all aspects of community oral health practice
5. All oral health care must be informed by evidence; life-long learning and access to quality research findings are critical to EBP
B. Research—continual search for new knowledge using the scientific method; systematic and objective inquiry through

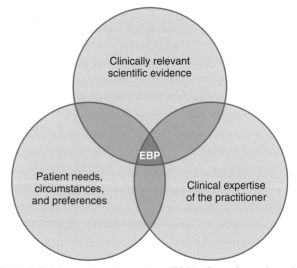

FIG 20-2 Evidence-based practice (EBP). (Data from American Dental Association, Center for Evidence-Based Dentistry: Critical summaries and plain language summaries, April 2014. http://ebd.ada.org/~/media/EBD/Files/WEBSITE_Operations_Manual_April%202014.ashx; and Forrest JL, Miller SA: Evidence-based decision making. In Darby ML, Walsh MM: *Dental hygiene theory and practice,* ed 4, St Louis, 2015, Elsevier Saunders.)

laboratory, field, and clinical investigations that lead to discovery or revision of knowledge, resulting in improvements in health and health care delivery
C. Scientific method—methods used in any type of research that increase the likelihood that information gathered will be relevant, reliable, and unbiased (Fig. 20-4)

Systematic
review w/
meta analysis;
Cochrane reviews*

Systematic review
w/o meta analysis

One or more
randomized controlled trials

Well-designed cohort studies

Well-designed case control studies

Cross-sectional studies; uncontrolled experimental studies

Case series

Opinions of respected authorities, based on clinical experience;
reports of expert committees; descriptive surveys; case reports

Non-human (animal) research

* The gold standard of evidence (best clinical evidence available) is at least one published systematic
review of multiple, well-designed studies of the type that is best to answer the research question.

FIG 20-3 Ranking of evidence for EBP. (Data from Icahn School of Medicine at Mount Sinai, Levy Library: Evidence-based medicine tutorial, 2013. http://libguides.mssm.edu/hierarchy; Oxford Centre for Evidence-Based Medicine: OCEBM 2011 levels of evidence. http://www.cebm.net/wp-content/uploads/2014/06/CEBM-Levels-of-Evidence-2.1.pdf.)

Identification and statement
of the problem

Formulation of a hypothesis

Collection, organization,
and analysis of data

Formulation of conclusions

Verification, rejection or
modification of the hypothesis

FIG 20-4 Steps of the scientific method.

D. Categories of community oral health research
  1. Epidemiologic research to determine the presence and distribution of disease in the population and factors that relate to the occurrence of disease within the population
  2. Clinical trials and tests of techniques and products to prevent and control disease
  3. Research in educational techniques and the behavioral sciences related to oral health education
  4. Evaluation of community oral health programs

E. Risk versus causality
  1. *Risk* identifies attributes that are associated with a disease, from case-control and cohort studies (Table 20-5); *causality* identifies factors that have been demonstrated to be causally related, from randomized controlled clinical trials (RCTs))
  2. Risk is established with analytic studies; causality is established with experimental studies; causality can be inferred with high-quality longitudinal analytic studies
F. Three classifications of epidemiologic research (Table 20-6)
G. Experimental research
  1. Requirements for an experimental study
    a. Use of a control group
    b. Control of extraneous variables
    c. Randomization (random assignment to groups)
    d. Control of errors in measurement to increase validity and reliability
    e. Manipulation of the independent variable
    f. Measurement of the dependent variable
    g. Occurrence of the independent variable before the dependent variable in the design
  2. A representative sample is required to allow for generalization (also called *inference*); replication studies (repeated studies with different samples) are frequently conducted to compensate for the poor generalizability (low external validity) resulting from the use of small convenience samples; multiple-site studies broaden the representation of the population and improve the generalizability of findings

TABLE 20-5 Types of Risk Attributes

Risk Attribute	Modifiable	Type of Analytic Study	Application
Risk factor (strong indication of risk)	Yes	Cohort/longitudinal or case control/retrospective	Causal role is inferred; should be an important consideration in making recommendations
Risk indicator (weaker indication of risk)	Yes	Cross-sectional	Possible causal role; causal role may be incorrectly assumed; should be applied with care when making recommendations
Demographic risk factor (also called risk marker or risk predictor)	No	Cross-sectional; case control	No causal role; not important in making individual recommendations to control the factor but indicates greater need to control modifiable risk factors and risk indicators; should be considered to identify target populations for dental public health programs

TABLE 20-6 Classifications of Epidemiologic Research

Type of Research	Definition	Types of Studies	Classification	Use/Purpose
Descriptive	Involves description, documentation, analysis, and interpretation of data to evaluate a current event or situation; does not test a hypothesis	Survey	Cross-sectional	Establish prevalence
Analytic (also called observational or developmental)	Encompasses observation of a disease or condition to identify determinants of the disease by showing relationships or associations between diseases and other factors; does not establish cause-and-effect relationship	Cohort: one group observed over time; can be compared to comparison group	Longitudinal, prospective	Establish incidence; determine risk
		Case control: two groups, one with disease (cases) and one without (controls), are compared to identify factors in their history that can be associated with the disease or condition	Retrospective	Determine risk; examine relationships among variables that cannot be studied prospectively because of ethical concerns about research participants
		Cross-sectional: representative cross section of the population (one group, but several subgroups) is observed at one point in time; disease attributes and potential risk attributes are associated	Cross-sectional	Identify risk indicators and risk predictors; cannot be used to confirm risk factors; establish prevalence
Experimental	Carefully designed study to test a hypothesis; involves manipulation of the supposed cause or controlling agent and observation of the result	Randomized clinical trial (RCT)—a well-controlled experimental study with humans	Longitudinal	Determine effectiveness of altering a factor or factors to establish cause-and-effect relationships (causality)
		Quasi-experimental—an experimental study that is not well controlled		

Data from Beatty CF: Oral epidemiology. In Nathe CN: Dental public health and research, ed 4, Upper Saddle River, NJ, 2015, Pearson.

3. Experimental study designs
   a. Pretest/posttest—the dependent variable is measured before and after introducing the independent variable; provides a baseline measure for comparison
   b. Posttest only—the dependent variable is measured only after introducing the independent variable; controls any possible effect of the pretest procedure on the dependent variable
   c. Split-mouth—procedure unique to oral health research in which each side of the mouth receives a different intervention; controls subject-related variables (variables that can change from one research participant to another)
   d. Crossover—each group receives a different intervention or control and, after a period, is switched over to the opposite treatment, with an intervening washout period during which no treatment is given, to eliminate the possibility of the first treatment affecting the second one; controls subject-related variables
   e. Time-series (repeated measures)—design in which the dependent variable is measured several times over a specific period, to determine whether the effect of the independent variable on the dependent variable holds over time
   f. Blind (or masking)—this refers to examiners measuring the dependent variable without knowing the group assignment, to eliminate bias; if *both* examiners and participants are unaware of the group assignments, it is called *double-blind*
   g. Designs can be combined; for example, a study can combine double-blind, pretest/posttest, split-mouth, and repeated-measures designs to test the effectiveness of an antimicrobial to reduce or control periodontal pocket depths over a long period

TABLE 20-7 Comparison of Clinical Trials and Epidemiologic Surveys

	Clinical Trial	Epidemiologic Survey
Populations	Experimental and control groups are specially constituted as representative samples from appropriate populations	Naturally occurring samples of target populations are usually studied
Sample size	Sample sizes are often small, particularly when "treatments" are more complicated	Fairly large sample sizes are used
Time frame	Trials are conducted over a period, usually varying from 1 week to 6 months to several years (e.g., dental caries research), depending on treatment involved and disease or condition measured, to compare treatment outcomes	Surveys are usually cross-sectional in design, measuring only one time; longitudinal designs are used occasionally
Methods	Although assessment methods may include indices, biomedical instruments, or physiologic measures, methods have validity, reliability, and clinical significance	Indices are used for assessment, to establish the disease level of selected populations, and to compare data from different populations
Data	Data generated from clinical trials are applicable to specific hypothesis testing	Data generated from surveys are used to establish underlying etiologic factors and derive possible preventive methods, leading to the development of hypotheses to be tested by controlled clinical trials

4. Comparison of clinical trials and epidemiologic surveys (Table 20-7)

H. Hypothesis—a predictive statement of the expected outcome or relationship among variables; answers the research question in a manner that is observable and measurable; hypotheses can exist for all types of studies, not just experimental
   1. Null hypothesis—negative statement of the hypothesis that assumes the absence of statistically significant differences between the sample groups; for example, statement that no difference exists in the effectiveness of the two treatments (experimental), or two variables are not associated (nonexperimental); this is the hypothesis that is statistically tested
   2. Research hypothesis—also called the *positive* or *alternative hypothesis*; positive statement of the hypothesis is in terms that express the opinion or prediction of the researcher; for example, a statement that a difference exists in the effectiveness of the two treatments (experimental), or two variables are associated (nonexperimental)

I. Variable—a state, condition, concept, construct, or event whose value is free to vary (e.g., height, dental caries rate, IQ, creativity); must be measurable
   1. Independent variable—in an experimental study, the treatment or intervention under study; condition that is manipulated or controlled by the investigator; the experimental variable; the experimental treatment
   2. Dependent variable—in an experimental study, the dependent variable is a measure of the outcome of manipulating the independent variable; it is measured to observe the effect of the independent variable
   3. Nonexperimental studies measure variables as well; in analytic studies, an attempt is made to determine the association or relationship of these variables, also called *factors*
   4. Extraneous variables—uncontrolled variables that may influence the dependent variable and influence (or confound) the outcome, thus interfering with accurate interpretation and producing invalid research results; can be present in all types of research studies

J. Sampling (Table 20-8)

1. Target or priority population—portion of the population to whom the researcher wants to generalize findings; all members of a specific group who possess a clearly defined set of characteristics
2. Sample—a portion of a specific population that, if properly selected, can provide meaningful information about the entire population; a sample is examined when the researcher cannot study an entire population or does not have the resources; a sample may be random or nonrandom and may be representative or nonrepresentative
3. Sample size
   a. Large sample, if selected properly:
      (1) Accurately represents a defined population
      (2) Increases the validity and reliability of collected data
      (3) Reduces the standard error of the sample mean
   b. Small sample
      (1) May be necessary, depending on the purpose of the research; for example, a pilot study
      (2) Results from a small study may not be generalized to target population and lead to inaccurate conclusions when inappropriate for the type of research
      (3) Small samples require specialized statistics (nonparametrics)

K. Group assignment—experimental and control groups are formed in an experimental study (Table 20-8); randomization of groups is best way to form groups to increase validity of the study

L. Pilot study—a study conducted with a small sample; often used as a trial run to test research design and methodology before initiating a full-scale study; can be conducted with any type of research

EPIDEMIOLOGY OF ORAL DISEASES AND CONDITIONS

A. Role of *Healthy People 2020* objectives
   1. Targets for various oral health diseases and conditions and the strategies to address them have been set in the *HP 2020* objectives for the U.S. population (see Table 20-2); these targets will drive community oral health programming for the decade 2010 to 2020

TABLE 20-8 Sampling and Group Assignment

Type of Sample or Group Assignment	Definition	Result
Random sample	Study participants are chosen independently of each other, with known opportunity or probability for inclusion; table of random numbers can be used	Increases external validity by controlling differences in study participants; yields a representative sample with a homogeneous population; allows for valid generalization of results to the population (reduced bias)
Stratified random sample	Study participants are randomly selected from an existing, known subdivided population; most representative sample for a heterogeneous population	Results in the sample proportionately and accurately representing the subgroups in the population; yields the most representative sample for a heterogeneous population
Systematic random sample	Selection of every nth member of the population from a list or file of the total population; the n depends on the size of the sample desired in relation to the population; for example, 10% is every tenth member of the population	Not strictly a random sample; it is considered to be random when the first member of the sample is selected randomly and the list or file is in random order
Convenience sample	Study participants are chosen on the basis of availability; used when access to the total population is not feasible for random sample selection	Introduces bias, which reduces validity of the sample and limits the generalizability of study results
Judgmental or purposive sample	Study participants are chosen by the researcher or someone else who has knowledge of the population; used when participants are needed that require specific disease levels and/or characteristics	Introduces bias, which reduces validity of the sample and limits the generalizability of study results
Experimental group	Sample group in an experimental study who is exposed to the experimental variable being studied (receives the independent variable)	Randomization (also called randomized group assignment) results in equivalent groups to control differences in groups; controls validity of study
Control group	Sample group in an experimental study who does not receive the experimental treatment (independent variable); receives a placebo, traditional or standard treatment, or no treatment	Provides a comparison group for a stronger study design; randomization (also called randomized group assignment) results in equivalent groups to control differences in groups; controls validity of study

2. Analysis of outcomes in relation to the *HP 2010* initiative indicated that significant progress was made in meeting oral health goals; most objectives moved toward, met, or exceeded their target; significant exceptions were the objectives to reduce dental caries and untreated dental caries in children, increase early detection of oral and pharyngeal cancer, and increase dental utilization (see Table 20-2)

3. Even though progress was made, disparities in oral health still exist; community programs and interventions aimed at reducing oral health disparities remain a high priority

B. Dental caries
   1. Occurrence in the population
      a. Dental caries is the most common chronic childhood disease; among 5- to 17-year-olds, it is five times more common than asthma, seven times more common than hay fever; one of the major reasons for hospitalization of children, and costly to treat
      b. The most commonly occurring type of caries is pit-and-fissure caries, followed by smooth-surface coronal caries and root caries; first and second molars are the most frequently affected teeth
      c. During the last half of the twentieth century, a substantially declining caries rates in all age groups was observed in the United States, including lower cumulative caries rates, less severe caries, substantially fewer carious lesions in anterior teeth, and fewer teeth lost as a result of caries

d. However, dental caries is still widespread, affects all age groups, and increased during the 2000 to 2010 in preschool-age (early childhood caries, or ECC; Table 20-9) and school-age children (see Table 20-2)

TABLE 20-9 Categorizing Early Childhood Caries* (ECC) and Severe Early Childhood Caries (S-ECC)

Age (years)	ECC	S-ECC
Younger than 6	1 or more DMFS[†] (cavitated or noncavitated)	
Younger than 3		Any sign of smooth-surface caries
Age 3		1 or more cavitated DMFS in maxillary anterior teeth OR 4 or more DMFS
Age 4		1 or more cavitated DMFS in maxillary anterior teeth OR 5 or more DMFS
Age 5		1 or more cavitated DMFS in maxillary anterior teeth OR 6 or more DMFS

Data from American Academy of Pediatric Dentistry (AAPD): Policy on early childhood caries (ECC): classifications, consequences, and preventive strategies, Chicago, 2014. http://www.aapd.org/policies/.
*The term *early childhood caries* replaces previously used terms such as *baby-bottle tooth decay, nursing caries, baby-bottle mouth,* and *baby-bottle caries.*
[†]*DMFS,* Decayed, missing, and/or filled primary tooth surfaces.

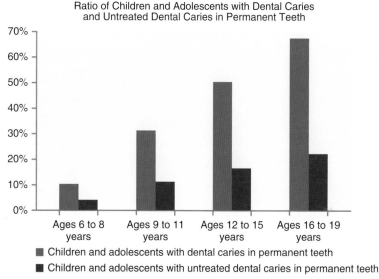

FIG 20-5 Ratio of dental caries to untreated dental caries in children and adolescents. (Data from National Institute of Dental and Craniofacial Research: Dental caries (tooth decay) in children (age 2 to 11), May 28, 2014. http://www.nidcr.nih.gov/DataStatistics/FindDataByTopic/DentalCaries/; and National Institute of Dental and Craniofacial Research: Dental caries (tooth decay) in adolescents (age 12 to 19), March 7, 2014. http://www.nidcr.nih.gov/DataStatistics/FindDataByTopic/DentalCaries/DentalCariesAdolescents12to19.htm#Table1.)

in the United States; Fig. 20-5 provides a summary of current dental caries in these age groups

e. These recent rates of dental caries are accompanied by increases in untreated caries for preschool-age and school-age children (see Table 20-2 and Fig. 20-5), the association between low dental utilization and higher caries rates in a population group is a significant concern

f. Increases in early childhood dental caries (ECC) and untreated caries in preschool-age children have raised concerns about the potential for a trend of increasing caries in older age groups in the future

g. Root surface caries rates have increased as a result of the aging population and because older adults are retaining their natural teeth; there is a new *Healthy People* objective for 2020 related to root surface caries (see Table 20-2)

2. Factors that have contributed to the general trend of lower caries rates

a. Use of fluorides, including water fluoridation, fluoride dentifrices, and other fluoride modalities is the most significant factor in the long term, primarily reducing smooth-surface caries; widespread use of fluorides has decreased state and regional differences in caries rates

b. More recently, dental sealants have contributed to reductions in pit-and-fissure caries

c. Greater emphasis on preventive care and increased dental utilization also contribute

3. Distribution varies for both coronal and root surface caries and untreated caries in different groups in the population (Table 20-10); this has implications for community programming

TABLE 20-10 Oral Disease Disparities by Age, Ethnicity, Socioeconomic Status (SES), and Dental Attendance*

Oral Disease	Age/Gender	Ethnicity[†]	SES[‡]	Dental Attendance
Dental caries (coronal caries)	Similar rates for male and female children in all ages groups Slightly higher DMFT rates and lower rates of untreated decay in female adults, possibly because of higher dental care utilization rates	Higher rates of caries and untreated caries in nonwhite ethnic groups, especially among children age 2-4 years and 6-8 years	Higher rates of caries and untreated caries among lower-SES cohorts at all ages; greatest disparity in preschool age (ECC) Up to three times as much caries and untreated caries in groups who are poorest and less than high school education of parents Higher prevalence of ECC also when child care is provided by low-SES individuals	Higher in groups with lower dental attendance
Root caries	Higher in males Lower rates of untreated root caries in females (generally higher dental care utilization rates)	ND	Higher in lower-SES cohorts	Higher in groups with lower dental attendance
Dental sealants	ND	Higher rates in non-Hispanic Caucasian children; associated with SES	Positive association of parents' educational level with children's sealant rates	Higher rates associated with higher dental utilization
Periodontal disease	More recession, severe CAL, and destructive periodontitis in men compared to women, all ages More gender-related temporary periodontal conditions in women resulting from hormonal changes Better oral hygiene in women Increase in rates of moderate and severe CAL, gingival recession, and deeper pocket depths with age; highest in older adults who keep their teeth Very low rates of mild and moderate CAL in children; uncommon in young children	Lower rates of CAL and gingivitis in non-Hispanic Caucasian groups; Mexican Americans Considerably more periodontal treatment in non-Hispanic Caucasians Lower rates of CAL and gingivitis in non-Hispanic Caucasian groups; Mexican Americans Considerably more periodontal treatment in non-Hispanic Caucasians	Substantially higher rates and severity with less education and decreasing family income Higher prevalence and severity in rural compared to urban areas because of SES differences More disparities in low-SES groups and those with low health literacy	Higher rates in populations with low dental attendance
Tooth loss	Higher rates with increasing age Similar rates for males and females	Lower rates in non-Hispanic Caucasian cohorts	Higher rates in lower-SES groups	Higher rates in populations with low dental attendance
Oral and pharyngeal cancer (OPC)	Higher rates with increasing age; median age of 62 at diagnosis and 67 at death Higher OPC rates and death rates among males Narrowing gender gap, attributed to increased and prolonged use of tobacco products by women	Lower rates of OPC and higher survival rates in non-Hispanic Caucasians	Lower rates of OPC and higher survival rates among higher SES groups, related to differences in high-risk behaviors	Lower rates of OPC and higher survival rates in groups with high dental care utilization
Cleft lip and palate	More isolated cleft palates in females More facial clefts in males	Higher rates in non-Hispanic Caucasian cohort compared with African American and Hispanic cohorts Highest rates in Asian and Native American populations	Differences associated with high-risk behaviors	ND
Malocclusion and orthodontic treatment	ND	ND	Disparities occur in treatment, depending on the SES	ND

TABLE 20-10 Oral Disease Disparities by Age, Ethnicity, Socioeconomic Status (SES), and Dental Attendance—cont'd

Oral Disease	Age/Gender	Ethnicity	SES	Dental Attendance
Temporomandibular joint disorders	More common in women than men	ND	ND	ND
Fluorosis	ND	Higher rates in non-Hispanic Caucasian groups as a function of SES	Higher rates in higher SES populations because of excessive use of fluorides	Associated with dental attendance, as a function of SES

Data from National Center for Health Statistics (NCHS): Healthy people 2010 final review: overview and selected findings, PHS Pub No 2012-1038, Hyattsville, Md, 2012, NCHS, http://www.cdc.gov/nchs/data/hpdata2010/hp2010_final_review.pdf; Department of Health and Human Services: Surgeon General report on oral health, Magnitude of the problem, updated April 3, 2014, http://www.nidcr.nih.gov/datastatistics/surgeongeneral/sgr/chap4.htm; Centers for Disease Control and Prevention: Disparities in oral health, July 10, 2013, http://www.cdc.gov/OralHealth/oral_health_disparities/; Li Y, Lee S, Hujoel P, et al: Prevalence and severity of gingivitis in American adults, Am J Dent,23(1):9-13, 2010, http://www.ncbi.nlm.nih.gov/pubmed/20437720; American Academy of Periodontology, CDC: Half of American adults have periodontal disease, 2014: Available at http://www.perio.org/consumer/cdc-study.htm; Eke PI, Dye BA, Wei L, et al: Prevalence of periodontitis in adults in the United States: 2009 and 2010, J Dent Res 91 (10):914-920, 2012, https://www.scribd.com/doc/132397066/Prevalence-of-Periodontitis-in-Adults-in-the-United-States-2009-and-2010-Full-Text-Available; Thornton-Evans G, Eke P, Wei L, et al: Periodontitis among adults aged ≥30years—United States, 2009–2010, MMWR 62(3 Suppl):129-135, November 22, 2013, http://www.cdc.gov/mmwr/preview/mmwrhtml/su6203a21.htm; National Cancer Institute, Surveillance, Epidemiology, and End Results (SEER) Program: SEER stat fact sheets: oral cavity and pharynx cancer, 2011, http://seer.cancer.gov/statfacts/html/oralcav.html; Agarwal MSS, Chopra SS, Jayan B, Verma MM: Epidemiology in orthodontics: a literature review, Orthod Cyber J, September 2013, http://orthocj.com/2013/09/epidemiology-in-orthodontics-a-literature-review/; National Institute of Dental and Craniofacial Research: TMJ (temporomandibular joint and muscle disorders), July 10, 2014, http://www.nidcr.nih.gov/oralhealth/topics/tmj/; and Centers for Disease Control and Prevention: Facts about cleft lip and cleft palate, April 23, 2014, http://www.cdc.gov/ncbddd/birthdefects/cleftlip.html.

ND, No differences documented; *DMFT,* decayed-missing-filled teeth; *ECC,* early childhood caries, *CAL,* clinical attachment loss.

*Health literacy is an underlying factor in disparities in the distribution of all oral diseases.

†In general, people who are non-Hispanic black, Hispanic, and American Indian and Alaska Native generally have the poorest oral health of any racial and ethnic groups in the United States.

‡In general, populations of low SES have much greater oral health disparities than higher-SES populations; low SES is the strongest predictor of poor oral health.

4. Risk and associated factors vary in the population and form the foundation of public health programs (see Chapters 13 and 16 for further discussion of risk factors for caries)
   a. Caries is a multifactorial, infectious, transmissible disease
   b. Low socioeconomic status (SES) of the family is the most powerful predictor of caries in young children; caries control programs should be targeted especially to low-SES populations
   c. Lack of access to water fluoridation is a critical risk factor
   d. Health education and health promotion efforts should be directed to preventive measures to reduce the risk factors
      (1) Reduce bacteria with good oral hygiene and antimicrobials
      (2) Reduce the amount and frequency of fermentable carbohydrates and other acidic foods and drinks in the diet
      (3) Routinely use fluorides and other chemotherapeutic measures to increase the resistance of the enamel to acid attack and enhance the protective nature of saliva
      (4) Place dental sealants to increase the caries resistance of pit-and-fissure surfaces
      (5) Eliminate carious lesions and restore cavitated teeth to eliminate bacteria and improve the individual's ability to remove plaque biofilm

5. Additional risk factors for ECC should be addressed in community programs focused on maternal and child health, especially in lower-SES populations
   a. Transmission of cariogenic bacteria from the caregiver to the young child; parental risk-related behaviors for ECC include infant feeding practices, whether the infant is breastfed or bottle-fed; delayed weaning from bottle feeding or breastfeeding; allowing a baby to fall asleep with a bottle
   b. High-cariogenic diet, including sugar drinks in the bottle or sippy cup and high sugar levels in other components of the diet
   c. ECC is also more common in situations where child care is provided by individuals with low oral health literacy or poor understanding of oral disease prevention
6. Other risk and associated factors for root caries to be considered in public health programs
   a. Root caries increases with age because of a greater likelihood of exposed cementum and other risk factors
   b. The increasing age of the population and decreasing tooth loss result in more available root surfaces to become carious
   c. Older adults exhibit greater use of medications that cause xerostomia, in which case saliva loses its protective capacity; multiple medications are especially a major risk factor for this

d. Increased sugar intake as sense of taste diminishes and eating habits change with age creates a greater risk of caries for older individuals

e. History of coronal caries and smoking are risk factors for root caries

f. Diminished manual dexterity may limit oral self-care

C. Dental sealants

1. Rates of sealed first and second molars have improved; further increase of these rates is an important *Healthy People* objective for 2020 (see Table 20-2)

2. Disparities occur in the rates of sealants in children (see Table 20-10)

3. Permanent molar teeth are most frequently sealed and are targeted in community-based sealant programs because of their greater susceptibility to caries; a new *Healthy People* objective for 2020 is to increase dental sealant application on primary teeth (see Table 20-2) because of the increase in dental caries in children over the past decade

4. Sealants are targeted at children; placement is recommended as soon as possible after tooth eruption

D. Periodontal diseases

1. Periodontal diseases manifest as different clinical entities, depending on aggressiveness, severity, rate of progression, systemic diseases present, hormonal influences, genetics, and other factors

2. Prevalence of periodontal diseases

a. The presence of periodontal diseases, either gingivitis or periodontitis or both, is almost universal, with over 70% of adults in all countries affected

(1) Worldwide data indicate prevalence of severe periodontitis in the range of 5% to 15% in almost all populations, regardless of economic development, oral hygiene, or dental care available

(2) Increased levels of prevalence and severity of periodontal diseases are found in areas of the world where generalized malnutrition is common

(3) Differences in periodontal disease levels between peoples of developed countries and developing countries are attributed to differences in oral hygiene levels

b. Variations in data related to the prevalence of periodontal diseases can be attributed to differences in study designs and measurement

c. Prevalence of moderate to severe destructive periodontitis in the United States in people age 45 to 74 is approximately 13% and has decreased over the previous decade (see Table 20-2); periodontitis is observed even in well-treated patients because of the influence of genetics and immune response

d. Milder forms of periodontitis are more common; over 90% of persons age 13 or older show signs of some clinical attachment loss (CAL) while still maintaining a functioning dentition

e. Although gingivitis has declined in recent years because of greater attention to oral hygiene, it is still present in the majority of the population

3. The distribution of periodontal diseases varies in the U.S. population according to demographic characteristics (see Table 20-10)

4. Risk and associated factors (see the section on "Epidemiology of Periodontal Diseases and Related Risks" in Chapter 14)

5. Tooth retention and tooth loss

a. Rate of complete tooth loss as a result of dental caries or periodontal disease in adults age 65 to 74 is 24%; approximately three fourths of adults age 45 to 64 have had no permanent tooth loss (see Table 20-2)

b. Rates are decreasing despite the aging U.S. population because of increased emphasis on preventive dentistry, greater use of fluorides, improved success with periodontal therapy, and higher dental care utilization rates, especially for preventive strategies

c. Smoking, early tooth loss, poor health, and low level of health literacy are risk factors for edentulism

d. Disparities exist in both edentulism and partial tooth loss (see Table 20-10)

6. Denture use

a. Current specific data on denture use are unavailable

b. Despite reductions in tooth loss, the number of denture wearers will remain significant because of the aging population; the need will continue for denture fabrication and related patient education and community oral health promotion programs with older adults

7. Oral and pharyngeal cancers

a. Occurrence

(1) In the United States, in 2011 an estimated 281,591 people were living with oral and pharyngeal cancers (cancers of the lips, tongue, buccal mucosa, floor of the mouth, and pharynx); estimates for 2014 are 42,440 cases of new oropharyngeal cancer diagnoses and 8390 deaths[1]

(2) Occurrence and site distribution within the mouth vary widely in different parts of the world

(3) Oral and pharyngeal cancers account for 2.5% of all cancers in the United States and 1.4% of all cancer deaths[1]

(4) The survival rate 5 years after diagnosis is 62.7%; the mortality rate varies according to the stage at diagnosis; those diagnosed in the earliest stage have an 82.7% 5-year survival rate versus 37.3% for those diagnosed in the latest stage;[1] the proportion of these cancers diagnosed at the earliest stage has decreased in the past decade (see Table 20-2)

(5) Disparities exist in the distribution of these cancers among different groups (see Table 20-10)

8. Causal and risk factors

a. Evidence is sufficient to infer a causal relationship between the use of tobacco and oropharyngeal cancers; a dose-response relationship exists between cigarette smoking and cancers of the lung, larynx, oral cavity, and urinary bladder in women

b. The major risk factors for oropharyngeal cancers include heavy alcohol consumption, tobacco use, combined alcohol and tobacco use (increases the risk two to four times compared with either factor alone), older age, and high levels of ultraviolet (UV) light exposure (i.e., sun exposure)

c. Other determinants include chronic inflammation, viral infections such as human papillomavirus (particularly HPV-16 and HPV-18), immunodeficiency, poor nutrition, occupational exposures, and genetics

9. *Healthy People 2020* goals directed at improving oropharyngeal cancer morbidity and mortality rates include increased screening by dentists and dental hygienists, increased detection in the early stage, and increased tobacco cessation counseling by dentists and dental hygienists; progress was made from 2000 to 2010 on increased screening, but ground was lost on early detection; no data were available for the frequency of tobacco counseling (see Table 20-2)

E. Cleft lip and palate

1. The CDC estimates that about 2650 babies are born with cleft palate and 4440 are born with cleft lip in the United States each year;[2] oral clefts are the most common class of congenital malformations in the United States; cleft lip is more common than cleft palate

2. Risk factors are important in relation to education for prevention; clefts are associated with maternal diabetes and thyroid disease, smoking, drug consumption (e.g., certain medications to treat epilepsy), nutritional deficiencies (e.g., folic acid deficiency), alcohol consumption, use of teratogenic agents (e.g., corticosteroids, drugs of abuse) during the early stages of pregnancy, and premature birth status

3. In the United States, 33 states have a system for recording and referring infants and children with cleft lips and cleft palates to craniofacial anomaly rehabilitative teams;[3] an HP 2020 objective is to increase this number (see Table 20-2)

4. Disparities exist for clefts in different population groups (see Table 20-10)

F. Malocclusion and orthodontic treatment

1. Although current epidemiologic data are not available for the United States, adequate basic information is available to demonstrate the prevalence of malocclusion and the need for orthodontic care; in general, the prevalence of malocclusion is considered to be increasing worldwide[4]

2. Malocclusions can occur from congenital or acquired crowding of the teeth or jaws; prolonged bottle feeding, thumb sucking, and other behaviors during development are attributed, which indicates a need for public health education programs for young mothers regarding feeding practices and the habits of young children in order to prevent malocclusion

3. No data are available on differences in distribution of malocclusion among population groups, but differences occur in frequency of orthodontic treatment (see Table 20-10)

G. Craniofacial injuries and tooth trauma

1. Crown fractures are the most common type of dental injury to the permanent dentition, and subluxation and avulsion are the most common injury to the primary dentition[5]

2. There is no single risk factor for dental trauma; causes of head and face injuries include accidental falls, assaults, sports-related and recreational activities, bicycle and automobile collisions, and work-related tasks and projects around the house; sports accidents account for 10% to 29% of all dental injuries in children[6]

3. One third of traumatic dental injuries could be prevented, according to treating dentists;[5] prevention depends on an understanding of the risk factors

4. Use of mouthguards, face guards, and helmets is recommended to prevent injuries during high risk contact sports,[6] but few sports have regulations that require their use; health promotion efforts regarding prevention of orofacial injuries should target parents; children, youth, college students, and adults involved in organized sports; coaches; and staff of school and sports organizations that influence policy decisions

5. Most injuries are treated in emergency rooms; education of medical personnel will increase the success of treatment of dental-related injuries; an *HP 2020* objective is to increase the number of states that have an oral and craniofacial health surveillance system (see Table 20-2)

H. Temporomandibular joint (TMJ) disease

1. It is estimated that 10 million Americans are affected by TMJ disorders[7]

2. Possible symptoms include pain in the jaw joint and muscles of mastication, jaw muscle stiffness, limited movement or locking of the jaw, painful clicking or crepitus in the TMJ, and a change in the occlusion; symptoms can be present even when individuals do not perceive a problem

3. Symptoms can be alleviated by eating soft foods, applying ice packs, avoiding extreme jaw movements such as wide yawning and gum chewing, short-term use of over-the-counter (OTC) or prescription pain medicines, and learning techniques to reduce stress; symptoms usually clear with minimal or no treatment; aggressive treatment is rarely recommended

4. Variations in distribution occur according to demographic characteristics (see Table 20-10)

I. Dental fluorosis

1. Description—chronic endemic form of enamel hypoplasia caused by ingesting excessive fluoride during the time of tooth formation in the late secretory to early maturation stage of enamel development; starts for central incisors as early as age 22 months, usually occurs at 24 months, and may occur as late as age 4 years; characterized by retention of enamel proteins and change in enamel matrix structure; defective calcification produces a white, chalky appearance of the enamel that may undergo brown discoloration and change of surface texture in more severe classifications

2. Dean's classification of dental fluorosis (see "Fluorosis Indices" in Table 20-11)—provides a description of fluorosis for survey purposes; other fluorosis indices, such as

TABLE 20-11	**Common Dental Indices Used in Community Oral Health and Oral Health Research**
Dental Index	**Interpretation**
Dental Caries Indices	
Decayed-Missing-Filled Teeth (DMFT) *Index:* complex irreversible index used to measure past and present coronal caries experience of a population with permanent teeth *D* indicates a carious tooth *M* indicates a tooth missing as a result of dental caries *F* indicates a filled tooth because of caries	DMF and def can be scored on teeth (DMFT and deft) or surfaces (DMFS and defs); scoring on teeth is recommended for survey work, and scoring on surfaces is recommended for clinical trials because it provides more sensitivity even though it has greater variability Total DMF (D+M+F) or dmf indicates cumulative caries experience; D provides information about morbidity and specific treatment needs; F and M provide information about dental utilization Programming needs can be determined by the total score as well as the scores within each category; e.g., high caries experience (DMF or dmf) indicates need for programs to prevent and control caries; high D or d indicates need for treatment programs; high M or m indicates need for education and earlier intervention; high F or f score indicates dental utilization Scores can be compared to evaluate program success; e.g., reduction of D or d and increase in F or f indicates a successful caries treatment program, and marked increase in D or d, DMF or dmf, or both, indicates failure of caries prevention program
deft Index: variation of the DMFT; is used to measure observable caries experience in primary teeth; the *d* and *f* symbols are the same as in the DMFT; however, *e* indicates the need for extraction (not extracted), and missing teeth are not considered	To control for variability of scoring missing teeth in children at the age of exfoliation, the def index does not score exfoliated or extracted teeth or surfaces, thus possibly underrepresenting caries experience
Root Caries Index (RCI): method for reporting the severity of root caries (decayed and filled exposed root surfaces)	The index is expressed as a percentage of decayed and filled root surfaces out of the population of at-risk root surfaces (those exposed to the oral environment as a result of gingival recession)
Gingivitis Indices	
Gingival Index (GI): reversible index based on severity of inflammation at the gingival margin; can be used to determine prevalence and severity of gingivitis in epidemiologic surveys as well as individual dentition; often used in controlled clinical trials of preventive or therapeutic agents	Results can be unreliable and difficult to replicate due to subjectivity of criteria (calibration is critical) SCORING CRITERIA: 0—Normal gingiva 1—Mild inflammation: slight change in color; slight edema; no bleeding on probing 2—Moderate inflammation: redness, edema, and glazing; bleeding on probing 3—Severe inflammation: marked redness and edema, ulceration; tendency to spontaneous bleeding INTERPRETATION OF GI: 0.1 to 1.0: Mild gingivitis 1.1 to 2.0: Moderate gingivitis 2.1 to 3.0: Severe gingivitis
Sulcus Bleeding Index (SBI): complex index designed to detect early symptoms of gingivitis; useful in short-term clinical trials; measured on probing	Results can be unreliable due to subjectivity of criteria (calibration is critical) Results are reported by frequency of each score SCORING CRITERIA: 0—Healthy appearance of papillary and marginal gingiva; no bleeding on sulcus probing 1—Apparently healthy papillary and marginal gingiva showing no change in color and no swelling; but bleeding from sulcus on probing 2—Bleeding on probing and change of color caused by inflammation; no swelling or microscopic edema 3—Bleeding on probing; change in color; and slight edematous swelling 4—Bleeding on probing; obvious swelling; may have change in color 5—Bleeding on probing; spontaneous bleeding; change in color; and marked swelling with or without ulceration
Gingival Bleeding Index (GBI): simple, easy-to-implement measure of the presence or absence of bleeding (dichotomous measure); measured with the use of floss	Index only provides information about bleeding, not about other parameters of gingivitis Dichotomous measure lacks sensitivity but has good reliability (easy to calibrate) SCORING CRITERIA: Results are reported by frequency of score based on presence (1) or absence (0) of bleeding
Eastman Interdental Bleeding Index (EIBI): simple, easy-to-implement measure of the presence or absence of bleeding (dichotomous measure); measured with the use of a triangular interdental stimulator	Index only provides information about bleeding, not about other parameters of gingivitis Dichotomous measure lacks sensitivity but has good reliability (easy to calibrate) SCORING CRITERIA: Results are reported by frequency of score based on presence (1) or absence (0) of bleeding
Periodontal Disease Indices	
Periodontal Disease Index (PDI): used to measure the presence and severity of periodontal disease, combining measures of reversible and irreversible disease within the same index	This index was first to introduce the current method of combining recession and pocket depth to determine clinical attachment loss (CAL) The six teeth scored by the PDI (numbers 3, 9, 12, 19, 25, and 28), referred to as the Ramfjord teeth (after Dr. Ramfjord, who developed the index), are considered sensitive for partial mouth scoring of periodontal conditions with other indices The PDI is no longer recommended because of the current understanding that gingivitis and periodontitis are two different disease entities; the various components are currently measured separately with other indices or measures

TABLE 20-11   Common Dental Indices Used in Community Oral Health and Oral Health Research—cont'd

Dental Index	Interpretation
Community Periodontal Index of Treatment Needs (CPITN): used as part of the Oral Health Surveys by the World Health Organization; facilitates rapid assessment of mean disease status of a population; the Periodontal Screening and Recording (PSR) Index developed by the American Dental Association for use in clinical practice uses the same codes and criteria; pockets are measured with a specially designed, lightweight probe with a 0.5-mm markings, a colored area to denote 3.5-mm to 5.5-mm depth, and a ball tip	Scores are reported as codes in six sextants of the mouth CRITERIA FOR SCORING CODES: *Code 0*—Line at colored area visible; no rough areas, no bleeding *Code 1*—Line at colored area visible with bleeding after probing *Code 2*—Line visible with bleeding and rough areas (calculus) *Code 3*—Colored area only partially visible (>3.5 mm) *Code 4*—Colored area completely disappears (>5.5 mm) By code for furcation involvement, mobility, mucogingival problem, marked recession, or all INTERPRETATION OF CODES (Treatment Needs): *Code* 0—Preventive care; biofilm control *Code* 1—Preventive care; biofilm control *Code* 2—Preventive care and calculus removal; biofilm removal *Code* 3—Comprehensive periodontal assessment and treatment plan (TP); counseling regarding TP; biofilm control *Code* 4—Comprehensive periodontal assessment and TP for nonsurgical periodontal therapy; counseling regarding TP; biofilm control
Community Periodontal Index (CPI): adaptation of the CPITN to measure periodontal status of a community; treatment need codes from the CPITN are eliminated; compared to the CPITN, the CPI measures periodontal status, whereas the CPITN reports periodontal treatment needs	Reported as CPI (periodontal status) codes and loss of attachment (LOA; same as CAL) codes SCORING CRITERIA FOR CPI PERIODONTAL STATUS CODES: *Code 0*—Entire colored band visible; healthy periodontal tissues: no bleeding *Code 1*—Entire colored band visible; bleeding on probing *Code 2*—Entire colored band visible; calculus present *Code 3*—Colored band partially hidden: 4-mm to 5-mm pockets *Code 4*—Colored band entirely hidden: >6-mm pockets If the cemento-enamel junction (CEJ) is visible or the CPI is 4, LOA codes 1 to 4 are used CRITERIA FOR LOA (CAL) CODES: *Code 0*—0 to 3 mm LOA—CEJ covered by gingival margin and CPI score of 0 to 3 *Code 1*—3.5 to 5.5 mm LOA; CEJ within the black band on probe *Code 2*—6 to 8 mm LOA; CEJ between top of black band and 8.5-mm mark on probe *Code 3*—9 to 11 mm LOA; CEJ between 8.5-mm and 11.5-mm marks on probe *Code 4*—LOA >12 mm; CEJ beyond highest mark (11.5 mm) on probe
Oral Hygiene Indices	
Simplified Oral Hygiene Index (OHI-S): reversible index used to measure oral hygiene status; useful to survey oral hygiene in a population; scores six teeth that represent the whole mouth, assessing them separately for debris and calculus, and yielding a DI-S score (debris index–simplified) and a CI-S score (calculus index–simplified), which are combined for the OHI-S score	SCORING CRITERIA FOR DI-S: 0—No debris or stain present 1—Soft debris covering not more than one third of exposed tooth surface or presence of extrinsic stains without debris regardless of surface area covered 2—Soft debris covering more than one third but not more than two thirds of exposed tooth surface 3—Soft debris covering more than two thirds of exposed tooth surface SCORING CRITERIA FOR CI-S: 0—No calculus present 1—Supragingival calculus covering not more than one third of exposed tooth surface 2—Supragingival calculus covering more than one third but not more than two thirds of exposed tooth surface or presence of individual flecks of subgingival calculus around cervical portion of tooth 3—Supragingival calculus covering more than two thirds of exposed tooth surface or a continuous heavy band of subgingival calculus around cervical portion of tooth INTERPRETATION OF OHI-S: 0.0 to 1.2: Good oral hygiene 1.3 to 3.0: Fair oral hygiene 3.1 to 6.0: Poor oral hygiene INTERPRETATION OF DI-S or CI-S: 0.0 to 0.6: Good oral hygiene 0.7 to 1.8: Fair oral hygiene 1.9 to 3.0: Poor oral hygiene

(Continued)

TABLE 20-11 Common Dental Indices Used in Community Oral Health and Oral Health Research—cont'd

Dental Index	Interpretation
Plaque Index (PlI): used to assess extent of soft deposits, measuring differences in thickness of debris only at the gingival margin of the tooth surface; useful in longitudinal studies and clinical trials	SCORING CRITERIA: 0—No plaque in gingival area 1—Film of plaque adhering to free gingival margin and adjacent area of tooth; plaque is noticed only by running probe across tooth surface 2—Moderate accumulation of soft deposits within the gingival margin, on adjacent tooth surface, or in both areas that can be seen with the naked eye 3—Abundance of soft matter within the gingival pocket, at the gingival margin, or both, and on the adjacent tooth surface INTERPRETATION OF PlI: 0: Excellent 0.1 to 0.9: Good 1.0 to 1.9: Fair 2.0 to 3.0: Poor
Patient Hygiene Performance (PHP): provides a simple, quick, overall oral hygiene assessment, scoring disclosed plaque biofilm in five sections of the tooth surface of six representative teeth; separately interproximal areas to evaluate interdental cleaning	SCORING CRITERIA: Plaque biofilm is scored as present (1) or absent (0) in each of the five areas; scores are combined for the tooth score or reported separately for evaluation of oral hygiene in specific areas INTERPRETATION OF PHP: 0: Excellent 0.1 to 1.7: Good 1.8 to 3.4: Fair 3.5 to 5.0: Poor
Turesky modification of the Quigley-Hein Plaque Index (TPl): provides an overall assessment of oral hygiene similar to the OHI-S but more sensitive because (1) the scale has more differentiation at the lower end, (2) all teeth are scored, and (3) disclosant is used; recommended for clinical trials of preventive and therapeutic agents	Teeth are disclosed; all teeth except third molars are evaluated; results can be unreliable because of subjectivity at the lower end of the scale; careful calibration is critical SCORING CRITERIA: Mesial, distal, and middle aspects of buccal and lingual surfaces of all teeth are scored on a scale of 0 to 5 0—No plaque 1—Separate flecks of plaque at the cervical margin 2—A thin continuous band of plaque (up to 1 mm) at the cervical margin 3—A band of plaque wider than 1 mm but covering less than one third of the tooth surface 4—Plaque covering at least one third but less than two thirds of the surface 5—Plaque covering two thirds or more of the surface
Modified Navy Plaque Index (MNPl): provides a detailed assessment of overall oral hygiene as well as effectiveness of interdental cleaning; similar to the PHP with more sensitivity as a result of the surfaces being divided into nine instead of five areas; useful to assess the value of oral health education programs and individuals' oral hygiene practices	Results can be unreliable because of the complexity of the index; requires careful calibration SCORING CRITERIA: Plaque biofilm is scored as present (1) or absent (0) in each of the nine areas; scores are combined for the tooth score or reported separately for evaluation of oral hygiene in specific areas, as follows: Whole mouth (all nine areas) Marginal (mesial, distal, and middle aspects of the marginal area) Approximal (mesial and distal contact areas)
Volpe-Manhold Index (VMl): measures extent of supragingival calculus on the lingual surfaces of mandibular anterior teeth for calculus clinical trials	Height of calculus is measured, which can be reported as a tooth score (possible range of 0 to 15) or whole-mouth score (possible range of 0 to 90) Large range of scores allows for more valid statistical analysis

Fluorosis Indices

Dental Index	Interpretation
Dean Fluorosis Index and *Community Fluorosis Index (CFI):* Dean developed the classification as categories only, referred to as Dean Fluorosis Index; later numbers ranging from 0 to 4 were added to denote the categories for surveillance purposes, and the index was referred to as the Community Fluorosis Index *Comparison to other fluorosis indices:* The Thylstrup-Fejerskov (TF) fluorosis index and Tooth Surface Index of Fluorosis (TSIF) are based on Dean's categories with expansion of categories to create greater sensitivity for research purposes	An individual is categorized by classification and prevalence of each category is reported in a population; the CFI of a population is assigned based on the mean of all scores of the study population; a classification of mild or less is not considered a cosmetic problem, and a CFI score of less than 0.6 is not considered a problem for the community SCORING CRITERIA: *Normal (0)*—Enamel presents the usual translucent semi-vitriform structure; the surface is smooth, glossy, and usually pale creamy white *Questionable (0.5)*—Enamel has slight aberrations from the normal translucency, ranging from a few white flecks to occasional white spots; this classification is used in when neither the *Very Mild* nor *Normal* classification is definitively justified *Very mild (1)*—Small, opaque, paper-white areas are scattered irregularly over the tooth but not involving as much as approximately 25% of the tooth surface; frequently included in this classification are teeth showing no more than about 1 to 2 mm of white opacity at the cusp tips of premolars or second molars

TABLE 20-11   Common Dental Indices Used in Community Oral Health and Oral Health Research—cont'd

Dental Index	Interpretation
	Mild (2)—White opaque areas in the enamel are more extensive but do not involve as much as 50% of the tooth
	Moderate (3)—All enamel surfaces of the teeth are affected, and surfaces subject to attrition show wear; brown stain is frequently a disfiguring feature
	Severe (4)—All enamel surfaces are affected; hypoplasia is so marked that the general form of the tooth may be affected; discrete or confluent pitting is a the major diagnostic sign of this classification; brown stains are widespread, and teeth often appear as if corroded
	SIGNICANCE OF CFI SCORES:
	0.0 to 0.4: Negative
	0.4 to 0.6: Borderline
	0.6 to 1.0: Slight
	1.0 to 2.0: Medium
	2.0 to 3.0: Marked
	3.0 to 4.0: Very marked

Data from Carranza FA, Forrest JL, Kenney EB, Klokkevold PR: Carranza's clinical periodontology, ed 12, St Louis, 2014, Elsevier Saunders; Hiremath SS: Textbook of preventive and community dentistry, ed 2, New Delhi, India, 2011, Elsevier India; Wilkins EM: Clinical practice of the dental hygienist, ed 11, Philadelphia, 2012, Lippincott, Williams and World Health Organization: Oral health/periodontal/country profiles, 2014. http://www.who.int/oral_health/databases/niigata/en/.

the Tooth Surface Index of Fluorosis and the Thylstrup-Fejerskov Fluorosis Index, are based on Dean's classification and are more sensitive for research purposes

3. Prevalence of dental fluorosis
   a. Less than one fourth of the population exhibit fluorosis, with the vast majority in the classifications "very mild" and "mild"; the prevalence is higher in younger groups, and the prevalence of fluorosis in young children may be increasing in the very mild to mild categories as a result of widespread use of fluorides
   b. Even children born and raised in optimally fluoridated communities can exhibit mild forms of fluorosis because of excess fluoride consumption from other sources
   c. Occurs in many parts of the world; considered a public health problem in East Africa, India, and Eastern Europe because of the severity; not considered a major public health problem in the United States at this time and is being addressed by the careful use of fluorides and the downward adjustment of the Public Health Service (PHS) recommended level of fluoride for water fluoridation
   d. Differences occur in the distribution of fluorosis in different groups (see Table 20-10)
4. Causes
   a. Ingesting water with naturally occurring excessive fluoride
      (1) 1 to 2 parts per million fluoride (ppm F) results in mild fluorosis; 2 to 4 ppm F results in moderate to severe fluorosis
      (2) The Environmental Protection Agency (EPA), which is responsible for the safety and quality of water, has set the maximum allowable limit for fluoride at 4 ppm F and a secondary limit at 2 ppm F (defluoridation is required at 4 ppm F and recommended at 2 ppm F)
      (3) Some communities do not have a community water supply; some members of the population depend on well water; fluoride levels of well water vary
   b. Children swallowing excessive amounts of fluoride-containing dentifrices—swallowing or overenthusiastic use of fluoridated toothpaste by young children is a concern; prudent use is "smear" or "rice-size" amount of toothpaste on the brush for children younger than age 3 years and a "pea-size" amount for children age 3 to 6 years; it is also recommended that toothpaste be placed on the toothbrush by an adult
   c. Inappropriate supplementation with fluoride tablets or fluoride-containing vitamins in children—mild to moderate fluorosis is associated with the use of fluoride supplements by children; use tends to be higher in children from higher-SES families
   d. Halo effect of secondary fluoride exposures to fluoride in processed foods and beverages, especially those that vary by water source, can occur even in nonfluoridated areas
      (1) Infant formula, especially soybean-based formulas, should be used in moderation in fluoridated communities
      (2) Fruit juices and drinks with moderate to high concentrations of fluoride consumed by children may contribute to fluorosis; in the United States; water and processed beverages can provide approximately 75% of a person's fluoride intake
      (3) Some bottled water manufactured in the United States contains an optimal concentration of fluoride; most contain less than 0.3 ppm fluoride
   e. Consumption of fluoridated water in combination with other significant dietary sources of fluoride
      (1) Combining systemic fluorides will increase the fluoride level above the optimum and cause fluorosis in children who are still in the stages of enamel

BOX 20-5 Recommendations to Reduce the Risk of Fluorosis

1. Counsel parents and caregivers regarding the use of fluoride toothpaste by young children, especially those younger than 2 years
2. Encourage parents to supervise the use of fluoride toothpaste among children younger than 6 years to reduce swallowing it
3. Promote the use of a small amount of toothpaste by young children
4. For children younger than 2 years, weigh the risk and benefits of recommending fluoride products, taking into consideration the fluoride level in the community drinking water, other sources of fluoride, and factors likely to affect susceptibility to tooth decay
5. Target mouth rinsing and application of high-concentration fluoride products to persons at high risk for dental caries
6. Target and judiciously prescribe fluoride supplements
7. Know the fluoride concentration in the primary source of drinking water in order to make appropriate recommendations
8. Use an alternative source of water for children age 8 and younger whose primary drinking water contains more than 2 parts per million fluoride (ppm F)
9. Label the fluoride concentration of bottled water
10. Collaborate with professional health care organizations, public health agencies, and suppliers of oral care products to educate health care professionals and the public
11. Identify effective strategies to promote adoption of recommendations for using fluoride

Data from Centers for Disease Control and Prevention: Community water fluoridation; Dental fluorosis, July 10, 2013. http://www.cdc.gov/fluoridation/faqs/dental_fluorosis/#a10.

development (up to age 8 years); education is needed to inform the public of the need to control early consumption of fluoride
    (2) Care must be taken to control young children inadvertently swallowing other sources of fluoride, such as toothpaste and mouthrinse
  5. Prevention of dental fluorosis
    a. The CDC has issued recommendations to reduce the risk of fluorosis (Box 20-5)
    b. Because of concerns about the increase in fluorosis in children, DHHS recently recommended reducing the optimal amount of fluoride per liter of water to reduce the possibility of children receiving too much fluoride, since there are now multiple other sources of fluoride; this updated recommendation is based on EPA and DHHS scientific assessments in 2011, which will also guide the EPA in determining whether to lower the maximum amount of fluoride allowed in drinking water; this currently recommended optimal level is 0.7 mg F per liter of water (0.7 ppm F)
    c. Prior to promoting a fluoride modality or combination of modalities, one must consider the group's risk for dental caries, fluoride history, current fluoride sources, and potential for dental fluorosis
    d. Actions and recommendations related to the optimal level of fluoride in drinking water and judicious use of other fluorides are in response to the need to control fluorosis; future assessment will determine the results of current measures to prevent fluorosis

MEASUREMENT OF DISEASES AND CONDITIONS IN ORAL EPIDEMIOLOGY

A. Dental index—abbreviated measurement tool used for data collection; measures the presence or degree of intensity of a disease or condition in a population; graduated numerical scale with defined upper and lower limits designed to facilitate summarizing or describing a disease or condition in the population, or for comparisons among populations; a higher number on the scale indicates more severe disease or condition; measured by clinical observation with an epidemiologic examination

B. Attributes of an ideal dental index
  1. Validity—accuracy of measuring what is intended to be measured
  2. Reliability—measures consistently at different times; reproducibility, stability of measurement
  3. Utility—clear, simple, and objective
  4. Sensitive to shifts in disease in either direction
  5. Acceptable to the individuals being measured
  6. Quantifiable; amenable to statistical analysis
  7. Clinically significant and meaningful

C. The index may assess disease that is a reversible condition, an irreversible condition, or a combination; therefore, indices are classified as:
  1. Reversible index—measures conditions that can be reversed (e.g., gingivitis, plaque biofilm, calculus)
  2. Irreversible index—measures cumulative conditions that cannot be reversed (e.g., dental caries, bone loss, fluorosis)

D. Some common dental indices are used in community oral health and oral health research (Table 20-11)

E. Index selection is determined by:
  1. Type of condition to be assessed, specific to the information of interest or the needs of the client or community
  2. Age of the population
  3. Purpose of the assessment (e.g., survey or clinical trial)

F. Other approaches to measurement in a population
  1. A disaggregated approach rather than an index is currently used on the NHANES and other surveys to assess periodontal conditions; gingival bleeding, recession, pocket depth, CAL, and calculus as a contributing risk factor are measured
  2. Basic Screening Survey (BSS) for surveillance
    a. A simple screening method currently used with adults, school-age children, and preschool-age children in national surveys
    b. Includes oral screening and an optional questionnaire
    c. Screeners may be nondental personnel to improve access to the population and reduce cost
    d. Assesses a variety of oral health conditions consistent with the Healthy People oral health objectives to monitor the success of these objectives and compare population groups
    e. Efficiently assesses dental caries using dichotomous measures (e.g., yes or no) to assess the absence or presence of untreated dental caries and dental caries

experience (at least one decayed, restored, or missing tooth) on a per-person basis, as opposed to use of more complex indices

  f. Regardless of condition being measured, results are reported as the following categories to assess need and referral for dental care:

    (1) None—no obvious oral health problem; routine care recommended

    (2) Early—observable oral health problem; early dental care (within several weeks) recommended

    (3) Urgent—signs or symptoms present (e.g., pain, infection, swelling, soft tissue ulceration) of longer than 2 weeks' duration; emergency dental care (within 24 hours) recommended

  g. Results will underestimate disease prevalence

G. Examiners or raters should use calibrated or standardized observational criteria in their use of an index or the BSS criteria; examiner reliability requires training on the use and interpretation of evaluative criteria and repeated use of the index

  1. Intra-rater (intra-examiner) reliability—each examiner repeats the scoring process using a data collection instrument; extent to which a rater remains consistent within himself or herself

  2. Inter-rater (inter-examiner) reliability—consistency exists between or among examiners; degree to which different raters obtain the same results when using the same data collection instrument

H. Potential errors in assessing disease

  1. Errors in sampling technique—use of nonrandomized samples, use of incorrect or inconsistent sampling technique, sample bias and too-small sample size can result in a nonrepresentative sample, particularly for subgroups of interest

  2. Errors in collecting and recording data—variation in assessment; lack of calibration; inconsistent or inaccurate data collection by the examiners; known or unknown bias; intended or unintended misleading or untruthful responses; lack of compliance of participants; incorrect documenting of data by recorders; and inaccurate data entry into the computer

  3. Errors in analyzing data—incorrect computation, incorrect selection of statistical tests, incomplete analysis, and invalid interpretation

PREVENTING AND CONTROLLING ORAL DISEASES AND CONDITIONS

Public Health Measures

A. Population-focused strategies to alleviate, reduce, or eliminate a health problem or issue that is an actual or potential cause of morbidity or mortality

B. Selection of strategy is based on the seven characteristics of an effective public health solution (see earlier section on "Basic Concepts"); several strategies may be implemented depending on the issue to be addressed

---

BOX 20-6   Ten Great Public Health Achievements—United States, Twentieth Century
1. Immunizations
2. Motor vehicle safety
3. Workplace safety
4. Control of infectious diseases
5. Decline in deaths from heart disease and stroke
6. Safer and healthier foods
7. Healthier mothers and babies
8. Family planning
9. Fluoridation of drinking water
10. Tobacco as a health hazard

Data from Centers for Disease Control and Prevention: Ten great public health achievements in the 20th century, 1900–1999, April 26, 2013. http://www.cdc.gov/about/history/tengpha.htm.

C. Examples of public health measures include vaccination, water purification, and water fluoridation (Box 20-6)

Measures for Preventing and Controlling Dental Caries

Refer to the sections on "Topical Fluorides and Fluoride Varnishes" and "Dentifrices and Prophylactic Pastes" in Chapter 13 and "Caries Management" in Chapter 16.

A. Water fluoridation (Table 20-12)

  1. Adjustment of the natural fluoride (F) concentration to optimal level

    a. 0.7 ppm F (same as 1 mg F/L water) was recommended by the DHHS in 2011 (see earlier discussion of dental fluorosis for the reason)

    b. This suggested level of fluoride is a nonenforceable recommendation from the PHS

    c. Some states have community fluoridation laws that are enforceable

    d. Partial exposure (lower than the recommended fluoride level) provides partial protection

    e. Level must be maintained to continue maximum benefits of fluoridation; benefits are lost when fluoridation is discontinued

  2. Fluoridation is one of the 10 most effective public health measures of the twentieth century (see Box 20-6); meets the requirements of a public health solution (see Box 20-1)

  3. Fluoridation does not have specific targets; it has the potential to reduce disparities by reaching everyone in the community

  4. Fluoridation is the most practical form of preventing caries in communities with established community water systems

  5. Fluoridation effectively prevents and controls dental caries in children and adults

    a. Is attributed with 20% to 40% caries reduction in the mixed dentition of children (8 to 12 years of age), 15% to 35% caries reduction in the permanent dentition of adolescents (14 to 17 years of age), and 20% to 40% reduction of coronal caries in adults

TABLE 20-12   Overview of Fluoride Delivery Modalities

Delivery Mechanism	Active Ingredient(s)	Intended Population	Indications for Use
Professionally Applied Fluoride			
Gels, foams, mouthrinses	2% NaF (920 ppm) *or* 1.23% APF (12,300 ppm) *or* 0.15% SnF (1000 ppm)	Any person with an elevated caries risk	APF and SnF no longer recommended for general population; may be indicated for high-risk, special-needs groups
Varnishes	5% NaF (22,600 ppm)	Any person with an elevated caries risk	Recommended as a more effective fluoride delivery mechanism due to sustainability in salivary solution
Self-Applied Fluoride			
Dentifrices	0.243% NaF *or* 0.76% MFP *or* 0.0454% SnF All are 1000 to 15000 ppm	Ages 2+ years Low to moderate caries risk	Most important delivery mode for fluoride due to consistent topical exposure; indicated as a preventive agent for all populations.
Fluoride Rx	NaF or APF; concentration % can vary depending on delivery modality and weight of individual	Any person with an elevated caries risk and/or lack of available community water fluoridation	*Children* 0.25-, 0.50-, or 1.0-mg NaF tablets, lozenges, liquids, and vitamin preparations for systemic use generally in children 6 months to 16 years; drops used with infants (see Table 20-13); school programs no longer recommended by the CDC *Adults* 1.1% NaF dentifrice, 0.5% NaF gel, or 0.15% SnF gel prescribed for topical use in individuals age 16 and older
Public Health Fluoride Programs			
Community water fluoridation	0.7 ppm F sodium silicofluoride (solid), NaF (solid), or hydrofluorosilicic acid (liquid)	Communities at large; municipal water system is required	Most cost-effective and efficient modality for bringing fluoride benefits to a community *Healthy People 2020* objective OH-13 goal = 79.6% of U.S population served by fluoridated water Fluoridation costs vary with size of community Primary benefit is topical exposure after tooth eruption
School water fluoridation	4.5 times optimum water concentration	School-age children in nonfluoridated communities	No longer emphasized because of increased presence of water fluoridation, multiple other sources of fluoride, and disadvantages of modality
School fluoride tablet programs	1-mg NaF chewable tablet, swished and swallowed	School-age children in unfluoridated communities	No longer emphasized because of increased presence of water fluoridation and other sources of fluoride
School fluoride mouthrinse programs	0.05% NaF (230 ppm): daily rinsing 0.2% NaF (920 ppm): weekly rinsing	School-age children in fluoridated and nonfluoridated communities	Limited use today because of increased presence of community water fluoridation; OTC mouthrinses in similar concentrations readily available for at-home use
Fluoride varnish programs (see Box 20-7)	5% NaF (22,600 ppm)	At-risk children, usually less than 6 years old; status of water fluoridation not a consideration	Recommended and widely popular with Head Start and other preschool-age programs as well as in public health well-baby clinics and pediatric medical offices because of effectiveness, minimal risk of ingestion, and ease of use
Other Fluoride Modalities			
Addition of fluoride to salt	250 ppm NaF	Countries lacking widespread municipal water supplies	Used with food preparation; distribution and equitable population exposure may vary; not used in United States or Canada
Addition of fluoride to milk	$\leq$4 ppm NaF or sodium monofluoride	School-age children in countries lacking widespread municipal water supplies	Studied in other countries but not used in United States or Canada due to extensive water fluoridation; effective but not ideal form of delivery

Data from American Dental Association: Fluoride and fluoridation, 2014, http://www.ada.org/en/public-programs/advocating-for-the-public/fluoride-and-fluoridation; Fluoride supplements, http://www.ada.org/en/member-center/oral-health-topics/fluoride-supplements; Fluoridation facts, 2005, http://www.ada.org/~/media/ADA/Member%20Center/FIles/fluoridation_facts.ashx; Centers for Disease Control and Prevention: Community water fluoridation, July 10, 2013, http://www.cdc.gov/fluoridation/; Guidelines and recommendations, April 14, 2014, http://www.cdc.gov/fluoridation/guidelines/index.htm/; and Texas Department of State Health Services: Happy child, bright smile: fluoride varnish manual, Pub No E08-13077, March 2009, http://www.dshs. state.tx.us/dental/default.shtm.

APF, Acidulated phosphate fluoride; *NaF,* sodium fluoride; *SnF,* stannous fluoride; *OTC,* over-the-counter; *sodium monofluorophosphate*

b. Benefits both primary and permanent teeth

c. Primarily benefits smooth surface caries; as DMFS (decayed, missing, and filled permanent surfaces) rates in a population are reduced by fluoride, the proportion of pit-and-fissure caries increases, even though the absolute number is reduced

d. Controls both coronal and root caries in older adults

e. Helps to control caries resulting from reduced salivary flow caused by medications

f. Has no known prenatal benefits

g. Benefits of fluoride accumulate; combination of water fluoridation with topical fluoride provides additional benefits (systemic programs should not be combined to avoid increase in fluorosis in the population)

h. Fluoride is the most effective means to prevent and control dental caries; a common misconception is that oral hygiene is the most effective means

6. Indirect benefits of fluoride include fewer missing teeth resulting in improved self-image, less complicated restorative procedures, pain reduction, decreased malocclusion, and decreased periodontal problems related to tooth loss, all of which lead to improved quality of life for the public; indirect benefits also include positive influence on the practice of dentistry and dental hygiene

7. Posteruption benefits—primary benefit of fluoridated water occurs after tooth eruption as a result of topical effects; preeruption effects are minor

a. Critical period for benefits in children is immediately after tooth eruption so that immature enamel of newly erupted teeth can uptake the fluoride (ages 6 months to 13 years)

b. Posteruption benefits rely on the fluoride being available in solution (via saliva) at the surface of the tooth; systemic fluoride is released into saliva and is available in saliva and plaque biofilm fluids

c. Fluoride inhibits demineralization by adsorbing to the carbonated hydroxyapatite crystals, protecting the enamel surface from dissolution by acids

d. Fluoride enhances remineralization of incipient caries by adsorbing during the continual demineralization-remineralization process; this is the primary action of fluoride for control of dental caries

e. When fluoridated water is consumed, saliva has a constant fluoride level, making it continually available for uptake by the enamel

f. Bound fluoride in plaque biofilm is released in response to the lowered pH level and taken up more readily by the demineralized enamel

8. Preeruption benefits—once thought to be the primary action, this is now understood to be a minor effect compared with the posteruptive action; fluoride is incorporated into the mineralized tooth structure during tooth development by the replacement of hydroxyapatite with fluorapatite during enamel formation

9. Most cost-effective and efficient method of bringing fluoride benefits to a community

a. A *Healthy People 2020* Oral Health objective calls for 79.6% of the U.S. population served by community water systems to have optimally fluoridated water; 72.4% of the population currently has fluoridated water (see Table 20-2)

b. Cost of fluoridation varies with the size of the community, water system, labor costs, and chemicals used; smaller communities experience higher costs because equipment and supplies required for smaller water systems are more costly

c. The approximate annual per-person cost of water fluoridation is 50 cents for communities of more than 20,000 residents, $1 for communities of 10,000 to 20,000 residents, and $3 for communities of less than 5000

d. Annual per-person savings of dental treatment costs range from $16 in small communities to $19 in large communities; every $1 invested yields $38 in savings of dental treatment costs; the approximate cost of providing fluoridation to an individual for a lifetime is equivalent to the national average cost to restore one carious lesion

e. Fluoridation is compatible with other water treatment processes; quality assurance protocol, including recommended annual training of personnel to prevent spills, is necessary; equipment or machinery used for community water fluoridation resembles that used to add other agents to water systems, facilitating training of water treatment personnel

10. Compounds used for water fluoridation

a. Any compound that forms fluoride ions in aqueous solution can be used; the selection depends on the number and accessibility of water sources and water quality

b. Most popular compounds used in fluoridation of water supplies include:
   (1) Sodium silicofluoride (solid)
   (2) Sodium fluoride (solid)—most commonly used and least expensive; byproduct of fertilizer manufacturing, which results in the claim of those opposed to fluoridation that it is a ploy to use waste
   (3) Hydrofluorosilicic acid (liquid)—most expensive

11. Extensive research has demonstrated the safety of fluoridation

a. It is noncarcinogenic (opponents claim it is carcinogenic)

b. Kidney failure is the only condition that requires consideration; kidney dialysis requires the use of mineral-free water

c. No valid research results have linked optimal levels of fluoride to any health problems

d. It is safe to the fetus; the U.S. Food and Drug Administration (FDA) does not recommend the use of fluoride during pregnancy because no known benefits exist, not because it is considered unsafe

12. Role of government agencies
    a. PHS provides funding through block grants and consultation to states
    b. CDC provides education to public and water operators and monitors water fluoridation as part of the NOHSS
    c. State oral health departments provide consultation and assistance to counties and cities attempting to fluoridate, training and monitoring for water system operators, and monitoring of water fluoridation within the state
    d. Local governments without state-mandated fluoridation decide whether or not to fluoridate, implement water fluoridation, and pay the ongoing costs of equipment and supplies
13. Legality of fluoridation—courts have upheld the constitutionality of water fluoridation
14. Promotion of water fluoridation
    a. Oral health care professionals are effective advocates for promoting water fluoridation within a community (Box 20-7)
    b. Ongoing education of individuals is required to encourage their continual support of fluoridation; fluoridation continues to be an issue with regard to wider public acceptance; individuals should be aware of their community fluoride water levels (information is available at My Water's Fluoride at http://apps.nccd.cdc.gov/MWF/Index.asp) and of the ways they have benefited from fluoridation in their communities

---

---

c. Three methods of implementing fluoridation:
   (1) Administrative decision—a community leader introduces the idea of community water fluoridation through appropriate government channels, and the idea is approved by the appropriate governing body (i.e., water board, public services director, mayor, city council)
   (2) Initiative petition or referendum—allows members of the community to vote for or against fluoridation of the water supply; the referendum should be a last resort to avoid a politically charged situation
   (3) Legislative action—mandate passed by state legislators that requires specified public water supplies to be fluoridated or allows health departments to order public water supplies to be fluoridated under certain conditions; it is generally recommended that the decision to fluoridate be made at the local level, although some states have mandatory fluoridation laws
d. Public attitudes toward water fluoridation are both positive and negative—only 20% of population opposed to fluoridation; the majority of Americans support fluoridation; the lack of organization and passivity on the part of the supporters of fluoridation make it easier for well-organized anti-fluoridationists to block its implementation or adoption
e. Opponents' arguments and tactics appeal to emotions and use of scare tactics
   (1) Suggest that water fluoridation is unconstitutional and violates individual freedom of choice
   (2) Create suspicion of government programs, officials, or both
   (3) Allege that fluoridation is overregulation by the government
   (4) Associate fluoridation with concerns about poor health, disease, and aging, based on anecdotal evidence and poorly designed research studies
   (5) Imply that water fluoridation is poisonous and causes health hazards
   (6) Claims that it causes fluorosis when nonfluoridated communities have lower levels of fluorosis than fluoridated communities
   (7) Tied it to environmental issues, such as addition of unnecessary chemicals to the water
   (8) Asserting that adults do not benefit from fluoridation, making it inappropriate for tax dollars appropriation
f. Strategies used to support water fluoridation
   (1) Outcomes from rigorous studies that provide the evidence base for fluoridation
   (2) Knowledge of the community (e.g., past efforts to introduce water fluoridation or discontinue water fluoridation)
   (3) Working with all community leaders, organizations, stakeholders, and members of the community having influence, such as newspaper editors

BOX 20-8 Steps to Implement Water Fluoridation in a Local Community to Avoid a Referendum

1. Form a citizen's community such as "Citizens for Healthy Teeth"; consider hiring a consultant or arrange for consultation from the state dental public health department
2. Know the facts: scientific basis for fluoridation, physiology, effectiveness, safety, cost of fluoridating community, anti-fluoridationists' tactics, charges and answers, legality of fluoridation, and history of local fluoridation
3. Identify and contact key community leaders to educate them and receive support for the issue
4. Gather endorsements from key community leaders to document support when meeting with the city council
5. Form a broad base of support beyond the dental and medical professions through the committee and endorsements
6. Educate the city council members on the issue, one-on-one, before the issue is brought before council meetings
7. Bring the issue formally before the city council only after support has been received from community leaders and individual council members
8. Attend council meetings to show support of the issue
9. Be prepared to testify at the city council meetings

or radio/television personalities; collaboration with other health care professionals

(4) Creating awareness of the methods, tactics, and nonscientific materials used by fluoridation opponents; recognition of the impact of incorrect information presented in print and electronic media

g. Steps to implement a fluoridation campaign (Box 20-8)

B. Dietary fluoride supplements (Table 20-12)
1. Dosage and age recommendations are available (Table 20-13); other available fluoride and related factors, such as risk, cooperation, age, and ability of the child, should also be considered
2. School-based fluoride supplement programs
   a. Yielded 30% reduction in dental caries
   b. Were cost-effective and efficient

c. Required parental consent and ongoing cooperation of highly motivated staff and parents made implementation cumbersome

3. Current public health recommendation to prevent fluorosis is to use fluoride supplements only with children age 6 years and older and only when fluoridated water is not being consumed; this targeted approach is based on the availability of multiple other sources of fluoride and balances caries reduction benefits of fluoride for high-risk children and its potential to cause fluorosis

4. At-home use has the disadvantage of dependence on adherence; increased client adherence may be achieved with combined fluoride-vitamin supplements

5. Controlled daily at-home use results in caries reduction similar to water fluoridation

6. Dietary supplements are not recommended for infants who are breast-fed; breast milk contains 0.0004 ppm F

7. Prenatal supplementation with fluoride is not recommended, although it is not harmful to the fetus; even though it crosses the placental barrier and enters the fetal circulation, benefits are minor, since mineralization of enamel is not advanced until after birth, and primary benefit of fluoride occurs after tooth eruption

8. Varnish programs (see Table 20-12)
   a. Studies show 45% caries reduction with public health programs
   b. Fluoride varnish programs have numerous advantages compared to other fluoride modalities (Box 20-9)
   c. Child positioning for examination and fluoride varnish application
      (1) Knee to knee – infants are held by parents in their laps, with the child's head on the parent's knees and the child's legs around the parent's waist, and the operator is knee to knee with the parent,

TABLE 20-13 Dietary Fluoride Supplementation Schedule (in mg F/day*)

Age	CONCENTRATION OF FLUORIDE IN THE WATER		
	<0.03 ppm	0.3 ppm to >0.6 ppm	>0.6 ppm
0 to 6 months	0	0	0
6 months to 3 years	0.25 mg	0	0
3 to 6 years	0.50 mg	0.25 mg	0
6 to 16 years	1.0 mg	0.50 mg	0

Data from American Academy of Pediatric Dentistry (AAPD): Guideline on fluoride therapy, 2014. http://www.aapd.org/media/Policies_Guidelines/G_FluorideTherapy.pdf.

*2.2 mg sodium fluoride (NaF) contains 1 mg fluoride ion; *ppm,* parts per million; 1.0 ppm, 1 mg/L.

BOX 20-9 Advantages of Public Health Fluoride Varnish Programs

- No special dental equipment required
- Professional dental cleaning not required before application
- Ease of application
- Dries immediately on contact with saliva
- Safety
- Well tolerated by all; especially convenient for use on infants, young children, and individuals with special needs
- Inexpensive
- Minimal training required for placement; nondental personnel can be trained
- Allows the ability to eat or drink immediately after application
- Prevents and reverses decay
- Shows caries reduction up to 45% compared with 30% to 35% for other fluoride systems

Data adapted from Texas Department of State Health Services: *Happy child, bright smile; fluoride varnish manual,* Pub No E08-13077, March 2009, http://www.dshs. state.tx.us/dental/default.shtm; and Centers for Disease Control and Prevention: Other fluoride products, July 10, 2013, http://www.cdc.gov/fluoridation/fluoride_products/.

treating the infant from behind; an alternate is to place the infant on an examination table and work from behind

    (2) Face to face—young children are seated in small school chairs, and the operator is seated directly facing the child, tilting the child's head back for good visibility; alternative positions are the child standing in front of the seated operator or the operator standing behind the seated larger child and working from above

  d. Varnish should be reapplied every 3 months in high-risk children and every 6 months in moderate-risk children

  e. CDC recommends programs with preschool-age children such as Head Start

  f. Educational program with parents and children should be included to increase adherence and address other aspects of caries prevention and control

C. School water fluoridation (see Table 20-12)

  1. Still in use in some communities with suboptimal fluoride levels, particularly rural areas where community water fluoridation is impossible; the extent of current practice is unknown; no longer recommended by the CDC because of the disadvantages

  2. This program reduced caries among schoolchildren by approximately 40%

  3. Disadvantages—children do not receive benefits until they begin school; exposure occurs only during the school year and on school days; benefits only schoolchildren; equipment for these small water systems have logistical problems and greater risk of spills

  4. To compensate for children drinking this water only when school is in session, it is fluoridated at 4.5 times the optimum concentration

D. Fluoridated salt (see Table 20-12)

  1. Addition of fluoride to table salt is a feasible way to deliver fluoride in countries lacking widespread municipal water systems (not the United States or Canada)

  2. Reduction in caries parallels rates found with water fluoridation

  3. Used in some other countries; WHO criteria include the inability to implement water fluoridation, low levels of fluoride in the diet and environment, lack of political will to introduce water fluoridation, centralized salt production, and appropriate package labeling

E. Fluoridated milk (see Table 20-12)

  1. The addition of fluoride to milk consumed in schools has been studied in several European countries (not the United States or Canada)

  2. Outcomes have shown protection from caries comparable with water fluoridation at the same concentration

  3. Disadvantages—only provides a single fluoride exposure on school days, requires refrigeration, and milk consumption declines with increasing age of child

F. Professionally applied topical fluoride (see Table 20-12 and the sections on "Topical Fluorides and Fluoride Varnishes" in Chapter 13 and "Fluorides" in Chapter 16)

  1. Professional application of topical F is the least cost-effective public health fluoride measure

  2. Sodium fluoride (NaF), stannous fluoride (SnF_2), and acidulated phosphate fluoride (APF) in gel, foam, and mouthrinse forms are no longer recommended by the CDC as a population-based strategy, although they may be indicated in high-risk populations in targeted clinical programs such as institutions for high-risk, special-needs groups

G. Fluoride mouthrinses in school-based public programs (see Table 20-12)

  1. Widely used at one time; still used in some areas, especially in developing countries

  2. Studies indicated a 20% to 35% reduction in caries; not cost-effective in combination with systemic fluoride

  3. Although highly successful, their use is limited today in the United States because of expansion of water fluoridation and availability of other sources of fluoride

  4. Disadvantages—required level of parental compliance and dependence on teachers and school nurses to administer the program

H. Fluoride dentifrices (see Table 20-12)

  1. Fluoride dentifrices are the most important fluoride vehicle on a global scale, providing 15% to 30% caries reduction in children over a 3-year period without water fluoridation; they are cost-effective and add to the effectiveness of water fluoridation and other sources of fluoride

  2. Their use is institutionalized in the United States, Canada, and other developed countries, accounting for over 90% of the market; this makes distribution as a public health measure unnecessary; public health distribution has value in developing countries where the population does not have access to F dentifrices

I. Other chemical therapies

  1. Xylitol

    a. Used in food and snack items as a noncariogenic sweetener; its use may reduce the incidence of dental caries in people with moderate or higher risk; additional research is needed

    b. Some studies have shown that xylitol is superior to other chemical therapies to interrupt the vertical transmission of dental caries from parent or caregiver to infants and the horizontal transmission among siblings; this use is no longer standard practice, and additional research is needed

    c. Recommended to be used in combination with topical fluoride

  2. Chlorhexidine gluconate

    a. Effective against *Streptococcus mutans*

    b. Recommended for individuals who are at high or extreme risk for caries

    c. CAMBRA (Caries Management by Risk Assessment) recommended regimen for caries control is 0.12% chlorhexidine gluconate rinsed for 1 minute daily for 1 week each month; additional research is needed

d. Loses effectiveness in the presence of lauryl sulfate or fluoride; rinse should be used about 30 minutes after toothbrushing with dentifrices that contain either compound

e. The American Dental Association recommends use of chlorhexidine-thymol combination varnish for control of root caries

3. Amorphous calcium phosphate (ACP)

a. Calcium and phosphate ions in ACP will prevent caries progression by enhancing enamel remineralization, occluding dentinal tubules, and increasing fluoride uptake in areas of demineralization; also reduces sensitivity

b. Should be used in combination with fluoride therapy

c. Recommended for use by individuals who are at high risk for caries

d. Contained in dentifrices and sensitivity relief products as well as professional-use products such as polishing paste and sealants

4. Casein phosphopeptides–amorphous calcium phosphate (CPP-ACP)—also known by the name *Recaldent*

a. Enhances the effects of fluoride and provides a supersaturated environment of calcium and phosphate for remineralization; also reduces sensitivity

b. Recommended to be used in combination with fluoride therapy

c. Recommended for use by individuals who are at high risk for caries

d. Some studies suggest long-term caries prevention effects; additional research is needed

e. Contained in chewing gum and pastes for professional application

5. Sodium bicarbonate

a. Claims are that it neutralizes acids produced by acidogenic bacteria and has antibacterial properties; recommended for individuals with xerostomia

b. Contained in chewing gum and dentifrice; can be rinsed by mixing 2 teaspoons baking soda with 8 ounces water

c. Aggressive use of fluoride therapy should be continued by individuals with xerostomia or other conditions that produce high oral acidity

6. Calcium sodium phosphosilicate (NovaMin)

a. Delivers calcium phosphorus, sodium, and silica to replace minerals lost to demineralization; should be used in combination with fluoride

b. Contained in dentifrices, mints, and chewing gums

c. Additional research is needed

7. Tricalcium phosphate

a. Protects calcium ions and frees phosphate ions to prohibit calcium from reacting prematurely with fluoride

b. Ingredient in Clinpro 5000 dentifrice

8. Probiotics

a. Noncariogenic bacteria replace and displace cariogenic bacteria

b. Promising results but additional research needed

J. Dental sealant programs (see the sections on "Pit-and-Fissure Sealants" in Chapter 13 and "Dental Sealants" in Chapter 16)

1. Sealants prevent caries in sound and noncavitated pits and fissures and reduce the rate of incipient carious lesions that progress to cavitation

2. Sealants reduce bacteria levels in cavitated lesions 100-fold and reduce lesions with any viable bacteria by 50%

3. Sealants are recommended in both fluoridated and nonfluoridated communities

4. The use of fluorides in conjunction with sealants is recommended so that both smooth surfaces and pit-and-fissure surfaces benefit

5. Sealant and fluoride programs are the most beneficial community-based dental disease-prevention programs; sealants are a critical component of disease prevention programs

6. Based on epidemiologic evidence, community-based sealant programs are justified for children, adolescents, and young adults, but not for other age groups

7. Sealant program settings may include schools, clinics, day care facilities, and community centers; a team approach is necessary for screening and treatment, including necessary support and cooperation from administrators, staff, teachers, parents, caregivers, and volunteers

8. Targeting school-based sealant programs

a. Schools are targeted that have high rates of children from low-SES groups who are at high risk of dental caries, as determined by the percentage of students eligible for free or subsidized lunch programs

b. Limited resources require that sealant programs use criteria that include risk of dental caries, availability of care, grade level of the targeted group (e.g., second and sixth grades), and teeth with deep pits and fissures

c. Teeth should be sealed within 6 months of eruption of first and second molars

9. The cost-effectiveness of community-based sealant programs is a result of the pattern of dental caries; the vast majority of dental caries in schoolchildren currently occurs in pits and fissures

10. Retention rates are:

a. Comparable for various oral health professionals who place sealants; cost-effectiveness depends on the use of nondentists to place sealants

b. Higher with four-handed technique; parent and staff volunteers can be trained to assist

11. Most third-party insurance payers cover sealants

12. An educational component is critical for parents and children of the targeted population to increase adherence to other aspects of caries prevention and control

13. CDC provides clinical guidelines for sealant use and recommendations for school-based sealant programs (Box 20-10)

K. Caries management by risk assessment

1. CAMBRA is the process of dealing with dental caries as an infectious disease by risk assessment and planned interventions or treatment based on that risk (see Chapter 15)

BOX 20-10 **CDC Recommendations for Sealant Use in Community Oral Health**

Clinical Recommendations

1. Sealants should be placed on pits and fissures of children's primary teeth when it is determined that the tooth, or the patient, is at risk of experiencing caries.
2. Sealants should be placed on pits and fissures of children's, adolescents', and adults' permanent teeth when it is determined that the tooth, or the patient, is at risk of experiencing caries.
3. Pit-and-fissure sealants should be placed on early (noncavitated) carious lesions in children, adolescents, young adults, and adults to reduce the percentage of lesions that progress.
4. Conditions that favor the placement of resin-based versus glass ionomer cement; resin-based sealants are the first choice of material for dental sealants.
5. Use of a bonding agent between the previously acid-etched enamel surface and the sealant material may enhance sealant retention.
6. Use of a bonding agent that excludes acid etching is not recommended.
7. Routine mechanical preparation of enamel before acid etching is not recommended.
8. When possible, a four-handed technique should be used for placement of sealants.
9. The oral health care professional should monitor and reapply sealants as needed to maximize effectiveness.

10. The manufacturer's instructions for sealant placement should be followed.

Recommendations for School-Based Sealant Programs

1. Seal pit-and-fissure tooth surfaces that are sound or have noncavitated lesions, prioritizing first and second permanent molars.
2. Unaided visual assessment is adequate prior to sealant placement to differentiate surfaces with the earliest signs of tooth decay from more advanced lesions.
3. Prior to assessment, dry the teeth with a cotton roll, gauze, or, when available, compressed air.
4. An explorer may be used to gently confirm cavitations; do not use a sharp explorer under force.
5. X-ray films are not needed solely for sealant placement.
6. A toothbrush can be used to help clean the tooth surface before acid etching; more complex cleaning methods are not recommended.
7. Use a four-handed technique with an assistant to increase retention.
8. Provide sealants to children even if follow-up examinations for every child cannot be guaranteed.
9. Evaluate sealant retention within 1 year.

Data from Beauchamp J, Caufield PW, Crall JJ, et al: Evidence-based clinical recommendations for the use of pit-and-fissure sealants: a report of the American Dental Association Council on Scientific Affairs, *J Am Dent Assoc* 139:257-268, 2008; Centers for Disease Control and Prevention (CDC): School-based dental sealant programs; and Gooch BF, Griffin SO, Gray SV, et.al: Preventing dental caries through school-based sealant programs: updated recommendations and reviews of evidence, *J Am Dent Assoc* 140:1356-1365, 2009. http://www.cdc.gov/oralhealth/dental_sealant_program/.

---

2. Risk is based on the balance of pathologic factors and protective factors; the level of risk is determined by professional judgment of this balance
3. Targeting community-based programs should be done according to the level of risk
   a. Parent or caregiver of a child belonging to a low-SES group automatically results in high risk for the child
   b. Current or recent caries experience places any-age individual at a high-risk level
   c. Xerostomia and special-needs status automatically result in an extreme-risk category

Measures for Preventing and Controlling Periodontal Diseases

A. No parallel to water fluoridation and other fluoride modalities exists for the prevention of periodontal diseases
B. A combination of meticulous self-care by individuals on a regular basis, elimination of high risk behaviors such as smoking, control of systemic diseases and conditions, and periodic periodontal maintenance therapy leads to improved gingival health, decreased attachment loss, and maintenance of natural dentition
   1. Various mechanical and chemical interventions prevent and control some periodontal diseases
   2. Gingivitis is controllable with mechanical oral prophylaxis and adequate oral hygiene to reduce or disrupt dental plaque biofilm
   3. Personal oral hygiene practices such as regular toothbrushing and interdental cleaning can be supplemented by OTC and prescription antimicrobial mouthrinses

4. Tobacco cessation aids in periodontal disease prevention, control, and progression
5. Health education informs persons about the relationship of systemic diseases (diabetes, heart disease, stroke, osteoporosis, stress, respiratory disease) and pregnancy to periodontal health
6. Addressing periodontal disease at the population level is complicated by role of genetic factors in destructive periodontal disease
C. Community activities could include:
   1. Public education to increase health literacy; for example, personal oral hygiene, control of behaviors that increase risk, regular professional oral care, and linking systemic and oral health
   2. Tobacco cessation programs and efforts
   3. Support of funding for and promotion of population-based research

Measures for Preventing and Controlling Other Oral Diseases and Anomalies

A. Oropharyngeal cancers
   1. A primary prevention technique for human papillomavirus–related oropharyngeal cancers is the HPV vaccine. Primary prevention for most oral and pharyngeal cancers is not available; avoiding known risk factors such as alcohol and tobacco is recommended
   2. Although overall cigarette use in the United States has declined over the last decade, tobacco prevention and cessation initiatives are still necessary because the use of smokeless tobacco, cigars, e-cigarettes, and hookahs has increased

3. Advocating for regular oral cancer screening and examinations
4. School-based prevention programs are important
   a. The rate of cigarette use among high school students has decreased steadily each year since 1997, but approximately 15% of high school students reported smoking in 2013; the use of cigar smoking and smokeless tobacco among high school students have remained unchanged[8]
   b. Recommendations for education of students—for example, programs and information from the CDC and the American Dental Hygienists Association (ADHA) Smoking Cessation Initiative Project
      (1) Focus on restricting social influences and environments that lead to tobacco use
      (2) Develop and enforce a school policy on tobacco use prevention, control, and cessation
      (3) Provide instruction on the short-term and long-term negative physiologic and social influences of tobacco, peer norms regarding tobacco use, and refusal skills
      (4) Deliver tobacco-use prevention education in kindergarten through twelfth grade; this instruction should begin no later than fifth grade, should be especially intensive in middle school, and reinforced in high school
      (5) Offer program-specific training and dialogue scripts to teachers and school nurses
      (6) Involve parents and families in support of school-based programs to prevent tobacco use
      (7) Support cessation efforts among students and all school staff who use tobacco; involve other associations and organizations such as parent-teacher associations (PTAs), American Association of Retired Persons (AARP), employers, and health insurers
      (8) Evaluate outcomes of tobacco-use prevention program at regular intervals
5. Tobacco cessation as a preventive intervention
   a. A *Healthy People 2020* objective is to provide tobacco cessation counseling by dentists and dental hygienists (see Table 20-2)
   b. Some health insurance policies provide tobacco cessation coverage
6. Secondary prevention consists of early detection (screening) and treatment
   a. Mass screening for oral cancers is costly
   b. Professionals should include oral cancer examinations as part of their assessment and teach self-examination techniques to clients; progress was made in the last decade (see Table 20-2)
7. Other recommended strategies
   a. Focus on populations at risk for use of smokeless tobacco (e.g., little league teams)
   b. Emphasize health warnings on posters, brochures, websites, products, and public service announcements that warn of hazards

   c. Urge people to regularly visit a professional oral health care provider for examination, advice, and assistance with quitting tobacco use
   d. Provide public education regarding signs and symptoms of oral cancer; promote regular self-examination
   e. Encourage use of QUIT phone lines
   f. Promote use of online smoking cessation assistance
   g. Support population-based research efforts and lobbying strategies
   h. Keep abreast of new information on tobacco cessation, such as from ADHA and CDC
   i. Advocate for policies related to controlling the sale and use of tobacco products
B. Craniofacial birth defects
   1. Cleft palate and cleft lip are among the most frequent birth defects
   2. Public health programs should emphasize awareness of risk and protective factors during pregnancy
      a. Prenatal care
      b. Good nutrition
      c. Tobacco use
      d. Alcohol consumption
      e. Drug abuse
      f. Teratogenic prescription drugs (e.g., drugs used to treat acne)
      g. Many occurrences cannot be linked to a direct behavioral link or cause
   3. Advocacy for policies related to improvement of surveillance and referral
C. Facial injury or trauma (see the section on "Mouth Protectors [Athletic Mouthguards]" in Chapter 13)
   1. Oral health education that focuses on preventive behaviors
   2. Increased public attention to the importance of head and facial protection
      a. Headgear and athletic mouth protectors during contact-sports activities
      b. Safety restraints in automobiles
      c. Helmets for bicycling, skateboarding, in-line skating (roller blading), and motorcycle use
      d. Measures to prevent injuries from falls in the home, including good lighting, nonskid flooring materials, and handrails
   3. Emphasis on education of parents, coaches, caregivers and policy makers
D. Tooth loss
   1. Oral health education focused on the value of keeping natural teeth and importance of early treatment of caries and periodontal diseases
   2. Advocacy for and policies that improve access to care for underserved populations
E. Problems related to denture use
   1. Oral health education focused on importance of and techniques used for denture cleanliness
   2. Policies related to denture identification during fabrication
   3. Health promotion programs for caregivers and staff of nursing homes to encourage assistance with oral hygiene

and denture care for older-adult denture wearers who need assistance

F. Fluorosis

1. Monitoring of safe water fluoridation practices; training of water treatment personnel
2. Promotion of policies related to removing excess fluoride from community water supplies
3. Oral health education of the public and other health professionals related to the safe use of fluorides

COMMUNITY INTERVENTION

A. Steps of dental hygiene process of care (ADPIE) are similar to those used in community programming in a circular approach continually to improve programs: assessment, determination of priorities (problem identification), planning, implementation, and evaluation (Fig. 20-6)
B. Community groups vary—programming principles can be applied to all groups and types of programs, although programs may need to be adapted for various priority populations based on culture and other demographic factors
C. Factors to consider in community programming—current health care system, workforce issues, resources, funding, geography, sociocultural background, SES, cultural and political climates, and oral health literacy
D. Community programming uses various strategies
1. Surveillance at national and state levels that:
    a. Provides information necessary for public health decision making
    b. Collects data on health outcomes, risk factors, and intervention strategies
    c. Can link current databases and address identified data gaps
    d. Identifies public health issues requiring immediate action
    e. Measures and monitors trends in the burden of disease
    f. Guides planning, implementation, and evaluation of programs

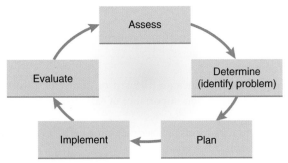

FIG 20-6 Use of ADPIE in community programming. Assessment, Determination of priorities (problem identification), (Data from Nathe CN: *Dental public health and research*, ed 4, Upper Saddle River, NJ, 2015, Pearson.)

g. May influence public policy and allocation of funds
    h. Includes important qualities of surveillance: simplicity, flexibility, data quality, representativeness, and timeliness
2. Survey
    a. A description of the defined population at a point in time
    b. Can be part of a needs assessment
3. Needs assessment that identifies:
    a. Extent and types of assets and challenges in a community
    b. Current system of services and programs available
    c. Extent of needs and resource utilization
E. Roles of dental hygienists in community health planning and practice
1. Program planner or initiator
2. Consultant and resource person
3. Service provider
4. Administrator or manager of a particular program or division
5. Researcher, including data collection
6. Educator and oral health promotion professional
7. Consumer advocate
8. Politician
9. Trainer—training others to provide a service is a more efficient use of resources
F. Several program planning models are used; elements common to community oral health initiatives include education, financing, and formative evaluation
1. Identify priority population
2. Assess the priority population
3. Collect, organize, and analyze data
4. Determine priorities
5. Develop a program plan
6. Implement the plan
7. Evaluate the program

Assessment and Problem Identification

A. Definition—multifaceted, organized, and systematic approach to identify a target group and define the extent and severity of the oral health care needs that are present
1. Priority group—group of individuals who are the focus of a particular oral health care service or program; may be identified by health professional or by group themselves
2. Use of a community-oriented primary care (COPC) philosophy of health planning—this is the community being involved in identifying its perceived needs and assigning priorities; also referred to as *community-based participation*
B. Data collection
1. Important to complete as part of the needs assessment before planning the intervention
2. Develop a community profile of the area where the target population is located if adequate needs assessment is not available

3. Identify ongoing types of programs or projects
   a. Purpose is to provide oral health services, education, disease prevention, research, or combination
   b. Community individuals and groups responsible for programs and success
   c. Locations or facilities where oral health care activities can occur
   d. Individuals, special equipment (e.g., mobile vans or portable equipment), facilities, coalitions, funding opportunities, and other resources to meet the oral health care needs of the target population
4. Assess current oral health status and needs
   a. Used to identify the extent and severity of need and in determining project aims and objectives
   b. Three basic approaches to documenting oral health status and needs:
      (1) Identify and use an assessment method to obtain specific data related to the proposed project or program

(2) Coordinate assessment with an agency or group such as an academic center or community-based agency that is seeking similar data about the target population
(3) Secondary data—research and collect secondary data from records of state or local health care agencies, dental or medical programs, and public health or related agencies
5. Various data collection methods can be used (Table 20-14)
   a. Method used is influenced by the type of information or data needed
   b. Types of data collected for assessment affects assessment methods used
      (1) Baseline data—data collected before program implementation; used for problem identification, planning, and evaluating a program; it is compared to outcomes data to evaluate success of program; baseline data is also called *pretest data* in research

TABLE 20-14 Data Collection Methods and Applications

Data Collection Method	Instrument	Indications	Advantages	Limitations
Direct observation of events, objects, people	Checklist, content analysis, evaluation forms, camera, tape recorder, videotape, thermometer, sphygmomanometer, rating and ranking scales	Used when subject recall may affect accuracy of data collection Used to study behavior Used to study psychomotor activity Used in experimental research	Observations can be made as they occur in the "natural" setting Observations can be made of behaviors that might not be reported by respondents	Time-consuming Difficulty in recording Factors that may interfere with the situation Difficulty in quantification of observations Expensive Observer-respondent interaction
Interview; face-to-face or telephone survey	Interview guide (interview schedule)	Used to obtain information on attitudes, beliefs, and opinions Used in a survey Used to gain information on past or present events Face-to-face method can be used for focus groups or one-on-one	Flexibility Questions can be clarified and explained Complete data can be collected Survey participants do not have to be able to read or write	Respondents may be inhibited to respond accurately and truthfully Time-consuming Expensive Interviewer may affect the responses Language barriers
Question-based survey: written or oral	Questionnaire, opinionnaire, email source; asking questions to seek specific information	Used for obtaining information on attitudes, beliefs, and opinions May be used to gain information on present conditions and past events Used to obtain information about existing status Used in planning	Ease of administration Relatively inexpensive Standardization of instructions and questions Economy of time Data can be gathered from a wide geographic area Data can reflect public opinion Vast amount of data can be collected Cross-sectional, generalized statistics can be obtained	Misinterpretation of questions by respondents If written, low return may bias results Superficiality of responses Incomplete data collection Honesty of respondent Control of extraneous variables is lacking

(Continued)

TABLE 20-14	Data Collection Methods and Applications—cont'd			
Data Collection Method	**Instrument**	**Indications**	**Advantages**	**Limitations**
Epidemiologic survey, screening survey	Dental indices	Used to study disease patterns in a population Used to evaluate the effectiveness of therapeutic or preventive treatments in a specific geographic area	Vast amount of data can be collected Cross-sectional, generalized statistics can be obtained Data are quantifiable Provides actual measure of health status	Difficulty in determining causation because of complexity of variables Time-consuming Expensive; requires trained and calibrated examiners
Records, documents	Reports of legislative bodies and state or city officials, deeds, wills, appointment records, dental charts, report cards	Used to study past events	Unbiased in terms of the investigator Inexpensive No subject-investigator interaction Convenience and economy of time	Incomplete records Accuracy of records may be unknown

Data from Beatty CF: Community oral health practice for the dental hygienist, ed 4, St Louis, 2017, Elsevier Saunders.

(2) Primary data—new data collected by various techniques (e.g., questionnaire, interview, direct observation, indices, records, documents)

(3) Secondary data—existing data previously collected by federal or state agencies, public policy organizations or other sources (e.g., Census Bureau, Gallup polls, Oral Health America)

(4) Qualitative data—nonnumerical descriptive data such as observations, perceptions, attitudes, and comments made

c. Multiple data collection methods can be used together based on program goals

d. Surveys—method used to assess knowledge, oral health status, oral health behavior, interests, values, and attitudes; can be done by use of questionnaire or interview

e. Oral health surveys—type of survey method used to collect information about oral health, disease status, and treatment needs for planning or monitoring oral health care needs

  (1) Can be accomplished with a clinical examination (primary data) or review of dental records (secondary data)

  (2) Existing survey data may be available for comparisons of target group to comparable groups or different geographic regions

    (a) National data from federal agencies responsible for monitoring health and oral health status, such as CDC and NOHSS

    (b) State-level surveillance data available from the CDC, NOHSS, or some state health departments

  (3) ASTDD and WHO are resources for guidelines for conducing and reporting results of an oral health survey

  (4) Four types of examinations and inspections are used in oral health surveys to measure dental caries (Table 20-15); the type used varies according to the index or measurement approach (see Table 20-11)

f. Special considerations are needed in planning oral health surveys

  (1) Cumulative nature of some diseases

  (2) Disease is age related

  (3) A significant percentage of the population is affected

  (4) Irreversible nature of some oral diseases

  (5) Trends in disease prevalence exist

  (6) Common oral diseases exist in all populations; prevalence may be higher in underinsured and uninsured, low-SES, and nonwhite and Hispanic populations

  (7) Standard measurements are used to assess many oral diseases (dental indices); subjectivity and potential for error are inherent in use of many dental indices

  (8) Surveying requires planning, calibration of examiners, and possibly pilot testing before implementation

C. Development of a community profile

  1. Community profile—provides information essential in planning a community health program; the rationale is to understand the environment in which the target population is located

  2. Not always necessary and depends on the scope of the proposed intervention; the comprehensive nature depends on resources and goals

  3. Size, location, and type of community dictate the type, amount, and comprehensiveness of information necessary for a community profile

TABLE 20-15   Types of Caries Examinations and Inspections

Type	Description	Advantages	Disadvantages
I	Complete examination—done with mouth mirror and explorer, adequate illumination, thorough radiographic survey, and additional tests as indicated	Comprehensive; designed for comprehensive treatment	Requires extensive time and personnel; expensive
II	Limited examination—done with mouth mirror, explorer, adequate illumination, posterior bitewing radiographs, and single periapical radiographs as indicated	Useful when program may include dental treatment for individuals	Requires time, personnel and expense
III*	Inspection—done with mouth mirror, explorer, and adequate illumination; used in the Basic Screening Survey	Useful in surveys; offers chance to establish rapport and plan motivational strategy for oral health instruction; provides baseline data	May be erroneously relied on as an examination; follow-up is required for referral
IV*	Screening—done with tongue depressor and available illumination	Useful for initial needs assessment in relation to program planning	Identifies only glaring needs for referral; follow-up is required

*Type III and Type IV are the most common methods used in dental public health.

4. General areas for inclusion can consist of:
   a. Community overview
      (1) Number of individuals in the population and distribution by income, age, education, employment rate, public assistance, health and dental insurance rates, and percentage of population receiving Medicare, Medicaid, or CHIP
      (2) Geographic location and boundaries, population setting and density (urban or rural), standard of living, homelessness
      (3) Ethnic background, cultural heritage, languages, customs, behaviors, beliefs
      (4) Diet, nutritional levels, nutrition programs
      (5) Amount, types, and influence of public services and utilities, including transportation schedules, routes, fares, and reliability
      (6) Informed-consent procedures and confidentiality of health records
      (7) Distribution of public and private schools and religious or faith-based organizations
      (8) Extent and type of community fluoride and sealant programs; fluoridation history
      (9) State and local statutes, public health codes, and related administrative rules and regulations
   b. Community leadership and organization; political atmosphere
      (1) Community, financial, and religious leaders, liaisons, and councils
      (2) Community power base for policy formulation
      (3) Governance structure (e.g., health council, city government, advisory board, school board, union); political environment
      (4) Grassroots individuals with political influence
      (5) Educational institutions providing professional education, resources, and support
      (6) Attitudes of all these entities toward oral health, acquired through interviews or surveys, is important in terms of whether they will be assets or barriers to the community programming process

   c. Financing and funding of health services
      (1) Local and state budget allocation procedures for oral health care programs
      (2) Funding sources (e.g., federal, state, or local funding; individual or third-party payment; private funds; foundations; grants; endowments)
      (3) Mechanism for requesting the necessary funding; the importance of the need for collaborative partners to successfully obtain funding must be determined
   d. Facilities, resources, and workforce
      (1) Location of space and facilities in the community or institution; U.S. Department of Labor Occupational Safety and Health Administration (OSHA) standard compliance
      (2) Availability and adequacy of equipment
      (3) Location of medical and health science centers, clinics, community health centers, and dental laboratories; ease of access
      (4) Number of licensed practicing dentists, dental hygienists, midlevel dental providers, dental assistants, laboratory technicians, medical personnel, or others experienced in working with target population
      (5) Consortia of health professionals, facilities, and resources (collaboration is important)
      (6) Barriers that limit access of the population to oral health care (e.g., cost, transportation, political climate of community, attitudes of leaders about oral health)
   e. Sometimes a community assessment is accomplished for overall community planning before identifying any specific group to target; in this case, population groups previously identified as being at high risk for oral health needs should be included in the community assessment
      (1) Preschool-age and school-age children
      (2) Intellectually, developmentally, and physically challenged persons
      (3) Chronically ill and medically compromised persons

(4) Older adults

(5) Pregnant women and infants

(6) Low-income and minority groups

(7) Residents of inner-city and rural communities

D. Analysis of data

1. Analysis includes organizing, evaluating, and interpreting data

2. Data analysis can range from simple to complex, using simple descriptive tabulations or advanced statistical tests

   a. Planner alone can analyze the data

   b. Statisticians and epidemiologists can be involved

   c. Computers

   d. Analysis of qualitative data requires special skills

   e. Economic analysis of existing programs, including a cost/benefit ratio

3. After analysis, population needs and priorities can be identified

   a. Formal and informal input is sought through meetings, focus groups, and social media

   b. Input is sought from various stakeholder groups

   c. Community representatives, partners, and advisory groups are consulted

   d. Consumers; political, religious, and financial leaders; and health care professionals may be included

4. An opportunity for dialogue is important to gain support

Program Planning

A. Definition—organized response to reduce or eliminate one or more problems; organized effort that includes the objective of reducing or eliminating one or more problems, performance of one or more activities, and use of resources

B. Elements of a program plan

1. Identification of program goals and objectives

2. Strategies and specific activities to meet objectives, including sequence and individuals responsible

3. Resources required—facilities, equipment, materials, personnel (employed and volunteer), with consideration of appropriateness, adequacy, effectiveness, and efficiency

4. Timetables and deadlines clearly outlined, with some flexibility

5. Projected budget and budget justification

6. Program promotion and marketing

7. Identification of strengths, weaknesses/challenges, opportunities, and threats (SWOT/SCOT analysis)

C. Goals and objectives

1. For each need prioritized, a goal with related objectives must be determined

   a. Goal—broadly based statement of what changes will occur as a result of the program; provides direction

   b. Objectives—specific statements that describe, in a measurable manner, the desired outcomes from program activities

   c. Most activities may deal with immediate goals, but intermediate and long-term goals must also be considered

   d. Objectives are stated in specific, measurable terms; SMART formula for developing objectives provides the necessary components of what, who, where, when, and how much

     (1) Specific: clearly states the objectives

     (2) Measurable: objectives can be evaluated

     (3) Appropriate: taking the identified needs of target population into consideration

     (4) Realistic or related: objectives that are achievable and related to anticipated outcomes

     (5) Time-bound: establishment of a timeline

D. Program activities

1. The dynamic, energy-using procedures carried out to achieve program objectives

2. Can be preventive, educational, treatment oriented, or research oriented

E. Promotion or marketing of program

1. Necessary for participation, recognition, and success of project

2. Varied promotion techniques

   a. Advisory committee composed of stakeholders (those who have a stake in the outcome of the program) and key leaders from the community

   b. Liaison with related groups

   c. Mass media (television and radio), printed media, banners, billboards, Web-based and special-interest publications and programs

   d. Smaller programs may use posters, flyers, invitations, newsletter announcements, and email

F. Implementation strategy development—the steps for implementing the program are outlined before beginning the implementation process

G. Evaluation plan—the evaluation plan should be in place before implementing the program to ensure its successful execution throughout and on completion of the program

Implementation

A. Implementation is the process of operationalizing the plan; the implementation strategy is employed to conduct the program

B. During implementation of the program, it is important to monitor the program activities, personnel, equipment, resources, and supplies to ensure smooth program operation

C. Ongoing formative evaluation throughout the program implementation provides opportunity to make program adjustments as needed; feedback mechanisms from personnel and participants are critical components of this formative evaluation

Health Education and Health Promotion

See also the sections on "Oral Health Education" and "Prevention-Oriented Health Models" in Chapter 16.

A. Related concepts

1. Health promotion—a broad concept referring to the process of enabling people and communities to increase their control over determinants of health and therefore improve their own health; includes wide range of

strategies that may include policies that prohibit sale of tobacco products to young people, product labeling to indicate the amount of sugar in a product, strategies to increase access to care, and educational interventions

2. Health education—the process in which the client is encouraged to become responsible for personal oral health and is informed of scientifically based methods for preventing dental disease

3. Health continuum—conceptualization of health status as perceived on a continuous scale from optimal health through illness and death

4. Prevention—health education is one means of primary prevention for both individuals and groups

5. Theories of health education and health promotion (Table 20-16)

a. Approaches to health promotion and health education strategies and interventions should be based on sound theories in order to result in desired changes in oral health status of individuals and communities

b. No single theory applies to all situations; theories can be combined to meet the needs of the situation; multi-dimensional approaches may be more effective for conditions with multiple social, behavioral, and biologic risk factors

c. These theories can help the professional move individuals through the stages of the learning ladder (progression of learning): unawareness, awareness, self-interest, involvement, action, and habit

d. Individual models should be used to design community oral health education programs; community

TABLE 20-16 Health Education and Promotion Theories

Theory	Key Points	Application Examples	Limitations
Individual Theories			
Health belief model (HBM)	Underlying foundation: when individuals have accurate information, they will make better health choices. Four health perceptions (beliefs) accepted in order: -Susceptibility to disease (risk) -Seriousness of disease -Effectiveness of intervention to control disease -Possibility of overcoming barriers (self-efficacy)	Presentations that provide health information. Providing clients with brochures and handouts of health information. Most knowledge-based oral health education programs are based on HBM	Just knowledge is not enough: information is essential but not sufficient. Does not provide tools needed for behavior change to occur. Behavior change is not so linear
Trans-theoretical model (stages of change)	State of readiness is required to change; follows step-by-step, orderly process of change through predictable stages: -Precontemplation -Contemplation -Preparation—think about making change at this stage -Action -Maintenance—more than 6 months of behavior change -Termination—as if old behavior never existed	Assessing one's state of readiness and position in the stages, then adapting education to the appropriate stage. Smoking cessation programs are based on stages of change. Useful for any health education strategy that involves progression through the stages, e.g., adoption of flossing behavior	Behavior change is not so linear. Research shows more success in immediate change (early stages) than in long-term change (maintenance and termination stages)
Theory of reasoned action	People make rational decisions based on behavioral intention; person's intent to change is strongest predictor of action. Behavioral intention is affected by one's personal behavioral beliefs and attitudes and social norms	Focus on or establishment of social norms for desired oral health behavior, e.g., children brushing at school, mother brushing with child, expression of concern for oral health by authority figures, appeal to social acceptability for teens. Soliciting behavioral intentions, e.g., to stop smoking on specific quit date	Does not deal with factual information. Focuses only on the emotional aspects and motivation of behavior
Social cognitive theory (SCT)	Knowledge, behavior, and environment act in a reciprocal (circular) manner to continually affect each other (multi-dimensional) and increase self-control over personal actions. Self-efficacy is belief that personal actions affect outcomes and predict health status. Self-efficacy is acquired through enactive attainment, verbal persuasion, observational learning, behavioral capability, and reinforcements	Using small successes to motivate behavior change, e.g., praise for increased frequency of flossing. Counseling that failure is part of the learning process. Using credible role models to tie learning to someone else's experience. Providing ongoing counseling. Reinforcing behavior. Encouraging self-initiated rewards and incentives. Personally modeling desired oral health behaviors and outcomes	Not a step-by-step model; sloppy. Self-efficacy varies for different health conditions

(Continued)

TABLE 20-16 Health Education and Promotion Theories—cont'd

Theory	Key Points	Application Examples	Limitations
Locus of control (LOC)	Perception of personal control over health status: -Internal LOC: personal actions determine health status -External LOC: others strongly influence health decisions and health status; can negate positive influence of knowledge -One's LOC tends to relate to all health issues	Counseling that focuses on individual's personal power over health decisions and health status	Perceptions can be deeply ingrained and emotionally driven
Sense of coherence (SOC)	Extent to which one has confidence that one's environment is predictable and that things will work out as well as can reasonably be expected; application to health is based on concept that disease is a continuum; stressors and tension (problems) move one along the continuum toward disease; individuals develop resources to reduce or manage stressors to move along the continuum toward health; resources consist of heredity, knowledge, finances, physical resources, friends, family, faith, etc., that help one view problems as manageable (have resources to cope), understandable (make sense), and meaningful (willing to use or spend resources to manage stressors); higher SOC is associated with better oral health	Helping people identify resources that are available to manage the stressors that relate to their oral health such as dental insurance; source of accurate information, trusted oral health care provider, access to healthy food, belief that oral health is important Focus on motivation	Cognitive, perceptual, and social model; does not include a focus on expanding knowledge of factual oral health information Time-consuming to implement

Community Theories

Theory	Key Points	Application Examples	Limitations
Community organization	Represents several theories that describe how community groups are assisted in identifying common problems or goals, mobilizing resources, and implementing strategies to reach the goals they have set collectively Accomplished through empowerment, community competence, participation and relevance, issue selection, and critical consciousness	Application on a small scale is involvement of the staff, parents, and even students in the ADPIE process of community programming in relation to an oral health program for the school	Requires time and effort to identify key influencers and involve the members of the community
Diffusion of innovation	Addresses how new ideas, products, practices, and services spread within a society Diffusion process consists of a spread of planned efforts to make the innovation become routine, taking into account the society's communication channels and social system Strategies are planned that address the characteristics of the innovation: relative advantage, compatibility, complexity, triability, and observability	Adoption of sealants, fluoride varnish, CAMBRA, and other innovative dental procedures by our society, including the profession	Requires a complex and comprehensive approach
Organizational change theory	A wide variety of forces make an organization resistant to change; these forces include how it operates, and its structure, culture and control systems A wide variety of forces also push an organization toward change; these include changing of tasks and the environment of the organization These two sets of forces always oppose each other; for an organization to change, it is necessary to find ways to increase the forces for change, decrease the resistance of change, or do both at the same time	Reorganizing the structure of the health system in the nation Reorganizing a community-based clinic to meet the changing needs of the population it serves Reorganizing a professional organization to influence its members in the direction of meeting population needs	Theory relates to the infrastructure of community oral health practice, not to health promotion Requires a complex and comprehensive approach Requires time and effort to change an organization

Data from Isman B: Health promotion and health communication. In Beatty CF: Community oral health practice for the dental hygienist, ed 4, St Louis, 2017, Elsevier Saunders; and Hollister MC: Health education and promotion theories. In Harris NO, Garcia-Godoy F, Nathe CN, editors: Primary preventive dentistry, ed 8, Upper Saddle River, NJ, 2014, Pearson.
ADPIE, Assessment, determination of priorities (problem identification), planning, implementation, and evaluation; *CAMBRA*, caries management by risk assessment.

models should be used to develop oral health promotion strategies that may include health education

6. Communication skills are critical to the effective implementation of health promotion and health education programs (see the section on "Client Management with Effective Communication" in Chapter 15)

7. Health education and health promotion programs must demonstrate cultural sensitivity to meet the needs of varied groups within the population; programs should be adapted to the culture of the target population

8. The health literacy of the target population must be considered for successful outcomes; almost two thirds of the U.S. population have less-than-adequate health literacy (Table 20-17)

B. Goals of health education
1. Improve knowledge of health topics
2. Foster motivation for changes in health behaviors
3. Result in outcomes of changed health behaviors
4. Ultimately to improve health status

C. Both direct and indirect processes impact oral health education
1. Formal activities include the deliberate provision of oral health education designed to elicit specific health promotion or disease prevention behaviors
2. Informal activities and environmental influences can impact the indirect or vicarious acquisition of oral health–related information and motivation that may lead to specific health promotion or disease prevention behaviors

D. Health education and health promotion are often integral parts of community activities; may be directed to:
1. Other health care professionals
2. Preschool, elementary, secondary, and college students
3. Educators
4. Special population groups and caregivers
5. Adult and older-adult groups
6. Institutionalized populations
7. Diverse population groups recently settled in the community

TABLE 20-17	Health Literacy	
Health literacy: "The degree to which individuals have the capacity to obtain, process, and understand basic health information and services needed to make appropriate health decisions."		
What is health literacy?	Health literacy is more than just knowledge about health topics; health literacy involves being able to:	
	-Find health information and health services and process the meaning and usefulness of the information and services	
	-Navigate the health care system, including filling out complex forms, locating providers and services, and making appointments	
	-Share personal information with providers, such as health history and current medications	
	-Engage in self-care and management of chronic disease	
	-Understand mathematical concepts such as probability and risk	
	-Apply numeracy skills such as calculating blood sugar levels, reading nutritional labels, and computing deductibles and copays	
Why is health literacy important?	Low health literacy is associated with:	
	-Poor health outcomes	
	-Less frequent utilization of preventive services	
	-Higher hospitalization rates	
	-Lower rates of having health insurance	
	-Higher overall health care costs	
Who is at risk for health literacy?	Low health literacy is most frequently seen in individuals who are:	
	-Older adults	
	-Racial and ethnic minorities	
	-Less educated, specifically less than a high school degree or GED; those with lower general literacy and numeracy skills	
	-Low socioeconomic status (SES)	
	-Nonnative English speakers	
	-Medically compromised	
	-Education, language, culture, access to resources, age, and general literacy and numeracy skills are all factors that affect a person's health literacy skills.	
How is health literacy improved?	Health professionals need to develop skills to:	
	-Understand how to provide useful information and services	
	-Consider which information and services work best for different situations and people so they can act	
	-Use plain language to communicate health information	
	-Convey information in the patient's or client's primary language, using a translator when needed	
	-Verify understanding of what people are explicitly and implicitly asking	
	-Take time to check a patient's or client's recall and comprehension of new concepts	
	-Provide assistance in learning basic numerical skills such as calculating dosages or understanding concepts such as risk	
	-Aid people in finding providers and services and filling out complex forms	

Data from Centers for Disease Control and Prevention: Health literacy, August 11, 2014, http://www.cdc.gov/healthliteracy/; and US Department of Health and Human Services, Office of Disease Prevention and Health Promotion: Quick guide to health literacy fact sheet, http://www.health.gov/communication/literacy/quickguide/factsbasic.htm.

E. Health education topics cannot be limited to oral hygiene instruction; topics might include:
 1. Preventive measures, such as appropriate use of fluorides, sealants, and xylitol
 2. Oral diseases and conditions (e.g., periodontal diseases, malocclusion, oropharyngeal cancers) and risk factors such as diet, systemic diseases, poor oral self-care behaviors, and infant-feeding practices
 3. Importance of routine assessment, prevention, and treatment
 4. Self-examination techniques
 5. Dental safety and dental emergencies (e.g., use of mouth protectors, procedures for avulsed tooth)
 6. Roles of various health professionals and their interrelationships
 7. Care of the oral cavity and dental prostheses
 8. Careers in dentistry and dental hygiene
 9. Becoming a discriminating dental consumer; oral health care products
 10. Effects of tobacco use on oral and systemic health
 11. Environmental factors affecting oral health (e.g., occupation-related concerns)
 12. Prenatal and postnatal oral health issues and recommendations; early childhood caries
 13. How to provide oral health care to those unable to care for themselves
 14. Oral and systemic disease links
 15. Topics reflected in current *Healthy People* objectives (see Table 20-2); *Healthy People 2020* website provides resources in the Tools Resources tab; ADHA, CDC, and other professional organizations also provide resources

Methods of Oral Health Education

A. Instructional methods
 1. Lecture—informative talk, prepared beforehand and given to a group; useful to introduce new topics, arouse interest in a subject, or review concepts
  a. Advantages
   (1) Can present many facts and ideas in a short period
   (2) Can convey information to large numbers of individuals
   (3) Preparation takes place before presentation
   (4) Allows instructor to determine aims, content, organization, pace, and direction of presentation
   (5) Integrates diverse materials and highlights various ideas and concepts in an orderly way
   (6) Can use media
   (7) Builds on foundational knowledge in subsequent presentations; allows for gradual development of complex or difficult concepts and theories
  b. Disadvantages
   (1) No active participation by the learner; encourages one-way communication; stifles creativity
   (2) Instructor must have effective writing, speaking, and modeling skills; poor presentation technique is a barrier to learning

   (3) Difficult to monitor student learning; requires a considerable amount of unguided student time outside the classroom
 2. Lecture-demonstration—informative talk that presents information supplemented by a demonstration to reinforce learning; can be used to introduce information and to demonstrate skills or techniques to supplement information
  a. Advantages
   (1) Illustrates information visually
   (2) Sets forth information in a complete format
   (3) Allows for concentration of attention and economical use of time
   (4) Useful for reinforcing material
   (5) May use models, computer-generated presentation, slides, videotapes, or other teaching tools; technology may allow larger number of participants to view a demonstration (e.g., viewing computer monitors)
  b. Disadvantages
   (1) Difficult for large groups to see a demonstration unless appropriate technology is used
   (2) Requires careful preparation for success; requires adequate equipment and facilities
 3. Discussion—group activity in which the student and teacher define a problem and seek a solution; an interaction between teachers and students to promote divergent thinking where closure is not expected; promotes understanding and clarification of concepts, ideas, and feelings; includes use of questions by the leader to stimulate interaction
  a. Advantages
   (1) Allows interaction among participants
   (2) Provides two-way communication between the group leader and members
   (3) Encourages individuals to contribute to the discussion
   (4) Engages participants in problem solving (higher-order learning)
   (5) Encourages teamwork, tolerance of divergent opinion, and development of interpersonal skills
   (6) Assists leader in directing the discussion
   (7) Can be focused on both cognitive and affective learning
  b. Disadvantages
   (1) Strong personalities can influence a group
   (2) Poor discussion leader may contribute to failure of the discussion
   (3) Nothing may be achieved; discussion may go in many directions without closure
   (4) May not be profitable if group members do not have appropriate background
 4. Discovery learning—uses a less direct questioning format to prod the learner into using logic or common sense to discover ideas or concepts; useful to build on foundational knowledge and introduce new concepts
  a. Advantages
   (1) Requires learner involvement
   (2) Requires application of knowledge (higher-level learning)

(3) Promotes critical thinking; motivates student to discover the "right answer"; several answers may be plausible

b. Disadvantages

(1) May be interpreted as guessing

(2) Need to guide learner so that correct information is concluded

5. Brainstorming—free sharing of ideas generated by unstructured group interaction; may have a well-defined, clearly stated problem to address; ideas recorded for future discussion but never analyzed for merit during session; useful for group identification of an issue or problem

a. Advantages

(1) Useful for youth and adult groups

(2) Encourages creativity

(3) Encourages application of knowledge

(4) Encourages contribution by all participants with no fear of a "wrong answer"

(5) Encourages people to build on others' ideas

b. Disadvantages

(1) Group dynamic may be influenced by stronger personalities

(2) Needs to be carefully managed so the purpose is not lost

(3) Not useful for actual sharing of information, just for problem identification or issue clarification

6. Web-based learning—uses a computer to present information in a method that can be interactive; includes use of the monitor to present photos, animation, video, print, and sound for lecture-demonstration and cases, discussion groups, online testing, and other online teaching methods

a. Advantages

(1) Provides an alternative medium to present information

(2) Accessible at all times if learner has access to a computer

(3) Can be updated

(4) Provides enhanced printed material

(5) Provides ready access to wealth of resources on the Internet

b. Disadvantages

(1) Some older adults and institutionalized persons may not have computer skills or access to appropriate technology

(2) Cost of equipment and linkages

7. Cooperative and collaborative learning activities—occur both inside and outside the classroom or learning environment, such as group activities and projects

8. Additional options

a. Field trips; virtual field trips

b. Panel discussions and debates

c. Problem-solving assignment

d. Symposium reporting

e. Distance learning

f. Computer simulations and modeling

g. Library research

h. Independent study

9. General principles for selection of oral health instructional methods

a. Oral health education should be focused on education and intervention, stressing skill acquisition and adoption of risk-reducing behaviors (evidence based)

b. Oral health education is more successful when characterized by active involvement of participants

c. A combination of teaching techniques should be used for best results to meet the needs of various learning styles and keep the interest of the audience

d. Various techniques are more suitable for different topics and for different age groups

B. Selection of media—vehicles of communication

1. Criteria for selection of media for instruction

a. Some priority populations may not have access to specific equipment, computers, or the Internet

b. Mass media can be used to create awareness

c. Material must be presented at a convenient time for the majority of participants

d. Media must be directed at participants' level of understanding

e. Size of participant group may affect the appropriateness of different types of media

f. Availability and familiarity with the operation of the educational technology are necessary

g. Environments vary in their conduciveness to the use of media and technology

2. Educational aids

a. Printed materials (e.g., pamphlets, books)

b. Photos, overheads, charts, posters, models, puppets, mobiles

c. Electronic, computer-generated presentations, slides, videotapes, CD-ROMs, DVDs

d. Boards—story, flannel, bulletin, magnetic

e. Science experiments

f. Computer-generated media

g. Mass media—useful to increase awareness; not as useful to motivate change of health behaviors

h. Radio and television (including cable)

i. Newspaper and magazine

j. Billboards

k. Advertisements

l. Distance education technologies (e.g., Internet, computerized instruction, Web-based tutorials, telecommunications, teleconferencing, iPods, discussion boards)

m. Social media

3. General principles for evaluation and selection of media

a. Specific purpose—arouse interest, provide information, develop attitudes, change behavior

b. Accuracy and relevancy

c. Based on scientific principles and rigorous research (evidence informed)

d. Target audience—appropriateness (reading level, use of pictures), attractiveness, audience appeal, gender and racially inclusive, culturally sensitive

e. Complexity of information and readability

f. Physical properties—illustrations, color, continuity, and style

Characteristics of Different Types of Learners

A. Groups of learners share commonalities; all groups are made up of individuals, so care must be taken not to generalize indiscriminately

B. Characteristics of adult learners

1. Goal orientation and relevancy orientation; need to know the reason to learn something

2. Driven by intrinsic motivation to learn

3. Interested in the immediacy of its application

4. Bring knowledge and experience to the learning situation

5. Come to the learning situation ready to learn

6. Possibly shy and apprehensive; do not respond as quickly as children do

7. Used to an authority system and can take direction

8. Enjoy a fun, warm, friendly and humorous learning environment

9. Respond well to personal attention, compliments, and reinforcement

10. Value being treated as equals; are put off if "talked down to," embarrassed, humiliated, or kept waiting

11. Are social; like to share stories and get to know each other

12. Prefer hands-on, practical, tangible, orderly, and predictable activities that include active involvement

13. Need a focus on transference of information (ability to use information in a new setting)

C. Suggestions for oral health education programs for low-literacy learners

1. Assess level of knowledge

2. Provide new information, building on and relating to what is already known

3. Have meaningful interactions; ask questions related to responses

4. Provide information through familiar and uncomplicated modes; use television, DVDs, radio, personal experience, demonstration, and oral explanation

5. Provide explicit information that is relevant to current needs

6. Limit the amount of information taught at one time

7. Limit written materials; use basic terminology; maintain a fifth-grade level, especially for written materials

D. Characteristics of young children as learners

1. Have undeveloped intrinsic motivation; respond to reinforcement and behavior modification

2. Have limited attention and concentration spans; a variety of activities are required to maintain attention

3. Have undeveloped problem-solving skills

4. Have a weak memory; repetition is required

5. Have limited life and learning experience; tend to accept information being presented at face value

6. Use concrete reasoning; are unable to understand abstract concepts; learning is better with hands-on and visual activities related to the tangible, such as demonstration and practice

7. Very young children are unable to read and write; lessons must use pictures

8. Have varied interests at different ages, based on their physical and emotional development and life experiences

9. Motivations are current interests and needs (e.g., young children's need for approval by teacher; adolescents' need for peer acceptance)

10. Respond well to oral health education geared to current level of development (e.g., tooth eruption, orthodontic treatment)

11. Do not possess fine motor coordination skills; recommended oral hygiene methods must be age appropriate (e.g., method of brushing, flossing)

12. Possess a social nature and interest in sharing stories when asked questions

13. Show lack of self-control; classroom management is required to control behavior

Oral Health Education Plan Development

A. Health education plan (lesson plan)—organization of topics, goals, objectives, learning experiences, and evaluation plan in relation to a central theme or problem; provides educators with an organized approach, which is vital in dynamic teaching for both student and teacher; includes all the elements of a program plan previously described

B. Assessment of needs—learner needs, oral health status, interests, and developmental level; teaching environment; availability of media; resources available to support the lesson; previous oral health learning experiences and current oral health knowledge and behavior

C. Prioritization of the learning needs of the audience to determine the purpose, aim, and rationale of the lesson

D. Planning the lesson

1. Goals—one or two recommended; general, broad statements of direction for the lesson

2. Instructional objectives—statement that describes the intended outcome, aim, or product of instruction; what a successful learner is able to do at the end of instruction; expected behavior; should be precise and measurable; useful for guiding instruction and evaluation; components of an effective, precise instructional objective include:

a. Performance—what a learner is expected to be able to do or demonstrate when the instructional event ends, using a verb that denotes an observable behavior or action; for example, "The client will demonstrate the modified Bass toothbrushing technique"

b. Conditions—the important conditions (if any) under which the performance is to occur; for example, "Given a soft-bristled toothbrush, the client will demonstrate the modified Bass toothbrushing technique on all tooth surfaces and on the tongue"

c. Criterion—the criterion of acceptable performance; a description of how well the learner must perform to be considered acceptable; for example, "Given a soft-bristled toothbrush, the client will demonstrate the modified Bass toothbrushing technique and remove all clinically visible plaque biofilm, as measured by the Plaque Index"

3. Identifying teaching strategies and learning experiences—should be based on the objectives and on the principles of learning and strategy selection previously explained

4. Identifying materials and media needed based on criteria described earlier; identifying resources for materials; allowing preparation time

5. Identifying and arranging for equipment required to present lesson

6. Planning follow-up activities and materials, such as handouts to send home to parents or caregivers

E. Implementing the lesson
1. Introduction, main activity or activities, closure or conclusion, and follow-up activities
2. Considering the learning needs of the audience during presentation
3. Preparing and practicing beforehand to control anxiety
4. Flexibility and adjustment of plans as needed

F. Evaluation of learning outcomes—should relate to objectives and to pretest and assessment procedures to provide basis for comparison; used for changes in future lessons and self-development as an educator

Health Education and Promotion Programs in the School Setting

A. The program should focus on a combination of strategies and efforts to reach parents, students, school personnel, and the community

B. The programs in school settings have the potential to reach significant numbers of participants

C. The school environment supports learning and reinforcement, ideally through an integrated curriculum, not isolated instances

D. The school program should be comprehensive, including efforts directed to improving the environment, providing education, and providing or promoting services (e.g., referrals, school-based sealant and fluoride programs)

E. Teachers can serve as role models

F. Success is enhanced by identifying responsible individual(s) (decision makers); involving parents for reinforcement at home; using community resources and personnel (e.g., agencies, other oral health care professionals); and evaluating and revising the program, when appropriate

G. The primary role of the dental hygienist is to be a resource, train teachers, work with the various groups to enhance the overall program, and manage and support the program, not to provide all the classroom instruction

PROGRAM EVALUATION

General Principles

A. Program evaluation is a key element of community oral health programs; should take place at all stages; consists of both formative and summative evaluation
1. Formative evaluation—ongoing evaluation during the program to assess processes; can lead to revisions to improve program success
2. Summative evaluation—evaluation of outcomes based on program objectives; provides comparison to needs assessment (baseline) data to determine success of the program

B. Program evaluation is applied research; research methods are used (see the earlier sections "Epidemiology and Research" and "Measurement of Diseases and Conditions in Oral Epidemiology")

C. Points to evaluate
1. Quality of program and personnel (formative)
2. Progress and effectiveness of activities—identify problems and solutions to assist in revisions and modifications to meet goals and objectives (formative)
3. Perceptions, attitudes, and participation of recipients of program (formative)
4. Systematic and regular evaluation of goals and objectives by using specific measurement instruments; outcomes assessment (summative)
5. Health status indicators of recipients of program (summative)

Use of Statistics

A. Data—numbers collected from measurements or counts
1. Continuous data—numerical data capable of being any value along a continuum (e.g., periodontal probe readings, blood pressure, time, temperature); can be expressed meaningfully as a fraction
2. Discrete data—numerical variables or data that are counted only in terms of whole numbers; for example, number of clients examined, number of children who had teeth sealed, and number of children with caries experience
3. Categorical data—division of data into categories with no numeric representation (e.g., SES, ethnic group membership, gender, school attended, grade in school)
4. Dichotomous data—categorical variable with only two groups (e.g., male/female, yes/no, bleeding/no bleeding, pass/fail)

B. Scales of measurement—data fall in one of four scales:
1. Nominal scale—observations belong to mutually exclusive classes or categories; for example, Republicans/Democrats, smokers/nonsmokers, normal/abnormal, place of residence, gender, and ethnic group membership
2. Ordinal scale—classes or categories that have ranking of characteristics in some empirical order; for example, class rankings of high school graduates; Likert

scales such as strongly disagree, disagree, agree, and strongly agree for patient satisfaction and other measures; most dental indices; periodontal classification; and SES

3. Interval scale—measurement scale characterized by equal intervals along the scale; has no absolute zero, such as a Fahrenheit thermometer; not useful in oral health research

4. Ratio scale—measurement scale characterized by equal intervals along the scale and the presence of an absolute zero, such as age, weight, height, DMF, number of sealants, and test scores; most dental indices are treated as ratio data

C. Statistics—science that describes, summarizes, analyzes, and interprets numerical data

    1. Statistic—numerical characteristic of a sample derived from the data collected

    2. Parameter—numerical characteristic of a population

D. Descriptive statistics—statistics used numerically to describe and summarize data collected (Box 20-11)

    1. Measures of central tendency—used to describe what is typical (the midpoint) in the sample group based on the data gathered (e.g., mean, median, and mode)

    2. Measures of dispersion—used to describe variability of scores in a distribution (e.g., range and standard deviation)

E. Correlation statistics—statistical measure for determining the strength of the linear relationship between two or more variables; used to associate variables and determine risk in analytic studies; correlation does not demonstrate causality (Box 20-11)

F. Summary presentation of descriptive and correlation statistics

    1. Frequency distribution table—table that summarizes the frequencies of data in the distribution; data are entered into a frequency distribution table before creating a graph

    2. Bar graph (or bar chart)—two-dimensional diagram used pictorially to display data that are discrete in nature, regardless of scale of measurement; bars do not touch

    3. Histogram—type of bar graph used to represent interval-scaled or ratio-scaled variables that are continuous in nature; bars touch each other

    4. Frequency polygon—line graph used to represent data that are continuous in nature; a histogram and a frequency polygon can be used to represent the same data; a frequency polygon can be easier to read than a histogram when more than one distribution is presented for comparison

    5. Polygon—a line graph that does not represent frequency data; for example, a line graph showing the progression of a Plaque Index score over time in a repeated-measures experimental study (this would also be called a time series graph)

    6. Pie graph (or pie chart)—used to display parts of a whole

---

BOX 20-11   Common Statistics in Community Oral Health

Descriptive Statistics

Descriptive statistics are used to describe data.

Mean—the arithmetic average; the sum of the values divided by the number of items

- Incorporates the value of each score
- Affected by extreme scores
- Used with interval or ratio data

Median—midpoint of a distribution, with 50% of the scores falling above it and 50% below it; scores of distribution are arranged in either ascending or descending order to locate the midpoint

- When the total number of scores is odd, the median is the middle score
- When the total number of scores is even, the two middle scores are added, then divided by 2
- Median can be a decimal
- Not affected by extreme scores
- Can be used with ordinal data; can be used with ratio data to avoid effect of extreme scores

Mode—the most frequently occurring score in a distribution

- Distribution may be unimodal, bimodal, multi-modal, or have no mode
- Can be used with nominal data

Range—the spread between the highest and the lowest scores in a distribution

- Easily determined
- Somewhat unreliable because it is determined by only two scores of the distribution
- Can be used with ordinal and higher data

Standard deviation (SD)—the positive square root of the variance

- The greater the dispersion or spread of scores around the mean of the distribution, the higher is the value of the SD and variance
- A small SD indicates that the distribution of scores is clustered closely around the mean; a large SD indicates that scores are dispersed widely around the mean

Correlation Statistics

Correlation statistics are used to associate variables and determine risk in analytic studies; correlation does not demonstrate causality.

- Correlation coefficient, r, ranging from +1.0 to −1.0; the sign indicates the direction of the correlation, and the number indicates the strength of the correlation
- Interpretation of correlation coefficient

    1. Direction of relationship

      - Positive—value of one variable increases as the value of the second also increases (e.g., presence of plaque biofilm and gingivitis); expressed as a positive number

      - Negative—inverse relationship between two variables; as the value of one increases, the other decreases, and vice versa (e.g., fluoride exposure and dental caries); expressed as a negative number

    2. Strength, regardless of direction of relationship

      - Very high: $r = 0.9$ to 1.0 (+ or −)

      - High: $r = 0.70$ to 0.89 (+ or −)

      - Moderate: $r = 0.50$ to 0.69 (+ or −)

      - Weak: $r = 0.26$ to 0.49 (+ or −)

      - Little if any: $r = 0$ to 0.25 (+ or −)

BOX 20-11 Common Statistics in Community Oral Health—cont'd

Inferential Statistics

Inferential statistics are used to test hypotheses, make inferences, and demonstrate causality.

Parametric Inferential Statistics

- The *t* test—determines if a statistically significant difference exists between two mean scores
- The *t* test for independent samples—data are from two sample groups drawn independently from a population (two independent groups); commonly known as *Student's t test*
- The *t* test for dependent samples—data are from two samples that are related (two groups that are matched for relevant variables or pretest and posttest from one group); also known as *t test for correlated samples* and *paired t test*; more sensitive than the *t* test for independent samples because groups are paired, eliminating a possible source of variance
- Analysis of variance (ANOVA)—used to analyze differences among three or more mean scores; used to examine the effects of two or more independent variables simultaneously within the same research design and to determine interactions among the variables in multiple sample groups
  F ratio—value that results when ANOVA is computed
  Result communicates if a difference exists somewhere among the mean scores; follow-up statistics are used to determine exactly where the difference lies

Variations of ANOVA include ANCOVA (analysis of covariance) to control for extraneous variables in a study design and MANOVA (multi-variate analysis of variance), which is used when multiple dependent variables are measured

Nonparametric Inferential Statistics

Chi-square test—used to determine if a statistically significant difference exists between frequencies of data (versus comparing mean scores as is done with parametrics); used with nominal data from two or more distributions with more than 5 scores in each one; has different versions for special applications

- One version is used with a single distribution of data to determine whether or not a significant difference exists between the observed number of cases within designated categories and the expected number of cases within designated categories according to the hypothesis (goodness of fit)
- Another version is used with two data sets to test the differences in the distributions of data (versus the differences in the mean scores)
- Another version is used to test the statistical significance of a correlation coefficient result

Other similar nonparametric statistics exist to test differences of data distributions that represent ordinal data, come from groups with more than 5 in each one, come from more than two groups, or a combination

Data from Beatty CF, Beatty CE: Biostatistics. In Nathe CN: *Dental public health and research,* ed 4, Upper Saddle River, NJ, 2015, Pearson.

7. Scattergram (or scatter plot)—a graph in which scores are plotted to show the relationship or association of two variables; visually shows the relationship represented by a correlation statistic
8. Advantages of tables and graphs—they provide a neat and organized way to present data, facilitate understanding and analysis of data at a glance, expedite review of data, enable comparisons, and ease recall of data

G. Distributions of data (Fig. 20-7)
   1. Normal (bell) curve—symmetrical distribution of scores in which the mean, median, and mode have the same value, and the scores fall within a standard relationship to the mean (standard deviation, SD)
      a. 68% of the scores fall between +1 and −1 SD of the mean
      b. 95% of the scores fall between +2 and −2 SD of the mean
      c. 99% of the scores fall between +3 and −3 SD of the mean
   2. Skewed distribution—one in which the distribution is asymmetrical
      a. Positive skew—mean has a higher value than the median and mode; the bulk of the scores are at the lower end of the distribution, and the tail of the curve is at the higher end
      b. Negative skew—mean has a lower value than the median and mode; the bulk of the scores are at the higher end of the distribution, and the tail of the curve is at the lower end

H. Inferential statistics—that branch of statistics used to infer research findings from the sample to the general population from whom the sample was taken; used to test

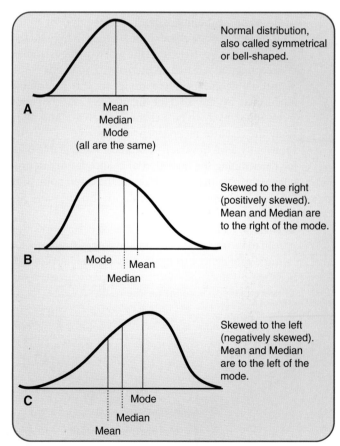

FIG 20-7 Distribution curves. (From Beatty CF: *Community oral health practice for the dental hygienist,* ed 4, St Louis, 2017, Elsevier Saunders.)

hypotheses, generalize results to a larger population of interest, and provide evidence of causality (see Box 20-11)

1. Parametric statistics—inferential statistical procedures that require the following assumptions about the population parameters:
   a. Data are interval or ratio scaled; dental indices are treated as ratio scaled even though many are ordinal scaled
   b. Population from which the data are taken is normally distributed (bell curve)
   c. Sample is large (i.e., n $\geq$ 30) and randomized
2. Nonparametric statistics—inferential statistical procedures used when the population parameters do not meet the assumptions required for parametric statistics
   a. Required if data are nominal or ordinal in nature
   b. Population from whom the sample is drawn does not have a normal distribution (has a skewed curve), or distribution is unknown
   c. Required with continuous data if sample size is small or skewed

I. Hypothesis testing
1. Definition—a formal decision-making process of testing a hypothesis using statistical significance and inference, followed by interpreting the statistical results
2. Null hypothesis is tested statistically to make the statistical decision
   a. Retaining the null hypothesis is equivalent to rejecting the research or alternative hypothesis
   b. Rejection of the null hypothesis is equivalent to the acceptance of the research or alternative hypothesis
   c. Failure to accept (rejecting) the null hypothesis implies accepting the research or alternative hypothesis
3. Statistical significance—according to the probability established by the level of significance, the obtained result is less likely to be a chance occurrence and more likely the result of the independent variable
4. Probability level (*p* value)—researcher's acceptable odds for determining the operation of chance factors in producing the obtained research result; the cutoff point used to reject or accept the null hypothesis; also known as *significance level* and *alpha value*
   a. Small *p* values indicate rare chance occurrences that lead to the rejection of the null hypothesis and provide more confidence that the statistical decision is correct
   b. Large *p* values indicate that chance occurrences are more likely to account for the result

   c. Maximum *p* value to reject the null hypothesis in oral health research is typically 0.05; *p* values of 0.01 and 0.001 indicate greater statistical significance
      (1) If the probability is 0.05 or less, the results obtained are reported as statistically significant
      (2) A probability result of greater than 0.05 ($p > 0.05$) indicates results are not statistically significant
5. Inferential statistics are used to test the hypothesis
6. Test statistics used to make the statistical decision depend on the size of the sample, the number of samples, the type of data, and other factors (see assumptions in the previous discussion of inferential statistics and Box 20-11)
7. Because statistical decision making is based on probability (chance), errors may occur (Fig. 20-8)
   a. Type I error—based on statistical results, the researcher rejects the null hypothesis and concludes that a statistically significant difference exists when, in fact, no true difference is present; rejecting a null hypothesis that is true
   b. Type II error—the researcher concludes that no statistically significant difference exists and accepts the null hypothesis when, in fact, a significant difference does exist; accepting a null hypothesis that is false
   c. The p value is set to control the acceptable rate of error, which depends on the clinical importance or significance of the question being researched
      (1) Type I errors lead to unwarranted change; for example, a client could receive ineffective treatment
      (2) Type II errors maintain status quo; for example, a client could miss out on treatment that could have been helpful or even lifesaving
   d. The potential for error is the reason why multiple studies are critical for evidence-based decision making

J. Clinical significance
1. Statistical decision making is not the sole means by which research findings are interpreted and applied; findings may have statistical significance without having clinical significance
2. Practical implications of research may or may not be inherent in research results; statistical significance does not necessarily indicate that results are important or meaningful; for example, the free gingival margin may have a statistically significant resorption of 1.0 mm, while the pocket depth is still 6.0 mm, so the resorption may not be meaningful in the overall periodontal outcome

| | | Null hypothesis is | |
		Accepted	Not accepted
Null hypothesis is actually	True	No error	Type I error ($p = \alpha$)
	Not true	Type II error ($p = \beta$)	No error

FIG 20-8 Type I and type II statistical errors.

Evaluating Professional Literature

A. Professional responsibility includes keeping current with new developments for evidence-informed decision making

B. Reviewing the professional literature is important for the contemporary dental hygienist in all roles
   1. It is necessary to review and study the literature before and during community programming
   2. It provides an impetus and evidence base for various types of community activities
   3. Journal articles, particularly randomized clinical trials, systematic reviews, and meta-analyses, serve as a source of current information for evidence-informed decision making

C. Reviewing the professional literature is a valuable means of continuing education

D. Scientific writing should be comprehensible for the average reader who is knowledgeable about the general area

E. Professional literature should be evaluated to ascertain the validity of results (Box 20-12)

PROVISION OF ORAL HEALTH CARE

Diverse Modes of Dental Practice in the United States

A. Dental care is delivered via a complex, fragmented system of care that consists of diverse modes of dental practice and multiple sources of funding (Table 20-18)

B. *Healthy People 2020* objectives (see Table 20-2) address the need for changes to the public health infrastructure to increase utilization

---

BOX 20-12 Criteria for Evaluating the Professional Literature

1. Overall description of the article
   • Concise and descriptive title
   • Descriptive abstract
2. Reputable and refereed journal
   • Editorial review board in place
   • Peer review of articles before publication
   • Affiliation with a learned society, professional group, specialty group, or reputable scientific publisher
   • Not a "popular" magazine sponsored by a cause or published by a commercial firm
   • Concisely written articles, using a scientific style
3. Currency of data published
   • Represents current knowledge, not outdated by more recent research
   • General guide of 5 years
4. Qualified author
   • Appropriate credentials to have knowledge of the topic
   • Expertise in a particular area supported by current or past position
   • Satisfactory reputation for well-conducted research
   • No affiliation with a commercial firm if the report is of product research
5. Funding of research
   • Evidence of finances and facilities to support the research if the article reports research results
   • No conflict of interest represented
6. References
   • Comprehensive, accurate, and reputable
   • Appropriate number of current references, according to the topic (older references may be indicated for historical purposes or because they are considered classic)
7. Clear, accurate, and complete description of the research problem
   • Clear purposes of the study
   • Inclusion of a thorough review of the literature
   • Adequate operational definitions of important terms and concepts
   • Adequate and clear statement of the hypotheses or objectives that follow directly from the problem statement

Methods
   1. Adequate description of the research design
   2. Appropriate for the type of study (descriptive, analytic, and experimental studies require different methods)

3. Adequate description of the characteristics of the population sampled and an outline of the allocation of groups if a clinical trial
4. Adequate description of the sampling techniques
5. Lack of bias in the selection or assignment of objects or persons in the sample
6. Control of variables that might influence the results
7. Evidence of comparability of experimental and control groups
8. Evidence of control of bias
9. Discussion of the limitations of the design
10. Use of tests and instruments that reasonably measure the factors under study
    • Use of valid and reliable measures (evidence of reliability is provided)
    • Control of conditions in which measurements are made
    • Control and reporting of the reliability of the examiners
    • Appropriate duration of the study
11. Data analysis
    • Inclusion of all the factors needed to test the hypotheses or achieve the objectives
    • Use of appropriate statistical tests
    • Description of general-purpose computer programs used for data analysis
    • Presentation of statistical results of hypotheses testing
    • Clear presentation of findings
    • Clear, easy-to-understand, and titled data tables and figures
    • Straightforward presentation of data
12. Discussion to highlight significant issues from the research
    • Interpretation of results
    • Clear discussion of the importance or clinical significance of the findings
    • Explanation of the strengths and limitations of the study
    • Report of any treatment or study complications and adverse effects
    • Discussion of the relationship of the results to previous studies
    • Discussion of the implications for practice or the profession
13. Conclusions
    • Clear
    • Supported by methods and findings

Data from Beatty CF: *Community oral health practice for the dental hygienist*, ed 4, St Louis, 2017, Elsevier Saunders; and Nathe CN: *Dental public health and research*, ed 4, Upper Saddle River, NJ, 2015, Pearson.

TABLE 20-18 Modes of Dental Practice

Practice Setting	Population Served	Financing	Utilization Patterns	Advantages	Disadvantages	Oral Health Personnel
Private practice (solo or group)	Midlevel to high-level socioeconomic status (SES) patients Tend to be located in areas of economic opportunity and desirable locations	Third-party private dental insurance Fee-for-service systems Some discounted-fee programs	Higher SES and dental insurance are associated with greater utilization of dental services Greater demand for esthetic services Higher tooth retention rate among those over age 65	Flexibility for patients and providers Providers determine practice philosophy Inherent economic incentive to be efficient Advantages of groups compared to solo include availability during nontraditional hours, provision of more varied services, quality assurance via built-in peer review and consultation, and availability of emergency care from partners	Serves limited population Difficult to monitor quality assurance	Single or multiple dentists and hygienists Limited experience to date with incorporation of midlevel providers into this model
Corporately managed dental practice	Low-level to midlevel SES patients May be located in urban or suburban areas	Third-party private dental insurance Public financing via Medicaid and CHIP Some discounted-fee programs	Greater utilization by children and adolescents up to age 21 (Medicaid and CHIP coverage) Higher rate of racial minority groups that correlates with SES status	Nontraditional hours Convenient locations Dentists are employees rather than owners Corporate benefits often available to employees Multiple payment options	Practice decisions usually made by corporate administrators Quality of care may suffer from focus on profit over patient care	Multiple dentists and hygienists No evidence of incorporation of midlevel providers into this model
Hospital dental clinic	Specific, medically compromised patient populations Located in or near public or private hospital facilities, military bases, Indian reservations	Public and private financing combined Medicaid/CHIP From patient and hospital funding sources	Special populations such as children who are medically compromised or have other disabilities; cancer patients; veterans Dental services often mandatory before medical procedures or surgery	Accessible to hospital patients who are unable to travel elsewhere Resources, personnel specifically oriented toward patients' special needs Utilize extensive quality assurance programs	Limited to hospital population, and in some cases, family members May require extensive travel for outpatients	Variety of providers, including dental/dental hygiene students and residents Strong inter-professional component Student participation often as a service learning opportunity Federally funded clinics may use USPHS, NHSC, or military personnel
Community-based clinics	Lower-SES patients Located in nontraditional settings in urban or rural areas May serve specific populations, e.g. migrant farm workers, Indian reservations School-based clinics serve high-risk schoolchildren	Public and private financing combined via Medicaid/CHIP, grants, donations, and patient fees Some are faith based with funding from related faith organization May utilize a sliding-fee scale based on income	Increased utilization of services among low-SES groups because of affordability and access For school-based clinics, increased utilization by children and adolescents	Ease of access Affordable care Providers are often bilingual Services may be deeply discounted, sometimes free	State practice acts may limit locations for some providers (RDHs, ADHPs, DHTs) Consistent financing may be difficult	Varity of providers, including midlevel providers Often includes strong inter-professional component Student participation often as a service learning opportunity Federally funded clinics may use USPHS, NHSC, or military personnel

TABLE 20-18 Modes of Dental Practice—cont'd

Practice Setting	Population Served	Financing	Utilization Patterns	Advantages	Disadvantages	Oral Health Personnel
Mobile clinics	Lower-SES populations Located in nontraditional settings, urban or rural areas Populations with limited mobility and transportation Patients in institutions or homebound, e.g., long-term care facilities	Public and private financing combined via grants, donations, and patient fees Medicaid/CHIP	Increased utilization of services for populations with poor access to care (homebound, long-term care facilities, homeless) Increased utilization for school-age children	Portability of care Increased flexibility with scheduling, delivering care Services may be deeply discounted, sometimes free	State practice acts may limit locations for some providers (RDHs, ADHPs, DHTs) Quality assurance measures may or may not be in place Consistent financing may be difficult Services may be limited	Variety of providers, including midlevel providers Student participation often as a service learning opportunity
Dental/dental hygiene educational clinics	Low-SES to midlevel-SES patients Located in educational institutions in or near metropolitan or urban areas	Public and private financing combined From patient and institutional funding sources	Increases utilization of services among lower-SES populations due to affordability of care Provide a safety net for lower-SES populations	High quality of care resulting from close oversight by institution Extensive quality assurance program	Limited flexibility with scheduling Lengthy appointments Multiple appointments often required Extensive travel required by most patients because of location	Dental and dental hygiene students and residents Faculty clinic may or may not be available

Oral Health Care Personnel Workforce

A. Types—dentist, dental assistant, dental hygienist, expanded-function dental hygienists and assistants, dental laboratory technician, denturist, other emerging midlevel practitioners in some states such as the dental therapist or dental therapist/hygienist

B. Supply and distribution of dentists
1. Supply is traditionally measured with a dentist-to-population ratio—not always an accurate reflection of supply because of location, population involved, community need, demand for dental services, and trends in use of other oral health care personnel to provide dental treatment services
2. The number of active dentists began to decline in 2000, has continued, and is projected to continue through 2020, influenced by retirement patterns and smaller annual number of graduates[9]
3. The American Dental Association (ADA) estimates that the national supply of dental services will increase as a result of a significant growth in dental productivity because of increased employment of allied dental professionals[9]
4. The dental profession has recognized the need to develop programs to resolve the problem of uneven distribution of dentists, which exists for various reasons:

a. Dentists have freedom to choose their practice location and tend to locate their practices in areas of economic opportunity, high demand for services, and desirable environments; most are drawn to suburban areas rather than rural and urban areas
b. Location of dental schools provides an abundant number of dentists in some areas and few in other areas; not all states have a dental school
c. Portability of license from state to state is needed to be able to relocate easily in response to geographic population shifts that result in changes in areas of high demand; a national dental licensing examination would provide greater portability
5. Inadequate supply and maldistribution of dental personnel results in *dental health professions shortage areas* (DHPSAs, or DHSAs), as defined by the federal government
a. Based on provider-to-population ratio (dentist/population ratio of 1:5,000);[10] access to care according to distance, time, and incomes at poverty level are also considered
b. In 2014, more than 49 million people were living in approximately 4900 DHPSAs, and the number of practitioners needed to achieve the recommended dentist/population ratio was over 7300;[10] number of

DHPSAs, number of people living in DHPSAs, and number of dentists required to remedy the shortage areas have increased steadily over the past decade;[11] federal incentives are available to attract dentists and dental hygienists to these areas

6. The dental profession has recognized the need to increase underrepresented minorities in the oral health care professions

a. Women are underrepresented in the profession; the number of women graduating from dental schools has gradually increased; currently approximately 50% of dental school students are female;[12] there is a need to evaluate the effect of this increasing shift of gender on the values, caring quality, patient orientation, and practice models of dentistry, as well as the number and distribution needed to meet the needs of the population

b. A continuing need exists to increase the diversity of the dental profession

c. Fig. 20-9 depicts current racial/ethnic distribution of dentists in the United States

d. Although *Healthy People 2010* targets were exceeded for representation of the Asian or Pacific Islander population in dentistry, representation for the black non-Hispanic population moved away from the target, and targets were not met for other minority groups in the dental profession[3]

e. The Indian Health Service (IHS) and the Health Resources and Services Administration (HRSA)

programs support diversification of the health care professions workforce through scholarships, repayment programs, and other incentives

f. The goal is to have diversity of oral health care personnel that is proportionate to the diversity of the population; projected data indicate movement toward this goal (Fig. 20-9)

C. Dental school enrollment

1. At 65 U.S. dental schools, located in 38 states, the Commonwealth of Puerto Rico, and the District of Columbia, representing a very slight increase over the past 10 years[13]

2. With 12,001 dental school applicants in 2010; current trend is an increase in the number of applicants[12] and the opening of new dental schools[14]

D. Supply of dental hygiene personnel

1. About 192,800 dental hygienists were employed in 2012, with a projected increase of 33% for 2012 to 2022[15]

2. About 335 accredited dental hygiene programs in the United States in 2014 offered a certificate, associate's or bachelor's degree, reflecting a 65.8% increase in number of programs since 1990; 7097 dental hygienists graduated in 2012; there are 55 degree completion programs and 22 dental hygiene master's programs[16,17]

3. More dental hygienists than dentists have graduated every year since 1991, and the difference has increased each year; projections are that this trend will continue[17]

4. States will continue to expand the scope of dental hygiene practice; practice settings will grow and less supervision will be required in order to meet the increasing demand for greater access to dental care at a more affordable cost

5. As an organized profession, dental hygiene has sought to help meet the oral health care needs of the population and improve access to care by:

a. Promoting higher levels of education within dental hygiene, such as baccalaureate, master's, and doctoral degree preparation

b. Establishing the dental hygienist as a primary care provider

c. Seeking direct reimbursement of dental hygienists and midlevel practitioners; in 2013, 15 states recognized and reimbursed dental hygienists as Medicaid providers[16]

d. Developing and supporting the advancement of new, nontraditional practice models, such as collaborative and independent practice as well as dental hygiene–based midlevel providers, to improve access to care for underserved populations and better meet the needs of community oral health care practice

e. Creating and developing the advanced dental hygiene practitioner model

(1) The concept of midlevel providers in dentistry has become a reality in the United States, possibly marking the beginning of a new era in dentistry in which high-quality, cost-effective dental care

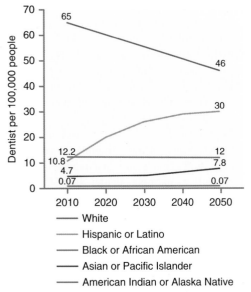

FIG 20-9 Racial/ethnic representation of dentists in the United States, 2010: actual and projected to 2050. (Data from American Dental Education Association: Dean's briefing book, 2013. http://www.adea.org/uploadedFiles/ADEA/Content_Conversion_Final/deansbriefing/ADEA_Deans_BB_2013_FINAL.pdf.)

can be provided for currently underserved groups in the population[18] (Table 20-19)

(2) Three states have now authorized dental therapists who function as midlevel providers;[18] in 2013, eight additional states considered a variety of related proposals,[16] and 15 states are currently considering legislation to allow midlevel providers[18]

f. Currently, 37 states in the United States allow dental hygienists to provide direct care to patients in at least one practice setting in the community without a dentist present, many of whom were authorized within the last 10 years; many of these states have collaborative dental hygiene practice models under various names that allow for unsupervised practice of dental hygiene[19] (Table 20-19)

g. Midlevel providers and other alternative practice models are able to increase access to care cost-effectively for population groups who do not have access to the traditional dental office, as well as expand access to dental care in DHSAs, especially in rural areas[18]

h. Some midlevel providers are dentistry based, whereas others are dental hygiene based; ADHA promotes the value of the dental hygiene–based model to build on the foundation of dental hygiene education and practice experience[20]

TABLE 20-19   Nontraditional Oral Health Care Personnel and Midlevel Providers

Models	Practice Settings	Status	Supervision	Education/ Qualifications	Scope of Services
Community dental health coordinator (CDHC)	Community health centers: clinics, schools, churches, senior citizen centers, Head Start programs in dental health (professional) shortage areas (DHSAs)	Developed by ADA and piloted in selected DHSAs, beginning in 2009; evaluation currently underway; ADA focus is to expand CDHC to DHSAs nationwide	Direct supervision; assists practicing dentist in triage of patients, addressing social, environmental, and health literacy issues	18-month training program piloted at select dental schools CDHC comes from the community, thus is accepted by the community and understands the culture of the community	Advocacy role to address social barriers to utilization of dental care; interviewing and counseling clients to enroll in government-funded dental programs, providing social support, and offering limited preventive services
Dental health aide therapist (DHAT)	Community health center clinics in rural Alaska villages	Program specific to Alaska; developed by the Alaska Native Tribal Health Consortium in 2003; DHATs practice in 42 other countries	General supervision; partners with dentist via teledentistry, including real-time video and radiologic oversight; refers to a dentist as needed	2-year training program; comes from the community served to better address social barriers to dental care utilization	Considered a midlevel provider; based on dentist's diagnosis and treatment plan, performs restorations, pulpotomies, prophylaxis, basic extractions, preventive services, and referral to dentist for care beyond DHAT's scope
Dental therapist (DT),* dental hygiene therapist (DHT),† and advanced dental therapist (ADT)†	Settings that serve low-income, uninsured, and underserved populations, DHSAs	DT and ADT established in 2009 in Minnesota (MN); Both programs in the state educate to the advanced dental therapist level.	Indirect supervision of DT in MN; direct supervision of DHT in ME; ADT can practice unsupervised in MN under collaborative agreement with a dentist	DHT: advanced training after licensure as dental hygienist in Maine ADT: MS or MDT awarded; graduates must practice as a DT for 2000 hours and pass an examination to be a certified as an ADT.	Considered midlevel providers; broad range of basic preventive and restorative treatment, minor surgical care, pain control; similar scope of practice for all levels
Independent practice for dental hygienists (IPDH)	Personal private offices, community settings	Limited number of states	Unsupervised; can own practice in one states	Licensed to practice dental hygiene; BS degree in some states; various years or hours of clinical dental hygiene experience in different states	Traditional scope of dental hygiene practice authorized in that state

(Continued)

TABLE 20-19	Nontraditional Oral Health Care Personnel and Midlevel Providers—cont'd				
Models	Practice Settings	Status	Supervision	Education/Qualifications	Scope of Services
Collaborative, affiliated, alternative, public health, or extended care practice of dental hygiene (various names in different states)	Private dental office, facilities and institutions, schools, homebound, community centers, public health clinics, DHSAs, serving low–socioeconomic status (SES), underserved populations	Numerous states	Unsupervised; must have collaborative agreement with a dentist for consultation, referral, and emergencies on file with the state dental board; in some states, patient must have a current referral from a dentist or physician	Licensed dental hygienist; various years or hours of clinical dental hygiene experience in different states; BS degree in some states; additional education and training in some states	Traditional scope of dental hygiene practice authorized in that state

Data from Academy of General Dentistry: Definitions of mid-level oral health care providers, http://www.agd.org/files/webuser/website/advocacy/definitionsmidlevelproviders.pdf; American Dental Association (ADA): About community dental health coordinators, 2014, http://www.ada.org/en/public-programs/action-for-dental-health/community-dental-health-coordinators; American Dental Hygienists Association: ADHA supports increased access to care, use of dental hygienists and midlevel providers to help deliver dental services, July 1, 2014, http://www.adha.org/resources-docs/ADHA_Supports_Increased_Access_to_Care_Use_of_Dental_Hygienists_and_Mid_level_Providers.pdf; ADHA: Direct access states, June 2014, https://www.adha.org/resources-docs/7513_Direct_Access_to_Care_from_DH.pdf; ADHA: The benefits of dental hygiene-based oral health provider models, July 2014, http://www.adha.org/resources-docs/75112_Hygiene_Based_Workforce_Models.pdf; American Student Dental Association: Midlevel providers, 2014, http://www.asdanet.org/midlevel-providers.aspx; Emmerling H, Standley E: The mid-level, RDH, June 1, 2011, http://www.rdhmag.com/articles/print/volume-31/issue-6/features/the-mid-level.html; and Minnesota Board of Dentistry: Advanced dental therapist scope of practice. http://www.dentalboard.state.mn.us/Portals/3/Licensing/Dental%20Therapist/ADTSCOPE.pdf; Dental therapists, 2014, http://www.dentalboard.state.mn.us/Licensing/ProcessingandApplications/DentalTherapistAdvDentalTherapist/tabid/1165/Default.aspx; University of Minnesota School of Dentistry: Dental therapy—a new profession, February 2014, http://www.dentistry.umn.edu/programs-admissions/dental-therapy/index.htm; University of Washington School of Medicine: Dentex dental health aide therapist program, http://depts.washington.edu/dentexak/; and Wides C, Bates T, Mertz E: Registered dental hygienists in alternative practice in California, 2009 descriptive report, Center for the Health Professions, University of California San Francisco, December 2011. http://www.futurehealth.ucsf.edu/Content/11660/2011_12_Registered_Dental_Hygienists_In_Alternative_Practice_in_California.pdf.

BS, Bachelor of science; *MS*, master of science.
*Dentistry based dental therapist/midlevel provider.
†Dental hygiene based dental therapist/midlevel provider.

i. More than 50 countries, including Canada, New Zealand, Australia, and the United Kingdom, use dental therapists[16]
j. Workforce issues should continue to be analyzed and adjustments made on the basis of retirement patterns of practicing dentists, availability of oral health care personnel, productivity improvement, population and economic growth, demand for and financing of dental care, and new models of midlevel oral health care practitioners
E. Gender and racial–ethnic group representation among dental hygienists
1. Primarily women—95.8% of students in 2012 were female[17]
2. Inadequate racial-ethnic group representation in the dental hygiene profession; 72.5% enrolled in 2012 were non-Hispanic white[17]

FINANCING ORAL HEALTH CARE

A. Oral health care financing in the United States is complex because of the dual involvement of the corporate sector and the public sector, as well as the presence of varied and multiple mechanisms of payment, sources of payment, types of insurance plans, and providers of insurance plans
B. This pluralistic system results in greater emphasis on individual responsibility for oral health care
C. The Patient Protection and Affordable Care Act (ACA) expanded dental coverage for children through Medicaid and state exchanges; some believe that the new benefits may not be sufficiently comprehensive or affordable[21]
D. Overall spending for dental services and out-of-pocket spending have continued to increase[22] and are forecasted to increase even more over the next 10 years[23]

Mechanisms of Payment for Dental Care

A. Payment by the individual or fee-for-service—two-party system (provider and client); less common today as third-party payment increases
B. Third-party payment—also called *insurance*
1. Payment for health care services by some agency other than the beneficiary (client or patient) of those services (e.g., insurance company, employer, government agency); designed to improve access to care and increase use of care

2. The dentist and the client are the first and second parties; the administrator of the finances is the third party (also known as the *carrier, insurer, underwriter,* or *administrative agent*) and may collect premiums, assume the financial risk, pay claims, and provide administrative services
3. Third-party plans can be private (a private insurance company or employer) or public (government program such as Medicaid, Medicare, or CHIP)
4. The purchaser of a private plan can be an organized private group such as a union or employer or a government agency
5. Reimbursement for insurance plans is done by a variety of mechanisms (Table 20-20)
6. Mechanisms are used by third-party carriers to control costs by discouraging overuse and protecting the third-party payer's ability to continue in business (Table 20-20)
C. Different types of insurance (benefits) plans
1. Although frequently referred to as "dental insurance," *benefits plan* is a more accurate term because, unlike medical insurance, it does not truly represent the concept of insurance; specific types of dental benefits plans fall into the two categories, fee-for-service and managed care (Table 20-21)
2. Fee-for-service—traditional system that provides freedom-of-choice arrangements under which clients are not limited in their selection of providers (called *open panel*), control of treatment decisions are maintained by the provider and beneficiary, and the provider is paid for each service rendered according to the fees established by the provider[24]
3. Managed care—cost-containment systems that restrict the type, level, and frequency of treatment; limit the client's freedom of choice to select a provider with financial benefits to use only certain providers; and control the level of reimbursement for services[24]
   a. Characterized by a comprehensive set of health care services, selected providers (called *closed panel*), and financial incentives to use selected providers
   b. Typified by internal programs to monitor the amount and quality of services provided (i.e., quality assurance)

TABLE 20-20 Mechanisms of Payment for Oral Health Care

Mechanism	Description
Individual Payment Methods	
Fee-for-service	Traditional two-party arrangement in which fee is set for a service and client is charged for service performed; declining method of payment as third-party payment becomes more prevalent
Barter system	The provider and client negotiate payment by exchanging goods or services without using money; still evident in some rural areas and developing countries
Encounter fee	A set fee each time a patient has a treatment encounter (comes in for treatment), regardless of the services provided; used by community programs as a discounted fee for clients with no dental insurance
Third-Party Reimbursement Methods	
Usual, customary, and reasonable (UCR) fee	Third-party payment based on an average of fees for the area; varies by geographic area and population size, and from carrier to carrier; most commonly used payment method in dentistry
Discounted fee	Third-party system in which fees lower than the area UCR are agreed to by a provider for members of a specifically identified group (students, older adults) or participants in a prepaid group; becoming more common in dentistry
Fee schedule	List of charges set by the third-party payer and agreed to by the provider who enrolls as a provider; provider is reimbursed by the third-party payer and cannot charge more; system used by Medicaid/CHIP
Table of allowances	List of covered services with an assigned dollar amount set by the third-party payer; providers are reimbursed by the third-party payer and can charge patients the difference between their fees and the fees set by the table of allowances
Capitation	A form of contracted care in which a provider receives a fixed payment from a third-party payer in exchange for all or most care needed by a group of patients during the contract period; method used by health maintenance organizations (HMOs); designed to increase preventive care; payment is made to the provider regardless of use by enrollees; effectiveness is in question; not typically used in dentistry
Direct reimbursement	Beneficiaries (clients or patients) are reimbursed by the employer or benefits administrator (e.g., insurance company) for a specified percentage of dental expenses on presentation of evidence of expenses
Methods Used to Control Costs	
Co-payment	Patient pays a fixed amount at each visit, and the remainder of the fee is covered by the third party; the purpose is to discourage overuse
Co-insurance	Similar to co-payment, but it is a percentage rather than a fixed amount; used by most dental insurance plans
Deductible	Patient must pay a required amount as an out-of-pocket expense before the insurance plan will pay
Annual limits (maximum coverage)	Insurance plan will pay only up to a specific dollar limit each year
Waiting period	Patient must wait specified length of time before coverage begins

TABLE 20-21 Dental Insurance (Benefits) Plans

Type of Plan	Provider	Description
Fee-for-Service		
Indemnity dental benefits plan	For-profit, commercial insurance companies	Traditional fee-for-service plan in which beneficiary (client or patient) can visit any provider (freedom of choice) and provider is free to set fees; includes co-insurance, deductible, and maximums; company reimburses client or provider based on fee profiles (similar to UCR); patient is responsibility for any difference between the benefit paid and the fee charged; can have some of the characteristics of managed care: (1) include a prepayment review and (2) require preauthorization and practice guidelines that may limit or discount payment for dental procedures; most expensive form of insurance
Direct reimbursement	Employers	Not a true insurance plan; self-funded plan that reimburses patients according to dollars spent on dental care, not type of treatment received; employers pay employees a percentage of actual treatments received, saving the cost of the middleman, the insurance plan administrator; allows freedom of choice and autonomy of decision making about treatment; includes an annual limit on the amount the employer sets aside to reimburse each employee; ADA's preferred method of financing dental treatment
Managed Care		
Preferred provider organization (PPO)	Health service and dental service corporations (not for profit), commercial insurance companies (for profit)	Dentist contracts with insurer to provide care at lower-than-average fees; insurer selectively directs patients to specific providers (preferred providers); patient can visit a dentist outside of the PPO and pay the difference (amount above the discounted fee); includes co-insurance, deductible, and maximum coverage; insurance company reimburses patient or dentist accepts payment directly from insurance company; less costly than traditional indemnity plan; variation is an exclusive provider organization (EPO), also known as exclusive provider arrangement (EPA), that does not cover out-of-network care
Dental health maintenance organization (HMO) (prepaid plan)	Health service and dental service corporations; commercial insurance companies; prepaid, large group practices	Beneficiaries must use one dentist or facility (plan does not pay if they go outside HMO); includes co-payment and possibly maximums but no deductibles; uses capitation; usually lowest-cost program; uncommon for dental benefits; dentists frequently limit number of HMO patients to offset loss of income; a variation is the point-of-service (POS) plans that are similar except that the beneficiary may seek care out of network
Dental discount plan	Employers, provider organizations; organization of corporate clinics	Providers join the plan by paying a fee and agreeing to offer discounted fees, then are listed as a member provider (way of recruiting patients); patients join the plan by paying a fee, receive a list of providers who are on the plan and a card to present to the member provider, and pay deeply discounted fees to member providers; not "true" insurance; no deductibles, no annual limits, no co-payments, no paperwork for the client or dentist for reimbursement, and no pre-qualifications
Individual practice association (IPA)	Association of independent dental providers	More of a business arrangement than a dental benefits plan; organization contracts with independent dentists to provide services to HMO patients for discounted fees or through capitation arrangement

Data from American Dental Association: The advantages of offering a dental benefits plan, 2014. http://www.ada.org/en/public-programs/dental-benefit-information-for-employers/insurance-and-financing.

c. Providers receive compensation in a predetermined form, such as fixed amount per program member or fixed amount per service

d. Results from increased costs of health care, the need to control costs, and the need to improve access to care for a large segment of the population without traditional dental insurance (benefits)

e. Views on managed care vary

(1) Managed dental care has not yet evolved to the extent of managed medical care; dental professional groups have expressed concern about closed-panel third-party approaches because clients are denied freedom of choice of dentists[24]

(2) An argument against the closed-panel approach relates to the quality of care provided, although charges of poor quality have not been substantiated

(3) Publically funded insurance is often administered through managed care programs (Table 20-21)

(4) Managed care is expected to increase because of the need to control the cost of dental care nationwide and greater governmental involvement in financing dental care; dental hygienists may contribute significantly in a managed care model because of the emphasis on prevention and on cost savings

Providers of Dental Benefits Plans

A. The variety of providers of dental benefits plans adds to the complexity of the pluralistic system of payment for dental care in the United States

B. The providers that offer different types of plans are explained in Table 20-21

Public Financing of Dental Care

A. Primarily addresses the needs of poor persons
  1. The percentage of persons living in poverty in 2013 was 14.5%, down slightly for the first time in 7 years; the poverty rate of children under age 18 years is considerably higher than other age groups; there is less poverty among the non-Hispanic white population, and rates vary by geographic region and metropolitan status[25]
  2. The significance of poverty rates in the population is the that low-SES groups experience a greater number of factors that are associated with poor health (determinants of health) and generally have poorer oral health status
B. Problems with public financing
  1. Fragmented; difficult to find and utilize resources
  2. Medicaid has been plagued by changing eligibility requirements, limitation of services, low allowable fees paid, delays in payment for services, and dentists' refusal to treat Medicaid clients
  3. Poor enrollment of dentists as providers—reasons given include low reimbursement rates, missed appointments by Medicaid clients, difficult treatment issues, too much bureaucratic paperwork, reluctance to have patients from low-SES groups in the reception room with other patients, and preference to provide charity care rather than Medicaid services

4. Many children who qualify are not enrolled in Medicaid/CHIP
5. Large numbers of additional adults and children will be insured with pubic insurance as a result of the ACA;[26] overall quality of care provided may be affected by the limitations of public insurance and the increased burden placed on providers accepting publically funded insurance programs
C. Strategies to address problems with public financing
  1. Recent increases in the services allowed and fees reimbursed by Medicaid
  2. Recent public health department initiatives to increase the number of Medicaid/CHIP dental providers
  3. Development of midlevel providers to make available a workforce who can provide care at a lower cost to society
D. Medicaid/CHIP—most public expenditures for dental care are from Medicaid or CHIP (Table 20-22)
  1. In 2013, more than 28 million children were enrolled in Medicaid and 5.7 million in CHIP, representing a reduction in the rate of uninsured children; even so, over 7 million children remain uninsured[27]
  2. The number of Medicaid recipients is expected to grow as a result of the ACA;[27] access to dental coverage for Medicaid-eligible adults is expected to decline because

TABLE 20-22 Public Funding of Oral Health Programs

Program	Description
Reimbursement to Providers for Services Provided	
Medicaid	Title XIX amendment of the Social Security Act passed in 1965; federal insurance program to provide access to health care to low-income and other special groups, for example, children of lawfully admitted immigrants, newborn children without insurance, children under Child Protective Services, and disabled individuals; funded via a partnership of federal and state governments; administered by the state; eligibility, designated expenditures, and authorized services vary from state to state
	Dental care is only mandatory for persons under 21 years of age; all states must provide oral health care services to Medicaid-eligible children as specified by the Early and Periodic Screening, Diagnosis, and Treatment (EPSDT) program (medical, dental, and vision care are mandatory); providers must enroll; patients must be enrolled in Medicaid and can only seek care from Medicaid providers; source of funding for local philanthropic, educational, and community programs that bill Medicaid for services provided to Medicaid beneficiaries
Children's Health Insurance Program (CHIP)	Joint federal-state program created by the Social Security Act in 1997, giving each state permission to offer health insurance to children up to age 19 from families with incomes above Medicaid level but too low to afford health insurance (up to 200% to 250% of federal poverty level); all states participate; state can establish the CHIP program as an extension of the Medicaid program or as a separate state program; jointly funded by state and federal governments; state administers program and determines eligibility requirements and available services; benefits must be at least equivalent to those provided under Medicaid; program varies from state to state
	Covers dental as well as medical care; nearly all states provide CHIP coverage for dental benefits; co-payments and co-insurance for certain treatments vary from state to state; patients must be enrolled in CHIP and use a CHIP provider
Medicare	Title XVIII amendment of the Social Security Act passed in 1965; federal insurance program to pay medical bills for insured persons age 65 years and older and certain disabled individuals; administered by the Centers for Medicare and Medicaid Services (CMS); no income limitations
	Dental care coverage is limited to services that have medical implications
Publicly Funded Programs	
Indian Health Service (IHS)	Federal funding of hospitals and clinics on reservations and in urban areas that serve Native Americans and Alaska Natives who are members of federally recognized tribes; IHS clinics are staffed by PHS officers; also pays for contracted care through private dental offices
Public Health Service (PHS)	

(Continued)

TABLE 20-22	Public Funding of Oral Health Programs—cont'd
Program	**Description**
	Federal funding of PHS officers who provide dental care for U.S. Coast Guard, federal prisons, and IHS facilities as well as selective defined groups such as migrant and seasonal farmworkers and homeless persons
Community Health Center Fund	Federal funding established by the Affordable Care Act (ACA) for expansion of local community-based health centers and clinics, to be used in combination with state funding
School-Based Health Center Capital (SBHCC) Program	Federal funding established by the ACA for expansion of school-based health centers and clinics, to be used in combination with state funding
Maternal and Child Health Services	Federal funding through the states for prenatal care for women and primary and preventive care for children; health and supportive services for special needs children; funding comes to the state via *block grants*
Women, Infants and Children (WIC) program	Federal funding of supplementation of food, health care referrals, and nutritional education for low-income pregnant women, mothers of infants and young children, and infants and children at nutritional risk; administered through the Department of Agriculture
Head Start program	Federal funding of oral health screening, oral hygiene activities, and weekly oral health curricula for children in Head Start, which is the federal preschool child development program administered by the Administration for Children and Families
Civilian Health and Medical Program of the Uniformed Services (CHAMPUS)	Health care services for military personnel and dependents; also provides a voluntary dental benefits program; requires participants to pay part of premiums
Crippled Children's Program	Federal and state funding of treatments for children with craniofacial deformities, cleft lip and palate, and certain other conditions
Ryan White Comprehensive AIDS Resources Emergency Act	Health professional education related to acquired immunodeficiency syndrome (AIDS)
Other federal governmental agencies	Responsible for the provision of dental services and oral health education to specific population groups, such as military personnel and their dependents, disadvantaged groups, and incarcerated persons; staffed by PHS officers; examples are Department of Defense (DoD); Department of Veterans Affairs (VA); Department of Justice, Bureau of Prisons (BoP); DHHS Health Resources and Services Administration (HRSA)
State programs	Vary from state to state; use state funds to provide care to particular populations; primarily provide programs to support health education and health promotion at state and local levels through health departments; treatment programs are provided for state institutions such as state prisons and residential facilities for intellectually challenged individuals
Other Funding of Community-Based Programs	
"Faith"-based programs	Clinics and school dental programs operated by churches and other faith-based institutions
Community clinics	Funded by local foundations, civic organizations, and community resources (e.g., United Way)
Programs operated by organized dental hygiene and dentistry	Head Start varnish programs and school- and community-based sealant programs (ADHA constituents and components); Give Kids a Smile (free dental care events sponsored by the ADA), Donated Dental Services (direct dental care), Bridge (preventive education services and screening by hygienists in facilities for developmentally challenged individuals), and House Calls (homebound dental care) conducted by the National Foundation of Dentistry for the Handicapped, an affiliate of the ADA

only about half of states offer dental benefits to adults, and capacity will be compromised by the increase in demand to serve children

3. Many children enrolled in the Medicaid/CHIP program do not receive dental services, which is related to the need to improve health literacy

E. Federal and state programs (Table 20-22)

F. Local programs
1. Funded through a variety of sources, including local health department funds; federally funded programs; national, state, and local foundations; faith-based organizations; and other local sources of funding (Table 20-22)
2. Collaboration must occur among public health agencies, nongovernmental organizations (NGOs), dental and dental hygiene associations and educational programs, community agencies, and volunteer groups to fund local community oral health care programs

G. Involvement of the federal government in health care financing has increased steadily, especially since 1965

1. Dental care has continued to be a small part, at best
2. Demand for services for the low-income population has increased at a time when available services are declining
3. The emergence of alternative health care plans as a result of the ACA provide future promise of more public funding of dental care
4. It is expected that future oral health care financing will continue the current varied and complex financing systems and pubic coverage for a large proportion of the population, primarily poor persons

NEED FOR, DEMAND FOR, AND UTILIZATION OF DENTAL SERVICES

A. Definition of terms (Table 20-23)

B. Current dental care utilization
1. Measured as the proportion of persons who visit a health care provider during a given year

TABLE 20-23 Terminology Related to Utilization

Term	Definition/Description
Demand	Volume and types of health care services that an individual or population desires to consume at some price level; measured by self-report surveys *Effective demand*—desire for care and ability to obtain care (client or community has access to care) *Potential demand*—desire for care and inability to obtain care (client or community lacks access to care)
Need	*Normative need*—usually professional judgment about the amount and types of health care services or medical care services required by an individual or community to attain or maintain some standard level of health; normative need defined as professionally determined; expressed in terms of a population or individual; includes specific needs identified through individual or community-based clinical assessment procedures *Perceived need* or *felt need*—defined as determined by the client or the community; can differ from normative need; clinically, perceived need can be referred to as a chief concern; measured with self-report surveys and interviews; health education is required to help a client or community to adjust perceived need to match normative need
Utilization	Proportion of the population who use dental services over a period; volume and types of services actually consumed; typically measured by dental attendance rates during the year

2. Less than half of the population visit the dental office each year, and this rate has remained relatively unchanged in the past decade (see Table 20-2)
3. Two *Healthy People 2020* objectives address the goal to increase utilization:
   a. Increase the use of the oral health care system by persons age 2 years and older
   b. Increase the receipt of preventive dental services by low-income children and adolescents
C. Dental public health officials support the inclusion of an oral health indicator to increase the proportion of children, adolescents, and adults who use the oral health care system each year[28]
D. Emergency department use as a safety net for preventable dental conditions has increased and is costly to hospitals and society[29]
E. Patterns of dental care utilization in this decade
   1. Gender—females continue to have more dental visits than males[3]
   2. Age—higher utilization in children than adults and older adults; slight increase in utilization for children and older adults and a decrease in adults[30]
   3. Race and ethnicity—utilization varies for racial and ethnic groups, mostly as a function of SES and culture; overall utilization is highest for the non-Hispanic white population, but disparities are less for utilization of preventive dental services by low-income children and adolescents, who are more likely to have dental benefits than other age groups[3]

   a. Culture and SES are associated with health literacy, which affects health decisions
   b. Hispanic Americans and African Americans have lower utilization rates than non-Hispanic whites[3]
   c. Native Americans residing on reservations receive care primarily through the IHS; traditionally, utilization has not been high but varies by location
4. Geographic location—utilization of dental care is lower in rural communities (both farm and nonfarm) than urban areas; suburban populations are the most frequent users
5. Region—utilization rates differ among states

Factors That Influence Dental Care Utilization and Oral Health Behaviors

A. Increase in public awareness of health and oral health, influenced by:
   1. New technologies such as telehealth, bioinformatics, and virtual reality
   2. Databases specifying the human, animal, and microbial genomes
   3. Strong emphasis on evidence-informed approaches to health care delivery
B. A person's level of adopting the wellness paradigm versus the health-disease paradigm
C. Compliance with recommendations varies as a result of:
   1. Beliefs—trust placed in a provider, health custom, or system of health care because of acceptance that something is true; personal or cultural beliefs about illness and wellness may then influence health behaviors
   2. Attitudes—patterns of mental views based on judgments of likes and dislikes (about health care systems, providers, or utilization); established because of prior experience
   3. Values—the importance or worth placed on health care and health practices; beliefs, attitudes, and values are all interrelated and affect each other; although difficult, beliefs, attitudes, and values related to oral health care and health practices can be changed over time through development of rapport, communication, persuasion, education, and new experiences
D. Access to dental insurance benefits—those with benefits are more likely to utilize care, and the type of dental benefits is associated with utilization
   1. More than one third of the U.S. population do not have dental benefits;[29] coverage varies by age: more than twice as many children have coverage than adults, and almost twice as many adults have coverage than older adults;[31] this represents an increase in coverage for children, a decrease for adults, and the same coverage for older adults compared to 10 years earlier[31]
   2. Of those who have dental benefits, a greater percentage have private dental coverage (almost 40% more children, five times more adults, and one and one-half times more older adults) compared to public insurance (e.g., Medicaid, CHIP); the number of children with public insurance has increased and is expected to continue to increase because of the ACA[31]

3. Utilization rates vary according to the type of insurance; rates are almost twice as high for those with private insurance compared to those with no insurance; those who have public insurance have higher utilization than those with no insurance but considerably lower use than those with private insurance[30]
4. Utilization for preventive visits increased in children over the last decade because of an increase in the number of children enrolled in Medicaid/CHIP[32]
5. Because the majority of dental benefits are private, a higher rate of coverage is associated with higher income levels[29]
6. Dental insurance coverage influences the types of services used; concerns exist about insurance companies and government agencies dictating the care provided based on guidelines for payment

E. Barriers to dental care utilization—factors that block or prevent access or ability to seek care or adopt healthy behaviors, thus reducing dental utilization (i.e., low oral health literacy); must be addressed to increase utilization within a population
1. Barriers not related to cost
   a. Lack of perceived need
   b. Access to care difficult or impossible
   c. Availability of providers (e.g., office hours, distribution of personnel)
   d. Types of services needed not being available because of practitioners' lack of skill or interest
   e. Geographic isolation
   f. Nonambulatory status (e.g., homebound or institutionalized)
   g. Lack of public transportation
   h. Values, attitudes, and beliefs
   i. Unfavorable view of dental personnel—lack of cultural sensitivity
2. Cost-related barriers
   a. Services not affordable
   b. Dental insurance benefits issues
      (1) Coverage limited or not available (see previous discussion on access)
      (2) Continuing lack of providers available to individuals with Medicaid/CHIP coverage[29]
      (3) A narrow insurance company definition of "medically necessary dental care" that sets limits on oral health care services available to many insured clients, including Medical Assistance in many states and especially older adults with Medicare coverage
   c. Lost wages resulting from time away from work; more critical than the perceived need for services
3. Social and psychological barriers
   a. Low value placed on dental care and facial appearance related to the oral cavity
   b. Unpleasant prior experience resulting in anxiety
   c. Emotional factors such as fear of dental care
4. Cultural barriers
   a. Language—client unable to find a provider who speaks his or her language or a qualified interpreter

b. History and tradition—no importance given to dental care in the client's culture
   c. Basic cultural beliefs about general and oral health, illness, disease, and health care model
   d. Failure to understand that a missed appointment can be costly and disruptive
   e. Difficulty in understanding the recommendations for dental care or dietary changes
   f. Few oral health care providers from minority groups—current emphasis of the dental profession is to increase diversity in the profession to enhance reaching minority population groups[33]

F. Most powerful predictors of dental care utilization are gender, SES (income and education), dentate status, availability of dental benefits, and overall economy

Shifts in Dental Care Utilization Patterns

A. Reported increase in examinations, preventive services, extractions, implants, and esthetic dentistry and slight decline in dentures
1. Resulting partially from the changing demographics of the population; persons over age 65 are the fastest-growing segment of the U.S. population and have higher tooth retention rates, resulting in their increased utilization of dental services; dentate individuals are more likely than edentulous individuals to visit the dentist
2. Each generation demands a different variety of services; older populations focus on restoration, periodontal treatment, prosthetics, and control and treatment of root caries; middle-age persons need some restorative and periodontal services or orthodontic services; children need more primary prevention and orthodontic services

B. Prevention
1. General interest in prevention has caused an increase in preventive dentistry services
2. The success of preventive interventions affects the types of future services required

C. The American society's interest in appearance and esthetics influences demand for restorative options, cosmetic dentistry, orthodontics, periodontal services, and dental implants

D. Increases in Medicaid/CHIP coverage for children have impacted the shift of services

E. Increased utilization is expected as a result of the ACA
1. Dental coverage is being offered through subsidized health insurance as a result of the ACA; expected to provide dental benefits for 3 million children and nearly 18 million adults
2. Parents who want dental coverage for their children can buy dental insurance–only policies
3. Young adults can stay on their parents' health insurance, which usually includes dental coverage, through age 26
4. Increase in public dental benefits resulting from the ACA will not necessarily bring about a proportional increase in dental utilization[30]

F. Increase in utilization and reduction of disparities in oral health care services require a multi-pronged approach
1. This includes oral health literacy of the population, improved access to care for underserved populations,

increased demand for preventive oral health care, and reduction of barriers to oral health care

2. Various interventions are needed that address all the core functions of public health, assessment, policy development, and assurance, using evidence-based approaches to health education, health promotion, and provision of services

ORAL HEALTH CARE CHALLENGES AFFECTING COMMUNITY ORAL HEALTH PRACTICE

A. Continuing significant burden of oral diseases and disorders in the U.S. population in the twenty-first century
1. Striking disparities in dental diseases and conditions, depending on income levels; unprecedented changes in demography and patterns of diseases and disorders
2. Effect of unintentional injuries on craniofacial tissues
3. Increases in systemic conditions that are associated with oral diseases and that compromise oral health
4. Prevalence of tobacco-related oral diseases beginning in adolescence
5. Increased prevalence of oral cancer among young adults associated with more common sexual practices in adolescents and young adults
6. An increase in caries prevalence and rates of untreated caries in preschool-age children over the last decade
7. Significant loss of school and work hours each year because of dental-related illnesses
8. Progressive and cumulative nature of oral diseases that become more complex over time

B. Trends in oral health care delivery
1. Continuing trend of low dental attendance, although utilization increases each year
2. Significant numbers of uninsured, low-SES children
3. Emphasis on increasing access to care for underserved population to decrease oral health disparities
4. Changes in health care financing, including greater involvement of public financing
5. Increase in the cost of oral health care
6. Inability of Medicaid and CHIP to fill the gaps in the provision of dental care to poor children (fewer than 50% of children covered by Medicaid and CHIP receive dental care)
7. Potential for increased utilization because of the aging population, combined with changes in oral disease patterns and a decline in total tooth loss in older adults
8. Continuing low rates of detecting oral cancer at early stages despite an increase in the reported rates of annual examinations for oral cancer
9. Broadening treatment options due to an emphasis on esthetics, adult orthodontics, and dental implants
10. Changes in science, technology, and therapeutics; availability of new biomaterials and biotechnology
11. Access to multiple information systems, including the Internet, computer-assisted technology, telehealth care, and distance education technology

12. Access to genetic information that will influence assessment of risk factors and care planning
13. A philosophy of "best practices," that is, determining which treatment will work for which clients and under what circumstances; an evidence-informed approach to dental and dental hygiene care based on risk assessment
14. Paradigm shift to a treatment model that focuses on nonsurgical, noninvasive, biologic, and pharmacologic interventions that are guided by genetics and risk assessment, requiring a shift in oral health care education, teaching, and outcome methodologies and a greater focus on lifelong learning for oral health care personnel
15. Greater emphasis on the use of validated health education, health promotion, and organizational theories for the individual and community-based focus of oral health education and promotion for preventive strategies
16. Coordination and collaboration of dental care and medical care
17. Greater orientation of the current society in general on oral disease prevention
18. A need to focus on making those who do not seek care aware of available dental care services, as well as implementing health promotion strategies to change their oral health behaviors
19. A need to focus on the control and prevention of early childhood caries, prevention of periodontal disease, control of tobacco use by young people, and early detection of oral cancer
20. An increase in the complexity of the oral health care delivery system because of the numerous, multifaceted arrangements for delivering services and financing care, the changes in supply and distribution of provider personnel, and the varying state laws regarding scope of practice for oral health practitioners and midlevel dental personnel

C. Redirected focus of dental personnel
1. Identify individuals currently not seeking care; for example, special population groups and low-income and minority individuals
2. Increase access to and availability of care; for example, vary office hours, offer care in nontraditional settings, improve payment and financing mechanisms, and continue to explore the use of midlevel practitioners
3. Develop creative solutions to meet increasing demands for dental care personnel during a period of natural retirement of an older dental profession, decreasing numbers of dentists, increasing numbers and increased educational levels of dental hygienists, and emergence of midlevel oral health care practitioners
4. Educate the public with an evidence-based focus on periodontal disease, caries, oral cancer, tobacco cessation, systemic health–oral health connection, and preventive interventions
5. Encourage professional lifelong learning to address current scientific understanding of oral diseases, the changing oral health care needs of the population, cultural competence and sensitivity, and technologies to assess and treat populations

6. Develop an understanding within the oral health professions about the demographic and ethnic changes in the population; cultivate cultural sensitivity and competence, and apply strategies to improve health literacy

7. Recognize dentistry's changing role, with an emphasis on diagnostic skills and evaluation

8. Accept dental hygienists' changing role as more autonomous, interdependent practitioners and as collaborators with other members of the oral health care team as well as interdisciplinary health care teams

9. Employ appropriate oral health care personnel; recognize the capabilities of all team members to increase access to care, and be aware that the current litigious society demands skilled practitioners and high-quality services

10. Make changes in oral health care delivery and oral health promotion that address the current status of oral health and recommendations made by relevant national agency reports

11. Incorporate scientific evidence into all aspects of oral health care practice

12. Use innovative collaborations and partnerships to promote oral health and solve oral health problems

13. Focus on local community needs

14. Develop multiple skills to function in many roles, with multidisciplinary approaches, and in diverse care delivery environments

D. Recommendations to reduce oral health and oral health care disparities

1. Through research, identify biomarkers that will facilitate early detection and diagnosis of disease

2. Conduct epidemiologic studies of populations to establish baselines for the incidence and prevalence of specific oral health problems and to assist in tracking, reducing, or eliminating identified health disparities

3. Conduct randomized controlled clinical trials to provide an evidence base for the effective prevention and management of health disparities

4. Carry out population-based research to understand the basis of health disparities

5. Place a high priority on efforts to reduce widespread disparities in oral health status and access to care

6. Increase measures to ensure oral health and access to care for children by correcting inadequate government policies, such as increasing Medicaid funding, implementing school sealant and fluoride varnish programs, fluoridating water supplies, and protecting the current status of fluoridated water supplies

7. Emphasize research and community oral health promotion programs that will result in decreasing incidence and prevalence rates of oral diseases and conditions for the entire population, as well as special emphasis on populations at high risk for these conditions

8. Restructure oral health care professional education programs to meet the critical requirement of preparing a workforce that is qualified in public health principles and practice

9. Focus on serving all Americans, regardless of SES, gender, and ethnic or racial group representation, in the recruitment of students and faculty, design and implementation of curricula, conduct of research, provision of services, and participation in community outreach

ETHICAL AND LEGAL ISSUES

See Box 20-13.

BOX 20-13 Ethical/Legal Issues Related to Community Oral Health*

General Ethical Issues
- Application to community as the "client"
- Weighing the needs of the individual and the community
- Application of principles of social justice, common good, human dignity, confidentiality, informed consent, nonmaleficence, beneficence, integrity and totality, competence and capacity, autonomy, and surrogacy to community oral health practice
- Encompassing professionalism, personal and professional ethics, and the role of the profession and the educational system in the context of the greater society

Ethical Practices in Action
- Focus by educational institutions to develop skilled, ethically and socially sensitive graduates committed to their professional obligation to community education and service
- Development and implementation of community-based models of education and service that may include alumni participation, local professional society participation, or both

- Commitment of educational institutions to incorporate community outreach activities as part of the professional curriculum; emphasis on a multidisciplinary approach with other health care students and providers
- Reinforcement of a lifelong commitment to the professional codes of ethics (ADHA, ADA) that suggest an ethical obligation to community oral health and well-being
- Development of strategies to develop cultural and linguistic competence through lifelong learning
- Expansion of minority representation in the profession
- Education of students about the career opportunities in federal, state, and local public health agencies and in other community organizations that provide oral health care services to various population groups (e.g., IHS, VA, local hospitals)
- Developing mechanisms that encourage and support a perspective of social responsibility
- Identification and development of mechanisms, such as scholarships and pay-back programs, to encourage minority and other health care providers to serve underserved populations

BOX 20-13   Ethical/Legal Issues Related to Community Oral Health—cont'd

- Increasing knowledge and awareness of community oral health issues, best practices, skills, and resources by obtaining information from journals, conferences, seminars, websites, and other means
- Promotion of evidence-informed decision making in relation to all aspects of community oral health practice, including scientific bases for disease control and prevention, as well as application of tested theories of organization, health promotion, and health education
- Setting standards of ethical conduct that reflects social responsibility to the community through oral health promotion, education, and practice
- Focusing of individual practitioners on social responsibility in their dental hygiene practice
- Serving on advisory boards to community oral health programs
- Volunteering in community service activities sponsored by local professional societies, educational institutions, and community organizations

- Participating in, encouraging the development of, and organizing community outreach events through private offices of employment
- Commitment to lifelong learning and evidence-based practice in relation to community oral health practice as well as clinical practice
- Providing leadership in the solution of local public health problems to improve the oral health of the local community

Legal Issues
- Effect of varying state laws related to scope of practice and supervision on the ability of various personnel to participate fully in community programs
- Emerging midlevel practitioners models of practice in some states; resulting differences among states in the ability to address access-to-care issues within the state and on a national level

*Refer to Chapter 22 for discussion of ethical principles.

Website Information and Resources

Source	Website Address	Description
American Dental Hygienists Association	http://adha.org	Data on the profession; information about careers in public health, midlevel providers, and advocacy
Association of State and Territorial Dental Directors	http://www.astdd.org	Access to state and territorial public health agencies of the United States, U.S. territories, and the District of Columbia; engaged in legislative, scientific, educational, and programmatic issues and activities on behalf of public health; provides best practices for current, effective community oral health programming
HealthyPeople.gov	http://www.healthypeople.gov/2020/topicsobjectives2020/overview.aspx?topicid=32	*Healthy People 2020* oral health objectives; overview of history and development, objectives, baseline measures, target outcomes, suggested interventions and resources, and methods to measure outcomes
National Maternal and Child Oral Health Resource Center	http://www.mchoralhealth.org/	A variety of resources to develop community oral health programs for young children, including publications, "how-to" guides, toolboxes, Head Start information, and grants
National Institute of Dental and Craniofacial Research	http://www.nidcr.nih.gov/	Variety of resources for information useful in community programming; includes links to *Oral Health in America: a Report of the Surgeon General*, *A National Call to Action to Promote Oral Health*, and *Healthy People 2020* objectives (history and development, objectives, baseline measures, target outcomes, suggestions for interventions and resources, methods to measure outcomes)

REFERENCES

1. National Cancer Institute: *Surveillance, epidemiology, and end results (SEER) program: SEER stat fact sheets: oral cavity and pharynx cancer*, 2011: http://seer.cancer.gov/statfacts/html/oralcav.html. Accessed October 1, 2014.

2. Centers for Disease Control and Prevention: *Birth defects*, August 14, 2012: http://www.cdc.gov/ncbddd/birthdefects/features/craniofacialdefects.html. Accessed October 2, 2014.

3. National Center for Health Statistics: *Healthy people 2010 final review: overview and selected findings*, PHS Pub No 2012-1038, Hyattsville, Md, 2012, NCHS. http://www.cdc.gov/nchs/data/hpdata2010/hp2010_final_review.pdf. Accessed October 1, 2014.

4. Agarwal MSS, Chopra SS, Jayan B, Verma MM: Epidemiology in orthodontics- a literature review, *Orthod Cyber J* September 2013. http://orthocj.com/2013/09/epidemiology-in-orthodontics-a-literature-review/. Accessed October 1, 2014.

5. Perheentupa U: *Epidemiology management and outcome of facial injuries, master's thesis*, Finland, 2014, University of Turku. http://www.doria.fi/bitstream/handle/10024/96674/Annales D1118Perheentupa.pdf?sequence=2. Accessed October 2, 2014.

6. American Academy of Pediatric Dentistry: Policy on prevention of sports-related orofacial injuries, *Oral Health Policies Reference Manual* 35(6):67–71, 2013: http://www.aapd.org/media/Policies_Guidelines/P_Sports.pdf. Accessed October 2, 2014.

7. National Institute of Dental and Craniofacial Research: *TMJ (temporomandibular joint and muscle disorders)*, July 10, 2014: http://www.nidcr.nih.gov/oralhealth/topics/tmj/. Accessed October 2, 2014.

8. Myers ML: New survey shows U.S. youth smoking rates fell to record low in 2013, June 12, 2014: *Campaign for Tobacco-Free Kids* (http://www.tobaccofreekids.org/press_releases/post/2014_06_12_cdc. Accessed October 10, 2014.

9. Valachovic RW: Current demographics and future trends of the dentist workforce, *The U.S. Oral Health Workforce in the Coming Decade*, February 9, 2009, Institute of Medicine Workshop. http://www.iom.edu/~/media/Files/Activity%20Files/Workforce/oralhealthworkforce/2009-Feb-09/1%20-%20Valachovic.ashx. Accessed October 4, 2014.

10. Health Resources and Services Administration: *Shortage designation: health professional shortage areas & medically underserved areas/populations*, June 19, 2014: http://www.hrsa.gov/shortage/index.html. Accessed October 7, 2014.

11. Health Resources and Services Administration: *Oral health workforce*: http://www.hrsa.gov/publichealth/clinical/oralhealth/workforce.html. Accessed October 4, 2014.

12. American Dental Education Association: *U.S. dental school applicants and enrollees, 2010 entering class (ADEA AADSAS application cycle 2010-11)*, 2012. file:///C:/Users/CHRIST~1/AppData/Local/Temp/ADEADentalSchoolAppEnrollees2010ClassExecSummaryTables.pdf. Accessed October 7, 2014.

13. Commission on Dental Accreditation: *DDS/DMD programs*, 2014: http://www.ada.org/en/coda/find-a-program/search-dental-programs/dds-dmd-programs. Accessed October 4, 2014.

14. Anderson EL: *Expansion in dental education: new schools*, 2011: http://www.dentalboards.org/PDFS/2011MidYearPresentations.pdf. Accessed October 4, 2014.

15. Bureau of Labor Statistics: *Occupational handbook: dental hygienists*, January 8, 2014: http://www.bls.gov/ooh/healthcare/dental-hygienists.htm#tab-6. Accessed October 5, 2014.

16. American Dental Hygienists Association: *Facts about the dental hygiene workforce in the United States*, 2013: http://www.adha.org/resources-docs/75118_Facts_About_the_Dental_Hygiene_Workforce.pdf. Accessed October 4, 2014.

17. American Dental Hygienists Association: *Dental hygiene education: curricula, program, enrollment and graduate information*, July 9, 2014: http://www.adha.org/sites/default/files/72611_Dental_Hygiene_Education_Fact_Sheet_0.pdf. Accessed October 4, 2014.

18. Pew Charitable Trusts: *Pew commends Maine for authorizing dental hygiene therapists*, April 29, 2014: http://www.pewtrusts.org/en/about/news-room/press-releases/2014/04/29/pew-commends-maine-for-authorizing-dental-hygiene-therapists. Accessed October 4, 2014.

19. American Dental Hygienists Association: *Direct access states*, June 2014: https://www.adha.org/resources-docs/7513_Direct_Access_to_Care_from_DH.pdf. Accessed October 7, 2014.

20. American Dental Hygienists Association: *The benefits of dental hygiene-based oral health provider models*, July 2014: http://www.adha.org/resources-docs/75112_Hygiene_Based_Workforce_Models.pdf. Accessed October 2, 2014.

21. Andrews A: Health law offers dental coverage guarantee for some children, *Kaiser health news*, January 14, 2013. http://www.kaiserhealthnews.org/features/insuring-your-health/2013/011513-michelle-andrews-on-kids-dental-care-coverage.aspx. Accessed October 5, 2014.

22. Centers for Medicaid and Medicare Services: *National health expenditures 2012 highlights*: https://www.cms.gov/Research-Statistics-Data-and-Systems/Statistics-Trends-and-Reports/NationalHealthExpendData/downloads/highlights.pdf. Accessed October 4, 2014.

23. Centers for Medicaid and Medicare Services: *National health expenditure projections 2012-2022 forecast summary*: http://www.cms.gov/Research-Statistics-Data-and-Systems-Statistics-Trends-and-Reports/NationalHealthExpendData/downloads/proj2012.pdf. Accessed October 7, 2014.

24. American Dental Association: *The advantages of offering a dental benefits plan*: http://www.ada.org/en/public-programs/dental-benefit-information-for-employers/insurance-and-financing. Accessed October 5, 2014.

25. US Census Bureau: Poverty: 2003 highlights. https://www.census.gov/hhes/www/poverty/about/overview/. Accessed October 7, 2014.

26. Helms AD: Putting teeth in health reform, *Kaiser health news*, September 2, 2014. http://www.kaiserhealthnews.org/stories/2014/september/02/putting-teeth-in-health-reform.aspx?referrer=search. Accessed October 5, 2014.

27. Rudowitz R, Artiga S, Arguello R: Children's health coverage: medicaid, CHIP and the ACA, *The Kaiser family foundation*, March 26, 2014. http://kff.org/health-reform/issue-brief/childrens-health-coverage-medicaid-chip-and-the-aca/. Accessed October 7, 2014.

28. Association of State and Territorial Dental Directors: *Healthy people 2020 oral health leading health indicator policy statement*, March 17, 2014: http://www.astdd.org/docs/hp-2020-oral-health-leading-health-indicator-march-17-2014.pdf. Accessed October 4, 2014.

29. US Senate Committee on Health: *Education, labor & pensions, subcommittee on primary health and aging (Bernard Sanders, Chairman): dental crisis in America: the need to expand access*, February 29, 2012: http://www.sanders.senate.gov/imo/media/doc/DENTALCRISIS.REPORT.pdf. Accessed October 5, 2014.

30. Nasseh K, Vujicic M: *Dental care utilization continues to decline among working-age adults, increases among the elderly, stable among children*, October 2013, American Dental Association, Health Policy Institute. http://www.ada.org/~/media/ADA/Science%20and%20Research/HPI/Files/HPIBrief_1013_2.ashx. Accessed October 5, 2014.

31. Vujicic M, Goodell S, Nasseh K: *Dental benefits to expand for children, likely decrease for adults in coming years*, April 2013, American Dental Association Health Policy Institute Research Brief. http://www.ada.org/~/media/ADA/Science%20and%20Research/HPI/Files/HPIBrief_0413_1.ashx. Accessed October 6, 2014.

32. US Government Accountability Office: *Dental coverage: information on coverage, payments, and fee variation*, September 6, 2013: http://www.gao.gov/products/gao-13-754. Accessed October 6, 2013.

33. American Dental Education Association: Need for diversity, *Dentistry* 101:2015: http://www.adea.org/GoDental/Dentistry_101/Need_for_diversity.aspx. Accessed April 15, 2015.

SUGGESTED READINGS

Beatty CF: *Community oral health practice for the dental hygienist*, ed 4, St Louis, 2017, Elsevier Saunders.

Gagliardi L: *Dental health education lesson planning and implementation*, ed 2, Long Grove, Ill, 2014, Waveland Press.

Institute of Medicine: *Advancing oral health in America*, Washington, DC, 2011, National Academies Press. http://www.iom.edu/Reports/2011/Advancing-Oral-Health-in-America.aspx.

Institute of Medicine: *Improving access to oral health care for vulnerable and underserved populations*, Washington, DC, 2011, National Academies Press. http://iom.edu/Reports/2011/Improving-Access-to-Oral-Health-Care-for-Vulnerable-and-Underserved-Populations.aspx.

Lamoreux D: Caries management: fluoride and nonfluoride caries-preventive agents. In Darby ML, Walsh MM, editors: *Dental hygiene theory and practice*, ed 7, St Louis, 2015, Elsevier Saunders.

Nathe CN: *Dental public health and research,* ed 4, Upper Saddle River, NJ, 2015, Pearson.

National Maternal and Child Oral Health Resource Center: A guide for developing and enhancing community oral health programs. http://www.aacdp.com/guide/.

US Department of Health and Human Services: *Oral health in America: a report of the surgeon general,* Rockville, Md, 2000, DHHS. http://www.nidcr.nih.gov/DataStatistics/SurgeonGeneral/.

US Department of Health and Human Services: *A national call to action to promote oral health,* NIH Pub No 03-5303, Rockville, Md, Spring 2003, DHHS, Public Health Service, National Institutes of Health, National Institute of Dental and Craniofacial Research. http://www.nidcr.nih.gov/DataStatistics/SurgeonGeneral/.

CHAPTER 20 REVIEW QUESTIONS

Answers and rationales to review questions are available on this text's accompanying Evolve site. See inside front cover for details.

evolve

TESTLET A

You have been employed as a public health dental hygienist in a local health department to provide educational presentations for the participants in the WIC program in a nonfluoridated community. The natural fluoride (F) concentration of the community water supply is 0.3 ppm F. One of your first assignments is to present an educational program on basic oral health practices for culturally diverse pregnant teens in three alternative high schools that have day care facilities.

Use Testlet A to answer questions 1 to 5.

1. **Which of the following roles of the dental hygienist is illustrated by this activity?**
   a. Administrator/manager
   b. Advocate
   c. Clinician
   d. Educator

2. **How much additional fluoride is required to bring the F concentration of the water supply to the optimal level?**
   a. 0.4 ppm F
   b. 0.7 ppm F
   c. 1 ppm F
   d. 0.4 to 0.9 ppm F

3. **What is the first step that should be accomplished to conduct this program?**
   a. Develop a lesson plan for the educational session for the pregnant teens
   b. Meet with the people involved to determine program goals and objectives

   c. Plan an educational presentation for the day care children
   d. Request funding for oral hygiene supplies from the local health department
   e. Select teaching strategies for the educational program

4. **Which index would be appropriate to determine the rate of pregnancy gingivitis in this population?**
   a. CPI
   b. CPITN
   c. GI
   d. PSR

5. **Which of the following agencies would be the BEST resource for program planning for this population?**
   a. National Maternal and Child Oral Health Resource Center
   b. DHHS Centers for Medicare and Medicaid
   c. Public Health Service
   d. DHHS Human Resources and Services Administration

TESTLET B

The director of the Vintage Retirement Center contacts the local dental hygiene society to provide a seminar on oral health and conduct oral cancer screenings for the purpose of improving the oral health of the residents. The facility has a population of 100 well residents between ages 60 and 78 who have a middle SES; 80% of the residents are dentate, with varying numbers of teeth present. The oral health assessment results reveal a mean PlI of 2.1, mean GI of 0.8, mean DMFT of 5.2, mean D of 2.0, RCI of 2.1, and untreated root caries of 1.5. Correlation analysis reveals a correlation coefficient of $r = 0.81$ for the relationship between the RCI and PlI of this group. About 70% of the residents report having a dental home where they receive routine dental care. Over 50% of them report signs and symptoms of xerostomia. A SMART objective is established to improve the oral hygiene within 6 months by a six-member team of volunteer members of the Dental Hygiene Society delivering an oral hygiene educational program for residents and staff, providing oral hygiene supplies, and following up with reminders and motivational techniques to enhance the residents' daily effective oral hygiene. The Society has a budget for community oral health that can be used to support the program.

Use Testlet B to answer questions 6 to 12.

6. **The correlation between the RCI and PlI demonstrates what relationship between root caries and plaque biofilm in this target population?**
   a. Moderate positive
   b. Strong negative
   c. Strong positive
   d. Weak negative
   e. Little if any

7. **What level of oral hygiene is revealed by the mean PlI?**
   a. No plaque present
   b. Slight plaque present

c. Moderate plaque present

d. Severe plaque present

e. Cannot be determined from the information provided

8. **What change in the DMFT scores would indicate that the needs are being met 5 years after implementation of a program?**

a. Decrease in the total DMFT score

b. Decrease in D, no change in M, and increase in F

c. No change in D, decrease in M, and increase in F

d. Decrease in D, increase in M, and increase in F

e. Both B and D could be acceptable indicators of success

9. **Which component of the SMART objective is missing?**

a. Achievable

b. Measurable

c. Relevant

d. Specific

e. Time-bound

10. **All the following preventive programs are indicated by the assessment results EXCEPT one. Which one is this *exception*?**

a. Educational presentation on basic oral hygiene

b. Referral for restorative treatment

c. Use of a 0.12% chlorhexidine rinse daily

d. Daily use of a higher-concentration fluoride dentifrice

11. **Which of the following programs should be planned to address one of the *Healthy People 2020* Oral Health objectives for this target population?**

a. Denture marking and educational presentation on denture care

b. Oral cancer screening and referral, as needed

c. Referral to a Medicaid provider for dental treatment

d. Screening of periodontal condition and referral, as needed

e. Treatment with fluoride varnish to control dentinal hypersensitivity

12. **What is the BEST measure of the success of this program?**

a. Administrative support for the program

b. Improved oral health indicators of the residents

c. Improved oral hygiene of the residents

d. Increased availability of oral hygiene supplies for the use by the residents

e. Increased oral health knowledge of the staff

TESTLET C

The human resources director of an urban county hospital is alarmed by the rising cost of employee health insurance premiums related to tobacco-associated health conditions. The administrator charges the occupational health director, a dental hygienist, with addressing the issue of employee tobacco consumption. Employee demographics for the hospital are as follows: 40% Caucasian, 38% African American, 12% Hispanic, and 10% Asian. The dental hygienist conducts an employee tobacco usage survey as part of the program planning process.

Analysis of the survey reveals mean cigarette usage per day of 4.6 for administrators, 19.6 for clerical support staff, 10.6 for nurses, 6.2 for physicians, and 19.8 for allied health technicians. Standard deviation is 2.2 cigarettes for all groups. Cigarette packs are known to contain 20 cigarettes. A computer-based educational program is planned for the initial intervention with the goal of reducing daily cigarette usage.

Use Testlet C to answer questions 13 to 17.

13. **Based on the survey results, which of the following is the highest-priority population to target with an intervention?**

a. Allied health technicians

b. Clerical support staff

c. Hospital administrators

d. Hospital patients

e. Nurses

f. Physicians

g. All the groups are equally important and should be targeted at the same time.

14. **Which of the following is the BEST instructional objective for this initiative?**

a. After completing the educational program, participants will understand the harmful effects of tobacco and how they contribute to oral and systemic diseases and conditions.

b. Participants will be able to list recommended methods to control cravings that can lead to failure.

c. Ninety percent of the staff will voluntarily participate in the program during the first month of availability.

d. On completion of the computer-based educational program, staff members will be able to correctly identify 80% of the harmful ingredients in tobacco.

15. **What is the MOST important cultural factor to consider when planning an intervention for this population?**

a. Age

b. Gender

c. Educational level

d. Ethnic background

e. Health literacy

16. **Which step of program planning is BEST represented by the survey described in the scenario?**

a. Analysis of needs

b. Collection of data

c. Determination of priorities

d. Implementation and strategy development

e. Program evaluation

17. **The data reported from the survey represent ordinal data. A pie chart is the most appropriate graphic representation of these results.**

a. Both statements are TRUE.

b. Both statements are FALSE.

c. The first statement is TRUE; the second statement is FALSE.

d. The first statement is FALSE; the second statement is TRUE.

TESTLET D

The director of a local nursing home has contracted with a public health dental hygienist to design an oral health protocol for the 300 residents. Currently, a registered nurse performs the intake oral examination. The majority of the residents are partially edentulous, have partial removable dentures, and require assistance with daily hygiene practices. The caregivers state that the residents have severe halitosis, trouble eating, and frequently lose their removable partial dentures. The dental hygienist observes that the caregivers are neglecting daily oral hygiene care and are not conducting oral cancer screenings. On the basis of these observations, the dental hygienist determines to carry out oral hygiene and oral cancer screening of all residents and introduce an educational component for the facility's caregivers and interested family members. Students from the local dental hygiene educational program are recruited to assist with the educational program. The caregivers' knowledge is measured prior to and a week following the educational program; these measures are compared to evaluate changes in knowledge. The caregivers' ability to conduct oral cancer screening is evaluated weekly for several weeks after the educational program. The success of the program will be evaluated by screening the residents again 1 year later to identify any lesions that have not been found during the year. If the data reveal lesions that have not been identified, the dental hygienist plans to work with the director of nursing to establish a new protocol for routine oral cancer screening by the registered nurses on staff. The dental hygienist secures funding from a local foundation for the equipment needed to screen the residents.

Use Testlet D to answer questions 18 to 23.

18. **What type of study is represented by evaluating the change of knowledge as a result of the educational component?**
    a. Case-control
    b. Correlational
    c. Crossover
    d. Pretest/posttest
    e. Time-series

19. **What type of data is being collected by the screening?**
    a. Qualitative and primary
    b. Qualitative and secondary
    c. Quantitative and primary
    d. Quantitative and secondary

20. **Which term BEST describes the extent of oral cancer lesions found at the 1-year evaluation screening?**
    a. Count
    b. Incidence
    c. Prevalence
    d. Proportion
    e. Rate

21. **Which core public health function is exemplified by the potential future establishment of a new program protocol?**
    a. Assessment
    b. Assurance
    c. Policy development
    d. Prevention

22. **The stakeholders involved in this program represent what level of public health involvement?**
    a. Local
    b. State
    c. National
    d. A combination of two or more levels

23. **What is the BEST method to use for the weekly evaluation of the caregivers' ability to conduct oral cancer screening in this program?**
    a. Administer a weekly written test over the cancer screening procedure
    b. Interview the residents about the caregivers' technique
    c. Observe the caregivers conducing oral cancer screening
    d. Survey the family members about the caregivers' technique

TESTLET E

A high dental caries rate has been reported by the school nurses in Head Start children in the county on the basis of the rate of toothaches and absences. The families are primarily Spanish-speaking Hispanic and East Indian migrant farmworkers. They reside in predominantly rural settings with individual well-water supplies. At an informational meeting, the Head Start dental health coordinator introduces the goal of the program to the Head Start family advocates. A team of dental hygiene students from the local college is asked to design a comprehensive program to address the problem of dental caries in this population. They begin by collecting baseline data using the deft, OHI-S, and GI and identify a high level of S-ECC.

Use Testlet E to answer questions 24 to 29.

24. **Which of the following is indicated by the second component of the caries index used in this program?**
    a. Decayed surface
    b. Decayed tooth
    c. Tooth that needs to be extracted because of the severity of decay
    d. Tooth that has been extracted because of decay
    e. Tooth that has naturally exfoliated

25. **Which of the following would be MOST appropriate to explain during the informational session?**
    a. Benefits of community water fluoridation
    b. Cause of early childhood caries
    c. Effectiveness of daily brushing
    d. Value of healthy food choices

26. **All the following would be an appropriate source of funding for this program EXCEPT:**
    a. CHIP
    b. Head Start grant
    c. Medicare
    d. Medicaid
    e. Private funding from a local foundation

27. **Which preventive program is indicated for this target population?**
    a. Distribution of fluoridated dentifrice
    b. Professional fluoride applications every 6 moths

c. School fluoride varnish program

d. School sealant program

e. Water fluoridation

28. **Which index would be appropriate to evaluate the improvement in the children's oral hygiene resulting from strategies introduced in this program?**

   a. OHI-S

   b. PHP

   c. PlI

d. Turesky modification of the Quigley-Hein Plaque index

e. Any of the above would be appropriate.

29. **Which of the following describes the level of ECC for the older age of this population?**

   a. No smooth-surface caries is present.

   b. No cavitated lesions are present on anterior teeth.

   c. Number of carious lesions is less than four.

   d. The number of carious lesions is greater than five.

TESTLET F

Dental hygiene students from a local program visit a geriatric day care called Camp Sunshine to implement a service learning project. These older adults are functionally independent, although they are medically compromised. Under faculty supervision, the students screen the older adult clients to identify denture cleanliness and teach them how to clean their dentures daily. The goals are to improve their oral health by cleaning their dentures or partial dentures, increase their awareness of the need for daily oral care, and empower them to clean their dentures. The students compute the mean scores of the denture cleanliness measure for future evaluation of the program outcomes. The educational program consists of three weekly visits to teach and provide practice in various aspects of denture care. During the

first weekly lesson, the students use motivational interviewing to identify the clients' current practices and intentions regarding daily denture cleaning. The students use this information to plan individualized instruction for each client. The students return in 6 months to measure denture cleanliness to evaluate the success of the program. Although the outcomes indicate improvement in cleanliness for the majority of the clients, the results are skewed as a result of a large number of them missing one of the weekly sessions because they came down with the flu that week. At the end of the program, the students prepare a final report in which they communicate the outcomes of the program to the facility director and propose funding of supplies by Camp Sunshine for future programs.

Use Testlet F to answer questions 30 to 35.

30. **Which of the following terms BEST describes the situation described related to the flu?**

   a. Cluster

   b. Endemic

   c. Epidemic

   d. Occurrence

   e. Pandemic

31. **Which of the following is an ethical responsibility of the students and faculty who are implementing this program?**

   a. Communicate oral findings to the staff of the facility

   b. Prepare a formal report of findings to submit to the health department

   c. Refer clients who have suspicious lesions identified during the program

   d. Take the dentures back to the dental hygiene clinic to clean them more thoroughly

32. **What is the BEST teaching method for the psychomotor learning in this program?**

   a. Demonstration

   b. Guided practice

   c. Lecture

   d. A video presentation

33. **Which health education and health promotion theory is BEST reflected by the strategies used in the educational program?**

   a. Health belief model

   b. Organizational change theory

   c. Social cognitive theory

   d. Trans-theoretical model (stages of change theory)

34. **Which statistic is BEST to determine the statistical significance of the improved denture cleanliness?**

   a. Analysis of variance (ANOVA)

   b. Chi-square

   c. Correlation coefficient

   d. The t test

35. **What is the BEST way for the students to provide the final report?**

   a. Discuss the results at a meeting with the administrators in which they provide a written proposal of the funding request

   b. Include in the written proposal a list of the clients with their baseline and posttest cleanliness scores

   c. Include in the written proposal tables and graphs that summarize the pretest and posttest denture cleanliness data

   d. Write a few paragraphs in the proposal that describe the statistical analysis of the pretest and posttest denture cleanliness data

---

TESTLET G

A local dental hygienists' association and a faith-based organization collaborate to target a school for a comprehensive oral disease prevention program. The school serves a population that consists of 50% Medicaid-eligible children, and 75% of them receive the school lunch program. The ethnic group representation is 15% Hispanic American, 5% African American, and 80% non-Hispanic white. The fluoride concentration of the community water is below the optimal level. A public health hygienist screens the children in preschool through grade 5 annually. Data for 2014 indicate a 22% urgent decay rate across all ages.

Further assessment reveals that many of the children are not seeing a dentist routinely. A sealant program is conducted in grades 2 and 5. Af luoride varnish program is conducted with the preschoolers and grade K, including two applications annually; these children are screened for dental caries with a tongue blade and available light at the time of each application. An educational program is designed to meet the needs of the children in this school. Finally, the team explores the option of a fluoridation campaign to achieve water fluoridation in this community.

Use Testlet G to answer questions 36 to 42.

36. Which of the following is a required action for this program?
   a. Phone call to each family to describe the program
   b. Presence of a dentist while the fluoride varnish is placed by hygienists
   c. Radiographs before placing sealants
   d. Written informed consent form signed by parents or legal guardians of all children who participate

37. What assessment classification is used with preschoolers and grade K in this program?
   a. Type I
   b. Type II
   c. Type III
   d. Type IV

38. What would have been the BEST means of identifying the reported decay rate?
   a. Basic Screening Survey (BSS)
   b. deft
   c. DMFT
   d. RCI

39. The same education materials can be used with participants in the other schools in the district, because the cultural diversity of this population represents the cultural diversity of the general U.S. population.
   a. Both the statement and the reason are correct and related.
   b. Both the statement and the reason are correct but NOT related.
   c. The statement is CORRECT, but the reason is NOT correct.
   d. The statement is NOT correct, but the reason is CORRECT.
   e. NEITHER the statement NOR the reason is correct.

40. What is the basis for deciding to target this school with this program?
   a. Convenience
   b. Cultural diversity of the school
   c. Random selection of the school
   d. SES of the children in the school

41. Which of the following should be done FIRST in this program?
   a. Contact key community leaders to obtain a broad base of support for fluoridation
   b. Determine the fluoride level of the community water supply
   c. Organize a massive community education program about the benefits and safety of fluoridation
   d. Schedule a referendum to allow the citizens to express their opinion about fluoridation
   e. Testify before the city council to convince them to fluoridate the water

42. Which of the following programs has the HIGHEST priority to further meet the needs of this population?
   a. Conduct a daily classroom fluoride rinse program
   b. Establish dental homes and refer children for treatment
   c. Make plans to implement school water fluoridation
   d. Plan a health fair for the children and the families

TESTLET H

A dental hygiene U.S. Public Health Services (USPHS)–commissioned core officer is assigned to an Indian Health Service (IHS) clinic to improve the oral care of pregnant women in an American Indian rural community with a population of 26,000. Approximately 20% of the pregnant women in this population develop gestational diabetes. When a woman first sees the physician in the clinic for prenatal care, she is referred to the dental clinic for a dental examination. Only 25% of the patients referred over the previous 6 months complied with the dental referral, scheduled an appointment, and received treatment. The community is not classified a "dental manpower shortage area" because of the staffing of this clinic and the existence of this program. A survey of the pregnant women served by this clinic reveals that the women do not realize their risk for diabetes, are unaware of the relationship between oral health status and diabetes, and do not understand the benefits of an oral health assessment in relation to their overall health and the health of their babies. For the purpose of discussing the problem and possible solutions, the dental hygienist arranges a meeting of the medical clinic director, the dental clinic director, the medicine man of the Indian tribe, and a dental clinic staff member who is a member of the tribe. This team sets a goal of doubling the rate of compliance with the dental referral to 30% within 6 months.

Use Testlet H to answer questions 43 to 47.

43. Which of the following is the BEST intervention to implement first to meet the goal of the program?
   a. Conduct a mailing program to remind pregnant women to schedule an appointment for a dental examination
   b. Develop an oral health screening program to be implemented during prenatal care visits
   c. Develop written educational materials for distribution during prenatal visits
   d. Document the oral condition of the women who have complied and received a dental examination
   e. Plan an educational presentation for the pregnant women on the relationship among oral health, systemic health, and the risks and consequences of diabetes

44. On the basis of the results of the survey, which health education theory is indicated as the foundation for an oral health education intervention to meet the goal?
   a. Health belief model
   b. Learning ladder
   c. Social cognitive theory
   d. Theory of reasoned action
   e. Trans-theoretical model (stages of change theory)

45. Lack of compliance with the dental referral could be a result of which TWO of the following factors?
   a. Cost of dental care
   b. Lack of available appointments
   c. Lack of transportation to the dental clinic
   d. Low dentist-to-population ratio
   e. Low health literacy

46. The dental referral by the medical clinic is an example of which characteristic of public health?
 a. Application of biostatistics to analyze population health problems
 b. Community rather than the individual as the client
 c. Multi-disciplinary team approach to solving public health problems
 d. Social responsibility for oral health

47. Which theory of health promotion is exemplified by this program?
 a. Community organization
 b. Diffusion of innovation
 c. Organizational change
 d. Sense of coherence

TESTLET I

Dental hygiene students conduct a study to compare the effectiveness of two nonalcohol mouthrinses, a 0.02% NaF rinse (Listerine Zero) and a 0.07% CPC rinse (Crest Pro Health), in controlling plaque biofilm and gingivitis. A sample of 136 healthy adult volunteers is taken from the university dental hygiene clinic. Only dentate adults with no to mild periodontitis are accepted to participate in the study. The study participants are qualified for inclusion in the study by their plaque biofilm forming potential and presence of mild gingivitis. Two groups are formed, and an unmarked bottle of mouthrinse is given to each participant. Study participants and examiners are unaware of the formula used by each participant. One group receives the 0.07% CPC mouthrinse, and the other group receives the 0.02% NaF mouthrinse. All other ingredients of both rinses are standardized. Two examiners are calibrated in the use of the PlI and GI to measure plaque biofilm at baseline, 2 months, and 4 months. The baseline PlI scores are used during group assignment to ensure that the two groups have equivalent oral hygiene.

Use Testlet I to answer questions 48 to 52.

48. What sampling technique is used for this study?
 a. Convenience sampling
 b. Judgmental or purposive sampling
 c. Random sampling
 d. Stratified random sampling
 e. Systematic sampling

49. The application of the PlI in this study is an example of which step in the scientific method?
 a. Collection, organization, and analysis of data
 b. Formulation of a hypothesis
 c. Identification and statement of the problem
 d. Verification, rejection, or modification of the hypothesis

50. Which of the following is a statement of the null hypothesis for this study?
 a. Neither mouthrinse is effective in controlling plaque and gingivitis.
 b. Plaque and gingivitis are strongly associated.
 c. The 0.02% NaF mouthrinse and the 0.07% CPC mouthrinse differ in ability to control plaque and gingivitis.

 d. There is no difference between the ability of the 0.02% NaF mouthrinse and the 0.07% CPC mouthrinse to control plaque and gingivitis.
 e. Which controls plaque and gingivitis better, the 0.02% NaF mouthrinse or the 0.07% CPC mouthrinse?

51. What type of study is reflected by the methods of this research study? Select FOUR types of studies from the following list.
 a. Analytic study
 b. Clinical trial
 c. Double-blind study
 d. Experimental study
 e. Posttest only study
 f. Retrospective study
 g. Time-series study

52. Which of the following is controlled by the procedures used with the examiners as they measure the plaque biofilm?
 a. Inter-examiner reliability
 b. Intra-examiner reliability
 c. Inter-examiner variability
 d. Intra-examiner variability

TESTLET J

The administrator of a group home for mentally challenged adults has received multiple complaints from the attending caregivers regarding the residents' oral health. Limited manual dexterity abilities of the residents require that they receive assistance with oral hygiene routines; yet complaints of severe resident halitosis and bleeding during normal oral hygiene routines have made the caregivers reluctant to provide assistance. Frustrated by a lack of staff compliance, the group home administrator contacts the local county public health dental hygienist, knowing that the county health department has a grant for oral care for this population. After gathering basic demographic information, the dental hygienist makes a visit to the home to determine the actual oral health status of the residents.

Use Testlet J to answer questions 53 to 57.

53. What is the BEST way for the dental hygienist to assess the actual oral hygiene routines in the group home?
 a. Assess the values of caregivers by conducting focus groups
 b. Measure the plaque biofilm and gingivitis scores of residents over time
 c. Observe the residents' ability to brush correctly

 d. Observe the caregivers' ability to brush correctly
 e. Survey the beliefs and attitudes of caregivers with a questionnaire

54. From initial observations, what *Healthy People 2020* objective is MOST applicable to this target group?
 a. Reduce untreated dental decay in children and adults
 b. Reduce gingivitis and destructive periodontal disease in adults

c. Increase detection of oral cancer lesions at stage I

d. Increase annual use of dental services by residents of long-term care facilities

55. **What known characteristics about this population can be utilized in a community profile? Select THREE characteristics from the following list.**

a. Age

b. Ethnicity

c. Source of funding

d. Gender

e. Geographic location

f. Literacy level

g. Population setting

56. **Which of the following is the BEST use of the dental hygienist in this situation?**

a. Conduct an educational program on daily oral hygiene care for the residents

b. Make available dental hygiene services for the residents using portable equipment

c. Present an in-service training program to the group home staff

d. Provide daily oral hygiene care for the residents

57. **Which of the following is an effective teaching strategy to raise the caregivers' compliance in this situation?**

a. Demonstrate to them the proper oral hygiene procedures

b. Provide a lecture for them on the importance of oral hygiene

c. Show them pictures of good oral health versus oral disease

d. Provide training on how to maintain personal oral hygiene skills for themselves

Medical Emergencies

Leslie Koberna

Dental hygienists must prevent and effectively manage medical emergencies that occur in the health care environment. Careful client observation and questioning during assessment will enable the dental hygienist to identify, prepare, and care for the client who experiences a medical complication. The ability to recognize signs and symptoms of medical disorders, prevent further complications through appropriate interventions, and manage a medical emergency is essential.

GENERAL CONSIDERATIONS[1–3]

A. Medical emergency
 1. A medical emergency means a client experiences an unforeseen, immediate, health-related difficulty that is potentially life threatening
 2. Medical emergencies require prompt recognition and action by the dental team to maintain the client's health and, at times, the client's life
B. Dental hygienist's legal responsibilities
 1. To provide timely, quality care according to current standards of practice
  a. The dental hygienist must be prepared for managing medical emergencies and adverse events in a health care environment; dental hygienists may be held liable if they lack knowledge and training in medical emergency management
  b. All dental hygienists should be current in medical emergency management, including basic life support (BLS)
 2. To maintain complete records of medical emergencies in the health care setting
  a. Documentation must describe the onset and management of the emergency, the client's vital signs, nature of the treatment performed and the client's response, type and dose of drugs administered, and the time when treatment was provided
  b. Thorough and complete records of medical emergencies are an important component of continuous quality improvement and protect the oral health care team in the event of legal action

MEDICAL HISTORY[1–3]

A. Reviewing a client's health history is the first step in preventing a medical emergency
B. A thorough health history, taken at the first appointment and updated at each subsequent appointment, reveals conditions that predispose a client to medical complications
C. Information obtained from the health history is used to modify the client's care plan and reduce the likelihood of the client experiencing a medical complication or emergency in the oral health care setting
D. If more information regarding the client's health status is needed, the dentist or the dental hygienist should consult the client's general physician before initiating treatment
E. The assessment and documentation of the client's vital signs (usually blood pressure, body temperature, pulse, respiration rate) provide information regarding the client's health status
F. The probability of a stress-induced medical emergency in the oral health care environment may be reduced by careful appointment planning, stress reduction protocol, good client rapport, and prescribed stress-reducing medication

VITAL SIGNS[1–5,8]

Basic Concepts

A. Vital signs refer to numerical values given to blood pressure, body temperature, pulse rate, and respiration rate; dental hygienists should explain the purpose of and the method for measuring vital signs to the client before initiating these procedures
B. Vital signs and a health history are used to determine a client's fitness to undergo oral health care procedures
C. Abnormal values and significant findings should be brought to the attention of the dentist, the client, and the client's physician
D. Vital sign values should be taken for each new client, at each recall appointment, and more frequently for clients with hypertension and other cardiac diseases

E. Vital signs should be compared to the baseline readings and monitored during an emergency; vital signs should be taken every 5 minutes for emergencies related to the heart, diabetes, adrenal insufficiency, drug-related emergencies, acute allergic reactions, and the postictal phase of seizures

F. Vital signs should be recorded in the client's chart

Blood Pressure

A. Definitions
  1. Blood pressure (BP)—the force exerted by blood on the walls of the blood vessels during the contraction and relaxation of the heart; BP depends on the heart's contractile force, peripheral vascular resistance, and vascular volume
     a. BP may increase with age or in response to exercise, stress, certain medications, smoking, and illness
     b. BP is recorded as millimeters of mercury (mm Hg), with the systolic pressure over the diastolic pressure; systolic (mm Hg)/diastolic (mm Hg)
  2. Systolic pressure—the force exerted during ventricular contraction (heart beat); the highest pressure in the cardiac cycle
  3. Diastolic pressure—the resting pressure, which occurs during ventricular relaxation (heart rest); the lowest pressure of the cardiac cycle
  4. Pulse pressure—the value obtained when diastolic pressure is subtracted from systolic pressure
  5. Hypertension—sustained, abnormally high BP
  6. Hypotension—sustained, abnormally low BP
B. Normal values
  1. Children—BP values vary based on age, height, and gender
  2. Adults—BP is considered normal when systolic reading is less than 120 mm Hg and diastolic less than 80 mm Hg
  3. Normal BP should be checked every 2 years in the dental office
  4. BP classifications and recommended management regimen for adults
     a. Prehypertension—clients with systolic reading between 120 and 139 mm Hg and/or diastolic reading between 80 and 89 mm Hg are considered to be prehypertensive; BP should be rechecked once a year
     b. Stage I hypertension—clients are considered to have stage 1 hypertension when systolic reading is between 140 to 159 mm Hg and/or diastolic reading is between 90 to 99 mm Hg; BP should be rechecked in 2 months
     c. Stage II hypertension—clients with systolic reading between 160 and 179 mm Hg and/or diastolic reading between 100 and 109 mm Hg are considered to have stage II hypertension and should be referred to a physician within 1 month
     d. Clients with systolic reading of 180 mm Hg or greater and/or diastolic reading of 110 mm Hg or greater should be referred to a physician for immediate care; activate the emergency medical services (EMS) system if the person is symptomatic (i.e., experiencing chest pain, shortness of breath, back pain, numbness/weakness, changes in vision, or difficulty speaking)

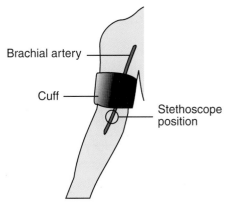

FIG 21-1 Stethoscope position for blood pressure (BP) measurement.

C. Equipment for measuring blood pressure
  1. Sphygmomanometer—an inflatable cuff and pressure gauge used to measure BP
  2. Stethoscope—an instrument used to listen to the sounds of the blood as it passes through the brachial artery (Fig. 21-1)
     a. The first sound heard through the stethoscope is the systolic BP, or Korotkoff sounds
     b. The last distinct sound heard is the diastolic BP

Body Temperature

A. Normal oral temperature for both adults and children ranges from 97°F to 99.6°F (36.1°C to 37.5°C)
B. Values higher than 101°F may indicate an active disease process; values above 99.6°F indicate a fever
C. Body temperature elevation may be caused by exercise, ingestion of hot food or drink, smoking, or a pathologic condition
D. Body temperature may be decreased because of starvation or shock
E. Body temperature varies during the day
  1. Lower in the morning, higher in the afternoon
  2. Fever of pyrexia is an abnormal elevation in body temperature

Pulse

A. Definition and basic concepts
  1. Pulse—the force of the blood through an artery created by the heart's contraction; each contraction creates a wave of blood that can be felt by gently pressing a superficial artery against underlying tissue
  2. Pulse is evaluated by rate (fast, slow), rhythm (regular, irregular), and quality (full or strong, thready or weak)
  3. Pulse rate is measured as the number of heartbeats per minute (beats/min)
  4. Pulse rate may increase because of exercise, certain drugs, anxiety, heat, eating, or disease
  5. Pulse rate may decrease because of sleep, certain drugs, fasting, or disease
B. Heart rate
  1. Heart rates of infants and children are more rapid than adult rates and vary based on age, gender, and size

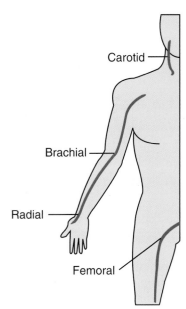

FIG 21-2 Location of pulse points.

2. Normal pulse rates for children age 1 to 10 years—60 to 140 beats/min
3. Normal pulse rates for children older than 10 years and adults—60 to 100 beats/min
4. Normal resting heart rate for adults ranges from 60 to 100 beats/min
   a. Bradycardia—less than 60 beats/min
   b. Tachycardia—greater than 100 beats/min
C. Determining the pulse rate
   1. Sites used for determining pulse rates (Fig. 21-2)
      a. Brachial pulse—located on the medial aspect of the antecubital fossa of the elbow
      b. Radial pulse—located on the lateral aspect of the wrist (thumb side) on the ventral surface
      c. Carotid pulse—located in the neck groove, just anterior to the sternocleidomastoid muscle
      d. Femoral pulse—located on the medial aspect of the upper thigh
   2. In emergency situations, the carotid pulse (which indicates that blood is flowing to the brain) is monitored
      a. Care is required in carotid palpation because vagal stimulation may occur, resulting in a decrease in BP or syncope
      b. It is important *not* to palpate the carotid arteries simultaneously because one or both may be partially occluded
   3. In nonemergency situations, the brachial or the radial pulse is monitored

Respiration Rate

A. Definitions and basic concepts
   1. Respiration is the inspiration and expiration of air by the body
   2. Respiration rate—the number of breaths taken by a person per minute; it is counted by the rise and fall of the chest
   3. When assessing a client's respiration, the depth (shallow, deep), rhythm (regular, irregular), rate, quality (labored, easy), breathing sounds (wet/noisy, clear), and client position during respiration should be evaluated
B. Factors that affect respiration
   1. Respiration rate may be increased as a result of exercise, pain, certain drugs, anxiety, shock, or disease
   2. Respiration rate may be decreased as a result of sleep, certain drugs, or disease
C. Normal respiration rate ranges
   1. Teens to adults—12 to 20 respirations per minute
   2. Preschool children—20 to 25 respirations/min
   3. Older children—15 to 25 respirations/min
D. American Society of Anesthesiologists (ASA) Physical Status (PS) Classification System (see Table 15-3 in Chapter 15)
   1. A system developed to determine risk for clients who will undergo surgery or anesthesia
   2. In dentistry, the following classifications are used:
      a. ASA 1 (PS1)—normal client without systemic disease; client can walk up flight of stairs, walk a quarter mile with little distress, and should be able to handle the stress of a dental appointment
      b. ASA 2 (PS2)—client with mild systemic disease or an ASA 1 client who demonstrates extreme anxiety; examples include clients who have controlled type 2 diabetes, asthma, or hypertension; should tolerate elective dental care
      c. ASA 3 (PS3)—patient with severe systemic disease with limited activity but functions normally; can climb stairs or walk a quarter mile with difficulty; examples include persons with stable angina, post–myocardial infarction (MI) or post–cerebrovascular accident (CVA), controlled type 1 diabetes, or chronic obstructive pulmonary disease (COPD); can have routine dental care but risk is increased
      d. ASA 4 (PS4)—patient with an incapacitating or life-threatening disease; cannot walk up a flight of stairs or walk a quarter mile; examples include persons with unstable angina, MI within 1 month, CVA within 6 months, uncontrolled type 1 diabetes; risk is too great, and elective care should *not* be performed

THE EMERGENCY KIT[2]

A. A basic medical emergency kit accessible to all treatment areas should be maintained and readily available for use
   1. Staff should be familiar with the content of the kit and its location
   2. An emergency kit should contain only the emergency medications the dentist and staff are trained to use (Table 21-1)
B. Emergency preparation
   1. Each member of the dental team should be current in BLS (cardiopulmonary resuscitation), including the use of an AED (automatic external defibrillator), and should be trained to recognize and manage common medical emergencies

TABLE 21-1   Medications Typically Supplied with Basic Medical Emergency Kit*

Drug	Route	Indication	Comments
Oxygen	Inhaled (nasal cannula, face mask, bag-valve-mask)	Respiratory distress, cardiac disease	Do not use in hyperventilation
Nitroglycerin	Sublingual	Angina pectoris	No more than three doses in 15 minutes; may cause a drop in blood pressure
Epinephrine pen	Subcutaneous	Acute allergic reaction; acute bronchospasm (asthma)	—
Bronchodilator (e.g., albuterol)	Inhaled	Bronchospasm (asthma)	—
Antihistamine (e.g., diphenhydramine)	Oral	Allergic reaction	May cause drowsiness in adults; may excite children
Glucose (nondiet soft drink; glucose tablet, honey sticks)	Oral	Hypoglycemia	—
Aspirin	Oral (chewable)	Analgesic, antipyretic, anti-inflammatory	Potentiates bleeding problems

*The drugs and equipment available in the dental office should reflect the training of the dentist and the staff. Only drugs and equipment that the dentist, the dental hygienist, and the staff are trained to use should be included in the medical emergency kit.

2. Each oral health care team member should have delegated responsibilities in the event of a medical emergency; simulations ensure each individual understands his or her role should a medical emergency arise

EMERGENCY CARE[1,2,4,6–8]

A. Definitions and basic concepts
 1. Stress reduction protocol
   a. Establish good client rapport
   b. Create a low-stress environment
   c. Possibly administer pretreatment medication
   d. Administer pain control
   e. Assess anxiety level
 2. Cardiopulmonary resuscitation (CPR)—BLS technique with the goal of providing oxygen to the brain, heart, and other vital organs until definitive medical treatment can be given; CPR requires assessment and basic skills in the management of the airway, breathing, and circulation
 3. Emergency medical system (EMS) —a coordinated community system that uses communication, transportation, prevention, education, trained personnel, emergency medical facilities, and other elements in providing emergency medical care
 4. Respiratory arrest—sudden cessation of breathing
 5. Cardiac arrest—sudden, unexpected cessation of the heartbeat and circulation
 6. Clinical death—cessation of the activity of the heart and of breathing; may be reversible through life support measures, especially if initiated within 4 to 6 minutes, or may progress to biologic death
 7. Biologic death—permanent cellular damage, particularly of the oxygen-sensitive brain cells, resulting from an inadequate supply of oxygen

B. Administering basic life support—cardiopulmonary resuscitation
 1. The steps in CPR are known as CAB:
   a. Circulation—the hygienist assesses the client's circulation and provides cardiac support by external cardiac compressions and defibrillation; first step in CPR
   b. Airway—the hygienist assesses the airway and establishes a clear air passage; second step in CPR
   c. Breathing—the hygienist assesses breathing and provides respiration through rescue breathing; third step in CPR
 2. Performing CPR
   a. Determine the client's level of consciousness
   b. Activate the emergency response system
   c. Attain an AED
   d. Place client in supine position
   e. Check pulse for less than 10 seconds; use carotid artery for adults, femoral artery for children ages 1 to 12, and brachial artery for infants
   f. If pulse not present
    (1) Begin compressions
      (a) Adult—administer 30 compressions at rate of 100 per minute and depress sternum 2 inches
      (b) Child (1 year to puberty)—administer 30 compressions at rate of 100 per minute and depress sternum 2 inches with heel of hand
      (c) Infant (under 1 year)—administer 30 compressions at rate of 100 per minute and depress sternum 1½ inches using 2 fingers between nipples
    (2) Administer 2 breaths
    (3) Continue cycle (compressions/breaths)
    (4) Check for pulse after every 4 cycles or 2 minutes
   g. Pulse is present—administer 10 to 12 rescue breaths per minute
C. Basic life support in late pregnancy
 1. Oxygen demands increase during pregnancy

2. Functional residual capacity of the lungs is decreased because of the upward displacement of the diaphragm; as a result, oxygen reserve is compromised when the pregnant woman is in the supine position, and cardiac output is decreased by 25%
3. To help alleviate the effects of the supine position on circulation, the uterus should be shifted toward the left side by placing a wedge under the right hip
4. Aspiration caused by delayed gastric emptying is a concern
5. Chest compressions for CPR should be performed higher than usual on the sternum, just above the center of the sternum, to accommodate the upward displacement of the diaphragm

D. Automated external defibrillator
1. Computerized device that analyzes cardiac rhythms and delivers an electric shock to the heart when appropriate; manual defibrillators and pediatric-capable AEDs are the preferred devices to be used on infants and children age 1 to 8 years
2. If available, an AED should be used as soon as possible in the CPR sequence, since early defibrillation increases the chances of survival for victims of sudden cardiac arrest
3. Considerations when using an AED
   a. Client should be kept dry
   b. Defibrillator pads should be placed at least 1 inch to the side of implanted pacemakers, not over the implanted pacemaker
   c. Transdermal medication patches in the area should be removed before placing AED

Administration of Oxygen

A. Basic concepts
1. During a medical emergency, the body's increased need for oxygen, or its diminished ability to obtain or use oxygen, may call for the administration of a higher concentration of oxygen than exists in regular air
2. Indications for oxygen administration include syncope, cardiac problems, and respiratory difficulties (with the exception of hyperventilation)
B. Equipment—portable oxygen unit consists of an oxygen tank (an E cylinder is recommended), regulator, tubing, a self-inflating resuscitation bag (Ambu bag used for high-flow oxygen, 10 to 15 liters per minute), a clear oxygen mask with a reservoir bag (covers face and nose; used for high-flow oxygen, 8 to 15 L/min), and a nasal cannula (used for low-flow oxygen, up to 6 L/min)
C. Place an unconscious client in the supine position; a conscious client can be seated in a comfortable position for administration of oxygen

MANAGEMENT OF MEDICAL EMERGENCIES
Obstructed Airway[2]

A. Basic concepts for conscious clients
1. An obstructed airway occurs when an object or foreign body prevents exchange of air during breathing

2. Foreign body obstruction may occur when eating, when unconscious (the tongue may block the pharynx), during resuscitation (aspiration of vomitus or blood), or during other events
B. Mild airway obstruction
1. Clients with mild airway obstruction can cough forcefully
2. Management—encourage spontaneous coughing and deep breathing
C. Severe airway obstruction with poor air exchange
1. Clients experiencing severe airway obstruction may exhibit a weak cough, cyanosis, high-pitched noises, increased difficulty breathing; may be unable to speak or breathe, clutching at the neck
2. Management
   a. Subdiaphragmatic abdominal thrusts (Heimlich maneuver) are administered to children and adults for severe foreign body airway obstruction
   b. Back blows and chest thrusts are performed on infants
   c. Blind finger-sweep is never performed
   d. For severe foreign body airway obstruction in a conscious woman in her last trimester of pregnancy, chest thrusts rather than abdominal thrusts are recommended

Unconscious Client[1,2,4]

A. Definitions and basic concepts
1. Unconsciousness—the inability to respond to stimuli, make purposeful movements, or gain awareness of events taking place
2. Levels of unconsciousness range from syncope (transient, simple fainting) to coma (prolonged, deep unconsciousness)
B. Causes
1. Diminished blood supply to the brain (inadequate cerebral circulation), altered quality of blood flow to the brain (metabolic disorder), central nervous system (CNS) disorder, or emotional disturbance.
2. Common causes of unconsciousness in the dental setting are psychogenic factors (fear, anxiety); treatment for this type of unconsciousness is aimed at increasing the amount of oxygenated blood received by the brain
C. Preventing loss of consciousness
1. Obtain a complete health history, evaluate vital signs, and determine client's dental stress level
2. Stress reduction protocols, premedication, and pain management for treating the anxious client
D. Managing unconsciousness
1. Assess the client's vital signs
2. Place client in supine position to facilitate cerebral blood flow
3. Implement CAB

Syncope (Fainting, Vasodepressor Syncope)[1-3,8]

A. Definition—sudden, transient loss of consciousness
B. Causes
1. Decreased cerebral function resulting from impaired circulation or altered metabolism

2. Psychogenic factors (anxiety, fear)
3. Nonpsychogenic factors (hypoglycemia, position change, heat)
C. Preventing syncope
   1. Obtain a complete health history to determine previous syncopal episodes, dental stress level, illness, if client has eaten, and other pertinent information
   2. Follow stress reduction protocol
   3. Clients who "feel faint" should be placed in the supine position
D. Signs and symptoms—three stages of syncope:
   1. Presyncope stage—client reports feeling of warmth in neck and face, not feeling well, weakness and nausea, lightheadedness, and tingling in the toes and fingers; observation of pallor or gray color of skin, dilated pupils, piloerection, hypotension, and tachycardia
   2. Syncope stage—client exhibits flaccid muscles, impaired consciousness, pallor, weak slow pulse, shallow breathing; unconsciousness of less than 5 minutes
   3. Postsyncope stage—client wakens and may report feeling weak and disoriented; BP and pulse rate return to normal
E. Managing syncope
   1. Presyncope
      a. Place client in supine position with legs slightly elevated; in most cases, this will prevent syncope
      b. Administer oxygen
      c. Consider postponing treatment
   2. Syncope
      a. Assess client
      b. Place client in supine position with legs slightly elevated
      c. Implement CAB
      d. Administer oxygen
      e. Monitor vital signs
      f. Place blanket over the client to keep warm
      g. Administer atropine (optional) for bradycardia
      h. For delayed recovery of 15 to 20 minutes, contact EMS
   3. Postsyncope
      a. Once recovers, client should remain in the supine position and rest for a time sufficient to prevent another episode
      b. Administer glucose (soft drink or orange juice) for associated hypoglycemia (optional)
      c. Determine cause of the syncope
      d. Someone should accompany client home
      e. Possible referral to physician

Orthostatic Hypotension or Postural Hypertension[1,2]

A. Definition—sudden drop in systolic BP of at least 20 mm Hg caused by a change in body position
B. Cause
   1. Sudden change from the supine to sitting or from sitting to standing position
   2. Prolonged bed rest, medications, prolonged standing, pregnancy, and age can affect the body's ability to adjust quickly to the impact of gravity on the cardiovascular system as body position changes

3. Addison's disease
4. Exhaustion and starvation
C. Signs and symptoms
   1. Client will report lightheadedness, blurred or darkened vision, and nausea
   2. Hygienist will observe pallor, syncope, and sweating
D. Prevention
   1. Slowly raise the client from the supine to the upright position
   2. Have the client change from the sitting position to the standing position slowly
E. Management of the emergency
   1. Assess the client
   2. Position the client back to the supine position with feet slightly elevated
   3. Implement CAB
   4. Administer oxygen if needed
   5. Monitor vital signs
   6. Raise the client slowly; provide assistance
   7. If recovery is delayed, EMS should be contacted

Shock[1-3,8]

A. Definition—circulatory system does not adequately circulate blood through body tissues, resulting in a lack of oxygen in the cells
B. The client experiencing shock may complain of thirst, restlessness, or anxiety
   1. May exhibit low BP; rapid, weak pulse; shallow, rapid respiratory rate
   2. Skin may be pale, cool, and clammy
   3. In severe cases, the victim may go into a coma
C. Management procedures for shock
   1. Place the client in the supine position with feet slightly elevated or Trendelenburg position
   2. Contact EMS
   3. Initiate CAB
   4. Administer oxygen
   5. Monitor vital signs
D. Types of shock
   1. Hypovolemic shock—most common type of shock
      a. Cause—severe hemorrhage or dehydration can lead to inadequate blood volume or venous return
      b. Signs and symptoms—dehydration, rapid thready pulse, cool clammy skin, decreased urine output, confusion, weakness, pallor
      c. Management—follow procedures listed earlier for shock
   2. Distributive shock or vasogenic shock—three types: anaphylactic, septic, neurogenic
   3. Anaphylactic shock
      a. Cause—acute allergic reaction; release of histamine results in sudden vasodilation throughout the body and bronchoconstriction
      b. Signs and symptoms—bronchoconstriction, difficulty in breathing, hypotension, respiratory arrest
      c. Management—follow procedures listed earlier for shock; in addition, administer epinephrine, histamine blockers, and corticosteroids

4. Septic shock
   a. Cause—infectious agent produces an acute systemic infection that prevents blood flow to the cells, tissues, and organs; often fatal; toxic shock syndrome is an example of septic shock
   b. Signs and symptoms—fever, vasodilation, increased cardiac output; tissue edema, pink and warm skin; hypotension; restlessness and anxiety; tachycardia; thirst; eventual respiratory failure
   c. Management—follow procedures previously listed for shock; in addition, administer intravenous (IV) fluids and antimicrobial therapy; client may need surgery
5. Neurogenic shock
   a. Cause—psychological or neurologic disorder or injury to the brainstem or spinal cord from disease, drugs, or trauma; causes loss of sympathetic nerve activity, impairing nerve impulses to the blood vessels, which in turn prevents vasoconstriction
   b. Signs and symptoms—hypotension, bradycardia, peripheral vasodilation
   c. Management—follow procedures previously listed for shock; in addition, administer phenylephrine or dopamine and epinephrine
6. Cardiogenic shock
   a. Cause—inadequate cardiac output to peripheral organs and tissues; common causes are MI, cardiac arrhythmias, and heart failure; occurs approximately 10 hours after an MI
   b. Signs and symptoms—hypotension, rapid weak pulse, cold clammy skin, peripheral cyanosis, chest pain, shortness of breath, reduced urine output, confusion
   c. Management—follow procedures listed earlier for shock; in addition, administer IV fluids and medications to restore heart rate and BP (beta blockers, vasodilators, and positive inotropes)
7. Obstructive shock
   a. Cause—obstruction of blood flow peripheral to the heart, as in arterial stenosis and pulmonary embolism; obstructive shock prevents the heart from beating
   b. Signs and symptoms—severe hypotension and dyspnea
   c. Management—follow procedures listed earlier for shock; in addition, remove or correct obstruction and administer IV fluids with caution

Asthma[1,2,8]

A. Definition—chronic inflammatory disease of the airway that causes reversible airway obstruction from hyperresponsiveness to stimuli, resulting in episodes of dyspnea, wheezing, and coughing
B. Types and causes
   1. Extrinsic or allergic asthma—caused by allergens outside the body (i.e., airborne, such as dust, foods, and drugs); bronchospasms occur within minutes of exposure
   2. Intrinsic asthma (also known as *nonallergic, idiopathic,* or *infective* asthma)—caused by nonallergic factors such as respiratory infections, psychological and physiologic stress, physical exertion, and environmental factors
   3. Additional categories in some textbooks include *exercise-induced, drug-induced,* and *infectious* asthma
C. Signs and symptoms—onset of a productive or a nonproductive cough, dyspnea (shortness of breath), tachypnea (increased respiratory rate), tachycardia (increased heart rate), anxiety and agitation, wheezing, cyanosis, chest tightening, nostril flaring, flushing
   1. Asthma occurs most often at night
D. Prevention of the emergency
   1. Identify clients at risk through thorough health history taking
   2. Ask probing questions related to asthma
   3. Implement stress reduction protocol
   4. Have the client take a prophylactic dose of bronchodilator before the appointment
   5. Encourage clients with asthma to bring their inhalers to all dental appointments
E. Management of an emergency related to asthma
   1. Position the client in the sitting position
   2. Initiate CAB
   3. Have the client administer own prescribed medications (bronchodilators); if not available, use bronchodilator from office emergency kit
   4. Administer oxygen if the episode continues
   5. Activate the EMS if the episode continues

Hyperventilation[2]

A. Definition—rapid breathing; often the result of pain, anxiety, or drugs; rapid breathing causes an excessive elimination of carbon dioxide, which results in respiratory alkalosis
B. Prevention of the emergency—implement stress reduction protocol
C. Signs and symptoms—tingling or numbness of extremities, giddiness, lightheadedness, dizziness, confusion, cold hands, heart palpitations, rapid respirations (25-30 breaths/min), rapid pulse
D. Management of the emergency related to hyperventilation
   1. Position the client in the upright position
   2. Initiate CAB
   3. Calm the client
   4. Have the client cup hands over mouth and nose and breathe slowly and deeply (only 4-6 breaths/min)
   5. Oxygen should *not* be administered

Cardiac Emergencies[1,2,8]

A. Cardiac emergencies have many causes and require immediate, definitive medical treatment
   1. Sudden, unexpected cessation of cardiac activity is called *cardiac arrest*; unless CPR/AED is promptly performed to maintain the heart's function and EMS contacted, biologic death may result
   2. A cardiac emergency may be caused by accidents (electric shock, drowning, trauma, asphyxiation) or coronary disease

B. Causes and pathophysiology—coronary disease and emergencies may result from a change in the heart's function (arrhythmia, hypertrophy, ischemia), blood vessels (atherosclerosis, arteriosclerosis), blood volume (shock, hemorrhage), or blood composition (anemia)

C. Prevention of a cardiac emergency
1. Identify clients at risk with thorough health history taking
2. Recognize signs and symptoms
3. Promptly refer the client to a physician
4. If coronary symptoms develop in the dental office, rapid access to EMS is indicated

D. Cardiovascular diseases
1. Hypertension—persistent BP elevation indicates the heart is working harder to supply blood through the arteries; the probability of a CVA (stroke), MI, congestive heart failure, and kidney disease may be increased because of a consistently elevated BP
   a. Signs and symptoms—may include headaches, dizziness, or no symptoms; consistent, elevated blood pressure readings
   b. Prevention of medical emergencies—for recommendations regarding treating clients with elevated blood pressure (see earlier discussion under the section "Blood Pressure")
2. Angina pectoris—a transient (temporary) ischemia (lack of oxygenated blood) of the myocardium (heart muscle), usually manifested by chest pain or discomfort; angina occurs because the heart requires more oxygen than the amount produced
   a. Signs and symptoms
      (1) Sudden onset of a dull chest pain or discomfort that may be described as a constant pressing, crushing, burning, or squeezing sensation
      (2) Pain may radiate to the shoulders (left is most common), arms, neck, mandible, or epigastrium
      (3) Pain is reproducible and predictable and may last 1 to 10 minutes
      (4) Pain may be precipitated by exertion, emotional stress, cold weather, or a heavy meal and may be accompanied by weakness and shortness of breath
      (5) Client may appear apprehensive, have labored breathing, or is sweating
      (6) Heart rate and BP are elevated
   b. Prevention
      (1) Schedule short, late-morning or early-afternoon appointments
      (2) Take a thorough health history, identifying clients with angina; discuss questions related to the angina episodes, cause, length of episode, medication, effectiveness of medication, frequency of episodes, and usual symptoms
      (3) Dismiss clients with unstable angina (pain is increasing in duration, intensity, and frequency) and refer to a physician
      (4) Place the client's nitroglycerin medication within easy reach of the clinician and client to use in the event of an emergency

(5) Use stress reduction protocol
(6) Monitor vital signs
(7) Administer low-flow oxygen during appointment
(8) Administer local anesthetic for pain control when needed (maximum of 2 carpules local anesthesia with 1:100,000 epinephrine, not to exceed 0.04 mg epinephrine)
(9) Administer nitrous oxide–oxygen (N_2O-O_2) to provide psychosedation
(10) Dismiss the client if he or she shows signs of fatigue, sweating, anxiety, or fidgeting

   c. Management of an emergency
      (1) If the client has no history of angina, follow the procedures listed later for myocardial infarction
      (2) Place patient in supine position
      (3) Implement CAB, as needed
      (4) Administer nitroglycerin
          (a) The client's nitroglycerin is preferred
          (b) Administer 1 nitroglycerin tablet or 1 to 2 metered sprays every 5 minutes; do not exceed three doses within 15-minutes
          (c) The client's discomfort should lessen within 2 to 4 minutes
          (d) If the client's discomfort has not decreased significantly after the first dose, the second dose should come from the office emergency kit
          (e) Nitroglycerin should not be taken if the client exhibits hypotension
      (5) Administer oxygen
      (6) Monitor the client's vital signs
      (7) If pain is not relieved within 10 minutes, the client requests EMS, or the pain returns, summon EMS and administer aspirin
      (8) If pain is relieved by rest and nitroglycerin, encourage rest, discontinue oral health services for that appointment, and refer the client for further evaluation by a physician
      (9) Treatment should be modified for the next visit to alleviate the client's stress

3. Myocardial infarction (MI)—diminished or interrupted supply of oxygenated blood to the heart that causes death (necrosis) of part of the heart muscle, resulting in impaired heart function and diminished cardiac output; if a large area of the heart is affected, the heart may be unable to function and may stop beating (cardiac arrest)
   a. Signs and symptoms
      (1) Chest pain, often described as a "crushing pressure," is the classic symptom of an MI; the pain often radiates to the arm (most frequently the left arm), neck, or mandible; the pain intensifies and lasts for more than 15 to 20 minutes; nitroglycerin, rest, and changing positions do not alleviate the pain
      (2) Client may have an ashen-gray appearance and may exhibit a cold sweat, nausea, vomiting, dyspnea, dizziness, weakness, and the feeling of impending doom

(3) Vital signs most often will present as a weak, thready, rapid pulse; low BP; and rapid, shallow respirations

(4) Women do not always present with chest pain but rather may experience more vague warning signs, such as fatigue, nausea, vomiting, dizziness, breathlessness, back pain, or deep throbbing in the left or right bicep or forearm

(5) A client who is developing signs of acute pulmonary edema will begin to have a slight dry cough; this will develop into a paroxysmal nocturnal dyspnea, asthmatic-type wheezing, pallor, sweating, frothy blood-tinged sputum, tachypnea, dyspnea, and a feeling of suffocation

b. Prevention for clients who have had a previous MI

(1) Take a thorough health history to identify clients at risk

(2) Clients who have had a previous MI should have vital signs checked at the start and at the end of each appointment

(3) Implement stress reduction protocol

(4) Administer oxygen at a flow rate of 3 to 5 L/min

(5) Administer N_2O-O_2 sedation to decrease the client's stress

(6) Maintain adequate pain control through administration of local anesthesia with 1:100,000 epinephrine

(7) Keep appointments short, and dismiss the client if he or she begins to appear anxious and is showing signs of increased stress

(8) Do not treat a client for the first 30 days after an MI

(9) Refer clients to their physician if they appear unable to handle the stress of a dental appointment

c. Management of an emergency

(1) Immediately activate the EMS if the client does not have a history of angina, or if client with history of angina is experiencing chest pains different than normal, or requests the EMS

(2) Position a conscious client according to client preference

(3) Implement CAB

(4) Monitor the client's vital signs (BP, heart rate/rhythm, respirations) every 5 minutes

(5) Administer oxygen at a flow rate of 4 to 6 L/min

(6) Administer nitroglycerin unless the client exhibits hypotension (systolic BP <90 mm Hg or <30 mm Hg below baseline); administer 1 nitroglycerin tablet; pain should decrease within 2 to 4 minutes if angina is the cause of the pain; pain will continue or return if the cause is an MI

(7) Administer aspirin (160-325 mg) to prevent thrombus formation

4. Congestive heart failure (CHF)—results when the heart is unable to pump an adequate amount of blood to meet the body's demands; precipitating factors include

hypertension, coronary artery disease (CAD), congenital and valvular heart disease, toxins, inflammatory disorders, and endocrinopathies

a. Signs and symptoms

(1) Client may complain of weakness, anxiety, shortness of breath, unexplained sudden weight gain, cough, and swelling of the ankles

(2) Client may present with edema, cyanosis, elevated BP, narrowed pulse pressure, tachycardia, increased respiratory rate, and prominent jugular veins

(3) Left ventricular failure causes respiratory distress with accompanying signs of weakness, fatigue, and dyspnea

(4) Right ventricular failure causes venous congestion with accompanying signs of cyanosis, coolness in the extremities, peripheral edema, and prominent jugular veins

b. Prevention of an emergency

(1) Identify clients at risk through a thorough health history

(2) Refer clients with symptomatic CHF (experience CHF symptoms during normal activities) for a medical consultation before elective dental care; clients who are asymptomatic and do not experience CHF symptoms during normal exertion may be seen for dental treatment

(3) Implement stress reduction protocol

(4) Administer low-flow oxygen at a rate of 3 to 4 L/min

(5) Position so that the client is comfortable, generally upright or semi-supine; if the client has orthopnea (inability to breath when reclined), needs to be sent for a medical referral

(6) Watch for signs of acute pulmonary edema (see earlier myocardial infarction discussion)

c. Management of acute pulmonary edema

(1) Contact EMS

(2) Position a conscious client according to client preference

(3) Calm the client

(4) Perform CAB as needed

(5) Administer oxygen at a high flow rate of 10 L/min

(6) Monitor vital signs every 5 minutes (BP, heart rate/rhythm, respirations)

(7) Perform a bloodless phlebotomy if symptoms of acute pulmonary edema are present—BP cuffs are used as tourniquets on three extremities (below shoulders and below the groin), always leaving one of the extremities without a cuff; the cuffs are inflated for 5 to 10 minutes, removed, and rotated

(8) Administer 2 or 3 nitroglycerin tablets or sprays every 5 to 10 minutes unless the client is hypotensive

5. Cardiac arrest or sudden cardiac death (SCD)—the unexpected cessation of heart and lung functions as a result of an electrical malfunction of the heart

a. Cardiac arrest is cardiopulmonary collapse caused by ventricular fibrillation, CAD, respiratory arrest, shock, drugs, arrhythmias, accidents, or anaphylaxis; some sources consider cardiac arrest and SCD to be the same, whereas other sources consider them to be different

b. Signs and symptoms
   (1) Client loses consciousness and has no pulse, BP, or respirations (clinical death)
   (2) A majority of clients will experience signs and symptoms before SCD, including chest pain, cough, shortness of breath, fainting, dizziness, palpitations, and fatigue
   (3) About 25% of those who experience SCD or cardiac arrest will have no signs or symptoms

c. Management of the emergency
   (1) Activate EMS
   (2) Position the client in supine position
   (3) Begin CAB
   (4) Implement defibrillation
   (5) Continue CAB and defibrillation until the EMS arrives

Allergic Reactions[1,2,8]

A. Allergic reactions occur from a wide range of physiologic responses caused by hypersensitivity to an allergen

B. Causes
   1. Allergic responses may be evoked by drugs, pollens, foods, chemicals, insect bites, and other factors
   2. When the body comes into contact with these substances, an antigen-antibody reaction occurs and results in an inappropriate response by the body's immune system

C. Preventing allergic reactions
   1. Take a thorough health history, which should reveal a previous history of allergic reactions to drugs or materials used in dental therapeutics
   2. Ask the client who has a prior history of an allergic reaction to describe its type and severity
   3. Refer the client with a suspected allergy for evaluation by a physician

D. Types of allergic reactions
   1. Delayed allergic reactions
      a. Signs and symptoms include skin manifestations such as erythema (redness), urticaria (hives), and angioedema (swelling) or respiratory reactions (respiratory distress, wheezing, dyspnea, angioedema) that occur hours or even days after contact with an allergen
      b. Treatment of delayed allergic reactions
         (1) Assess the need for CAB.
         (2) Administer antihistamine and/or oxygen if allergic reaction is severe
         (3) If the reaction persists, the client should be accompanied to a physician; if a delayed reaction becomes severe, epinephrine may need to be administered

   (4) If epinephrine is administered, EMS should be contacted
   2. Immediate reaction or anaphylaxis
      a. Immediate allergic reactions occur within 60 minutes of exposure to the antigen and are characterized by urticarial reactions (hives), abdominal cramps, diarrhea, nausea, angioedema, rhinitis (inflamed mucous membranes of the nose), respiratory distress (bronchospasms, dyspnea), cyanosis, and cardiovascular changes, including hypotension, rapid weak pulse, tachycardia, and arrhythmias, which may progress to cardiovascular collapse
      b. Types of immediate allergic reactions
         (1) Food allergies irritate the gastrointestinal tract
         (2) Bronchospasms affect the respiratory tract
         (3) Urticarial reactions affect the skin
         (4) Anaphylactic reactions can be localized (laryngeal edema) or generalized
      c. Treatment for immediate nonanaphylactic reactions
         (1) Assess for CAB
         (2) Monitor vital signs every 5 minutes
         (3) Administer an antihistamine and oxygen
         (4) Position a hypotensive client in the supine position
         (5) If the client exhibits signs of cardiovascular or respiratory distress, or if the heart rate, respirations, or BP change, administer epinephrine and contact EMS
      d. Treatment for bronchospasms
         (1) Position the client in the upright position
         (2) Assess for CAB
         (3) Summon EMS
         (4) Calm the client
         (5) Administer a bronchodilator
         (6) Administer an antihistamine
      e. Treatment of laryngeal edema
         (1) Position client according to client preference, generally upright
         (2) Assess for CAB; continue to monitor airway
         (3) Contact EMS
         (4) Administer 0.3 mL of 1:1000 epinephrine; repeat in 3 to 5 minutes if needed
         (5) Administer oxygen
         (6) Administer histamine blocker (diphenhydramine)
      f. Treatment for generalized anaphylaxis
         (1) Position the client in the supine position with feet elevated if hypotensive or unconscious
         (2) Implement CAB
         (3) Summon EMS
         (4) Administer 0.3 mL 1:1000 epinephrine in a preloaded syringe; administer a second dose if condition does not improve within 5 minutes; an additional dose can be administered at 5- to 10-minute intervals depending on cardiovascular response
         (5) Administer oxygen at a rate of 5 to 6 L/min
         (6) Administer antihistamine, 25 to 50 mg of diphenhydramine, orally (PO), intramuscularly (IM), or intravenously (IV)

(7) Administer corticosteroid, 100 mg of hydrocortisone, subcutaneously (SC), IM, or IV, once the client has improved

(8) Perform CPR as needed

(9) An insufficient dose of medication could cause anaphylaxis to return within 3 to 10 hours, known as *biphasic anaphylaxis*

Drug-Related Emergencies and Poisoning[1,2,4]

Basic Concepts

A. Drug-related emergencies include allergic response, overdose, psychogenic response (syncope or hyperventilation), idiosyncratic reaction, drug interactions, and complications in a client who is chemically dependent

B. A thorough health history should reveal the client's drug allergies, previous adverse reactions, or chemical dependency; these agents, materials, and drugs must be avoided during dental and dental hygiene care

Specific Reactions

A. Local anesthetic—result of psychogenic or allergic response, toxic overdose, or chemical intoxication

1. Psychogenic response—usually manifests as syncope or hyperventilation; generally the result of fear of the injection rather than a reaction to the local anesthetic agent; syncope and hyperventilation should be managed according to the criteria described earlier in related sections

2. Allergic reactions—occur more often with ester-type anesthetics (procaine); very rare and should be managed by the criteria established under the previous section on "Allergic Reactions"

3. Toxic overdoses—result from delayed biotransformation or elimination of the agent, excess total dose, or IV injection of the agent

   a. Prevention—client factors such as age, weight, and predisposing medical conditions and drug factors such as amount, rate of injection, and type of anesthetic used must be considered when administering local anesthesia

   b. Signs and symptoms—very talkative, agitated, anxious, confused, slurred speech; elevated BP, heart rate, and respiratory rate; client may complain of headache, dizziness, and disorientation and may lose consciousness; with moderate to high levels of local anesthetic, the client may have seizures, lose consciousness, and undergo respiratory arrest

   c. A mild overdose reaction generally occurs within 5 to 30 minutes of the injection

   d. Steps to manage a toxic overdose

   (1) Assess CAB

   (2) Administer oxygen, and ask the client to hyperventilate to lower arterial carbon dioxide tension ($PaCO_2$) levels; this will lower the risk of a seizure

   (3) Monitor vital signs every 5 minutes until the client has recovered

   (a) After recovery, the client should be assessed by a physician or hospital

   (b) If the client experiences a seizure with an anesthetic overdose reaction or has a severe overdose reaction (signs and symptoms occur during or immediately after administration of anesthetic), the following steps should be followed:

   [1] Place the client in the supine position

   [2] Summon EMS

   [3] Assess CAB

   [4] Administer oxygen, and have the client hyperventilate

   [5] Monitor the client's vital signs every 5 minutes

   [6] Administer an anticonvulsant IV if needed; if an anticonvulsant has been administered, EMS should be contacted

4. Chemically dependent client

   a. Prevent emergencies by identifying the chemically dependent client and adjusting the dental treatment accordingly

   b. Cocaine-intoxicated client

   (1) Do not administer anesthetic containing epinephrine within in 24 hours of cocaine use

   (2) If cardiac arrest occurs after administration of an anesthetic containing epinephrine, follow the management procedures listed earlier for cardiac arrest (SCD)

B. Fluoride poisoning

1. Some oral health care products contain enough fluoride to be hazardous, especially to children

   a. 1 ounce of topical fluoride gel or one 8-ounce tube of fluoridated toothpaste could be life threatening to a small child

   b. A lethal dose of fluoride for a child is 500 to 1000 mg, depending on the child's weight and size

2. Signs and symptoms of fluoride overdose

   a. Nausea, abdominal pain, excessive salivation, thirst, vomiting, and diarrhea within 30 minutes of ingestion

   b. Burning sensation in the oral cavity and a sore tongue may also be present

   c. In severe cases, muscle cramping, bronchospasm, and cardiac arrest may occur

3. Treatment of acute fluoride poisoning (for adults and children age 6 years and older)

   a. Administer ipecac syrup to induce vomiting (only if client has a gag reflex, is conscious, and is not convulsing)

   b. Administer milk or 1% calcium gluconate or calcium chloride PO

   c. Activate the EMS

   d. Implement CAB

   e. N_2O-O_2 oversedation

   f. Sign—lethargy

   g. Management of emergency

   (1) Increase O_2 intake and decrease N_2O intake

   (2) Assess CAB

Cerebrovascular Accident (CVA)[2,8]

A. CVA, or stroke, results when the supply of oxygen to the brain cells is disrupted by ischemia, infarction, or hemorrhage of the cerebral blood vessels; co-contributing factors include tobacco use, hypertension, diabetes mellitus, and CAD

B. Prevention
   1. Take a thorough health history, and evaluate vital signs to help identify clients at risk for a CVA
   2. Do not alter anticoagulant medication before dental care for post-CVA clients
   3. Post-CVA clients should not be seen for at least 6 months after CVA or TIA
   4. Post-CVA clients with systolic readings above 160 mm Hg and diastolic readings above 95 mm Hg should be referred to their physician for an immediate consultation and should not be seen for dental treatment
   5. Stress reduction protocol should be followed
      a. Appointments should be short and scheduled for midmorning
      b. N_2O-O_2 can be administered; a pulse oximeter should be used to monitor oxygen saturation (So_2) levels
      c. Light oral sedation (benzodiazepines) can be administered; CNS suppressants should not be taken
      d. Pain control should be monitored; a local anesthetic with 1:100,000 or 1:200,000 epinephrine can be given in limited amounts

C. Signs and symptoms
   1. Clients could experience sudden weakness on one side (hemiparesis), difficulty of speech, temporary loss of vision (especially in one eye), unexplained dizziness, altered level of consciousness, shortness of breath, nausea, sudden severe headache, and confusion
   2. A client experiencing CVA may have an elevated BP and cardiac arrhythmias (irregular heartbeats)

D. Treatment
   1. Conscious client
      a. Position the client upright
      b. Activate EMS
      c. Assess CAB
      d. Monitor the client's vital signs every 5 minutes (heart rate, rhythm, BP)
      e. Administer oxygen
      f. Do not administer CNS depressants
   2. Unconscious client
      a. Place client in the supine position with feet elevated unless BP is noticeably elevated, in which case, place the client in the semi-Fowler position (supine position with head and chest elevated)
      b. Continue to monitor the vital signs (heart rate, rhythm, BP, respirations)

E. Transient ischemic attacks (TIAs)
   1. TIAs, or "mini-strokes," can present with similar symptoms as a stroke; however, the client recovers within 10 minutes
   2. Because of a high risk for future strokes, a TIA requires immediate referral to a physician for preventive treatment

Seizures and Convulsive Disorders[1,2,8]

A. Seizures and convulsive disorders are the result of changes in brain function
   1. Seizures—characterized by alterations in consciousness, motor function, and sensory perceptions; usually have a rapid onset and brief duration (1 to 3 minutes)
   2. Convulsions—involuntary contractions of the voluntary muscles
   3. Epilepsy or seizure disorder—condition characterized by recurrent seizures and convulsions

B. Preventing seizures
   1. Thorough health history should identify an individual with a history of seizures or convulsive disorders
   2. Ask questions that address causes, type, and severity of seizure and the aura the client experiences prior to a seizure
      a. If a client has a history of seizures, determine if medications have been prescribed to control seizures and if the client has taken the required medication before the appointment
   3. Short appointments scheduled early in the day may reduce the likelihood of a seizure in the oral health care setting
   4. Administration of N_2O-O_2 with at least 20% oxygen is recommended for the apprehensive client with seizure disorders
   5. Benzodiazepines for oral conscious sedation may also be effective for clients who are less apprehensive
   6. Administration of local anesthesia is the most likely cause of a seizure in a nonepileptic client in the dental setting; care should be taken in the administration, dose, and type of anesthesia administered
   7. Alcohol can precipitate a seizure; therefore a client who has a history of seizures should not be seen for dental care if alcohol has been consumed

C. Types of seizures
   1. Convulsive—generalized tonic-clonic (grand mal) seizure
      a. Signs and symptoms include an aura (change in taste, smell, or sight precedes the seizure), loss of consciousness (may be several minutes), an epileptic cry (sudden expulsion of air through glottis), involuntary tonic-clonic muscle contractions, altered breathing, and sometimes involuntary defecation or urination
      b. After the seizure, respirations should spontaneously return, muscles relax, and consciousness returns; the person may have a headache or muscle aches and may be drowsy or disoriented
   2. Nonconvulsive—absence (petit mal) seizure
      a. Signs and symptoms are sudden momentary loss of awareness without loss of postural tone and a blank stare for up to 90 seconds, although the individual may twitch or blink
      b. The person is usually unaware of the seizure
   3. Complex partial (psychomotor) seizure—signs and symptoms may include an aura, purposeless movements, and loss of awareness lasting for only a few minutes

D. Management of seizure
1. Convulsive seizure— three phases:
   a. Prodromal phase—marked by the presence of an aura
      (1) Prepare for the seizure
      (2) Remove all dental equipment and removable appliances from the client's mouth
      (3) Place the client in the supine position with legs elevated
      (4) Clear the area of all sharp and dangerous objects
   b. Ictal phase—the tonic-clonic phase of the seizure
      (1) Make no attempts to restrain the client or place any objects in the mouth
      (2) Protect the client's head, if needed, by placing a soft item under the head
      (3) Assess and establish an airway
      (4) Monitor vital signs, and assess CAB, as needed
      (5) Activate EMS
      (6) Prevent injury
   c. Postictal phase—most dangerous phase of the seizure; the body experiences a generalized depression that affects the central nervous, respiratory, and cardiovascular systems; death can occur during this phase
      (1) Keep the client in supine position
      (2) Continue CAB
      (3) Monitor vital signs every 5 minutes (BP, respirations, heart rate)
   d. Management of an emergency involving a convulsive seizure
      (1) Place the client in the supine position with feet elevated
      (2) Remove all objects that could harm the client
      (3) Lightly restrain the client to protect from injury
      (4) Consider contacting EMS
      (5) Assess CAB
      (6) Once seizure ceases, administer oxygen at a flow rate of 5 to 6 L/min
      (7) Assess CAB
      (8) Monitor vital signs (BP, heart rate, respirations)
      (9) Reassure the client when consciousness returns
      (10) Allow the client to recover
      (11) Assess the client to send home, to physician, or to hospital
2. Status epilepticus
   a. Grand mal (tonic-clonic) seizure that lasts longer than 5 minutes
   b. Contact EMS if not already contacted
   c. Assess CAB
   d. Once seizure ceases, administer oxygen at a flow rate of 5 to 6 L/min
   e. Administer anticonvulsant drug IV and 50% dextrose IV
3. Nonconvulsive seizure in the oral health care setting
   a. Terminate the dental procedure
   b. Closely observe the client
   c. Reassure the client when the seizure has concluded
   d. Discharge the client when he or she has recovered
   e. If the seizure lasts longer than 5 minutes, contact EMS
   f. Assess CAB

Diabetes Mellitus[1,2,8]

A. Definition—characterized by elevated levels of blood glucose resulting from an impaired ability to produce or use the hormone insulin
B. Four types of diabetes
1. Type 1, or insulin-dependent, diabetes mellitus usually occurs in young persons and is more likely to precipitate a diabetic emergency known as *ketoacidosis* or *diabetic coma*; primarily hereditary or genetic
2. Type 2, or non–insulin-dependent, diabetes mellitus usually occurs in adulthood and rarely results in an emergency situation; clients with type 2 diabetes may become insulin dependent; type 2 is a milder form of diabetes than type 1
3. Gestational diabetes occurs during pregnancy
4. Impaired glucose tolerance, also known as *prediabetes*; these clients are at risk for developing diabetes and cardiovascular disease
C. Emergencies related to diabetes may result from two different situations:
1. Client has too much insulin (hyperinsulinism), resulting in hypoglycemia (low blood sugar); blood glucose levels are below 50 mg/dL
   a. Typical causes are increased insulin dosage, missed meal, vomiting, or excessive exercise
   b. Hypoglycemia can lead to *insulin shock*
2. Client has inadequate insulin, resulting in hyperglycemia (high blood sugar); blood glucose levels are above 250 mg/dL
   a. Hyperglycemia can lead to ketoacidosis and diabetic coma
   b. Occurs most often with type 1 diabetes from inadequate insulin levels, infection, or MI
   c. Can occur with type 2 diabetes from stress, epinephrine therapy, or medication
   d. Emergency situations develop slowly and generally take more than 48 hours from the onset of signs and symptoms
D. Prevention
1. A thorough health history is essential to prevent diabetic emergencies in the oral health care setting; factors to determine when taking the health history include the type and severity of diabetes and the client's medications and their frequency, duration, and dosage; medical consultation may be necessary
2. Clients whose diabetes is not under control or who exhibit the signs and symptoms listed next should postpone elective dental and dental hygiene care
3. Establish that the client's medications have been taken according to prescriptions, and that the client has eaten meals according to schedule on the day of the appointment
4. Minimize the client's stress and anxiety in the dental office
5. Appointments should be scheduled to ensure that the client is rested and that the client's meal and medication schedules are not interrupted; morning appointments are best, 1 to 1½ hours after breakfast

E. Signs and symptoms
   1. Clients with uncontrolled diabetes may be experiencing xerostomia, infection, poor healing, increased incidence and severity of caries, candidiasis, gingivitis, periodontal disease, periapical abscesses, or burning mouth syndrome
   2. Signs and symptoms of hypoglycemia may occur suddenly or gradually; clients experience an altered state of consciousness (confusion, anxiousness, incoherence, uncooperative or bizarre behavior), hunger, headache, pale moist skin, hyperthermia, dizziness, weakness, trembling, tonic-clonic movements, normal or depressed respirations, hypotension or loss of consciousness; if left untreated, will lead to coma and death
   3. Signs and symptoms of conscious clients experiencing diabetic ketoacidosis or impending diabetic coma include the "classic" signs of polydipsia (excessive thirst), polyuria (excessive urination), polyphagia (excessive hunger), nausea, vomiting, dry flushed skin, deep and rapid respirations (Kussmaul respirations or air hunger), weak and rapid pulse, and a "fruity" breath odor; blurred vision, hypotension, and unconsciousness may follow; if left untreated, will lead to coma and death
F. Management of the emergency
   1. Regardless of the cause of the emergency, a diabetic client is treated based on consciousness or unconsciousness, *not* on hyperglycemia or hypoglycemia; all diabetic emergencies are treated based on the assumption the emergency is hypoglycemia
   2. Treatment for the conscious client
      a. Place the client in a comfortable position
      b. Assess CAB and perform BLS as needed
      c. Administer oral carbohydrates and sugars (orange juice, candy bar, soft drink), 3 to 4 ounces every 5 to 10 minutes
      d. Observe for 1 hour before dismissing client
   3. Treatment for the unconscious client
      a. Place the client in supine position with feet slightly elevated
      b. Assess CAB and perform BLS as needed
      c. Activate EMS
      d. Administer oxygen, 5 to 6 L/min flow rate
      e. Administer 5% dextrose IV, or glucagon 1 mg IM; administer 0.5 mg of 1:1000 epinephrine if dextrose or glucagon is not available
      f. Monitor vital signs every 5 minutes

Acute Adrenal Insufficiency, or Adrenal Crisis[2,8]

A. Definition
   1. Adrenal crisis is a life-threatening situation
   2. Clients having adrenal insufficiency may go into cardiac arrest or shock
B. Causes
   1. Acute adrenal insufficiency (adrenal crisis) occurs when the adrenal gland is unable to produce enough cortisol to enable the body to respond to a stressful situation, either physical or psychological
   2. In the dental office, stress from surgical procedures or severe anxiety of dental and dental hygiene care can cause acute adrenal insufficiency

   3. Results from:
      a. An abrupt withdrawal of exogenous administration of glucocorticosteroids
      b. Primary adrenal insufficiency (Addison's disease)
      c. Secondary adrenal insufficiency, which occurs when the body is unable to produce cortisol because of prolonged exogenous glucocorticosteroid use and therefore cannot meet the increased demand for cortisol during a time of stress
C. Prevention—clients who are extremely anxious or who will be undergoing surgical procedures and who are at risk for adrenal suppression should be given two to four times their normal dose of glucocorticosteroids on the day of the appointment
D. Signs and symptoms
   1. Clients will exhibit confusion; weakness; lethargy; abdominal, lower back, and leg pain; extreme fatigue; wet, clammy skin; headache; nausea; and vomiting
   2. The cardiovascular system will deteriorate; pulse may be rapid and weak; the client may develop hypotension, followed by shock-like symptoms and unconsciousness or coma
E. Management of emergency
   1. Activate the EMS
   2. Place the client in supine position with feet slightly elevated
   3. Implement CAB; open and maintain the airway
   4. Monitor vital signs every 5 minutes (BP, heart rate)
   5. Administer high-flow oxygen at rate of 5 to 10 L/min
   6. Administer 100 mg of glucocorticosteroid or 4 mg of dexamethasone IV
   7. May need to also administer a vasopressor drug (epinephrine 1:1000, 0.05 mL) if client is unconscious
   8. Transport to hospital via EMS

Aspirated Materials[2]

A. Dental materials and instruments may be aspirated during oral health care because of the client's position, diminished responses caused by drugs, and diminished "oral awareness" caused by local anesthesia
B. Prevention of aspiration of materials can be accomplished through use of a rubber dam during many dental procedures
C. If a client is already reclining in the dental chair and aspirates an object into the oropharyngeal area, lower the back of the chair, and place client on his or her left side, using gravity to assist the client's efforts to dislodge the object; encourage coughing; however, the client may want to sit upright
D. If an object is aspirated into the trachea, activate the EMS; manage as mild or severe obstruction; the client may want to sit upright to facilitate breathing and coughing
E. If an object that has been swallowed cannot be located, the client must be escorted to seek further medical evaluation; a chest x-ray film may be indicated to rule out aspiration into a lung
   Unless specifically noted, client positioning was determined by the client's preference. Although not stated, dental treatment was discontinued at the onset of all emergencies.

CONCLUSION

This chapter is only an approximate guideline for some common medical emergencies encountered in dental hygiene practice. Dental professionals should use standard operating protocols to manage emergencies and review or practice them regularly. Please consult current textbooks and journals for detailed information, and refer to the American Heart Association and American Red Cross for current protocol and training in BLS, ACLS, and EMS (see "Website Information and Resources").

Website Information and Resources

Source	Website Address	Description
eMedicine, Inc.	http://emedicine.medscape.com/emergency_medicine	Medical emergency reference
American Academy of Family Physicians	www.aafp.org	Health topic search and health information handouts and links to health-related sites; search under client care
American Heart Association	http://www.heart.org/HEARTORG/	National directory of resources related to heart diseases
Nemours Center for Children's Health Media	www.kidshealth.org	First-aid and safety section; also contains articles and fact sheets on a variety of health topics
Medline Plus Encyclopedia	http://www.nlm.nih.gov/medlineplus/encyclopedia.html	Links to A.D.A.M Medical Encyclopedia with over 4,000 articles
	http://www.nlm.nih.gov/medlineplus/	Link to many health related topics
Mayo Clinic	http://www.mayoclinic.org/diseases-conditions/	Link to Mayo Clinic's comprehensive guide of health-related topics

REFERENCES

1. Grimes E: *Medical emergencies: essentials for the dental professional,* ed 2, Boston, 2014, Pearson.
2. Malamed S: *Medical emergencies in the dental office,* ed 7, St Louis, 2015, Mosby Elsevier.
3. Pickett F, Gurenlian J: *Preventing medical emergencies: use of the medical history,* Baltimore, 2009, Lippincott Williams & Wilkins.
4. Bowen DM, Walsh MM: Medical emergencies. In Darby ML, Walsh MM, editors: *Dental hygiene theory and practice,* ed 4, St Louis, 2015, Elsevier.
5. US Department of Health and Human Services: *Seventh report of the Joint National Committee on Prevention, Detection, Evaluation, and Treatment of High Blood Pressure (JNC 7),* NIH Pub No 03-5231, May 2003.
6. American Heart Association: *BLS for healthcare providers: student manual,* Dallas, 2011, AHA.
7. Hazinski F, editor: *American Heart Association guidelines for CPR and ECC 2010,* Dallas, 2010, AHA.
8. Little J, Falace D, Miller C, Nelson R: *Dental management of the medically compromised client,* ed 8, St Louis, 2013, Elsevier.

CHAPTER 21 REVIEW QUESTIONS

Answers and rationales to review questions are available on this text's accompanying Evolve site. See inside front cover for details.

evolve

1. **Which of the following emergencies occurs when the cells do not receive enough oxygen because blood is not circulating through the tissues adequately?**
   a. Hypertension
   b. Shock
   c. Asthma
   d. Hyperventilation
2. **Which automated external defibrillator (AED) can be used on infants and children ages 1 to 8 years?**
   a. Manual
   b. Adult automatic
   c. Pediatric-capable
   d. All the above
3. **How frequently can nitroglycerin be administered for the treatment of angina?**
   a. 1 tablet every 5 minutes, not to exceed 3 tablets in 15 minutes
   b. 2 or 3 tablets every 5 minutes
   c. 1 tablet every 10 minutes, not to exceed 3 tablets in 30 minutes
   d. 2 or 3 tablets every 10 minutes
4. **Your client has had a cerebrovascular accident (CVA). How long before his next dental hygiene appointment should you have him discontinue his anticoagulant?**
   a. The morning of the appointment
   b. 2 days
   c. 4 days
   d. He should continue to take his anticoagulant.
5. **Your client has indicated a fear of injections and begins to breathe rapidly, complains of tingling or numbness, and is experiencing tachycardia. Your client most likely is experiencing:**
   a. Hypertension
   b. Hyperventilation

c. Congestive heart failure

d. Shock

6. **Heart rates of infants and children are slower than an adult's normal heart rate, and pediatric rates will vary based on age, gender, and size.**

   a. Both statement are TRUE.

   b. Both statements are FALSE.

   c. The first statement is TRUE; the second statement is FALSE.

   d. The first statement is FALSE; the second statement is TRUE.

7. **Which of the following is the most common type of shock and can be caused by dehydration from vomiting and diarrhea?**

   a. Cardiogenic shock

   b. Distributive shock

   c. Hypovolemic shock

   d. Neurogenic shock

8. **Your client is asymptomatic but presents with blood pressure of 168/107 mm Hg. What should you do?**

   a. Send home and reschedule for a morning appointment in 2 weeks

   b. Refer to the client's physician for a consultation before seeing

   c. Provide hygiene and refer to the client's physician to be seen within 1 month

   d. Activate the EMS to have your client taken to the hospital

9. **Clients receiving glucocorticosteroid therapy should NOT be seen for elective dental care. They should postpone treatment until they have discontinued glucocorticosteroids for at least 1 year.**

   a. Both statements are TRUE.

   b. Both statements are FALSE.

   c. The first statement is TRUE; the second statement is FALSE.

   d. The first statement is FALSE; the second statement is TRUE.

10. **In addition to administering 0.3 mL of 1:1000 epinephrine and additional doses if needed, which of the following is also administered to treat anaphylactic shock?**

    a. Oxygen at a rate of 5 to 6 mL/min

    b. Antihistamine (25-50 mg of diphenhydramine)

    c. Corticosteroid (100 mg of hydrocortisone)

    d. All the above

11. **All the following management procedures should be utilized to prevent an angina attack for a client with a history of angina EXCEPT:**

    a. Short appointments scheduled in the late morning or early afternoon

    b. Do not see a client with unstable angina, and refer to his or her physician

    c. Administer low-flow oxygen

    d. Use local anesthetic for pain control; maximum 4 carpules of 1:100,000 epinephrine

12. **Treatment for shock includes placing the client in the supine position and monitoring vital signs. Treatment for shock also includes administering IV fluids.**

    a. Both statements are TRUE.

    b. Both statements are FALSE.

    c. The first statement is TRUE; the second statement is FALSE.

    d. The first statement is FALSE; the second statement is TRUE.

13. **Oxygen is used for all the following emergencies EXCEPT:**

    a. Hyperventilation

    b. Syncope

    c. Angina

    d. Shock

14. **If your client's blood pressure is 125/85 mm Hg, you should check BP every:**

    a. 6 months

    b. Year

    c. 2 years

    d. You only need to take a baseline measurement.

15. **Stress reduction protocol includes which of the following?**

    a. Creating a low-stress environment

    b. Administering a premedication (optional)

    c. Establishing good client rapport

    d. All the above

16. **Your diabetic client complains that he is very thirsty and nauseated, and you notice he is flushed, is taking deep rapid breaths, and his breath has a fruity odor. First, you realize he is suffering from hyperglycemia. Second, you know the BEST way to manage this emergency is to administer insulin.**

    a. Both statements are TRUE.

    b. Both statements are FALSE.

    c. The first statement is TRUE; the second statement is FALSE.

    d. The first statement is FALSE; the second statement is TRUE.

17. **Match the six types of shock to their corresponding causes (a to f).**

    _____ 1. Hypovolemic shock

    _____ 2. Neurogenic shock

    _____ 3. Cardiogenic shock

    _____ 4. Anaphylactic shock

    _____ 5. Septic shock

    _____ 6. Obstructive shock

    a. Obstruction of blood flow prevents the heart from beating

    b. Inadequate cardiac output to the peripheral organs and tissues

    c. An acute systemic infection prevents blood flow to the cells, tissues, and organs

    d. Vasoconstriction results from impaired nerve impulses to the blood vessels or loss of sympathetic nerve activity

    e. Inadequate blood volume

    f. Histamine release causes sudden vasodilation

18. **Which of the following is the result of excessive loss of carbon dioxide?**

    a. Asthma

b. Hyperventilation
c. Orthostatic hypotension
d. Shock

19. **During his appointment, your client is appears flushed, anxious, and short-tempered. He begins to cough and wheeze, is experiencing dyspnea, and begins to appear cyanotic. The emergency your client is experiencing is related to which of the following?**
    a. Asthma
    b. Congestive heart failure
    c. Overdose reaction to local anesthetic
    d. Angina

20. **Emergencies involving diabetic patients occur MOST frequently with which type of diabetes?**
    a. Type 1
    b. Type 2
    c. Gestational
    d. Impaired glucose tolerance

21. **Nitroglycerin is contraindicated for emergency treatment of angina or congestive heart failure when the client has which of the following?**
    a. Hypoglycemia
    b. Hyperglycemia
    c. Hypotension
    d. Hypertension

22. **Which of the following phases of a seizure poses the greatest risk for a client?**
    a. Prodromal
    b. Ictal
    c. Postictal
    d. All phases pose equal risk.

23. **The FIRST step in preventing a medical emergency is to:**
    a. Take the client's vital signs
    b. Create a stress-free environment
    c. Become familiar with the client's health history
    d. Place the client in the supine position

24. **When should EMS be activated when treating an emergency involving an asthmatic client?**
    a. At the beginning of the emergency
    b. As soon as CAB has been assessed
    c. After a bronchodilator and oxygen have been administered
    d. If the bronchodilator fails to stop the asthma attack

25. **Your client is becoming very talkative and anxious; these are signs of N$_2$O-O$_2$ oversedation. Management for oversedation of N$_2$O-O$_2$ includes increasing the client's oxygen intake and decreasing his nitrous oxide intake.**
    a. Both statements are TRUE.
    b. Both statements are FALSE.
    c. The first statement is TRUE; the second statement is FALSE.
    d. The first statement is FALSE; the second statement is TRUE.

26. **Match the six types of shock with the corresponding signs and symptoms (a to f).**
    ____ 1. Cardiac shock
    ____ 2. Anaphylactic shock
    ____ 3. Septic shock
    ____ 4. Obstructive shock
    ____ 5. Hypovolemic shock
    ____ 6. Neurogenic shock
    a. Difficulty breathing, hypotension, bronchoconstriction, respiratory arrest
    b. Severe hypotension and dyspnea
    c. Rapid thready pulse, cool clammy skin, confusion, weakness, pallor, dehydration, decreased urine output
    d. Peripheral cyanosis, chest pain, shortness of breath, hypotension, confusion, rapid weak pulse, cold clammy skin
    e. Tissue edema, pink warm skin, fever, vasodilation, tachycardia, restlessness and anxiety, thirst, increased cardiac output, eventual respiratory failure
    f. Hypotension, bradycardia, peripheral vasodilation

27. **During an emergency involving a toxic overdose of a local anesthetic, how frequently will vital signs be monitored?**
    a. Constantly
    b. Every 5 minutes
    c. Every 10 minutes
    d. At the beginning and end of the appointment

28. **Normal respiration rates for adults and children are 12 to 20 respirations a minute; normal rates for teens are between 20 and 25 respirations a minute.**
    a. Both statements are TRUE.
    b. Both statements are FALSE.
    c. The first statement is TRUE; the second statement is FALSE.
    d. The first statement is FALSE; the second statement is TRUE.

29. **How long after a CVA can a client be seen for dental care?**
    a. Immediately
    b. 1 month
    c. 3 months
    d. 6 months

30. **Which of the following statements is NOT correct concerning a woman in the last trimester of pregnancy?**
    a. Chest compressions should be performed above the center of the sternum.
    b. Chest thrusts should be performed for a foreign body obstruction.
    c. Oxygen demands increase.
    d. While in the supine position, the client's left hip should be elevated to displace the uterus in order to increase cardiac output and oxygen reserve.

31. **Systolic pressure is measured when the heart is relaxed. Pulse pressure is the difference between diastolic and systolic pressure.**
    a. Both statements are TRUE.
    b. Both statements are FALSE.
    c. The first statement is TRUE; the second statement is FALSE.
    d. The first statement is FALSE; the second statement is TRUE.

32. It may be beneficial to have your asthmatic clients take a prophylactic dose of a bronchodilator prior to a dental appointment. In the event of an emergency with an asthmatic client, position the client in the supine position.
    a. Both statements are TRUE.
    b. Both statements are FALSE.
    c. The first statement is TRUE; the second statement is FALSE.
    d. The first statement is FALSE; the second statement is TRUE.

33. All the following increase body temperature EXCEPT:
    a. Exercise
    b. Smoking
    c. Shock
    d. Pathologic condition

34. Your client has no history of angina and begins to experience a crushing, squeezing pain in his chest and down his left arm. The pain is not subsiding with movement. What should you do FIRST?
    a. Administer 1 nitroglycerin tablet, wait 5 minutes, and if pain does not subside, administer a second tablet
    b. Administer 2 nitroglycerin tablets, wait 5 minutes, and administer 1 more tablet
    c. Administer oxygen
    d. Summon EMS

35. Which of the following is the BEST way to stop hyperventilation?
    a. Have the client cup the hands over the mouth and nose and take slow, deep breaths
    b. Have the client breathe into a paper bag
    c. Administer low-flow oxygen
    d. Administer high-flow oxygen

36. All the following can cause an increase in heart rate EXCEPT:
    a. Fasting
    b. Exercise
    c. Anxiety
    d. Heat

37. Your client is elderly, fairly sedentary, and is taking medications for hypertension. His blood pressure at the beginning of the appointment is 140/90 mm Hg. He has been in the supine position for 45 minutes. When you raise the chair to the upright position, he begins to feel lightheaded and nauseated. You notice him sweating and becoming pale. You check his BP again, and it is now 115/85 mm Hg. What is your client experiencing?
    a. Hypertension
    b. Orthostatic hypotension
    c. Syncope
    d. Hypotension

38. The new American Heart Association guidelines for CPR are:
    a. Airway, circulation, breathing
    b. Airway, compressions, breathing
    c. Circulation, airway, breathing
    d. Compressions, airway, breathing

39. Your post-CVA client has a blood pressure of 165/97 mm Hg. What is the protocol care?
    a. Check your client's BP at the end of the appointment
    b. Monitor your client's BP every 5 minutes
    c. Refer your client for an immediate consultation with the physician
    d. Continue as you normally would, since there is no concern

40. During an emergency, which of the following pulse points is used to determine a client's pulse rate?
    a. Brachial
    b. Radial
    c. Carotid
    d. Femoral

41. Clients experiencing syncope should be placed in the supine position, and aromatic ammonia should be administered.
    a. Both statements are TRUE.
    b. Both statements are FALSE.
    c. The first statement is TRUE; the second statement is FALSE.
    d. The first statement is FALSE; the second statement is TRUE.

42. Which of the following should be monitored when checking respirations?
    a. Rhythm
    b. Rate
    c. Breathing sounds
    d. All the above

43. Body temperatures are higher in the:
    a. Early morning
    b. Late morning
    c. Early afternoon
    d. Late afternoon

44. A transient ischemia of the heart is known as:
    a. Cardiogenic shock
    b. Anaphylactic shock
    c. TIA
    d. Angina

45. A heart rate of 105 is considered:
    a. Normal
    b. Bradycardia
    c. Tachycardia

46. How long after a dose of nitroglycerin should angina pain lessen?
    a. Instantly
    b. 2-4 minutes
    c. 5-8 minutes
    d. 10-15 minutes

CASE A

Your client is a 61-year-old man who is 5'5" tall and weighs 220 pounds. His vital statistics are blood pressure (BP) 175/108 mm Hg, pulse 98, and respirations 20. He is under the care of a physician. He was hospitalized 3 months ago for a heart attack. Three years ago, he had a pacemaker placed as an outpatient. He is currently being treated for hypertension and heart disease.

Use Case A to answer questions 47 to 53.

47. **How frequently should vital signs, including BP, be taken for your client?**
    a. Frequency of vital signs monitoring depends on the BP guidelines; follow the BP classification
    b. Every year
    c. Before each appointment
    d. Before and after each appointment

48. **How soon after your client's myocardial infarction could he be scheduled for his hygiene recall appointment?**
    a. 1 month
    b. 3 months
    c. 6 months
    d. The amount of time does not matter

49. **Based on this client's BP, he has stage II hypertension. He should be dismissed and told to see his physician immediately.**
    a. Both statements are TRUE.
    b. Both statements are FALSE.
    c. The first statement is TRUE; the second statement is FALSE.
    d. The first statement is FALSE; the second statement is TRUE.

50. **All the following procedures are considered to be preventive care for a client with a previous myocardial infarction EXCEPT:**
    a. Schedule short appointments
    b. Administer oxygen with a flow rate of 8 to 12 L/min
    c. Administer N_2O-O_2 sedation
    d. Maintain adequate pain control through the administration of no more than 2 carpules of lidocaine with 1:100,000 epinephrine

51. **Your client begins to complain of a crushing feeling in his chest; he appears ashen gray and begins to exhibit a cold sweat and dyspnea. He complains of nausea, dizziness, and weakness, and he thinks he is going to die. First, you realize your client may be experiencing a myocardial infarction. Second, you should immediately contact the EMS and implement CAB.**
    a. Both statements are TRUE.
    b. Both statements are FALSE.
    c. The first statement is true; the second statement is FALSE.
    d. The first statement is false; the second statement is TRUE.

52. **Which of the following should be administered to your client?**
    a. Oxygen (4-6 L/min)
    b. Nitroglycerin (1 tablet every 5 minutes, not to exceed 3 tablets in 15 minutes)
    c. Aspirin (160-325 mg)
    d. All the above

53. **You have been monitoring your client's vital signs and assessing CAB, and he goes into cardiac arrest. You will have to use the defibrillator. Where will you put the electrodes?**
    a. Directly over the pacemaker
    b. The opposite side of the pacemaker
    c. One inch to the side of the pacemaker

d. The defibrillator cannot be used on a client with a pacemaker

Your retired 82-year-old client has been coming to see you for many years. He is 5'10" tall and weighs 250 pounds. His vital signs are blood pressure 150/95 mm Hg, pulse 83, and respirations 20. He is under the care of a physician and being treated for angina, heart failure, and diabetes. Today your client has an ashen color, and when you shake his hand, it feels very cold. During the health history interview, he informs you that his ankles have been swelling. He presses on his ankle, and it remains pitted. On the head and neck exam, you notice a prominent jugular vein.

Use Case B to answer questions 54 to 58.

54. **What is the MOST likely cause of your client's symptoms?**
    a. Angina
    b. Diabetes mellitus
    c. Left ventricular failure
    d. Right ventricular failure

55. **What is the treatment regimen for your client on this visit?**
    a. Normal hygiene appointment
    b. Shortened hygiene appointment because the longer appointments will increase his stress
    c. Reschedule for next week, when he is exhibiting less symptoms
    d. Refer your client to his physician before you see him again

56. **When your client has been cleared by his physician to receive dental care, you can take measures to help prevent an emergency. Positioning your client in the upright or semi-supine position is one measure. Another measure is to administer low-flow oxygen at a rate of 3 to 4 L/min.**
    a. Both statements are TRUE.
    b. Both statements are FALSE.
    c. The first statement is TRUE; the second statement is FALSE.
    d. The first statement is FALSE; the second statement is TRUE.

57. **While working on the maxillary arch, you notice your client has a slight dry cough and is beginning to wheeze. He coughs into a tissue, and you notice his sputum is frothy and tinged with blood, and he develops dyspnea. First, you realize your client is experiencing acute pulmonary edema. Second, you should immediately contact EMS, calm your client, and implement CAB.**
    a. Both statements are TRUE.
    b. Both statements are FALSE.
    c. The first statement is TRUE; the second statement is FALSE.
    d. The first statement is FALSE; the second statement is TRUE.

58. **Once the EMS has been contacted, which of the following should be administered to your client?**
    a. Oxygen
    b. Nitroglycerin
    c. Morphine
    d. All the above

Ethical and Legal Issues

*Pamela Zarkowski**

Understanding and applying legal and ethical principles protects the provider (dental hygienist), the client, the employer, and the employee. Dental hygienists make decisions that are influenced by laws and ethics. At times, these decisions are clear; at other times, ethical dilemmas create conflict with employers, colleagues, or clients. Dental hygienists must be cognizant of the laws governing the employer-employee relationship and influencing the responsibilities and rights of the parties involved. This chapter reviews the laws and ethics most closely associated with the dental hygiene profession.

ETHICAL CONSIDERATIONS

A. Definitions
   1. Ethics—the science of human duty; correlate motives and attitudes with moral actions and values
   2. Professional ethics—rules or standards governing conduct of members of a profession
   3. Bioethics—ethical and moral implication of new biologic discoveries and biomedical advances
B. Ethical theories
   1. Are the foundation of ethical analysis; explain moral principles
   2. Provide a basis for ethical rule, policy development, or both
   3. Assist in the resolution of ethical dilemmas
C. Three major theories
   1. Teleologic/utilitarian ethics (John Stuart Mill)—comprise rules for conduct based on consequences of action; an action is considered right or wrong on the basis of its usefulness; useful actions bring about the greatest good for the greatest number of individuals
      a. Act utilitarianism—examines a situation and determines which course of action will bring about the greatest happiness or least harm and suffering to an individual regardless of personal feelings or societal constraints such as laws
      b. Rule utilitarianism—searches for the greatest happiness and seeks public agreement to define nature of

happiness; considers the law and fairness; an action is considered right if it conforms to a rule; the rule should have positive results in a wide range of situations
   2. Deontologic ethics (Immanuel Kant)—focus on the morality of the act rather than the situation or consequences of actions; one would say, "It's the principle of the thing"; a person's intention, not the consequences of the action, is key; three important elements: applied universally to all individuals, unconditional, and demand an action
      a. Act deontology—based on personal moral values of the individual making the decision and considers the ethical principles involved in an action in light of the circumstances; for example, avoid the truth if it is harmful
      b. Rule deontology—based on the belief that certain standards for ethical decisions are of greater value than an individual's moral values; considers the principles and rules in general as they apply to types of actions
   3. Virtue ethics (Aristotle and Plato)—focus on character traits and excellence of character; evaluate ethical dilemma by asking, "Is this what a virtuous person would do?"
   4. Other theories
      a. Situational ethics—course of action determined by:
         (1) The unique characteristics of each individual
         (2) The relationship between the health care provider and the client
         (3) The most humanistic action in a given circumstance
      b. Principalism—focuses on ethical principles, including autonomy, veracity, beneficence, nonmaleficence, and justice
      c. Professional codes of ethics—designed in a rule-making format; may include aspirational statements, usually directs decision making among professionals more than ethical theories
D. Universal principles
   1. Veracity—truthfulness; mutual responsibility for the client and the provider; for example, the client must be truthful to receive appropriate care, and the provider must provide truthful information so that the client can exercise his or her autonomy

*Pamela Zarkowski and the publisher acknowledge the past contribution of Judith A. Davison to this chapter.

2. Autonomy—personal liberty; individuals are free to make decisions regarding their own health; respect for the individual autonomy of others is basic to the health care provider–client relationship; informed consent and informed refusal is basic to autonomy (see discussion on informed consent later in this chapter)
3. Beneficence—the provider's duty is a commitment to the health and welfare of the client above all other considerations; duty to prevent or remove harm and promote good
4. Nonmaleficence—the provider's duty not to use the treatment to injure or wrong the client; inflict no harm
5. Fidelity (role fidelity)—health care providers are required to provide services within the scope of their practice; ethics require that health care providers practice within the constraints of the role assumed within the health care environment; the provider is expected to follow through with commitments
6. Confidentiality—based on an individual's right to privacy; for example, a client has the right to expect all his or her medical records and communications to be kept confidential
7. Justice—fair and equitable treatment of clients

PROFESSIONALISM

Defining a Profession

A. Characteristics of a profession
   1. Special advanced education or preparation
   2. Identifiable membership
   3. Strong service orientation
   4. Promotion of a body of knowledge in the field (research and theory development)
   5. Autonomy of practice
   6. Self-regulation
   7. The recognized authority with societal sanction
   8. Primarily intellectual nature of the work
   9. Adherence to a code of ethics
B. Code of ethics
   1. Historical evidence of Western medical ethics traced to guidelines outlining the duties of physicians
   2. Early evidence included oaths and rabbinic and Christian sources
   3. Common themes include:
      a. Respecting autonomy
      b. Preventing harm
      c. Protecting confidentiality
   4. Hippocratic Oath—fifth century BCE; statement of principles guiding the professional conduct of physicians
      a. Interpreted to advocate, "Above all, do no harm," or "First, do no harm" (The phrase is not found in the original code)
      b. Protected the rights of the patients
      c. Admonished physicians to maintain patient confidentiality
      d. Placed needs of patient above those of society
      e. Placed an obligation on physicians to teach the next generation of physicians

5. Ethical codes for health care professionals continue to be evaluated and revised to reflect:
   a. Current practice issues
   b. Protections for population groups that are subjects in research investigations
   c. Identification of impaired health care providers
   d. Professional responsibilities
   e. Use of social media
6. Common elements of codes
   a. Self-imposed—the health care professional self-assesses and determines compliance; range of sanctions from a professional organization or licensing agency for lack of compliance
   b. Set rules governing behavior—the professional uses them as a framework for action
   c. Serving to protect the public—on the basis of ethical principles that support actions to benefit the client and prevent harm
   d. Striving to enhance the profession—adherence to code characterizes a profession
   e. Providing a framework for ethical decision making
7. American Dental Hygienist's Association (ADHA) Code of Ethics and the Canadian Dental Hygienists Association (CDHA) Code of Ethics
   a. Identify and describe ethical principles to guide the oral health care provider
   b. State the obligations and responsibilities of the dental hygienist
      (1) Personal and professional obligations and responsibilities
      (2) Obligations and responsibilities to the public and the scientific community
8. Codes of Ethics—compare all codes
   a. For the ADHA's Code of Ethics, visit the website at https://www.adha.org/resources-docs/7611_Bylaws_and_Code_of_Ethics.pdf (also see Appendix C)
   b. For the CDHA's Code of Ethics, visit the website at http://www.cdha.ca/CDHA/The_Profession/Resources/Code_of_Ethics.aspx
   c. For the American Dental Association's Code of Professional Responsibility and Conduct (revised April 2012), visit the website at http://www.ada.org/~/media/ADA/About%20the%20ADA/Files/code_of_ethics_2012.ashx
9. Client's Bill of Rights—outlines client expectations and provides guidelines for provider conduct; the client has the right to:
   a. Respectful, competent, and considerate care irrespective of ethnicity, gender, national origin, age, or disability
   b. Receive current, accurate, and complete information regarding diagnosis, treatment, and prognosis
   c. Receive information necessary to give informed consent or informed refusal before treatment; be informed of the consequences of refusing treatment
   d. Confidentiality regarding all communications, consultations, and records except when permission has been granted to submit this information to others

e. Obtain information relating to the credentials of all providers rendering services

f. Reasonable continuity of care

g. Examine and receive accurate copies of professional services and fees

h. Receive treatment from health care professionals who act within the limits of their professional licenses (scope of practice) and adhere to the standard of care in delivering services

10. Types of professional credentials
   a. Licensure—state regulation of professionals
      (1) Granted by a state agency or board
      (2) Limits practice to:
         (a) Responsibilities and behaviors prescribed by law in the state practice act in the United States or determined by the provincial practice act in Canada
         (b) Responsibilities and behaviors delineated by rules and regulations
      (3) Authorized practice by professionals meeting specified qualifications
      (4) Failure to meet responsibilities and expected behaviors may result in fines, suspension, or removal of license
      (5) Status of provider's license available to public; may indicate current license status (e.g., active, pending, suspended)
      (6) The purpose is to protect the public from unqualified or unethical providers
   b. Registration—qualified professionals listed in a directory
      (1) Dental hygiene is a self-regulated profession in most Canadian provinces, and registration is a provincial responsibility (e.g., College of Dental Hygienists of Ontario http://www.cdho.org/Registration.asp)
      (2) A certificate of registration to practice is issued only to those who meet established standards of qualification and practice
   c. Certification—state or national recognition
      (1) Recognition by a nongovernmental agency (e.g., a professional association)
      (2) Identification of professionals who have met specified qualifications

ETHICAL ISSUES IN PUBLIC POLICY

A. Ethical issues and public policy
   1. Distributive justice—fair allocation of resources involved
      a. Macro-allocation of resources—based on public needs (e.g., water fluoridation)
      b. Micro-allocation of resources—based on individual needs (e.g., fluoride varnish treatment)
   2. Distributive justice or allocation of scarce resources—determination of who should receive treatment when all cannot be treated; services may be allocated on basis of:
      a. Equity—all persons receive equal treatment

      b. Need—treatment allocated on the basis of prioritized needs
      c. Effort—treatment allocated to those who have earned it
      d. Contribution—treatment allocated to those who are making a contribution to society
      e. Merit—treatment allocated to those who are most deserving
   3. Influenced by principles of human dignity and human rights and contributing to the common good
   4. Current health policy debates
      a. Question of whether public health funds should be used for:
         (1) Financial assistance and care of the disadvantaged or seniors
         (2) Financial assistance and care for undocumented immigrants
         (3) Financial support for victims of:
            (a) Acute or chronic diseases
            (b) Personal choices (e.g., tobacco use, risky lifestyle)
         (4) Provision of health care services
            (a) Appropriate range of services provided
            (b) Impact of public versus private funding on the:
               [1] Consumer and taxpayer
               [2] Provider
               [3] Third-party payer
               [4] Government (local, state, federal, or all)
            (c) Concerns about authority in treatment decisions
            (d) Tele–health care
            (e) Expanded scope of practice for midlevel providers
            (f) Delegation of responsibility to nonhealth providers
      b. Research
         (1) Identification of appropriate decision makers to identify and prioritize research agendas, especially for controversial topics (e.g., stem cell research)
         (2) Identification of sources of financial support (e.g., what proportion of the national budget should be allocated to health care and research)

B. Public policy
   1. A system of plans of action, regulatory measures, laws, and funding priorities concerning a specific topic or issue
   2. Promulgated by a governmental entity or its representatives
   3. Public policy is typically embodied in constitutions, legislative acts, and judicial decisions

C. Creating public health policy
   1. Goal—assessment of a variety of actions and consequences to solve identified societal problem
   2. Action—a decision by all members of society or their elected representatives (e.g., public vote vs. state legislature passing statute regarding mandatory use of seat belts)

3. Analysis—determining which policy among alternatives best achieves the goal, how policy should be implemented, or how to evaluate what is currently being done
D. Policy makers—usually legislators, members of executive branch of government, and government officials who write regulations
E. Policy analysts—provide policy makers with information required to determine the impact of past and current public policies; determine whether new policy should be implemented or present policy or no policy should continue
F. Examples of community-based programs requiring public policy analysis
   1. Federal or state partnerships to provide oral health services
   2. Fluoridation initiatives (e.g., community water fluoridation and school fluoride programs)
   3. Caries prevention programs such as dental sealant or fluoride varnish programs in public health settings
   4. Provision and funding of oral health care services by non-dental personnel
G. Policy makers may seek input from professionals or professional associations; health-related professional associations frequently hire lobbyists to influence government policy makers
H. Distinctions between ethics and law
   1. Laws are societal mandates, whereas ethics are professionally based
   2. Ethical principles and legal doctrine are related
      a. Ethical principles integral to federal and state legislation that is enacted
         (1) Obligation to obtain informed consent (client autonomy)
         (2) Health Insurance Portability and Accountability Act (HIPAA) regulations (confidentiality)
         (3) Discrimination protections for clients with specific disease states such as human immunodeficiency virus (HIV) infection (justice)
         (4) Tort regulation (nonmaleficence)
         (5) Occupational Safety and Health Administration (OSHA) regulations (beneficence)
      b. Ethical issues inherent in the litigation of cases
   3. Ethical duties are usually greater than legal duties; for example, a health care provider who is acquitted in civil or criminal court after being charged with illegal conduct did not necessarily act ethically
   4. Compliance with the law sometimes mandates unethical conduct—health care providers are ethically and legally bound to keep confidential all client communications and records; however, the law makes exceptions and requires disclosure to appropriate authorities in specific situations (e.g., in cases of suspected child or elder abuse or threats of inflicting bodily harm to another person or self)
   5. Personal values not necessarily congruent with professional ethics or the law—under law, individuals have a right to control their own bodies; this includes the right

to refuse medical or dental treatment; health care providers must honor this right despite their own personal values
   6. Differentiating between ethics and law (Table 22-1)

LEGAL CONCEPTS

A. Law defined
   1. Rules and regulations that govern society
   2. Reflects society's attitudes, mores, and needs; therefore, law is constantly changing to meet the requirements and expectations of society
B. Sources of law
   1. U.S. Constitutional law
      a. Constitutional law—supreme law of the land; both state and federal laws must be consistent with the U.S. Constitution
      b. The U.S. Constitution establishes the organization of the federal government and places limitations on the federal government through the Bill of Rights (first 10 amendments to the U.S. Constitution)
      c. Delineates the specific powers of the federal government to the:
         (1) Executive branch (Office of the President)
         (2) Legislative branch (U.S. Congress)
         (3) Judicial branch (U.S. Supreme Court)
      d. Powers not specifically granted to the federal government are the powers of state government

TABLE 22-1   Differentiating Between Ethics and Law

	Ethics	Law
Definition	Individual interpretation of the nature of right and wrong and rules of conduct	Rules and regulations by which society is governed set forth in a formal and legally binding manner
Source	Internalized; individual nature and beliefs	Externalized rules and regulations of society
Emphasis	Individual moral behavior for the good of the individual within society	Social behaviors that are good for society as a whole
Conduct	Motives and reasons why the individual behaves the way he or she does	Overt conduct of the individual; what a person actually did or failed to do
Sanctions	Professional organization—expulsion from the organization	Judicial and administrative bodies—criminal sanctions such as fines and imprisonment imposed by the courts; civil sanctions such as monetary damages imposed by the courts; disciplinary sanctions such as fines, license suspension, or license revocation by a board of dentistry

e. Each state has its own constitution that grants powers and places limitations on the powers of the state government
2. Statutory law
   a. Laws made by the legislative branch of government (federal, state, and local governments)
   b. State dental practice acts are examples of statutory laws
3. Administrative law
   a. Administrative agencies are given the authority to oversee the specific laws or statutes to ensure that the intent of the law is enforced
   b. Administrative laws are the results of decisions of administrative agencies; for example, state boards of dentistry and the College of Dental Hygienists of Ontario implement rules and regulations to enforce the law
   c. Administrative agencies may conduct investigations and hearings and may issue decisions that suspend or revoke the license of a dentist, dental hygienist, or dental assistant; decisions of administrative agencies may be appealed through the state court system to determine whether:
      (1) The agency complied with the regulation
      (2) Evidence supports the agency's decision
      (3) The agency exceeded its authority
      (4) The delegation of power to the agency was proper
      (5) The agency followed proper procedures
      (6) The agency acted in an arbitrary or capricious manner
4. Judicial law
   a. Determined by courts (state, provincial, and federal), which interpret legal issues in dispute
   b. *Stare decisis*[1] (Latin, meaning "let the decision stand")—doctrine of law whereby the court will base its decision on previous case law (a prior case with similar facts); the previous case must be from the same jurisdiction (state); emphasizes the importance of legal precedent

   c. Landmark decisions—court decision that departs from precedent; for example, new technology may require different conclusions based on the same facts
   d. *Res judicata*1 (Latin, meaning "a thing or matter settled by judgment")—legal doctrine that applies when a legal ruling has been made by a competent court of jurisdiction, and no appeals are possible; prevents parties from taking the same issues to different courts
C. Classifications of law (Fig. 22-1)
   1. Common law and civil law—two concepts of legal thought, one from England (common law) and one from Europe (civil law)
      a. Common law—general principles derived from decisions in case law using the concept of precedent
      b. Civil law—civil code system developed by legislature, based on rules and regulations; enforced through the court system and protects the legal rights of private persons
      c. Level of proof—preponderance of evidence; the greater weight of the evidence required in a civil (noncriminal) lawsuit for jury or judge without a jury to decide in favor of one side or the other
   2. Criminal law—relates to acts considered offensive to society as a whole
      a. Classifications of crimes
         (1) Misdemeanors—usually involve fines of less than $1000 or imprisonment for less than 1 year, or both; examples include vandalism, trespassing, and reckless driving
         (2) Felonies—serious crime; usually involve punishment ranging from fines of more than $1000 or imprisonment of more than 1 year (or both); receiving a death sentence depending on the crime committed and the jurisdiction (state); examples include robbery, illegal drug use or sale, and battery

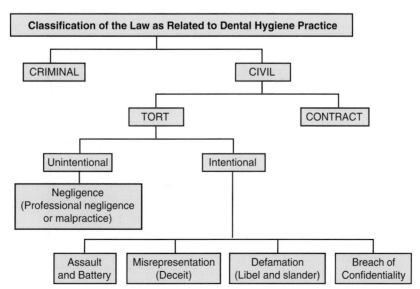

FIG 22-1 Classifications of law as it relates to dental hygiene practice.

b. Certain violations of law may be considered both criminal and civil; for example, if a client loses his or her life resulting from gross negligence of a dental hygienist, the estate of the deceased person could bring civil charges such as wrongful death against the hygienist, and the state may bring criminal action such as manslaughter against the hygienist

c. Level of proof—"beyond a reasonable doubt" required to determine innocence or guilt in a criminal case; the level of certainty a jury must have to find a defendant guilty of a crime

D. Primary individuals involved in a lawsuit
1. Plaintiff—party bringing the lawsuit
2. Defendant—party against whom the lawsuit is filed
3. Attorney—individual serving as an advocate for either the plaintiff or the defendant
4. Expert witness—explains specialized information to jurors; possesses appropriate credentials and expertise
5. Lay witness—testifies as to facts for judge and jury
6. Dental hygienist as a witness (lay or expert)
   a. Expert qualifications based on education, licensure or certification, experience, and publications
   b. Expertise to testify as to standard of care for dental hygiene
   c. Familiarity with the state or provincial dental practice act
   d. Knowledgeable about all records (written or electronic) relating to the controversy
   e. Knowledge of office, agency, or institutional policy and procedure where (and at the time) the incident occurred
7. Cannot be lay witness if named in lawsuit

E. Due process and equal protection
1. Due process—protects the public from arbitrary actions of the state; the law must apply to all persons equally; elements of due process
   a. The law, as applied, must be reasonable and definite
   b. Fair procedures must be followed in enforcing the law; for example, the state may not arbitrarily take away a license to practice dental hygiene; the hygienist must first be given notice of the violation, a hearing, and an opportunity to respond before license revocation or suspension is imposed
2. Equal protection—equal protection clause of the Fourteenth Amendment to the U.S. Constitution protects individuals from state action; states may not enforce laws based solely on classification of persons such as race, age, gender, religion, national origin, or disability

F. Judicial process
1. Questions of law or fact—usually the jury determines what is fact from the evidence admitted by the court; the judge determines questions of law
2. Jurisdiction of the courts—authority of the court to determine the controversy; for example, the bankruptcy court may not hear divorce cases
3. State courts
   a. Trial courts—courts with trial jurisdiction; usually handle cases such as traffic, probate, family matters,

arraignments for felonies, small claims, juvenile, and criminal misdemeanors
   b. Appellate courts—courts with trial, appellate, civil, and criminal jurisdiction; usually with a monetary restriction (plaintiff must request a fair minimum amount)
   c. State supreme court—appellate jurisdiction only
4. Federal courts
   a. Federal district courts—courts with trial jurisdiction; hear only matters that involve federal law or parties with diversity of citizenship (residents of different states)
   b. U.S. Courts of Appeal—courts with appellate jurisdiction only
   c. U.S. Supreme Court—court with appellate jurisdiction only; decisions cannot be overturned by any other court (state or federal); decisions can only be changed by new congressional legislation or subsequent Supreme Court decisions

G. Statute of limitations
1. Each state (or province) has a statute (law) that delineates specific periods within which a lawsuit must be filed after the event that caused the action; after that period, the right to initiate a lawsuit is lost
2. In tort actions, time may be measured from the time of the injury or harm or may be measured from when the plaintiff discovers the injury; periods vary from state to state

H. Case law—case law comprises the decisions, or the interpretations made by judges while deciding on the legal issues before them which are considered common law or as an aid for interpretation of a law in subsequent cases with similar conditions; case law is used by attorneys to support their views to favor their clients; it also influences the decisions of the judges; it is public record (occasionally court records are sealed)
1. Legal decisions available in publications appropriate for the level of the court where the case was tried; most decisions of state appellate courts are published in regional reports
2. Citations—references to legal authority that provide key information about the case; for example, in the following citation, *Edwards v Penn. Dental Examining Board*, 454, A2d 218 (1983): Edwards is the plaintiff (party bringing the lawsuit), the Dental Board is the defendant (party against whom the lawsuit is filed), 454 is the volume number of A2d (second series of the Atlantic Regional Reporter); 218 is the page number; and 1983 is the year the case was decided

CIVIL LAW AND THE DENTAL HYGIENIST

A. A lawsuit can be filed against an oral health care provider in two areas of civil law:
1. Contract violation
2. Tort violation

B. Contract law[1]—a contract is an agreement between two or more consenting and competent parties to do or not to do a legal act for which sufficient consideration exists; breach of contract occurs if either party fails to comply with the terms of the contractual obligations

1. Two methods to create a contract:
   a. Implied contract through signs, inaction, or silence; also called *apparent*
   b. Express contract entered through oral or written communication
2. The contract exists between a client and a health care provider when the client agrees to a specific treatment
3. Contractual responsibilities of the provider to the client
   a. Possess proper license and certification
   b. Exercise reasonable skill, care, and judgment in diagnosis and treatment
   c. Use standard drugs, materials, and techniques
   d. Complete the treatment in a reasonable time
   e. Never abandon the client
   f. Complete procedures consented to by the client
   g. Provide adequate instructions
   h. Refer appropriately
   i. Maintain confidentiality and client privacy
   j. Maintain an appropriate level of knowledge and skill
   k. Practice within the scope of practice; never exceed the defined scope
   l. Maintain accurate records
   m. Comply with all laws regulating practice
   n. Practice in a manner consistent with a code of ethics
4. Contractual obligations of the client
   a. Pay a reasonable fee in a reasonable time
   b. Cooperate in care
   c. Keep appointments
   d. Provide accurate history and information
   e. Follow instructions
   f. Keep the dental provider aware of status
   g. Follow home care instructions
5. Client-practitioner relationship—contractual; both are free to enter or decline the relationship; a practitioner may decline to undertake treatment of a client unless the practitioner has agreed to treat the client by participating in a specific dental insurance plan or the practitioner is employed by another who makes treatment decisions; if the practitioner offers services to the public, he or she may not refuse to treat clients because of race, color, gender, religion, national origin, disability, or any other basis that would constitute invidious discrimination; being bound to the code of ethics assumes a preexisting relationship between the client and practitioner
6. Termination of the client-practitioner relationship may be by:
   a. The client
   b. The practitioner, after giving the client notice and an opportunity to secure an alternative source of future treatment
7. Abandonment[1]—failure of a health care professional to provide services after the professional has established a relationship with the client; duty to the client to complete all treatment started; clients may be dismissed from future treatment

C. Tort law[1]—deals with civil wrongs committed against a person or a person's property; wrongful conduct
1. Unintentional torts
   a. Negligence and malpractice
      (1) Negligence—failure to use such care as a reasonable person would use under similar circumstances
      (2) Malpractice—wrongful acts of professional persons; usually failure to meet the standard of care or failure to foresee consequences that one with his or her particular skills and education should foresee
   b. Elements of negligence or malpractice, which must be shown in order for a lawsuit to go forward
      (1) Duty owed to the client (the plaintiff)
      (2) Breach of the duty by the professional or the defendant
      (3) Harm to the client (the plaintiff)
      (4) Causation—harm must be caused by breach of duty; foreseeability, that is, the event may reasonably be expected to cause the result
   c. Standard of care—the degree of care that a reasonably prudent professional should exercise; minimum requirements of acceptable client care; for example, practicing within the rules and regulations of the state or provincial dental practice act
   d. Damages (awarded to the defendant; to restore injured party)
      (1) Special damages—actual expenses
      (2) Nominal damages—at the court's discretion (could be $1)
      (3) General damages—part of harm; difficult to determine (e.g., can include pain and suffering)
      (4) Contract damages—for breach of contract
      (5) Punitive damages—to punish deliberately wrongful conduct (usually not covered by liability insurance)
      (6) States may place a cap on the maximum allowable damages that can be paid
   e. *Res ipsa loquitur*[1] (Latin, meaning "the thing speaks for itself")—legal doctrine that permits the plaintiff to prove negligence or malpractice without proving fault; no expert testimony required if the plaintiff shows a particular result occurred and would not have occurred except for someone's negligence
      (1) The type of injury does not occur unless negligence has occurred
      (2) The injury is caused by something or someone under exclusive control of defendant
      (3) The injury was not caused by plaintiff by contributing to own injury in any manner (no contributory negligence)
   f. Defenses to unintentional torts (protect defendant from liability)—not limited to, but include:
      (1) Statute of limitations—time limit for initiating lawsuit has passed
      (2) Comparative or contributory negligence—injured party is held responsible for a portion or all of the

injury (states or provinces differ regarding degree of responsibility)

(3) Release—signed during the settlement of claim to prevent future claims

(4) Immunity—protection from prosecution; for example, the action may fall within a state's Good Samaritan law

(5) Defense of fact—no causation exists

2. Intentional tort—an act must be willful; the defendant must have intended to cause the harm or injury; the act must have been a substantial factor in bringing about the injury

   a. Assault—any action that places one in fear of bodily harm (e.g., threatening behaviors)

   b. Battery—intentional infliction of offensive or harmful bodily contact; unwanted touching

   c. Defamation—communication to a third person of an untrue statement about another person

      (1) Libel—written defamation (e.g., untrue or unflattering statement entered into a client's record)

      (2) Slander—spoken defamation (e.g., discussing an employer in a derogatory manner while dining in a restaurant and being overheard by a third person)

   d. Invasion of privacy—protects one's right to privacy

      (1) Intrusion on seclusion—invasion of a private place or affairs of another; must be highly offensive to a reasonable person

      (2) Appropriation—use of another's name or likeness for financial gain (e.g., unauthorized photographs of dental clients used in a research article or textbook)

      (3) Publicity of private life—publicizing details of another person's private life; must be highly offensive to a reasonable person; health care professionals must not disclose a client's information without written authorization (e.g., no disclosure of client information over the phone or via email or to client's relatives, including spouse or friends)

      (4) False light—putting another person before the public eye in a false light; highly offensive to a reasonable person

   e. Infliction of mental distress—outrageous conduct that causes emotional distress; behavior must be beyond standards of rudeness; behavior was intended to cause mental distress and actually did cause mental distress (e.g., publicly revealing client's nonpayment; notifying neighbors or relatives of nonpayment)

   f. Fraud or intentional misrepresentation—intentional perversion of truth (misrepresentation) for the purpose of gaining another person's trust and reliance whereby that person suffers harm or loss as a result of trusting and relying (e.g., never guarantee treatment outcomes)

   g. Interference with advantageous relations—generally prevents an individual from interfering with the gainful employment of another; name and definitions may vary from state to state; giving a former employee a poor reference is not a basis for this tort

   h. Wrongful discharge—illegal termination of an employee; most dental hygienists are hired without employment contracts and are employees-at-will; they can be fired for any reason except:

      (1) If reason for firing was against federal and/or state anti-discrimination laws (e.g., pregnancy of employee)

      (2) If firing is against public policy (e.g., sexual harassment or "whistleblower" cases)

      (3) Office policy and procedures (oral and written) may be considered an implied employment contract (e.g., office manual must address the issue in controversy)

   i. Defenses against intentional torts are not limited to, but include:

      (1) Statute of limitations—whether the time limit for initiating lawsuit has passed

      (2) Privilege—person making the statement has the duty to do so; for example, dental hygienists are often required by state law to report cases of suspected child abuse; in that case, they are not held legally liable for doing so

      (3) Disclosure statutes (state and federal)—permit access to client records by specific individuals or agencies without client consent (e.g., workers' compensation statutes allow for such access to client information if a claim is filed)

      (4) Consent—oral, implied by law (e.g., during emergencies, when a client is not capable of consent) or apparent (e.g., client sits in dental chair and opens mouth for an examination)

      (5) Self-defense or defense of others—behavior is justified to protect self or others from harm; if force is necessary, one may use only the amount of force necessary for protection (reasonable force)

      (6) Necessity—allows personal property to be confiscated (e.g., weapon)

3. Informed consent—from concept of battery and individual rights to make choices regarding own body

   a. Content—legal requirements vary from state to state; in general, a client must have information that a reasonable person would find material in making a decision regarding treatment

   b. Client should be told in a language or format that the client can understand

   c. Specifically, client must be informed of:

      (1) Diagnosis

      (2) Proposed treatment and benefits

      (3) Risks regarding proposed treatment and chances of success

      (4) Alternative forms of treatment; and benefits; risks associated with the alternatives offered

      (5) Prognosis if treatment is refused

      (6) Provided with an opportunity to ask questions

(7) Needs to sign a consent form indicating that the client fully understands the information provided (minimum to no technical language on form, or explanation provided if technical language is used)

d. Competency of consent
   (1) Client must be of legal age and mentally competent (able to understand material facts)
   (2) Consent must be based on knowledge and understanding and voluntary (cannot force someone to consent to a procedure)
   (3) Minors and incompetent adults
      (a) Parents or legal guardian must sign for a child; children of divorced parents may have specific requirements for consent related to divorce decree
      (b) Emancipated minor (individual is not a legal adult; most states define adult as 18 years or older) may sign for themselves; teenager can obtain emancipation by:
         [1] Proving independence from parental control to the court; legal process involved
         [2] Being legally married
         [3] Enlisting in one of the U.S. Armed Forces
      (c) Legal guardians or health care decision maker must sign for incompetent adults

e. Informed refusal[2,3]—client may refuse treatment; to refuse
   (1) Client must be provided with same type information as provided informed consent; include general and oral health risks
   (2) Documentation of refusal, including information provided to client, must be placed in the client's record
   (3) Client, operator, and witness signature recommended

D. Dental practice acts
   1. Statutes regulating the dental professions; in all legal jurisdictions (e.g., states and the District of Columbia or provinces)
   2. Enacted by state or provincial legislature; grant authority to a board of dentistry (board of dental examiners or other administrative agency) to adopt rules and regulations for dentistry, dental hygiene, and dental assisting and for dental laboratory technologists and denturists
      a. Rules and regulations must be consistent with the statute
      b. A board may not waive provisions unless specifically authorized to do so by statute
   3. Practice acts are enacted to protect the public; boards of dentistry or other agencies grant licenses to individuals to engage in a specific profession after demonstrating a minimal level of competence to perform the responsibilities required of the profession

4. Composition of dental boards—usually elected or appointed officials
   a. Dentists
   b. Dental hygienists
   c. Consumers
   d. Others (e.g., lawyers, dental assistants, denturists)
5. Board duties
   a. Regulate applications for licensure
   b. Implement mechanisms for measuring competence of applicants, that is, credentials, examinations, mandatory continuing education or other certifications
   c. Implement mechanisms for investigating complaints made against practitioners
   d. Grant and revoke licenses
   e. Draft laws pertaining to the dental professions for the legislature
   f. Design rules and regulations pertaining to the dental professions
   g. Monitor educational standards
   h. Monitor other procedures related to licensure (e.g., licensure renewal, continuing education requirements)
6. Elements of dental practice act (vary from jurisdiction to jurisdiction)
   a. Requirements for licensure and renewal to show minimum competence
      (1) Minimum age and education
      (2) Character references
      (3) Examinations (regional, written) required
      (4) Continuing education requirements for relicensure
      (5) Evidence of specific requirements (e.g., current CPR certification)
      (6) Exemptions—"grandfather" clauses (e.g., licensure of dental hygienists trained in jurisdictions where preceptorship is legal)
      (7) Provisions for licensure across jurisdictions
         (a) Reciprocity—agreements between states for recognition of licensure from another state
         (b) Endorsement—granting of licensure if the applicant is licensed in another state and can present specific documents or credentials, and the states' requirements were the same or similar
         (c) Licensure by examination—when no reciprocity or endorsement is granted by states
         (d) Licensure by waiver—when a step toward licensure can be omitted (e.g., waiver of the clinical examination requirement)
      (8) Disciplinary action—boards have this authority with the power to enforce licensure requirements
         (a) License revocation or refusal to renew
         (b) License suspension
         (c) Probation
         (d) Reprimand—public or private
   b. Requirements for practice—defines scope of practice, that is, legally permissible tasks or procedures (Table 22-2)

TABLE 22-2 Dental Hygiene Practice Act Overview: Permitted Functions and Supervision Levels by State

Function	AL	AK	AZ	AR	CA	CO	CT	DE	DC	FL	GA	HI	ID	IL	IN	IA	KS
Prophylaxis	D	G/A	G/A	G/A[1]	G/A	A	G/A	G	G	G	D	D/G	G	G	D/G	G/A	G/A
X-ray films	D	G/A	G/A	G	G/A	A	G/A	G	G	G	D	D/G	G	G	D/G	G/A	G
Local anesthesia		G/A	D	D	D	G	D		D	D		D	G	D	D	D	D
Topical anesthesia	D	G/A	G/A		G/A	A	G/A	G	G	G		D/G	G	G		G/A	G/A
Fluoride	D	G/A	G/A	G/A[1]	G/A	A	G/A	G	G	G/A[4]	D	D/G	G	G	D/G	G/A	G/A
Pit/fissure sealants	D	G/A	G/A	G/A[1]	G/A	A	G/A	G	G	G/A	D	D/G	G	G	D	G/A	G
Root planing	D	G/A	G/A	D	G/A	A	G/A	G	G	D	D	D/G	G	G	D	G/A	G
Soft tissue curettage	D	G/A	G	D	G/A	G	G/A	G	G	D	D	D/G	G	G	D	G/A	G
Administer N$_2$O	D	G	G	D	D	D		G	D	D	D		D	D			G
Study cast impressions	D	D	G	D	D	D	G/A	G	G	D	D	D/G	D		D	D	G
Place perio dressings	D	G	D	G	G/A	A	G/A	G	D	D	D	D/G	D		D	G	G
Remove dressings	D	G	D		G/A	G	G/A	G	D	G	D	D/G	G	G	D	G	G
Place sutures			D		G/A	G						D/G					
Remove sutures	D	G	G		G/A	G	G/A	G	D	G	D	D/G	G	G	D	G	G
DH diagnosis							G										
Treatment planning						A											
DH assessment						A											
Prescriptive authority					G/A											G	G/A

Function	KY	LA	ME	MD	MA	MI	MN	MS	MO	MT	NE	NV	NH	NJ	NM	NY	NC
Prophylaxis	G	D/G	G/A	G	G/A	G/A	G/A	D	G/A	G/A	G/A	G/A	G/A	D/G	G/A	G	D/G
X-ray films	G	D/G	G	G	G/A	G/A	G/A	D	G	G/A	G	G/A	G	D/G	G/A	G	D/G
Local anesthesia	D	D	D	D	D	D	G		D	D	D	D/G	D	D	D/G	D	
Topical anesthesia	D	D/G	G/A	G	G/A	G/A	G		G	G/A	G	G/A	G	D	D	G	D/G
Fluoride	G/A	D/G	G/A	G	G/A	G/A	G/A	D/G[4]	G/A	G/A	G/A	G/A	G/A	D/G	G/A	G	D/G
Pit/fissure sealants	G/A	D/G	G/A	G	G/A	G/A	G/A	D	G/A	G/A	G/A	G/A	G/A	D/G	G	G	
Root planing	G/A	D	G/A	G	G/A	G/A	G/A	D	G	G/A	G/A	G/A	G/A	D/G	G	G	D/G
Soft tissue curettage			G/A	G	G/A	D	G	D	G	G/A	G/A	G/A			G	G	
Administer N$_2$O	D[1]	D[1]		D		D	G	D	D			D/G	D	D		D	
Study cast impressions	G	D	G/A	G	G/A	G/A	G		G	G/A		G/A	G	D	G	D	D/G
Place perio dressings	G	D	D	G	G/A	G/A	G		G	G/A		G/A		D	G	D	
Remove dressings	G	D	G/A	G	G/A	G/A	G		D	G	G	G/A	G	D	G	D	D/G
Place sutures																	
Remove sutures	G	D	G/A	G	G/A	G/A	G		G	G	G	G/A	G	D	G	D	D/G
DH diagnosis																	
Treatment planning												G/A					
DH assessment																	
Prescriptive authority															G/A		

Function	ND	OH	OK	OR	PA	RI	SC	SD	TN	TX	UT	VT	VA	WA	WV	WI	WY
Prophylaxis	G	G/A	G	G/A	G/A	G/A	G	G	G	G/A	G	G/A	G/A⁵	G/A	G/A	G/A	G
X-ray films	G	G	G	G/A	G/A	G/A	G	G	G	G/A	G	G/A	G	G	G	G	G
Local anesthesia	D	D	D	G	D	D	D	D	D		D	D	D³	D	D	D	D
Topical anesthesia	G	G	G	G/A	G/G	G/A	D	G	G	G/A	G	G/A		G	G	G	G
Fluoride	G	G/A	G	G/A	G/G	G/A	G	G	G	G/A	G	G/A	G/A⁵	G/A	A	G/A	G
Pit/fissure sealants	G	G/A	G	G/A	G/A	G/A	D/G	G	G	G/A	G	G/A	G/A⁵	G/A	G	G/A	D
Root planing	G²	G	G	G/A	G/A	G/A	D/G	G	G	G/A	G	G/A	G	G/A	G	G/A	G
Soft tissue curettage	G²	D	G	G/A				G	D		G			D/A			
Administer N₂O	D	D	D	D	D	D	D	D	D		D		D³	D			D
Study cast impressions	G	G	G	G/A	D	D	D		D	G/A	G	G	G	G	G	G	G
Place perio dressings	G	G	G	G/A	D	D				G/A	G	G	G	D	D	D	D
Remove dressings	G	G	G	G/A	D	D	D		D	G/A	G	G	G	D	D	D	D
Place sutures																	
Remove sutures	G	D	G	G/A	D	D	D		D	G/A	G	G	G	D	D	D	G
DH diagnosis				A													
Treatment planning	G			A													
DH assessment																	
Prescriptive authority				G/A													

D—Direct Supervision levels; dentist needs to be present.

G—General Supervision levels; dentist needs to authorize prior to services, but need not be present.

A—Direct Access Supervision levels; hygienist can provide services as she or he determines appropriate without specific authorization.

Two letters denote separate supervision levels depending on setting Private/Public.

DH, Dental hygiene.

Footnotes apply to both settings if applicable.

Disclaimer: Information based on ADHA staff research. This document should not be considered a legal document.

¹Rules pending,

²On direct order.

³On patients 18 years or older.

⁴Public health supervision applies to fluoride varnish only.

⁵Participating in remote supervision pilot program.

(1) List regulations—many states have a list of legal tasks delegated to dental hygienists

(2) Open provision—some states have a general statement of what cannot be delegated; tasks delegated are at the discretion of the supervising dentist

c. Legally problematic areas (scope of practice)

(1) If a negligent act presents a scope-of-practice issue, a dental hygienist's actions should be within the scope of practice for the particular jurisdiction; procedures billed to the insurance company must be performed by the appropriately licensed professional, or the state insurance board also could take action

(2) When the standard of care changes or increases because of the type of procedure performed or the addition of a legally recognized duty; for example, a dental hygienist administering a local anesthetic agent would be held to the same standard of care as a comparably trained professional such as a dentist

(3) When issues arise relating to use of new technology that may not yet be addressed in the dental practice act (e.g., use of lasers to fuse deep pits and fissures)

(4) Wide variations exist from state to state in the scope of dental hygiene practice; for example, practicing in a new jurisdiction where the dental practice act is more restrictive does not always allow the dental hygienist to deliver the treatment he or she was trained to perform or is competent to provide in another jurisdiction

d. Supervision (varies from state to state, and province to province)

(1) General supervision and assignment—licensed dentist authorizes the procedures on the basis of his or her diagnosis and treatment plan; need not be physically present when procedures are performed; some states require that the dentist or a designated dentist be available for consultation, if needed

(2) Indirect or close supervision—licensed dentist authorizes procedures and remains in dental facility while procedures are being performed

(3) Direct and immediate supervision—licensed dentist diagnoses the condition to be treated, authorizes procedures to be performed, and remains on premises while treatment is being performed, before the client is dismissed; some states do not require a dentist to approve the work before dismissal

(4) Personal supervision—licensed dentist provides a service for a client and authorizes an auxiliary to aid treatment by concurrently performing supportive procedures

(5) Unsupervised practice—services may be performed by a licensed dental hygienist without the supervision of a licensed dentist

(6) States are diverse in requirements for dental hygienists

(a) Forty-seven states allow general supervision, which does not require that a dentist be physically present during traditional dental hygiene procedures in offices

(b) Thirty-seven states allow direct access, which means that the dental hygienist can initiate treatment on the basis of his or her assessment of a client's needs without the specific authorization of a dentist to treat the client and without the presence of a dentist and can maintain a provider-client relationship (Box 22-1 and Fig. 22-2)

(c) Forty-five states permit dental hygienists to administer a local anesthetic agent (Table 22-3 and Fig. 22-3); all states except Oregon require the administration of a local anesthetic agent to be completed under direct supervision

(d) Thirty states and Washington D.C. permit dental hygienists to administer nitrous oxide–oxygen (N_2O-O_2) analgesia (Table 22-4 and Fig. 22-4)

(e) Thirty-five states allow dental hygienists to perform restorative procedures (Table 22-5)

7. State dental hygiene committee

a. Seventeen states have dental hygiene committees

b. These committees assist in varying degrees in the regulation of dental hygiene practice (Box 22-2)

8. Alabama dental hygiene practice and education

a. The state practice act allows only direct supervision of dental hygienists

b. Prohibits performance of restorative functions by dental hygienists (see Table 22-4)

c. Prohibits administration of a local anesthetic agent or N_2O-O_2 analgesia by a dental hygienist

d. Has unique educational and licensing procedures for dental hygienists

(1) Alabama Dental Hygiene Program, since 1919

(2) Only such preceptorship program in the United States

(3) Eligibility—1-year employment as a dental assistant, followed by an educational program that includes basic science and clinical theory

(4) Dentists are "preceptors," who provide on-the-job training in the dental office

(5) Program replaces formal dental hygiene education from an accredited academic program; graduates are not eligible to take the National Board Dental Hygiene Examination; therefore, their practice is limited to Alabama

(6) Graduates are not eligible for membership in the American Dental Hygienists Association

9. Updating dental practice acts

a. Revision or amendments made by state legislatures

BOX 22-1   States Where Dental Hygienists Can Provide Direct Access (Direct Access States)

For purposes of this document, "direct access" means that the dental hygienist can initiate treatment based on his or her assessment of a client's needs without the specific authorization of a dentist, treat the client without the presence of a dentist, and can maintain a provider-client relationship.

Alaska 2008
AS 08.32.115

Collaborative Agreement:
Hygienist may provide services according to terms of collaborative agreement. Dentist's presence, diagnosis, or treatment plan is not required unless specified by agreement. Care under the agreement can be provided in settings outside a dentist's "usual place of practice" (e.g., private dental office).
Special Requirements: Hygienist must have minimum of 4000 hours of clinical experience within preceding 5 years. Agreement must be approved by state board of dental examiners.
Services: Agreement can authorize nearly the entire dental hygiene scope of practice (e.g., client education, prophylaxis, sealants, x-ray films).
Notes:
- Dentists are limited to 5 or less collaborative agreements with dental hygienists.

Arizona 2006
32-1289B
Dental hygienist working under contract for schools, public health settings, and institutions may screen and apply fluoride unsupervised.

Arizona 2004
Sec. 32-1281 H, 32-1289

Affiliated Practice Agreement:
A dental hygienist with a written affiliated practice agreement may perform dental hygiene services on clients who meet certain financial criteria and are enrolled in a federal, state, county or local health care program. Written agreement must be submitted to state board of dental examiners. Hygienists must refer clients for additional treatment by a dentist within 12 months of first treatment.
Special Requirements: Hygienist must have 5 years of practice experience and must have been actively engaged in dental practice for at least 2000 hours in the preceding 5 years.
Services: The agreement must outline practice settings and services provided (nearly all of dental hygiene scope except root planing, local anesthesia, and nitrous oxide administration are allowed).
Notes:
- Direct Medicaid reimbursement allowed.

Arkansas 2010
Sec. 17-82-701

Collaborative Agreement:
A dental hygienist with a Collaborative Care Permit I or II who has entered into a collaborative agreement may perform dental hygiene services on children, senior citizens, and persons with developmental disabilities in long-term care facilities, free clinics, hospitals, Head Start programs, residence of homebound clients, local health units, schools, community health centers, and state and county correctional institutions. Hygienist must have written agreement with no more than one dentist.
Special Requirements: Must have malpractice insurance.Collaborative Care Permit I: hygienist must have 1200 hours of clinical practice experience or must have taught dental hygiene courses for 2 of the proceeding 3 years.Collaborative Care Permit II: hygienists must have 1800 hours of clinical practice

experience or has taught dental hygiene courses for 2 of the proceeding 3 years and has completed 6 hours of continuing education (CE) courses.
Services: Collaborative Care Permit I may provide prophylaxis, fluoride treatments, sealants, dental hygiene instruction, assessment and other services in scope if delegated by consulting dentist to children in public settings without supervision or prior examination.Collaborative Care Permit II may provide prophylaxis, fluoride treatments, sealants, dental hygiene instruction, assessment, and other services in scope if delegated by the consulting dentist to children, senior citizens, and persons with developmental disabilities in public settings without supervision or prior examination.

California 2002
Sec 1763 (a) 2002
Any dental hygienist may provide screening and apply fluorides and sealants without supervision in government-created or government-administered public health programs.

California 1998
Sec. 1774, 1775

Registered Dental Hygienist in Alternative Practice (RDHAP):
RDHAPs may provide unsupervised services for homebound persons or at schools, residential facilities, institutions, and in dental health professional shortage (DHPS) areas. RDHAPs can offer a client care for up to 18 months and provide additional care if the client obtains a prescription from a dentist or physician.
Special Requirements: RDHAP must have a bachelor's degree (or equivalent), 3 years of clinical experience, completion of additional 150 clock hours in designated courses, and pass exam. RDHAP must provide board with documentation of an existing relationship with at least one dentist for referral, consultation, and emergency services.
Services: All services permitted under general supervision, including prophylaxis, root planing, pit-and-fissure sealants, charting, and examination of soft tissue.
Notes:
- Direct Medicaid reimbursement is allowed.

Colorado 1987
Sec. 12-35-122.5

Unsupervised Practice:
There is no requirement that a dentist must authorize or supervise most dental hygiene services. Hygienist may also own a dental hygiene practice.
Special Requirements: None.
Services: Hygienist can provide dental hygiene diagnosis; take x-ray films; remove deposits, accretions, and stains; do curettage without anesthesia; apply fluorides and other recognized preventive agents; administer topical anesthetic; and perform oral inspection and charting. Local anesthesia requires general supervision.
Notes:
- Direct Medicaid reimbursement allowed.

Connecticut 1999
Section 20-126 I

Public Health Dental Hygienist:
Dental hygienists with 2 years of experience may practice without supervision in institutions, public health facilities, group homes, and schools.
Special Requirements: Hygienist must have at least 2 years of experience.
Services: Hygienist can provide oral prophylaxis; remove deposits, accretions, and stains; perform root planing; apply sealants; and do assessment, treatment planning, and evaluation.

(Continued)

BOX 22-1   **States Where Dental Hygienists Can Provide Direct Access (Direct Access States)—cont'd**

Notes:
- Direct Medicaid reimbursement allowed.

Florida 2011
Section 466.003. 466.024

Dental hygienists may provide services without the physical presence, prior examination, or authorization of a dentist, provided that a dentist or physician gives medical clearance before performance of prophylaxis in "health access settings." A dentist must examine a client within 13 months following prophylaxis, and an exam must take place before additional oral services may be performed.

Health access settings are a program of the Department of Children and Family Services, the Department of Health, the Department of Juvenile Justice, a nonprofit community health center centers, a Head Start centers, a Federally Qualified Health Center (FQHC), a school-based prevention program, or a clinic operated by an accredited dental or dental hygiene program.

Services: Dental charting, take vital signs, record histories, apply sealants and fluorides (including varnish), and perform the prophylaxis.

Notes:
- The setting operating the program may bill a third party for reimbursement of the hygienist's services.
- The hygienist must maintain professional liability insurance.

Idaho 2004
I.C. 54-903 (9)/54-904

Extended Access Endorsement:
Hygienist can provide services in a hospital, long-term care facility, public health facility, health or migrant clinic, or other board-approved setting if the dentist affiliated with setting authorizes services.

Special Requirements: Hygienist must be an employee of the facility or obtain Extended Care Permit; ECP requires 1000 hours experience in last 2 years.

Services: As determined by authorizing dentist.

Iowa 2004
Rule 650-10.5 (153)

Public Health Dental Hygienist:
Hygienist may administer care based on standing orders and a written agreement with a dentist.

Services can be administered in schools, Head Start settings, nursing facilities FQHCs, public health vans, free clinics, community centers, and public health programs.

Special Requirements: Hygienist must have 3 years of clinical experience and must submit an annual report to the state department of health noting the number of clients treated and services administered.

Services: All services in the dental hygiene scope (except local anesthesia and nitrous) may be provided once to each client. To offer repeat services other than assessment, screening, and fluoride, a dentist must examine the client.

Kansas 2003/2012
Sec. 65-1456

Extended Care Permit (ECP) I, II, and III:
Hygienist may practice without the prior authorization of a dentist if the hygienist has an agreement with sponsoring dentist who will monitor his or her practice. Examples of settings are schools, Head Start programs, state correctional institutions, local health departments, indigent care clinics, and in adult care homes, hospital long-term units, or at the home of homebound persons on medical assistance. The ECP I permit authorizes treatment on children in various limited-access categories, whereas the EPT II permit is for seniors and persons with developmental disabilities. ECP III permit authorizes hygienists to treat a wider range of clients, including underserved children, seniors, and developmentally disabled adults, and to provide more services than ECP I and II.

Special Requirements: Hygienist must have 1200 clinical hours or 2 years of teaching in last 3 years for ECP I and 1600 hours or 2 years of teaching in last 3 years plus 6-hour course for ECP II. Hygienist must also carry liability insurance and must be paid by dentist or facility. ECP III requires 2000 hours clinical experience plus 18 clock hours of board-approved course.

Services: ECP I and II provide prophylaxis, fluoride treatments, dental hygiene instruction, assessment of the client's need for further treatment by a dentist, and other services if delegated by the sponsoring dentist. ECP III can additionally provide atraumatic restorative technique, adjustment and soft reline of dentures, smoothing sharp teeth with handpiece, local anesthesia in setting where medical services available, and extraction of mobile teeth.

Notes:
- Dentist can only monitor 5 practices.

Kentucky 2010
313.040

Volunteer Community Health Settings:
A dental hygienist may provide the services listed below without the supervision of a dentist in volunteer community health settings.

Services: Hygienist can provide dental hygiene instruction, nutritional counseling, oral screening with subsequent referral to a dentist, fluoride application, demonstration of oral hygiene technique, and sealants.

Maine 2008
Sec. B-1. 32 MRSA c. 16, sub-c. 3-B

Independent Practice Dental Hygienist:
A dental hygienist licensed as an independent practice dental hygienist may practice without supervision by a dentist in all settings.

Special Requirements: Hygienist must possess a bachelor's degree from a Commission on Dental Accreditation (CODA)–accredited dental hygiene program and 2000 work hours of clinical practice during the 2 years preceding the application or possess an associate degree from a CODA-accredited dental hygiene program and 6000 work hours of clinical practice during the 6 years preceding the application. They are also required to provide a referral plan to clients in need of additional care by a dentist.

Services: Hygienist may interview patients and record complete medical and dental histories, take and record the vital signs of blood pressure, pulse and temperature, perform oral inspections, recording all conditions that should be called to the attention of a dentist; perform complete periodontal and dental restorative charting; perform all procedures necessary for a complete prophylaxis, including root planing; apply fluoride to control caries; apply desensitizing agents to teeth; apply topical anesthetics; apply sealants; smooth and polish amalgam restorations, limited to slow-speed application only; cement pontics and facings outside the mouth; take impressions for athletic mouthguards and custom fluoride trays; place and remove rubber dams; place temporary restorations in compliance with the protocol adopted by the board; and apply topical antimicrobials, excluding antibiotics, including fluoride, for the purposes of bacterial reduction, caries control, and desensitization in the oral cavity. The independent practice dental hygienist must follow current manufacturer's instructions in the use of these medicaments.

BOX 22-1 States Where Dental Hygienists Can Provide Direct Access (Direct Access States)—cont'd

Maine 2001
Rule 02 313 Chap. 1. Sec. 4

Public Health Dental Hygienist:
Hygienist may provide services in a public or private school, hospital, or other, nontraditional practice setting under a public health supervision status granted by the dental board on a case-by-case basis. The hygienist may perform services rendered under general supervision. The dentist should have specific standing orders and procedures to be carried out, although the dentist need not be present when the services have been provided. A written plan for referral or an agreement for follow-up shall be provided by the public health hygienist recording all conditions that should be called to the attention of the dentist. The supervising dentist shall review a summary report at the completion of the program or once a year.
Special Requirements: A dental hygienist must apply to the board to practice providing such information the board deems necessary. The board must take into consideration whether the program will fulfill an unmet need, whether a supervising dentist is available, and that the appropriate public health guidelines and standards of care can be met and followed.
Services: All services that can be provided under general supervision. Dentist's diagnosis for sealants is not needed in public health or school sealant programs.
Notes:
- Direct Medicaid reimbursement allowed.

Maryland 2010/2014
10.44.21.10

General Supervision:
A dental hygienist may practice dental hygiene under the general supervision of a dentist in a long-term care facility in accordance with this regulation. A dental hygienist practicing under the general supervision of a licensed dentist in a long-term care facility must have a written agreement with the supervising dentist that clearly sets forth the terms and conditions under which the dental hygienist may practice.
Special Requirements: A dental hygienist must hold an active license to practice dental hygiene in the State, hold a current certificate evidencing Health Care Provider Level C Proficiency, or its equivalent, in cardiopulmonary resuscitation, have at least 2 years of active clinical practice in direct client care, and ensure that the long-term care facility where the dental hygienist will practice under general supervision has:
  (a) A written medical emergency plan in place
  (b) Adequate equipment, including portable equipment and appropriate armamentarium, available for the appropriate delivery of dental hygiene services
  (c) Adequate safeguards to protect the client's health and safety
Services: Limit dental hygiene tasks and procedures to toothbrush prophylaxis, application of fluoride, dental hygiene instruction, and other duties as may be delegated, verbally or in writing, by the supervising dentist.

Massachusetts 2009
Chap. 112, Sec. 51.

Public Health Dental Hygienist:
Hygienist may provide dental hygiene services without the supervision of a dentist in public health settings, including, and not limited to, hospitals, medical facilities, schools, and community clinics. Prior to providing services, a public health dental hygienist must have a written collaborative agreement with a local or state government agency or institution, or licensed dentist that states the level of communication with the dental hygienist to ensure client health and safety. Public health dental hygienists must provide clients with a written referral to a dentist and an assessment of further dental needs.
Special Requirements: Hygienist must have at least 3 years of full-time clinical experience practicing in a public health setting and any other training deemed appropriate by the department of health.
Services: Hygienist can provide full scope of dental hygiene practice services allowed under general supervision in the private office, including prophylaxis, root planing, curettage, sealants, and fluoride.
Notes:
- Direct Medicaid reimbursement allowed.

Michigan 2005
Sec. 333.16625

PA 161 Dental Hygienist:
Hygienist with grantee status can practice in a public or nonprofit entity, or a school or nursing home that administers a program of dental care to a dentally underserved population. Collaborating dentist need not be present for or authorize treatment, but hygienist must have continuous availability of direct communication with a dentist to establish emergency protocol and review client records.
Special Requirements: Hygienist must apply to the state department of community health for designation as grantee health agency.
Services: Hygienist can provide full scope of dental hygiene services allowed under general supervision, including prophylaxis, sealants, and fluoride treatments.

Minnesota 2001
Section 150A. 10, Subd. 1a

Collaborative Practice:
Hygienist must enter into a written collaborative agreement with a licensed dentist that designates authorization for the services provided by the dental hygienist (agreement need not be submitted to state). Collaborative practice hygienist can be employed or retained by a health care facility, program, or nonprofit organization.
Special Requirements: Hygienist must have at least 2400 hours of clinical experience in the preceding 18 months or a career total of 3000 hours, including a minimum of 200 hours of clinical practice in 2 of the past 3 years. Hygienist must also meet additional CE requirements.
Services: Collaborative practice hygienist can administer prophylaxis, application of topical preventive and prophylactic agents, application of sealants, fluoride varnishes, coronal polishing, preliminary charting, x-ray films, and root planing.
Notes:
- Direct Medicaid reimbursement allowed.

Missouri 2001
Statute 332.311.2

Public Health Dental Hygienist:
Hygienist may provide services without supervision in public health settings to Medicaid-eligible children and can be directly reimbursed by Medicaid.
Special Requirements: Hygienist must have 3 years of experience.
Services: Hygienist can provide oral prophylaxis, sealants, and fluorides.
Notes:
- Direct Medicaid reimbursement allowed.

(Continued)

Montana 2003
Sec. 37-4-405

Public Health Dental Hygienist/Limited Access Permit (LAP):
Dental hygienists may obtain an LAP to practice under public health supervision in a variety of federally funded health centers and clinics, nursing homes, extended care facilities, home health agencies, group homes (elderly, disabled, youth), Head Start programs, migrant work facilities, and local and state public health facilities. Public health supervision means the hygienist can provide services without the authorization of a dentist provided the hygienist follows protocols to be established by the board and refers any clients needing dental treatment.
Special Requirements: Hygienist must have 2400 hours experience in the last 3 years; 3000 hours over career with 350 hours each of the last 2 years. An additional 12 hours CE every 2 years and liability insurance are also required.
Services: Hygienist can provide prophylaxis, fluoride, root planing, sealants, polishing of restorations, x-ray films for diagnosis by a dentists, and oral cancer screening.
Notes:
- Direct Medicaid reimbursement allowed.

Nebraska 2007
Sec. 71-193.18

Public Health Dental Hygienist:
The Department of Health may authorize an unsupervised RDH to provide public health–related services in a public health setting or a health care or related facility.
Special Requirements: Hygienist must have 3000 hours experience in at least 4 of last 5 years. Hygienist must also have professional liability insurance.
Services: Hygienist can perform prophylaxis for a healthy child, pulp vitality testing, and preventive measures, including fluorides and sealants.
Notes:
- Direct Medicaid reimbursement allowed.

New Hampshire 1993
Rule 302.02(d); 402.01 (c)

Public Health Supervision:
Hygienist may treat clients in public or private school, hospital or institution, or residence of a homebound client. Supervising dentist must authorize hygienist to provide services (i.e., standing orders) but need not be present for care.
Special Requirements: None.
Services: Hygienist can provide instruction in oral hygiene, topical fluorides, and oral prophylaxis; assess medical/dental history; do periodontal probing/charting; and apply sealants.

New Mexico 2007
Sec. 61-5-C
No supervision required for any dental hygienist to apply fluorides, and remineralization agents.

New Mexico 1999/2011
Sec. 61-5A-4D, Rule 16.5.17

Collaborative Practice:
Hygienist can practice in any setting with collaborative agreement and can own or manage a collaborative dental hygiene practice. Hygienist must enter into a written agreement with one or more collaborative dentist(s), which must contain protocols for care. Hygienist must refer clients for annual dental exam.
Special Requirements: Hygienist must have 2400 hours of active practice in preceding 18 months or 3000 hours in 2 of the past 3 years.
Services: Collaborative practice hygienist can provide a dental hygiene–focused assessment, x-ray films, oral prophylaxis, fluoride treatments, assessment for and application of sealants, root planing, and may prescribe and administer and dispense topically applied fluoride and antimicrobials, depending on the specific services allowed in agreement with collaborating dentist.
Notes:
- Dentist may not collaborate with more than 3 hygienists.
- Direct Medicaid reimbursement allowed.

New York 2005
Rules Sec. 61.9

General Supervision:
Hygienist can initiate client care in any public or private setting. Dentist must authorize (i.e., issue standing orders) for dental hygienist and be available for consultation, diagnosis, and evaluation.
Services: Hygienist can provide prophylaxis, root planing, fluoride treatments, client education, charting, and x-ray films without a prior dental examination, the presence of a dentist, or need to refer to a dentist.

Nevada 1998
Sec. 631.287

Public Health Dental Hygienist:
Dental hygienists may obtain approval to work as public health dental hygienists in schools, community centers, hospitals, nursing homes, and such other locations as the state dental health officer deems appropriate without supervision.
Special Requirements: Special endorsement from the dental board. Submissions of protocol to describe the methods a hygienist will use to provide services.
Services: May provide most hygiene services and may administer local anesthesia and nitrous oxide in a facility with certain equipment and dentist authorization.
Notes:
- Direct Medicaid reimbursement allowed.

Ohio 2010
Sec. 4715.363

Oral Health Access Supervision Permit Program:
Dental hygienists who possess an oral health access supervision permit may provide dental hygiene services through a written agreement with a dentist in public health settings, including, and not limited to, health care facilities, state correctional institutions, residential facilities, schools, shelters for victims of domestic abuse or runaways, foster homes, nonprofit clinics, dispensaries, and mobile dental clinics. Before providing services, a dental hygienist with an oral health access supervision permit must have a written agreement with a dentist, who possesses an oral health supervision permit, that states the dentist has evaluated the dental hygienist's skills and has reviewed and evaluated the client's health history. The dentist need not be present or examine the client before the dental hygienist may provide care. The collaborating dentist must perform a clinical evaluation of the client before the dental hygienist may provide subsequent care. The evaluation may be done using electronic communication.
Special Requirements: Two years and a minimum of 3000 hours of clinical experience; minimum of 24 CE credits during the 2 years before applying for the

BOX 22-1 States Where Dental Hygienists Can Provide Direct Access (Direct Access States)—cont'd

Oral Health Access Supervision Permit, including a course on identification and prevention of potential medical emergencies; and completed an oral health access supervision permit class approved by the board.

Services: Prophylactic, preventive, and other procedures a dentist can delegate to a hygienist, except definitive root planing, definitive subgingival curettage, administration of local anesthesia, and other procedures specified in rules adopted by the board.

Ohio 2013
House Bill 59 (amendment adopted; not yet codified)

The requirement for a dentist to perform an examination and diagnose a client before the client receives dental hygiene services through a program operated by a school district or other specified entity does not apply when the only services to be provided are the placement of pit-and-fissure sealants.

Oklahoma 2003
Sec. 328.34 C

General Supervision:
Hygienist may provide services outside the private dental office for a client not examined by the dentist. Dentist must authorize care in writing.

Special Requirements: Hygienist must have at least 2 years of experience.
Services: Most dental hygiene services, including sealants, fluorides, and prophylaxis, to a client one time before a dental exam.

Oregon 2011
Sec 680.205

Expanded Practice Dental Hygienist (EPDH)
Replaces Limited Access Permit (LAP); adds services to clients below federal poverty level and other settings approved by the board to EPDH practice settings; adds limited prescriptive authority, local anesthesia, temporary restorations, and dental assessments to unsupervised EPDH scope if EPDH has agreement with a dentist; requires insurance reimbursement of EPDHs.

Oregon 1997
Sec. 680.200
Rule 818-035-0065

Limited Access Permit (LAP):
Dental hygienists who have obtained an LAP may initiate unsupervised services for clients in a variety of limited-access settings such as extended care facilities, facilities for mentally ill or disabled persons, correctional facilities, schools and preschools, medical offices or offices operated or staffed by a nurse practitioner midwives or physician assistants, and job training centers. Hygienist must refer the client annually to a licensed dentist available to treat the client.

Special Requirements: Hygienist must have 2500 hours of supervised dental hygiene practice and has completed 40 hours of board-approved courses in an accredited dental hygiene program or completed a board-approved course of study that includes at least 500 hours of dental hygiene practice on clients with limited access while under direct faculty supervision. Hygienist must also have liability insurance.

Services: LAP hygienists can provide all dental hygiene services; however, some services (local anesthesia, pit-and-fissure sealants, denture relines, temporary restorations, radiographs, nitrous oxide) must be supervised by a dentist. Hygienist may prescribe fluorides and assess the need for sealants.

Notes:
- Direct Medicaid reimbursement allowed.

Pennsylvania 2007
Sec. 2 (Definitions), Sec. 11.9

Public Health Dental Hygiene Practitioner:
Dental hygienists who are certified as public health dental hygiene practitioners may provide care in a variety of public health settings without the supervision or prior authorization of a dentist.

Special Requirements: Hygienist must have 3600 hours experience and liability insurance. Hygienist must also complete 5 hours of continuing education in public health during each licensure period.

Services: Dental hygienists in the state are authorized to provide educational, preventive, therapeutic, and intraoral services, including complete prophylaxis and sealants.

Rhode Island 2006
Sec. 5-31.1-6.1

General Supervision:
Dental hygienists working under a dentist's general supervision can initiate dental hygiene treatment to residents of nursing facilities. Dental hygienists working in nursing facilities can treat clients, regardless of whether or not the client is a patient of record, as long as documentation of services administered is maintained and necessary referrals for follow-up treatment are made.

Special Requirements: None.

Services: Hygienist can initiate dental hygiene services, including oral health screening assessments, prophylaxis, fluoride treatments, charting, and other duties delegable under general supervision.

South Carolina 2003
Sec. 40-15-110 (A) (10)

General Supervision:
Hygienists employed by, or contacted through, the Department of Health and Environment Control (DHEC) may provide services under general supervision that does not require prior examination by a dentist in settings such as schools or nursing homes.

Special Requirements: Hygienist must carry professional liability insurance.
Services: Hygienist employed by, or contacted through, the DHEC may provide prophylaxis, fluorides, and sealants.

South Dakota 2011
Sec 36-6A-40

Collaborative practice was enacted, but the rules needed to implement are pending. It will enable a dental hygienist actively engaged in clinical practice for 2 of the last 3 years to enter into a collaborative agreement with a dentist to provide preventive and therapeutic services to a client for up to 13 months before the dentist must evaluate the client.

Services: To be established in rules.

Tennessee 2013
Sec. 63-5-109

Dental hygienists may apply dental sealants or topical fluoride to the teeth of individuals in a setting under the direction of a state or local health department, without requiring an evaluation by a dentist prior to such application, under a protocol established by the state or a metropolitan health department.

Texas 2001
Sec. 262.1515

(Continued)

BOX 22-1   States Where Dental Hygienists Can Provide Direct Access (Direct Access States)—cont'd

General Supervision:

Hygienist may provide services for up to 6 months without dentist seeing the client. Services may be performed in school-based health center, nursing facility, or community health center. Hygienist must refer the client to a dentist after treatment and may not perform a second set of services until the client has been examined by a dentist.

Special Requirements: Hygienist must have at least 2 years of experience.

Services: No limitations; dentist must authorize services in writing.

Vermont 2008
Rule 10.2

General Supervision Agreement:

Hygienist may provide services in a public or private school or institution under the supervision of a dentist through a general supervision agreement. The agreement authorizes the hygienist to provide services, as agreed to between the dentist and the dental hygienist. The agreement does not require physical presence of the dentist but stipulates that the supervising dentist review all client records.

Special Requirements: Hygienist must have 3 years licensed clinical practice experience.

Services: Hygienist can provide sealants, fluoride varnish, prophylaxis and x-ray films; periodontal maintenance is allowable to clients with mild periodontitis.

Virginia 2009
Sec. 54.1-2722

Remote Supervision:

Virginia Pilot Project seeks to assess the impact that dental hygienists practicing in an expanded capacity under remote supervision have on increasing access to dental health care for underserved populations. Hygienist will refer clients without a dental provider to a dentist with the goal of establishing a dental home. Hygienists must enter into a remote supervision agreement with a licensed dentist and maintain regular, periodic communication (14-day intervals) with the licensed dentist (protocol must be submitted to Department of Health).

Special Requirements: Hygienists must have 2 years of experience and must be employed by the Department of Health.

Services: Hygienists can provide initial examination of teeth and surrounding areas, prophylaxis, scaling, sealants, topical fluoride, education services, assessments, and screening.

Washington 2007
Sec. 18.29.056

Off-Site Supervision:

Hygienist can provide care to clients in "senior centers" if hygienist has a written agreement with dentist to provide "off-site" supervision.

Special Requirements: Hygienist must have 2 years of clinical experience. Hygienist must collect client data to submit to the Department of Health.

Services: Hygienist can provide prophylaxis, root planing, curettage, and apply preventive agents.

Washington 2001
Sec. 18.29.220

Public Health Dental Hygienist:

Dental hygienists who are school endorsed may assess for and apply sealants and fluoride varnishes and perform prophylaxis in community-based sealant programs carried out in schools.

Special Requirements: Sealant/Fluoride Varnish Endorsement from Department of Health. Hygienist must submit data to the Department of Health concerning patient demographics, treatment, reimbursement, referrals, etc.

Washington 1984
Sec. 18.29.056

Unsupervised Practice:

Unsupervised practice in hospitals, nursing homes, home health agencies, group homes (elderly, handicapped, or youth), state institutions under Department of Health and Human Services (DHHS), jails, and public health facilities, provided the hygienist refers the client to a dentist for dental treatment and needed care.

Special Requirements: Hygienist must have 2 years clinical experience within the last 5 years.

Services: Hygienist can provide prophylaxis, application of typical preventive or prophylactic agents, polishing and smoothing of restorations, root planing, and curettage.

Notes:
- Direct Medicaid reimbursement allowed.

West Virginia 2008
Sec. 5-1-8.5

Public Health Dental Hygienist:

Hygienist may provide care in hospitals, schools, correctional facilities, jails, community clinics, long-term care facilities, nursing homes, home health agencies, group homes, state institutions under DHSS, public health facilities, homebound settings, and accredited dental hygiene education programs. Dentist must authorize hygienist to provide care (i.e., standing orders) but need not be present have previously seen the client.

Special Requirements: Hygienist must have 2 years and 3000 hours of clinical experience and take six additional CE hours. Hygienist and dentist must submit annual written report of care to state board of dental examiners.

Services: Hygienist can provide patient education, nutrition counseling, and oral screening with referral to dentist; apply fluoride and sealants; and offer complete prophylaxis (pursuant to a collaborative agreement or written order).

Wisconsin 2007
Sec. 447.06

The statute does not require the presence or supervision of a dentist in a public or private school, a dental or dental hygiene school, or a facility owned by a local health department.

Special Requirements: None

Services: Hygienist can provide prophylaxis, root planing, screening, treatment planning, sealants, and delegable duties.

Notes:
- Direct Medicaid reimbursement allowed.

From the American Dental Hygienists Association, 2014. https://www.adha.org/resources-docs/7524_Current_Direct_Access_Map.pdf.

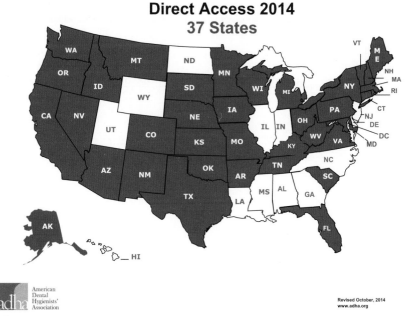

FIG 22-2 States in which dental hygienists can provide direct access. (From the American Dental Hygienists' Association. https://www.adha.org/resources-docs/7524_Current_Direct_Access_Map.pdf.)

b. Sunset laws—set review of the entire act at a fixed interval (e.g., every 7 years, to keep act updated and relevant to society); if not completed by legislature by designated date or if found to no longer serve its function to society, the act will automatically expire (thus the term *sunset*)

10. Due process requirements for disciplinary action—if a complaint is filed against a professional, with the licensing board, the licensee has a right to:
    a. Receive a clear statement of charges
    b. Question opposing witnesses
    c. Produce witnesses and give testimony (answer charges)
    d. The services of an attorney
    e. Receive a firm conclusion based on the evidence
    f. Contest the board's decision at a court of law
    g. If these rights are not provided, the board's decision could be reversed by a court of law

11. Practicing without a license—penalties vary from state to state
    a. Criminal charges—usually result in a fine (~$50 to $500) or imprisonment (usually not to exceed 60 days), or both
    b. Civil suits—may be filed for monetary damages by individuals who have been harmed
    c. Criminal or civil actions, or both, may be brought against the unlicensed person

12. Reporting professional violations—failure to report a violation is grounds for disciplinary action; failure to report is considered unprofessional conduct; reporting a violation requires the following:
    a. Facts must be documented in writing with complete description of violation

b. Report must list other witnesses and clients involved, if applicable

13. National Practitioner Data Bank (NPDB)
    a. Created by the U.S. Department of Health and Human Services (DHHS) in 1990
    b. Purpose—electronic repository that collects information on adverse licensure actions, certain actions restricting clinical privileges, and professional society membership actions taken against physicians, dentists, and other practitioners
    c. Medical and dental regulatory boards are required to report certain actions taken against licensees
    d. Health care entities such as hospitals are required to report certain disciplinary action taken against staff members
    e. Licensees are not required to report incidents
    f. Access to data bank information
       (1) Individuals, who may request their own record
       (2) State licensing boards
       (3) Researchers, health care entities (e.g., hospitals, nursing homes)
       (4) Professional societies
       (5) Attorneys
    g. The law prohibits the release of information in the NPDB to the public

14. Health Care Integrity and Protection Data Bank (HIPDB)
    a. Combats fraud and abuse in health insurance and health care delivery
    b. Flagging system used to alert users
    c. Intended to augment, not replace, traditional forms of review and investigation, serving as an important supplement to a review of a practitioner's, providers, or supplier's past actions

TABLE 22-3   Local Anesthesia Administration by Dental Hygienists: State Chart

State and Year Implement	Supervision Required	Block and/or Infiltration	Education Required	Exam Required	Implement Language in Statute or Rules	Legal Requirements for Local Anesthesia Courses (hours)?
AK 1981	General	Both	Specific	Yes—WREB	Statute	16 didactic 6 clinical 8 lab
AZ 1976	Direct	Both	Accredited	Yes—WREB	Statute	36 total; 9 types of injections
AR 1995	Direct	Both	Approved and Accredited	No	Statute	16 didactic 12 clinical
CA 1976	Direct	Both	Course taken as part of dental hygiene program or course approved by Dental Hygiene Committee of California	No	Rules	16 didactic 3 clinical 8 types of injections listed
CO 1977	General	Both	Accredited	No	Statute	12 didactic 12 clinical
CT 2005	Direct	Both	Accredited	No	Statute	20 didactic 8 clinical
DC 2004	Direct	Both	Board approved	No	Rules	20 didactic 12 clinical
FL 2012	Direct	Both	Accredited	No	Statute	30 didactic 12 clinical
HI 1987	Direct	Both	Accredited	Yes—exam given by course	Statute	39 didactic and clinical 50 injections
ID 1975	General	Both	Accredited	Yes—board approved	Statute	No
IA 1998	Direct	Both	Accredited	No	Rules	
IL 2000	Direct	Both	Accredited	No	Statute	24 didactic 8 clinical
IN 2010	Direct	Both	Accredited	Yes—NERB local anesthesia exam or equivalent state or regional exam	Rules	15 didactic 14 clinical Permit required
KS 1993	Direct	Both	Accredited and board approved	No	Statute	12 total
KY 2002	Direct	Both	Accredited and board approved	Yes—written exam given by course	Statute	32 didactic 12 clinical
LA 1998	Direct	Both	Accredited	Yes—board approved	Rules	72 total; minimum of 20 injections
MA 2004	Direct	Both	Accredited	Yes—NERB written exam by NERB	Statute	35 total; at least 12 clinical

State and Year Implement	Supervision Required	Block and/or Infiltration	Education Required	Exam Required for Certificate?	Implement Language in Statute or Rules	Legal Requirements for Local Anesthesia Courses?
ME 1997	Direct	Both	Accredited	Yes—board administered	Rules	40 total; minimum of 50 injections
MD 2009	Direct	Both	Accredited and board approved	Yes—NERB	Rules	20 didactic 8 clinical
MN 1995	General	Both	Accredited	No	Rules	No
MO 1973	Direct	Both	Accredited and board approved	No	Rules	No
MI 2002	Direct	Both	Accredited	Yes—state or regional board–administered written exam (NERB)	Statute	15 didactic 14 clinical
MT 1985	Direct	Both		Yes—WREB	Statute	No
ND 2003	Direct	Both	Accredited	No	Rules	Course must include clinical and didactic components, but no specific hourly requirements.

State and Year Implement	Supervision Required	Block and/or Infiltration	Education Required	Exam Required for Certificate?	Implement Language in Statute or Rules	Legal Requirements for Local Anesthesia Courses?
NE 1995	Direct	Both	Approved	No	Statute	12 didactic 10 types of injections listed 12 clinical
NH 2002	Direct	Both	Accredited	Yes—NERB local anesthesia exam	Statute	20 didactic 12 clinical
NV 1982	Direct General	Both	Accredited and approved	No	Rules	No
NM 1972	Direct General	Both	Accredited and approved	Yes—WREB	Statute	24 didactic 10 clinical
NJ 2008	Direct	Both	Accredited and board approved	Yes—NERB local anesthesia	Rules	20 didactic 12 clinical Including a minimum of 20 hours monitored administration of local anesthesia
NY 2001	Direct	Infiltration	Accredited	No	Statute	30 didactic 15 clinical and lab
OH 2006	Direct	Both	Accredited	Yes—written regional or state exam	Statute	15 didactic 14 clinical
OK 1980	Direct	Both	Approved	No—exam given by course	Rules	20 total
OR 1975	General	Both	Accredited or approved	No	Rules	No
PA 2009	Direct	Both	Accredited and approved	No	Rules	30 Didactic and Clinical Permit; must renew
RI 2005	Direct	Both	Accredited	Yes—NERB	Statute	20 didactic 12 clinical
SC 1995	Direct	Infiltration	Approved	Yes—board	Statute	No
SD 1992	Direct	Both	Accredited and approved	No	Statute	No
TN 2004	Direct	Both	Accredited and approved	No	Rules	24 didactic 8 clinical
UT 1983	Direct	Both	Accredited	Yes—WREB	Statute	No
VT 1993	Direct	Both	Accredited	Yes—board administered	Statute	24 total
VA 2006	Direct	Both *Only on clients over age 18	Accredited	Yes—accredited program Board of another jurisdiction accepted	Statute	36 didactic-clinical
WA 1971	Direct	Both	Approved	Yes—WREB	Statute	10 listed injections
WI 1998	Direct	Both	Accredited	No	Statute	10 didactic 11 clinical
WV 2003	Direct	Both	Board approved	NERB local anesthesia exam or equivalent state or regional exam	Statute	12 didactic 15 clinical
WY 1991	Direct	Both	Approved	Yes	Rules	No

Accredited—Course must be provided within a Commission on Dental Accreditation (CODA)–accredited dental hygiene (DH) program or an institution housing a CODA program.
Approved—Course must be approved by the state licensing agency
Specific—Course is specified in law.
Direct Supervision—means the dentist must be present.
General Supervision—means dentist need not be present.
NERB, Northeast Regional Board of Dental Examiners, Inc.; *WREB*, WREB: A National Dental and Dental Hygiene Testing Agency.
Data compiled from 51 practice acts/rules.

STATES WHERE DENTAL HYGIENISTS MAY ADMINISTER LOCAL ANESTHESIA

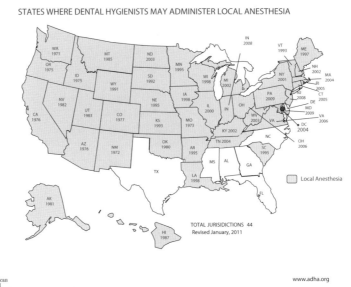

FIG 22-3 States in which dental hygienists can administer local anesthesia. (From the American Dental Hygienists Association. http://www.adha.org/resources-docs/7521_Local_Anesthesia_by_State.pdf.)

DENTAL RECORDS AND RECORD KEEPING

A. Purpose of dental records
 1. Provides all privileged parties with information; method of communication with dental and other medical providers
 2. Tool for quality assessment and management
 3. Documents assessment findings, treatment, care provided, and outcomes
 4. Serves as an important document in third-party relationships
 5. Provides evidence of compliance with state record-keeping requirements
 6. Resource in forensic identification
 7. Reference in litigation and provides information for the client and provider
 8. Useful in research
B. Written record management
 1. Adheres to state dental practice or state medical records guidelines, if required
 2. Legible and written in black ink or ballpoint, not pencil
 3. Consistent style for all entries; uniformly spaced
 4. Corrections and additions clearly explained
 5. Deletions noted by single line through entry
 6. Signed and initialed by appropriate operator
C. Electronic dental records
 1. Same record-keeping principles as for paper records
 2. System should include protections from tampering
 3. Courts accept as documentation
D. Client records—must be clear, complete, and accurate and include:
 1. Client identification data—client's name, address, employment, home and cell telephone numbers, Social Security number, birth date, emergency contact, physician's name and phone number, financial information; legal guardian information, if appropriate
 2. Consent forms—informed consent and informed refusal
 3. Health, pharmacologic, and dental histories—before treatment, updated at each visit, signed and dated by the client and oral health care professional
 4. Referrals—referrals made to other professionals, reports of tests, or reports from other providers
 5. Clinical observations—intraoral and extraoral examination results, findings of pathology, periodontal evaluation, radiographs, study models, diagnostic photographs
 6. Progress or treatment notes—chronologic notation of treatment, pretreatment procedures, unusual incidents or circumstances, diagnosis and care plans, oral hygiene recommendations, client noncompliance, postoperative instructions, telephone conversations with the client or other health care providers, medications taken or prescribed with dosage, client's missed or canceled appointments
 7. Failure to maintain or store dental records for a specified period may violate state dental practice acts; considered medical malpractice in some jurisdictions in a court of law
 8. Records also include radiographs, photographs, and models
 9. State regulations or statutes may delineate specific costs for duplication of records
E. Confidentiality—client confidentiality is protected by federal and state laws; state laws often regulate the disclosure of substance abuse, mental health history, human immunodeficiency virus/acquired immunodeficiency syndrome (HIV/AIDS) status; improper disclosure can result in liability for breach of fiduciary duty, breach of implied contract, or invasion of privacy

TABLE 22-4 Nitrous Oxide Administration by Dental Hygienists

State	Year Enacted	Statute or Rules	Education	Permit or Certificate
Alaska	1997	Rules	3 clinical/3 didactic hours CPR	No
Arizona	1976	Rules	36 hours, included in local anesthesia course	No
Arkansas	1994	Rules	Minimum of 4 hours	No
California	1974	Rules	Board-approved course	No
Colorado	1997	Statute	16 hours	Yes
District of Columbia	2004	Rules	32 hours total	Yes
Idaho	1979	Rules	Degree completion or accredited	No
Illinois	1999	Rules	14 hours	No board certification, but 12-hour course required; must provide proof of completion
Iowa	2001	Rules	Board-approved course or part of degree	No
Kansas	1994	Statute	Board-approved course 12 hours	No
Kentucky	2002	Statute	2 hours clinical, in addition to 32 hours of local anesthesia course and 12 hours of practical demonstration	Yes
Louisiana	2010	Statute	Rules pending	Yes
Maine	2006	Rules	8 hours didactic 8 hours clinical CODA-accredited or board-approved course and exit exam	Yes
Michigan	2004	Statute	4 didactic hours 4 clinical hours	Yes
Minnesota	1995	Rules	16 hours of clinical-didactic CPR	No
Missouri	1994	Rules	Course that provides proof of competence	Yes
Nevada	1982	Statute	Board-approved course or part of degree	Yes
New Hampshire	2006	Statute	8 hours didactic 6 hours clinical	Yes
New Jersey	2008	Rules	7 didactic hours 7 clinical hours CPR	Yes
New York	2001	Statute	30 didactic hours 15 clinical hours	Yes
Ohio	2010	Rules	4 didactic hours 2 clinical hours, written exam Clinical evaluation	Yes
Oklahoma	1975	Rules	12 hours completed in board-approved course	No
Oregon	1975	Rules	14 hours in nitrous oxide administration CPR	Yes
Rhode Island	2011	Rules	4 didactic hours 4 clinical hours CPR	
South Dakota	1992	Rules	Board-approved course	Yes
Tennessee	2000	Rules	Board-approved course	Yes
Utah	1983	Statute		Yes
Virginia	2006	Statute	8 hours didactic and clinical	Yes
*on patients aged 18 and older only				
Washington	1971	Rules	Didactic-clinical competency	No

CODA, Commission on Dental Accreditation; *CPR,* cardiopulmonary resuscitation.
*Most states require dentist to be present. Please check with the state licensing agencies for specific information on any one state.

1. Health Insurance Portability and Accountability Act (HIPAA)
   a. Purpose—this federal act allows employees to move their health insurance when changing jobs and is in place to develop standards for health information, provide greater safeguards regarding privacy of protected health information (PHI), and reduce health care fraud and abuse
   b. Protects health information by establishing transaction standards for the exchange of health information, security standards, and privacy standards for the use and disclosure of individually identifiable health information (IIHI)
   c. PHI includes all individually identifiable health information that is:
      (1) Sent or stored in any form

States Where Dental Hygienists Can Administer Nitrous Oxide

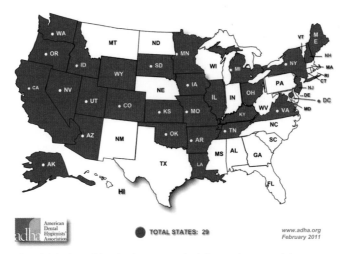

TOTAL STATES: 29

www.adha.org
February 2011

FIG 22-4 States in which dental hygienists can administer nitrous oxide–oxygen analgesia. (From the American Dental Hygienists Association. http://www.adha.org/resources-docs/7522_Nitrous_Oxide_by_State.pdf.)

TABLE 22-5 Dental Hygienists Restorative Duties by State

State	Apply Cavity Liners and Bases	Place and Remove Temporary Restorations	Place and Remove Temporary Crowns	Place, Carve, and Finish Amalgam Restoration	Place and Finish Composite Resin Silicate Restoration	Requirements
AK				Allowed*	Allowed*	Board-approved course WREB or equivalent exam
AL	Allowed*	Allowed*	Place only*	Prohibited	Prohibited	
AR				Prohibited	Prohibited	Program
AZ		Place*				
CA	Allowed*	Allowed*	Allowed*	Allowed* Requires RDAEF license	Allowed* Requires RDAEF license	
CO						
CT		Prohibited		Prohibited	Prohibited	
DC	Prohibited	Allowed		Prohibited	Prohibited	
DE		Prohibited	Prohibited	Prohibited	Prohibited	
FL	Allowed	Allowed	Allowed	Prohibited	Prohibited	
GA	Allowed*		Allowed*			
HI				Prohibited	Prohibited	
IA	Allowed*	Allowed*				
ID	Allowed*		Place only*	Allowed	Allowed	Restorative endorsement WREB or equivalent restorative exam.
IL				Prohibited	Prohibited	
IN						
KS						
KY	Allowed*		Allowed*	Allowed*	Allowed*	Proof of competency.
LA				Prohibited	Prohibited	
MA	Prohibited	Remove only*	Allowed*	Prohibited	Prohibited	
MD		Allowed	Allowed	Prohibited	Prohibited	
ME		Allowed	Allowed*	Allowed*	Allowed*	Board-approved EFDA program

TABLE 22-5 Dental Hygienists Restorative Duties by State—cont'd

State	Apply Cavity Liners and Bases	Place and Remove Temporary Restorations	Place and Remove Temporary Crowns	Place, Carve, and Finish Amalgam Restoration	Place and Finish Composite Resin Silicate Restoration	Requirements
MI	Allowed*	Allowed*	Allowed	Allowed*		Registered dental assistant took approved course
MN		Allowed*	Allowed*	Allowed	Allowed*	Board-approved course to place and adjust permanent restorations
		Note: MN also permits registered dental hygienist (RDH) to place, contour, and adjust glass ionomer.				
MO		Allowed*		Allowed*	Place only*	Proof of competency
MS						
MT		Allowed*		Prohibited	Prohibited	
NC	Allowed*	Place only*				
ND	Prohibited	Allowed*	Allowed*	Prohibited	Prohibited	
NE				Prohibited	Prohibited	
NH	Allowed	Allowed	Allowed*	Place		Expanded Duty course
NJ		Allowed*				
NM		Allowed	Allowed	Allowed	Allowed	EFDA certification
NV		Place only	Allowed			
NY		Allowed*		Allowed*	Allowed*	Approved course
OH		Allowed*		Place only	Place only	
OK		Place only				
OR				Allowed*	Allowed*	Board-approved course WREB or equivalent exam; restorative function endorsement
PA	Allowed*			Allowed*	Allowed*	
RI		Allowed		Prohibited	Prohibited	
SC				Prohibited	Prohibited	
SD		Place only		Prohibited	Prohibited	
TN	Allowed	Allowed		Place only		Restorative Function Permit
TX	Prohibited	Prohibited	Prohibited	Prohibited	Prohibited	
UT						
VA						
VT						Training in expanded function
WA		Allowed*	Allowed*	Allowed*	Allowed*	Restorative services in curriculum of Washington Dental Hygiene programs WREB restorative required for dental hygiene license
WI		Place only				Replacement of temporary restorations in emergency situations only
WV	Allowed*	Allowed*	Allowed			
WY		Place only		Allowed (with Expanded Permit [EP] certificate)	Allowed (with EP certificate)	Expanded Function certificate no longer offered, but existing certificates honored

This chart is for comparative purposes only. If information does not indicate whether one of the functions is prohibited or allowed, no assumptions should be made.

Disclaimer: Information based on American Dental Hygienists Association (ADHA) staff research of state statutes and legislation. This document should not be considered a legal document.

RDAEF, Registered Dental Assistant in Expanded Functions; *EFDA,* Expanded Functions Dental Assistant; *WREB,* WREB: A National Dental and Dental Hygiene Testing Agency.

*Can do services by virtue of inclusion in dental assistants' scope of practice. Please check practice act for education requirements.

BOX 22-2 Dental Hygiene Participation in Regulation

The following states have dental hygiene advisory committees or varying degrees of self-regulation for dental hygienists.

1. Arizona

   The Arizona advisory committee consists of one dentist and one dental hygienist from the board, plus four additional dental hygienists and one public member. The committee serves as a forum for discussion of dental hygiene issues and advises the board on rules and proposed statute changes concerning dental hygiene education, regulation, and practice. In addition, the committee evaluates continuing education (CE) classes for expanded functions and monitors dental hygienists' compliance with CE requirements.

2. California

   The Dental Hygiene Committee of California is a self-regulating dental hygiene committee in conjunction with the Department of Consumer Affairs. The committee consists of four dental hygienists, four public members, and one dentist appointed by the governor.

3. Connecticut

   Connecticut is unique. Dental hygiene is directly under the Department Public Health. Although there is no standing dental hygiene committee, if there is a need to address rules or disciplinary matters, the department director has the ability to appoint an ad hoc committee of dental hygienists.

4. Delaware

   Delaware's advisory committee is appointed by the governor and consists of three dental hygienists. The committee writes the examination for dental hygiene licensure, in conjunction with the dental board. In addition, the committee votes with the board on issues of dental hygiene licensure by credentials, disciplinary decisions, CE requirements for dental hygiene licensure, disciplinary action involving dental hygienists, and issues involving the policy and practice of dental hygiene, but not the scope of practice.

5. Florida

   Florida has both dental hygiene and dental assisting councils. The dental hygiene council is composed of four dental hygienists, one of whom sits on the board, and one dentist member of the board. The council is expected to develop all dental hygiene rules to submit to the board for its approval.

6. Iowa

   Beginning in 1999, both dental hygienists on the dental board and one of the dentists became a dental hygiene committee of the board. This committee has the power to make all rules pertaining to dental hygiene. The board will be required to adopt those rules and enforce the committee rules.

7. Maine

   Maine has a subcommittee on dental hygiene. The subcommittee consists of five members: one dental hygienist, who is a member of the board; two dental hygienists appointed by the governor; and two dentists, who are members of the board and appointed by the board president. The duties of the subcommittee are to perform an initial review of all applications for licensure as a dental hygienist, submissions relating to continuing education of dental hygienists, and all submissions relating to public health supervision status of dental hygienists.

8. Maryland

   Maryland's advisory committee consists of three dental hygienists, one dentist, and one public member, all of whom are full voting members of the dental board. The committee was created during sunset review as a compromise to the creation of a separate dental hygiene regulatory board. According to statute, all matters pertaining to dental hygiene must first be brought to the committee for its review and recommendation.

9. Michigan

   This six-member committee, comprising two dental hygienists, two dentists, one dental assistant, and one public member, considers matters related to the dental hygiene profession and makes recommendations to the full board of dentistry. All members of the committee are voting members on the board. The existence of the committee is not mandated by state rules or statutes, but instead is a committee appointed by the chairperson of the board.

10. Missouri

    A five-member advisory commission, composed of the dental hygienist on the dental board and four dental hygienists appointed by the governor, was created by the state legislature in 2001. The commission makes recommendations to the board concerning dental hygiene practice, licensure, examinations, discipline, and educational requirements.

11. Montana

    In 2002, the dental board assigned both dental hygienist members and one dentist member to be a standing committee to consider and address dental hygiene issues in a timely manner. The committee formulates specific recommendations to bring to the entire board for action.

12. Nevada

    Legislation in 2003 added a third dental hygienist to the dental board who, together with a dentist appointed by the board, constitute a dental hygiene committee who may formulate recommendations on dental hygiene rules for the board and may be assigned additional duties by the board.

13. New Mexico

    New Mexico has a board of dental health care comprising five dentists, two dental hygienists, and two public members. A dental hygiene committee is composed of five dental hygienists, two public members, and two dentists. The committee selects two of its dental hygiene members to serve as the dental hygienists on the board. The board's public members and two of its dentist members are the dentist and public members of the committee. The committee adopts all the rules pertaining to dental hygiene and is also responsible for the discipline of dental hygienists. The board enforces the dental hygiene committee's rules.

14. New Hampshire

    The New Hampshire Dental Hygienists' Committee is a five-member advisory committee composed of one dental hygienist member of the board, one dentist member of the board, and three dental hygienist members appointed by the governor. The Committee proposes rules concerning the practice, discipline, education, examination, and licensure of dental hygienists. The rules proposed by the Committee may be accepted by the Board of Dental Examiners for adoption.

15. Oklahoma

    The dental hygiene advisory committee is composed of the dental hygiene board member and four dental hygienists appointed by the board.

16. Oregon

    Under its authority to create standing committees, the Oregon dental board has appointed a committee composed of three dentists, three dental hygienists, and one nondental health care provider to advise the board concerning dental hygiene issues.

17. Texas

    In 1995, a dental hygiene advisory committee composed of three dental hygienists and two public members appointed by the governor and one dentist appointed by the board was established. All rules relating to the practice of dental hygiene must be submitted to the committee for review 30 days prior to board adoption. The committee has been responsible for researching and developing rules for licensure by credentials and the application of tetracycline fibers. Legislation in 2003 gave the committee the authority to propose specific rules for board action.

18. Washington

    The state of Washington has a uniform disciplinary code that applies to all health professions and creates the regulatory bodies to implement each practice act. Dentistry and dental hygiene have separate practice acts. Dentists are regulated by the Dental Quality Assurance Commission (an independent dental board with no dental hygiene members). Dental hygienists are regulated by the Department of Health, but the statute requires that the Department develop rules and definitions to implement the dental hygienist act in consultation with the Dental Hygiene Examining Committee. The committee is composed of three dental hygienists and one public member appointed by the department

(2) Identifies the client or can be used to identify the client

(3) Created or received by a covered entity

(4) About the client's past, present, or future treatment and payment for services

d. Three major areas addressed relating to requirements for privacy and confidentiality of health information (effective April 14, 2003)

  (1) Privacy standards

    (a) Client notification of privacy policies of office or institution

    (b) Written acknowledgment of receipt of notice of privacy policies

    (c) Written and signed authorization and consent

  (2) Client's rights

    (a) Right to inspect and copy confidential health care information

    (b) Right to amend confidential information in the client record

    (c) Right to obtain a list of disclosures of PHI

    (d) Right to confidential communication

    (e) Right to complain to the practice, to the DHHS Secretary, or to both

  (3) Administrative requirements

    (a) Develop policies, procedures, and documentation

    (b) Provide notice of privacy policy to clients

    (c) Designate a privacy officer and a contact person to receive complaints

    (d) Implement complaint systems

    (e) Provide training for employees

    (f) Execute business associate contracts

    (g) Mitigate any breach of confidentiality

2. Exceptions to nondisclosure of client information—original client records should never be released

a. Client consent—with written authorization only, specifying name of the client, name of the person authorized to disclose the information, amount and type of information to be released, name of the person or entity to receive the information, the date information is to be released, the date authorization expires, and the client's signature

b. Relevant copies of a client's medical records may be released to the court where the client's medical condition is put in issue by filing a lawsuit[4]

c. Duty to disclose—state reporting statutes may require release of client information (e.g., in cases of child or elder abuse); state statutes identify health care providers who are obligated by law to report suspected cases of abuse; statutes also provide immunity from civil liability for health care providers involved in reporting suspected abuse, unless it can be proved that a false report had been made, and the person knew that the report was false; access statutes allow for release of client information with no client authorization required (e.g., workers' compensation statutes)

3. PHI in electronic form is sometimes referred to as ePHI, which can include client information in an email, in an electronic file, or on a CD or memory stick

4. Health Information Technology for Economic and Clinical Health (HITECH); enacted as part of the American Recovery and Reinvestment Act of 2009; signed into law on February 17, 2009

a. Expands HIPAA's privacy and security provisions

b. Requires covered entities to provide notice of any breaches or unauthorized disclosures of PHI

EMPLOYER AND EMPLOYEE RIGHTS AND RESPONSIBILITIES

A. Employment

1. Employer—person, business, or organization that hires and compensates one or more workers; engages the services of an individual

2. Employee—person who is hired to provide services to a company on a regular basis in exchange for compensation

3. Status

a. At will; individual can be hired or terminated without notice

  (1) Employees without a contract

  (2) Should a dispute arise relating to termination of employment, courts often examine the office policy and procedure manual in determining an implied contract

b. Contract—a legally binding agreement between two or more parties

  (1) Elements (to be enforced by a court)

    (a) Offer—one party proposes a bargain

    (b) Acceptance—the other party agrees to the proposed bargain

    (c) Consideration—one party gives up something of value, and the other party makes a promise in exchange for that something of value

    (d) Mutuality—parties must reach an agreement or understanding

    (e) Legal capacity—all parties must have legal capacity (i.e., must be the age of majority and mentally competent)

  (2) Contract must be for a lawful purpose

  (3) Breach of contract—failure of performance of a contractual agreement by one or more parties

    (a) Remedies for breach of contract

      [1] Specific performance (the court requires performance of the contract)

      [2] Monetary damage

      [3] Injunctions (the court orders a party to refrain from specific behavior)

  (4) Employment contracts (Box 22-3)

    (a) Define duties and responsibilities of the position; location and hours

    (b) Define salary and benefits

    (c) Describe notice and termination requirements

    (d) Provide written description of understanding between the parties

BOX 22-3   Employment Contract Terms

An employment contract describes the conditions of employment, including wages, hours, and type of work. Depending on the level of employment, the responsibility of the new employee, and the nature of the business, the conditions of employment should be detailed regarding the following elements:

Parties, including the name of the employer and the entity and the name of the employee

Time and place: hours of employment and location

Duties: general and specific, scope of practice, if appropriate

Term and conditions of employment

Compensation, including salary, bonus pay, vacation, sick leave, continuing education policies and reimbursement, and professional memberships

Benefits, including disability, medical, life insurance, and retirement plan

Termination provisions

4. Independent practitioner—one who provides services directly to the public; dental hygienists who perform as independent practitioners may do so only in a state where it is allowed by the dental practice act; a dental hygienist as an independent practitioner must follow the state's (province's) dental practice act and regulations (Box 22-4)

5. Independent contractor—contracted by another person, company, or agency to produce a certain result, but not subject to the control of the employer and may do the work in a manner he or she selects; a dental hygienist as an independent contractor must follow both Internal Revenue Service (IRS) rules and the state's dental practice act and regulations

BOX 22-4   Independent Practice

There is virtually no legal guidance—even in the laws of states which allow it—about what "independent practice" means. If one equates it with other health practices, one would expect that the practice is a business entity that can be sold to another, can be directly reimbursed for services, and has patients of record.

Four states that have specific authorization in the practice act law allowing a hygienist to own a dental hygiene practice: Colorado (any hygienist), Maine (hygienists licensed as independent dental hygiene practitioners), New Mexico (hygienists in collaborative practice) and California (RDHAPs, registered dental hygienists in alternative practice). In several other states, including Washington and Oregon, where dental hygienists may practice with no or little supervision in various types of settings outside the dental office, dental hygienists do own dental hygiene businesses.

If you are interested in what business ownership options are available in a state other than these, you need to review the practice laws to see whether there is an actual or implied prohibition. Some state practice acts specify or strongly imply that a dental hygienist must be employed or must be an independent contractor. Others define owning, operating, or managing a dental practice as the practice of dentistry.

Keep in mind that supervision issues are different from worker status (employee vs. independent contractor) and business option issues. Supervision concerns the degree of oversight of client treatment that the practice law requires. Even owners of dental hygiene practices in Colorado and Maine must have an agreement with a dentist to provide supervision for some services; New Mexico practitioners need to practice in an agreed protocol with a collaborating dentist, and patients of California RDHAPs need a prescription from a dentist or physician to obtain dental hygiene services.

6. Vicarious liability—one party is responsible for another's action; *respondeat superior* (Latin, meaning "let the master answer"), an employer is legally responsible for the wrongs committed by an employee acting within the scope of his or her employment; dentist employer may be held responsible for negligent acts of a dental hygienist
   a. Vicarious liability or negligent retention may shield a dental hygienist from liability in tort cases
   b. Dental hygienists are liable for their actions
7. Negligent hiring and retention—employer can be held liable for acts or omissions of employees if the client can show that the employee was incompetent and the employer knew or should have known

B. Employment laws—offer protections for employer and employee
   1. Equal Employment Opportunity Commission (EEOC)—enforces federal laws passed to prevent discrimination in the workplace; investigates complaints and assists an individual or the Department of Justice in bringing a lawsuit
   2. Title VII of the Civil Rights Act of 1964—forbids discrimination against employees by federal, state, and local governments, by employers with 15 or more employees, and by labor organizations, if the basis of discrimination is race, color, national origin, religion, or gender
   3. Civil Rights Act of 1991—expanded rights under federal anti-discrimination law
   4. Sexual harassment—"unwelcome sexual conduct that is a term of employment"[5] is considered sexual discrimination and is prohibited under Title VII
      a. *Quid pro quo* (Latin, meaning "something for something") sexual harassment[6] criteria
         (1) The employee was in a "protected group" (a subordinate position)
         (2) The employee encountered unwelcome sexual advances or requests for sexual favors
         (3) Conduct was sexually motivated (e.g., hostile acts toward an individual because of his or her gender)
         (4) Harassment must affect a "tangible aspect of the job," such as salary, benefits, and promotions
      b. Hostile work environment as sexual harassment criteria—"verbal or physical conduct of a sexual nature that has the purpose or effect of creating an intimidating, hostile, or offensive work environment"[7]
         (1) Created by the words or conduct of an employer, colleague, vendor, or client
         (2) Examples
            (a) Unwanted touching
            (b) Suggestive comments about one's appearance
            (c) Display of sexually suggestive objects or pictures
            (d) Use of diminutive terms such as "honey" or "cutey"
         (3) Employer has legal duty to take action to stop or prevent sexual harassment
         (4) Sexual harassment may occur between members of the opposite sex or members of the same sex

5. Age Discrimination in Employment Act of 1967 (ADEA)—forbids discrimination against persons over age 40 by federal, state, and local governments and by employers with 20 or more employees

6. Equal Pay Act of 1963 (EPA)—illegal to pay lower wage to employees of one gender if the jobs have equal responsibility, working conditions, requirements for mental or physical effort, and requirements in experience, education, or training

7. Uniformed Services Employment and Reemployment Rights Act of 1994 protects civilian job rights and benefits for veterans and members of Reserve components

8. Occupational Safety and Health Act of 1970 (OSHA)—see Chapter 10

   a. The dental profession must comply with all General Industry standards[8] of primary importance to the dental practice, such as OSHA's Bloodborne Pathogens Standard (1991)

   b. Requirements for employers—employers must:
      (1) Identify employees at risk
      (2) Provide personal protective equipment to employees (e.g., gloves, protective eyewear, masks)
      (3) Provide hepatitis B vaccinations to employees
      (4) Provide safety needles for the workplace
      (5) Provide puncture-proof containers for sharps
      (6) Ensure that standard precautions are practiced in the work environment
      (7) Provide prompt treatment to employees who have needlestick or other exposures (includes immediate medical screening and follow-up treatment)
      (8) Provide annual employee education relating to bloodborne diseases

   c. OSHA amended the Bloodborne Pathogens Standard[6] (2001)—stricter requirements to prevent needlesticks and other exposures to blood (http://www.osha.gov/SLTC/bloodbornepathogens/); employers covered by the standards must:
      (1) Provide safety needles
      (2) Maintain a log of needlestick or other injuries to employees
      (3) Enlist the assistance of employees who provide direct client care to prevent needlestick and other exposures by seeking input regarding equipment selection and work practices
      (4) State OSHA laws—if a state has a health and safety law that meets or exceeds federal OSHA standards, enforcement of the law is assumed by the state rather than by a federal agency
      (5) Twenty-five states, Puerto Rico, and the Virgin Islands have OSHA-approved state plans that cover public and private sector employees; five states have plans that cover only public sector employees; and the states have adopted their own standards and enforcement policies; for the most part, these states adopt standards that are identical to federal OSHA; however, some states have adopted different standards applicable to this topic or may have different enforcement policies; contact state agency for copy of the safety and health standards (state plans, see https://www.osha.gov/dcsp/osp/states.html)

9. Family and Medical Leave Act of 1993 (FMLA)—protects job security for women and men by allowing unpaid leave for medical reasons (e.g., care of a child, spouse, or parent; birth; adoption; or serious illness); updated January 19, 2009, to include military family leave entitlements

10. Pregnancy Discrimination Act of 1978 (PDA)—protects rights of pregnant women in the workplace; maternity-related medical conditions must be treated as all other medical conditions

    a. FMLA and Americans with Disabilities Act (ADA) both require an employer to grant medical leave to an employee in certain circumstances; FMLA and Title VII both have requirements governing leave for pregnancy and pregnancy-related conditions

    b. FMLA covers private employers with 50 or more employees within a 75-mile radius of the workplace; ADA and Title VII cover private employers with 15 or more employees; only those private employers with 50 or more employees are covered concurrently by FMLA, ADA, and Title VII

    c. State and local government employers are covered by ADA and FMLA, regardless of the number of employees; state and local government employers are covered by Title VII, but only if they have 15 or more employees

11. Americans with Disabilities Act (ADA of 1990)—prohibits discrimination against qualified applicants and employees on basis of disability

    a. Must be a mental or physical impairment that substantially limits one or more of the major life activities

    b. Disabilities include visual and hearing impairments, epilepsy, HIV-positive status, and AIDS

    c. Employer must make reasonable accommodations for employee

    d. Updated by the ADA Amendments Act of 2008 and expanded list of major life activities protected by the Act (http://www.ada.gov/pubs.adastatute08mark.htm#12102)

12. Fair Employment Statutes—many federal employment laws apply to workplaces with as many as 50 employees (e.g., FMLA); therefore, most do not apply to dentistry; most states have passed statutes that enhance these federal laws; each state's statutes differ; contact specific state's attorney general for information

13. Workers' compensation: insurance program regulated by each state's insurance commission; employer must purchase insurance through an insurance company to protect employees should they become seriously ill or injured as a result of conditions in the workplace; programs vary from state to state; employees are covered on first date of employment, and benefits include medical expenses and income

RISK MANAGEMENT AND AVOIDING LITIGATION

A. Concepts
1. Risk management—clinical and administrative activities undertaken to identify, evaluate, and reduce the risk of injury to clients, staff, and visitors
2. Risk assessment
    a. Evaluation of personnel, policies, and protocol to identify and address risk factors
    b. Strategies
        (1) Personnel evaluations; conducted by employer or peer review
        (2) Office audits
            (a) Review and updating of staff handbook
            (b) Assessment of policies related to client care (e.g., record keeping, referral policies, documentation)
            (c) Evaluation of equipment (e.g., condition)
            (d) Protocol reviews (e.g., accident protocol)
            (e) Personnel assessment (e.g., current licenses, communication style)
    c. Identified risks are addressed and remedied
B. Individual risk management
1. Maintain a current license and certifications, if required (e.g., CPR certification)
    a. Be knowledgeable of state dental practice act and statutes or guidelines impacting health care providers
    b. Comply with state guidelines, federal guidelines, or both for infection control, record keeping, reporting requirements, confidentiality, and other specified mandates
2. Obtain membership in a professional association such as ADHA or CDHA that provides legal updates through various publications
3. Provide evidence-informed care in all aspects of client care activities
4. Maintain competence by participation in continuing education; continuing education is mandatory in 47 states; from a legal perspective, it is advisable to document current competency with tasks routinely performed and those within the scope of practice
5. Possess knowledge of legally protected employee rights and responsibilities
    a. Use legal or state or federal resources that provide guidance
    b. Document in detail any incidents occurring in the workplace
    c. Seek legal advice, if necessary
6. Purchase professional liability insurance; keep the policy current
    a. Policy classifications
        (1) Occurrence-based policy—covers injuries arising out of incidents that occurred during the time the insurance was in effect, even if cancelled at a later date (preferred type)

        (2) Claims-made policy—covers injuries occurring and reported during the period in which the policy premiums are paid and in force
    b. Declaration—states policyholder's personal data (name, address, occupation) and limits of liability coverage (dollar figure for each claim and aggregate for policy period)
    c. Exclusions—liabilities not covered by policy; usually injuries resulting from criminal behavior, those involving alcohol or drug abuse on the part of health care provider, or cases involving practice beyond the scope of one's license
    d. Injuries covered—listed in policy (e.g., bodily injury, defamation, invasion of privacy)
    e. Supplemental coverage—lost earnings
    f. Conditions—subrogation of rights, policyholder's right to hire counsel versus insurance company's right to retain counsel
        (1) Policyholder's interest and insurance company's interest may be in conflict
        (2) A conflict of interest could also arise if a health care provider relies on the employer's insurance for liability coverage; protection is broader with an individual policy; an employer's policy provides coverage only when acting within the scope of employment; if the health care provider (by his or her action or failure to act) was liable for the client's injury, the employer (or his or her insurance company) may bring an indemnity claim and recover a portion of dollar amount awarded by the court to the client
C. Professional risk management
1. Maintain knowledge of professional and legal responsibilities related to the provision of oral health care services
2. Be familiar with and adhere to the professional code of ethics (ADHA Code of Ethics and CDHA Code of Ethics)
3. Maintain a professional and respectful relationship with employers, colleagues, and clients
4. Provide accurate and appropriate communication to clients, verbally and in writing; poor record keeping can contribute to a poor outcome in a lawsuit
5. Maintain confidentiality—obtain proper written authorization from the client before release of any client information; ensure that any disclosure is covered by a reporting or access law and is appropriately followed
6. Document informed consent or informed refusal in client record before treatment
7. Ensure that all progress notes and client records are complete, accurate, factual, legible, unaltered, and promptly recorded; failure to do so is considered malpractice; a client's record may be obtained by an opposing party in a lawsuit
8. Be familiar with professional guidelines, including ADHA Standards for Clinical Dental Hygiene
9. Remain up-to-date on state or provincial dental hygiene practice acts and regulations

Website Information and Resources

Legal Resources	Website Address	Description
Find Law	www.findlaw.com	Provides resources to learn about the law, find a lawyer, and find answers to legal questions and legal forms
9to5 National Office	9 to5 National Headquarters 207 E. Buffalo Street, Suite 211 Milwaukee, WI 53202 T: (414) 274-0925 Fax: (414) 272-2870 http://www.9to5.org	National organization dedicated to putting working women's issues on the public agenda; 9to5's constituents are low-wage women, women in traditionally female jobs, and those who have experienced any form of discrimination; committed to, among other objectives, eliminating workplace discrimination through educating women about legal rights on the job, monitoring enforcement agencies, and expanding anti-discrimination laws
American Dental Hygienists Association	444 N. Michigan Avenue, Suite 3400 Chicago, IL 60611 T: 312-440-8900 www.adha.org	Largest professional association representing dental hygienists
National Practitioner Data Bank and Health Care Integrity and Protection Data Bank	http://www.npdb.hrsa.gov/	U.S. Department of Health and Human Services (DHHS), Health Resources and Services Administration (HRSA), Bureau of Health Professions (BHPr), Division of Practitioner Data Banks (DPDB) is responsible for the management of the National Practitioner Data Bank and the Health Care Integrity and Protection Data Bank
U.S. Equal Employment Opportunity Commission	http://www.eeoc.gov/ contact/index.cfm Charge filing process 1-800-669-4000, info@eeoc.gov	Responsible for enforcing federal laws that make it illegal to discriminate against a job applicant or an employee because of the person's race, color, religion, gender (including pregnancy), national origin, age (40 or older), disability or genetic information; it is also illegal to discriminate against a person because the person complained about discrimination, filed a charge of discrimination, or participated in an employment discrimination investigation or lawsuit Work is conducted at the headquarters and at 53 field offices throughout the United States
Occupational Safety and Health Administration Seeking legal advice from a qualified attorney is also recommended; the State Bar Association provides referrals to an attorney for legal services in a particular location	200 Constitution Avenue NW Washington, DC 20210 T: 1.800.321.OSHA (6742) www.osha.gov	Ensures safe and healthful working conditions for working persons by setting and enforcing standards and by providing training, outreach, education, and assistance

Ethics Resources	Website Address	Description
Center for Health Policy and Ethics, Creighton University Medical Center	www.chpe.creighton.edu	A multi-disciplinary group of scholars dedicated to the study and teaching of ethical dimensions of health care and health policy; also offer roundtables, lectures, and courses
Center for Law, Ethics and Health, University of Michigan School of Public Health	www.sph.umich.edu/cleh	An interdisciplinary research center to examine the influence of law and ethics on the health care and public health system; provides publications and other resources
Berman Bioethics Institute, Johns Hopkins University	www.bioethicsinstitute.org	Provides education, conducts research, and provides leadership for the understanding of ethical issues in health care; trains mentors and future leaders in the field of bioethics, health and science
Center for Ethics and Leadership in the Health Professions, Regis University	www.ethicsandleadership.org	Provides educational and consulting services and ethics simulations; provides services to professionals and contributes to the national dialogue on health care through scholarship and professional activities

REFERENCES AND LEGAL CITATIONS

1. Garner BA: *Black's law dictionary*, ed 10, 2014, Thomson West.
2. *Norwood Hospital v Munoz*, 564 NE 2d 1017, 1991.
3. *Thor v Superior Court*, 855 P2d 375, 21 Cal. Rept. 2d 357, 1993.
4. *Harlan v Lewis*, 141 F.D.R. 107, 109, n5.
5. 729 CRF, § 1604.11(a).
6. 29 CRF 1910.1030, Occupational exposure to bloodborne pathogens, needlestick and other sharps injuries; Final rule, *Fed Reg* 66:5317–5325, January 18, 2001.
7. *Harris v Forklift Sys. Inc.*, 510 US 17, 1993.
8. 29 CRF 1910.

SUGGESTED READINGS

American Dental Hygienists Association: *Standards for clinical dental hygiene practice, 2008*: Chicago, 2008, ADHA http://www.adha.org/resources-docs/7261_Standards_Clinical_Practice.pdf. Accessed October 25, 2014.

American Dental Hygienists Association: *Bylaws—codes of ethics, 2010:* Chicago, 2010, ADHA http://www.adha.org/resources-docs/7611_Bylaws_and_Code_of_Ethics.pdf. Accessed October 15, 2014.

Beemsterboer PL: *Ethics and law in dental hygiene,* ed 2, St Louis, 2010, Saunders.

Canadian Dental Hygienists Association: *Codes of ethics, 2002:* Ontario, 2002, CDHA http://www.cdho.org/reference/english/codeofethics_pocketmanual.pdf. Accessed October 15, 2014.

Darby ML, Walsh MM: *Dental hygiene theory and practice,* ed 4, St Louis, 2014, Saunders.

CHAPTER 22 REVIEW QUESTIONS

Answers and rationales to review questions are available on this text's accompanying Evolve site. See inside front cover for details.

evolve

1. The dental hygienist obtains a new client's consent to obtain dental records from a previous dental provider. In reviewing the record, it appears the client was not truthful concerning his health history. Which of the following ethical principles did the client violate?
   a. Autonomy
   b. Beneficence
   c. Justice
   d. Veracity

2. A new dental office manager distributes guidelines to staff dental hygienists indicating that client appointments will be reduced by 50%. The dental hygienist is concerned about the substandard care that will be delivered because of lack of adequate time. Which of the following ethical principles is violated by this request?
   a. Informed consent
   b. Acts of mercy and charity; promoting the good
   c. Provision of care within the scope of practice
   d. Fairness and equity
   e. Obligation not to inflict harm

3. A front desk staff person at a dental clinic receives a telephone call from an insurance company representative who is seeking health-related information about a client. The person is concerned about sharing information without the client's consent. Which of the following ethical principles is guiding the front desk person in her decision making?
   a. Respecting the client's privacy
   b. Acts of mercy and charity; promoting the good
   c. Provision of care within the scope of practice
   d. Fairness and equity
   e. Do not inflict harm intentionally
   f. Truthfulness and honesty

4. A state has a dental hygiene board that oversees the practice of dental hygiene, disciplinary matters, and licensure requirements. This reflects a profession's obligations to:
   a. Provide guidance and a framework for regulating practice
   b. Protect the public
   c. Ensure dental hygienists practice legally and ethically
   d. All the above

5. After a client's assessment and data collection, a dentist determines that referral to a periodontist is necessary for the client to receive appropriate treatment. The dental hygienist does not agree and does not give the client a referral slip for a periodontist. Which of the following BEST describes this situation?
   a. Risk of losing the client
   b. Failing to fulfill a duty that results in harm
   c. Justice
   d. A difference of opinion

6. A client does not take premedication as instructed before dental treatment. Which of the following BEST describes this situation? :
   a. Contributory negligence
   b. Standard negligence
   c. Defamation
   d. An expressed contract

7. A state law requires that a dental malpractice case must be filed against a dental provider within 2 years from the time the client was treated by the provider. This time limit refers to:
   a. An area of law that governs actions of administrative agencies of government
   b. An area of law that protects people, property, and privacy
   c. An area of law that protects society
   d. A maximum period allowed before filing a lawsuit
   e. Standard provider protections and guidelines

8. A dentist describes an unusual case study in his practice that is published in the state dental society journal with pictures of the client. The client contacts the office upset about the use of the photographs. Which of the following violations of privacy occurred?
   a. Implied contract
   b. Paternalism
   c. Informed consent
   d. Appropriation

9. A 16-year-old client informs you that he no longer lives with his parents, identifying himself as an "emancipated minor." However, the parents continue to pay for his dental treatment. Which of the following statements BEST describes the situation?
   a. A declaration is sufficient to create emancipated status.
   b. Client needs only to be physically separated from parents.
   c. Client is not emancipated because of financial connection with parents.
   d. Specific conditions must be met for an individual less than 18 years old to become emancipated.

10. A state's dental practice act is revised and mandates that dental providers take at least one continuing education course on pain management as a requirement for license renewal. This action falls within which board duty?

a. Description by dental practice act or policies and procedures

b. Authority to revoke or suspend licenses

c. Required continuing education that supports maintaining competence

d. Credentialing

11. A dental hygienist is scheduled to provide treatment to clients when the dentist is not in the office. The dental hygienist only performs those procedures within the accepted scope of practice as described in the dental practice act. This type of supervision falls within which type of arrangement?

a. General supervision

b. Indirect supervision

c. Direct supervision

d. Unsupervised practice

12. A dental hygienist relocates to another state and practices dental hygiene without obtaining a license in that state. Which of the following may be a consequence of practicing without a license?

a. Patient abandonment

b. Violation of tort law

c. A civil and/or criminal lawsuit

d. Breach of contract

13. A client writes an article in the newspaper containing false statements about her dental hygienist's care and treatment. What tort does this describe?

a. Defamation

b. Slander

c. Libel

d. Beneficence

14. A boating accident results in victims requiring positive identification. A request is made to a dental office to provide dental records, and the office agrees to assist in the process. which of the following functions is the record satisfying?

a. Resource in forensic identification

b. Documentation used in a lawsuit and reviewed by plaintiff and defendant attorneys

c. Source of data collection for analysis

d. Allowed sharing of patient information with all providers

e. Documentation of information to assess quality control and risk management information

15. During a PTA meeting, a client makes false statements about his dentist. The statement has a negative effect on the provider's reputation in the community. Which of the following intentional torts does this BEST describe?

a. Battery

b. Defamation

c. Libel

d. Slander

e. Miscommunication

16. A client is provided with a prescription for an antibiotic after dental treatment but fails to have the prescription filled and take the medication as directed. The client experiences a serious infection and is hospitalized. The client sues the dental provider, but the legal determination is that the injured individual is responsible for a portion of the injury suffered. What is the legal concept being used as part of the dental provider's defense?

a. Creating apprehension about harmful or offensive touching or contact

b. Individual contributed to the harm suffered

c. Legal permission to provide health care

d. The harm speaks for itself; duty of care

17. A dental hygienist observes clinical findings that may indicate child abuse. Her employer refuses to report the abuse and suggests if the dental hygienist does take action, she may lose her job. The dental hygienist decides to report the abuse. Which of the following ethical concepts do the dental hygienist's actions BEST follow?

a. Action will bring greatest happiness or least harm

b. Seek greatest happiness and public agreement

c. Basis in personal moral values of individual decision making

d. Standards greater than individual morals

18. Which of the following from the ADHA Code of Ethics provides guidance to the dental hygienist about obligations to report cases of suspected abuse or violence against adults and children?

a. Most states require dental providers to report child and adult abuse

b. Situation described not related to personal circumstances

c. Actions that promote well-being and professional development and expertise

d. Supporting patient information confidentiality and HIPAA compliance

19. After a discussion with a client concerning proposed dental hygiene treatment, including alternatives, risks and benefits, and outcomes, the client accepts and signs an informed consent form. Which of the ethical principles guiding oral health care did the process of obtaining informed consent satisfy?

a. Autonomy

b. Beneficence

c. Fair and equitable care

d. Reliability or trustworthiness does not apply to the process of informed consent

e. Truthfulness

20. Faculty in a dental hygiene program collaborate with the local dental hygiene group on a research investigating the impact of a new mouthrinse on burning mouth syndrome in perimenopausal women. Which of the following characteristics of a profession does this research project support?

a. Formal education, credentials, and licensure

b. Charitable and community-based activities impacting oral health

c. Contribution to research and creating evidence-based outcomes

d. Peer review

e. Ethical codes guide decision making

21. **A client bill of rights provides:**
    a. Specific recommendations regarding oral health services
    b. A paper or electronic dental record
    c. List of services provided for client information or insurance purposes
    d. A framework that guides patient expectations
    e. Scope of practice for oral health providers

22. **The Hippocratic Oath is an example of an early ethical code that advocates health providers should do no harm. Which universal ethical principle BEST supports this recommendation?**
    a. Autonomy
    b. Nonmaleficence
    c. Justice
    d. Beneficence
    e. Veracity

23. **A state dental board or dental hygiene committee monitors the behavior of licensed oral health care providers and recommends sanctions for individuals who violate a state dental practice act because:**
    a. Sanctions are mandated by the principles in the code of ethics
    b. There is no federal mandate
    c. Dental boards are created to protect the citizens of a state
    d. Accrediting agencies mandate this oversight

24. **A city council votes to allocate health department funds for a dental sealant program. After consultation with appropriate individuals, the council determines children enrolled in either a hot lunch program or a state-funded program for medical services for children from low-income families should receive the sealants. On which principle of allocation of resources is this determination based?**
    a. An individual's contribution to society
    b. Prioritized needs
    c. Individuals receiving treatment because they have earned it
    d. Individuals receiving equal services
    e. The most deserving individuals receiving services

25. **A dental hygienist has allegations of professional misconduct reported to the state board. A hearing is conducted, and the dental hygienist has an opportunity to hear and respond to the allegations. These actions BEST demonstrate which of the following?**
    a. Right to communicate one's ideas and opinions
    b. Protection of an individual from discrimination
    c. Protected right for notification of detailed charges and response
    d. Illegal activity based on race, gender, national original, color, religion, or disability
    e. Written or spoken untrue statement

26. **A dentist examines a client, develops a treatment plan, and obtains informed consent. The client nods in agreement and indicates that she will be making further appointments. On the basis of the dentist's and client's actions, which of the following may exist?**
    a. Contract established through written communication
    b. Implied contract established through nonverbal communication
    c. A specific ethical obligation
    d. Contract between an insurer and insured

27. **A dental hygienist recently relocated to a state and is seeking to apply for a dental hygiene license. The license application asks the applicant to indicate whether he or she has been convicted of any felonies. A felony is:**
    a. A violation of the scope of practice defined by a dental or dental hygiene board
    b. Description of a misdemeanor
    c. A crime punishable by death or imprisonment of at least 1 year
    d. Description of a civil rights violation

28. **A dental provider and a client discuss a proposed dental hygiene treatment plan. The written plan outlines the treatment, the fees, the risks and benefits, the client's financial obligations, and the expectations of the provider concerning the client's responsibilities. The provider and client sign the treatment plan. This situation BEST describes:**
    a. The written terms of the planned treatment imply a contract exists between the client and provider
    b. Supported by the ethical principle of justice
    c. There is no agreement between parties, thus no contractual agreement
    d. Agreement between an insurer and insured individual

29. **A dental office employs a dental hygiene student approximately 6 months before graduation. The dentist in the office was scheduled to provide a maintenance visit with a client. However, an emergency client is also waiting to be assessed for care. The dentist asks the dental hygiene student to provide a "quick cleaning." Which area of jurisprudence does the dentist's action fall under?**
    a. Case law is formulated by judge or determined by court decisions.
    b. Failure to remain current and use evidence-based therapies is not an area of jurisprudence.
    c. Professional negligence is a failure to perform a clinical action.
    d. Administrative law prohibits nonlicensed individuals from performing functions clearly defined by the scope of practice for a licensee.

30. **The trial for a dental hygienist alleged to have committed negligence is complete. The judge prepares to give the jury instructions pertaining to the level of proof the jury must consider to make their decision about the guilt or innocence of the defendant. Which of the following is needed to convict the defendant?**
    a. Unanimous agreement of all jurors
    b. A preponderance of evidence
    c. The level a reasonable person finds useful to reach a conclusion
    d. Information or items presented in court must prove or disprove an allegation

31. **A client's contractual responsibilities include all the following EXCEPT:**

a. Keeping appointments, making timely cancellations, or rescheduling appointments

b. Providing accurate and truthful information to the provider and following recommendations and instructions regarding accepted treatment

c. Obligation to pay for dental services

d. Providing accurate and complete health history information

e. Compliance with a 6-mouth dental hygiene recare interval

32. A new client presents to a dental office for treatment. Client demographic and clinical data are collected and reviewed by the dentist and the dental hygienist, who together determine the case is too complex for the office to manage and suggest the client seek another provider. The client is informed that he will not be accepted into the practice. Which statement BEST describes this situation?

a. Abandonment

b. Dental office is not obligated to treat all clients as long as the decision is not made for a discriminatory reason

c. Risk management

d. Breach of contract

33. A dental hygienist has demonstrated behaviors that include purposefully using a loud voice and waving syringes and handpieces in a threatening manner. The dental hygienist is aware of the actions and their potential impact on a client. Which of the following intentional torts may the dental hygienist be accused?

a. Assault

b. Battery

c. Loss of or damage to a person's rights, property, or mental well-being

d. Defamation

e. Negligence

34. Adam is scheduled for sealants on his four first molars. His record indicates he is somewhat uncooperative during dental appointments. As the appointment progresses, the dental hygienist and the dental assistant become increasingly aggravated at Adam's uncooperative actions. At one point, the assistant holds Adam's hands down, and the dental hygienist firmly takes Adam's chin to position his face. At the end of the appointment, red marks are seen on Adam's hands and cheeks. As he enters the reception area, Adam's mother looks at her son and says to the assistant, "What did you do to my son?" Which of the following might the dental hygienist and the assistant be accused?

a. Action that results in apprehension or threat of harm

b. Intentional offensive or harmful physical contact

c. Loss of or damage to a person's rights, property, or mental well-being

d. Intentional perversion of the truth to gain a person's trust

e. Failure to exercise care expected of a reasonably prudent provider

35. All the following are key elements of obtaining an informed refusal EXCEPT one. Which one is the *exception*?

a. An oral refusal is considered a legal agreement

b. Explanation and justification for the recommended treatment and alternatives

c. Documentation as to why the client is refusing treatment

d. The risks of refusing treatment

e. Signature of client, provider, and witness

36. The dental hygienist is performing root planing and scaling and removes a portion of a client's amalgam during the procedure. The dental hygienist fails to inform the client, who later experiences pain and swallows a portion of the remaining restoration. The intentional tort committed is:

a. Malpractice

b. Misrepresentation

c. Negligence

d. Breach of contract

37. A dentist is accused of a serious criminal violation against a client. After the trial, the jury will be asked to judge the facts and make a decision based on which of the following standards?

a. Level of proof must be beyond a reasonable doubt.

b. A majority of jurors is needed for a conviction.

c. In regulatory discipline cases, a state board or agency has the burden of proof.

d. The victim must be compensated.

38. Dr. Miller recently joined a private practice as a partner. The office staff can check email or order supplies using the Internet from a computer in the staff lounge. The mostly female staff use the lounge to eat lunch. During lunch, Dr. Miller frequently logs on to read his email. He usually reads his email, laughs out loud, and without anyone asking, proceeds to read some of the jokes, poems, and "stories" out loud. Most of the jokes would be considered crude or inappropriate. Which workplace law is being violated?

a. Affirmative action

b. Sexual harassment

c. Occupational Safety and Health Act of 1970 (OSHA)

d. Americans with Disabilities Act

39. A dental hygienist is terminated from a full-time position in a dental office with 25 employees. The dental hygienist recently turned 65 and suspects the reason for the termination is based on age. Which of the following federal regulations provides legal protection for the employee?

a. Age Discrimination Act

b. Civil Rights Act of 1964

c. Occupational Safety and Health Act

d. The state's dental practice act

40. The level of care a reasonably prudent practitioner would provide in the same or similar circumstances BEST describes:

a. Informed consent

b. Harm-avoidance model

c. Paternalism

d. Standard of care

e. Risk management

41. **To assist in maintaining competence and reduce the risks of malpractice allegations, it is advisable for a dental provider to:**
    a. Maintain membership in a professional organization
    b. Participate in continuing education courses
    c. Purchase malpractice liability insurance
    d. Understand legally protected employee rights

42. **A client requests and is allowed to review his or her dental record. Which of the following regulations supports this?**
    a. Health Insurance Portability and Accountability Act (HIPAA)
    b. Occupational Safety and Health Act of 1970
    c. Patient Bill of Rights
    d. Fraud, Waste, Abuse
    e. Clients do not have a legal right to review their record

43. **A dental hygienist realizes that an entry made 2 days ago in a client's dental record incorrectly recorded the number of carpules that were used for anesthesia. The dental hygienist obtains the record to correct the entry. Which is the appropriate method to make a correction?**
    a. It is not advisable to delete or obliterate any entry.
    b. Provider should white-out the incorrect entry.
    c. Provider should use a pen to draw a line through incorrect entry and is allowed to make corrections and note reason for the correction.
    d. Provider should insert the correct entry above or below a previously recorded entry.

44. **A dental provider accepts a client and during the course of treatment decides not to complete the treatment because of an antagonistic relationship with the client. To legally terminate a client, which of the following steps must be followed?**
    a. A client must be given 2 weeks to find another dentist.
    b. Client dismissal requires formal written notification.
    c. Client may be given a referral, but this is not necessary.
    d. Client termination is the process of verbally notifying the client that the provider-client relationship is formally ended.

45. **A dental provider seeking to obtain informed consent discusses a client's diagnosis, proposed treatment including risks and benefits; and anticipated outcomes of the treatment; allows the client to ask questions; and provides answers. Which element of informed consent is lacking?**
    a. Photographs and diagrams pertinent to the treatment plan

b. A witness present for signing of the informed consent form

c. Alternative options for treatment with a description of benefits and risks

d. Payment plans available

46. **Legislation is passed in a state to allow dental hygienists to administer local anesthetic agents under the direct supervision of a dentist. Direct supervision usually requires that a licensed dentist has authorized the procedure and that the dentist:**
    a. Be available via a pager or cell phone
    b. Give oversight to the dental hygienist
    c. Be present on the premises
    d. Evaluate the procedure within a given number of days

47. **Which of the following expanded HIPAA privacy and security provisions require notification of breaches or unauthorized disclosures of protected health information?**
    a. Health Care Reform Act
    b. Health Information Technology Economic and Clinical Health Act (HITECH)
    c. Medical Injury Compensation Reform Act
    d. Occupational Safety and Health Act
    e. Patient Protection and Affordable Care Act

48. **All the following are recommended personal risk management strategies EXCEPT:**
    a. All licenses and certifications should be up-to-date.
    b. Clinical decisions and care should be based on scientific, evidence-based information.
    c. Lifelong learning and participation in continuing education courses contribute to competent care.
    d. Dental providers are responsible for their own decision making and the consequences of that decision making.
    e. Liability insurance provides financial protection for the provider.

49. **A dental hygienist is informed that the employment situation is "at will." This situation is BEST described as:**
    a. The hygienist's willingness to work for an employer
    b. An employment status that someone can be hired or fired without cause
    c. A form of insurance that protects professionals from incurring the full cost of defending allegations of negligence
    d. A form of insurance providing wage replacement and medical benefits to employees injured in the course of employment in exchange for not suing the employer

PREFIXES

a-, ab-, abs- From; away; departing from normal
ad- Addition to; toward; nearness
amb-, ambi- Both; ambidextrous, having the ability to work effectively with either hand
amphi- On both sides
ampho- Both
an- Negative; without or not
ana- Upper, away from
andro- Signifying man; human
ant-, anti- Against
ante-, antero- Front; before
bili- Pertaining to bile
brady- Slow
brom-, bromo- A stench
broncho- Pertaining to the bronchi
cac- Bad
cardi-, cardio- Pertaining to the heart
cata- Down or downward
cervico- Pertaining to the neck
circa- About
circum- Around
co- With or together
con- Together with
contra- Opposite; against
demi- Half
di- Twice
dia- Through
dialy- To separate
en- In
end-, endo-, ento- Inward; within
ep-, epi- On; in addition to
ex- Out; away from
exo- Without; outside of
extra- Outside of; in addition to
fibro- Pertaining to fibers
gaster-, gastr-, gastro- Pertaining to the stomach
hemi- Half
hemo- Pertaining to the blood
hepat-, hepatico-, hepato- Pertaining to the liver
heter-, hetero- Denoting other; relationship to another
homeo- Denoting likeness or resemblance
homo- Denoting sameness
hyal-, hyalo- Transparent
hyper- Above; excessive; beyond
hypo- Below; less than

ideo- Pertaining to mental images
idio- Denoting relationship to one's self or to something separate and distinct
in- Not; in; inside; within; also intensive action
infra- Below
inter- In the midst; between
intra- Within
intro- In or into
iso- Equal or alike
juxta- Of close proximity
karyo- Pertaining to a cell's nucleus
kypho- Humped
laryngo- Pertaining to the larynx
medi- Middle
myelo- Pertaining to the spinal cord or bone marrow
omni- All
ovari-, ovario- Pertaining to the ovary
per- Through; by means of
peri- Around; about
post- Behind or after
postero- Pertaining to the posterior
pre- Before
pro- Before, in front of
pseudo- False
re- Back; again (contrary)
retro- Backward
semi- Half
steato- Fatty
sub- Under; near
syn- Joined together
trans- Across; over
un- Not; reversal

SUFFIXES

-able, -ible, -ble The power to be
-ad Toward; in the direction of
-aemia, -emia Pertaining to blood
-age Put in motion; to do
-agra Denoting a seizure; severe pain
-algia Denoting pain
-ase Forms the name of an enzyme
-blast Designates a cell or a structure
-cele Denoting a swelling
-centesis Denoting a puncture
-ectomy A cutting out
-esthesia Denoting sensation

-**facient** That which makes or causes

-**gene**, -**genesis**, -**genetic**, -**genic** Denoting production; origin

-**gog**, -**gogue** To make flow

-**gram** A tracing; a mark

-**graph** A writing; a record

-**iasis** Denoting a condition or pathologic state

-**id** Denoting shape or resemblance

-**ite** Of the nature of

-**itis** Denoting inflammation

-**logia** Denoting discourse, science, or study of

-**oid** Denoting form or resemblance

-**oma** Denoting a tumor

-**osis** Denoting a morbid process

-**ostomosis**, -**ostomy**, -**stomy** Denoting an outlet; to furnish with an opening or mouth

-**plasty** Denoting molding or shaping

-**rhaphy** Denoting suturing or stitching

-**rhea** Denoting a flow or discharge

-**rrhagia** Denoting a discharge; usually bleeding

-**scope**, -**scopy** Generally an instrument for viewing

-**tomy** Denoting a cutting operation

-**trophy** Denoting a relationship to nourishment

COMBINING FORMS

aer-, **aero-** Denoting air or gas

alge-, **algesi-**, **algo-** Pertaining to pain

allo- Other; differing from the normal

anomalo- Denoting irregularity

arthro- Pertaining to a joint or joints

brevi- Short

celio- Denoting the abdomen

centro- Center

cheil-, **cheilo-** Denoting the lip

chol-, **chole-**, **cholo-** Pertaining to bile

chondr-, **chondri-** Pertaining to cartilage

chrom-, **chromo-** Pertaining to color

cole-, **coleo-** Denoting a sheath

colp-, **colpo-** Pertaining to the vagina

cranio- Pertaining to the cranium of the skull

crymo-, **cryo-** Denoting cold

crypt- To hide; a pit

cyano- Dark blue

cyclo- Pertaining to a cycle

cysto- Pertaining to a sac or cyst

cyto- Denoting a cell

dacryo- Pertaining to the lacrimal glands

dactylo- Pertaining to digits

dent-, **dento-** Pertaining to teeth

derma-, **dermat-** Pertaining to skin

desmo- Pertaining to a bond or ligament

dextro- Right

diplo- Double; twofold

dorsi-, **dorso-** Pertaining to the back

duodeno- Pertaining to the duodenum

electro- Pertaining to electricity

encephalo- Denoting the brain

entero- Pertaining to the intestines

episio- Pertaining to the vulva

eso- Inward

esthesio- Pertaining to feeling or sensation

facio- Pertaining to the face

gangli-, **ganglio-** Pertaining to a ganglion

geno- Pertaining to reproduction

gero-, **geronto-** Denoting old age

giganto- Huge

gingivo- Pertaining to the gingiva or gum

gloss-, **glosso-** Pertaining to the tongue

gluco- Denoting sweetness

glyco- Pertaining to sugar

gnath-, **gnatho-** Denoting the jaw

gon- Denoting a seed

grapho- Denoting writing

hapt-, **hapte-**, **hapto-** Pertaining to touch or a seizure

helo- Pertaining to a nail or callus

hist-, **histio-**, **histo-** Pertaining to tissue

holo- Pertaining to the whole

hydr-, **hydro-** Denoting water

hygro- Denoting moisture

hyl-, **hyle-**, **hylo-** Denoting matter or material

ileo-, **ilio-** Pertaining to the ileum

ipsi- Denoting self

irido- Pertaining to a colored circle

iso- Equal

jejuno- Pertaining to the jejunum

kerato- Pertaining to the cornea

kino- Denoting movement

labio- Pertaining to the lips

lacto- Pertaining to milk

laparo- Pertaining to the loin or flank

latero- Pertaining to the side

leido-, **leio-** Smooth

leuk-, **leuko-** Denoting deficiency of color

lip-, **lipo-** Pertaining to fat

litho- Denoting a calculus

macr-, **macro-** Large; long

mast-, **masto-** Pertaining to the breast

meg-, **mega-** Great; large

meli- Sweet

meningo- Denoting membranes; covering the brain and the spinal cord

micr-, **micro-** Small in size or extent

mono- One

morpho- Pertaining to form

multi- Many

my-, **myo-** Pertaining to muscle

myc-, **mycet-** Denoting a fungus

myringo- Denoting the tympanic membrane or the eardrum

myx-, **myxo-** Pertaining to mucus

narco- Denoting stupor

naso- Pertaining to the nose

necro- Denoting death

neo- New

nephr-, **nephro-** Denoting the kidney

normo- Normal or usual
oculo- Denoting the eye
odyno- Denoting pain
oleo- Denoting oil
onco- Denoting a swelling or mass
onycho- Pertaining to the nails
oo- Denoting an egg
opisth-, opistho- Backward
ophthal-, ophthalmo- Pertaining to the eye
optico- Pertaining to the eye or vision
orchi-, orcho- Pertaining to the testes
oro- Pertaining to the mouth
ortho- Straight; right
oscillo- Denoting oscillation
osteo- Pertaining to the bones
ot-, oto- Denoting an egg
palato- Denoting the palate
patho- Denoting disease
pedia-, pedo- Denoting a child
perineo- Combining form for the region between the anus and the scrotum or vulva
phago- Denoting a relationship to eating
pharyngo- Pertaining to the pharynx
phleb-, phlebo- Denoting the veins
phon-, phono- Denoting sound
phot-, photo- Pertaining to light
phren- Pertaining to the mind
picr-, picro- Bitter
pilo- Denoting hair
plasmo- Pertaining to plasma or the substance of a cell
pneuma-, pneumono-, pneumoto- Denoting air or gas
pod-, podo- Denoting the foot
poly- Many
proct-, procto- Denoting the anus and rectum
psych-, psycho- Pertaining to the mind
ptyalo- Denoting saliva
pubio-, pubo- Denoting the pubic region
pulmo- Denoting the lung
pupillo- Denoting the pupil
py-, pyo- Denoting pus
pyel-, pyelo- Denoting the pelvis
pyloro- Pertaining to the pylorus
recto- Denoting the rectum
rhin-, rhino- Denoting the nose
salpingo- Denoting a tube, specifically the fallopian tube
schizo- Split
sclero- Denoting hardness
scoto- Pertaining to darkness
sero- Pertaining to serum
sialo- Pertaining to saliva or the salivary glands
sidero- Denoting iron
sinistro- Left
somato- Denoting the body
somni- Denoting sleep
spasmo- Denoting a spasm
spermato-, spermo- Denoting sperm
sphero- Denoting a sphere; round

sphygmo- Denoting a pulse
splen-, spleno- Denoting the spleen
staphyl-, staphylo- Resembling a bunch of grapes
steno- Narrow; short
sterco- Denoting feces
steth-, stetho- Pertaining to the chest
stomato- Denoting the mouth
sym-, syn- With; along
tacho-, tachy- Swift
tarso- Pertaining to the flat of the foot
terato- Denoting a marvel, prodigy, or monster
thoraco- Pertaining to the chest
thrombo- Denoting a clot of blood
toxico-, toxo- Denoting poison
tracheo- Denoting the trachea
trichi-, tricho- Denoting hair
ur-, uro-, urono- Pertaining to urine
varico- Denoting a twisting or swelling
vaso- Denoting a vessel
veno- Denoting a vein
ventri-, ventro- Denoting the abdomen
vertebro- Pertaining to the vertebra
vesico- Denoting the bladder
viscero- Denoting the organs of the body
vivi- Denoting alive
xantho- Denoting yellow
xero- Denoting dryness

TERMINOLOGY FREQUENTLY USED TO DESIGNATE BODY PARTS OR ORGANS

anus Anal, ano-
arm Brachial, brachio-
blood Hem-, hemat-
chest Thoracic, thorax
ear Auricle, oto-
eye Ocular, oculo-, ophthalmo-
foot Pedal, ped-, -pod
gallbladder Chole-, chol-
head Cephalic, cephalo-
heart Cardium, cardiac, cardio-
intestines Cecum, colon, duodenum, ileum, jejunum
kidney Renal, nephric, nephro-
lip Cheil-
liver Hepatic, hepato-
lungs Pulmonary, pulmonic, pneumo-
mouth Oral, os, stoma, stomat-
muscle Myo-
neck Cervix, cervical, cervico-
penis Penile
rectum Rectal
skin Derma, integumentum
stomach Gastric, gastro-
testicle Orchio-, orchi-, orchido-
urinary bladder Cysti-, cysto-
uterus Hystero-, metra
vagina Vulvo, vaginal

Professional Organizations of Interest to Dental Hygienists

Academy of General Dentistry
560 W. Lake Street, Sixth Floor
Chicago, IL 60661
Phone: (888) 243–3368
Fax: (312) 335–3443
http://www.agd.org

American Academy of Pediatric Dentistry
211 E. Chicago Avenue, Suite 1600
Chicago, IL 60611
Phone: (312) 337–2169
Fax: (312) 337–6329
http://www.aapd.org
aapdweb@aapd.org

American Association for Dental Research
1619 Duke Street
Alexandria, VA 22314
Phone: (703) 548–0066
Fax: (703) 548–1883
http://www.aadronline.org
research@iadr.com

American Association of Public Health Dentistry
3085 Stevenson Drive, Suite 200
Springfield, IL 62703
Phone: (217) 529–6941
Fax: (217) 529–9120
http://www.aaphd.org
info@aaphd.org

American Dental Association
211 E. Chicago Avenue
Chicago, IL 60611
Phone: (312) 440–2500
Fax: (312) 440–2800
http://www.ada.org

American Dental Education Association
655 K Street, NW, Suite 800
Washington, DC 20001
Phone: (202) 289–7201
Fax: (202) 289–7204
http://www.adea.org

American Dental Hygienists Association
444 N. Michigan Avenue, Suite 3400
Chicago, IL 60611
Phone: (312) 440–8900
http://www.adha.org

American Public Health Association
800 I Street NW
Washington, DC 20001
Phone: (202) 777–2742
Fax: (202) 777–2534
http://www.apha.org
comments@apha.org

Association of Schools of Allied Health Professions
122 C Street, NW, Suite 650
Washington, DC 20001
Phone: (202) 237–6481
Fax: (202) 237–6485
http://www.asahp.org

Canadian Dental Association
1815 Alta Vista Drive
Ottawa, Ontario
Canada K1G 3Y6
Phone: (613) 523–1770
Fax: (613) 523–7736
http://www.cda-adc.ca/
reception@cda-adc.ca

Canadian Dental Hygienists Association
1122 Wellington Street W
Ottawa, Ontario
Canada K1Y 2Y7
Phone: (613) 224–5515 or (800) 267–5235
Fax: (613) 224–7283
http://www.cdha.ca
info@cdha.ca

Canadian Public Health Association
404–1525 Carling Avenue
Ottawa, Ontario
Canada K1Z 8R9
Phone: (613) 725–3769

Fax: (613) 725–9826
http://www.cpha.ca
info@cpha.ca

Centers for Disease Control and Prevention
1600 Clifton Road
Atlanta, GA 30329
Phone: (800) 232–4636 or (888) 232–6348
http://www.cdc.gov
cdcinfo@cdc.gov

FDI World Dental Federation
Avenue Louis Casaï 51
P.O. Box 3
1216 Geneve-Cointrin
Switzerland
Phone: 41 22 560 81 50
Fax: 41 22 560 81 40
http://www.fdiworldental.org
info@fdiworldental.org

Hispanic Dental Association
3910 South IH-35, Suite 245
Austin, Texas 78704
Phone: (512) 904–0252
http://www.hdassoc.org
hdassoc@aol.com

International Association for Dental Research
1619 Duke Street
Alexandria, VA 22314
Phone: (703) 548–0066
Fax: (703) 548–1883
http://www.iadr.com
research@iadr.com

International Association for Disability and Oral Health
Spoorstraat 94
6591 GV Gennep
Netherlands
http://www.iadh.org

International Federation of Dental Hygienists
100 South Washington Street
Rockville, MD 20850
Phone: (240) 778–6790
Fax: (240) 778–6112
http://www.ifdh.org
coordinator@ifdh.org

National Center for Dental Hygiene Research & Practice
USC School of Dentistry
925 W. 34th Street
Los Angeles, CA 90089
Phone: (213) 740–8669
Fax: (213) 740–1072
http://www.usc.edu/hsc/dental/dhnet/

National Dental Hygienists' Association/National Dental Association
6411 Ivy Lane, Suite 703
Greenbelt, MD 20770
Phone: (202) 588–1697
Fax: (240) 297–9181
http://www.ndaonline.org
admin@ndaonline.org

Special Care Dentistry Association
330 North Wabash Avenue, Suite 2000
Chicago, IL 60611
Phone: (312) 527–6764
Fax: (312) 673–6663
http://www.scdaonline.org
SCDA@SCDAonline.org

World Health Organization
Avenue Appia 20
1211 Geneva 27
Switzerland
Phone: 41 22 791 21 11
Fax: 41 22 791 31 11
http://www.who.int
info@who.int

American Dental Hygienists Association and Canadian Dental Hygienists Association Codes of Ethics

THE AMERICAN DENTAL HYGIENISTS' CODE OF ETHICS*

1. Preamble

As dental hygienists, we are a community of professionals devoted to the prevention of disease and the promotion and improvement of the public's health. We are preventive oral health professionals who provide educational, clinical, and therapeutic services to the public. We strive to live meaningful, productive, satisfying lives that simultaneously serve us, our profession, our society, and the world. Our actions, behaviors, and attitudes are consistent with our commitment to public service. We endorse and incorporate the Code into our daily lives.

2. Purpose

The purpose of a professional code of ethics is to achieve high levels of ethical consciousness, decision making, and practice by the members of the profession. Specific objectives of the Dental Hygiene Code of Ethics are:

- To increase our professional and ethical consciousness and sense of ethical responsibility.
- To lead us to recognize ethical issues and choices and to guide us in making more informed ethical decisions.
- To establish a standard for professional judgment and conduct.
- To provide a statement of the ethical behavior the public can expect from us.

The Dental Hygiene Code of Ethics is meant to influence us throughout our careers. It stimulates our continuing study of ethical issues and challenges us to explore our ethical responsibilities. The Code establishes concise standards of behavior to guide the public's expectations of our profession and supports existing dental hygiene practice, laws, and regulations. By holding ourselves accountable to meeting the standards stated in the Code, we enhance the public's trust on which our professional privilege and status are founded.

3. Key Concepts

Our beliefs, principles, values, and ethics are concepts reflected in the Code. They are the essential elements of our comprehensive and definitive code of ethics, and are interrelated and mutually dependent.

*Reprinted with permission from the American Dental Hygienists Association (www.adha.com).

4. Basic Beliefs

We recognize the importance of the following beliefs that guide our practice and provide context for our ethics:

- The services we provide contribute to the health and well-being of society.
- Our education and licensure qualify us to serve the public by preventing and treating oral disease and helping individuals achieve and maintain optimal health.
- Individuals have intrinsic worth, are responsible for their own health, and are entitled to make choices regarding their health.
- Dental hygiene care is an essential component of overall healthcare and we function interdependently with other healthcare providers.
- All people should have access to healthcare, including oral healthcare.
- We are individually responsible for our actions and the quality of care we provide.

5. Fundamental Principles

These fundamental principles, universal concepts, and general laws of conduct provide the foundation for our ethics.

Universality

The principle of universality assumes that if one individual judges an action to be right or wrong in a given situation, other people considering the same action in the same situation would make the same judgment.

Complementarity

The principle of complementarity assumes the existence of an obligation to justice and basic human rights. It requires us to act toward others in the same way they would act toward us if roles were reversed. In all relationships, it means considering the values and perspective of others before making decisions or taking actions affecting them.

Ethics

Ethics are the general standards of right and wrong that guide behavior within society. As generally accepted actions, they can be judged by determining the extent to which they promote good and minimize harm. Ethics compel us to engage in health promotion/disease prevention activities.

Community

This principle expresses our concern for the bond between individuals, the community, and society in general. It leads us to preserve natural resources and inspires us to show concern for the global environment.

Responsibility

Responsibility is central to our ethics. We recognize that there are guidelines for making ethical choices and accept responsibility for knowing and applying them. We accept the consequences of our actions or the failure to act and are willing to make ethical choices and publicly affirm them.

6. Core Values

We acknowledge these values as general guides for our choices and actions.

Individual Autonomy and Respect for Human Beings

People have the right to be treated with respect. People have the right to informed consent prior to treatment, and they have the right to full disclosure of all relevant information so that they can make informed choices about their care.

Confidentiality

We respect the confidentiality of client information and relationships as a demonstration of the value we place on individual autonomy. We acknowledge our obligation to justify any violation of a confidence.

Societal Trust

We value client trust and understand that public trust in our profession is based on our actions and behavior.

Nonmaleficence

We accept our fundamental obligation to provide services in a manner that protects all clients and minimizes harm to them and others involved in their treatment.

Beneficence

We have a primary role in promoting the well-being of individuals and the public by engaging in health promotion/disease prevention activities.

Justice and Fairness

We value justice and support the fair and equitable distribution of healthcare resources. We believe all people should have access to high-quality, affordable oral healthcare.

Veracity

We accept our obligation to tell the truth and assume that others will do the same. We value self-knowledge and seek truth and honesty in all relationships.

7. Standards of Professional Responsibility

We are obligated to practice our profession in a manner that supports our purpose, beliefs, and values in accordance with the fundamental principles that support our ethics. We acknowledge the following responsibilities:

To Ourselves as Individuals ...

- Avoid self-deception, and continually strive for knowledge and personal growth.

- Establish and maintain a lifestyle that supports optimal health.
- Create a safe work environment.
- Assert our own interests in ways that are fair and equitable.
- Seek the advice and counsel of others when challenged with ethical dilemmas.
- Have realistic expectations of ourselves and recognize our limitations.

To Ourselves as Professionals ...

- Enhance professional competencies through continuous learning in order to practice according to high standards of care.
- Support dental hygiene peer-review systems and quality-assurance measures.
- Develop collaborative professional relationships and exchange knowledge to enhance our own lifelong professional development.

To Family and Friends ...

- Support the efforts of others to establish and maintain healthy lifestyles and respect the rights of friends and family.

To Clients ...

- Provide oral healthcare utilizing high levels of professional knowledge, judgment, and skill.
- Maintain a work environment that minimizes the risk of harm.
- Serve all clients without discrimination and avoid action toward any individual or group that may be interpreted as discriminatory.
- Hold professional client relationships confidential.
- Communicate with clients in a respectful manner.
- Promote ethical behavior and standards of care by all dental hygienists.
- Serve as an advocate for the welfare of clients.
- Provide clients with the information necessary to make informed decisions about their oral health and encourage their full participation in treatment decisions and goals.
- Refer clients to other healthcare providers when their needs are beyond our ability or scope of practice.
- Educate clients about high-quality oral healthcare.

To Colleagues ...

- Conduct professional activities and programs, and develop relationships in ways that are honest, responsible, and appropriately open and candid.
- Encourage a work environment that promotes individual professional growth and development.
- Collaborate with others to create a work environment that minimizes risk to the personal health and safety of our colleagues.
- Manage conflicts constructively.
- Support the efforts of other dental hygienists to communicate the dental hygiene philosophy of preventive oral care.
- Inform other healthcare professionals about the relationship between general and oral health.

- Promote human relationships that are mutually beneficial, including those with other healthcare professionals.

To Employees and Employers …

- Conduct professional activities and programs, and develop relationships in ways that are honest, responsible, open, and candid.
- Manage conflicts constructively.
- Support the right of our employees and employers to work in an environment that promotes wellness.
- Respect the employment rights of our employers and employees.

To the Dental Hygiene Profession …

- Participate in the development and advancement of our profession.
- Avoid conflicts of interest and declare them when they occur.
- Seek opportunities to increase public awareness and understanding of oral health practices.
- Act in ways that bring credit to our profession while demonstrating appropriate respect for colleagues in other professions.
- Contribute time, talent, and financial resources to support and promote our profession.
- Promote a positive image for our profession.
- Promote a framework for professional education that develops dental hygiene competencies to meet the oral and overall health needs of the public.

To the Community and Society …

- Recognize and uphold the laws and regulations governing our profession.
- Document and report inappropriate, inadequate, or substandard care and/or illegal activities by any healthcare provider to the responsible authorities.
- Use peer review as a mechanism for identifying inappropriate, inadequate, or substandard care and for modifying and improving the care provided by dental hygienists.
- Comply with local, state, and federal statutes that promote public health and safety.
- Develop support systems and quality-assurance programs in the workplace to assist dental hygienists in providing the appropriate standard of care.
- Promote access to dental hygiene services for all, supporting justice and fairness in the distribution of healthcare resources.
- Act consistently with the ethics of the global scientific community of which our profession is a part.
- Create a healthful workplace ecosystem to support a healthy environment.
- Recognize and uphold our obligation to provide pro bono service.

To Scientific Investigation …

- We accept responsibility for conducting research according to the fundamental principles underlying our ethical beliefs in compliance with universal codes, governmental standards, and professional guidelines for the care and management of experimental subjects. We acknowledge our ethical obligations to the scientific community:
- Conduct research that contributes knowledge that is valid and useful to our clients and society.
- Use research methods that meet accepted scientific standards.
- Use research resources appropriately.
- Systematically review and justify research in progress to ensure the most favorable benefit-to-risk ratio to research subjects.
- Submit all proposals involving human subjects to an appropriate human subject review committee.
- Secure appropriate institutional committee approval for the conduct of research involving animals.
- Obtain informed consent from human subjects participating in research that is based on specifications published in Title 21 Code of Federal Regulations Part 46.
- Respect the confidentiality and privacy of data.
- Seek opportunities to advance dental hygiene knowledge through research by providing financial, human, and technical resources whenever possible.
- Report research results in a timely manner.
- Report research findings completely and honestly, drawing only those conclusions that are supported by the data presented.
- Report the names of investigators fairly and accurately.
- Interpret the research and the research of others accurately and objectively, drawing conclusions that are supported by the data presented and seeking clarity when uncertain.
- Critically evaluate research methods and results before applying new theory and technology in practice.
- Be knowledgeable concerning currently accepted preventive and therapeutic methods, products, and technology and their application to our practice.

THE CANADIAN DENTAL HYGIENISTS ASSOCIATION CODE OF ETHICS

"Dental hygienists believe that oral health is an integral part of a person's overall health, well-being, and quality of life."

Table of Contents

Preamble
Summary of the Main Principles in the Code
Principle I: Beneficence
Principle II: Autonomy
Principle III: Privacy and Confidentiality
Principle IV: Accountability
Principle V: Professionalism
Appendix A: Ethical Challenges/Problems
Appendix B: Reporting Suspected Incompetence or Unethical Conduct
Appendix C: Decision—Procedure
References

Preamble

Dental hygienists believe that oral health is an integral part of a person's overall health, well-being, and quality of life. The profession of dental hygiene is devoted to promoting optimal oral health for all. Dental hygiene has an identified body of knowledge and a distinctive expertise which dental hygienists use to serve the needs of their clients and promote the public good.

The Code of Ethics sets down the ethical principles and ethical practice standards of the dental hygiene profession. The principles express the broad ideals to which dental hygienists aspire and which guide them in their practice. The standards provide more specific direction for conduct. They are more precise and prescriptive as to what a given principle requires under particular circumstances. Clients, colleagues, and the public in general can reasonably expect dental hygienists to be guided by, and to be accountable under, the principles and standards articulated in this Code.

The purpose of the Code of Ethics is to

- Elaborate the ethical principles and standards by which dental hygienists are guided and under which they are accountable;
- Serve as a resource for education, reflection, self-evaluation, and peer review;
- Educate the public about the ethical principles and standards of the profession; and,
- Promote accountability.

The Code of Ethics is a public document that augments and complements the relevant laws and regulations under which dental hygienists practise. By elaborating on the profession's ethical principles and standards, the Code promotes accountability and worthiness of the public's trust.

The Code of Ethics applies to dental hygienists and dental hygiene students in all practice settings including, but not limited to, private practice, institutions, research, education, administration, community health, and industry.

Interpretation and application of the Code in specific circumstances requires individual judgment. Several aids are appended to the Code to assist in this.

Summary of the Main Principles in the Code

The fundamental principle underlying this Code is that the dental hygienist's primary responsibility is to the client, whether the client is an individual or a community.

Principle I: Beneficence

Beneficence involves caring about and acting to promote the good of another. Dental hygienists use their knowledge and skills to assist clients to achieve and maintain optimal oral health and to promote fair and reasonable access to quality oral health services.

Principle II: Autonomy

Autonomy pertains to the right to make one's own choices. By communicating relevant information openly and truthfully, dental hygienists assist clients to make informed choices and to participate actively in achieving and maintaining their optimal oral health.

Principle III: Privacy and Confidentiality

Privacy pertains to the individual's right to decide the conditions under which others will be permitted access to his or her personal life or information. Confidentiality is the duty to hold secret any information acquired in the professional relationship. Dental hygienists respect the privacy of clients and hold in confidence information disclosed to them, subject to certain narrowly defined exceptions.

Principle IV: Accountability

Accountability pertains to the acceptance of responsibility for one's actions and omissions in light of relevant principles, standards, laws, and regulations and the potential to self-evaluate and to be evaluated accordingly. Dental hygienists practise competently in conformity with relevant principles, standards, laws and regulations, and accept responsibility for their behavior and decisions in the professional context.

Principle V: Professionalism

Professionalism is the commitment to use and advance professional knowledge and skills to serve the client and the public good. Dental hygienists express their professional commitment individually in their practice and communally through their professional associations and regulatory bodies.

Principle I: Beneficence

Beneficence involves caring about and acting to promote the good of another. Dental hygienists use their knowledge and skills to assist clients to achieve and maintain optimal oral health and to promote fair and reasonable access to quality oral health services.

Standards for Principle I

Dental hygienists:

1a. provide services to their clients in a caring and respectful manner, in recognition of the inherent dignity of human beings;

1b. provide services to their clients with respect for their individual needs and values and life circumstances;

1c. provide services fairly and without discrimination, in recognition of fundamental human rights;

1d. put the needs, values, and interests of their clients first and avoid exploiting their clients for personal gain;

1e. seek to improve the quality of care and advance knowledge in the field of oral health through such activities as quality assurance, research, education, and advocacy in the public arena.

Principle II: Autonomy

Autonomy pertains to the right to make one's own choices. By communicating relevant information openly and truthfully, dental hygienists assist clients to make informed choices and to participate actively in achieving and maintaining their optimal oral health.

Standards for Principle II

Dental hygienists:

2a. actively involve clients in their oral health care and promote informed choice by communicating relevant information openly, truthfully, and sensitively in recognition of the client's needs, values, and capacity to understand;

2b. in the case of clients who lack the capacity for informed choice, actively involve and promote informed choice on the part of the client's substitute decision-makers, involving the client to the extent of the client's capacity;

2c. honour the client's informed choices, including refusal of treatment, and regard informed choice as a precondition of treatment;

2d. do not rely upon coercion or manipulative tactics in assisting the client to make informed choices;

2e. recommend or provide only those services they believe are necessary for the client's oral health or as consistent with the client's informed choice.

Note: Critical elements of informed choice include disclosure (i.e., revealing pertinent information, including risks and benefits); willingness (i.e., the choice is not coerced or manipulated); and capacity (i.e., the cognitive capacity to understand and process the relevant information). "Informed choice" encompasses what is sometimes referred to as "informed consent."

Principle III: Privacy and Confidentiality

Privacy pertains to the individual's right to decide the conditions under which others will be permitted access to his or her personal life or information. Confidentiality is the duty to hold secret any information acquired in the professional relationship. Dental hygienists respect the privacy of clients and hold in confidence information disclosed to them, subject to certain narrowly defined exceptions.

Standards for Principle III

Dental hygienists:

3a. demonstrate regard for the privacy of their clients;

3b. hold confidential any information acquired in the professional relationship and do not use or disclose it to others without the client's express consent, except:

    3b.i as required by law

    3b.ii as required by the policy of the practice environment (e.g., quality assurance)

    3b.iii in an emergency situation

    3b.iv in cases where disclosure is necessary to prevent serious harm to others

    3b.v to the guardian or substitute decision-maker of a client, in these cases, disclose to others only as much information as is necessary to accomplish the purpose for the disclosure;

3c. may infer the client's consent for disclosure to others directly involved in delivering and administering services to the client, provided there is no reason to believe the client would not give express consent if asked;

3d. obtain the client's express consent to use or share information about the client for the purpose of teaching or research;

3e. inform their clients in advance of treatment about how they will use or share their information, in particular about any uses or sharing that may occur without the client's express consent;

3f. promote practices, policies, and information systems that are designed to respect client privacy and confidentiality.

Principle IV: Accountability

Accountability pertains to the acceptance of responsibility for one's actions and omissions in light of relevant principles, standards, laws, and regulations and the potential to self-evaluate and to be evaluated accordingly. Dental hygienists practise competently in conformity with relevant principles, standards, laws and regulations, and accept responsibility for their behaviour and decisions in the professional context.

Standards for Principle IV

Dental hygienists:

4a. accept responsibility for knowing and acting consistently with the principles, standards, laws and regulations under which they are accountable;

4b. accept responsibility for providing safe, quality, competent care including, but not limited to, addressing issues in the practice environment within their capacity that may hinder or impede the provision of such care;

4c. take appropriate action to ensure first and foremost the client's safety and quality of care when they suspect unethical or incompetent care;

4d. practise within the bounds of their competence, scope of practice, personal and/or professional limitations, and refer clients requiring care outside these bounds;

4e. inform the dental hygiene regulatory body when an injury, dependency, infection, condition, or any other serious incapacity has immediately affected, or may affect over time, their continuing ability to practise safely and competently;

4f. promote workplace practices and policies that facilitate professional practice in accordance with the principles, standards, laws and regulations under which they are accountable.

Principle V: Professionalism

Professionalism is the commitment to use and advance professional knowledge and skills to serve the client and the public good. Dental hygienists express their professional commitment individually in their practice and communally through their professional associations and regulatory bodies.

Standards for Principle V

Dental hygienists:

5a. uphold the principles and standards of the profession before clients, colleagues, and others;

5b. maintain and advance their knowledge and skills in dental hygiene through continuing education and the quality of the care they provide through ongoing self-evaluation and quality assurance;

5c. advance general knowledge and skills in the field of oral health by supporting, participating in, or conducting ethically approved research;

5d. participate in professional activities such as meetings, committee work, peer review, and participation in public forums to promote oral health;

5e. participate in mentoring, education, and dissemination of knowledge and skills in oral health care;

5f. support the work of their professional associations and regulatory bodies to promote oral health and professional practice;

5g. inform potential employers about the principles, standards, laws and regulations to which they are accountable and determine whether employment conditions facilitate professional practice accordingly;

5h. collaborate with colleagues in a cooperative, constructive, and respectful manner toward the primary end of providing safe, competent, fair, quality care to clients;

5i. communicate the nature and costs of professional services fairly and accurately.

Appendix A: Ethical Challenges/Problems

No code of ethics can be expected to resolve definitively all ethical challenges or problems that may arise in practice. The analysis below is intended to help dental hygienists understand the nature of ethical challenges or problems and thereby better resolve them.

Ethical challenges or problems faced by practicing dental hygienists tend to fall into the categories of ethical violations, ethical dilemmas, and ethical distress.

Ethical violations: when dental hygienists fail to meet or neglect their specific ethical responsibilities as expressed in the Code's standards. An example would be a dental hygienist who recommends unnecessary treatment in order to achieve personal gain at the expense of the client.

Ethical dilemmas: when one or more ethical principles conflict either with other ethical principle(s) or with self-interest(s) and no apparent course of action will satisfy both sides of the dilemma. An example would be a client with a hip prosthesis who may refuse to be premedicated prior to receiving invasive dental treatment. In this case, the principle of autonomy conflicts with the principle of beneficence.

Ethical distress: when dental hygienists experience constraints or limitations in relation to which they are or feel powerless and which compromise their ability to practise in full accordance with their professional principles or standards. An example would be a dental hygienist who is expected by the employer to complete dental hygiene treatment in a length of time insufficient to render quality care or to provide an acceptable level of infection control.

This Code is a useful guide in helping dental hygienists to identify, work through, and put into words ethical issues in light of their responsibilities as articulated in the Code's principles and standards, and to decide on an ethically responsible course of action. It is important to realize that some challenges or problems are perceived to be primarily ethical in nature when, in fact, they arise less from conflicting principles than from poor communication or lack of information. Reflecting on a perceived challenge or problem in light of the Code can help determine to what extent the problem or challenge is truly rooted in conflicting ethical principles, and to what extent it can be resolved by improved communication or by new information.

The Code provides clear direction for avoiding ethical violations. When a course of action is mandated by a standard in the Code or by a principle where there exists no opposing principle, ethical conduct requires that course of action.

In the case of ethical dilemmas and ethical distress, the Code cannot always provide a clear direction. The resolution of dilemmas often depends on the specific circumstances of the case in question. Total satisfaction by all parties involved may not be achieved. Resolution may also depend on which opposing ethical principle is considered to be more important, a matter on which reasonable people may disagree. Ethical distress often arises in situations where the dental hygienist is significantly limited by factors beyond his or her immediate control that may not be resolvable in the specific context.

In all cases, dental hygienists are accountable for how they conduct themselves in professional practice. Even in situations of ethical dilemma or distress where the Code does not prescribe a specific course of action, the hygienist can be expected to give account of his or her chosen action in light of the principles and standards expressed in the Code. Ultimately, dental hygienists must reconcile their actions with their consciences in caring for clients.

Appendix B: Reporting Suspected Incompetence or Unethical Conduct

The first consideration of the dental hygienist who suspects incompetence or unethical conduct in colleagues or associates is the welfare of present clients and/or potential harm to future clients. Adherence to the following guidelines could be helpful:
1. First, confirm the facts of the situation.
2. Ensure you are familiar with existing protocols in the practice setting for reporting incidents, incompetence, or unethical care and follow those protocols.
3. Document and report issues that cannot be resolved within the practice setting and report to the appropriate authority or regulatory body.

The dental hygienist who attempts to protect clients threatened by incompetent or unethical conduct should not be placed in jeopardy (e.g., loss of employment). Colleagues and professional organizations are morally obligated to support dental hygienists who fulfil their ethical obligations under the Code.

Appendix C: Decision—Procedure
Guidance Regarding the Process for Resolving Ethical Challenges

Ethical problems or challenges arise in a variety of contexts and require thoughtful analysis and careful judgment. The following guide may be useful to assist dental hygienists faced with an ethical challenge, recognizing that other stakeholders may need to be involved in resolving the matter. Talking with or getting advice from others at any step on the way to a decision can be very helpful.
1. Identify in a preliminary way the nature of the challenge or problem. What is the issue? What kind of issue is it? What ethical principles are at stake?

2. Become suitably informed and gather information (e.g., talk to others to find out the facts; research relevant policy statements) relevant to the challenge or problem, including:
   a. Factual information about the situation. What has happened? What is the sequence of events?
   b. Applicable policies, laws or regulations. Does a workplace policy address the issue? What does the Code say? What does law or regulation say?
   c. Who are the relevant stakeholders? How do they view the situation?

3. Clarify and elaborate the challenge or problem after getting this information. Now that you are better informed, What is the issue? What ethical principles are at stake? What stakeholders need to be consulted or involved in resolving the challenge or problem?

4. Identify various options for actions, recognizing that the best option may not be obvious at first and realizing it may require creativity or imagination.

5. Assess the various options in light of applicable policy, law or regulation, being as clear as possible in your mind of the pluses and minuses of each option as assessed in this light.

6. Decide on a course of action, mindful of how you would justify or defend your decision in light of the applicable policy, law or regulation, if you are called to account.

7. Implement your decision as thoughtfully and sensitively as possible, communicating a willingness to explain or justify the reasons for taking it.

8. Assess the consequences of your decision. Evaluate the process you used to arrive at the decision and the decision itself in light of those consequences. Did things turn out as you thought they would? Would you do the same thing again? What went wrong? Or, what went right?

In all of this, bear in mind that reasonable people can disagree about what is the right thing to do when faced with an ethical challenge or problem. If you cannot be certain whether you have made the right decision, you can at least have some assurance that you came to your decision in a responsible way. The test for this is whether you are able to defend your decision in light of relevant laws, principles, and regulations, and to defend the process by which you came to your decision. Reference to the above guidelines will help in this.

In addition, there is a very rich literature on ethics that can be very helpful for thinking through ethical challenges and problems in dental hygiene or for ongoing professional education and development.

Dental hygienists may also find it useful to familiarize themselves with various ethical theories, which tend to guide or orient ethical thinking along different lines. The main ethical theories current today are briefly described below:

- Deontology guides ethical thinking in terms of duties and rights, which the philosopher Immanuel Kant grounds in the fundamental imperative to act in relation to others according to principles that apply universally to all people, and that one would also wish for others to apply in their actions in relation to oneself.
- Utilitarianism guides ethical thinking in terms of harms and benefits, which the philosopher J.S. Mill grounds in the fundamental imperative to promote the greatest good for the greatest number.
- The ethic of care guides ethical thinking in terms of preserving and enhancing relationships and service to others. This theory derives from the work of Carol Gilligan, who found in her research that this style of ethical thinking tends to be more associated with females than with males.
- Virtue ethics guides ethical thinking in terms of habits of acting and assesses actions in terms of virtues and vices of character. This theory derives from the work of the philosopher Aristotle, who emphasized that ethics cannot be reduced to rules or formulas and held that the person of good character (the "good man") is the ultimate standard of right and wrong and should be emulated by others as a role model.
- Feminist ethics guides ethical thinking in terms of sensitivity to the power or political dimension of human interaction. The philosopher Susan Sherwin grounds feminist ethics in the allegiance to those who are oppressed, vulnerable, or disadvantaged and the imperative to improve their situation.

This is by no means a complete listing of ethical theories, nor is the richness of these theories captured in the condensed descriptions given. Moreover, considerable controversy exists not only among these theories but also among adherents of each theory.[1]

---

[1]Reprinted with permission from the American Dental Hygienists' Association homepage (www.adha.com).

REFERENCES

American Dental Hygienists Association: *Code of ethics for dental hygienists,* Chicago, 1995, ADHA.

Canadian Dental Assistants Association: *CDAA code of ethics,* Ottawa, 2000, CDAA.

Canadian Dental Association: *Code of ethics,* Ottawa, August 1991, CDA.

Canadian Dental Hygienists Association: *Code of ethics,* Ottawa, July 1997, CDHA.

Canadian Dental Hygienists Association: *Dental hygiene: client's bill of rights,* Ottawa, October 2001, CDHA.

Canadian Medical Association: *Code of ethics of the Canadian Medical Association,* Ottawa, 1997, CMA.

Canadian Nurses Association: *Code of ethics for registered nurses,* Ottawa, March 1997, CNA.

College of Dental Hygienists of British Columbia: *Code of ethics,* Victoria, March 1, 1995, CDHBC.

Canadian Dental Hygienists Association
1122 Wellington Street W
Ottawa, ON K1Y 2Y7
Telephone (613) 224–5515 or (800) 267–5235
Fax (613) 224–7283
www.cdha.ca

Note: Page numbers followed by *b* indicate boxes, *f* indicate figures and *t* indicate tables.

Numbers

3 As (analgesic/antipyretic/anti-inflammatory), 337
3- to 7-day food record or diary, 384
5-Fluorouracil (5-FU), 352

A

Abandonment, 713
Abbreviations, Latin, 326t
Abdominopelvic cavity, 55, 56f
Abducens nerve (CN VI), 122
Abscesses, 433
Absence (petit mal) seizure, 699
Absolute refractory period, 76, 548
Absorption, 327
Abutment, 500
Academy of General Dentistry, 746
Acarbose (Pre-cose), 349
Acceptance, 482
Access, to oral health care, 568
Accessory nerve (CN IX), 123
Accessory structures, 61
Accountability, 751–752
Acetylcholine, 72, 330
Acid-fast stain, 258
Acidogenic bacteria, 364
Acidulated phosphate fluoride (APF), 503
Acquired deformities, 433–436.
    See also Periodontium.
Acquired immunodeficiency syndrome (AIDS), 234b, 268
Acrylic appliances, 415–416
Acrylic denture bases, 416
Act deontology, 707
Act utilitarianism, 707
Actinomyces israelii, 266t
Action mechanism, 550
Action potential, 548
Activation, 525
Active listening, 482
Active site, 60
Active transport, 20, 59, 361
Activity, in weight management, 379
Acute adrenal insufficiency, 701
Acute disease, 625t
Acute inflammation, 177–181, 178f.
    See also Inflammation.
    chemotaxis in, 179
    mediators
        arachidonic acid, 180
        chemical, 179, 179t
    outcomes of, 181
    phagocytosis in, 179
    vascular changes in, 177, 178f
Acute lymphoblastic leukemia (ALL), 231

Acute myeloblastic leukemia (AML), 231
Acyclovir, 287t, 343
ADA. *See* American Dental Association (ADA).
Adaptation, 525
Addison anemia, 228
Adenohypophysis (anterior pituitary), 82
Adenosine triphosphate (ATP), 259, 378
Adenovirus, 264t
ADEX. *See* American Board of Dental Examiners (ADEX).
ADHA. *See* American Dental Hygienists Association (ADHA).
ADHD. *See* Attention deficit hyperactivity disorder (ADHD).
Adipose-derived stem cells (ASCs), 185
Administration, routes of, 326
Administration for Children and Families (ACF), 621b
Administrative law, 711
Administrative requirements, 733
Adolescence, 387
Adrenal crisis, 348, 701
Adrenal glands, 84
Adrenal insufficiency, acute, 701
Adrenergic agents, 328–329, 328f, 329t
    adverse reactions of, 328
    drug interactions of, 329
    pharmacologic effects of, 328
    therapeutic uses of, 329
    as vasoconstrictors, 329
Adrenergic agonists, 328, 350
β_2-Adrenergic agonists, 350
β-Adrenergic blocker antagonists, 330
α-Adrenergic blockers, 329–330
Adrenergic drug, 552
Adrenergic neuronal agonists and antagonists, 330
α-Adrenergic receptors, 553
β-Adrenergic receptors, 553
Adrenocorticosteroids (steroids), 348, 348t
    for asthma, 351
Adrenocorticotropic hormone, 363
Adult stem cells, 185
Advanced dental therapist (ADT), 669t
Advanced instrumentation techniques, 535–536
Advanced root instrumentation, 523
Advancing Oral Health in America, 623
Adverse reactions, 327–328
    pharmacokinetics and, 327–328
    receptors and, 328
    side effects, 327
Aerobic bacteria, 262

AFSCs. *See* Amniotic fluid-derived stem cells (AFSCs).
Age, pain and, 548
Age Discrimination in Employment Act (ADEA) of 1967, 735
Aggressive periodontitis, 431–432.
    See also Periodontitis.
Agonist agents, 328
Agonist-antagonist agents, 338
Agranulocytes, 115
AIDS. *See* Acquired immunodeficiency syndrome (AIDS).
Air polishing, conventional supragingival, 537
Airborne microbes, reduction of, 308
Airway, obstructed, 692
Alabama dental hygiene practice and education, 718
Albendazole, 287t
Alcohol abuse and dependence, 353, 594
Alcoholism, 366
Alcohol-related neurodevelopmental disorders (ARND), 571
Alkylating agents, 352
ALL. *See* Acute lymphoblastic leukemia (ALL).
Allergic contact dermatitis, 306, 467
Allergic reactions, 327, 697–698
Allergy, 270f
Allopurinol (Zyloprim), 339
"All-or-none" principle, 76
Allosteric effectors, 60
Alloys. *see also* Biomaterials.
    casting, 412–413
    chromium, 413
    porcelain-fused-to-metal, 413–414
Alternative hypothesis, 629
Aluminum discs, 159f
Alveolar bone, 43–44
    components of, 44f
Alveolar mucosa, 131t
    examination of, 470
Alveolar process, 429, 429f
    of mandible, 112
    of maxillae, 110
Alveolar ridges, examination of, 470
Alzheimer's disease, 574–575
Amalgam
    dental, 399–401, 399–400f
    tattoo, 246, 246f
Amantadine, 287t
Ameloblasts, 36f, 377
    depositing hydroxyapatite crystals, 41f
Amelogenesis, process of, 40
Amelogenesis imperfecta, 240–241, 240–241f

American Academy of Pediatric Dentistry, 746

American Association for Dental Research, 746

American Association of Public Health Dentistry, 746

American Board of Dental Examiners (ADEX), 1, 9

American Dental Association (ADA)
  Code D9215, 549
  contact data for, 746
  standards of
    biomaterials, 398
    dental hygiene process as, 458

American Dental Education Association, 746

American Dental Hygienists Association (ADHA)
  code of ethics of, 748–750
  contact data for, 746
  dental hygiene process, 458
  Practice Act overview, 716t

American National Standards Institute (ANSI), 398

American Public Health Association, 746

American Society of Anesthesiologists (ASA), 464
  physical status classification system and stress reduction protocols, 465t

Americans with Disabilities Act (ADA of 1990), 735

Amine hormones, 80

Amino acid pool, 367

Aminobisphosphonates, 352

Aminoglycosides, 342

AML. See Acute myeloblastic leukemia (AML).

Amniotic fluid-derived stem cells (AFSCs), 185

Amorphous calcium phosphate, 504, 647

Amoxicillin, 285t

Amphetamine, 329t, 353

Amphotericin B, 287t

Ampicillin, 285t

Amprenavir (AP), 272

Anabolic hormones, 363

Anabolism, 368

Anaerobic bacteria, 295

Analgesic nephropathy, 338

Analgesics, 337, 337t
  acetaminophen (n-acetyl-p-aminophenol), 338
  aspirin, 337
  general considerations for, 337
  gout drugs, 339
  nonsteroidal anti-inflammatories
    adverse reactions to, 338
    agents (NSAIAs), 338
    drugs (NSAIDs), 331t, 338
  opioid (narcotic), 338–339, 339t
  salicylates, 337

Analytic research, 628t

Anaphase, of mitosis, 21

Anaphylactic shock, 693

Anaphylaxis, 697

Anastomosis, 115

Anatomic crown, 129

Anatomic nomenclature, 53–55, 107, 108f

Anatomical position, 107

Anatomy and physiology, 53–106
  basic concepts in, 53–55
    anatomic nomenclature in, 53–55
    body cavities, 55, 56f
    levels of organization in, 53, 54f
  body systems and components, 61–103
  cells, 55–61. See also Cells.
  dental, 134–142
    clinical oral structures, 129, 130–131f, 131t
    dentition, 134, 136t
    eruption, 142–143
    interarch relationships, 143–147
    intra-arch relationships, 143–147
    periodontium, 428f.
      See also Periodontium.
    review questions for, 148, 148–149b, 148–149f
    terminology for, 129–134
    website information and resources for, 147b
  head and neck, 107–128
    bones of, 109–112
    circulatory system and, 115–117.
      See also Circulatory system.
    glands of, 118–119
    lymphatic system and, 117–118, 117f
    muscular system and, 112–114.
      See also Muscular system.
    nervous system and, 119–123.
      See also Nervous system.
    osteology, 107–112. See also Osteology.
    paranasal sinuses of, 112
    review questions for, 123–128, 127b
    temporomandibular joint, 114–115, 114f
    website information and resources for, 123b
  review questions for, 103, 104–106b
  tissues, 61

Anemia
  Addison, 228
  aplastic, 229–230
    primary, 229
    secondary, 229
  Biermer, 228
  Cooley, 229–230
  iron deficiency, 228–229, 229f
  pernicious, 228
  primary, 228
  sickle cell, 227–228, 227–228f

Anesthesia stages, 561
  and planes, 334

Anesthetic agents
  general, 334–335
  local. See Local anesthetic agents
  specific, 334–335

Aneurysmal bone cyst, 226

Angina pectoris, 587, 695

Angiogenesis, 182

Angle, Edward H., 145

Angled shank, 518

Angular cheilitis, 247, 247f

Angulation, 525, 525f

Anode, 153

Anodontia, 244

Anorexia bulimia, 574

Anorexia nervosa, 380, 574

ANSI. See American National Standards Institute (ANSI).

Antagonist, 328

Anterior middle superior alveolar (AMSA) nerve block, 558

Anterior superior alveolar (ASA) nerve, 120, 120t

Anthropometric analysis, 381

Antiacne agents, 331t

Antianginal agents, 344

Antiarrhythmics, 344–347
  antianginal agents, 344
  anticoagulants, 344–345
  anticonvulsants, 346–347, 346t
  antihypertensives, 344, 345t
  diuretics, 344

Antibacterial agents, 285t

Antibiotics, premedication guidelines for, 464t

Anticholinergic agents, 331, 331t

Anticoagulants, 344–345
  warfarin (Coumadin), 344–345

Anticonvulsants, 331t, 346–347, 346t

Antidepressants, 331t, 347–348

Antidiabetic agents, 329

Antidiarrheal, 331t

Antidiuretic hormone, 83

Antiemetics, 351–352

Antifungal agents, 287t, 343

Antihistamines, 331t

Antihypertensives, 331t, 338, 344, 345t

Anti-infectives (antibiotics), 339–343
  aminoglycosides, 342
  antifungal agents, 343
  as antineoplastic agent, 352
  antituberculosis agents, 343
  antiviral agents, 343
  cephalosporins, 341
  clindamycin, 341
  general considerations for, 339–340
  general dental concerns for, 340
  general side effects of, 340
  macrolides, 341
  metronidazole, 342–343
  penicillins, 340–341
  quinolones, 342
  sulfonamides, 342
  tetracyclines, 341–342

Anti-inflammatories
    adverse reactions to, 338
    nonsteroidal anti-inflammatory agents
        (NSAIAs), 338
    nonsteroidal anti-inflammatory drugs
        (NSAIDs), 331*t*, 338
Antimetabolites, 352
Antimicrobial substances, 267
Antinauseants, 331*t*
Antineoplastic agents, 352–353
Antiparasitic agents, 287*t*
Antiparkinson drugs, 331*t*
Antipsychotics, 331*t*, 347, 347*t*
Antiretroviral drugs, 343
Antispasmodics, 331*t*
Antituberculosis agents, 343
Antiviral agents, 287*t*, 343
Anxiety and pain management, 547–566
    armamentarium for, 548–549
        cartridge in, anesthetic, 549,
           549*f*
        needle in, 548, 548*f*
        record keeping and documentation in,
           549
        syringe in, anesthetic, 549, 549*f*
    Computer-controlled local anesthesia
        delivery device (CCLADD) in,
        556–559, 558*t*
        Basic CCLADD procedure and,
           556–558
        components of, 556
        injection administration with,
           558–559
        vs. traditional syringe, 558*t*
    local anesthetic agents for, 550–553
        biotransformation of, 550–551
        calculations for, 552
        chemical structure of, 550, 551*t*
        comparison of, 551*t*
        maximum recommended dose (MRD)
           for, 552
        mechanism of action of, 550
        metabolism of, 550–551
        potency of, 550
        topical, 552
        toxicity of, 550
        vasoconstrictors, 552–553, 552*t*
    nitrous oxide-oxygen in, conscious
        sedation with, 559
        advantages and disadvantages of, 562
        anesthesia stages for, 561
        chemistry of, 559
        contraindications to, 562
        equipment for, 562
        indications for, 562
        pharmacology of, 561
        physiology of, 561
        record keeping and documentation for,
           562
        safety measures for, 562
        signs and symptoms of, 562
        synonymous terms in, 559

Anxiety and pain management *(Continued)*
    pain characteristics and physiology in,
        547–548, 548*f*
    review questions for, 563, 565*b*
    trigeminal nerve, mandibular division of,
        554–556
        block injections for, 556, 557*t*
        innervation of, 554–555
    trigeminal nerve, maxillary
        division of, 554
        block injections for, 554, 555*t*, 556*f*
        innervation of, 554
    website information and resources for, 563*b*
Apex, 107, 129
Aphthous pharyngitis, 209–210, 210*f*
Aphthous ulcers
    major. *See* Major aphthous ulcers
    minor, 205–206, 206*f*
        recurrent aphthous stomatitis,
           205–206
        recurrent ulcerative stomatitis (RUS),
           205–206
Apical convergence, 139*f*
Aplastic anemia, 229–230
    primary, 229
    secondary, 229
Apoptosis, 179
Appellate courts, 712
Appendicular skeleton, 64–66, 65*f*
Appliances, 415–416, 500
Applied epidemiology, 624
Appropriation, 714
Arachidonic acid, 180
Arachnoid, 76, 76*f*
Arbovirus, 264*t*
Arc, reflex, 77
Arches, 143–147
Area-specific curet, 522*f*, 522–523.
        See also Curet.
Aristotle, 707
Arm muscle circumference, 381
Armamentarium, 548–549
ARND. *See* Alcohol-related
        neurodevelopmental disorders
        (ARND).
Arrested caries, 471
Arrhythmias, cardiac, 586
Arteries, 26
Arthritis, 580–581, 580*t*
Artificial fats, 370
ASA. *See* American Society of
        Anesthesiologists (ASA).
Ascaris lumbricoides, 287*t*
Ascomycota, 263
Asepsis, 300
    maintaining, in oral health care
        environment, 308–311
Aspartame, 365
Aspergillus, 263
Aspirated materials, 701
Aspirin, 337
Assault, 714

Assessment
    of community intervention, 650–654, 651*t*,
        653*t*
    of dentition, 471–474, 474*b*
    extraoral, 468–471
    as function of public health, 620
    human needs theory and, 458, 460–461*f*
    intraoral, 468–471
    oral hygiene, 476
    periodontal, 472*t*, 475
    periodontal instrumentation for, 518–546.
        See also Periodontal instrumentation.
    radiographic evaluation for, 475–476
    risk factor, 476–477. *See also* Risk factors.
Assignment, 718
Association of Schools of Allied Health
        Professions, 746
Assurance
    as function of public health, 620
    quality, 162
Asthma
    agents for, 350–351
    emergencies, 694
Ataxia, 578
Athetosis, 578
Athletic mouthguards, 417
Atlas, 112
Atropine, 331, 331*t*
Attention deficit hyperactivity disorder
        (ADHD), 573
Attorney, 712
Attribution theory, 491
Aura, 575
Auricular lymph nodes, assessment of, 469
Auriculotemporal nerve, 121
Auscultation, in extraoral and intraoral
        assessment, 468
Autism spectrum disorders (ASD), 572–573
Autolysis, 57
Automated external defibrillator, 692
Autonomic nervous system (ANS) agents,
        328–334
    β-adrenergic blocker antagonists, 330
    α-adrenergic blockers, 329–330
    adrenergic neuronal agonists and
        antagonists, 330
    parasympathomimetic (cholinergic), 328*f*,
        330–332
    sympathetic (adrenergic), 328–329, 328*f*, 329*t*
    xerostomia-producing drug groups, 331*t*
Autonomic reflex, 77
Autonomy, 708, 751
Autophagy, 57
Autoregulation, 90
Axial positioning, 143, 144*f*
Axial skeleton, 64–65, 109–112
    cranial bones, 109
    ethmoid bone, 109*f*, 110
    facial bones, 110, 111*f*
    frontal bone, 109, 109*f*
    neck bones, 112
    neurocranium, 109

Axial skeleton (Continued)
    occipital bone, 109f, 110
    parietal bones, 109, 109f
    sphenoid bone, 110
    temporal bones, 109
    viscerocranium, 110, 111f
Axis, 112
Axon, 75, 75f
Azithromycin, 285t, 341

B
Bacillary dysentery, 277
Bacillus anthracis, 266t
Bacillus fusiformis, 205
Backward caries, 471
Bacteria, 263. See also Microbiology and
        immunology.
    Firmicutes, 263
    Gracilicutes, 263
    of human importance, 266t
    Mendosicutes, 263
    Tenericutes, 263
Bacterial plaque, 290–291
Bacterial production, 261f
Bacteriophages, 264
Balanced, low-calorie diet, 379
Bar graph, 662
Barbiturates, 336
    abuse of, 353
    adverse reactions to, 336
    intermediate-acting, 336
    long-acting, 336
    pharmacologic effects of, 336
    short-acting, 336
    therapeutic uses of, 336
    ultrashort-acting, 335
Barrier-free environment, 568
Barriers
    disease, 267
    to oral health care, 569–570
Basal ganglia, 78
Basal metabolic rate (BMR), 378
Bases
    cement, 405–406, 405f
    denture, acrylic, 416
Basic life support (BLS), 688
Basic CCLADD Procedure, 556–558
Basic screening, 625t
Basic Screening Survey (BSS), 640
Basidiomycota, 263
Basophils, 115
Battery, 714
Beam intensity, 155
Beam quality, 154
Beam quantity, 154
Behavior change theory, 490–493
Behavior modification, in weight
        management, 379
Behçet syndrome, 212, 212f
Bell's palsy, 579, 579f
Beneficence, 708, 749, 751

Benefits plans, 671
    providers of, 672, 672t
Benign intraosseous neoplasms, 199–201
    characteristics of, 199
    chondroma, 200
    exostosis, 201
        torus mandibularis, 201, 201f
        torus palatinus, 201, 201f
    odontogenic myxoma, 200–201, 200f
    odontoma, 201, 202f
    osteoma, 199–200, 200f
Benign migratory glossitis, 247, 247f
Benign mixed tumor, 219–220, 220f
Benign mucous membrane pemphigoid,
        206–207, 207f
Benign oral lesions
    characteristics of, 193
    hemangioma, 194–195, 195f
    irritative fibroma, 193, 194f
    lipoma, 195, 195f
    papilloma, 193, 194f
    soft tissue origins of, 193–195
    traumatic fibroma, 193, 194f
    verruca vulgaris, 193–194, 194f
    wart, 193–194, 194f
Benzocaine, 333
Benzodiazepine receptor agonists, 336
Benzodiazepines, 331t, 335–336, 336t, 346
Bicarbonate, 367
Bidigital palpation, 468
Biermer anemia, 228
Biguanides, 349
Bilateral palpation, 468
Bile acid sequestrant, 349
Bimanual palpation, 468
Biochemistry, 360–393
    review questions for, 390, 393b
    web site information and resources for, 390b
Bioelectrical impedance, 382
Bioethics, 707
Biohazard symbol, 314f
Biologic death, 691
Biologic properties, 398. See also Biomaterials.
Biologic value (BV), 367
Biomaterials, 394–426
    applications of, 394
    classification of, 394
    general considerations for, 394
    preventive and restorative, direct, 399–409
        amalgam, dental, 399–401, 399–400f
        bonding agents, 403–405, 403–404f
        cement applications, 406
        cement bases, 405–406, 405f
        cement liners, 405
        cements, orthodontic, 406
        composites, dental, 401–402, 401f
        dentifrices, 408–409
        dressings, surgical, 406
        fluoride varnishes, 407–408
        fluoride-releasing restorative materials,
            406–407, 406f, 408f
        fluorides, topical, 407–408

Biomaterials (Continued)
        gingival tissue packs, 406
        infiltrants, 403
        pastes, prophylactic, 408–409
        sealants, pit-and-fissure, 402–403
        sealers, root canal, 406
        whitening agents, 409
    preventive and restorative, indirect,
            409–420
        alloys, casting, 412–413
        alloys, chromium, 413
        alloys, porcelain-fused-to-metal,
            413–414
        appliances, acrylic, 415–416
        athletic mouthguards, 417
        cast materials, 411–412, 411t
        cements, crown-and-bridge, 415, 415t
        ceramics, dental, 414–415
        denture bases, acrylic, 416
        denture cleansers, 417
        denture soft liners, 417
        denture teeth, 416
        die materials, 411–412, 411t
        implants, dental, 418–419
        impression materials, 409–410, 410t
        investment materials, 412
        model materials, 411–412, 411t
        mouth protectors, 417
        provisional materials, 410–411
        restorations, computer-assisted design/
            computer-assisted machining, 418
        solders, dental, 413
        tissue engineering, 419–420
        veneers, 417–418
        waxes, 412
    properties of, 395–398
        biologic, 398
        chemical, 395
        electrical, 395
        electrochemical, 396, 396f
        mechanical, 396, 397–398t, 397f
        physical, 395
        thermal, 395, 395f
    review questions for, 420
    structure of, 394
    website information and resources for, 420b
Biotransformation, 327
    of local anesthetic agents, 550–551
Bipolar neurons, 29f
Bitewing radiographs, 164, 164f
Black hairy tongue, 248, 248f
Blastocyst, embryology, 31
Blind, 628
Block injections, for trigeminal nerve
    mandibular, 556, 557t
    maxillary, 554, 555t, 556f
Blood, 26–27, 85
    characteristics of, 86
    components of, 27, 86, 86f
    groups, 87
    transport of gases of, 95
Blood analysis, 381

Blood disorders, 227–233
  anemia. *see also* Anemia.
    Addison, 228
    aplastic, 229–230
    Biermer, 228
    Cooley, 229–230
    iron deficiency, 228–229, 229f
    pernicious, 228
    primary, 228
    sickle cell, 227–228, 227–228f
  characteristics of, 227
  hemophilias, 233
  human immunodeficiency virus (HIV), 233–234. *See also* Human immunodeficiency virus (HIV).
  leukemia, 231–232. *See also* Leukemia.
  neutropenia, cyclic, 231, 231f
  Plummer-Vinson syndrome, 228–229, 229f
  polycythemia, 230
  purpura, 232–233
  thalassemia, 229–230
Blood dyscrasias, 346
Blood glucose
  energy from, 378
  reactions of, 362
  sources of, 361
Blood pressure
  classification of, 466t
  medical emergencies and, 689, 689f
Blood supply, 429–430
Blood vessels, 26
Blood-brain barrier (BBB), 77
Blurred images, 166, 167f
Board duties, 715
Board examinations
  administration of, 9–10
  client recruitment and, 10–11
  clinical facilities for, 10
  clinical testing and, 9
  content of, 14
  ethical and legal issues in, 12–14
  examiner selection and training, 9–10
  formats of, 11–12
  forms for, 10
  instruments for, 10
  Joint Commission on National Dental Examinations (JCNDE) and, 4
  licensure, 1–2
  National Board Dental Hygiene Examination (NBDHE) and, 4–9
  preparing for, 1–15
  results of, 12
  review questions for, 15
  state boards of dentistry and, 2–4
  website information and resources for, 14b
Body cavities, 55, 56f
Body mass index (BMI), 378, 378t
Body membranes, 61
Body part designations, 745. *See also* Medical terminology.
Body temperature, 689

Body tissues, clinical examination of, 381
Bonding agents, 403–405, 403–404f
Bone, 24–26
  formation, stages of, 26f
  tissue, microscopic morphology of, 25f
Bone cysts. *see also* Cysts.
  aneurysmal, 226
  hemorrhagic, 226
  simple, 226
  Stafne, 226–227, 227f
  static, 226–227, 227f
  traumatic, 226, 227f
Bone destruction patterns, in periodontitis, 438, 438f
Bone marrow-derived stem cells (BMSCs), 185
Bony depressions, 108
Bony openings, 108
Bony prominences, 108
Bordetella pertussis, 266t
Borrelia vincentii, 205
Botulism, 277
Bound ribosomes, 56
Brachial plexus, 77
Bradycardias, 586
Brain, 74, 77–78, 77f
  deformity of, 583
Brainstorming, for oral health, 659
Branchial cleft cyst, 222–223, 223f
Brand names, 325
Breach of contract, 733
Bronchitis, 585
Bronchospasms, treatment for, 697
Brucella spp., 266t
Brush biopsy, 509–510, 509f
  laboratory findings in, 510
Brushes
  interdental, 497–498, 497f
  single-tufted, 495
  toothbrushes
    maintenance of, 496
    manual, 494
    power, 495
Buccal block, 120t
Buccal frena, 131t
Buccal mucosa, 130f, 131t
  assessment of, 470
Buccal nerve, 121
Bulimia, 380, 574
Bupropion (Zyban), 354
Burden of disease, 624
  and community oral health practice, 677

C
Caffeine, 353
Calcitonin, 84
Calcium sodium phosphosilicate (NovaMin), 647
Calculations, for local anesthetic agents, 552
Calculus
  dental, 530
  removal of, steps for, 526–527, 526f

Calibration, 625t
Calorimetry, 378
CAMBRA. *See* Caries management by risk assessment (CAMBRA).
Canadian Dental Association, 746
Canadian Dental Hygienists Association
  code of ethics, 750–754
  contact information for, 746
Canadian Public Health Association, 746
Canal, pulp, 129
Cancers, 588–589, 589f
  carcinoma, squamous cell, 217–218, 218–219f
  oral, 634
    brush biopsy for, 509–510, 509f
    detection of, diagnostic tools for, 509–510
    examination technique for, 508–509
    high-risk factors of, 508
    other devices and oral examination for, 510
    risk assessment of, 508–509
  pharyngeal, 634
Candida, 263
Candidiasis, 274
Canines, 135, 136t. *See also* Dentition.
Cannon disease, 215
Carbamazepine (Tegretol), 346, 348
Carbohydrates, 360–366
  absorption of, 361, 362f
  biologic role and functions of, 364
  complex, 360
  definition of, 360
  digestion of, 361, 361t
  metabolism of, 361, 363f
  in oral biology, 364
  in persons with disease conditions, 365, 366t
  requirements for, 365
  simple, 360
  structure of, 360
Carboxylases, 60
Carcinoma, squamous cell, 217–218, 218–219f
Cardiac arrest, 691, 696
Cardiac cycle, 88, 89f
Cardiac emergencies, 694–697
Cardiac muscle, 30
Cardiogenic shock, 694
Cardiopulmonary resuscitation (CPR), 690–691
Cardiovascular agents, 343
  digitalis glycosides, 343
Cardiovascular disease (CVD), 371
  questions regarding, 464
Cardiovascular system, 85–91, 87f
Care plans, 129, 442–443
Caries, dental, 291–292, 291f, 381, 471, 630, 630t, 631f
  classification of, 474
  dietary modifications for, 365, 366t, 387
  distribution of, 631, 632t

Caries, dental *(Continued)*
examinations and inspections, types of, 653t
indices for, 636t
lower rates of, factors contributing to, 631
management of, 502–504, 647
caries management by risk assessment (CAMBRA) in, 502
fluoride in, 502–504. *See also* Fluorides.
xylitol in, 504
measures for preventing and controlling, 641–648, 642t, 644–645b
occurrence of, 630
rampant, 387
risk factors for, 476, 477t, 633
Caries activity tests, 386
Caries management by risk assessment (CAMBRA), 502
Carious lesions, 471, 531
Carotid artery, 115, 116f
Carpal bones, 65, 66f
Carrier-mediated passive transport, 58t. *See also* Facilitated diffusion.
Cartilage, 24, 108
Cartilaginous joints, 67, 70f
Cartridge, anesthetic, 549, 549f
Caruncle, sublingual, 131t
Case law, 711
Case presentation, 481
Case-control research, 628t
Casein phosphopeptides-amorphous calcium phosphate (CPP-ACP), 647
Casting
alloys, 412–413
materials, 411–412
Catabolic hormones, 363
Catabolism, 368
Cataracts, 576
Catecholamines, 84, 328
Cathode, 153
Cauda equina, 77
Caudal structures, 107
Causality, *vs.* risk, 627, 628t
Cefotaxime, 285t
Ceftizoxime, 285t
Ceftriaxone, 285t
Celecoxib (Celebrex), 338
Cell-derived mediators, 179
Cells, 17f, 55–61
blood components, 27
connective tissue, 23
eukaryotic, 259, 260t
growth and reproduction of, 61
internal environment and homeostasis, 20
membrane, 17
movement of substances through, 58–59
metabolism, 59–61
anabolism, 60
catabolism, 60
enzymes in, role of, 59
prokaryotes, 256, 260t
regulation of, 262–263

Cells *(Continued)*
replication, 21–31
specialization of, 16
structure of, 55–58, 57f
synthesis activities of, 18
transport, 20
Cellulose, 360
Cement. *see also* Biomaterials.
applications of, 406
bases, 405–406, 405f
crown-and-bridge, 415, 415t
liners, 405
orthodontic, 406
Cementoblasts, 377
Cementocytes, 377
Cemento-dentin junction (CDJ), 134
Cemento-enamel junction (CEJ), 43, 129, 139, 139f
Cementoma, 236
Cementum, 43f, 129, 429
formation, 36, 42f
tooth tissue, 42–43
Centers for Disease Control and Prevention (CDC), 318, 621b, 747
National Center for Health Statistics (NCHS), 624
ten great public health achievements, 641b
Centers for Medicare and Medicaid Services (CMS), 621b
Central giant cell granulomas, 197–198, 198f
Central nervous system (CNS), 27
infections of, 284–285
symptoms associated with lesions in, 582t
Central Regional Dental Testing Service, Inc. (CRDTS), 2b
Centrally-acting agents, muscle relaxants, 336
Centrioles, 20
Centromere, 61
Cephalosporins, 285t, 341
Ceramics, dental, 414–415
Cerebellum, 78
Cerebral lobes, 78
Cerebral palsy, 578–579, 578–579f
Cerebrospinal fluid (CSF), 77
Cerebrovascular accident (CVA), 587–588, 588t, 699
Cerebrum, 78
Cervical lesion levels, functional significance of, 584t
Cervical line, 129
Cervical lymph nodes, assessment of, 469
Cervical plexus, 77
Chamber, pulp, 129
Channel-mediated passive transport, 58t
Cheeks, 131t
Cheilitis, angular, 247, 247f
Cheilosis, 381
Chemical dependency, 592–594
Chemical disinfectants, 310
Chemical fibromatosis, 202–203, 203f
Chemical names, 325

Chemical properties, 395. *See also* Biomaterials.
Chemical synapses, 76
Chemokines, 179t, 181
Chemotaxis, 179
Chemotherapeutic agents, 285–287, 285t, 287t, 504–505
Cherubism, 235–236
Chest cavity, 55, 56f
CHF. *See* Congestive heart failure (CHF).
Chickenpox, 274
Children
dental hygienists working with, 493b
prevention principles for, 492–493
Children's Health Insurance Program (CHIP), 620, 673
Chlorhexidine gluconate, 646
Chlorines, 310t
Chloroquine, 287t
Cholera, 277
Cholesterol, 370
Cholinergic agents, 330–332
Chondroitin sulfate, 361
Chondroma, 200
Chorda tympani nerve, 122
Christmas disease, 233
Chromatids, 61
Chromatin, 18
Chromium alloys, 413. *See also* Alloys.
Chromosomes, 18
Chronic alcohol abuse and dependence, 594
Chronic caries, 471
Chronic disease, 625t
Chronic hyperplastic pulpitis hyperplasia, 198, 198f
Chronic inflammation, 181–182
Chronic lymphocytic leukemia (CLL), 232
Chronic myeloid leukemia (CML), 232
Chronic obstructive pulmonary disease (COPD), 585
Chronic pancreatitis, 371
Chronic periodontitis, 431, 293b, 293. *See also* Periodontitis.
Chylomicrons, 370
Cicatricial pemphigoid, 206–207, 207f
Ciliophora, 264
Cingulum, 134, 135f
Ciprofloxacin, 285t
Circle of Willis, 77
Circular compression, 468
Circulatory system, 89–91, 115–117
blood
components of, 115
supply, to head and neck, 115
classification and function of, 115
descriptive terminology in, 115
infections of, 280–281
microbial diseases of, 281
vascular system of, 115
Circumvallate papillae, 131t
CITA. *See* Council of Interstate Testing Agencies (CITA).

Citations, 712
Citric acid cycle, 60
Civil action, 725
Civil law, 711–727
Civil Rights Act
    of 1964 (Title VII), 734
    of 1991, 734
Civil suits, 725
Claims-made policy, 736
Clarithromycin, 285t, 341
Clasp, 500
Cleansers, denture, 417
Clear (blank) radiographs, 161
Cleft involvement, classifications of, 577
Cleft lip or palate, 577–578, 578f, 635
Client care
    maintaining oral health care environment
        after, 313–318
    maintaining treatment area during,
        311–313
Client records, 728
Client-clinician relationship, 492
Client-practitioner relationship, 713
Client-related controls, 301
Clients
    adherence to preventive regimen, factors
        influencing, 492
    consent, 733
    contractual responsibilities of, 713
    rights of, 733
    selection for, 387
    with special needs, dietary considerations
        for, 389
    support systems of, 492
Clindamycin, 285t, 341
Clinical attachment levels (CALs), 529,
    529f
Clinical competencies, clinical examination
    format and, 11
Clinical crown, 129
Clinical death, 691
Clinical examinations, future trends in, 13
Clinical impression, 189
Clinical oral structures, 129, 130f, 131t
    review questions for, 148, 148–149b,
        148–149f
Clinical trials, vs. epidemiologic surveys, 629t
Clinician, position of, 523–524, 523f
Clonazepam (Clonopin), 346
Close supervision, 718
Clostridium spp., 266t
Clotrimazole (Mycelex), 343
Clotting system, 180
Cluster, 625t
Cocaine, 353
Coccidioides, 263
Coccidioidomycosis, 276
CODA. See Commission on Dental
    Accreditation (CODA).
Code of ethics
    American Dental Hygienists Association,
        748–750

Code of ethics (Continued)
    Canadian Dental Hygienists Association,
        750–754
Coenzymes, 363
Cognitive challenges, 570, 570–571f
Coherent scatter, 154
Cohort research, 628t
Colchicine, 339
Cold sore, 208, 208f
Collagen fibers, 23
Collimation, 156
Combining forms, 744–745. See also Medical
    terminology.
Comfort, 482
Commensalism, 263
Commission on Dental Accreditation
    (CODA), 1
Commissure, labial, 131t
Common law, 711
Communication, and process of care, 482
Community, principle of, 748–749
Community dental health coordinator
    (CDHC), 669t
Community Fluorosis Index (CFI), 636t
Community intervention, 650–661, 650f
    assessment and problem identification in,
        650–654, 651t, 653t
    health education and health promotion in,
        654–658
        characteristics of different types of
            learners in, 660
        methods of, 658–660
        in school setting, 661
        theories of, 655t
    implementation in, 654
    planning, 654
    role of dental hygienist in, 650
    strategies in, 650
    surveillance in, 650
Community oral health planning and
    practice, 619–687
    basic concepts of, 619–623
        access, 620
        community, 620
        community health, 620
        community oral health, 620
        dental public health, 619
        health, 619
        health determinants, 619
        national documents, 621
        oral health, 619
        prevention, 620
        private vs. community health, 620,
            620t
        public health, 619
        public health problem, criteria for
            identification of, 620
        wellness, 619
    challenges affecting, 677–678
    community intervention, 650–661, 650f
        assessment and problem identification
            in, 650–654, 651t, 653t

Community oral health planning and practice
    (Continued)
        health education and health promotion
            in, 654–658, 655t, 657t
        implementation in, 654
        methods of oral health education in,
            658–660
        planning in, 654
        role of dental hygienist in, 650
        strategies in, 650
        surveillance in, 650
    epidemiology, 623–626
        characteristics of, 624, 625f
        concepts in, 625t
        definitions of, 623, 624b
        measurement concepts in, 625t
        measurement of diseases and conditions
            in, 624
        of oral diseases and conditions, 629–640,
            630t, 631f, 632t
        and research, 626–629, 628t
        uses of, 624, 624b
    ethical and legal issues in, 678, 679b
    financing oral health care in, 670–674
        mechanisms of payment in, 670–672,
            671t
        providers of dental benefits plans in, 672
        public, 673–674, 673t
    preventing and controlling oral diseases in,
        641–650
        measures for dental caries, 641–648,
            642t, 644–645b
        measures for other oral diseases and
            anomalies, 648–650
        measures for periodontal diseases, 648
        public health measures in, 641
    program evaluation, 661–665
        general principles of, 661
        of professional literature, 665, 665b
        statistics in, 661–664, 662b, 663f
    provision of oral health in, 665–670
        dental practice, diverse modes of,
            665–666, 666t
        personnel workforce in, 667–670, 668f,
            669t
    review questions for, 681, 681–686b
    utilization, of dental services, 674–677, 675t
        patterns of, shifts in, 676–677
    website information and resources for,
        679b
Community oral health research, categories
    of, 627
Community Periodontal Index (CPI), 636t
Community Periodontal Index of Treatment
    Needs (CPITN), 636t
Community profile, 652
Comparative negligence, 713
Competition, 263
Complement system, 267
Complementarity, principle of, 748
Complex partial (psychomotor) seizure, 699
Complex shank, 518

Complexity of therapy, 492
Composites, dental, 401–402, 401f
Compton scatter, 154
Computer-assisted design/computer-assisted machining (CAD/CAM), 418
Computer-controlled local anesthesia delivery system, 556–559, 558t
    Basic CCLADD procedure and, 556–558
    components of, 556
    injection administration with, 558–559
    vs. traditional syringe, 558t
Concavity, 129
Concrescence, 242, 243f
Concreteness, 482
Conductive hearing loss, 576
Confidentiality, 708, 728, 749, 751–752
Confocal-scanning laser microscopy, 257
Congenital heart disease, 585–586
Congenital syphilis, 283f
Congestive heart failure (CHF), 587, 696
Conjugation, 263
Conjunctiva, 78
Connective tissue, 22–26
    components of, 23–24
    fibers, 45f
Conscious sedation, with nitrous oxide-oxygen, 559
    advantages and disadvantages of, 562
    anesthesia stages for, 561
    chemistry of, 559
    contraindications to, 562
    equipment for, 562
    indications for, 562
    pharmacology of, 561
    physiology of, 561
    record keeping and documentation for, 562
    safety measures for, 562
    signs and symptoms of, 562
    synonymous terms in, 559
Consent, 714
    competency of, 715
    informed, 481
    vs. informed refusal, 715
Constitutional law, 710
Contact area, 134
Contact information, regional testing agencies and, 2b
Continued-care, 483
Continuous conduction, 76
Contract
    damages, 713
    elements of, 733
    employment, 733
    law, 712
Contracture, 183
Contralateral structures, 107
Contrast, 160
Contributory negligence, 713
Control group, 630t
Controlling oral malodor, 499–500
Convenience sample, 630t
Conventional supragingival air polishing, 537

Convulsion, 575
Convulsive disorders, 699–700
Convulsive seizures, 699–700
Cooley anemia, 229–230
COPD. See Chronic obstructive pulmonary disease (COPD).
Coronal plane. See Frontal plane.
Coronary heart disease, 586–587
Corynebacterium diphtheriae, 266t
Council of Interstate Testing Agencies (CITA), 2b
Count, 625t
Counter-dislodgement forces, 388
Courts of Appeal, 712
COX-1 and COX-2, 180
Cranial bones, 109
Cranial cavity, 55, 56f
Cranial nerves (CN), 30, 78, 119
    cranial nerve I (olfactory nerve), 119
    cranial nerve II (optic nerve), 119
    cranial nerve III (oculomotor nerve), 119
    cranial nerve IV (trochlear nerve), 119
    cranial nerve V (trigeminal nerve), 119. See also Trigeminal nerve.
    cranial nerve VI (abducens), 122
    cranial nerve VII (facial), 122, 122f
    cranial nerve VIII (vestibulocochlear nerve), 122
    cranial nerve IX (glossopharyngeal nerve), 122
    cranial nerve X (vagus nerve), 123
    cranial nerve XI (accessory nerve), 123
    cranial nerve XII (hypoglossal nerve), 123
Cranial structures, 107
Craniofacial birth defects, measures for, 649
Craniofacial injuries, 635
CRDTS. See Central Regional Dental Testing Service, Inc. (CRDTS).
C-reactive protein (CRP), 181
Cribriform plate, 110
Criminal action, 725
Criminal charges, 725
Criminal law, 711
Crisis, adrenal, 701
Cromolyn sodium, 351
Crossbites, 146
Crossover, 628
Cross-sectional plane. See Transverse plane.
Cross-sectional research, 628t
Crown-and-bridge cements, 415, 415t
Crowns, 129
    characteristics of, 136t
    lingual inclination of, 140f
Cryptococcus neoformans, 263
Cumulative trauma disorders, 482
Curet
    advance, designs for, 523
    area-specific, 522–523, 522f
    universal, 522, 522f

Curve of Spee, 143
Curve of Wilson, 143
Curved shank, 518
Cushing syndrome, 348
Cusp, 134
Cuspal inclines, 134
Cutaneous membranes, 61
Cutaneous wound healing, 183, 184f
CVA. See Cerebrovascular accident (CVA).
Cyclic neutropenia, 231, 231f
Cyclin-dependent kinases (CDKs), 61
Cyclins, 61
Cystic fibrosis, 371, 584–585
Cysts, 220–221
    classification of, 220
    developmental, 221–223
        dermoid, 223
        lymphoepithelial, 222–223, 223f
        nonodontogenic, 221–222, 222f
        thyroglossal tract/duct cysts, 222, 222f
    odontogenic, 223–227
        dentigerous, 224–225, 225f
        follicular, 224–225, 225f
        keratocyst, 223–224
        lateral periodontal, 223, 224f
        mucocele, 225–226
        necrotizing sialometaplasia, 226, 226f
        oral soft tissue injuries, 225–226
        primordial, 224
        ranula, 225, 225f
    periapical, 220, 220f
    radicular, 220, 220f
    residual, 220–221, 221f
    root-end, 220, 220f
    true, 220
Cytodifferentiation, tooth development, 34–35
Cytogenetic analysis, 187
Cytokines, 179t
Cytomegalovirus (CMV) infections, 281
Cytoplasm, 17, 56
Cytoskeleton, 56, 57f
Cytosol, 56

D
Dactinomycin, 352
Damages, 713
Dark radiographs, 161, 161f
Dark roller lines, 162
Darkfield microscopy, 257
Darunavir, 272
Data, 661
    analysis of, 654
    collection, 458, 650
        methods for, 651t
    distribution of, 663, 663f
De novo synthesis, 368
Deamination, 368
Dean Fluorosis Index, 636t
Decarboxylases, 60

Decayed-Missing-Filled Teeth (DMFT) Index, 636t
Deciduous dentition, 141
Decision making, evidence-based, 129, 479
Decision-procedure, 753–754
Decongestants, 331t
Decontamination area, 315
Deep, as directional term, 107
Defamation, 714
Defendant, 712
Defense of fact, 714
Deficient scar formation, 183
Deformities, periodontium.
        see also Periodontium.
    acquired, 433–436
    developmental, 433–436
Degradation, 179
Dehydrogenases, 60
Delayed cutaneous hypersensitivity skin tests, 381
Delayed tooth eruption, 570f
Delta hepatitis, 280
Demographic risk factors, 628t
Dendrite, 75, 75f
Dens evaginatus, 243, 244f
Dens in dente, 242–243, 243–244f
Dens invaginatus, 242–243, 243–244f
Dense connective tissue, 22
Density, of x-ray image, 160
Dental amalgam, 399–401, 399–400f
Dental anatomy, 134–142. See also Anatomy and physiology.
    clinical oral structures, 129, 130–131f, 131t
    dentition, 134, 136t
    eruption, 142–143
    interarch relationships, 143–147
    intra-arch relationships, 143–147
    review questions for, 148, 148–149b, 148–149f
    terminology for, 129–134
    website information and resources for, 147b
Dental biofilm, bacterial, 438–440
Dental biomaterials. See Biomaterials.
Dental boards, 715
Dental caries, 291–292, 291f, 630, 630t, 631f
    distribution of, 631, 632t
    examinations and inspections, types of, 653t
    high incidence of, 570f
    indices for, 636t
    lower rates of, factors contributing to, 631
    management of, 647
    measures for preventing and controlling, 641–648, 642t
    occurrence of, 630
    radiographic appearance of, 171, 171f
    risk and associated factors of, 633
Dental ceramics, 414–415

Dental composites, 401–402, 401f
Dental fluorosis, 635
    causes of, 639
    indices for, 636t
    measures for, 650
    prevalence of, 639
    prevention of, 640
    recommendations to reduce risk of, 640b
Dental health aide therapist (DHAT), 669t
Dental health care personnel, infection control procedures for, 302–308
Dental health professions shortage areas (DHPSAs), 667
Dental hygiene licensure, 1–2
    clinical examinations for, 3f
    regional testing agencies and, 2b
Dental hygiene paradigm, 458
Dental hygiene personnel, supply of, 668
Dental hygiene therapist (DHT), 669t
Dental hygienist
    civil law and, 712–727
    dental hygiene board examinations and, 1, 3–4
    direct access states, 719b, 725f
    roles of, 623
        in community intervention, 650
Dental implants, 418–419, 452–453
    definition of, 501
    design of, 452
    endosseous, 452
    goals of, 453
    instrumentation of, 535–536
    limiting factors for, 452
    maintenance of, 501–502
    management of, 453
    transosteal, 453
    types of, 452
Dental index, 636t, 640
Dental laboratory, infection control for, 313
Dental mirror, 519–520
Dental papilla, 35
Dental plaque biofilm detection, 493–494
Dental practice acts, 715, 716t, 718
Dental public health, 619
Dental radiographs, guidelines for prescribing, 158t
Dental records, 728–733
Dental sac, 35
Dental school enrollment, 668
Dental sealants, 505–507, 634, 647, 648b
    application guidelines for, 506–507
    contraindications to application of, 506
    general considerations for, 505
    indications for application of, 505–506
    school-based, 647
Dental services, utilization of, 674–677, 675t
    patterns of, shift in, 676–677
Dental solders, 413
Dental stem cells, 185
Dental therapist (DT), 669t
Dental tissues, concepts relating to, 21

Dental unit water, 311
    asepsis and, 310
    improving quality of, 311
Dental unit water lines (DUWLs), 308
Dental water jet, 498
Dental x-ray film, 157–161
    image characteristics, 159–160, 160t
    processing, 160–161
Dentifrices, 408–409, 498–499
    selection of, guidelines for, 499
    therapeutic and active ingredients of, 499
    use of, guidelines for, 499
Dentigerous cysts, 224–225, 225f
Dentin, 38–39, 129
    formation, 35–36
    pulp and, 40
Dentinal hypersensitivity
    assessment of, 510
    desensitization methods for, 511–512
    desensitizing agents for, 511
    desensitizing treatments for, types of, 511
    etiology of, 511–512
    pain
        mechanism, 511
        stimuli, 511
Dentinogenesis imperfecta, 241, 241f
Dentist, supply and distribution of, 667, 668f
Dentition
    assessment of, 471–474, 474b
    comparison, 141f
    mixed, 142, 145
    permanent, 134, 136t, 142
    primary, 141–142
Dentition charting, 471, 474b
Dento-enamel junction (DEJ), 134
Dentogenesis, process of, 38
Dento-gingival junction, 46–47
    formation, 36
Dentures
    bases, acrylic, 416
    cleansers for, 417
    definition of, 500
    hyperplasia, denture-induced, 196–197, 197f. See also Hyperplasia.
    liners, soft, 417
    teeth, 416
    use of, 634
        problems related to, measures for, 649
Deontologic ethics, 707
Deoxyribonucleic acid (DNA), 60
    replication, 61
Department of Defense (DoD), 621b
Dependent variable, 629
Depolarization, 548
Depressants, 353
Depression, 147
Dermatitis, 306
Dermis, 61
Dermoid cysts, 223
Descriptive research, 628t

Desensitizing
    agents for, 511
    treatments, types of, 511
Design
    computer-assisted design/computer-assisted machining, 418
    of dental implants, 452. *See also* Dental implants.
    of instrument, 518–519
        characteristics of, 519
Desmosomes, in cells, 16
Determinants, 624
Deuteromycota, 263
Developmental challenges, 570, 570–571*f*
Developmental cysts, 221–223
    dermoid, 223
    lymphoepithelial, 222–223, 223*f*
    nonodontogenic, 221–222, 222*f*
    thyroglossal tract/duct cysts, 222, 222*f*
Developmental groove, 134
Developmental research, 628*t*
DHCP-related controls, 301
Diabetes, 366
    dietary recommendations for, 366
    glycemic management for, 467*b*
    signs and symptoms of, 366
    type 1, 366
    type 2, 366
Diabetes mellitus, 348
    agents for, 348–349
        insulin, 349
        oral hypoglycemic agents, 349
    emergencies, 700–701. *See also* Medical emergencies.
    special care needs and, 590–592, 591*t*, 592*f*
Diagnosis
    differential, 188–189
    preliminary, 189
    process of care and, 469*f*, 478, 478*f*
Diazepam (Valium), 346
Didanosine, 272, 287*t*
Die materials, 411–412, 411*t*
Diencephalon, 78
Diet, computerized analysis of, 386
Dietary aids, 379
Dietary fluoride supplements, 641, 645, 645*t*
Dietary Guidelines for Americans, 383
Dietary intake, methods for assessment of, 382–386
Dietary modifications, 381
    for specific dental conditions, 387–388
    types of, 379
Dietary Reference Intake (DRI), 382
Dietary sugars, 388
Dietary sweeteners, 364, 364*t*
Differential diagnosis, 188–189
Differential staining procedures, 257, 257*t*
Diffuse scleroderma, 581
Diffusion, 58
    facilitated, 361
    membrane transport and, 20

Diffusion *(Continued)*
    passive, 361
Diffusion hypoxia, 334
Digastric muscle, 113
Digestive system, 96–97, 96*f*
Digital imaging, 162–163
Digital palpation, 468
Digitalis glycosides, 343
Digoxin, 338
Dilaceration, 241, 242*f*
Diphtheria, 275
Direct access states, 719*b*, 725*f*
Direct digital imaging, 163
Direct observation, in extraoral and intraoral assessment, 468
Direct preventive and restorative materials, biomaterials, 399–409.
        See also Biomaterials.
    amalgam, dental, 399–401, 399–400*f*
    bonding agents, 403–405, 403–404*f*
    cement
        applications, 406
        bases, 405–406, 405*f*
        liners, 405
        orthodontic, 406
    composites, dental, 401–402, 401*f*
    dentifrices, 408–409
    dressings, surgical, 406
    fluoride
        fluoride-releasing restorative materials, 406–407, 406*f*, 408*f*
        varnishes, 407–408
    gingival tissue packs, 406
    infiltrants, 403
    pastes, prophylactic, 408–409
    sealants, pit-and-fissure, 402–403
    sealers, root canal, 406
    topical, 407–408
    whitening agents, 409
Direct supervision, 718
Direct-acting drugs, 330
Disaccharides, 360
Disciplinary action, 715
Disclosing agents, 493–494
Disclosure statutes, 714
Discovery learning, for oral health, 658
Discussion, for oral health, 658
Diseases
    barriers to, 267
    mechanisms of spread and prevention of, 302*t*
    of periodontium, 430–436.
        See also Periodontics.
        abscesses, 433
        classification of, 430
        deformities, acquired, 433–436
        epidemiology of, 434–436
        gingival, 430–431
        immunology and microbiology of, 292–294, 293*b*
        necrotizing, 432–433
        periodontitis, aggressive, 431–432

Diseases *(Continued)*
        periodontitis, associated with endodontic lesions, 433
        periodontitis, chronic, 431
        risks of, 434–436
    prevention of, legal and ethical issues in, 320, 320*b*
    skin, 210–213
        Behçet syndrome, 212, 212*f*
        characteristics of, 210
        erythema multiforme, 210–211, 211*f*
        pemphigus vulgaris, 212–213, 213*f*
        Stevens-Johnson syndrome, 211–212, 211*f*
    transfer, 265–287, 301*f*
    transmission, 300–302
Disinfection, 300
    categories of, 309*t*
    surface, chemical agents for, 310*t*
Distal, as directional term, 107
Distal tooth surfaces, 134
Distortion, 160, 160*t*
Distributive shock, 693
Diuretics, 331*t*, 344
Docosanol (Abreva), 343
Documentation, and process of care, 483–484
Dopamine-norepinephrine reuptake inhibitors, 347
Doppler flowmetry, laser, 512
Dorsal cavity, 55, 56*f*
Dorsal structures, 107
Dorsum, of the tongue, 130*f*
Dosage
    effective dose (ED), 325, 326*f*
    forms of, 327
    lethal dose (LD), 325
    log dose-response curve, 325, 326*f*
    pediatric dose, 327
    variables, 327
Double-blind, 628
Down syndrome, 571–572, 572*f*
Doxycycline, 285*t*, 342
DPP-4 inhibitors, 349
Dressings
    periodontal, 451
    surgical, 406
Drug Enforcement Administration (DEA), 325
    schedules used in dentistry (I-V), 326*t*
Drugs. *see also* Pharmacology.
    action of, 325–327
    distribution of, 327, 328*f*
    drug-induced gingival enlargement, 202–203, 203*f*, 575, 576*f*
    use of, during pregnancy, 353–354
Dry-heat sterilization, 316
Dual-energy x-ray absorptiometry (DEXA), 382
Duchenne's muscular dystrophy, 582*t*
"Ductless glands". *See* Endocrine glands.
Due process, 712, 725
Dumping syndrome, 366, 371

Dura mater, 76, 76f
Duration, 325
Duty to disclose, 733
Dysplasia
    ectodermal, 244
    familial white folded, 215
    fibrous, 234–236
        cementoma, 236
        characteristics of, 234
        cherubism, 235–236
        monostotic, 235
        osteitis deformans, 236
        Paget disease, 236
        periapical cemento-osseous, 236
        polyostotic, 235
Dysrhythmias, cardiac, 586

E
Eastman Interdental Bleeding Index (EIBI),
        636t
Eating disorders, 380, 574
Eating disorders not otherwise specified
        (EDNOS), 380
Ebner's glands, 38
ECM deposition, 183
Ectodermal dysplasia, 244
Ectopic beats, isolated, 586
Edentulism, 387
Edrophonium (Tensilon), 330
Efavirenz (EFV), 272
Effective dose, 325, 326f
Effective teaching, concepts of, 492
Efficacy, 326, 327f
Elastic cartilage, 24
Elastic fibers, 23
Electrical properties, 395.
        See also Biomaterials.
Electrical pulp tester, 512
Electrical synapses, 76
Electrical testing devices, traditional, 512
Electrochemical corrosion, 396f, 396.
        See also Biomaterials.
Electromagnetic energy spectrum, 153f
Electron microscopy, 258
Electron transport system (ETS), 60
Elevation, 147
Embrasure, 134
Embryology
    general, 31–33
    histology and, 16–52
    review questions for, 48, 48b, 50b
Embryonic stem cells, 184
Emergencies, medical. See Medical
        emergencies.
Emergency kit, 690–691
    medications typically supplied
        with, 691t
Emergency medical system (EMS), 691
Emetics, 351–352
Emetine, 287t
Emotion, pain and, 548
Emotional disturbance, 573

Empathy, 482
Emphysema, 585
Employer vs. employee rights, and
        responsibilities, 733–735, 734b
Employment, 733
Employment contracts, 733, 734b
Employment laws, 734
Enabling, 353
Enamel, 129
    clinical appearance of, 241
    formation, 35–36
    hypocalcification of, 240
    hypomaturation of, 240
    hypoplasia of, 240
    hypoplastic-hypomaturation of, 241
    organ, layers of, 35f
    rod, 41, 41f
    tooth tissues, 40–42
Encapsulated nerve endings,
        definition of, 30
End point, of instrumentation, 532
Endemic, definition of, 625t
Endochondral ossification, 25, 107
Endocrine agents, 348–350
    adrenocorticosteroids, 348, 348t
    diabetes mellitus agents, 348–349
    estrogens and progesterones, 350
    oral contraceptives, 350
    thyroid agents, 349–350
Endocrine disorders, 236–238
    characteristics of, 236
    hyperparathyroidism, 236–237, 237f
    Langerhans cell disease, 238, 238f
    osteomalacia, 237
    rickets, 237
Endocrine glands, 80
    of neck, 119
Endocrine system, 80–85
    gastric and intestinal mucosa, 85
    glands of
        adrenal, 84
        parathyroid, 84
        pineal, 83
        pituitary, 82–83
        thymus, 85
        thyroid, 83–84
    gonads, 85
    heart and, 85
    hormones of, 80–82
    pancreatic islets of, 85
    placenta, 85
    prostaglandins in, 82
Endocytosis, 59
Endodontic lesions, periodontitis associated
        with, 433. See also Periodontitis.
Endoplasmic reticulum, 19–20, 56, 57f
Endorsement, 715
Endosseous implants, 452. See also Dental
        implants.
Endothelial progenitor cells (EPCs), 182
Endotoxins, 267
End-stage renal disease, 594–595

Energy
    for activity, 378
    for basal metabolism, 378
    measurement of, 378
    thermic effect of food, 378
Energy balance, 377–380
    energy-producing systems in, 378
Engineering, tissue, 419–420
Engineering controls, 300
Engulfment, 179
Entamoeba histolytica, 264, 287t
Enteric infections, 277
Enteric plexuses, 75
Enterobius vermicularis, 287t
Enterococcus spp., 285t
Enterovirus, 285
Entrance, furcation, 129
Entry inhibitors, 272
Environmental Protection Agency (EPA),
        310, 318, 639
Eosinophilic granuloma, 238, 238f
Eosinophils, 115, 177
Epidemic, definition of, 625t
Epidemiologic examination, 625t
Epidemiologic survey, vs. clinical trials, 629t
Epidemiology
    applied, 624
    characteristics of, 624, 625f
    concepts in, 625t
    definitions of, 623, 624b
    of diseases
        oral, 623–626, 629–640, 630t, 631f, 632t
        periodontium, 434–436
    measurement concepts in, 625t
    measurement of diseases and conditions in,
        640–641
    and research, 626–629, 628t
    uses of, 624, 624b
Epidermis, 61
Epidermophyton, 263
Epilepsy, 371
Epinephrine, 90, 329, 329t, 363
Epithelial cells, 377
Epithelial membranes, 61
Epithelial tissues, 22, 62
    classification of, 23f
Epstein-Barr virus (EBV), 281
Epulis fissuratum, 196–197, 197f
Equal Employment Opportunity
        Commission (EEOC), 734
Equal Pay Act (EPA) of 1963, 735
Equal protection, 712
Equilibrium, hearing and, 79, 79f
Eradication, 625t
Ergonomic hazards, prevention of, 482
Ergonomics, 482
Errors
    film-processing, 161–162
    focal through positioning, 167, 168f
    radiographic, 166–169
Eruption, 142–143
Erythema infectiosum, 275

Erythema migrans, 247, 247f
Erythema multiforme, 210–211, 211f
Erythema multiforme major, 211–212, 211f
Erythrocytes, 115
Erythromycin, 285t, 341
Escherichia coli, 266t
Essential fatty acids (EFAs), 371
Estrogen, 350
Ethanol, for energy, 378
Ethical challenges/problems, 753
　guidance regarding the process for
　　resolving, 753–754
Ethical considerations, 707–708
　bioethics, 707
　codes of ethics, 708
　　of American Dental Association's Code
　　　of Professional Responsibility and
　　　Conduct, 708
　　of American Dental Hygienists
　　　Association, 708, 748–750
　　of Canadian Dental Hygienists
　　　Association, 708, 750–754
　of community oral health planning and
　　practice, 679b
　of process of care, 484
　professionalism, 708–709
　public policy, 709–710
　review questions for, 738
　theories of, 707
　　deontologic, 707
　　situational ethics, 707
　　teleologic, 707
　　utilitarian, 707
　　virtue, 707
　universal principles, 707
　vs. legal considerations, 710, 710t
　web resources for, 737b
Ethics, 707
　definition of, 707
　principle of, 748
　vs. law, 710, 710t
Ethosuximide, 346
Ethylene oxide gas sterilization, 316
Eubacteria, 256
Eukaryotic cell structure, 259, 260t
Evaluation, 482–483
　of health history, 459–468
Evidence-based decision making, 479
Evidence-based practice (EBP), 626, 626–627f
Examination anxiety, managing, 8b
Examination procedure
　extraoral, 468–469
　intraoral, 470–471
Examination review committee, clinical
　　testing and, 9
Excessive scar formation, 183
Excitability, of cells, 16
Excitation, 547
Excitatory neurotransmitter, 76
Excretion, 328
Exemptions, 715
Exocrine glands, of head, 118

Exocytosis, 59, 59t
Exostosis, 201
　torus mandibularis, 201, 201f
　torus palatinus, 201, 201f
Exotoxins, 266
Experimental group, 630t
Experimental research, 628t
　designs for, 628
Expert witness, 712
Explorer, 520–521, 520f
　clinical assessment with, 530–531
Exposure, to radiation, 156–157
Express contract, 713
Extended lower shank, 518
External ear, 79
Extracellular matrix (ECM), 182
Extraneous variable, 629
Extraoral assessment, 468–471
Extraoral film, screens used with, 159
Extraoral radiographic examinations, types
　　of, 165–166
Extraoral technique errors, 167–169
Extreme bruxism, 579, 579f
Extrinsic stains, 536
Extrinsic tongue muscles, 114
Eyes
　components of, 78, 79f
　examination of, 468
　infections of, 285
　visual impairment and, 576
Eyewear
　protective, 307
　types of, 307

F

Face, examination of, 468
Facial artery, 115, 116f
Facial bones, 110, 111f
Facial development, 32, 33f
Facial injury or trauma, measures for, 649
Facial nerve (CN VII), 122, 122f
Facial tooth surfaces, 134
Facial vein, 116
Facilitated diffusion, 58, 58t, 361
Facio-scapulo-humeral muscular dystrophy,
　　582, 582t
Factors, 629
Fainting, 692–693
Fair employment statutes, 735
Fairness, 749
False light, 714
Familial white folded dysplasia, 215
Family and Medical Leave Act of 1993
　　(FMLA), 735
FAS. *See* Fetal alcohol syndrome (FAS).
FASD. *See* Fetal alcohol spectrum disorders
　　(FASD).
Fat, as energy source, 378
Fatigue, pain and, 548
Fat-soluble vitamins, 372
Fauces, 131t
FDI World Dental Federation, 747

Federal courts, 712
Federal district courts, 712
Fédération Dentaire Internationale (FDI),
　　398
Fee-for-service, 671
Felonies, 711
Femur, 66, 67f
Fenfluramine, 379
Fetal alcohol spectrum disorders (FASD),
　　571, 571f
Fetal alcohol syndrome (FAS), 571
Fever, 267
Fever blister, 208, 208f
Fiber, 363
　diameter of, 547
　excessive dietary, 364
　insoluble, 363
　periodontal ligament, 45
　soluble, 363
　specific, 363
Fibrinogen, 181
Fibroblast emigration, 183
Fibroblasts, 377
Fibrolipoma, 195
Fibromatosis, gingival, 201–203
　characteristics of, 201–202
　chemical, 202–203, 203f
　hereditary, 202
　irritative, 202
Fibromyalgia syndrome (FMS), 581
Fibrosis, 183
Fibrous cartilage (fibrocartilage), 24
Fibrous dysplasia, 234–236
　cementoma, 236
　characteristics of, 234
　cherubism, 235–236
　monostotic, 235
　osteitis deformans, 236
　Paget disease, 236
　periapical cemento-osseous, 236
　polyostotic, 235
Fibrous joints, 67, 69f
Fibrous matrix, of connective tissue, 23
Fibula, 66, 67f
Fidelity, 708
Fifth disease, 275
"Fight-or-flight" response, 119
Filaments, 20
File, periodontal, 521–522
Filiform papillae, 131t
Filtration, 59, 100
Financing, of oral health care, 670–674
　mechanisms of payment in, 670–672, 671t
　providers of dental benefits plans in, 672
　public, 673–674, 673t
Firmicutes, 263
Fissure, 134
Fixed-membrane-receptor hypothesis.
　　See Second messenger mechanism.
Fixed-prosthesis maintenance, 501
Flagellar staining, 258
Floor, of mouth, examination of, 470

Flora, oral
   development of, 290
   normal, 288–290, 289*t*
Flosses, 496–497, 497*f*
Flossing
   aids for, 497
   improper, 497
   technique for, 497
Fluconazole (Diflucan), 343
Flucytosine, 287*t*
Fluid mosaic model, of cell, 17*f*
Fluorescence microscopy, 257
Fluoridated milk, 642*t*, 646
Fluoridated salt, 642*t*, 646
Fluorides, 502–504, 631.
      See also Biomaterials.
   application of, 503–504
      amorphous calcium phosphate in, 504
      guidelines for client preparation, 503
      self-applied, 504
      tray systems for, 503–504
      xylitol, for dental caries prevention, 504
   considerations for, 502
   dentifrices, 642*t*, 646
   ingested, 502
   materials, fluoride-releasing restorative, 406–407, 406*f*, 408*f*
   mouthrinse, 642*t*, 646
   poisoning, 698
   for professional application
      agents for, 503
      indications for, 503
   topical, 407–408
   varnishes, 407–408, 503
Fluoxetine, 379
Fogged radiographs, 161, 161*f*
Foliate papillae, 131*t*
Folic acid analog, 352
Follicular cyst, 224–225, 225*f*
Follow-up care, 451
Food and Drug Administration (FDA), 318, 325, 398
Food flavors, 388
Food poisoning, 277
Food record diary, 381
Food texture, 388
Food-frequency questionnaires, 381
Foot, 66, 68*f*
Foramen, 129
Fordyce granules, 247, 247*f*
Fossa, 134
Francisella tularensis, 285*t*
Frankfort plane, positioning errors, 167, 168*f*
Fraud, 714
Free base, 332*f*
Free nerve endings, definition of, 30
Free ribosomes, 56
Frenum, 131*t*
Frequency distribution table, 662
Frequency polygon, 662

Frontal bones, 109, 109*f*
Frontal nerve, 120
Frontal plane, 55, 55*f*, 107, 108*f*
Frontal process, of maxillae, 110
Frontal sinuses, 112
Fructose, 360
Fructose intolerance, 365
Full-mouth survey, 165, 165*f*
Functional shank, 518, 519*f*
Fungal diseases, 263
Fungal infections, 273, 276
Fungi, 256, 287*t*
Fungiform papillae, 131*t*
Furcal concavity, 129
Furcation, 129, 475
   involvement, 530, 530*f*
Fusion, tooth, 242, 242*f*
Fusobacterium, 289

G

Galactose, 360
Galactosemia, 365
Gallbladder, 370
Gallbladder disease, 371
Ganciclovir, 287*t*, 343
Ganglia, 75, 119
Gap junctions, in cells, 16
Gardner syndrome, 199
Gastric mucosa, 85
Gastric ulcers, 371
Gastroesophageal reflux disease, agents for, 351
Gastrointestinal agents, 351–352
   affecting gastrointestinal motility, 351
   emetics and antiemetics, 351–352
   histamine (H_2-) blockers, 351
   proton pump inhibitors, 351
Gastrointestinal tract, infections of, 277–280
Gemination, 242, 243*f*
Gender, pain and, 548
Gene, 60
General anesthetics, 334–335
   anesthesia stages and planes in, 334
   specific agents, 334–335
General concepts, for pathology, 182, 185
   differential diagnosis of, 188–189
   genetics, 185–188
   genomics, 185
   regeneration and wound healing, 182–184, 182*f*
   regenerative medicine, 184–185
   review questions for, 190
   website information and resources for, 189*b*
   wound healing and regeneration, 182–184, 182*f*
General damages, 713
General supervision, 718
Generalized tonic-clonic seizures, 699
Generic names, 325

Genetics, 185–188
   chromosomes, 186
   genes and DNA sequences, 185
   genetic counseling referrals and, 187
   mutations, 186
   single-gene disorders, 186
Genioglossus muscle, 114
Geniohyoid muscle, 114
Gentamicin, 285*t*
Genuineness, 482
Geographic tongue, 247, 247*f*
German measles, 275
Germicidal chemicals, 309*f*
"Ghost teeth", 244, 245*f*
Giant cell granulomas. *see also* Granulomas.
   central, 197–198, 198*f*
   peripheral, 197, 197*f*
Giardia lamblia, 287*t*
Gingiva, 131*t*, 427–428, 428*f*
Gingival Bleeding Index (GBI), 636*t*
Gingival diseases, 430–431
Gingival enlargement, drug-induced, 202–203, 203*f*
Gingival fiber groups, 45
Gingival fibromatosis, 201–203
   characteristics of, 201–202
   chemical, 202–203, 203*f*
   hereditary, 202
   irritative, 202
Gingival margin, 131*t*
Gingival tissue packs, 406
Gingivitis, 381
   indices for, 636*t*
   therapy for, 480
Glands
   adrenal, 84
   endocrine, 80
      of neck, 119
   exocrine, of head, 118
   of head and neck, 118–119
   lacrimal, 78, 119
   mammary, 102
   parathyroid, 84, 119
   pineal, 83
   pituitary, 82–83
   salivary, 118
   sebaceous, 62
   sudoriferous, 62
   thymus, 85, 119
   thyroid, 83–84, 119, 119*f*
Glandular fever, 210
Glandular tissue, 22
Glaucoma, 576
Glial cells, 30
Globulomaxillary cyst, 221, 222*f*
Glossitis, 381
Glossopalatine arch, 131*t*
Glossopharyngeal nerve (CN IX), 122
Gloves, 305
   protocol for, 305
   risks associated with, 305
   types of, 305, 306*t*

Glucagon, 363
Glucocorticoids, 348
Glucose, 360
α-Glucosidase inhibitors, 349
Glycemic management, 467*b*.
        See also Diabetes mellitus.
Glycogen, 360
Glycogenesis, 362
Glycolipids, 361, 369
Glycolysis, 60, 362
Glycoproteins, 361
Golgi complex, 18–19, 19*f*, 57, 57*f*
Gonads, 85
Gonococcal glossitis, 281*f*
Gonorrhea, 281, 281*f*
Gout, 369
Governmental agencies
        and infection control, 318–320
        state board of dentistry and, 3
Gracilicutes, 263
Gram-positive *vs.* gram-negative bacteria,
        257*t*
"Grandfather" clauses, 715
Granulocytes, 115
Granulomas, 195–199
        characteristics of, 195
        epulis fissuratum, 196–197, 197*f*
        giant cell
                central, 197–198, 198*f*
                peripheral, 197, 197*f*
        hyperplasia
                chronic hyperplastic pulpitis, 198, 198*f*
                denture-induced, 196–197, 197*f*
                inflammatory, 196–197
                papillary, palate, 196, 196*f*
        papillomatosis, palatal, 196, 196*f*
        periapical, 199, 199*f*
        pulp polyp, 198, 198*f*
        pulpal, 198
        pyogenic, 195–196, 196*f*
        resorption, internal, 198–199, 199*f*
Gray matter, 75, 76*f*, 77
Greater palatine (GP) nerve, 120*t*, 121
Greater petrosal nerve, 122
Grills, 501
Griseofulvin, 287*t*
Groove, 134
Ground substance, in connective tissue, 24
Group assignment, 629, 630*t*
Growth hormone, 363

H
Haemophilus influenzae, 266*t*
Hair, 61
        infection of, 273–275
Hairy leukoplakia, 272*f*
Half-life (t½), 326
Halogenated hydrocarbons, 335
Hand hygiene, 304
Hand-activated instruments, 519–523
        advanced root in, 523
        area-specific curet as, 522–523, 522*f*

Hand-activated instruments *(Continued)*
        classifications of, 519
        dental mirror as, 519–520
        explorer as, 520–521, 520*f*
        periodontal file as, 521–522
        probe as, 520, 520*t*
        sharpening of, 532, 533*t*
        sickle scaler as, 521, 521*f*
        steps for calculus removal with, 526–527,
                526*f*
        universal curet as, 522, 522*f*
        use of, 519*t*
Handle, 518
Hand-Schüller-Christian disease, 238
Hantavirus pulmonary syndrome, 277
Hard palate, 131*f*, 131*t*. See also Palate.
        examination of, 470
Haversian systems. See Osteons.
Hazardous waste removal service, 314
Head and neck, anatomy and physiology of,
                107–128
        bones of, 109–112
        circulatory system, 115–117.
                See also Circulatory system.
        glands of, 118–119
        lymphatic system, 117–118, 117*f*
        muscular system, 112–114
        nervous system, 119–123. *See also* Nervous
                system.
        osteology, 107–112. *See also* Osteology.
        paranasal sinuses, 112
        review questions for, 123–128,
                127*b*
        temporomandibular joint of, 114–115,
                114*f*
        website information and resources for,
                123*b*
Health belief model, 491
Health Care Integrity and Protection Data
                Bank (HIPDB), 725
Health continuum, 655
Health determinants, 619
Health education, 654–658
        characteristics of different types of learners
                in, 660
        goals of, 657
        methods of, 658–660
        plan development for, 660–661
        in school setting, 661
        selection of media for, 659
        theories in, 655*t*
        topics for, 658
Health history, 459
        blood pressure classification in, 466*t*
        evaluation of, 459–468
        form for, 459
        glycemic management in, 467*b*
        information, 463–468
        Physical Status Classification System for,
                465*t*
        screening questions for, 460–463, 462*f*,
                463*t*

Health Information Technology for
                Economic and Clinical Health
                (HITECH), 733
Health Insurance Portability and
                Accountability Act (HIPAA), 484, 729
Health literacy, 492, 657*t*
Health promotion, 654–658
        in school setting, 661
        theories in, 655*t*
Healthy People 2020, 621
        objectives and targets of, 622*t*
        and oropharyngeal cancer, 635
        role of, 629
Hearing
        and equilibrium, 79, 79*f*
        impairment, 576–577, 577*t*
Hearing loss, 576, 577*t*
Heart, 87, 87*f*
        diseases of, 280–281
        endocrine role of, 85
Heat sterilization methods, comparison of,
                316*t*
Helicobacter peptic disease syndrome, 277
Helminths (worms), 256
Hemangioma, 194–195, 195*f*
Hemidesmosomes, in cells, 16
Hemispheres, of brain, 78
Hemophilias, 233, 590
Hemorrhagic bone cyst, 226
Hemostatic additive, 329
Heparin, 361
Hepatitis
        hepatitis A virus, 277, 279*t*
        hepatitis B virus, 278, 279*t*
        hepatitis C virus, 279*t*, 280
        hepatitis D virus, 279*t*, 280
        hepatitis E virus, 279*t*, 280
        hepatitis G virus, 280
        immunoglobulins, 279*t*
        non-ABCDE, 279*t*
Hepatitis B vaccine, 303
Hepatotoxicity, 338
Hereditary gingival fibromatosis, 202
Hereditary opalescent dentin, 241, 241*f*
Herpangina, 209–210, 210*f*
Herpes, 207–209
        herpes labialis, 208, 208*f*, 274*f*
        herpesvirus, 264*t*
        primary herpetic gingivostomatitis,
                207–208, 207*f*
        zoster (shingles), 208–209, 209*f*
Herpetic keratitis, 285
Hertwig's root sheath, 36
Heteropolysaccharides, 361
Hexoses, 360
Hierarchy of needs, Maslow's, 490–491,
                491*f*
High-density lipoproteins (HDLs), 370
High-fiber diet, 379
Hippocratic Oath, 708
Hispanic Dental Association, 747
Histamine (H$_2$-) blockers, 351

Histamines, 179t
Histogram, 662
Histology, 16–52. *See also* Embryology.
　basic tissues, 21–31
　cell replication and, 21–31
　general
　　　cells, 16–18
　　　inclusions, 18–20
　oral
　　　soft tissue, 36–38
　　　supporting tissues, 43–47
　　　tissues of the tooth, 38–43
　　　tooth development, 33–36
　review questions for, 48, 48b, 50b
　website information and resources for, 47b
Histoplasma, 263
History, 459
　blood pressure classification in, 466t
　evaluation of, 459–468
　form for, 459
　glycemic management in, 467b
　information, 463–468
　Physical Status Classification System for,
　　　465t
　screening questions for, 460–463, 462f,
　　　463t
Home irrigation, 500
Homeostasis, cells and, 20
Horizontal angulation, 166, 167f
Horizontal plane, 107, 108f.
　　　See also Transverse plane.
Hormones, 80–82, 352
　amino acid derivative, 80
　anabolic, 80
　classification of, 80
　function of, 80
　glycoprotein, 80
　mechanism of action of, 80
　nonsteroid, 80
　peptide, 80
　protein, 80
　regulation of, secretion, 82
　secreted by the adenohypophysis, 83
　sex, 80
　steroid, 80
　tropic, 80
Horns, pulp, 129
Hostile work environment, 734
24-hour recall method, 381, 384
Human behavior principles, 490
Human immunodeficiency virus (HIV),
　　　233–234
　acquired immune deficiency syndrome
　　　(AIDS) and, 234b
　antiviral agents, 287t
　CDC classification system for, 270
　dietary considerations for infection with,
　　　389
　incidence and prevalence of, 272
　oral lesions associated with, 233, 234b
　oral manifestations of, 272
　transmission of, 233

Human needs theory, 458, 460–461f
Human T lymphotropic virus (HTLV), 264t
Humerus, 65, 66f
Hyaline cartilage, 24
Hyaluronic acid, 361
Hydrases, 60
Hydrocarbons, halogenated, 335
Hydrochloric acid, 367
Hydrogenases, 60
Hydrogenation, 369
Hydrolyzing enzymes, 60
Hygiene assessment, oral, 476
Hyoglossus muscle, 114
Hyoid bone, 112
Hyoid muscles, 113
Hyperglycemia, 349
Hyperkeratosis, 217, 217f
Hyperlipoproteinemias, 371
Hyperparathyroidism, 236–237, 237f
Hyperplasia. *see also* Granulomas.
　chronic hyperplastic pulpitis, 198, 198f
　denture-induced, 196–197, 197f
　inflammatory, 196–197
　papillary, palate, 196, 196f
Hypersensitivity, 270f
　assessment of, 510
　desensitization methods for, 511–512
　desensitizing agents for, 511
　desensitizing treatments for, types of, 511
　etiology of, 511–512
　pain
　　　mechanism, 511
　　　stimuli, 511
Hypertension, 465, 466t, 586, 695
　postural, 693
Hypertensive disease, 586
Hypertensive heart disease, 586
Hyperthyroidism, 329, 349
Hypertonic solution, 20, 58
Hyperventilation, 694
Hyphae, 263
Hypnotic-sedative medications, 335–339, 335b
　barbiturates, 336
　benzodiazepines, 335–336, 336t
　general considerations for, 335
　nonbarbiturate nonbenzodiazepines,
　　　336–337
Hypocalcification, enamel, 240
Hypodontia, 244, 244f
Hypoglossal nerve (CN XII), 123
Hypoglycemia, 349
　reactive, 366
Hypoglycemic agents, 349
Hypomaturation, enamel, 240
Hypoplasia, enamel, 240
Hypoplastic-hypomaturation, enamel, 241
Hypotension, orthostatic, 693
Hypothalamus, 78
Hypothesis, 629
　null, 629
　research, 629
　testing of, 664

Hypothyroidism, 349
Hypotonia, 578
Hypotonic solution, 20, 58
Hypovolemic shock, 693

I
Ideal body weight (IBW), 379
Ideal occlusion, 145
Idiosyncrasy, 327
IFDH. *See* International Federation of Dental
　　　Hygienists (IFDH).
Imagery, 129
Imipenem, 285t
Immediate supervision, 718
Immune system, 92–93, 92f
　duality of, 268f
　questions regarding, 465
Immunity, 714
Immunizations, 303
Immunodeficiency, 267–273
Immunoglobulin (Ig), classes of, 93
Immunoglobulin G (IgG), 179
Immunology terms, 269b
Imperfect fungi, 263
Implants, dental, 418–419, 452–453
　definition of, 501
　design of, 452
　endosseous, 452
　goals of, 453
　identification of, 474
　instrumentation for, 535–536
　limiting factors for, 452
　maintenance of, 501–502
　management of, 453
　transosteal, 453
　types of, 452
Implementation, in process of care,
　　　481–482
Implied contract, 713
Impression materials, 409–410, 410t
Improving Access to Oral Health Care for
　　　Vulnerable and Underserved
　　　Populations, 623
Incidence, 625t
Incisal guidance, 147
Incisal tooth surfaces, 134
Incisive block, 120t
Incisive canal cyst, 221
Incisive nerve, 122
Incisive papilla, 131t
Incisor(s), 135, 136t
Incompetence, reporting suspected, 753
Incomplete penetrance, 186
Independent contractor, 734
Independent practice for dental hygienists
　　　(IPDH), 669t
Independent practitioner, 734, 734b
Independent variable, 629
Indian Health Service (IHS), 621b
Indices, 476
Indinavir (IDV), 272
Indirect digital imaging, 163

Indirect preventive and restorative materials, 409–420. *See also* Biomaterials.
  alloys
    casting, 412–413
    chromium, 413
    porcelain-fused-to-metal, 413–414
  appliances, acrylic, 415–416
  athletic mouthguards, 417
  cast materials, 411–412
  cements, crown-and-bridge, 415, 415t
  ceramics, dental, 414–415
  denture
    bases, acrylic, 416
    cleansers, 417
    soft liners, 417
    teeth, 416
  die materials, 411–412, 411t
  implants, dental, 418–419
  impression materials, 409–410, 410t
  investment materials, 412
  model materials, 411–412
  mouth protectors, 417
  provisional materials, 410–411
  restorations, computer-assisted design/
    computer-assisted machining, 418
  solders, dental, 413
  tissue engineering, 419–420
  veneers, 417–418
  waxes, 412
Indirect supervision, 718
Indirect-acting drugs, 330
Individual risk management, 736
Induced pluripotent stem cells (iPs), 185, 185t
Infections. *see also* Microbiology and
    immunology.
  of central nervous system, 284–285
  of circulatory system, 280–281
  control of, 300
    dental laboratory in, 313
    dental unit water and, 311
    evaluation programs in, 319–320, 319t
    governmental agencies and, 318–320
    procedures for dental health care
      personnel, 302–308
  of eye, 285
  factors related to, 301f
  of gastrointestinal (GI) tract, 277–280
  of hair, 273–275
  of nails, 273–275
  opportunistic, 295
  of oral cavity, 288–295
  oral-facial tissue, 294–295
  periapical, 294–295
  of reproductive system, 281–284, 281f
  of respiratory tract, 275–277
  of skin, 273–275
  urinary tract, 284
Infectious diseases
  development of, 300
  diagnosis and management of, 187
Infectious mononucleosis, 210
Infectious waste, regulated, 314
Infective endocarditis, 280

Inference, 627
Inferior alveolar (IA) nerve, 120t, 122
Infiltrants, 403
Inflammation, 267
  acute, 177–181, 178f
    chemotaxis in, 179
    mediators, arachidonic acid, 180
    outcomes of, 181
    phagocytosis in, 179
    vascular changes in, 177, 178f
  cardinal signs of, 177
  cells involved in, 177, 178f
    eosinophils, 177
    lymphocytes, 177
    mast cells, 177
  chronic, 181–182
  principal mediators of, actions of, 179t
  types of, 177
Inflammatory hyperplasia, 196–197.
    See also Hyperplasia.
Inflammatory tumors, 195–199
  characteristics of, 195
  epulis fissuratum, 196–197, 197f
  giant cell
    central, 197–198, 198f
    peripheral, 197, 197f
  hyperplasia
    chronic hyperplastic pulpitis, 198,
      198f
    denture-induced, 196–197, 197f
    inflammatory, 196–197
    papillary, palate, 196, 196f
  papillomatosis, palatal, 196, 196f
  periapical, 199, 199f
  pulp polyp, 198, 198f
  pulpal, 198
  pyogenic, 195–196, 196f
  resorption, internal, 198–199, 199f
Infliction of mental distress, 714
Influenza virus infection, 276
Informed consent, 714
  and process of care, 481
Informed refusal, 715
Informed refusal form, 481
Infrabony pocket, 437f
Infrahyoid muscle group, 114
Infraorbital (IO) nerve, 120,
    120t, 554
Ingested fluorides, 502
Inhalers, 350
Inhibitory neurotransmitter, 76
Initial care plan, 442–443
Inner ear, 79
Inner enamel epithelium (IEE), 35
Innervation
  of periodontium, 429–430.
    See also Periodontium.
  of trigeminal nerve
    mandibular division, 554–555
    maxillary division, 554
Instrument
  design for, 518–519
    characteristics, 519

Instrument *(Continued)*
  hand-activated, 519–523
    advanced root in, 523
    area-specific curet as, 522–523, 522f
    classifications of, 519
    dental mirror as, 519–520
    explorer as, 520–521, 520f
    periodontal file as, 521–522
    probe as, 520, 520t
    sharpening of, 532, 533t
    sickle scaler as, 521, 521f
    steps for calculus removal with,
      526–527, 526f
    universal curet as, 522, 522f
    use of, 519t
  mechanized, tip area of, 534f
  parts of, 518, 519f
  processing of, 314
  tip design for, 533
Instrumentation, periodontal
  advanced, techniques in, 535–536
  for assessment, 527–531
    clinical, using periodontal probes,
      528–530
    with dental explorer, 530–531
    with periodontal probes, 527, 527f
    probing technique in, 527–528
  concepts in, 531–532
    end point of, 532
    nonsurgical, rationale for, 531–532
    overhang removal, rationale for, 532
    preparation of, steps for, 532
    terminology in, 531
  ethical, legal, and safety issues in, 537
  principles of, 523–526
    activation, 525
    adaptation, 525
    angulation, 525, 525f
    clinician position, 523–524, 523f
    stabilization, 524–525, 524f
    strokes, 526
  review questions for, 538, 538–539b,
    541–543b
  selective stain removal in, 536–537
  ultrasonic and sonic, 532–535
  website information and resources for,
    538b
Insulin, 349
Insurance, 670
  types of, 671, 672t
Integumentary system, 61–62
Intentional misrepresentation, 714
Intentional tort, 714
Interarch relationships, 143–147
Intercellular substances, tissue components,
    21
Intercuspation, 145, 145f
Interdental alveolar bone, 44
Interdental brushes, 497–498, 497f
Interdental plaque biofilm control,
    496–498
  cleaning methods for, factors to consider
    when selecting, 496, 496f

Interdental tip, 498
Interdental wedges, 498
Interdigitation, 145, 145f
Inter-examiner (rater) reliability, 625t, 641
Interference with advantageous relations, 714
Interferons, 267
Interfurcal area, 129
Intermediate-acting drugs
    barbiturates, 336
    insulin, 349
Internal environment, of cell, 20
Internal resorption, 198–199, 199f
Internal Revenue Service (IRS), 734
International Association for Dental Research, 747
International Association for Disability and Oral Health, 747
International Federation of Dental Hygienists (IFDH), 13–14, 747
International numbering system, 139
International requirements, for dental hygiene board examinations, 13–14
International Standards Organization (ISO), 398
Interneurons, 30
Interpersonal communication, 482
Interphase, of mitosis, 21
Interradicular alveolar bone, 44
Interstitial fluid, 91
Interview, health history information from, 467
Intestinal mucosa, 85, 370
Intra-alveolar pocket, 437
Intra-arch relationships, 143–147
Intrabony pocket, 437
Intra-examiner (rater) reliability, 625t, 641
Intramembranous ossification, 25, 107
Intramuscular (IM) administration, 326
Intraoral assessment, 468–471
Intraoral film, components of, 159
Intraoral radiographic examinations, types of, 164–165
Intraoral radiographic techniques, 163, 163f
Intraoral technique errors, 166–167
Intraosseous neoplasms, benign, 199–201
    characteristics of, 199
    chondroma, 200
    exostosis, 201
        torus mandibularis, 201, 201f
        torus palatinus, 201, 201f
    odontogenic myxoma, 200–201, 200f
    odontoma, 201, 202f
    osteoma, 199–200, 200f
Intrapersonal communication, 482
Intravenous (IV) administration, 326
Intrinsic stains, 536
Intrinsic tongue muscles, 114
Intrusion on seclusion, 714
Invasion of privacy, 714
Investment materials, 412
Iodine number, 369
Iodophors, 310t

Iodoquinol, 287t
Ionization, degree of, 327
Ipratropium bromide (Atrovent), 351
Iris, 78
Iron deficiency anemia, 228–229, 229f
Irreversible index, 640
Irrigation, oral, 500
Irritant contact dermatitis, 306, 467
Irritative fibroma, 193, 194f
Irritative fibromatosis, 202
Ischemic heart disease, 586–587
Isomerases, 60
Isotonic solution, 20, 58
Isthmus, faucial, 131t
Itraconazole (Sporanox), 343

J
Jaw, osteonecrosis of, 352
JCNDE. See Joint Commission on National Dental Examinations (JCNDE).
Joint Commission on National Dental Examinations (JCNDE), 4
Joints, 67–68
Judgmental sample, 630t
Judicial law, 711
Jugular veins, internal and external, 116
Junction
    of surfaces, 134
    of tooth tissues, 129
Junctional epithelium, 47, 47f
Justice, 708, 749

K
Kant, Immanuel, 707
Kaposi's sarcoma, 273f
Karyotypes, 187
Keratin sulfate, 361
Ketamine, 335
α-Keto acid, 368
Ketoconazole, 287t, 343
Ketone production, 370
Kidneys, 97–98, 98f
    functions of, 100
Killing and degradation, 179
Kilovoltage peak (kVp), 153
Kinin system, 180
Kinins, 179t
Klebsiella spp., 266t
Krause's end bulbs, 80, 81t
Krebs cycle, 60, 362
Kwashiorkor, 369

L
Labeling, 568
Labial commissure, 131t
Labial frenum, 131t
Labial mucosa, 130f, 131t
    examination of, 470
Lacrimal bones, 110, 111f
Lacrimal glands, 78, 119
Lacrimal nerve, 120
Lactase, 361
Lactose, 360

Lactose intolerance, dietary modifications for, 365
Lamina dura, 44
Lamivudine, 287t
Landmark decisions, 711
Langerhans, islets of, 85
Langerhans cell disease, 238, 238f
Large intestine, in digestion of carbohydrates, 361
Laryngeal edema, treatment for, 697
Larynx, 94
    assessment of, 468
Laser Doppler flowmetry, 512
Lateral periodontal cyst (LPC), 223, 224f
Lateral structures, 107
Latex allergy, 306, 467
    procedures for management of persons with, 306
Latin abbreviations, 326t
Law
    classification of, 711, 711f
    definition of, 710
    sources of, 710
    vs. ethics, 710, 710t
Laws and legislation
    Age Discrimination in Employment Act of 1967 (ADEA), 735
    Civil Rights Act
        of 1964 (Title VII), 734
        of 1991, 734
    disclosure statutes, 714
    Equal Employment Opportunity Commission (EEOC), 734
    Equal Pay Act (EPA) of 1963, 735
    fair employment statutes, 735
    Family and Medical Leave Act of 1993 (FMLA), 735
    Health Information Technology for Economic and Clinical Health (HITECH), 733
    Health Insurance Portability and Accountability Act (HIPAA), 729
    Occupational Safety and Health Act of 1970 (OSHA), 735
    pharmacology-related, 325, 326t
    Practice Act overview, 716t
    Uniformed Services Employment and Reemployment Rights Act of 1994, 735
Laxatives, 351
Lay witness, 712
Lean body mass, 377
Lecture-demonstration, for oral health, 658
Lectures, for oral health, 658
Legal issues, 707–742
    in disease prevention, 320, 320b
    employer vs. employee rights, 733–735, 734b
    fundamentals of
        administrative law, 711
        case law, 711–712
        classification of, 711, 711f

Legal issues *(Continued)*
 common law, 711
 constitutional law, 710
 criminal law, 711
 due process, 712
 equal protection, 712
 judicial law, 711
 judicial process, 712
 lawsuit participants, 712
 level of proof, 711
 statute of limitations, 712
 statutory law, 711
 litigation avoidance strategies, 736
 of process of care, 484
 record keeping, 728–733
 risk management, 736
 web resources for, 737*b*
Legally problematic areas, 718
Legionella pneumophila, 266*t*
Legionnaires disease, 275
Legislations. *See* Laws and legislation.
Lens, 78
Leprosy, 273
Leptospira spp., 266*t*
Lesions, endodontic, periodontitis associated with, 433. *See also* Periodontitis.
Lesser palatine nerve, 121
Lethal dose (LD), 325
Letterer-Siwe disease, 238
Leukemia, 231–232, 589–590, 590*f*
 acute, 231–232, 232*f*
  lymphoblastic (ALL), 231
  myeloblastic (AML), 231
 characteristics of, 231
 chronic, 232
  lymphocytic (CLL), 232
  myeloid (CML), 232
Leukocyte products, release of, 179
Leukocytes, 115
 lysosomal components of, 181
Leukocytosis, 181
Leukoderma, 214
Leukotrienes, 179*t*
Level of proof, 711
Levonordefrin (Neo-Cobefrin), 329, 329*t*
Libel, 714
Licensure, 715
 by examination, 715
 future trends in, 13
 by waiver, 715
Lichen planus, 215–217, 216*f*
Lidocaine, 333
Life span approach, to care, 567, 568*t*
Ligament, periodontal, 428–429
Light microscopes, 257
Light radiographs, 161, 161*f*
Lignin, 361
Limb girdle muscular dystrophy, 582*t*
Limbic system, 78
Limiting factor, 553
Line angle, 134
Linea alba, 214, 214*f*

Liners
 cement, 405
 denture, soft, 417
Lingual artery, 115, 116*f*
Lingual frenum, 131*t*
Lingual mandibular bone concavity, 226–227, 227*f*
Lingual nerve, 122
Lingual thyroid nodule, 33
Lingual tonsils, 118, 131*t*
Lingual tooth surfaces, 134
Lingual veins, 131*t*
Linnaeus, Carolus, 256
Lipid solubility, 327
Lipids (fats), 369–371
 absorption and transport of, 370
 biologic role and functions of, 371
 compound, 369
 definition of, 369
 derived, 370
 dietary modifications for disease, 371
 digestion of, 370
 metabolism of, 370
  regulators of, 370
 nutritional requirements, 371
 simple, 369
Lipogenesis, 362, 370
Lipoma, 195, 195*f*
Lipoproteins, 369
Lipoxins, 180
Lips, 131*t*
 examination of, 470
Liquid chemical sterilants, 316
Liquid formulas (protein), 379
List regulations, 716
Listeria monocytogenes, 285*t*
Lithium, 338, 348
Litigation avoidance strategies, 736
Local anesthetic agents, 332–334, 332*f*, 334*t*, 550–553
 administration regulations for, 718, 726*t*, 728*f*
 adverse reactions, 333
 allergic reactions to, 333
 armamentarium for, 548–549
  cartridge in, anesthetic, 549, 549*f*
  needle in, 548, 548*f*
  record keeping and documentation in, 549
  syringe in, anesthetic, 549, 549*f*
 biotransformation of, 550–551
 calculations for, 552
 chemical structure of, 550, 551*t*
 chemistry of, 332
 comparison of, 551*t*
 compositions of, 333
 computer-controlled delivery system of. *See* Computer-controlled local anesthesia delivery device (CCLADD)
 dental hygiene considerations for, 333
 drug interactions of, 333
 injection sites for administration of

Local anesthetic agents *(Continued)*
 mandibular, 120*t*
 maxillary, 120*t*
 injection-free, 333
 maximum recommended dose (MRD) for, 552
 mechanism of action of, 332, 550
 metabolism of, 332, 550–551
 pharmacokinetics of, 332
 potency of, 550
 reactions of, 698
 reversal agent, 334
 topical, 333, 552
 toxicity of, 550
 vasoconstrictors, 552–553, 552*t*
Local anesthetic reversal agents, 334
Localized scleroderma, 581
Locus of control, 491
Log dose-response curve, 325, 326*f*
Long-acting agents
 barbiturates, 336
 insulin, 349
Longitudinal, definition of, 625*t*
Loose connective tissue, 23
Low-carbohydrate, high-protein diet, 379
Low-density lipoproteins (LDLs), 370
Lower respiratory system infections, 275–277
Lower (terminal) shank, 518, 519*f*
Low-fat diet, 379
Lumbar lesion levels, functional significance of, 584*t*
Lumbosacral plexus, 77
Lyme disease, 273
Lymph, 26–27, 117, 429–430
Lymph nodes, 117
 assessment of, 468
Lymphatic system, 27, 91–93, 91*f*, 117–118, 117*f*
Lymphatic vessels, 117
Lymphocytes, 115, 177
Lymphoepithelial cyst, 222–223, 223*f*
Lysergic acid diethylamide (LSD), 353
Lysosomes, 18, 57, 57*f*

M

mA. *See* Milliamperage (mA).
Macrodontia, 245
Macroparasites, 256
Magnification, 160, 160*t*
Mainstreaming, 568
Maintenance therapy, 482
Major aphthous ulcers, 206–210
 benign mucous membrane pemphigoid, 206–207, 207*f*
 cicatricial pemphigoid, 206–207, 207*f*
 glandular fever, 210
 herpangina, 209–210, 210*f*
 herpes, 207–209
 infectious mononucleosis, 210
 Mikulicz aphthae, 206, 206*f*
 mucous membrane pemphigoid, 206–207, 207*f*

Major aphthous ulcers (*Continued*)
  periadenitis mucosa necrotica recurrens, 206, 206*f*
  pharyngitis, aphthous, 209–210, 210*f*
  recurrent scarifying ulcerative stomatitis (RSUS), 206, 206*f*
  Sutton disease, 206, 206*f*
Malignant hyperthermia, 333
Malnutrition, 380–381
Malocclusion, 145, 146*f*, 571*f*, 635
Malodor, oral, 499–500
Malpractice, 713
Maltase, 361
Maltodextrim, 370
Maltose, 360
Managed care, 671
Mandible, 111, 111*f*
  assessment of, 468
  radiographic anatomy of, 170, 170*f*
Mandibular division, of trigeminal nerve, 554–556
  block injections for, 556, 557*t*
  innervation of, 554–555
Mandibular labial frenum, 131*t*
Mandibular nerve, 121, 121*f*
Manual palpation, 468
Manual scrubbing technique, 315
Manual toothbrushes, 494
Marasmus, 369
Maraviroc, 272
Margin, gingival, 131*t*
Marginal ridge, 134
Margination, 178
Marijuana (cannabis), 353
Masking, 628
Masks, 306
Maslow's hierarchy of needs, 490–491, 491*f*
Masseter, assessment of, 468
Mast cells, 177
Mastigophora, 264
Materials, 394–426
  applications of, 394
  classification of, 394
  general considerations for, 394
  preventive and restorative, direct, 399–409
    amalgam, dental, 399–401, 399–400*f*
    bonding agents, 403–405, 403–404*f*
    cement applications, 406
    cement bases, 405–406, 405*f*
    cement liners, 405
    cements, orthodontic, 406
    composites, dental, 401–402, 401*f*
    dentifrices, 408–409
    dressings, surgical, 406
    fluoride varnishes, 407–408
    fluoride-releasing restorative materials, 406–407, 406*f*, 408*f*
    fluorides, topical, 407–408
    gingival tissue packs, 406
    infiltrants, 403
    pastes, prophylactic, 408–409
    sealants, pit-and-fissure, 402–403

Materials (*Continued*)
    sealers, root canal, 406
    whitening agents, 409
  preventive and restorative, indirect, 409–420
    alloys, casting, 412–413
    alloys, chromium, 413
    alloys, porcelain-fused-to-metal, 413–414
    appliances, acrylic, 415–416
    athletic mouthguards, 417
    cast materials, 411–412
    cements, crown-and-bridge, 415, 415*t*
    ceramics, dental, 414–415
    denture bases, acrylic, 416
    denture cleansers, 417
    denture soft liners, 417
    denture teeth, 416
    die materials, 411–412, 411*t*
    implants, dental, 418–419
    impression materials, 409–410, 410*t*
    investment materials, 412
    model materials, 411–412
    mouth protectors, 417
    provisional materials, 410–411
    restorations, computer-assisted design/computer-assisted machining, 418
    solders, dental, 413
    tissue engineering, 419–420
    veneers, 417–418
    waxes, 412
  properties of, 395–398
    biologic, 398
    chemical, 395
    electrical, 395
    electrochemical, 396, 396*f*
    mechanical, 396, 397–398*t*, 397*f*
    physical, 395
    thermal, 395, 395*f*
  restorative, radiographic appearance of, 171, 171*f*
  structure of, 394
  website information and resources for, 420*b*
Maxilla, 110, 111*f*
  radiographic anatomy of, 169, 169*f*
Maxillary artery, 116
Maxillary division, of trigeminal nerve, 554
  block injections for, 554, 555*t*, 556*f*
  innervation of, 554
Maxillary fourth molar, 245
Maxillary labial frenum, 131*t*
Maxillary nerve, 120, 120*f*
Maxillary paramolar, 245
Maxillary tuberosity, 131*t*
Maximum (safe) dose (MD), 329
Maximum permissible dose (MPD), 157
Maximum recommended dose (MRD), for local anesthetic agents, 552
Measles, 275
  German, 275

Measurement, methods of, 256–258
Measures, for public health, 641
Mebendazole, 287*t*
Mechanical properties, of biomaterials, 396, 397–398*t*, 397*f*
Mechanized instrument, active tip area of, 534*f*
Medial structures, 107
Median mandibular cyst, 221
Median palatine cyst, 221
Median plane, 107
Median sulcus, 131*t*
Mediastinum, 55, 56*f*
Medicaid, 620, 673
Medical consultation, request for, 462*f*
Medical emergencies, 688–706
  acute adrenal insufficiency, 701
  adrenal crisis, 701
  allergic reactions, 697–698
  asthma, 694
  cardiac, 694–697
  care, 691–692
  cerebrovascular accident (CVA), 699
  dental hygienist's legal responsibilities, 688
  diabetes mellitus, 700–701
  drug-related, 698
  emergency kit, 690–691
  general considerations in, 688
  history in, 688
  hyperventilation, 694
  obstructed airway management, 692
  orthostatic hypotension, 693
  oxygen administration, 692
  poisoning, 698
  postural hypertension, 693
  review questions for, 702–706, 705–706*b*
  seizures and convulsive disorders, 699–700
  shock, 693–694
  syncope, 692–693
  transient ischemic attacks (TIAs), 699
  unconscious client, 692
  vital signs, 688–690
    blood pressure, 689, 689*f*
    body temperature, 689
    pulse, 689–690, 690*f*
    respiration rate, 690
  website information and resources for, 702*b*
Medical terminology, 743–745
  body part designations, 745
  combining forms, 744–745
  prefixes, 743
  suffixes, 743–744
Medications
  analgesics, 337, 337*t*
    acetaminophen (*n*-acetyl-*p*-aminophenol), 338
    general considerations for, 337
    gout drugs, 339
    nonsteroidal anti-inflammatory agents (NSAIAs), 338

Medications (*Continued*)
 nonsteroidal anti-inflammatory drugs
  (NSAIDs), 331*t*, 338
 opioid (narcotic), 338–339, 339*t*
 salicylates (aspirin), 337
antiarrhythmics, 344–347
 antianginal agents, 344
 anticoagulants, 344–345
 anticonvulsants, 346–347, 346*t*
 antihypertensives, 344, 345*t*
 diuretics, 344
antifungal agents, 287*t*
anti-infectives, 339–343
 aminoglycosides, 342
 antifungal agents, 343
 antituberculosis agents, 343
 antiviral agents, 343
 cephalosporins, 341
 clindamycin, 341
 general considerations for, 339–340
 macrolides, 341
 metronidazole, 342–343
 penicillins, 340–341
 quinolones, 342
 sulfonamides, 342
 tetracyclines, 341–342
antineoplastic agents, 352–353
antiparasitic agents, 287*t*
antiviral agents, 287*t*
autonomic nervous system agents,
  328–334
 α-adrenergic blocker, 329–330
 β-adrenergic blocker antagonists, 330
 adrenergic neuronal agonists and
  antagonists, 330
 local anesthetic agents, 332–334, 332*f*,
  334*t*
 parasympathetic (cholinergic), 328*f*,
  330–332
 sympathetic (adrenergic), 328–329, 328*f*,
  329*t*
 xerostomia-producing drug groups in,
  331*t*
cardiovascular agents, 343
 digitalis glycosides, 343
emergencies, drug-related, 698
endocrine agents, 348–350
 adrenocorticosteroids, 348, 348*t*
 agents for diabetes mellitus, 348–349
 estrogens and progesterone, 350
 oral contraceptives, 350
 thyroid agents, 349–350
gastrointestinal agents, 351–352
 affecting gastrointestinal motility, 351
 emetics and antiemetics, 351–352
 histamine (H₂-) blockers, 351
 proton pump inhibitors, 351
general anesthetics, 334–335
 anesthesia stages and planes in, 334
 specific agents, 334–335
general considerations for, 325–328
 adverse reactions, 327–328

Medications (*Continued*)
 agencies, 325
 definitions, 325
 drug action, 325–327
 legislations, 325, 326*t*
 nomenclature, 325, 326*t*
listing of current, 467
local anesthetic reversal agents, 334
psychotherapeutic agents, 347–348
 antidepressants, 347–348
 antipsychotics, 347, 347*t*
respiratory system agents, 350–351
 agents for asthma in, 350–351
sedative-hypnotic, 335–339,
  335*b*
 barbiturates, 336
 benzodiazepines, 335–336, 336*t*
 general considerations for, 335
 nonbarbiturate nonbenzodiazepines,
  336–337
smoking cessation and, 354
substance abuse and, 353
 definitions in, 353
 drugs, 353
Mediterranean anemia, 229–230
Medium-chain fatty acids, 370
Medulla oblongata, 77, 77*f*
Meglitinides, 349
Meiosis, 61
Meissner's corpuscles, 80, 81*t*
Melanin, 129
Melatonin receptor agonist, 336
Membership, in regional testing agencies, 2*b*,
  9
Membrane potential, 75
Membrane transport, of cells, 16, 20
Meninges, 76
Meningocele, 583
Meningomyelocele, 583
Mental block, 120*t*
Mental illness, 573
Mental nerve, 122
Mentalis muscle, assessment of, 468
Merkel discs, 81*t*
Mesial tooth surfaces, 134
Mesiodens, 245
Messenger RNA (mRNA), 18, 262
Metabolic pathways, 262
Metabolic syndrome (MetS), 466
Metabolism, 327
 anabolic hormones in, 363
 anabolism in, 368
 of carbohydrates, 361, 363*f*
 catabolic hormones, 363
 catabolism in, 368
 of local anesthetic agents, 550–551
 nitrogen balance in, 368
 transamination in, 368
Metaphase, of mitosis, 21
Metformin (Glucophage), 349
Methamphetamine abuse, and addiction,
  239–240

Methicillin, 285*t*
Methotrexate (MTX), 337–338
Methylphenidate (Ritalin), 329*t*
Methylxanthines, 351
Metronidazole, 285*t*, 342–343
Mezlocillin, 285*t*
Miconazole, 287*t*
Microbiology and immunology, 256–299
 bacteria, 263
  Firmicutes, 263
  Gracilicutes, 263
  of human importance, 266*t*
  Mendosicutes, 263
  Tenericutes, 263
 cell regulation, 262–263
 cell structure/function
  eukaryotic, 259, 260*t*
  helminths (worms), 256
  prokaryotic, 258–259, 260*t*
 chemotherapeutic agents, 285–287, 285*t*,
   287*t*
 disease barriers and, 267
 disease transfer and, 265–287
 fungi, 263–264
 immunodeficiency, 267–273
 infections
  central nervous system, 284–285
  circulatory system, 280–281
  eye, 285
  gastrointestinal (GI) tract, 277–280
  hair, 273–275
  nails, 273–275
  reproductive system, 281–284, 281*f*
  respiratory tract, 275–277
  skin, 273–275
  urinary tract, 284
 measurement methods for, 256–258
 metabolism for, 262–263
 microorganisms, 256–265
  binomial nomenclature for, 256
  genetics of, 263
  growth and cultivation of, 259–262
  medically important, 256
  relationships of, 263
 observation methods for, 256–258
 of oral cavity, 288–295
  bacterial plaque, 290–291
  dental caries, 291–292, 291*f*
  opportunistic infections, 295
  oral flora, development of, 290
  oral flora, normal, 288–290, 289*t*
  oral-facial tissue infections, 294–295
  periapical infections, 294–295
  periodontal diseases, 292–294, 293*b*
 prokaryotes, 256, 260*t*
 protozoa, 264
 review questions for, 296, 298*b*
 virulence factors and, 266–267
 viruses, 256, 264–265, 264*t*, 287*t*
 website information and resources for,
   296*b*
Microdontia, 245, 246*f*

Microorganisms, 256–265
    binomial nomenclature for, 256
    medically important, 256
    metabolism of, 262–263
    relationships of, 263
Microscopy
    confocal-scanning laser, 257
    darkfield, 257
    electron, 258
    fluorescence, 257
    phase-contrast, 257
Microspora, 264
Microsporum, 263
Microtubules, 20
Microvasculature, 26–27
    increased permeability of, 178
Midbrain, 77, 77f
Middle ear, 79
Middle superior alveolar (MSA) nerve, 120,
    120t
Mikulicz aphthae, 206, 206f
Mill, John Stuart, 707
Milliamperage (mA), 153
Mineralocorticoids, 84, 348
Minerals, 372–375
    chemistry and general functions of, 372
    classification, 372
    definition of, 372
    effects on oral cavity, 373t
Minimal threshold stimulus, 547
Mirror, dental, 519–520
Misdemeanors, 711
Mitochondria, 19, 19f, 57
Mitosis, 61
    phases of, 21f
Mixed dentition, 142, 145
Mobility, of teeth, 475
Model materials, 411–412
Modified Navy Plaque Index (MNPI), 636t
Molars, 136t, 139. See also Dentition.
    parts of, 133f
Molds, 256
Monoamine oxidase inhibitors (MAOIs),
    329, 347
Monocytes, 115, 179
Mononucleosis, infectious, 210
Monostotic fibrous dysplasia, 235
Moraxella, 289t
Morbidity, 625t
Morphodifferentiation, in tooth
    development, 34
Morphology, root, 129–151. See also Dental
    anatomy.
Mortality, 625t
Motility, gastrointestinal, agents affecting,
    351
Motivation, in human behavior principles,
    490
Motivation theories, 491
Motivational interviewing, evidence-based
    approach, 492
Motor disorders, 578

Motor neurons, 75, 119
Mounting, film, 169
Mouth, and digestion of carbohydrates,
    361
Mouth protectors, 417
Mouthrinses, 504–505
Mucobuccal fold, 131t
Mucocele, 225–226
Mucogingival examination, 529
Mucogingival line, 131t
Mucopolysaccharides, 361
Mucor, 263
Mucosa, 130f, 131t
    classifications of, 38
    gastric and intestinal, 85
    oral, 36–38
    of tongue, 38
Mucous membrane pemphigoid, 206–207,
    207f
Mucous membranes, 61
Mucus, extravasation, 225–226
"Mulberry molars" of congenital syphilis,
    283f
Multifactorial approach, 624
Multifactorial inheritance disorders,
    187
Multiple sclerosis, 581–582, 582t
Multi-polar neurons, 29, 29f
Muscarinic receptors, 330
Muscle contraction, 31
Muscle fiber, 31f
Muscle relaxants, 331t, 336
Muscle tissues, 30–31, 62
Muscular dystrophies, 582, 582t
Muscular system, 69–74, 112–114
    anatomy of, 69–74, 71f
    cervical muscles, 113
    descriptive terminology in, 112
    facial expression muscles, 112
    hyoid muscles, 113
    mastication muscles, 113, 113f
    muscles
        head and neck, 70
        lower limb, 70
        trunk, 70
        upper limb, 70
    and posture, 70–71
    skeletal muscle, 69
        function of, 71–73
        organs, functions of, 72f, 73
        structure of, 69–74, 72f
    sternocleidomastoid muscle, 113
    tongue muscles, 114
    trapezius muscle, 113
Musculoskeletal system, questions
    regarding, 466
Mutases, 60
Mutations, 263
Myasthenia gravis, 579–580
Myasthenic crisis, 579
Mycelium, 263
Mycobacterium leprae, 266t

Mycobacterium tuberculosis, 266t
Mycoplasmal pneumonia, 276
Myelin, 75, 75f, 581
Myelin sheath, 30
Myelomeningocele. See Meningomyelocele.
Mylohyoid muscle, 114
Mylohyoid nerve, 122
Myocardial infarction (MI), 587, 695
Myotonic muscular dystrophy, 582t
MyPerioIDSM PST, 187
MyPerioPathSM, 187
Myxoma, odontogenic, 200–201, 200f
Myxoviruses, 264t

N
Nails, 62
    infection of, 273–275
Nasal administration, 326
Nasal bones, 110, 111f
Nasociliary nerve, 120
Nasolabial cyst, 221
Nasolacrimal duct, 78
Nasopalatine canal cyst, 221
Nasopalatine (NP) nerve, 120t, 121
Natal teeth, 244
National Board Dental Hygiene Examination
    (NBDHE), 4–9. See also Board
    examinations.
    application process for, 6
    eligibility for, 6
    examination day guidelines, 6
    format of, 4–5
        case-based item, 6
        cause and effect item, 5
        competencies and, 4
        completion item, 5
        Dental Hygiene Test Specifications, 4
        item, 5–6
        negative item, 5
        paired true-false item, 5
        question item, 5
        testlet item, 5–6
    future trends in, 9
    multiple-choice tests, guidelines
        for, 8–9
    preparing for, 7–8
    results of, 6–7
National Call to Action to Promote Oral
    Health, 621
National Center for Dental Hygiene Research
    & Practice, 747
National Center for Health Statistics (NCHS),
    624
National Dental Hygiene Certification Board
    of Canada (NDHCB), 14
National Dental Hygienists' Association/
    National Dental Association, 747
National documents, 621
National Health and Nutrition Examination
    Survey (NHANES), 624
National Institute of Dental and Craniofacial
    Research, 567

National Institutes of Health (NIH), 621*b*
National Oral Health Surveillance System (NOHSS), 624
National Practitioner Data Bank (NPDB), 725
National Society for Genetics Counselors (NSGC), 188
Nationality, pain and, 548
NBDHE. *See* National Board Dental Hygiene Examination (NBDHE).
NDHCB. *See* National Dental Hygiene Certification Board of Canada (NDHCB).
Necessity, 714
Neck bones, 112
Necrotizing periodontal diseases, 432–433
Necrotizing sialometaplasia, 226, 226*f*
Necrotizing ulcerative gingivitis (NUG), 205, 205*f*, 381
Needle, 548, 548*f*
Needs theory, human, 458, 460–461*f*
Negative reversal, 625*t*
Negative staining, 258
Negligence, 713
Negligent hiring and retention, 734
Neisseria gonorrhoeae, 266*t*, 285*t*
Neisseria meningitides, 266*t*, 285*t*
Neoplasia, oral, 217–218
Neostigmine (Prostigmin), 330
Nerve, 119
Nervous system, 74–80, 74*f*, 119–123
  action potentials in, 75–76
  autonomic, 27, 75, 78, 119
  brain of, 74, 77–78, 77*f*
  cellular organization of, 75–76
  central, 74, 119
  classification and function of, 119
  cranial nerves, 119, 78. *See also* Cranial nerves.
  descriptive terminology, 119
  local anesthetic agent administration for, injection sites of, 120*t*
  parasympathetic, 119
  peripheral, 75, 119
  somatic, 75
  special senses in, 78–80
  spinal cord of, 76–77, 76*f*
  structure of, 75, 75*f*
  sympathetic, 119
  synaptic transmission in, 76
Nervous tissues, 62
Net protein utilization (NPU), 367
Neurilemma, 75
  definition of, 30
Neurocranium, 109
Neurogenic shock, 694
Neuroglia, 75
  definition of, 30
Neurohypophysis (posterior pituitary), 83
Neuroleptanalgesia, 335

Neurologic disorders, questions regarding, 467
Neurons, 29, 29*f*, 119
Neuropeptides, 181
Neurotransmitters, 30
  types of, 76
Neutral sodium fluoride (NaF), 503
Neutrophils, 115, 179
Nevirapine (NVP), 272
Nevus, white sponge, 215
Niclosamide, 287*t*
Nicotine, 353
  reduction systems for, 354
  stomatitis, 213–214, 214*f*
Nicotinic receptors, 330
Nitric oxide (NO), 179*t*, 181
Nitrogen balance, 368
Nitrogen mustards, 352
Nitrosureas-carmustine (BiCNU), 352
Nitrous oxide-oxygen (N$_2$O-O$_2$)
  administration regulations, 718, 729*t*, 730*f*
  analgesia, 334
    administration of, 334
    advantages of, 334
    adverse effects of, 334
    contraindications to, 334
    disadvantages of, 334
  conscious sedation with, 559
    advantages and disadvantages of, 562
    anesthesia stages for, 561
    chemistry of, 559
    contraindications to, 562
    equipment for, 562
    indications for, 562
    pharmacology of, 561
    physiology of, 561
    record keeping and documentation for, 562
    safety measures for, 562
    signs and symptoms of, 562
    synonymous terms in, 559
Nociceptors, 80, 81*t*, 547
Nodes of Ranvier, 75, 75*f*
Nominal damages, 713
Nonbarbiturate nonbenzodiazepines, 336–337
Nonconvulsive seizure, 700
Nonmaleficence, 708, 749
Nonnutritive sweeteners, 365
Nonodontogenic cysts, 221–222, 222*f*
Nonshivering thermogenesis, 378
Nonspecific immunity, 92, 267
Nonsterile (examination) gloves, 306*t*
Nonsteroid hormones, 80
  mechanism of action, 82
Nonsteroidal anti-inflammatories
  adverse reactions to, 338
  agents (NSAIAs), 338
  contraindications to, 338
  drug interactions in, 338
  drugs (NSAIDs), 331*t*, 338
  therapeutic use of, 338

Nonsurgical periodontal therapy (NSPT), 443, 444*t*
Nonthrombocytopenic purpura, 233
Nonverbal behaviors, 482
Noradrenergic drugs, for weight loss, 379
Norepinephrine, 90, 328–329
Norepinephrine-serotonin modulator-mirtazapine, 348
Normal (bell) curve, 663, 663*f*
Normal occlusion, 145
Normalization, 568
Norwalk virus and Norwalk-like virus, 280
Nose, examination of, 468
Nucleolus, 18
Nucleus, 18, 57, 57*f*
Null hypothesis, 629
  testing of, 664
Nursing bottle syndrome, 471
Nutrient data file, 386
Nutrients
  deficiencies in, 380
    manifestations of, 381
  effects on oral cavity, 373*t*
  effects on oral tissues and role in tooth formation, 376*t*
  essential, six major classes of, 360–377
    carbohydrates, 360–366
    lipids (fats), 369–371
    minerals, 372–375
    proteins, 366–369
    vitamins, 371–372
    water, 376–377
  overconsumption of, 380
  role of, in host defense system, 388
  and specialized cells of oral tissues, effects of, 377
Nutrition, 360–393
  review questions for, 390, 393*b*
  web site information and resources for, 390*b*
Nutritional assessment and counseling, 380–389
  complete, 381–382, 382*f*
  daily guide to food choices in, 384*t*
  dietary considerations for immunocompromised clients, 388–389
  dietary modifications for specific dental conditions in, 387–388
  for malnutrition, 380–381
  methods for, 382–386
  techniques for, 386–387
Nutritional Screening and Assessment of Dietary Intake Questionnaire, 384, 385*f*
Nutritive sweeteners, 364
Nystatin, 287*t*, 343

O

Oatrim, 370
Obesity
  carbohydrates in, 365
  lipids for, 371

Oblique ridge, 134
Observation methods, 256–258
Observational research, 628t
Obstructed airway management, 692
Obturator, 500
Occipital lymph nodes, assessment of, 468
Occlusal convergence, 139f
Occlusal plane, curves of, 143, 144f
Occlusal radiograph(s), 164, 164f
Occlusal tooth surfaces, 134, 134f
Occlusal trauma, 448
Occlusion, 145, 146f
    assessment of, 471
Occupational exposure report, 312b
Occupational Safety and Health Act of 1970,
    735
Occupational Safety and Health
    Administration, 303, 318
Occurrence, 625t
Occurrence-based policy, 736
Oculomotor nerve (CN III), 119
Odontoblastic process, 38f
Odontoblasts, 36f, 377
Odontodysplasia, 244, 245f
Odontogenic cysts, 223–227
    dentigerous, 224–225, 225f
    follicular, 224–225, 225f
    keratocyst, 223–224
    lateral periodontal, 223, 224f
    mucocele, 225–226
    necrotizing sialometaplasia, 226, 226f
    oral soft tissue injuries, 225–226
    primordial, 224
    ranula, 225, 225f
Odontogenic keratocyst, 223–224
Odontogenic myxoma, 200–201, 200f
Odontoma, 201, 202f
Older adults, special needs of, 595–596, 595f
Olestra, 370
Olfaction, in extraoral and intraoral
    assessment, 468
Olfactory nerve (CN I), 119
Olfactory sense, 80
Oligosaccharides, 360
Omohyoid muscle, 114
Onset, 325
Open bite, 146
Open contacts, 143
Open provision, 718
Operon, 262
Ophthalmic nerve, 120
Opioid (narcotic) analgesic agents, 338–339,
    339t
    abuse of, 353
    adverse reactions to, 339
    drug interactions with, 339
    pharmacologic effects of, 338
    therapeutic uses of, 339
Opportunistic infections, 295
Optic disc, 78
Optic nerve (CN II), 119
Oral administration, 326

Oral (PO) administration, 326
Oral and maxillofacial radiology, 152–176
    dental x-ray film, 157–161
        image characteristics of, 159–160, 160t
        processing, 160–161
    digital imaging and, 162–163
    film mounting, 169
    film-processing errors and, 161–162,
        161–162f
    general considerations in, 152–155
        radiation physics, 152–154, 153–154f
        x-radiation, 152, 154–155
    quality assurance in, 162
    radiation biology and, 155–157
        measurements and sources, 156, 156–157f
        protection, 156–157, 158t, 159f
    radiographic errors in, 166–169
        extraoral technique, 167–169, 168f
        intraoral technique, 166–167, 166–167f
    radiographic interpretation in, 169–172,
        169–172f
    review questions for, 172, 172b, 173–174f
    techniques in, 163–166
        extraoral radiographic examinations,
            165–166, 165f
        intraoral radiographic, 163, 163–165f
    website information and resources for, 172b
Oral and maxillofacial surgery, 387
    dietary modifications for, 388
Oral cancer, 387, 634
    brush biopsy for, 509–510, 509f
        laboratory findings in, 510
    detection of, diagnostic tools for, 509–510
    dietary considerations for, 388
    examination technique for, 508–509
    high-risk factors of, 508
    other devices and oral examination for, 510
    risk assessment of, 508–509
Oral cavity
    bacterial genera found in, 289t
    bacterial plaque, 290–291
    dental caries, 291–292, 291f
    immunology and microbiology of, 288–295
        oral flora, normal, 288–290, 289t
    opportunistic infections, 295
    oral flora, development of, 290
    oral-facial tissue infections, 294–295
    periapical infections, 294–295
    periodontal diseases, 292–294, 293b
    soft tissue of, 36–38
        classifications of mucosa, 38
        oral mucosa, 36–38
    tooth emerging into, 47f
Oral contraceptives, 340, 350
Oral epithelium, structure of, 37f
Oral flora
    development of, 290
    normal, 288–290, 289t
Oral health
    dietary guidelines for, 383
    promotion of, and disease prevention and
        control

Oral health (Continued)
    ethical, legal, and safety issues in, 513
    review questions for, 514, 515–516b
    website information and resources for,
        513b
Oral health care
    challenges in, affecting community oral
        health practice, 677–678
    delivery, trends in, and community oral
        health practice, 677
    environment and promotion of infection
        control, 308–318
    financing of, 670–674
        mechanisms of payment in, 670–672, 671t
        providers of dental benefits plans, 672
        public, 673–674, 673t
    infection control and prevention of disease
        transmission in, 300–324, 321b
        review questions for, 321, 321b
        website information and resources for,
            320b
    maintaining asepsis, 308–311
    pathogenic agents important in, 301t
    provision of, 665–670
        dental practice, diverse modes of,
            665–666, 666t
        personnel workforce in, 667–670, 668f,
            669t
Oral Health in America: A Report of the
    Surgeon General, 621
Oral health surveys, 652, 653t
Oral histology. see also Histology.
    supporting tissues
        alveolar bone, 43–44, 44f
        dento-gingival junction, 46–47
        periodontal ligament, 44–46
    tooth development, 33–36
        cytodifferentiation, 34–35
        dentin formation, 35–36
        enamel formation, 35–36
        morphodifferentiation, 34
    tooth tissues
        cemento-enamel junction, 43
        cementum, 42–43, 42–43f
        dentin, 38–40
        enamel, 40–42, 41f
        pulp, 39–40
Oral hygiene
    assessment of, 476
    indices for, 636t
Oral hypoglycemic agents (sulfonylureas),
    349
Oral irrigation, 500
Oral lesions, benign, 193–195. See also Benign
    oral lesions.
Oral malodor, controlling, 499–500
Oral mucosa, 36–38, 130f, 131t
Oral pathology, 193–255
    aphthous ulcers, 205–210, 206f
    benign intraosseous neoplasms, 199–201
    benign lesions, 193–195
    benign mixed tumor, 219–220, 220f

Oral pathology *(Continued)*
blood dyscrasias, 227–233
cysts, 220–221
developmental, 221–223
odontogenic, 223–227
dysplasia, fibrous, 234–236
endocrine disorders, 236–238
gingival fibromatosis, 201–203
granulomas, 195–199
human immunodeficiency virus (HIV),
233–234
inflammatory tumors, 195–199
neoplasia, 217–218
pleomorphic adenoma, 219–220, 220f
review questions and answers for, 248,
248b, 249–252f, 250b
skin diseases, 210–213
soft tissue conditions, 246–248
tongue abnormalities, 247–248
teeth abnormalities, 238–245
ulcerative diseases, 203–205
website information and resources for, 248b
white lesions, 213–217
Oral soft tissue conditions, 246–248
mucous membrane abnormalities,
246–247
skin abnormalities, 246–247
tongue abnormalities, 247–248
Oral soft tissue injuries, 225–226
Oral structures, clinical, 129, 130f, 131t
Oral tissues
clinical examination of, 381
specialized cells of, effects of nutrients on,
377
Oral trauma, example of, 579, 579f
Oral-facial tissue infections, 294–295
Organelles, 56
Orlistat, 379
Oropharyngeal cancers, measures for, 648
Oropharynx
assessment of, 470
soft palate and, 131f
Orthodontic band, 501
Orthodontic bracket, 501
Orthodontic cements, 406
Orthodontic treatment, 635
Orthodontic wire, 501
Orthodontics, dietary modifications for,
388
Orthostatic hypotension, 693
Osmosis, 58, 58t
membrane transport and, 20
Osmotic pressure, 20
Osteitis deformans, 236
Osteoarthritis, 580t
Osteocytes, 377
Osteology, 107–112
axial skeleton. *See* Axial skeleton
bony depressions, 108
bony openings, 108
bony prominences, 108
cartilage, 108

Osteology *(Continued)*
ossification
endochondral, 107
intramembranous, 107
skeletal articulations, 108
Osteoma, 199–200, 200f
Osteomalacia, 237
Osteonecrosis of the jaw (ONJ), 352
Osteons, 63
Outer enamel epithelium (OEE), 34
Outlines, comparison of, 139f
Overbite, 143, 145f
Overdenture, 500
Overgloves, 306t
Overhangs, 474
removal of, rationale for, 532
Overjet, 143, 145f
Oxidases, 60
β-Oxidation, 370
Oxidation-reduction enzymes, 60
Oxidative phosphorylation, 362
Oxygen administration, 692
Oxytalan fibers, 23
Oxytocin, 83

P
Pacinian corpuscles, 80, 81t
Packaging area, 315
Packs, gingival tissue, 406
Paget disease, 236
Pain
definition of, 547
fibromyalgia syndrome in, 581
intensity of, 548
perception of, 547
reaction, 547
Pain and anxiety management, 547–566
armamentarium for, 548–549
cartridge in, anesthetic, 549, 549f
needle in, 548, 548f
record keeping and documentation in,
549
syringe in, anesthetic, 549, 549f
Computer-controlled local anesthesia
delivery device (CCLADD) in,
556–559, 558t
Basic CCLADD procedure and,
556–558
components of, 556
injection administration with,
558–559
vs. traditional syringe, 558t
local anesthetic agents for, 550–553
biotransformation of, 550–551
calculations for, 552
chemical structure of, 550, 551t
comparison of, 551t
maximum recommended dose (MRD)
for, 552
mechanism of action of, 550
metabolism of, 550–551
potency of, 550

Pain and anxiety management *(Continued)*
topical, 552
toxicity of, 550
vasoconstrictors, 552–553, 552t
nitrous oxide-oxygen in, conscious
sedation with, 559
advantages and disadvantages of, 562
anesthesia stages for, 561
chemistry of, 559
contraindications to, 562
equipment for, 562
indications for, 562
pharmacology of, 561
physiology of, 561
record keeping and documentation for,
562
safety measures for, 562
signs and symptoms of, 562
synonymous terms in, 559
pain characteristics and physiology in,
547–548, 548f
review questions for, 563, 565b
trigeminal nerve, mandibular division of,
554–556
block injections for, 556, 557t
innervation of, 554–555
trigeminal nerve, maxillary division of,
554
block injections for, 554, 555t, 556f
innervation of, 554
website information and resources for, 563b
Pain mechanism, 511
Pain stimuli, 511
Pain-reaction threshold, 547
Palatal development, 32
Palatal-anterior superior alveolar (P-ASA)
nerve block, 559
Palate, 131t, 131f
cleft, 577–578, 578f
papillary hyperplasia, 196, 196f
"pipe smokers", 213
Palatine bones, 111
Palatine fovea, 131t
Palatine processes, 111
Palatine raphe, 131t
Palatine tonsils, 118
Palpation, in extraoral and intraoral
assessment, 468
Palsy
Bell's, 579, 579f
cerebral, 578–579, 578–579f
Pan-American Health Organization (PAHO),
621
Pancreas, 367, 370
Pancreatic islets, 85
Pancreatic juices, 361
Pandemic, definition of, 625t
Panoramic radiograph(s), 165, 165f
Papillae, 131t
Papillary hyperplasia, palate, 196, 196f
Papilloma, 193, 194f
Papillomavirus, 264t, 275

Paradigm, 458
Paranasal sinuses, 112
Paraphrasing, 482
Paraplegia, 583
Parasites, 287t
Parasitism, 263
Parasympathetic division, 29
Parasympathetic ganglia. *See* Terminal ganglia.
Parasympathetic nervous system (PANS), 328f, 330
Parasympathomimetic (cholinergic) agents, 328f, 330–332
Parathyroid glands, 84, 119
Parenteral administration, 326
Parietal bones, 109, 109f
Parietal membranes, 61
Parkinson's disease, 580
Parotid glands, examination of, 469
Parotid lymph nodes, assessment of, 469
Parotid papilla, 131t
Parotid salivary gland, 118
Partial anodontia, 244, 244f
Partial fetal alcohol syndrome (PFAS), 571
Passive diffusion, 361
Passive transport processes, 58, 58t
Pastes, prophylactic, 408–409
Patella, 66, 67f
Pathogens
  Bacillus fusiformis, 205
  Borrelia vincentii, 205
Pathology
  general, 177–192
    differential diagnosis of, 188–189
    genetics of, 185–188
    inflammation, 177–182
    regeneration and wound healing of, 182–184, 182f
    regenerative medicine in, 184–185
    review questions for, 190
    website information and resources for, 189b
  oral, 193–255
    aphthous ulcers, 205–210, 206f
    benign intraosseous neoplasms, 199–201
    benign lesions, 193–195
    benign mixed tumor, 219–220, 220f
    blood dyscrasias, 227–233
    cysts, 220–221
    developmental cysts, 221–223
    dysplasia, fibrous, 234–236
    endocrine disorders, 236–238
    gingival fibromatosis, 201–203
    granulomas, 195–199
    human immunodeficiency virus (HIV), 233–234
    inflammatory tumors, 195–199
    neoplasia, 217–218
    odontogenic cysts, 223–227
    pleomorphic adenoma, 219–220, 220f

Pathology *(Continued)*
    review questions and answers for, 248, 248b, 249–252f, 250b
    skin diseases, 210–213
    soft tissue conditions, 246–248
    teeth abnormalities, 238–245
    ulcerative diseases, 203–205
    website information and resources for, 248b
    white lesions, 213–217
Pathoses, 188
Pathways
  anesthetic, 556–558
  metabolic, 262
Patient Hygiene Performance (PHP), 636t
"Pavementing", 178
Pectin, 361
Pediatric dose, 327
Pemphigus vulgaris, 212–213, 213f
Penicillins, 285t, 340–341
  adverse effects of, 340
  extended-spectrum, 340–341
  penicillin G, 340
  penicillin V, 340
  penicillinase (β-lactamase)-resistant, 340
  pharmacokinetics of, 340
  stability of, 340
Penicillium, 263
Pentoses, 360
Pepsin, 367
Perception, tactile, 129
Perfringens poisoning, 277
Periadenitis mucosa necrotica recurrens, 206, 206f
Periapex, 129
Periapical cemento-osseous dysplasia, 236
Periapical cysts, 220, 220f
Periapical infections, 294–295
Periapical radiograph, 164f
Pericardial cavity, 55, 56f
Perimylolysis, 239
Periodontal diseases, 293b
  causal and risk factors for, 634
  and denture use, 634
  dietary modifications for, 365, 366t, 387
  identification of the bacterial cause, 294b
  measures for preventing and controlling, 648
  and oral and pharyngeal cancers, 634
  prevalence of, 634
    indices for, 636t
  principal bacteria associated with, 294b
  radiographic appearance of, 172, 172f
  risk assessment, 508
  tooth retention and tooth loss in, 634
Periodontal file, 521–522
Periodontal instrumentation
  advanced, techniques in, 535–536
  for assessment, 527–531
    clinical, using periodontal probes, 528–530

Periodontal instrumentation *(Continued)*
    with dental explorer, 530–531
    with periodontal probes, 527, 527f
    probing technique in, 527–528
  concepts in, 531–532
    end point of, 532
    nonsurgical, rationale for, 531–532
    overhang removal, rationale for, 532
    preparation of, steps for, 532
    terminology in, 531
  ethical, legal, and safety issues in, 537
  principles of, 523–526
    activation, 525
    adaptation, 525
    angulation, 525, 525f
    clinician position, 523–524, 523f
    stabilization, 524–525, 524f
    strokes, 526
  review questions for, 538, 538–539b, 541–543b
  selective stain removal in, 536–537
  ultrasonic and sonic, 532–535
  website information and resources for, 538b
Periodontal ligament, 44–46, 428–429
Periodontal ligament (PDL) injection, 559
Periodontal pocket formation, 437, 437f
Periodontal probes. *see also* Probe.
  assessments with, 527, 527f
  clinical assessment using, 528–530
Periodontics, 427–457
  assessments for, 440–442, 472t, 475
    documentation for, 440
    indices, 440
  bacterial dental biofilm, 438–440
  dental implants in, 452–453
    design of, 452
    endosseous, 452
    goals of, 453
    limiting factors for, 452
    management of, 453
    transosteal, 453
    types of, 452
  periodontium changes, disease-associated, 436–438
    pathogenesis of, 436
    periodontal pocket formation, 437, 437f
    stages of, 436
  periodontium diseases in, 430–436
    abscesses, 433
    classification of, 430
    deformities, acquired, 433–436
    deformities, developmental, 433–436
    epidemiology of, 434–436
    gingival diseases, 430–431
    necrotizing, 432–433
    periodontitis, aggressive, 431–432
    periodontitis, as systemic disease manifestation, 432
    periodontitis, chronic, 431
    periodontitis associated with endodontic lesions, 433

Periodontics *(Continued)*
risks of, 434–436
systemic effects of, 442
periodontium features in, 427–430
alveolar process, 429, 429f
anatomy of, 428f
blood supply, 429–430
cementum, 429
gingiva, 427–428, 428f
innervation, 429–430
lymph, 429–430
periodontal ligament, 428–429
radiographic, 429, 429f
postoperative care, 451–452
client instructions and education, 451
follow-up care, 451
periodontal maintenance, 451–452
review questions for, 454
risk factors in, 476
treatment, 442–451
additional clinical interventions, 448–450
care plan, initial, 442–443
gingival curettage, 448
healing following, 450
nonsurgical periodontal therapy, 443, 444t
occlusal trauma, 448
periodontal dressings and, 451
surgical interventions, 449–450
sutures and, 450–451
website information and resources for, 453b
Periodontitis
aggressive, 431–432
associated with endodontic lesions, 433
chronic, 431
as systemic disease manifestation, 432
therapy for, 480
Periodontium
diseases of, 430–436
abscesses, 433
classification of, 430
deformities, developmental, 433–436
epidemiology of, 434–436
gingival, 430–431
immunology and microbiology of, 292–294
periodontitis, aggressive, 431–432
periodontitis, as systemic disease manifestation, 432
periodontitis, chronic, 431
periodontitis associated with endodontic lesions, 433
risks of, 434–436
systemic effects of, 442
features of, 427–430
alveolar process, 429, 429f
anatomy of, 428f
blood supply, 429–430
cementum, 429
gingiva, 427–428, 428f

Periodontium *(Continued)*
innervation, 429–430
lymph, 429–430
periodontal ligament, 428–429
radiographic, 429, 429f
Peripheral giant cell granulomas, 197, 197f
Peripheral nervous system (PNS), 27
Peritoneum, 61
Permanent dentition, 134, 136t
development of, 142
Pernicious anemia, 228
Perpendicular plate, 110
Personal protective equipment (PPE), 300, 305
Personal supervision, 718
PFAS. *See* Partial fetal alcohol syndrome (PFAS).
Phagocytosis, 59, 59t, 92, 267
membrane transport and, 20
Pharmacodynamics, 325
Pharmacokinetics, 327–328
Pharmacology, 325–359
analgesics, 337, 337t
acetaminophen (*n*-acetyl-*p*-aminophenol), 338
general considerations for, 337
gout drugs, 339
nonsteroidal anti-inflammatory agents (NSAIAs), 338
nonsteroidal anti-inflammatory drugs (NSAIDs), 331t, 338
opioid (narcotic), 338–339, 339t
salicylates (aspirin), 337
antiarrhythmics, 344–347
antianginal agents, 344
anticoagulants, 344–345
anticonvulsants, 346–347, 346t
antihypertensives, 344, 345t
diuretics, 344
anti-infectives, 339–343
aminoglycosides, 342
antifungal agents, 343
antituberculosis agents, 343
antiviral agents, 343
cephalosporins, 341
clindamycin, 341
general considerations for, 339–340
macrolides, 341
metronidazole, 342–343
penicillins, 340–341
quinolones, 342
sulfonamides, 342
tetracyclines, 341–342
antineoplastic agents, 352–353
autonomic nervous system agents, 328–334
α-adrenergic blocker, 329–330
β-adrenergic blocker antagonist, 330
adrenergic neuronal agonists and antagonists, 330
local anesthetic agents, 332–334, 332f, 334t

Pharmacology *(Continued)*
parasympathomimetic (cholinergic), 328f, 330–332
sympathetic (adrenergic), 328–329, 328f, 329t
xerostomia-producing drug groups in, 331t
cardiovascular agents, 343
digitalis glycosides, 343
drug use during pregnancy and, 353–354
endocrine agents, 348–350
adrenocorticosteroids, 348, 348t
agents for diabetes mellitus, 348–349
estrogens and progesterone, 350
oral contraceptives, 350
thyroid agents, 349–350
gastrointestinal agents, 351–352
affecting gastrointestinal motility, 351
emetics and antiemetics, 351–352
histamine (H_2-) blockers, 351
proton pump inhibitors, 351
general anesthetics, 334–335
anesthesia stages and planes in, 334
specific agents, 334–335
general considerations for, 325–328
adverse reactions, 327–328
agencies, 325
definitions, 325
drug action in, 325–327
legislations, 325, 326t
nomenclature, 325, 326t
local anesthetic reversal agent, 334
in nitrous oxide-oxygen conscious sedation, 561
psychotherapeutic agents, 347–348
antidepressants, 347–348
antipsychotics, 347, 347t
respiratory system agents, 350–351
for asthma, 350–351
review questions for, 355, 355–357b, 359b
sedative-hypnotic medications, 335–339, 335b
barbiturates, 336
benzodiazepines, 335–336, 336t
general considerations for, 335
nonbarbiturate nonbenzodiazepines, 336–337
smoking cessation and, 354
substance abuse, 353
definitions, 353
drugs, 353
website information and resources for, 354b
Pharmacotherapy, 325
Pharmacy, 325
Pharyngeal cancers, 634
Pharyngeal tonsils, 118, 131t
Pharyngitis, aphthous, 209–210, 210f
Pharyngopalatine arch, 131t
Pharynx, 97
Phase-contrast microscopy, 257
Phencyclidine (PCP), 353

Phenylephrine (Neo-Synephrine), 329*t*
Phenylketonuria (PKU), 369
Phenytoin (Dilantin), 346
Philtrum, 131*t*
Phospholipids, 369
Phosphorylating enzymes, 60
Photoelectric effect, 154
Physical dependence, 353
Physical properties, 395
Physical Status Classification System, 465*t*
Physiology, of pain, 547–548, 548*f*
Physostigmine (Eserine), 330
Phytic acid, 364
Pia mater, 76, 76*f*
PICO mnemonic, 479, 479*t*
Picornaviruses, 264*t*
Pie graph, 662
Piercing, oral, 470
Pigmentation, melanin, 129, 246, 246*f*
Pilot study, 629
Pineal gland, 83
"Pink tooth", 199
Pinocytosis, 59, 59*t*
  membrane transport and, 20
Pinworm, 287*t*
Pioglitazone (Actos), 349
"Pipe smoker's palate", 213
Piperazine, 287*t*
Pit, 134
Pit-and-fissure caries, 471
Pit-and-fissure sealants, 402–403
Pituitary gland, 82–83
Placenta, 85
Plaintiff, 712
Planes, anatomic, 53, 55*f*, 107, 108*f*
Planning and practice strategies
  basic concepts of, 619–623
    access, 620
    community, 620
    community health, 620
    dental public health, 619
    health determinants, 619
    national documents, 621
    oral health, 619
    prevention, 620
    private *vs.* community health, 620, 620*t*
    public health, 619
  challenges affecting, 677–678
  community intervention in, 650–661, 650*f*
    assessment and problem identification in, 650–654, 651*t*, 653*t*
    health education and health promotion in, 654–658, 655*t*, 657*t*
    implementation in, 654
    methods of oral health education in, 658–660
    planning in, 654
    role of dental hygienist in, 650
    strategies in, 650
    surveillance in, 650
  epidemiology, 623–626
    characteristics of, 624, 625*f*

Planning and practice strategies *(Continued)*
    concepts in, 625*t*
    definitions of, 623, 624*b*
    measurement concepts in, 625*t*
    measurement of diseases and conditions in, 640–641
    of oral diseases and conditions, 629–640, 630*t*, 631*f*, 632*t*
    and research, 626–629, 628*t*
    uses of, 624, 624*b*
  financing oral health care in, 670–674
    mechanisms of payment, 670–672, 671*t*
    providers of dental benefits plans in, 672
    public, 673–674, 673*t*
  preventing and controlling oral diseases in, 641–650
    measures for dental caries, 641–648, 642*t*, 644–645*b*
    measures for other oral diseases and anomalies, 648–650
    measures for periodontal disease, 648
    public health measures in, 641
  in process of care, 479–481, 480*t*
  program evaluation in, 661–665
    general principles of, 661
    of professional literature, 665, 665*b*
    statistics in, 661–664, 662*b*, 663*f*
  provision of oral health care in, 665–670
    dental practice, diverse modes of, 665–666, 666*t*
    personnel workforce in, 667–670, 668*f*, 669*t*
    utilization of dental services in, 674–677, 675*t*
    patterns of, shifts in, 676–677
Plant alkaloids, 352
Plant viruses, 264
Plaque, 581
  accumulation, scattered, 581
  and gingival indices, 494
Plaque Index (PlI), 636*t*
Plasma, 55, 57*f*, 115
Plasma membrane, 17
Plasma proteins, 180
Plasma-derived mediators, 179
Platelet adhesiveness, 337
Platelet-activating factor (PAF), 179*t*
Platelets, 86, 115
Plato, 707
Pleomorphic adenoma, 219–220, 220*f*
Pleura, 61
Pleural cavity, 55, 56*f*
Plexus, 115
Plica fimbriata, 131*t*
Plummer-Vinson syndrome, 228–229, 229*f*
Pneumococcal pneumonia, 275
Pneumocystis, 263
Pneumonia
  mycoplasmal, 276
  pneumococcal, 275

Pockets, periodontal, 437, 437*f*
Point angle, 134
Poisoning, 698
Policy, classifications of, 736
Policy development, as function of public health, 620
Polishing
  adverse effects of, 536
  contraindications to, 536
Polyarthritis, 580
Polycythemia, 230
  characteristics of, 230
  primary, 230
  relative, 230
  secondary, 230
  vera, 230
Polygon, 662
  frequency, 662
Polymerase chain reaction (PCR), 187
Polymorphonuclear leukocyte (PMN), 177
Polyoma-papilloma, 264*t*
Polyostotic fibrous dysplasia, 235
Polyps, pulp, 198, 198*f*
Pons, 77, 77*f*
  pneumotaxic center in, 96
Pontic, 500
Population at risk, 625*t*, 628*t*
Porcelain-fused-to-metal (PFM) alloys, 413–414. *See also* Alloys.
Position
  anatomical, 107
  of clinician, 523–524, 523*f*
Position-indicating device (PID), alignment problems, 166, 167*f*
Positive hypothesis, 629
Posterior superior alveolar (PSA) nerve, 120*t*, 121, 554
Postnatal chromosome analysis, 187
Postoperative care, 451–452
Postsyncope stage, 693
Posttest only, 628
Postural hypertension, 693
Potency, 326, 327*f*, 550
Potential osmotic pressure, 58
Power interdental cleaning devices, 498
Power toothbrushes, 495
Power-driven polisher, 537
Poxviruses, 264*t*
Practicing without a license, 725
Pralidoxime (2-PAM/Protopam), 331
Praziquantel, 287*t*
Predation, 263
Predictive value, 625*t*
Prefixes, 743. *See also* Medical terminology.
Pregnancy, 387
  drug use during, 353–354
Pregnancy Discrimination Act (PDA) of 1978, 735
Preliminary diagnosis, 189
Premolars, 135, 136*t*
Prenatal chromosome analysis, 187

Pressure receptors, 81t
Presyncope stage, 693
Pretest/posttest, 628
Prevalence, 625t
Prevention, 655
Preventive and restorative materials.
    see also Biomaterials.
    direct, 399–409
        amalgam, dental, 399–401,
            399–400f
        bonding agents, 403–405, 403–404f
        cement applications, 406
        cement bases, 405–406, 405f
        cement liners, 405
        cements, orthodontic, 406
        composites, dental, 401–402, 401f
        dentifrices, 408–409
        dressings, surgical, 406
        fluoride varnishes, 407–408
        fluoride-releasing restorative materials,
            406–407, 406f, 408f
        fluorides, topical, 407–408
        gingival tissue packs, 406
        infiltrants, 403
        pastes, prophylactic, 408–409
        sealants, pit-and-fissure, 402–403
        sealers, root canal, 406
        whitening agents, 409
    indirect
        alloys, casting, 412–413
        alloys, chromium, 413
        alloys, porcelain-fused-to-metal,
            413–414
        appliances, acrylic, 415–416
        athletic mouthguards, 417
        cast materials, 411–412
        cements, crown-and-bridge, 415, 415t
        ceramics, dental, 414–415
        denture bases, acrylic, 416
        denture cleansers, 417
        denture soft liners, 417
        denture teeth, 416
        die materials, 411–412, 411t
        implants, dental, 418–419
        impression materials, 409–410, 410t
        investment materials, 412
        materials, 409–420
        model materials, 411–412
        mouth protectors, 417
        provisional materials, 410–411
        restorations, computer-assisted design/
            computer-assisted machining, 418
        solders, dental, 413
        tissue engineering, 419–420
        veneers, 417–418
        waxes, 412
Preventive care planning, 490
Prilocaine, 332–333
Primaquine, 287t
Primary anemia, 228
Primary aplastic anemia, 229
Primary deficiency, 380

Primary dentition, 141
    development of, 142
Primary herpetic gingivostomatitis, 207–208,
        207f, 284f
Primary polycythemia, 230
Primary radiation, 154
Primary teeth, 141f, 143f
Primordial cyst, 224
Principal fiber groups, 45
Principalism, 707
Prion, 256
Priority population, 629
Privacy, 751–752
Privacy standards, 733
Private vs. community health, 620, 620t
Privilege, 714
Probability level (p value), 664
Probe, 520
    markings, examples of, 520t
    periodontal
        assessments with, 527, 527f
        clinical assessment using, 528–530
Probenecid (Benemid), 337, 339
Probing
    bleeding on, 528
    periodontal, 475
    technique in, 527–528
Probiotics, 647
Problem identification, in community
        intervention, 650–654, 651t, 653t
Process of care, 458–489
    algorithm for, 459f
    assessments in
        of dentition, 471–474, 474b
        extraoral, 468–471
        human needs theory and, 458, 460–461f
        intraoral, 468–471
        oral hygiene, 476
        periodontal, 472t, 475
        radiographic evaluation for, 475–476
        risk factor, 476–477
    case presentation and, 481
    communication and, 482
    concepts of, 458–459
    dental hygiene paradigm and, 458
    diagnosis in, 469f, 478, 478f
    documentation and, 483–484
    ethical issues of, 484
    evaluation and, 482–483
    evidence-based decision making in, 479
    health history in, 459
        blood pressure classification in, 466t
        evaluation of, 459–468
        form for, 459
        glycemic management in, 467b
        information, 463–468
        Physical Status Classification System for,
            465t
        screening questions for, 460–463, 462f,
            463t
    implementation in, 481–482
    informed consent and, 481

Process of care (Continued)
    legal issues of, 484
    planning in, 479–481, 480t
    prognosis in, 478–479
    review questions for, 486, 486–487b
    safety issues of, 484
    as standard of practice, 458
    website information and resources for,
        484b
Processing, of DNA, 61
Professional associations, state board of
        dentistry and, 3
Professional ethics, 707
Professional literature, evaluation of, 665,
        665b
Professional organizations, of interest, to
        dental hygienists, 746–747
Professional risk management, 736
Professionalism, 708–709, 751–753
Progesterone, 350
Prognosis, process of care and, 478–479
Program evaluation, 661–665
    general principles in, 661
        of professional literature, 665, 665b
    statistics in, 661–664, 662b, 663f
Progressive irreversible brain disorder, 574
Prokaryotes, 256, 260t
Prokaryotic function, 258–259
Proliferation, 183
Properties, biomaterials, 395–398.
        See also Biomaterials.
Prophase, of mitosis, 21
Prophylactic pastes, 408–409
Proprietary (trade) name, 325
Proprioceptive sensations, 80
Prospective, 625t
Prostaglandins, 82, 179t
Prostate gland, 101
Prostheses, fixed and removable, care of,
        500–502
Prosthetic appliances, 474
Prosthodontics, dietary modifications for,
        388
Protease inhibitors (PIs), 272
Proteases, 179t
Protected health information (PHI), 733
Protective (barrier) clothing, 307
Protective eyewear, 307
Protectors, mouth, 417
Protein digestibility-corrected amino acid
        score (PDCAAS), 367
Protein efficiency ratio (PER), 367
Proteins, 366–369
    binding of, 327
    classifications of, 366
        biologic, 367
        chemical, 366
        structure, 367
    complementary, 367
    complete, 367
    compound, 366
    definition of, 366

Proteins *(Continued)*
  dietary modifications for disease, 369
  digestion of, 367
  as energy source, 378
  functions of, 368
  incomplete, 367
  metabolic regulation and, 368
  metabolism of, 367
  quality of, 367
  requirements for, 369
  simple, 366
  synthesis of, 18, 262
Proteus spp., 266*t*
Protozoa, 256
Protrusion, 147
Provider, contractual responsibilities
  of, 713
Provision, of oral health care, 665–670
  dental practice, diverse modes of, 665–666,
    666*t*
    personnel workforce in, 667–670, 668*f*,
      669*t*
Provisional materials, 410–411
Proximal, as directional term, 107
Proximal tooth surfaces, 134
Pseudocysts, 226–227
  aneurysmal, 226
  hemorrhagic, 226
  lingual mandibular bone concavity,
    226–227, 227*f*
  simple, 226
  Stafne, 226–227, 227*f*
  static, 226–227, 227*f*
  traumatic, 226, 227*f*
Pseudoephedrine (Sudafed), 329*t*
Pseudomonas aeruginosa, 266*t*
  infections, 273
Psilocybin, 353
Psittacosis, 285*t*
Psychedelics, 353
Psychological dependence, 353
Psychological disorders, questions regarding,
  467
Psychotherapeutic agents, 347–348
  antidepressants, 347–348
  antipsychotics, 347, 347*t*
Pterygomandibular raphe, 131*t*
Pterygopalatine nerves, 554
Public financing, 673–674, 673*t*
Public health, 619
  core functions of, 620
  governmental levels of, 621, 621*b*
  measures for, 641
Public Health Service (PHS), 621*b*
Public health solution, 620, 620*b*
Public policy, 709–710
Publicity of private life, 714
Pulp, 129
  polyp, 198, 198*f*
  tissue, 39–40
    dentin and, 40
Pulpal granulomas, 198

Pulpal vitality testing, 474
  devices, 512–513
  laser Doppler flowmetry in, 512
  thermal testing in, 512–513
  traditional electrical testing devices in, 512
Pulse, 689–690, 690*f*
Pumping, 59*t*
Punitive damages, 713
Pupil, 78
Purine antagonists, 352
Purposive sample, 630*t*
Purpura, 232–233
  characteristics of, 232
  nonthrombocytopenic, 233
  thrombocytopenic, 232
Pyogenic granuloma, 195–196, 196*f*.
  See also Granulomas.
Pyrazinamide, 285*t*
Pyrimethamine, 287*t*
Pyrimidine antagonists, 352

Q
Quadriplegia, 583
Quality assurance, 162
Quasi-experimental research, 628*t*
Quaternaries, dual or synergized, 310*t*
Questionnaires, health history information
  from, 467
Questions, health history, 460–463, 463*t*
Quid pro quo, 734
Quinacrine, 287*t*
Quinolones, 342

R
Radiation biology, 155–157
  measurements and sources, 156,
    156–157*f*
  protection, 156–157, 159*f*
Radiation physics, 152–154, 153–154*f*
Radicular cysts, 220*f*, 220. *See also* Cysts.
Radiographic features, of periodontium, 429,
  429*f*
Radiography
  history information from, 463
  process of care and, 475–476
Radiology, 152–176
  dental x-ray film, 157–161
    image characteristics of, 159–160, 160*t*
    processing, 160–161
  digital imaging and, 162–163
  film mounting, 169
  film-processing errors and, 161–162,
    161–162*f*
  general considerations in, 152–155
    radiation physics, 152–154, 153–154*f*
    x-radiation, 152, 154–155
  quality assurance in, 162
  radiation biology and, 155–157
    measurements and sources, 156, 156–157*f*
    protection, 156–157, 158*t*, 159*f*
  radiographic errors in, 166–169
    extraoral technique, 167–169, 168*f*

Radiology *(Continued)*
    intraoral technique, 166–167, 166–167*f*
  radiographic interpretation in, 169–172,
    169–172*f*
  review questions for, 172, 172*b*, 173–174*f*
  techniques in, 163–166
    extraoral radiographic examinations,
      165–166, 165*f*
    intraoral radiographic, 163, 163–165*f*
  website information and resources for,
    172*b*
Radiolucent, 160
Radiopaque, 160
Radius, 65, 66*f*
Rainbow® Stabilizing System, 609*f*
Raltegravir, 272
Rampant caries, 471
Ramus, 112
Rancidity, 369
Random sample, 630*t*
  stratified, 630*t*
  systematic, 630*t*
Ranula, 225, 225*f*
Rapid-acting insulin, 349
Rate, 625*t*
Ratio, 625*t*
Reactive hypoglycemia, 366
Reactive oxygen species, 179*t*
Recaldent, 647
Receptor placement, 166, 166*f*
Receptors, 328
Recessive inheritance
  autosomal, 186
  X-linked, 186
Reciprocity, 715
Recombinant DNA, 187
Recommended Dietary Allowance (RDA),
  382
Record keeping requirements, 728–733
  electronic, 728
  purpose of, 728
  written, 728
Rectal administration, 326
Recurrent aphthous stomatitis, 205–206
Recurrent caries, 471
Recurrent scarifying ulcerative stomatitis
  (RSUS), 206, 206*f*
Recurrent ulcerative stomatitis (RUS),
  205–206
Redistribution, 327
Reduced penetrance, 186
Reevaluation, 483
Reflective responding, 482
Reflex arc, 77
Refractory period, 548
  absolute, 76
Regeneration and wound healing, 182–184,
  182*f*
Regenerative medicine, 184–185
Regional Clinical Board Examinations,
  preparing for, 12–13
Relative polycythemia, 230

Relative refractory period, 548
Release, 714
Reliability, 625*t*
Removable-prosthesis maintenance, 501
Reoviruses, 264*t*
Repair process, 182
Replication, of cell, 21–31
Repolarization, 548
Reporting professional violations, 725
Reproduction, of cells, 16
Reproductive system, 101–103
    female, 102–103
    infections, 281–284, 281*f*
    male, 101–102
Res ipsa loquitur, 713
Res judicata, 711
Research, 626
    community oral health, 627
    and epidemiology, 626–629, 628*t*
    experimental, 627
Research hypothesis, 629
Resident flora, 304
Resistance, 340
Resorption, internal, 198–199, 199*f*
Respect, 482
Respiration rate, 690
Respiratory arrest, 691
Respiratory disease, questions regarding,
    466
Respiratory system, 93–96, 93*f*
    agents, 350–351
    infections, 276*t*
        lower, 275–277
        upper, 275
    lower respiratory tract, 94
    physiology of, 94–96
    upper respiratory tract, 94
Responsibility, principle of, 749
Responsiveness, 482
Resting membrane potential, 76
Resting nerve cell membrane, 547
Restorations, 474
    biomaterials for, computer-assisted
        design/computer-assisted
        machining, 418
    dental hygienist duties for, 718, 730*t*
Reticular activating system, 78
Reticular formation, 77
Reticulin fibers, 23
Retina, 78
Retinitis pigmentosa, 576
Retrolental fibroplasia, 576
Retromolar area, 131*t*
Retromolar triangle, 112
Retrospective, 625*t*
Retrovirus, 264*t*
Retrusion, 147
Reversal, definition of, 625*t*
Reversed film, 167, 167*f*
Reversed polarity, 548
Reversible index, 640
Reye syndrome, 337

Rheumatic fever, 280
Rheumatoid arthritis, 580*t*
Rhinovirus, 276*t*
Rhizopus, 263
Ribavirin, 287*t*
Ribonucleic acid (RNA) analysis, 187
Ribosomal RNA (rRNA), 18
Ribosomes, 18*f*, 56, 57*f*
Ribs, 65
Rickets, 237
Ridge, 134
Rifampin, 285*t*
Ringworm infections, 273
Risk, *vs.* causality, 627, 628*t*
Risk factors
    assessment of, 476–477, 736
    for caries, 476, 477*t*
    definition of, 476
    management, 736
    for oral and pharyngeal cancer, 476
    for periodontium disease, 434–436
    for systemic disease, 476
Root canal sealers, 406
Root caries, 474
Root-end cysts, 220*f*, 220. See also Cysts.
Roots
    advanced instrumentation for, 523
    characteristics of, 136*t*, 140, 140*f*
    furcation, 129
    morphology, 129–151
Rotavirus, 280
Roundworm, 287*t*
RSUS. *See* Recurrent scarifying ulcerative
    stomatitis (RSUS).
Ruffini's corpuscles, 80, 81*t*
Rugae, 131*t*
Rule deontology, 707
Rule utilitarianism, 707
RUS. *See* Recurrent ulcerative stomatitis
    (RUS).

S

S. mutans, 364
Sac fungi, 263
Saccharomyces, 263
Safety issues, of process of care, 484
Sagittal plane, 55, 55*f*, 107, 108*f*
Salicylates, 337
Salicylism, 337
Salivart, 331
Salivary amylase (ptyalin), 361
Salivary duct openings, 131*t*
Salmonella spp., 266*t*
Salmonellosis, 277
Salt, 332*f*
Salutatory conduction, 76
Sample, 629
Sample size, 629
Sampling, 630*t*
Saquinavir, 287*t*
Sarcomastigophora, 264
Saturated fatty acids, 369

Scaler, sickle, 521, 521*f*
Scar formation, 183
Scatter radiation, 154
Scattergram, 663
Schaeffer-Fulton spore stain, 258
Schedules I-V, 326*t*
School setting, health education and health
    promotion in, 661
Scientific method, 626, 627*f*
Sclera, 78
Scleroderma, 581
Scope of practice, 718
Screening questions, 463*t*
Sealants, 402–403. See also Biomaterials.
Sebaceous glands, 62
Second messenger mechanism, 82
Secondary aplastic anemia, 229
Secondary deficiency, 380
Secondary radiation, 154
Secondary union, 183
Sedation, conscious. *See* Conscious
    sedation.
Sedative-hypnotic medications, 335–339,
    335*b*
    barbiturates, 336
    benzodiazepines as, 335–336, 336*t*
    general considerations for, 335
    nonbarbiturate nonbenzodiazepines,
        336–337
Seizure disorders, 575–576, 576*f*
Selective polishing, 481
Selective serotonin reuptake inhibitors
    (SSRIs), 348
Selective stain removal, 536–537
Self-applied fluorides, 504
Self-defense, 714
Self-disclosure, 482
Sensation, 78
Senses, special, 78–80
Sensitivity, 625*t*
Sensorineural hearing loss, 577
Sensory neurons, 75, 119, 547, 548*f*
Sepsis, 181
Septic shock, 694
Serotonergic drugs, for weight loss, 379
Serotonin, 179*t*
Serotonin and norepinephrine reuptake
    inhibitors, 348
Serotonin modulators, 348
Serous membranes, 61
Serum amyloid A protein (SAA), 181
SES. *See* Socioeconomic status (SES).
Sexual harassment, 734
Shank, 518, 519*f*
Sharpening, of hand-activated instruments,
    532, 533*t*
Sharpey's fibers, 46
Sharpness, 160, 160*t*
Shigella spp., 266*t*
Shigellosis, 277
Shingles, 208–209, 209*f*, 275
Shock, 693–694

Short-acting drugs
  barbiturates, 336
  insulin, 349
Short-chain fatty acids, 370
Shunts, types of, 584*f*
Sialometaplasia, necrotizing, 226, 226*f*
Sibutramine (Meridia), 379
Sickle cell
  anemia, 227–228, 227–228*f*
  disease, 588
  trait, 588
Sickle scaler, 521, 521*f*
Side effects, 327
Signatures, genetic, 187
Simple bone cyst, 226. *See also* Cysts.
Simple diffusion, 58, 58*t*
Simple shank, 518
Simplesse, 370
Simplified Oral Hygiene Index (OHI-S), 636*t*
Single-food (monotonous) diet, 379
Single-gene disorders, 186
Single-tufted brushes, 495
Sinuses, paranasal, 112
SIRS. *See* Systemic inflammatory response
    syndrome (SIRS).
Situational ethics, 707
Skeletal articulations, 108
Skeletal (striated) muscle, 30
Skeletal system, 62–68, 62*f*
  bone, microscopic structure of, 63
  bone marrow, 63–64
  bone tissue, 63
  divisions of, 64–66
    appendicular, 65–66
    axial, 64–65
  joints, 67–68
  regulation of blood calcium level in, 64
Skeleton, axial. *See* Axial skeleton.
Skewed distribution, 663, 663*f*
Skin, 61
  color, 61
  diseases of, 210–213
    Behçet syndrome, 212, 212*f*
    characteristics of, 210
    erythema multiforme, 210–211, 211*f*
    pemphigus vulgaris, 212–213, 213*f*
    Stevens-Johnson syndrome, 211–212,
      211*f*
  examination of, 468
  infection of, 273–275
Skinfold thickness measurements, 381
Slander, 714
SLE. *See* Systemic lupus erythematosus (SLE).
Small intestine, in digestion
  of lipids, 370
  of proteins, 367
Smooth muscle, 30
  stimulation, 330
Smooth surface caries, 474
Societal trust, 749
Socioeconomic status (SES), 625*t*
Sodium bicarbonate, 647

Soft liners, denture, 417
Soft palate, 131*f*, 131*t*. *See also* Palate.
  examination of, 470
Soft tissue
  conditions, 246–248
    mucous membrane abnormalities,
      246–247
    skin abnormalities, 246–247
    tongue abnormalities, 247–248
  injuries, 225–226
  origins, benign lesions, 193–195
Solders, dental, 413
Solubility, 327
Somatic reflex, 77
Somatic sensory receptors, classification of, 81*t*
Somatic stem cells, 185
Sonic instruments, 533
Southern Regional Testing Agency, Inc.
    (SRTA), 2*b*
Spastic-type cerebral palsy, 578*f*
Special Care Dentistry Association, 747
Special care needs
  dental hygiene care for clients with,
      567–618
  dental hygienist and individuals
      with, 568
  dental management considerations for,
      596, 597*t*, 608–610*f*
  general definitions of, 568
  incidence and prevalence of individuals
      with, 567, 568*t*
  life span approach to care for, 567, 568*t*
  normalization goals for persons with,
      568–569
  potential barriers to oral health care,
      569–570
  review questions for, 610, 614–615*f*, 617*f*
  specific conditions, 570–596
    alcohol abuse and dependence, chronic,
      594
    alcohol-related neurodevelopmental
      disorders, 571
    Alzheimer's disease, 574–575
    arrhythmias, cardiac, 586
    arthritis, 580–581, 580*t*
    asthma, bronchial, 585
    attention deficit hyperactivity disorder,
      573
    autism spectrum disorders, 572–573
    Bell's palsy, 579, 579*f*
    cancer, 588–589, 589*f*
    cerebral palsy, 578–579, 578–579*f*
    cerebrovascular accident, 587–588,
      588*t*
    chemical dependency, 592–594
    chronic obstructive pulmonary disease,
      585
    cleft lip or palate, 577–578, 578*f*
    congenital heart disease, 585–586
    congestive heart failure, 587
    coronary heart disease, 586–587
    cystic fibrosis, 584–585

Special care needs *(Continued)*
    developmental and cognitive challenges,
      570, 570–571*f*
    diabetes mellitus, 590–592, 591*t*, 592*f*
    Down syndrome, 571–572, 572*f*
    dysrhythmias, cardiac, 586
    eating disorders, 574
    emotional disturbance, 573
    end-stage renal disease, 594–595
    fetal alcohol spectrum disorders, 571,
      571*f*
    fetal alcohol syndrome, 571
    fibromyalgia syndrome, 581
    hearing impairment, 576–577, 577*t*
    hemophilias, 590
    hypertensive disease, 586
    ischemic heart disease, 586–587
    leukemia, 589–590, 590*f*
    mental illness, 573
    multiple sclerosis, 581–582, 582*t*
    muscular dystrophies, 582, 582*t*
    myasthenia gravis, 579–580
    older adults, 595–596, 595*f*
    Parkinson's disease, 580
    partial fetal alcohol syndrome, 571
    scleroderma, 581
    seizure disorders, 575–576, 576*f*
    sickle cell disease, 588
    spina bifida, 583–584, 584*f*
    spinal cord injuries, 582–583, 583–584*t*
    stroke, 587–588, 588*t*
    thyroid disease, 592, 592*t*, 593*f*
    visual impairment, 576
  website information and resources for,
      610*b*
Special damages, 713
Special senses, 78–80
  equilibrium, 79, 79*f*
  eye, components of, 78, 79*f*
  hearing, 79, 79*f*
  olfactory sense, 80
  proprioceptive sensations, 80
  tactile sensation, 80, 81*t*
  tongue, 80
Specific immunity, 92–93
Specific receptor theory, 332
Specificity, 625*t*
Specimen preparation, 257
Sperm, 101
Spina bifida, 583–584, 584*f*
Spina bifida occulta, 583
Spinal cord, 74, 76–77, 76*f*
  cross section of, 27*f*
Spinal cord injuries, 582–583, 583–584*t*
Spinal nerves, 77
Spinal reflexes, 77
Spirillum, 258
Split-mouth, 628
Spoken defamation, 714
Sporothrix, 263
Spots, radiographs with, 162, 162*f*
Squamous cell carcinoma, 217–218, 218–219*f*

SRTA. *See* Southern Regional Testing Agency, Inc. (SRTA).
Stabilization, during instrumentation, 524–525, 524*f*
Stafne bone cyst, 226–227, 227*f*
Stain
  assessment of, 474
  removal of, selective, 536–537
Staining, 257, 257*t*
Standard of care, 713
Standard precautions, 301
Standards, 482
Staphylococcal food poisoning, 277
Staphylococcal infections, 273
Staphylococcus aureus, 266*t*, 285*t*
Starch, 360
Stare decisis, 711
State boards of dentistry, 2–4
State Clinical Board Examinations, preparing for, 12–13
State courts, 712
State dental hygiene committee, 718, 732*b*
State practice act, dental hygiene licensure and, 1
State supreme court, 712
Static bone cyst, 226–227, 227*f*
Static electricity artifacts, 162, 162*f*
Stationary relationships, 143
Statistical significance, 664
Statistics, 661–664, 662*b*, 663*f*
  clinical significance of, 664
  correlation, 662
  data in, 661
  descriptive, 662
  distributions of data in, 663, 663*f*
  errors in, 664, 664*f*
  hypothesis testing in, 664
  inferential, 663
  scales of measurement in, 661
  summary presentation of, 662
Status, 625*t*
Status epilepticus, 575, 700
Statute of limitations, 713–714
Statutory law, 711
Stavudine (d4T), 272
Stellate reticulum (STR), 35
Stem cells
  adult, 185
  types of, 185*t*
Sterile (surgical) gloves, 306*t*
Sterilization, 301, 315
  failure, 317
  methods, 315
  verification of, 317
Sterilization area procedures, 315
Sterilizing chemicals, 309*t*
Sternocleidomastoid muscle, 113
Sternohyoid muscle, 114
Sternothyroid muscle, 114
Steroid hormones, 80, 363
  mechanism of action, 82

Steroids, 370
  adrenocorticosteroids, 348, 348*t*
Sterols, 263, 370
Stevens-Johnson syndrome, 211–212, 211*f*
Stimulants, 353
Stimulus, 547
Stomach, in digestion
  of carbohydrates, 361
  of lipids, 370
  of proteins, 367
Stomatitis, 381
  gingivostomatitis, primary herpetic, 207–208, 207*f*
  nicotine, 213–214, 214*f*
  recurrent
    aphthous, 205–206
    ulcerative (RUS), 205–206
Storage area, 315
Stratified random sample, 630*t*
Stratum intermedium (STI), 35
Streptococcal infections, 273
Streptococcus mutans, 266*t*
Streptococcus pneumoniae, 266, 266*t*
Streptococcus pyogenes, 266*t*
Streptococcus viridans, 266*t*
Streptomycin, 285*t*
Stress, reduction protocols for, 465*t*
Stroke, 587–588, 588*t*
Structures, oral, clinical, 129, 130*f*, 131*t*
Styloglossus muscle, 114
Stylohyoid muscle, 114
Subcrestal pocket, 437
Subcutaneous (SC, SQ) administration, 326
Sublingual administration, 327
Sublingual caruncle, 131*t*
Sublingual folds, 131*t*
Sublingual salivary gland, 118
Submandibular glands, examination of, 469
Submandibular salivary gland, 118
Submental glands, examination of, 469
Substance abuse, 353
Successional lamina, 35
Sucrase, 361
Sucrose, 360
Sudden cardiac death (SCD), 696
Sudoriferous glands, 62
Suffixes, 743–744. *See also* Medical terminology.
Sugar, analysis and evaluation of, 386
Sugar alcohols, 365
Sulcus Bleeding Index (SBI), 636*t*
Sulfonamides ("sulfa" drugs), 342
Summation, 76
Sunset laws, 725
Superficial structures, 107
Supernumerary teeth, 244–245, 245*f*
Supervised neglect, 482
Supervision, 718
Supplemental groove, 134
Supporting tissues
  alveolar bone, 43–44, 44*f*
  dento-gingival junction, 46–47

Supporting tissues *(Continued)*
  periodontal ligament, 44–46
Supportive therapy, 482
Supra-alveolar pocket, 437
Supracrestal pocket, 437
Suprainfection, 340
Supreme Court, 712
Surface disinfection, chemical agents for, 310*t*
Surface epithelia, 22
Surfaces, of tooth, 134
Surfactant, 310
Surgical dressings, 406
Surgical therapy, 379
Surround® Toothbrush, 610*f*
Surveillance, 624
  in community intervention, 650
Sutton disease, 206, 206*f*
Sutures, 450–451
Symbiosis, 263
Sympathetic agents, 328–329, 328*f*
  adverse reactions of, 328
  drug interactions of, 329
  pharmacologic effects of, 328
  therapeutic uses of, 329
  as vasoconstrictors, 329
Sympathetic autonomic nervous system (SANS), 328–329
Sympathetic division, 29
Sympathetic ganglia, 78
Sympathetic nerves, 28*f*
Sympathomimetic amine, 552
Symphysis, 112
Synapse, definition of, 30
Synaptic transmission, 76
Syncope, 692–693
Syncope stage, 693
Synergism, 80
Synovial joints, 67, 70*f*
Synovial membranes, 61
Synthesis, in cells, 16, 18
Synthetic phenolics, 310*t*
Syntrophism, 263
Syphilis, 282, 282*f*
  congenital, 283*f*
  primary, chancre lesion of, 283*f*
Syringe
  anesthetic, 549, 549*f*
  traditional, *vs.* CCLADD, 558*t*
Systematic random sample, 630*t*
Systemic disease, risk factor for, 476
Systemic inflammatory response syndrome (SIRS), 181
Systemic lupus erythematosus (SLE), 214–215, 215*f*
Systems, body, 61–103

T

Tachycardias, 586
Tactile perception, 129
Tactile sensation, 80, 81*t*
Target population, 629

Tattoo, amalgam, 246, 246*f*
TB. *See* Tuberculosis (TB).
Teeth. *See* Tooth.
Teleologic ethics, 707
Telodendria, 75*f*
Telophase, of mitosis, 21
Temperature, body, 689
Temporal bones, 109
Temporalis muscle, assessment of, 468
Temporomandibular joint (TMJ), 114–115, 114*f*
  assessment of, 468
Temporomandibular joint disease, 635
Ten Great Public Health Achievements-United States, Twentieth century, 641*b*
Tenericutes, 263
Tentative diagnosis, 189
Teratogenic effect, 327
Terbinafine, 287*t*
Terminal ganglia, 78
Terminology, medical, 743–745
  body part designations, 745
  combining forms, 744–745
  prefixes, 743
  suffixes, 743–744
Tetanus, 273
Tetracaine, 333
Tetracycline, 285*t*
Tetracycline stain, 240
Thalamus, 78
Thalassemia, 229–230
Therapeutic index (TI), 325
Therapeutic polishing, 481
Thermal properties, 395, 395*f*
Thermal testing, 512–513
Thermic effect of food (TEF), 378
Thiabendazole, 287*t*
Thiazolidinediones, 349
Thin tissue layers, 61
Thirst response, 377
Thoracic (chest) cavity, 55, 56*f*
Thoracic lesion levels, functional significance of, 584*t*
Three As (analgesic/antipyretic/anti-inflammatory), 337
Thrombocytopenic purpura, 232
Thymus gland, 85, 119
Thyroglossal tract/duct cysts, 222, 222*f*
Thyrohyoid muscle, 114
Thyroid agents, 349–350
Thyroid crisis, 329
Thyroid disease, 592, 592*t*, 593*f*
Thyroid gland, 83–84, 119, 119*f*
  assessment of, 469
Thyroid storm, 329, 348
Thyroxine, 363
TIAs. *See* Transient ischemic attacks (TIAs).
Tibia, 66, 67*f*
Ticarcillin (Ticar), 285*t*
Tight junctions, in cells, 16
Time-series, 628

Tiotropium bromide (Spiriva), 351
Tip
  frequency, 534
  instrument, design for, 533
  interdental, 498
Tissue fluid, tissue components, 21
Tissue hormones. *See* Prostaglandins.
Tissues, 21–31, 61
  binding to, 327
  and body membranes, 62
  connective, 22–26, 62
    membranes, 61
  engineering, 419–420
  epithelial, 22
  muscle, 30–31
  nerve, 27–30
    components of, 29–30
  packs, gingival, 406
  remodeling, 183
  tooth, 38–43
Title VII of the Civil Rights Act of 1964, 734
TMJ. *See* Temporomandibular joint (TMJ).
TNF. *See* Tumor necrosis factor (TNF).
Tobacco cessation interventions, 507–508
Tobacco use interventions, 507–508
Tolerance, 326
Toluidine blue-O staining, 258
Tomes' process, enamel formation and, 36
Tongue, 80, 97
  abnormalities of, 247–248
    benign migratory glossitis, 247, 247*f*
    black hairy tongue, 248, 248*f*
    erythema migrans, 247, 247*f*
    geographic tongue, 247, 247*f*
  anatomy of, 130*f*, 131*t*
  development of, 32–33
  examination of, 470
  muscles of, 114
  surfaces of, 107
Tonsillar recess, 131*t*
Tonsillar region, 131*t*, 131*f*
Tonsils, 117–118, 131*t*
Tooth
  anatomy, radiographic, 169, 169*f*
  anomalies, 571*f*
  classes of, 135
  development of, 33–36, 34*f*
    cytodifferentiation, 34–35
    dentin formation, 35–36
    enamel formation, 35–36
    morphodifferentiation, 34
    sequential cellular interactions in, 35
  form, 139, 140*f*
    considerations for, 140
  loss, 634
    measures for, 649
  parts of, 129
  retention, 634
  surfaces of, 134
  tissues of, 34*f*
    cemento-enamel junction, 43
    cementum, 42–43, 42–43*f*

Tooth (*Continued*)
  dentin, 38–40
  enamel, 40–42, 41*f*
  pulp, 39–40
  trauma, 635
Tooth abnormalities, 238–245
  developmental defects, 240–241
    amelogenesis imperfecta, 240–241, 240–241*f*
    anodontia, 244
    concrescence, 242, 243*f*
    dens evaginatus, 243, 244*f*
    dens in dente, 242–243, 243–244*f*
    dens invaginatus, 242–243, 243–244*f*
    dentinogenesis imperfecta, 241, 241*f*
    dilaceration, 241, 242*f*
    fusion, 242, 242*f*
    gemination, 242, 243*f*
    hypodontia, 244, 244*f*
    macrodontia, 245
    microdontia, 245, 246*f*
    natal teeth, 244
    supernumerary teeth, 244–245, 245*f*
    tooth numbers, 244–245
    of tooth shape, 241–244
    of tooth size, 245
  drug-induced, 239–240
    methamphetamine abuse and addiction, 239–240
    tetracycline stain, 240
  tooth structure loss, 238–239
    abfraction, 239
    abrasion, 238–239, 239*f*
    attrition, 238, 239*f*
    erosion, 239, 240*f*
Toothbrushes
  maintenance of, 496
  manual, 494
  power, 495
Toothbrushing
  effectiveness, factors in, 495–496
  improper, 496
  manual, methods of, 494–495
Toothpicks, 498
Topical administration, 326
Topical anesthetic, 552
Topical fluorides, 407–408. *See also* Fluorides.
Tort, 712
Tort law, 713
Torus mandibularis, 201, 201*f*
Torus palatinus, 201, 201*f*
Total body water, 376
Touch receptors, 81*t*
Toxic overdoses, 698
Toxic reaction, 327
Toxic shock syndrome (TSS), 283
Toxicity, 550
Toxicology, 325
Toxoplasma gondii, 287*t*
Trade (proprietary) name, 325
Traditional electrical testing devices, 512
Transamination, 368

Transcription, 60, 262
Transduction, 263
Transfer
    disease, 265–287
    energy storage and, 262
Transfer RNA (tRNA), 18
Transformation, 263
Transient flora, 304
Transient ischemic attacks (TIAs), 699
Transitional dentition, 142
Translation, 60
Transmission, of disease, 300–302
Transmission electron microscope, 258
Transmission-based precautions, 301
Transosteal implants, 453. *See also* Dental
    implants.
Transport processes
    active, 59, 59*t*
    passive, 58, 58*t*
Trans-theoretical model, 491
Transverse plane, 55, 55*f*
Transverse ridge, 134
Trapezius muscle, 113
Traumatic bone cyst, 226, 227*f*.
    See also Cysts.
Traumatic fibroma, 193, 194*f*
Traumatic ulcers, 203–205, 204*f*
Tray systems, 503–504
Trench mouth, 205, 205*f*
Trend, 625*t*
Treponema pallidum, 266*t*
Triad, epidemiologic, 624, 625*f*
Trial courts, 712
Triangular ridge, 134
Tricalcium phosphate, 647
Tricarboxylic acid cycle (TCA), 362
Trichophyton, 263
Trigeminal nerve (CN V), 119
    divisions of, 120
        mandibular nerve, 121
        maxillary nerve, 120
        ophthalmic nerve, 120
    mandibular division of, 554–556
        block injections for, 556, 557*t*
        innervation of, 554–555
    maxillary division of, 554
        block injections for, 554,
            555*t*, 556*f*
        innervation of, 554
Trimethoprim-sulfamethoxazole, 285*t*
Trioses, 360
Trochlear nerve (CN IV), 119
Trophozoite, 264
True fats, 369
Trunk, root, 129
Trypsin, 367
Tubal tonsils, 118
Tuberculin skin test (TST), 304
Tuberculosis (TB), 276, 304, 343
Tubules, 20
Tumor, benign mixed, 219–220, 220*f*
Tumor necrosis factor (TNF), 181

Tumor-node-metastasis (TNM) staging
    system, 218, 219*b*
Turesky modification of the Quigley-Hein
    Plaque Index (TPI), 636*t*
Typhoid fever, 277
Tzanck cells, 213

U

Ulcerative diseases, 203–205
    characteristics of, 203
    necrotizing ulcerative gingivitis (NUG),
        205, 205*f*
    traumatic ulcers, 203–205, 204*f*
    trench mouth, 205, 205*f*
    Vincent's infection, 205, 205*f*
Ulna, 65, 66*f*
Ultrashort-acting barbiturates, 335
Ultrasonic devices, 532–533
Ultrasound methods, 382
Umbilical cord blood stem cells (UCBSCs),
    185
Unconsciousness, 692
Underwater weighing, 382
Unethical conduct, reporting suspected, 753
Uniformed Services Employment and
        Reemployment Rights Act of 1994, 735
Unintentional torts, 713
Unipolar neurons, 29*f*, 30
Universal curet, 522*f*, 522. *See also* Curet.
Universal Numbering System, 139, 471.
        See also Dentition.
Universal principles, 707
Universality, principle of, 748
Unprotected eyes, risks for, 307
Unregulated medical waste, 314
Unsaturated chemical vapor sterilization, 316
Unsaturated fatty acids, 369
Unsupervised practice, 718
Upper respiratory system infections, 275
Urea cycle, 368
Urinary bladder, 99, 99*f*
Urinary system, 97–101, 99*f*
    physiology of, 100
Urinary tract infections, 284
Urine analysis, 381
USDA MyPlate, 382*f*, 384, 386
Utilitarian ethics, 707. *See also* Ethical
        considerations.
Utility gloves, 306*t*
Uvula, 131*t*

V

Vagus nerve (CN X), 123
Validity, 625*t*
Valproate, 348
Valproic acid (Depakene, Depakote), 346
Values, in human behavior principles, 490
Vancomycin, 285*t*
Varenicline (Chantix), 354
Variable, 629
Variable expressivity, 186
Varicella, 264*t*

Varicella zoster virus (VZV), 208, 274
Variola, 264*t*
Varnish programs, 642*t*, 645, 645*b*
Varnishes, fluoride, 407–408.
        See also Fluorides.
Vascular endothelial growth factor (VEGF),
        183
Vascular system, 115
Vasoactive amines, 180
Vasoconstrictors, 552–553, 552*t*
    adrenergics as, 329
Vasodepressor syncope, 692–693
Vasodilation, 178
Vasogenic shock, 693
VEGF. *See* Vascular endothelial growth factor
        (VEGF).
Veins, 26
VELscope, 510
Veneers, 417–418
Venous drainage, of head and neck, 116
Venous sinus, 115
Ventral cavity, 55, 56*f*, 57*t*
Ventral structures, 107
Veracity, 707, 749
Verbal behaviors, 482
Vermillion zone, 131*t*
Verruca vulgaris, 193–194, 194*f*
Versions, 143
Vertebral cavity, 55, 56*f*
Vertebral column, 64, 64*f*
Vertical angulation, 166, 166*f*
Very-low-density lipoproteins (VLDLs), 370
Vestibule, 131*t*
Vestibulocochlear nerve (CN VIII), 122
Vibrio cholerae, 266*t*
Vicarious liability, 734
Vincent's infection, 205, 205*f*
Viral hepatitis, 278–279*t*
Viral infections, 274, 276, 276*t*, 284
Virtue ethics, 707. *See also* Ethical
        considerations.
Virulence factors, microbial, 266–267
Viruses, 256, 264–265, 264*t*, 287*t*
Visceral membranes, 61
Viscerocranium, 110, 111*f*
Visual examination, 188
Visual impairment, 576
Vital signs, 467, 688–690
    blood pressure, 689, 689*f*
    body temperature, 689
    pulse, 689–690, 690*f*
    respiration rate, 690
Vitalometer, 512
Vitamin K, 345
Vitamins, 371–372
    classification of, 371
    definition of, 371
    effects on oral cavity, 373*t*
    effects on oral tissues and role in tooth
        formation, 376*t*
    fat-soluble, 372
    general functions of, 372

Vitamins *(Continued)*
   nutritional requirements for, 372
   water-soluble, 372
Vitreous body, 78
ViziLite, 510
Volatile solvents, abuse of, 353
Volpe-Manhold Index (VMI), 636*t*
Vomer, 111
Von Ebner glands, 118
von Willebrand's disease, 233
VZV. *See* Varicella zoster virus (VZV).

W

Waist circumference, 379
Warfarin (Coumadin), 337, 340, 344–345
Warmth, 482
Warts, 275
   oral, 193–194, 194*f*
Waste disposal, 314
Waste management, 314
Water, 376–377
   balance of, 377
   biologic role and functions of, 376
   definition of, 376
   regulation of, 377
   requirements for, 377
   total body, 376
Water fluoridation, 641, 642*t*, 644–645*b*
   benefits of
      indirect, 643
      posteruption, 643
      preeruption, 643
   compounds used for, 643
   methods of implementing, 644
   promotion of, 644
   public attitudes towards, 644
   role of government agencies in, 644
   safety of, 643
   school, 642*t*, 646

Water jet, dental, 498
Water-soluble vitamins, 372
Waxes, 369, 412
WBCs. *See* White blood cells (WBCs).
Web-based learning, for oral health, 659
Wedges, interdental, 498
Weight control, 377–380
Weight loss, prescription drugs for, 379
White blood cells (WBCs), 86, 115
White lesions, 213–217
   Cannon disease, 215
   characteristics of, 213
   familial white folded dysplasia, 215
   hyperkeratosis, 217, 217*f*
   leukoderma, 214
   lichen planus, 215–217, 216*f*
   linea alba, 214, 214*f*
   nicotine stomatitis, 213–214, 214*f*
   systemic lupus erythematosus (SLE), 214–215, 215*f*
   white sponge nevus, 215
White matter, 75, 76*f*, 77
White sponge nevus, 215
Whitening agents, 409
WHO. *See* World Health Organization (WHO).
Whooping cough, 276
Withdrawal, 353
Withdrawal reflex, 77
Work practice controls, 301
Workers' compensation, 735
Working diagnosis, 189
Working end, 518
World Health Organization (WHO), 621, 747
Worms (helminths), 256
Wound healing and regeneration, 182–184, 182*f*
Wound strength, 183

WREB: A National Dental and Dental Hygiene Testing Agency, 2*b*
Written defamation, 714
Written record management, 728
Wrongful discharge, 714

X

Xero-lube, 331
Xerostomia-producing drug groups, 331*t*
X-linked recessive inheritance, 186
X-radiation
   characteristics of, 154–155
   discovery of, 152, 153*f*
   production of, 153, 154*f*
X-rays, 152
   film, dental, 157–161
   image characteristics, 159–160, 160*t*
   machine, 152
   with matter, interactions of, 154
   tube, 153
      diagram of, 154*f*
   types of, 153
Xylitol, 365, 646
   for dental caries prevention, 504

Y

Yellow-brown stained radiographs, 162
Yersinia pestis, 266*t*

Z

Zalcitabine, 287*t*
Zidovudine, 272, 287*t*
Zone, vermillion, 131*t*
Zygomatic arch, 110
Zygomatic bones, 110, 111*f*
Zygomatic nerve, 120, 554
Zygomatic process, 111
Zygomycota, 263